M. Hohenfellner · R.A. Santucci (Eds.) Emergencies in Urology

M. Hohenfellner · R.A. Santucci (Eds.)

Emergencies in Urology

With 312 Figures and 161 Tables

Springer

Markus Hohenfellner, MD
Professor and Chairman
Department of Urology
Heidelberg University, Medical School
69120 Heidelberg, Germany

Richard A. Santucci, MD
Chief of Urology, Detroit Receiving Hospital
Associate Professor, Wayne State University School of Medicine
4160 John R., Suite 1017
Detroit, MI 48201, USA

ISBN 978-3-540-48603-9 Springer-Verlag Berlin Heidelberg New York

Library of Congress Control Number: 2006938751

Springer is a part of Springer Science+Business Media
http://www.springer.com

Printed in Germany

Editor: Dr. Ute Heilmann
Desk Editor: Meike Stoeck
Copy-editing: WS Editorial Ltd, Shrewsbury, UK
Illustrations: Stephan Spitzer, Frankfurt, http://www.medizillu.de and
Reinhold Henkel, Heidelberg, http://reinholdhenkel.illustration.de
Production Editor: Joachim W. Schmidt

Cover design: eStudio Calamar, Spain

Typesetting: FotoSatz Pfeifer GmbH, D-82166 Gräfelfing
Printed on acid-free paper – 24/3150 – 5 4 3 2 1 0

To Ulrike and Christine

Preface

Emergencies in medicine are difficult on two fronts: they may challenge both the health of the patient and the skills of the doctor in charge. If the latter, the former may deteriorate rapidly. Thus, the definition of an emergency indeed depends on who is facing it. As we mature along our clinical pathways of education, training, and experience, the risk of going through a personal professional emergency is continuously reduced. Nevertheless, throughout our medical career, accurate self-assessment and subsequent control of our actions remain our most important qualities. This is true especially for anybody who endeavors into a surgical field.

This book focuses on both kinds of emergencies. It works to facilitate anticipation of potential situations, and therefore allow their competent management. This aim has only become possible with the support of some of the most distinguished urologists for this project. They contributed their rich experience not only in the classical form of textbook chapters but also by narrating their personal Armageddons as open-styled vignettes. These short stories are an impressive proof that persistent awareness and education are essential elements of a successful professional life. They also relay a golden rule to all of our readers, who still have the privilege to call somebody if needed: if in doubt – just do it. The so-called four big Cs: climb, communicate, confess, and comply are the basic actions for any pilot in distress and they may just be as applicable for any doctor facing a difficult situation that may exceed his experience and abilities. Our pride must be to consistently achieve the same result: *salus aegroti suprema lex* – only the best for our patients.

At this point, we want to extend our sincere thanks to the authors who have participated in this book. All of them are extremely busy, internationally renowned clinicians. Nonetheless, their effort and dedication to make *Emergencies in Urology* possible have surpassed all expectations, not only by the superb quality of the manuscripts but also by the timeliness and enthusiasm of their cooperation.

Special thanks are also extended to Stephan Spitzer, whose outstanding art and understanding of the author's picturesque suggestions created many of the ever-so-crucial illustrations.

The editors wish to thank the publishers at Springer-Verlag for a fantastic job. We are especially indebted to our Desk Editor, Meike Stoeck, who was in nearly daily contact with us for years. She helped us immeasurably to stay on time, on the job, and on focus. The final result has been inestimably improved by her efforts.

Markus Hohenfellner
Richard A. Santucci

The artwork in this volume was kindly sponsored by:

Astellas	81606 München, Germany
Ethicon	22861 Norderstedt, Germany
Farco-Pharma GmbH	50670 Köln, Germany
SIEMENS Medical Solutions	91052 Erlangen, Germany
KARL STORZ GmbH & Co. KG	78532 Tuttlingen, Germany
Takeda Pharma GmbH	52066 Aachen, Germany
Richard Wolf GmbH	75438 Knittlingen, Germany

The Editors

Markus Hohenfellner, MD

Dr. Hohenfellner is Professor of Urology and Chair of The Department of Urology of the University of Heidelberg, Medical School. His institution is consequently organized to function in a high-level interdisciplinary environment and addresses all the contemporary clinical challenges: urologic oncology, minimally invasive surgery, reconstructive surgery, pediatric urology, lower urinary tract dysfunction, stone disease, and andrology.

Dr. Hohenfellner is chairman of the EAU Working Group on Urologic Trauma. He is also the chief representative of the German Urological Association to establish guidelines on Urologic Trauma.

Richard A. Santucci, MD, FACS

Dr. Santucci is the Chief of Urology at the Detroit Receiving Hospital, one of the nation's first Level I trauma centers and the only hospital built from the ground up to serve as a trauma hospital. He is an Associate Professor at Wayne State University and is a widely published expert in the field of trauma and emergency urology.

Dr. Santucci also serves as the Director of the Center for Urologic Reconstruction at Detroit Receiving Hospital. The Center is a regional referral center for difficult cases in urologic reconstruction, including urethral injury, urethral stricture, and complex reconstructive problems of the bladder, ureters and kidneys.

Contents

List of Contributors

Arap, Marco A., MD
Assistant Professor of Urology
University of São Paulo
School of Medicine
Av. Dr. Eneas de Carvalho Aguiar 255
05422-970, São Paulo, SP, Brazil

Arap, Sami, MD
Professor Emeritus of Urology
University of São Paulo
School of Medicine
Av. Dr. Eneas de Carvalho Aguiar 255
05422-970, São Paulo, SP, Brazil

Bader, Pia, MD
Urologische Klinik, Städtisches Klinikum Karlsruhe
Moltkestraße 90
76133 Karlsruhe, Germany

Beck, Stephen D.W., MD, FACS
Assistant Professor of Urology
Department of Urology
Indiana University
Indiana Cancer Pavilion
535 N Barnhill Dr
Indianapolis, IN 46202, USA

Bella, Anthony J., MD, FRCSC
Clinical Instructor and American Urological Association
Foundation Robert J. Krane Scholar
University of California, San Francisco
400 Parnassus Ave, A633
San Francisco, CA 94143-0738, USA

Berger, Ingrid, MD
Resident for Urology
Department of Urology and Andrology
Donauspital
Langobardenstraße 122
1220 Vienna, Austria

Boccon-Gibod, Laurent, MD
Professor of Urology
Hôpital Bichat
Clinique Urologique
46 rue Henri Huchard
Paris 75018, France

Brant, William O., MD
Northstar Urology
PO Box 40,000
Vail, CO 81658, USA

Burkhard, Fiona, MD
Klinik und Poliklinik für Urologie
Universitätsspital Bern
Inselspital
Freiburgstrasse
3010 Bern, Switzerland

Buse, Stephan, MD
Member of the Faculty
Department of Urology
University of Heidelberg, Medical School
69120 Heidelberg, Germany

Chapple, Christopher R., BSc, MD, FRCS, FEBU
Professor of Urology
Section of Female and Reconstructive Urology
and Urodynamics
Dept. of Urology
Royal Hallamshire Hospital
Glossop Road
Sheffield, S10 2JF, UK

Cook, Anthony, BSc, MD, FRCSC, FAAP
Assistant Clinical Professor
Division of Pediatric Surgery
University of Calgary
Pediatric Urology Fellowship Director
Alberta Children's Hospital
Calgary, Alberta

Dall'Era, Marc A., MD
Dept. of Urology
University of Washington School Medicine
Seattle, WA 98125, USA

Diemer, Thorsten, MD
Universitätsklinikum Gießen und Marburg GmbH
Klinik und Poliklinik für Urologie und
Kinderurologie
Rudolf-Buchheim-Straße 7
35385 Gießen, Germany

Donatucci, Craig F., MD
Associate Professor and Vice-Chair
Deptartment of Surgery
Division of Urology
Duke University Medical Center
DUMC 3274
Durham, NC 27710, USA

Elliot, Sean P., MD
Professor of Urology
Fellow in Urologic Trauma and Reconstruction
San Francisco General Hospital
1001 Potrero Avenue, 3A-20
San Francisco, CA 94110, USA

Foster, Richard S., MD, FACS
Professor of Urology
Department of Urology
Indiana University
Indiana Cancer Pavilion
535 N Barnhill Dr
Indianapolis, IN 46202, USA

Fradet, Yves, MD
Département de Chirurgie (Urologie)
Hotel Dieu Hospital
11 Côte du Palais
Québec, Québec G1R 2J6, Canada

Frohneberg Detlef, MD
Professor of Urology
Urologische Klinik, Städtisches Klinikum Karlsruhe
Moltkestraße 90
76133 Karlsruhe, Germany

Gettman, Matthew T., MD
Mayo Clinic
Department of Urology
200 First Street, SW
Rochester, MN 55905, USA

Ghoneim, Mohamed A., MD
Professor of Urology
Urology and Nephrology Center
Mansoura University
Mansoura, Egypt

Gilfrich, Christian, MD
Department of Urology
University of Heidelberg, Medical School
69120 Heidelberg, Germany

Gil-Vernet, José M., MD
Professor and Chair of Urology
Chair of Urology
Centro Medico Teknon
Vilana, 12
08022 Barcelona, Spain

Gracia, Maurice M., MD
Chief Resident
Dept. of Urology
400 Parnassus Ave, A-633
San Francisco, CA 94143-0738, USA

Günther, Rolf W., MD
Dept. of Diagnostic Radiology
University Hospital
University of Technology
Pauwelsstraße 30
52074 Aachen, Germany

Haferkamp, Axel, MD
Associate Professor of Urology
Senior Faculty
Department of Urology
Heidelberg University, Medical School
69120 Heidelberg, Germany

Hartung, Rudolf, MD
Professor Emeritus of Urology
Urologische Klinik und Poliklinik
Technische Universität München
Ismaninger Str. 22
81675 Munich, Germany

Hermieu, Jean Francois, MD
Hôpital Bichat
Clinique Urologique
46 rue Henri Huchard
Paris 75018, France

Heyns, Christiaan F., MD
Department of Urology
University of Stellenbosch and Tygerberg Hospital
P.O. Box 19063
Tygerberg 7505
South Africa

Hohenfellner, Markus, MD
Professor and Chairman
Department of Urology
Heidelberg University, Medical School
69120 Heidelberg, Germany

Hohenfellner, Rudolf, MD
Professor Emeritus of Urology
Department of Urology
Johannes Gutenberg University
Langenbeckstraße 1
55101 Mainz, Germany

Ikoma, Fumihiko, MD
Professor Emeritus of Urology
18-27, Higashiyama-cho
659-0091 Ashiya, Japan

Jacobs, Micah, MD
The Department of Urology
Lahey Clinic
Burlington, MA 01805, USA

Jacobsen, Niels-Erik B., MD, FRCSC
Fellow, Urologic Oncology
Department of Urology
Indiana University School of Medicine
Indiana Cancer Pavilion
535 N Barnhill Dr
Indianapolis, IN 46202, USA

Jordan, Gerald H., MD
Professor of Urology
Eastern Virginia Medical School
400 W. Brambleton Ave., # 100
Norfolk, VA 23510, USA

Jünemann, Klaus-Peter, MD
Professor and Chairman
Klinik für Urologie und Kinderurologie
Universitätsklinikum Schleswig-Holstein, Campus Kiel
Arnold-Heller-Straße 7
24105 Kiel, Germany

Kavoussi, Louis R., MD
The Department of Urology
Johns Hopkins Hospital
600 N. Wolfe Street, Suite 161
Jefferson Street Building
Baltimore, MD 21287, USA

Khoury, Antoine Elie, MBBCH, FRCSC
Professor
Department of Surgery
The University of Toronto
Division of Urology
Hospital for Sick Children
555 University Avenue
Toronto, ON M5G 1X8, Canada

Kitrey, Noam D., MD
Department of Urology
Sheba Medical Center
Tel-Hashomer
52621 Ramat-Gan, Israel

Krieger, John N., MD
Department of Urology
University of Washington School of Medicine
Seattle, WA 98125, USA

Libertino, John, A., MD
Lahey Clinical Medical Center
41 Mall Rd.
Burlington, MA 01805-0001, USA

Lue, Tom F., MD
Professor of Urology
Department of Urology
400 Parnassus Ave, A-633
San Francisco, CA 94143-0738, USA

Månsson, Wiking MD, PhD
Department of Urology
University Hospital
22100 Lund, Sweden

Martin, Eike, MD
Professor and Chairman
Department of Anesthesiology
University of Heidelberg, Medical School
Im Neuenheimer Feld 110
69120 Heidelberg, Germany

Martínez-Piñeiro, José A., MD, PhD
Professor of Urology
Clinica La Luz, Former Head
Department Urology
Hospital Universitario La Paz
Avenida de San Luis 95
Madrid 28033, Spain

Martínez-Piñeiro, Luis, MD, PhD, FEBU
Urology Department
La Paz University Hospital
Paseo Castellana 261
28046 Madrid, Spain

Master, Viraj A., MD, PhD
Assistant Professor
Department of Urology
Emory University
1365 Clifton Road, N.E., Building B
Atlanta, GA 30322, USA

McAninch, Jack W., MD
Professor of Urology, Chief of Urology
San Francisco General Hospital
1001 Potrero Avenue, 3A-20
San Francisco, CA 94110, USA

Mor, Yoram, MD
Department of Urology
Sheba Medical Center
Tel-Hashomer
52621 Ramat-Gan, Israel

Motsch, Johann, MD
Professor of Anesthesiology
Department of Anesthesiology
University of Heidelberg, Medical School
Im Neuenheimer Feld 110
69120 Heidelberg, Germany

Mundy, Tony, AR
Professor of Urology
Trust Headquarters
University College London Hospitals
NHS Foundation Trust
250 Euston Road
London NW1 2PG, UK

Muntener, Michael, MD
Department of Urology
Johns Hopkins Hospital
600 N. Wolfe Street
Baltimore, MD 21287, USA

Nadu, Andrei, MD
Department of Urology
Sheba Medical Center
Tel-Hashomer
52621 Ramat-Gan, Israel

Olsson, Carl A., MD
Columbia University Medical Center
Department of Urology
Herbert Irving Pavilion
161 Fort Washington Ave.
New York, NY 10032, USA

Pansadoro, Vito, MD
Professor of Urology
Vincenzo Pansadoro Foundation
Via Aurelia 559
00165 Rome, Italy

Patterson, Jacob M., MBCHB, MRCS
Section of Female and Reconstructive Urology
and Urodynamics
Dept. of Urology
Royal Hallamshire Hospital
Glossop Road
Sheffield, S10 2JF, UK

Perez-Castro, Ellendt E., MD
Department of Urology
C/General Rodrigo, 8
28003 Madrid, Spain

Perovic, Sava, MD
Department of Urology
University Children's Hospital
Tirsova 10
11000 Belgrade, Serbia and Montenegro

Pfitzenmaier, Jesco, MD
Associate Professor
Department of Urology
University of Heidelberg
Im Neuenheimer Feld 110
69120 Heidelberg, Germany

Plas, Eugen, MD
Associate Professor of Urology and Andrology
Department of Urology and Ludwig Boltzmann
Institute for Urology and Andrology
Hietzing Hospital
Wolkersbergenstr. 1
1130 Vienna, Austria

Pontes, J. Edson
Department of Urology
Wayne State University
4160 John P. Denort, 41 I 48201, USA

Romero, Frederico R., MD
The Department of Urology
Johns Hopkins Hospital
600 N. Wolfe Street, Suite 161
Jefferson Street Building
Baltimore, MD 21287, USA

Santucci, Richard A., MD, FACS
Associate Professor
Wayne State University School of Medicine
Department of Urology
4160 John R., Suite 1017
Detroit, MI 48201, USA

Schiefer, Hans Gerd, MD
Professor
Medizinische Mikrobiologie
Universitätsklinikum Gießen und Marburg
Schubertstraße 1
35392 Gießen, Germany

Schlenker, Boris, MD
Urologische Klinik und Poliklinik
Klinikum der Universität München – Großhadern
Ludwig-Maximilians-Universität München
Marchioninistraße 15
81377 Munich, Germany

Schramm, Christoph, MD
Department of Anesthesiology
University of Heidelberg, Medical School
Im Neuenheimer Feld 110
69120 Heidelberg, Germany

Schumacher, Martin C., MD
Klinik und Poliklinik für Urologie
Universitätsspital Bern
Inselspital
Freiburgstrasse
3010 Bern, Switzerland

Segura, Joseph W., MD
Mayo Clinic
Department of Urology
200 First Street, SW
Rochester, MN 55905, USA

Seitz, Michael, MD
Urologische Klinik und Poliklinik
Klinikum der Universität München – Großhadern
Ludwig-Maximilians-Universität München
Marchioninstraße 15
80336 Munich, Germany

Serafetinides, Ephraim, MD
Department of Urology
General Hospital 'Asklipieion' Voula
Vas. Pavlou 1
16673 Voula, Greece

Shokeir, Ahmed A., MD, PhD, FEBU
Urology and Nephrology Center
Mansoura University
Mansoura, Egypt

Skinner, Donald G., MD
Chairman and Professor of Urology
Department of Urology
University of Southern California
USC/Norris Cancer Center
1441 Eastlake Avenue
Los Angeles, CA 90089-9178, USA

Stackl, Walter, MD
Professor of Urology
Urologische Abteilung Rudolfstiftung
Juchgasse 25
1030 Vienna, Austria

Stein, John P., MD, FACS
Associate Professor of Urology
Department of Urology
University of Southern California
USC/Norris Cancer Center
1441 Eastlake Avenue
Los Angeles, CA 90089-9178, USA

Stief, Christian, MD
Professor of Urology
Urologische Klinik und Poliklinik
Klinikum der Universität München – Großhadern
Ludwig-Maximilians-Universität München
Marchioninstraße 15
80336 Munich, Germany

Studer, Urs E., MD
Professor of Urology
Klinik und Poliklinik für Urologie
Universitätsspital Bern
Inselspital
Freiburgstrasse
3010 Bern, Switzerland

Theron, Pieter D., MD
Department of Urology
University of Stellenbosch and Tygerberg Hospital
P.O. Box 19063
Tygerberg 7505, South Africa

Tiguert, Rabi, MD
Centre de recherche l'Hotel-Dieu Quebec
Centre hospitalier universitaire de Quebec
11, Cote-du-Palais, Quebec G1R2J6, Canada

Trigo-Rocha, Flavio, MD
Associate Professor of Urology
Division of Urology
Sao Paulo University
Sao Paulo, Brazil

Türkeri, N. Levent, MD, PhD
Professor of Urology
Marmara University Hospital
Department of Urology
Tophaneliolu Cad. No. 13–15
Altunizade 34662
Istanbul, Turkey

Vaughan, Darracott Edwin Jr, MD
Department of Urology
Weill Cornell University
525 East 68th Street
New York, NY 10021, USA

Walsh, Thomas J., MD, MS
Dept. of Urology
University of Washington School Medicine
Seattle, WA 98125, USA

Wefer, Björn, MD
Klinik für Urologie und Kinderurologie
Universitätsklinikum Schleswig-Holstein
Campus Kiel
Arnold-Heller-Str.7
24105 Kiel, Germay

Weidner, Wolfgang, MD
Professor of Urology
Universitätsklinikum Gießen und Marburg GmbH
Klinik und Poliklinik für Urologie und
Kinderurologie
Rudolf-Buchheim-Straße 7
35385 Gießen, Germany

Wildberger, Joachim E., MD
Dept. of Diagnostic Radiology
University Hospital
University of Technology
Pauwelsstraße 30
52074 Aachen, Germany

Wimpissinger, Florian, MD, FEBU
Urologische Abteilung Rudolfstiftung
Juchgasse 25
1030 Vienna, Austria

Wolf, J. Stuart, Jr., MD
Professor of Urology
University of Michigan
1500 E. Medical Center Dr.
TC 3875
Ann Arbor, MI 48109-0330, USA

Wotkowicz, Chad, MD
Department of Urology
Lahey Clinic
Burlington, MA 01805, USA

Yoon, Gerald H., MD
Department of Urology
University of Southern California
USC, Norris Cancer Center
1441 Eastlake Avenue
Los Angeles, CA 90089-9178, USA

Zantl, Niko, MD
Associate Professor of Urology
Urologische Klinik und Poliklinik
Technische Universität München
Ismaninger Str. 22
81675 Munich, Germany

Urologic Emergencies: Overview

S.P. Elliott, J.W. McAninch

Compared to other surgical fields there are relatively few emergencies in urology. For this reason we may become unaccustomed to caring for the acutely ill patient. Therefore, it is important to keep certain guiding principles in mind when confronted with a patient with an emergent urologic condition.

First, remember that emergencies in urology are rarely life-threatening. Even some of the most concerning conditions such as pyonephrosis or renal trauma are urgent but usually not emergent. Remembering this principle will prevent one from making rushed decisions about management. Important questions to consider before acting are:

1. Is the patient well enough to undergo an operation?
2. Will an operation improve the situation or is a minimally invasive approach or patience a better course of action?
3. Have you considered possible concomitant pathology or injuries?
4. Should you involve a general surgeon, internist, or intensivist in the patient's care?
5. Would additional imaging be helpful?

By no means should an urgent problem go untreated but taking a couple of minutes to think through these questions could avoid misguided therapy.

Second, as mentioned above, avail yourself of imaging of the genitourinary tract. Radiology should be considered an extension of the physical exam in urology since many of the structures are difficult to examine by palpation. Contrast-enhanced computerized tomography of the abdomen and pelvis with delayed imaging of the urinary collection system plays a critical role in the evaluation and management of abdominal trauma involving the urinary system, ultrasound is often indispensable in the differentiation of orchitis and testicular torsion, and a cystogram diagnoses a bladder perforation as intraperitoneal or extraperitoneal. In each of these examples, findings on radiographic imaging will significantly alter one's choice of management. The urologist should be familiar with the options for imaging and the interpretation of those images.

Third, and perhaps most important, do not be afraid to involve other urologists or other services in the care of the patient, particularly if you are unfamiliar with the management of the acutely ill patient. As alluded to above, many of us have an office-based practice and perform mostly short-stay surgery. If one is uncomfortable managing an acutely ill patient one should not allow pride to prevent one from consulting a colleague early in the patient's hospital course.

2 The Clinical Approach to the Acutely Ill Patient

S. Buse, R. Santucci, M. Hohenfellner

2.1 Diagnosis

2.1.1 The Use of Guidelines and Algorithms

The first step in the management of urologic emergencies is to recognize the clinical significance. One must distinguish among genuinely life-threatening problems such as urosepsis or kidney rupture, urgent problems such as testicular torsion, and merely troublesome conditions such as cystitis in a healthy young woman. This may be more easily said than done. The practitioner is challenged both by the broad spectrum of urologic emergencies and by the even more numerous possible diagnoses mimicking urologic symptoms. For example, a patient with a long history of renal colic may present with acute flank pain, tachycardia, tachypnea, and hypotension. If renal ultrasound is normal (lack of upper tract dilatation) and urinalysis reveals no microhematuria, abdominal ultrasonography and/or computed tomography (CT), as indicated in a diagnostic algorithm, will lead to the correct diagnosis of ruptured abdominal aneurysm.

A useful source of immediate, compact information for clinicians is found in published clinical guidelines (e.g., from the European Association of Urology [EAU][Lynch et al. 2005], the American Urological Association [AUA][Montague et al. 2003], or others often based upon the classification for urologic trauma formulated by the American Association for the Surgery of Trauma [Baker et al. 1974; Moore et al. 1989]). Most preferable are guidelines classified by the level of evidence: S1 guidelines representing an informal consensus of experts, S2 a formal consensus, and S3 a formal consensus adhering to evidenced-based medicine, with the elaboration of clinical algorithms. Guidelines in this form are widely used in other fields such as emergency medicine (e.g., cardiovascular resuscitation, initial management of trauma patients) and are increasingly used in urology.

Algorithms lead the doctor through the different potential situations arising during a urologic emergency and communicate in a clear and rapid way how to proceed to the next step. Because they are presented in a stepwise fashion and are logical, they are often easy to memorize. The branching design of algorithms creates decision trees, and the management pathway cannot be continued until the proper test is ordered or the diagnostic solution found. Algorithms therefore provide what is essential and unique to emergency medicine: a simultaneity of diagnosis and therapy.

2.1.2 The Emergency Setting

The emergency setting is characterized by continuous and rapid changes in the patient, and thus the assessment can seldom be deemed complete. Accordingly, repeated checks of the patient and of the working hypothesis are warranted. It is also important to evaluate the results of each step in the therapeutic process.

The current availability of high-tech diagnostic tools does not supplant the need for a urologist who is able to identify the salient facts in the history and findings on physical examination, as these are the bases for the correct management choice. The urologist must also be skilled in extracting the relevant results from technical or laboratory tests and in integrating these into the given management pathway.

2.2 History

Urologic emergencies, even if life-threatening (e.g., sepsis or hemodynamically relevant postoperative bleeding), should not hinder history taking of the acute event. Information to elicit includes concurrent illness or operation (e.g., previous nephrectomy in a patient with traumatic kidney rupture), medication (e.g., fever in neutropenic patients after chemotherapy requires a different therapeutic approach), and (crucially) allergy. Any minimal delay in therapy is offset by the avoidance of any potential iatrogenic complication, possibly adding a second emergency to the one already under evaluation. The AMPLE history (Allergies, Medications, Past medical history, time of Last meal, Events preceding the injury) used in trauma surgery can be used as a template in traumatic and even nontraumatic emergencies. Other elements of the urgent history include localization, time dimension, intensity and mitigating/inducing factors of the current problem. Some patients may not be able to report their condition themselves. In young children, patients with dementia, and those who are severely ill (urosepsis or polytrauma) or whom we are asked to treat intraoperatively, the history may be obtained from family members, the rescue staff, or the operating team.

The importance of history taking in urologic emergency is illustrated by a prospective study (Eskelinen et al. 1998) addressing its accuracy in acute renal colic. The combination of gross hematuria, loin tenderness, pain lasting less than 12 h, and decreased appetite–all information easily available from history–detected renal colic with a sensitivity of 84% and a specificity of 98%.

2.3 Physical Examination

2.3.1 Primary Survey

In emergency urology, many decision trees branch on the vital signs of blood pressure, pulse rate, respiratory rate, temperature, and general assessment of the patient (i.e., toxic or well appearing). These should be available from nursing personnel before any history taking by the doctor; if not, they must be obtained quickly (and updated frequently). After the vital signs, the initial assessment follows. Although urologists will be tempted to emphasize the genitourinary physical examination, elements of airway, breathing, circulation, disability (neurologic) and exposure (environmental), making up the ABCs, must be assessed (even briefly) in emergency cases before getting down to the U for urology! The authors have witnessed patients with impressive gunshot wounds to the genitalia that completely diverted primary caregiver attention from chest gunshot wounds that ultimately required emergency thoracotomy.

The urologist will be better able to make use of modern diagnostic tools and management algorithms in a purposeful manner once the urologic history and physical examination are complete. They should not be bypassed. A prospective controlled study addressing the predictive value of abdominal examination in the diagnosis of abdominal aortic aneurysm, for instance, reported a negative predictive value higher than 90% for aneurysms of 4 cm and a positive predictive value over 80% for those larger than 5 cm (Vendatasubramaniam et al. 2004). Another group (van den Berg et al. 1999) compared the detection of groin hernia by different diagnostic tools and physical examination. Interestingly, physical examination achieved a sensitivity of 75% and a specificity of 96%. In patients with acute abdominal pain (Bohner et al. 1998), the variables with the highest sensitivity for bowel obstruction were distended abdomen, decreased bowel sounds, history of constipation, previous abdominal surgery, vomiting, and age over 50 years. The authors of this study calculated that, if only those patients presenting two of these variables had undergone imaging, radiography could have been avoided in 46% without loss of diagnostic accuracy.

2.3.2 Secondary Survey

After vital signs and the initial assessment, the secondary assessment is conducted. If possible, the physical examination should be conducted in a systematic way in a fully exposed patient. In trauma patients, the risk of hypothermia must be considered even in the warmer months; nevertheless, it should not hinder complete exposure for examination and it will be reduced by warm infusions and by covering with external warming devices after assessment (ATLS Manual 2004a). With the exception of life-threatening emergencies requiring immediate evaluation and therapy, the secondary assessment should include organ systems other than those assumed to be affected. This will allow the discovery of physical signs not necessarily linked to the working hypothesis, as well as those arising from any additional disease (e.g., discovering a melanoma in a patient presenting with renal colic).

The reduced interrater reliability (Close et al. 2001) or accuracy (Weatherall and Harwood 2002) of some physical tests should not lead to a dismissal of the physical examination as a whole. For example, blood at the urethral meatus is only 50% predictive of posterior urethral distraction injury, and a high-riding prostate is only 33% predictive, but they are nonetheless useful features of the assessment. It remains the task of universities and training programs to support the teaching of these basic physical examination skills and their successful incorporation into diagnostic and therapeutic algorithms.

2.4 Laboratory Testing

Before trusting any laboratory value, one should always verify that the results actually stem from the patient and that laboratory or collection error has not occurred. Even in modern hospital systems, laboratory values are not completely reliable and blood or urine samples may have been exchanged. This is particularly important in episodes of mass casualty with numerous traumatized patients arriving simultaneously at the emergency room (ATLS Manual 2004b). In all cases, laboratory values that appear erroneous or do not make sense should be quickly rechecked before irrevocable steps are taken in the patient's care. Blood drawn from a vein above an intravenous infusion, for example, may show a very low hematocrit level indicating massive blood loss, but if the patient appears well and has normal vital signs the value might best be rechecked rapidly before acting.

In the management of emergencies, the time required for a particular test to return a result is a relevant issue. Diagnostic tools that are faster but less accurate may be substituted. For example, a patient with a suspected pulmonary embolus and a positive d-dimer blood test in the emergency room (fast but not 100% accurate) may be started on heparin while awaiting a more definitive spiral CT of the chest or angiogram. This provides the soonest effective therapy.

A peculiarity in urologic laboratory testing is found in the analysis of dipstick versus microscopic versus microbiological (culture) urine analysis. Culture results, particularly, will not be available for 48–72 h. It is imperative, however, to have collected a sample before starting empiric antibiotic treatment. The safest plan is to consider a complete urinalysis to consist not only of a dipstick test but also microscopic analysis and, if there are any nitrates or white blood cells present, an automatic Gram-positive and Gram-negative microbiologic culture.

Dipstick tests are quick but give both false-positive and false-negative results in the presence of some physicochemical urine properties as well as certain drugs. Blood detection might be hindered by captopril or vitamin C intake and leukocyte esterase by elevated specific gravity, glycosuria, proteinuria, and oxidating drugs, including some cephalosporins, tetracycline, and gentamicin (Simerville et al. 2005).

The sensitivity of dipstick urinalysis ranges from 91% to 96% for microscopic hematuria, 72% to 97% for abnormal leukocyte esterase, and 19% to 48% for nitrites; specificity ranges from 65% to 99%, 41% to 86%, and 92% to 100%, respectively(Simerville et al. 2005). Under the pressure of cost containment, numerous studies have addressed the diagnostic value of dipstick testing in the emergency room. Two prospective observational studies concluded that, in women with suspected UTI, over- and undertreatment rates were similar for various test cut-off values for urine dipstick and microscopic urine analysis (Lammers et al. 2001) and that microscopy prompted changes in only 6% of patients with suspected UTI and in none with suspected microhematuria (Jou and Powers 1998). On the other hand, Leman (2002) calculated that microscopy improved the specificity for UTI in women presenting to the emergency room. More importantly, the study revealed the dipstick urinalysis to be susceptible to systemic bias for UTI, resulting in different sensitivity and specificity values in patients with different clinical manifestations (Lachs et al. 1992; Grosse et al. 2005). In short, although the value of microscopy may be controversial in the general emergency room setting, it is not so in the urologic emergency room. In this specific population, many with severe or recurrent UTI, the practice of obtaining microscopy in addition to dipstick urinalysis is warranted.

2.5 Imaging

2.5.1 Sonography

History, physical examination and laboratory tests are usually completed by various imaging procedures. In Europe, the easiest test to access is commonly sonography; in the US it is probably CT. Sonography allows the evaluation of the size and position of the kidneys, parenchymal width, and the detection of masses, calculi (especially over 3 mm) (Heinz-Peer and Helbich 2001) and calcifications. Moreover, it is possible to diagnose urinary tract dilatation and assess the grade of hydronephrosis. In the lower urinary tract, sonography can show bladder tumors, clots, and bladder stones. Finally, after micturition the residual volume can be calculated.

Emergency indications for formal renal ultrasound include renal colic, renal failure, acute renal infection, urinary retention, and the detection of complications in renal transplant patients, as well as the exclusion of important nonurologic differential diagnoses such as spleen or liver rupture. However, because of the overwhelming diagnostic advantages of CT (Fowler et al. 2002; Sheafor et al. 2000), renal ultrasound is likely the second best choice for imaging calculi in suspected colic, except in children and pregnant women.

Emergency vascular evaluation by Doppler or duplex sonography is indicated in the acute scrotum to detect testicular torsion: the ultrasound finding of decreased or absent testicular flow achieves a sensitivity of up to 90% and a specificity of over 98% (Karmazyn et al. 2005). Emergency duplex sonography is also applicable for the detection of renal venous thrombosis (as a second choice after CT in patients who are pregnant or allergic to iodinated contrast) and perfusion disorders complicating renal transplantation, trauma, or urologic surgery.

2.5.2 Plain Abdominal Films

Although less useful, plain abdominal films (KUB) include information about the size and position of the kidneys, of the psoas shadow (poor identification may be a manifestation of retroperitoneal hematoma from a ruptured aortic aneurysm), and of intestinal gas distribution (e.g., postoperative ileus) and can aid the search for calculi and organ calcification, free intraabdominal gas, and bone pathology. For more than half a century, the plain abdominal film was the only tool available to detect urolithiasis. However, because of its limited accuracy for the direct detection of stones (Haddad et al. 1992; Levine et al. 1997; Mutgi et al. 1991), it is indicated only in follow-up of conservatively managed urolithiasis, of fragmentation results after lithotripsy (in combination with sonography), and for missed calculi after ureterorenoscopy (Grosse et al. 2005). Its advantages include availability, rapidity, and the ease of image evaluation even by a nonradiologist. Its only secondary effect is a small degree of radiation exposure, which is generally not a contraindication except in pregnant women and perhaps young children.

2.5.3 Intravenous Pyelography

Intravenous pyelography (IVP) allows additional qualitative analysis over KUB. It can determine the secretory function of each kidney, the presence of delay in filling of the renal pelvis (found in urinary obstruction), the post-void residual volume, and can describe the genitourinary anatomic pathology. Until 1995, IVP was the mainstay in the diagnosis of renal colic, but it has since been supplanted by helical CT. Its drawbacks are its generally lower sensitivity, the risk of forniceal rupture because of osmotic diuresis from contrast in the presence of occluding calculi, and the relatively long time to obtain the several images required for a complete IVP study. In some hospital systems, although the patient may be billed more for a CT scan than for an IVP (say US $ 2,000 for a noncontrast CT of the abdomen and pelvis versus US $ 650 for an IVP), the actual cost to the institution is much lower for CT. The specificities of IVP and helical CT for urolithiasis appear to be similar (Niall et al. 1999; Reiter et al. 1999).

Further disadvantages of IVP include the potential to mask stones through the secreted contrast product, the risks of iodinated contrast (including allergic reaction up to anaphylaxis), and an eventual induction of thyrotoxicosis in patients with clinically silent hyperthyroidism. The possibility of impaired renal function from IVP dye and the contraindication to injection in those with significant renal insufficiency cannot be forgotten. It is not without its benefits, however, and there are some situations in which IVP is actually preferred, as in the need for precise anatomic planning before complex ureteroscopy or percutaneous nephrolithotomy (Grosse et al. 2005).

2.5.4 Computed Tomography

Computed tomography is the gold standard in most urologic emergencies, including urolithiasis and renal trauma in the context of polytrauma. It is also useful in the exclusion of postoperative complications such as hemorrhage, abscess, or ileus (Balthazar 1994), or differential diagnoses such as abdominal aortic aneurysm (Hirsch et al. 2006).

The use of the nonenhanced helical CT to detect urolithiasis has been established since the ninetees (Liu et al. 2000; Miller et al. 1998) and has now mostly displaced IVP (Dalla Palma 2001). The sensitivity, depending on calculus size, amounts to nearly 100% (Liu et al. 2000; Catalano et al. 2002; Fielding et al. 1997; Hamm et al. 2002). CT detects even nonradiolucent calculi, with the exception of stones composed of the protease-inhibitor indinavir (used to treat HIV). It can also predict the chances of spontaneous calculus discharge by its accurate size measurement and by the inverse correlation of the intensity of perinephric stranding with spontaneous discharge (Sandhu et al. 2003a, b).

Generally, exposure to radiation from CT is higher than with IVP, although newer low-dose nonenhanced helical CT protocols achieve radiation doses in the same range as IVP with comparable accuracy to standard CT imaging (Hamm et al. 2002).

CT urography (CT scan without, then with, contrast, followed by delayed images showing the urinary excretion phase) reaches an accuracy of 100% in the detection of urolithiasis and it permits assessment of the retroperitoneum and renal vessels, facilitating the differentiation from other causes of acute flank pain. Its major drawbacks are its long duration, high radiation dose, and the necessity for contrast with the attendant potential secondary effects.

In the hemodynamically stable trauma patient, CT is the gold standard, as it accurately defines the location and severity of injuries, allowing a conservative surgical approach if appropriate. It also provides a view of the entire abdominal viscera, retroperitoneum and pelvis. Hemodynamic instability still mandates immediate operative exploration in patients with suspected renal trauma (Kawashima et al. 2001). Intraoperatively, a single-shot IVP can be obtained to image renal injury (Nicolaisen et al. 1985).

In the setting of hemodynamic stable polytrauma patient, CT cystography is an excellent alternative to conventional retrograde cystography (Deck et al. 2000), when necessary. Also, it allows the diagnosis of ureteral lesions resulting in contrast extravasation. In cases of persistent strong suspicion with negative CT, IVP or retrograde ureteropyelography (Lynch et al. 2005) should be adopted. To detect urethral injury, the recommended imaging method is still retrograde urethrography (Lynch et al. 2005).

2.5.5 Magnetic Resonance Imaging

Because of its excellent anatomic accuracy, MRI has become irreplaceable in modern uroradiology, but most indications concern oncology and only rarely is it used to evaluate urologic emergencies. An exception worth mentioning is the evaluation of penile rupture (when history and examination are unclear).

In MRI urography, the T2-weighted sequences are used to create an accurate anatomic representation of the urogenital organs and for the detection and analysis of hydronephrosis and hydroureters independent of renal function. T1-weighted contrast-enhanced MRI allows the analysis of excretory renal function and the evaluation of urinary outflow in the upper urogenital tract. MRI urography is particularly useful in the diagnosis of congenital disturbances in children (Nolte-Ernsting et al. 2001). The avoidance of iodinated contrast also makes MRI the primary choice in patients allergic to contrast material.

2.5.6 Chest X-Ray

For a more comprehensive view of the patient, to exclude nonurologic differential diagnoses (e.g., basal pneumonia with low posterior intercostal pain mimicking pyelonephritis) or complications of urologic disorders (e.g., lung metastases in testicular cancer), chest-x-ray should also be considered. In any case, an interdisciplinary diagnostic and therapeutic approach should always be adopted to optimize patient management.

References

ATLS Manual (2004a) Advanced trauma life support for doctors, 7th edn. American College of Surgeons, Chicago, pp 18, 76

ATLS Manual (2004b) Advanced trauma life support for doctors, 7th edn. American College of Surgeons, Chicago, p 80

Baker SP, O'Neill B, Haddon W Jr et al (1974) The injury severity score: a method for describing patients with multiple injuries and evaluating emergency care. J Trauma 14:187

Balthazar EJ (1994) For suspected small-bowel obstruction and an equivocal plain film, should we perform CT or a small-bowel series? AJR Am J Roentgenol 163:1260

Bohner H, Yang Q, Franke C et al (1998) Simple data from history and physical examination help to exclude bowel obstruction and to avoid radiographic studies in patients with acute abdominal pain. Eur J Surg 164:777

Catalano O, Nunziata A, Altei F et al (2002) Suspected ureteral colic: primary helical CT versus selective helical CT after unenhanced radiography and sonography. AJR Am J Roentgenol 178:379

Close RJ, Sachs CJ, Dyne PL (2001) Reliability of bimanual pelvic examinations performed in emergency departments. West J Med 175:240

Dalla Palma L (2001) What is left of i.v. urography? Eur Radiol 11:931

Deck AJ, Shaves S, Talner L et al (2000) Computerized tomography cystography for the diagnosis of traumatic bladder rupture. J Urol 164:43

Eskelinen M, Ikonen J, Lipponen P (1998) Usefulness of history-taking, physical examination and diagnostic scoring in acute renal colic. Eur Urol 34:467

Fielding JR, Steele G, Fox LA et al (1997) Spiral computerized tomography in the evaluation of acute flank pain: a replacement for excretory urography. J Urol 157:2071

Fowler KA, Locken JA, Duchesne JH et al (2002) US for detecting renal calculi with nonenhanced CT as a reference standard. Radiology 222:109

Grosse A, Grosse CA, Mauermann J et al (2005) [Imaging techniques and their impact in treatment management of patients with acute flank pain]. Radiologe 45:871

Haddad MC, Sharif HS, Shahed MS et al (1992) Renal colic: diagnosis and outcome. Radiology 184:83

Hamm M, Knopfle E, Wartenberg S et al (2002) Low dose unenhanced helical computerized tomography for the evaluation of acute flank pain. J Urol 167:1687

Heinz-Peer G, Helbich T (2001) [Urological and nephrological emergency-value of diagnostic imaging]. Wien Med Wochenschr 151:560

Hirsch AT, Haskal ZJ, Hertzer NR et al (2006) ACC/AHA 2005 Practice Guidelines for the management of patients with peripheral arterial disease (lower extremity, renal, mesenteric, and abdominal aortic): a collaborative report from the American Association for Vascular Surgery/Society for Vascular Surgery, Society for Cardiovascular Angiography and Interventions, Society for Vascular Medicine and Biology, Society of Interventional Radiology, and the ACC/AHA Task Force on Practice Guidelines (Writing Committee to Develop Guidelines for the Management of Patients With Peripheral Arterial Disease): endorsed by the American Association of Cardiovascular and Pulmonary Rehabilitation; National Heart, Lung, and Blood Institute; Society for Vascular Nursing; TransAtlantic Inter-Society Consensus; and Vascular Disease Foundation. Circulation 113:e463

Jou WW, Powers RD (1998) Utility of dipstick urinalysis as a guide to management of adults with suspected infection or hematuria. South Med J 91:266

Karmazyn B, Steinberg R, Kornreich L et al (2005) Clinical and

sonographic criteria of acute scrotum in children: a retrospective study of 172 boys. Pediatr Radiol 35:302
Kawashima A, Sandler CM, Corl FM et al (2001) Imaging of renal trauma: a comprehensive review. Radiographics 21:557
Lachs MS, Nachamkin I, Edelstein PH et al (1992) Spectrum bias in the evaluation of diagnostic tests: lessons from the rapid dipstick test for urinary tract infection. Ann Intern Med 117:135
Lammers RL, Gibson S, Kovacs D et al (2001) Comparison of test characteristics of urine dipstick and urinalysis at various test cutoff points. Ann Emerg Med 38:505
Leman P (2002) Validity of urinalysis and microscopy for detecting urinary tract infection in the emergency department. Eur J Emerg Med 9:141
Levine JA, Neitlich J, Verga M et al (1997) Ureteral calculi in patients with flank pain: correlation of plain radiography with unenhanced helical CT. Radiology 204:27
Liu W, Esler SJ, Kenny BJ et al (2000) Low-dose nonenhanced helical CT of renal colic: assessment of ureteric stone detection and measurement of effective dose equivalent. Radiology 215:51
Lynch TH, Martinez-Pineiro L, Plas E et al (2005) EAU guidelines on urological trauma. Eur Urol 47:1
Miller OF, Rineer SK, Reichard SR et al (1998) Prospective comparison of unenhanced spiral computed tomography and intravenous urogram in the evaluation of acute flank pain. Urology 52:982
Montague DK, Jarow J, Broderick GA et al (2003) American Urological Association guideline on the management of priapism. J Urol 170:1318
Moore EE, Shackford SR, Pachter HL et al (1989) Organ injury scaling: spleen, liver, and kidney. J Trauma 29:1664
Mutgi A, Williams JW, Nettleman M (1991) Renal colic. Utility of the plain abdominal roentgenogram. Arch Intern Med 151:1589
Niall O, Russell J, MacGrego, R et al (1999) A comparison of noncontrast computerized tomography with excretory urography in the assessment of acute flank pain. J Urol 161:534
Nicolaisen GS, McAninch JW, Marshall GA et al (1985) Renal trauma: re-evaluation of the indications for radiographic assessment. J Urol 133:183
Nolte-Ernsting CC, Tacke J, Adam GB et al (2001) Diuretic-enhanced gadolinium excretory MR urography: comparison of conventional gradient-echo sequences and echo-planar imaging. Eur Radiol 11:18
Reiter WJ, Schon-Pernerstorfer H, Dorfinger K et al (1999) Frequency of urolithiasis in individuals seropositive for human immunodeficiency virus treated with indinavir is higher than previously assumed. J Urol 161:1082
Sandhu C, Anson KM, Patel U (2003a) Urinary tract stones: Part II: current status of treatment. Clin Radiol 58:422
Sandhu C, Anson KM, Patel U (2003b) Urinary tract stones: Part I: role of radiological imaging in diagnosis and treatment planning. Clin Radiol 58:415
Sheafor DH, Hertzberg BS, Freed KS et al (2000) Nonenhanced helical CT and US in the emergency evaluation of patients with renal colic: prospective comparison. Radiology 217:792
Simerville JA, Maxted WC, Pahira JJ (2005) Urinalysis: a comprehensive review. Am Fam Physician 71:1153
Van den Berg JC, de Valois JC, Go PM et al (1999) Detection of groin hernia with physical examination, ultrasound, and MRI compared with laparoscopic findings. Invest Radiol 34:739
Venkatasubramaniam AK, Mehta T, Chetter IC et al (2004) The value of abdominal examination in the diagnosis of abdominal aortic aneurysm. Eur J Vasc Endovasc Surg 27:56
Weatherall M, Harwood M (2002) The accuracy of clinical assessment of bladder volume. Arch Phys Med Rehabil 83:1300

3 New Developments in Anesthesia

J. Motsch, Ch. Schramm, E. Martin

3.1 Perioperative Cardiac Complications

Major cardiac complications presenting as myocardial infarction, myocardial ischemia, cardiac failure, or life-threatening dysrhythmias contribute significantly to perioperative morbidity and mortality. Preventive strategies are of major importance since even despite adequate treatment these events are associated with poor outcome.

3.1.1 Myocardial Ischemia

According to Poldermans and Boersma (2005), the incidence of a perioperative myocardial infarction is 0.185% in the United States. Approximately 50,000out of 27 million patients who are given anesthesia for surgical procedures annually suffer perioperative myocardial infarction. The cause is a prolonged mismatch between myocardial oxygen demand and supply owing to the stress of surgery or as the result of a sudden rupture of a vulnerable plaque followed by thrombus formation and coronary artery occlusion.

Beta-blockers decrease the myocardial oxygen demand by reducing heart rate and myocardial contractility. Additionally they modulate the adrenergic activity leading to decreased levels of fatty acids, thus resulting in a shift in myocardial metabolism toward glucose uptake (Schouten et al. 2006). To identify patients who might benefit from a perioperative beta-blocker therapy, Lindenauer et al. (2005) conducted a retrospective cohort study on 782,969 patients using the validated Revised Cardiac Risk Index (RCRI) (Lee et al. 1999) to stratify patients as low cardiac risk (RCRI 0 and 1) and as high cardiac risk (RCRI 2, 3, 4 or more). The study demonstrated that perioperative beta-blocker therapy is associated with a reduced risk of in-hospital death among high risk, but not low-risk patients undergoing major noncardiac surgery.

According to the meta-analysis of Schouten et al. (2006), in 1,077 patients with noncardiac surgeries, perioperative administration of beta-blockers lowers the risk of myocardial ischemia by 65% ($p<0.001$), the risk of myocardial infarction by 56% ($p=0.04$), and the surrogate risk of cardiac death and nonfatal myocardial infarction by 67% ($p=0.002$). Administration of beta-blockers should be commenced prior to surgery, a dose-titration has to be carried out up to the induction of anesthesia, and a lifelong continuation of beta-blocker therapy is recommended in high-risk patients. The optimum time interval to start treatment with beta-blockers before surgery has not yet been defined by studies. The choice of the beta-blocker is of minor importance, since no specific beta-blocker demonstrated a superior effect in the perioperative setting. The side effects of perioperative administration of beta-blockers are a 4.3-fold increased risk of bradycardia ($p=0.006$), but hypotension, atrioventricular block, pulmonary edema, and bronchospasm are not significantly associated with perioperative beta-blocker therapy. The following contraindications should be kept in mind prior to commencement of beta-blocker therapy: bradycardia, second or third degree atrioventricular block, sick sinus syndrome, and acute heart failure. Patients with asthma bronchiale have to be carefully evaluated as to whether they may benefit from primary protective cardiac effects or are harmed by side effects.

For a practical pathway concerning the perioperative beta-blocker therapy, please refer to Fig. 3.1.

3.1.2 Arrhythmias

Cardiac arrhythmias contribute significantly to morbidity and mortality in the perioperative period. Although the knowledge on antiarrhythmic drug use in nonsurgical settings is expanding rapidly, data on the use of these agents perioperatively are still scarce.

Antiarrhythmic pharmacology is focused on the cardiac ion channels and adrenergic receptors for management of arrhythmias in adults during surgery and anesthesia. Virtually all drugs that modulate heart rhythm work through the adrenergic receptor/second messenger system through one or more ion channels. Generally three classes of ion channels have to be considered based on the cation they conduct: sodium (Na^+), calcium (Ca^{2+}), and potassium (K^+) channels. Although ion channels as molecular targets are distinctive, the drug receptor sites are highly homologous, causing some class overlap associated with antiarrhythmic therapy. Table 3.1 lists the molecular targets of antiarrhythmic agents used perioperatively.

Table 3.1. Classification of antiarrhythmic drugs

Receptor	Class	Drugs
Na^+, K^+ channels	IA	Amiodarone, procainamide, ajmaline, quinidine
Na^+ channels	IB	Lidocaine, phenytoin, mexiletine[a], tocainide[a]
	IC	Propafenone
Beta-adrenoceptors	II	Esmolol, amiodarone, propranolol, atenolol, sotalol[a]
K^+ channels	III	Bretylium, ibutilide, sotalol[a], dofetilide[a]
Ca^{2+} channels	IV	Verapamil, diltiazem, amiodarone

[a] Orally (only commercially available form)

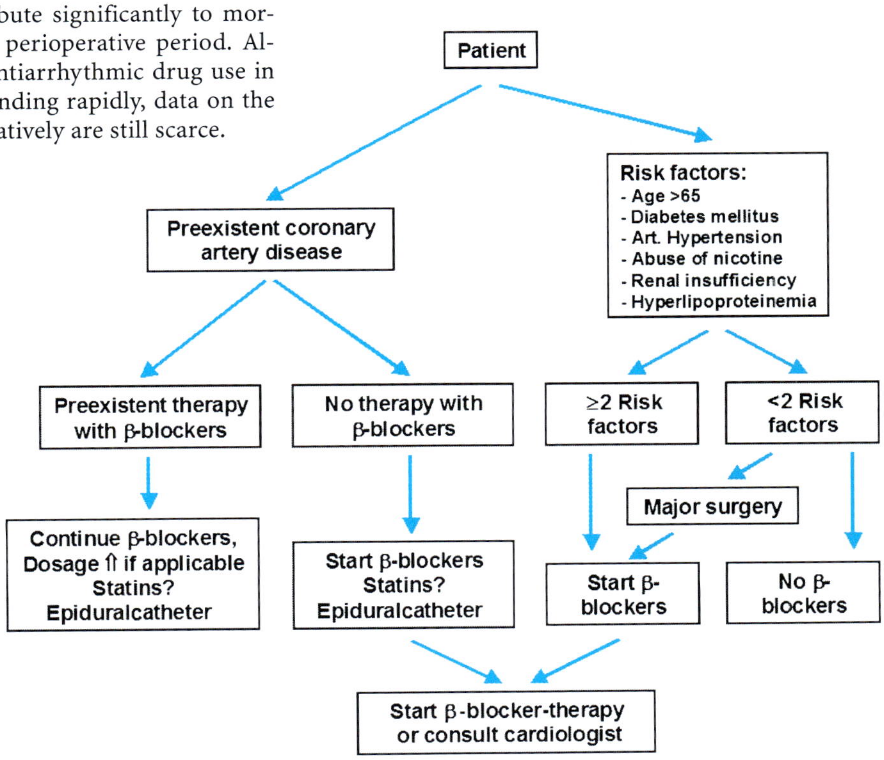

Fig. 3.1. Perioperative therapy with β-blockers. Patients with good left-ventricular function (LVF) receive metoprololsuccinate 95 mg once per day; patients with impaired LVF receive 47.5 mg once per day. For contraindications and further explanations see text. Modified from Teschendorf 2006

Perioperative arrhythmias are caused by physiologic and pathologic disturbances or by pharmacologic drug effects. Physiologic disturbances include hypoxemia, hypercapnia, acidosis, hypotension, hypovolemia, electrolyte imbalances, adrenergic stimulation (light anesthesia), vagal stimulation, and mechanical irritation (chest tube, pulmonary artery catheter). Pathologic cardiac disturbances include myocardial ischemia, infarction, acute heart failure, pulmonary embolism, and micro- or macrocirculatory shock. Therapy with proarrhythmic drugs must also be considered when arrhythmias occur perioperatively.

The primary indications for antiarrhythmics are compromised hemodynamics due to critical tachycardias or bradycardias with impaired cardiac output. Another indication is the increased risk for cardiac death due to malignant or potentially malignant arrhythmias. Since all of the antiarrhythmic drugs also bear a proarrhythmic effect, treatment with antiarrhythmics may harm the patient, as was demonstrated in the Cardiac Arrhythmia Suppression Trial (CAST). Therefore, a thorough risk–benefit analysis is mandatory prior to long-term treatment with antiarrhythmics. Generally, the primary aim of antiarrhythmic therapy is to treat the underlying condition such as coronary heart disease or acute heart failure and not to cure symptoms.

In the perioperative setting, arrhythmias are observed quite commonly. Since in the operating room environment there are many reversible causes that predispose patients to arrhythmias, these conditions should be treated before considering pharmacological antiarrhythmic strategies. But in some patients perioperative arrhythmias pose the potential for rapidly developing life-threatening events necessitating immediate treatment.

3.1.2.1
Bradycardia

Bradycardia is defined as a heart rate below 60 beats per minute. In trained athlete patients as well as in patients with excessive beta-blocker therapy, the heart rate can drop below 40 beats per minute with no symptoms. When low cardiac output is associated with bradycardia, the following stepwise therapeutic approach is indicated, where continuously the next step should be taken on failure of the previous step:

- Start with the administration of a parasympatholytic drug such as atropine up to 3 mg intravenously.
- Then administer a beta-adrenergic drug, e.g., epinephrine in boluses of 10 μg i.v.
- Thereafter consider the application of a transient pacemaker, either as an external transthoracic stimulation with pads or via an esophageal stimulation probe.

When an external pacemaker is not available, a defibrillator with its stimulation mode may be used in case of emergency. Alternatively, internal stimulation with a temporary transvenous-inserted sterile stimulation probe is the treatment of choice in severe heart block.

3.1.2.2
Supraventricular Tachyarrhythmias

Various adverse physiological phenomena can evoke supraventricular tachyarrhythmias in anesthetized or critically ill patients. For management of the surgical patient, a thorough but rapid consideration of potential causes is required, because correction of reversible conditions may prevent life-threatening conditions. Antiarrhythmic therapy should only be considered after these etiologies have been excluded or in cases of extreme hemodynamic instability.

The origin of supraventricular tachyarrhythmias lies in the area of the atria, the sinus node, or the atrioventricular node (AV node).

- Paroxysmal supraventricular tachyarrhythmia *with* preexcitation is caused (most commonly) by congenital short-circuit conductive fibers leading to a bypass of the regular excitation from the sinus node over the atria to the AV node.

Wolff-Parkinson-White syndrome (WPW) is the most common preexcitation syndrome with the so-called Kent fiber being the accessory conductive fiber. In type A WPW syndrome, ECG recordings show a positive delta wave in V1 and Q waves in II, III, and aVF. In type B WPW syndrome, a negative delta wave is recorded in V1 of the ECG. The delta wave is defined as a slow upslope of the R in the widened QRS complex. The PQ interval is below 0.12 s. WPW syndrome is potentially life-threatening, because an atrial fibrillation with the fast conducting accessory Kent fiber may lead to ventricular tachycardia or ventricular fibrillation. For treatment, a short trial of vagal stimulation may be attempted initially by the Valsalva maneuver or massage of the carotid sinus. On failure, the antiarrhythmic ajmalin 50 mg is administered by slow intravenous injection under ECG monitoring. As an alternative, amiodarone, procainamide, or flecainide should be considered.

It should be noted that patients with accessory pathways may also develop atrial fibrillation. These patients are at increased risk for developing ventricular fibrillation when treated with classic AV-nodal blocking agents (digitalis, calcium channel blockers, beta-blockers, adenosine), because these agents reduce the accessory bundle refractory period.

- A type of paroxysmal supraventricular tachyarrhythmia (PSVT) *without* preexcitation is the AV node reentry tachycardia. In two-thirds of patients, it is caused by a congenital defect of the cardiac conductive system, in one-third of patients, it is caused by a prolapse of the mitral valve, hyperthyroidosis, or other cardiac diseases. The ECG trace shows a heart rate of 180–200 beats/min, small QRS complexes, and a missing P wave. The symptomatic therapy consists of adenosine (6 mg bolus, after 3 min 12 mg bolus), verapamil (5 mg slow intravenous injection over 10 min), or overdrive pacing in circulatory stable patients. In unstable patients with a threat of cardiogenic shock, an electroconversion is indicated with initially 200 J, on failure with higher energy of 360 J. If the patient is conscious, a short-acting hypnotic such as etomidate or propofol should be used for sedation during the electroconversion. Causal therapy is high-frequency catheter ablation.

- Atrial fibrillation (AF) is the most common type of supraventricular tachyarrhythmia. The prevalence is about 0.5% of the adult population, but at age greater than 60 years, the prevalence is 4%. The etiology is primary or idiopathic in patients without cardiac disease or secondary due to a cardiac disease such as mitral valve disease, coronary heart disease, or due to extracardial causes such as arterial hypertension or alcohol-toxic effects on the heart ("holiday-heart"). The irregular conduction in the AV node leads to a tachyarrhythmia of the ventricles with frequencies of 100–150 beats/min. Treatment strategies include frequency control, conversion into sinus rhythm, and prophylaxis of recurrence. The frequency control is achieved by administering digitalis and verapamil (calcium channel blocker). ECG-triggered cardioversion is performed under short sedation with an initial energy of 100 J. It may be advisable to first establish a therapeutic level of an antiarrhythmic agent that maintains sinus rhythm (i.e., amiodarone, procainamide) in order to minimize the risk of SVT recurrence following electrical cardioversion. It is important to anticoagulate the patient before the cardioversion, if the AF persists longer than 48 h because intracardiac thrombi may have been formed. Thrombi formation can be checked by TTE (transthoracic echocardiography) or by TEE (transesophageal echocardiography). As an alternative, a drug-induced chemical cardioversion may be considered.

For intraoperative and postoperative patients developing new-onset AF who are stable and rate-controlled, pharmacological cardioversion of SVT is questionable. The 24-h rate of spontaneous conversion to sinus rhythm exceeds 50% and many patients who develop SVT under anesthesia will remit spontaneously before or during emergence. Moreover, the antiarrhythmic agents with long-term activity against atrial arrhythmias have limited efficacy when used for rapid pharmacologic cardioversion. Improved rates have been seen with amiodarone, but further studies have to confirm this because of the potential for undesirable side effects. Finally, it should be kept in mind that in recent-onset perioperative SVT, reversible causes should be excluded or resolved before considering pharmacological antiarrhythmic therapies.

3.1.2.3 Ventricular Tachyarrhythmias

Morphology (monomorphic vs polymorphic) and duration (sustained vs nonsustained) characterizes ventricular arrhythmias. Nonsustained ventricular tachycardia (NSVT) is defined as three or more premature ventricular contractions that occur at a rate exceeding 100 beats/min and last 30 s or less without hemodynamic compromise. The origin of ventricular premature beats is below the bifurcation of the HIS fibers. Usually the sinus node is not stimulated backwards. This leads to a compensatory pause, which is felt by the patient as an extra beat of the heart. These arrhythmias are routinely seen in the absence of cardiac disease and may not require drug therapy in the perioperative period. In contrast, in patients with structural heart disease, these nonsustained rhythms do predict subsequent life-threatening ventricular arrhythmias. However, antiarrhythmic drug therapies in patients with structural heart disease may worsen survival. When nonsustained ventricular arrhythmias occur during or after major operations, early or late mortality of patients with preserved left ventricular function is not influenced. These patients usually do not require antiarrhythmic drug therapy. However, as in SVT, these arrhythmias may signal reversible etiologies that should be treated. For example, potassium- and magnesium-serum levels should be checked and elevated digitalis levels should be excluded.

Sustained ventricular tachycardia (VT) presents as monomorphic or polymorphic. In monomorphic VT, the amplitude of the QRS complex remains constant, while in polymorphic ventricular tachycardia the QRS morphology continually changes.

Ventricular tachycardia is characterized as a regular tachycardia of 100–200 beats/min with bundle-branch-block-like deformed, widened ventricular complexes. The underlying etiology is idiopathic, severe organic cardiac disease, intoxication of digitalis or treatment with other antiarrhythmics, or the Brugada syndrome (congenital mutation of the sodium channel). The underlying mechanism for monomorphic VT is formation of a re-entry pathway, e.g., around scar tissue from a healed myocardial infarction.

This is a life-threatening condition and immediate action is required. Although lidocaine has traditionally been the primary drug therapy for all sustained ventricular arrhythmias, i.v. amiodarone is now also recommended for treatment of perioperative-occurring monomorphic VT.

Treatment strategies for sustained polymorphic ventricular tachycardia depend on the duration of the QT interval during a prior sinus rhythm. In the setting of a prolonged QT interval (torsades de points), emphasis is taken at reversal of QT prolongation. In addition to QT-prolonging antiarrhythmic drugs (class IA or III), a number of other medications used in the perioperative period may evoke QT prolongation and torsades de points. The management of torsades de points includes i.v. magnesium sulfate (2–4 g), repleting potassium, maneuvers increasing the heart rate (atropine, temporary atrial or ventricular pacing). Hemodynamic collapse requires asynchronous DC countershocks. When antiarrhythmic therapy is deemed necessary, i.v. amiodarone may be considered, because it bears the lowest risk of triggering torsades de points.

Unstable ventricular tachycardia and ventricular fibrillation are life-threatening arrhythmias in the operating room. The most important first maneuvers in patients who experience VF perioperatively are nonpharmacological: rapid defibrillation (360 J monophasic or 200 J biphasic), and correction of reversible etiologies. Amiodarone i.v. (300 mg) should be considered as pharmacological intervention in addition to other measures taken during resuscitation (Thompson and Balser 2004).

A new therapeutic option for the treatment of VT is the implantation of antitachycardic pacemakers. The implantable cardioverter defibrillator (ICD) is used in patients with increased risk of sudden cardiac death due to ventricular fibrillation in recurrent ventricular tachyarrhythmias or history of VF (ventricular fibrillation) with significantly impaired ventricular function. For supraventricular tachyarrhythmia, termination of the reentry mechanisms can be achieved by overdrive pacing with a stimulation frequency above the tachycardic frequency, programmable electrostimulation to terminate circulating impulses through premature impulses, or atrial high-frequency stimulation for the conversion of atrial flutter (Herold et al. 2006).

For an overview of the antiarrhythmic therapy, please refer to Fig. 3.2.

3.1.3 Acute Heart Failure

The acute heart failure (AHF) is defined as the rapid onset of symptoms and signs secondary to abnormal cardiac function. It may occur with or without previous cardiac disease. The cardiac dysfunction can be related to systolic or diastolic dysfunction, abnormalities in cardiac rhythm, or preload and afterload mismatch. It is often life-threatening and requires urgent treatment.

3.1.3.1 Etiology

In the perioperative setting, AHF poses a serious threat to the patient, because these patients have a very poor prognosis. The 60-day mortality rate was 9.6% and the combined rate for mortality and rehospitalization was 35.2% in the largest randomized trial to date (Cleland et al. 2003). The most common cause of AHF in the elderly is coronary heart disease, whereas in the younger population it is caused by dilatative cardiomyopathy, arrhythmia, congenital or valvular heart disease, or myocarditis (see Table 3.2).

3.1.3.2 Diagnosis

The diagnosis of AHF is primarily based on clinical findings, electrocardiogram (ECG), laboratory tests, chest x-ray, and echocardiography.

An impaired right ventricular function may be suspected if prominent jugular veins are present. To a cer-

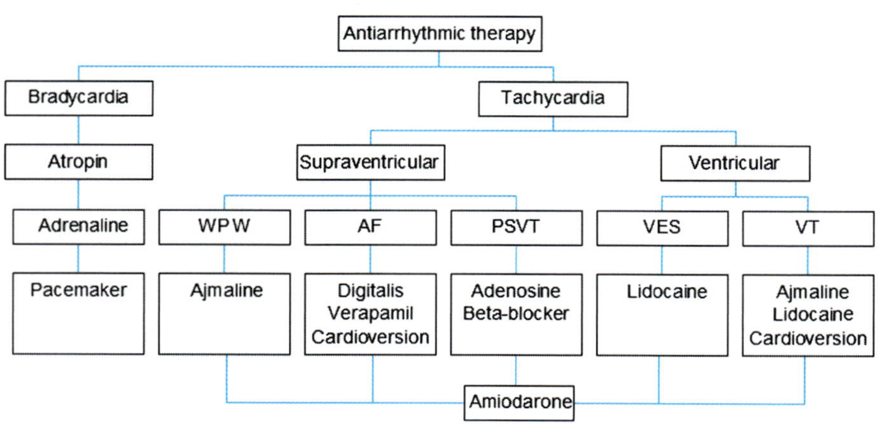

Fig. 3.2. Pathway for antiarrhythmic therapy. *WPW* Wolff-Parkison-White syndrome, *AF* atrial fibrillation, *PSVT* paroxysmal supraventricular tachycardia, *VES* ventricular extrasystole, *VT* ventricular tachycardia. Modified from Herold et al. (2006)

Table 3.2. Causes and precipitating factors in acute heart failure

Decompensation of preexisting chronic heart failure (e.g., cardiomyopathy)
Acute coronary syndromes: myocardial infarction/unstable angina with large extent of ischemia and ischemic dysfunction; mechanical complication of acute myocardial infarction; right ventricular infarction
Hypertensive crisis
Acute arrhythmia (ventricular tachycardia, ventricular fibrillation, atrial fibrillation or flutter, other supraventricular tachycardia)
Valvular regurgitation/endocarditis/rupture of chordae tendineae, worsening of preexisting valvular regurgitation
Severe aortic valve stenosis
Acute severe myocarditis
Cardiac tamponade
Aortic dissection
Postpartum cardiomyopathy
Noncardiovascular precipitating factors: lack of compliance with medical treatment, volume overload, infections, particularly pneumonia or septicemia, severe brain insult, after major surgery, reduction in renal function, asthma, drug abuse, alcohol abuse, pheochromocytoma
High output syndromes: septicemia, thyrotoxic crisis, anemia, shunt syndromes

Modified from Nieminen (2005)

tain extent, measurement of the central venous pressure (CVP) allows quantification of the amount of congestion. The normal range of the CVP is 4–12 cm H_2O. Caution is necessary in the interpretation of high measured values of central venous pressure in AHF, as this may be a reflection of decreased venous compliance together with decreased right ventricular (RV) compliance even in the presence of inadequate RV filling. If the left ventricular function is impaired, wet rales in the lung fields are present during chest auscultation.

A chest x-ray confirms the diagnosis of left ventricular failure and allows the differential diagnosis to inflammatory or infectious lung diseases. Additionally the chest x-ray is used for follow-up of improvement or unsatisfactory response to therapy.

The ECG usually shows pathologic signs in patients with AHF. It determines the etiology of the AHF and may indicate strain of the left or right ventricle or the atria, acute coronary syndromes, arrhythmias, perimyocarditis, and preexisting conditions such as left or right ventricular hypertrophy or dilated cardiomyopathy.

The recommended laboratory test in AHF include arterial blood gas analysis (BGA), venous oxygen saturation, plasma B-type natriuretic peptide (BNP), and standard tests such as blood count, platelet count, urea, electrolytes, blood glucose, and creatinine phosphokinase. The arterial BGA allows assessment of oxygenation (p_aO_2), adequacy of respiratory function (pCO_2), and acid–base balance (pH). Venous oxygen saturation is determined by oxygen supply, oxygen consumption of the body and regional circulation. It is useful as an estimate of the total body oxygen supply–demand balance. Another useful laboratory test is the plasma BNP, which is released from the cardiac ventricles in response to increased wall stretch and volume overload. The decision cut-off point is proposed as 100 pg/ml.

Echocardiography is used in AHF to evaluate the functional and structural changes of the heart and to assess acute coronary syndromes. Additional information is gathered by echo-Doppler studies, which can estimate pulmonary artery pressures (from the tricuspid regurgitation jet) and left ventricular preload.

Additional diagnostic procedures such as angiography, CT scan, or scintigraphy may be indicated according to the etiology of the AHF.

3.1.3.3 Therapy

If the diagnosis of AHF is verified, the patient must be treated in specialized wards such as emergency units, chest pain units, or intensive care units. The physicians should be trained and should follow guidelines.

If immediate resuscitation is necessary, basic and advanced life support (BLS/ALS) is applied according to the applicable guidelines.

The patient in distress or pain requires treatment with a sedative or analgesic agent. In this context, morphine is recommended in the early stage of the treatment, when a patient is admitted with severe AHF presenting with the signs of restlessness and shortness of breath (dyspnea). Additional effects of morphine include venodilation, mild arterial dilation, and reduction of the heart rate. Intravenous boluses of 3 mg (2–5 mg) are recommended and may be repeated as needed.

To achieve adequate tissue oxygenation, an arterial oxygen saturation of greater than 95 % is favorable. It is important to realize that increased concentrations of oxygen to patients without evidence of hypoxemia may cause harm, because hyperoxemia can be associated with reduced coronary blood flow, reduced cardiac output, increased blood pressure, and increased systemic vascular resistance. When arterial oxygen saturation is too low, oxygen supply via a face mask with reservoir bag is effective to increase inspiratory oxygen concentration. In case of failure, ventilatory support without endotracheal intubation is supplied as noninvasive ventilation: continuous positive airway pressure (CPAP) or biphasic positive airway pressure (BiPAP). If acute respiratory failure by AHF-induced respiratory muscle fatigue does not respond to vasodilators, oxygen therapy and noninvasive ventilation, the trachea has to be intubated and mechanical ventilation of the lungs commenced.

During bradycardia-induced AHF, external or internal pacing restores an adequate heart rhythm. Cardiac arrhythmias or tachycardia can cause AHF. Since antiarrhythmic drugs and beta-blocking agents such as metoprolol have negative inotropic properties, they should be used with extreme caution in AHF. However, in patients with acute myocardial infarction, who stabilize after having developed AHF, beta-blockers should be initiated early.

In patients with AHF and absence of hypotension (mean blood pressure above 70 mmHg) vasodilators are indicated. The primary pharmacologic treatment options include nitrates such as glyceryl trinitrate or isosorbide dinitrate, sodium nitroprusside, and the new agent nesiritide (atrial natriuretic peptide). The nitrates relieve pulmonary congestion without compromising stroke volume or increasing myocardial oxygen demand in acute left heart failure, particularly in patients with acute coronary syndrome. Their effect is limited to 16–24 h primarily due to development of tolerance. Sodium nitroprusside is indicated in patients with severe heart failure and in patients with predominantly increased afterload such as hypertensive heart failure or acute mitral regurgitation due to ruptured papillary muscle as a complication of severe myocardial infarction. The substance should be used cautiously, invasive monitoring of blood pressure is usually required, and toxicity of the cyanide metabolites should be taken into account. The new drug nesiritide is a recombinant human brain peptide, which is identical to the endogenous hormone produced by the ventricle (see description above). Nesiritide has venous, arterial, and coronary vasodilatory properties, reducing preload and afterload and thereby increasing cardiac output without direct inotropic effects. Calcium antagonists are contraindicated in AHF; ACE inhibitors are not indicated in the early stabilization phase of patients with AHF.

If the patients show symptoms of AHF secondary to fluid retention, diuretics are indicated. Usually loop diuretics such as furosemide or torasemide are administered. Hydrochlorothiazide (HCT) or spironolactone is added to loop diuretics in patients that are refractory to loop diuretics alone; a concomitant alkalosis is treated with acetazolamide. In refractory renal failure, hemodialysis or hemofiltration is initiated.

If the preload is low, a fluid challenge is indicated, but should be administered with extreme caution.

After executing all of the therapeutic steps mentioned above, the adequacy of cardiac output is assessed by reversal of metabolic acidosis, venous oxygen saturation, and clinical signs of adequate organ perfusion. The application of catecholamines or phosphodi-

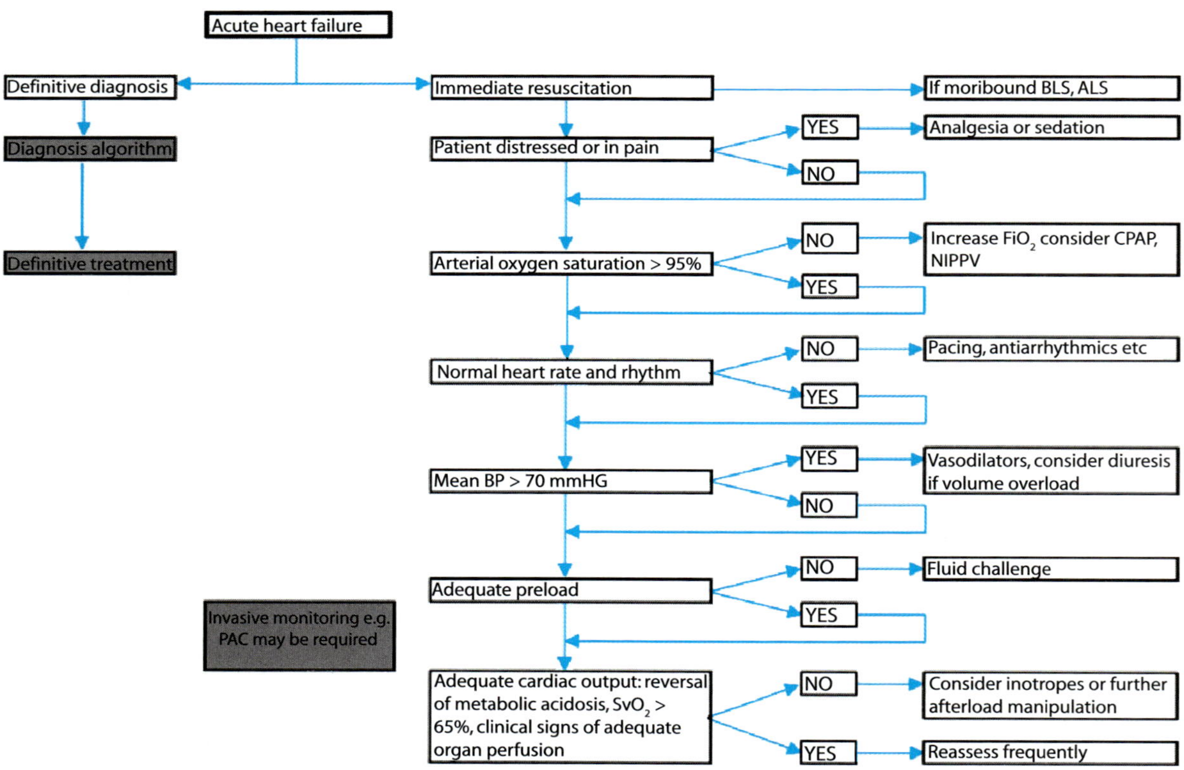

Fig. 3.3. Flow chart for immediate goals in treatment of the patients with acute heart failure. In coronary artery disease, the patient's mean blood pressure (mBP) should be higher to ensure coronary perfusion, mBP> 70, or systolic > 90 mmHg. *BLS* basic life support, *ALS* advanced life support, *CPAP* continuous positive airway pressure, *NIPPV* noninvasive positive pressure ventilation. From Nieminen et al. (2005)

esterase inhibitors as inotropic agents is indicated in persistent heart failure, if tissue hypoperfusion does not suspend under the therapy described previously; but one must pay particular attention to these patients as catecholamines increase the oxygen consumption of the heart.

Dopamine incorporates dose-dependent properties of action on the receptors: it stimulates dopamine receptors at low doses (<2 μg/kg/min), beta-adrenergic receptors at medium doses (2–5 μg/kg/min), and alpha receptors at high doses (>5 μg/kg/min). Dopamine may be used as an inotropic (>2 μg/kg/min i.v.) in AHF with hypotension. Infusion of low doses of dopamine (≤2–3 μg/kg/min i.v.) may be used to improve renal blood flow and diuresis in decompensated heart failure with hypotension and low urine output. However, if no response is seen, the therapy should be terminated, because no controlled trials regarding its long-term effects on renal function and survival have been conducted and concerns regarding its potential untoward effects on pituitary function, T cell responsiveness, gastrointestinal perfusion, chemoreceptor sensitivity, and ventilation have been raised.

Dobutamine stimulates beta1 receptors and beta2 receptors in a 3:1 ratio. The effect is a positive inotropic and chronotropic action as well as peripheral vasodilation. To increase cardiac output, dobutamine is initiated with an infusion rate of 2–3 μg/kg/min, which can be increased up to 20 μg/kg/min. After 24–48 h, beta-receptor tolerance decreases the effect of dobutamine. The indication for dobutamine is evidence of peripheral hypoperfusion (hypotension, decreased renal function) with or without congestion or pulmonary edema refractory to volume replacement, diuretics, and vasodilators at optimal doses.

Phosphodiesterase inhibitors such as enoximone and milrinone have a site of action distal of the beta receptors, which results in persistent inotropic, lusitropic, and peripheral vasodilatory effects even in the presence of beta-blockers. Therefore, they are preferred to dobutamine in patients with concomitant beta-blocker therapy. In severe heart failure, a combination of phosphodiesterase inhibitors with epinephrine or norepinephrine is indicated in order to provide sufficient cardiac output with adequate perfusion pressure.

The new substance levosimendan (calcium sensitizer) has two main mechanisms of action: calcium sensitization of the contractile proteins, responsible for positive inotropic action, and smooth muscle potassium channel opening, responsible for peripheral vasodilatation. It is indicated in patients with symptomatic low cardiac output heart failure secondary to cardiac systolic dysfunction without severe hypotension.

If the combined administration of inotropic substances and a fluid challenge fail to relieve the symptoms of AHF, a potent vasopressor such as epinephrine is indicated. Norepinephrine may be considered in right heart failure or in combination with phosphodiesterase inhibitors (Fig. 3.3) (Nieminen et al. 2005).

3.2 Deep Vein Thrombosis and Pulmonary Embolism

3.2.1 Risk Factors

Perioperative thromboembolic disease and pulmonary embolism contribute to morbidity and mortality in urological patients. Venous thromboembolism is a multifactorial disease involving clinical risk factors as well as genetic and environmental interactions. It is uncommon in the young, but after 40 years of age the incidence doubles with each decade of life. Hereditary risk factors include factor V Leiden mutation, G20210A prothrombin gene mutation, and deficiencies in protein C, protein S, and antithrombin. Hereditary and/or acquired risk factors are hyperhomocysteinemia and elevated levels of factor I, VIII, and IX. Acquired risk factors include malignancy, hospitalization/immobility, surgery, venous trauma, estrogen therapy, pregnancy, and the presence of antiphospholipid antibodies. Especially operations at the prostate activate the coagulation cascade. These patients are therefore prone to develop deep veins thrombosis and thrombosis in the pelvic vein bearing an increased risk of pulmonary embolism.

It is important to identify patients with risk factors for venous thromboembolism and pulmonary embolism and patients with contraindications for the regular prophylaxis, because routine surveillance and screening are not cost-effective in the perioperative setting, as they do not reduce symptomatic venous thromboembolism or fatal pulmonary embolism. In most cases, it is not necessary to initiate specific diagnostic procedures to identify the exact cause of the thrombophilia, but rather attach importance to a consequent perioperative antithrombotic strategy. Therefore, prevention using the standard protocol for prophylaxis is far more preferable. Anticoagulants are the first choice in the prevention of perioperative thromboembolic disease. There are widespread differences in the use of prophylaxis, however, although guidelines were published recently (Geerts et al. 2004).

One exception of the above-mentioned approach is a deficiency of antithrombin or protein C, which is usually known by the patient. After a targeted evaluation, a specific therapy with substitution of the deficient factor might by useful (Dempfle 2005).

According to a prospective study in 99 cancer patients by Sarig et al. (2005), F.V and F.VIII are elevated and can lead to acquired protein C resistance. These au-

Table 3.3. Risk factors for thromboembolic complications

Hereditary	Factor V Leiden mutation G20210A prothrombin gene mutation Protein C deficiency Protein S deficiency Antithrombin III deficiency
Hereditary and/or acquired	Hyperhomocysteinemia Anticardiolipin antibodies Lupus anticoagulant Elevation of F.I or F.VIII or F.IX
Acquired	Surgery requiring more than 30 min of anesthesia, especially cancer surgery Malignancy Fracture of pelvis, femur, or tibia Age > 40 years History of venous thromboembolism Obesity Pregnancy or recent delivery Estrogen therapy Prolonged immobilization, nursing home confinement Cerebrovascular incident Congestive heart failure Permanent pacemaker, internal cardiac defibrillator Chronic in-dwelling central venous catheter Inflammatory bowel disease Hypertension Cigarette smoking Long-haul air travel Activated protein C resistance

Modified from Motsch et al. (2006)

thors assume that acquired protein C resistance can serve as a possible risk factor for thromboembolic complications in cancer patients, but this needs to be further evaluated. In general, cancer is a major risk factor for developing thromboembolic complications. Therefore from the surgeon's point of view, it has been raised that patients presenting with the first episode of thromboembolic disease should always be screened for cancer. It should always be kept in mind that patients with prostate cancer are at increased risk for thrombosis or Trousseau syndrome, which is a manifestation of a chronic disseminated intravascular coagulopathy and clinically presents as a migratory superficial phlebitis. Table 3.3 summarizes the risk factors for thromboembolic complications.

3.2.2 Medical History

To reveal an increased risk for thromboembolism, the examiner should pay special attention to the following conditions in the patient's medical history: deep venous thrombosis, thrombophlebitis, pulmonary embolism, myocardial infarction, angina pectoris, other signs of coronary disease, cardiac arrhythmias, occlusion of arterial vessels, embolic events, strokes, prolonged ischemic deficits, anticoagulatory therapy, unexpected or allergic reactions to anticoagulants, immobilization before surgery, influenza-like diseases, and other conditions that initiate an acute phase reaction. Additionally, the medical history of relatives is important in order to detect a thrombophilic disposition: venous thromboembolism, arterial occlusion, cerebral ischemia, transitional neurologic deficits, and relatives with continuous anticoagulatory medication.

3.2.3 Therapy

After careful evaluation of the individual patient, an individual assessment of the degree of risk for perioperative thromboembolic complications is applied. Based on this evaluation, the appropriate prophylaxis is selected.

The basic preventive perioperative therapy against thromboembolism consists of early mobilization and the use of graduated elastic compression stockings. However, the backbone of specific strategies for perioperative prevention of venous thromboembolism is treatment with anticoagulants. The old drug, unfractionated heparin, is characterized by serious adverse effects and by large interindividual variability necessitating close monitoring. The new anticoagulants have a more predictable action, higher efficiency and are easier to handle because they no longer require routine monitoring, but effective antagonists are mostly lacking.

Although there are widespread differences in the use of prophylaxis, the following recommendations, which are based on recently published guidelines can be suggested. According to these guidelines (Motsch et al. 2006), low molecular weight heparins (LMWH) ≤3,400 U once daily or unfractionated heparin (UFH) 5,000 U every 8 h should be administered to general surgery patients without any additional risk factors for venous thromboembolism. High-risk patients should receive LMWH >3,400 U daily. Cancer patients should be treated as patients at high risk. Therefore, LMWH greater than 3,400 U should be administered twice daily and continued for 28 days. For patients with prolonged postoperative intensive care unit treatment and with delayed recovery, a surveillance by venous ultrasonography should be considered, because of the high incidence of venous thrombosis in patients staying in intensive care units.

New agents, such as fondaparinux, idraparinux are superior to the standard treatment in the prevention of venous thromboembolism after high-risk major orthopedic surgery and for initial treatment of patients with venous thromboembolism. In orthopedic patients, the risk of venous thromboembolism was reduced by approximately 55%. Although major bleeding occurred

Table 3.4. Risk stratification and therapy recommendations in pulmonary embolism

Risk category	Hemodynamic function	Therapy recommendations
1	Stable, no right ventricular dysfunction	Anticoagulation, using LMWH (or UFH) or fondaparinux
2	Stable, signs of right ventricular dysfunction	Anticoagulation, in some cases thrombolysis
3	Shock	Thrombolysis, except for strong contraindications
4	Cardiopulmonary resuscitation	Thrombolysis

Modified from Motsch et al. (2006)

more frequently, the incidence of critical bleeding was comparable to patients receiving LMWH (enoxaparin). Such superior prophylactic effects of fondaparinux could not be confirmed in 2,297 patients undergoing abdominal surgery when compared to dalteparin in a double-blind study. Data for prophylaxis in major urologic operations are lacking. Therefore, these new anticoagulants such as fondaparinux need to be evaluated for the perioperative urologic setting.

Inferior vena cava filters are not advisable for long-term treatment, because they pose a nidus for recurrent thrombi, but may be considered as temporary retrievable filters in selected cases, when patients cannot receive anticoagulation.

If pulmonary embolism is present, the therapy is stratified according to the severity of the disease, ranging from the use of anticoagulants to thrombolysis (see Table 3.4).

3.3 Shock

3.3.1 Intraoperative and Postoperative Hemorrhage

In the case of massive perioperative hemorrhage, the administration/substitution of large quantities of crystalloid and colloid solution and blood products is required to maintain an adequate circulating volume with a sufficient organ and tissue perfusion.

The preparation for red blood cells is usually a leukocyte-depleted erythrocyte concentrate extracted from a whole blood donation. Another product is fresh frozen plasma (FFP), which is also extracted from a whole blood donation. FFP needs to be warmed for about 40 min at 37 °C, until it can be used. This long delay can be bridged in very urgent cases with readily available coagulation factors such as Prothrombin factor II, Proconvertin factor VII, Christmas-Factor (factor IX), Stuart-Prower-Factor (factor X) concentrate (PPSB), antithrombin 3 (AT III), fibrinogen, and recombinant factor VIIa. The third column of blood component therapy are platelets, which are available as a pool concentrate from four whole blood donations or as an apheresis preparation from one donor.

Other solutions to maintain an adequate intravascular volume are colloidal solutions such as hydroxyethyl starches, gelatin, and dextran, which remain for a longer period in the intravascular system. Crystalloid solutions such as ringer's lactate or normal saline have a disadvantage in severe hemorrhage in that they distribute throughout the extracellular space, e.g., to fill up 1 l of lost blood 3–4 l of crystalloid solution is needed for replacement.

A new approach for fluid resuscitation in severe hypovolemic shock in emergency medicine is to combine a hypertonic solution (e.g., 7.5 % sodium chloride solution) with hyperoncotic solutions (e.g., 6 % Hydroxy ethyl starch [HES]) to mobilize the interstitial fluid to

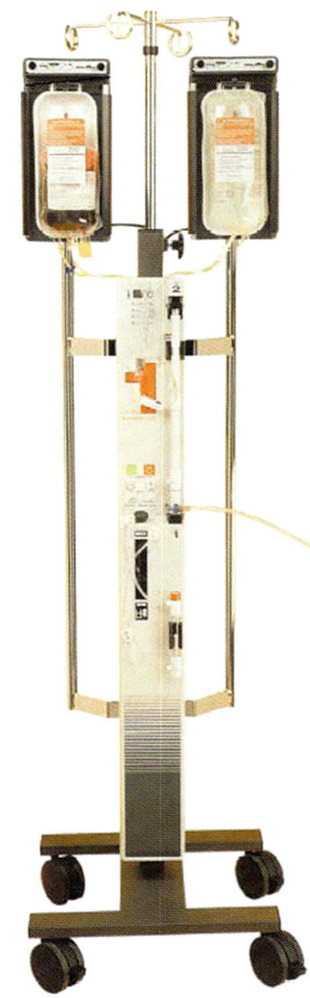

Fig. 3.4. High-flow blood and fluid warmer, System 1025, Level 1 (Level 1, Inc. 2006)

increase the intravascular volume. Since the dosage necessary is only 3 – 4 ml/kg of body weight in adults, this effective procedure is called small-volume resuscitation.

For the administration of fluid quantities required per time, large-bore intravenous cannulas of the highest possible diameters are useful. The diameter of appropriate peripheral cannulas is 14 gauge placed in the v. basilica or v. jugularis externa or 12-Fr catheters in the v. jugularis interna, v. subclavia, or v. femoralis. Special high-flow infusion lines and three-way-stop cocks should be used as well: because of the large diameter they allow the high required flows for fluid resuscitation. Fluid warming with special devices is advisable in order to prevent hypothermia with consecutive deterioration of the coagulation system and negative cardiac side effects. Pressure is applied to the infusion bags by compressing the infusion bags with a manually or automatically driven pressure bag. Figure 3.4 shows an example of a high-flow blood and fluid warmer, where up to 1,100 ml/min of fluid can be administered to the patient.

3.3.2 Anaphylaxis

The anaphylactic reaction (AR) is defined as an immediate humoral reaction due to preformed membrane-adherent immunoglobulins IgE, which lead to the release of histamine and other mediators. Anaphylaxis is the worst possible variant of an AR. The incidence for a severe intraoperative AR is 1 : 6,000 to 1 : 28,000.

Triggers for perioperative AR include neuromuscular blocking agents (60 % – 70 %), latex (18 %), colloidal solutions (5 %), barbiturates, antibiotics, opioids, protamine, ethylene oxide, blood transfusions, and methylmethacrylate (bone cement). Cross reactions such as penicillin – cephalosporin or sulfonamide – loop diuretics should be considered, as the AR to one substance may also implicate the AR to the other substance.

3.3.2.1 Symptoms and Treatment

The symptoms vary from a light cutaneous reaction (degree 0) to cardiopulmonary arrest (degree 4). Symptoms and treatment of each stage are described below.

Degree 0 is a localized cutaneous reaction (urticaria). Discontinuing of the trigger substance, reassurance, and in most cases the establishment of an intravenous line is indicated.

Degree 1 is a light general reaction with the following symptoms: disseminated cutaneous reaction (flush, pruritus, generalized urticaria), reaction of the mucous membranes, edema (nose, conjunctivitis), and general symptoms (cephalgia, restlessness, vomiting). The therapeutic measure include discontinuation of the triggering agent, reassurance, placement of an intravenous line, fluid resuscitation (500 ml), corticosteroids (e.g., 250 mg prednisolone), and antihistaminics (e.g., 0.1 mg/kg dimethindene in combination with 5 mg/kg cimetidine).

Degree 2 is a pronounced general reaction (pulmonary and/or cardiovascular reaction), dysregulation of the circulatory system (tachycardia, hypotension, arrhythmias), Quincke edema, laryngeal edema, dyspnea, beginning bronchospasm, and urge for defecation and urination. The treatment consists of the discontinuation of the allergen, intubation, and mechanical ventilation in good time, intravenous line and fluid resuscitation (500 – 1,000 ml). Epinephrine should be administered in boluses of 5 – 50 μg i.v., corticosteroids and antihistaminics should be administered as described above, and bronchospasmolytics be administered as needed (inhalative beta-2-mimetics such as terbutaline, fenoterol, salbutamol, and intravenous theophylline 5 mg/kg i.v.).

Degree 3 is characterized by a general reaction with shock, bronchospasm, and unconsciousness. In addition to the measures taken in degree 2 anaphylactic reactions, mechanical ventilation should be provided with 100 % oxygen, fluid resuscitation with 1,000 – 2,000 ml crystalloid and colloid solution, epinephrine (initial bolus 5 – 100 μg, followed by continuous infusion starting with 0.01 μg/kg/min effect-adjusted, dopamine infusion (3 – 7 μg/kg/min), prednisolone 500 – 1,000 mg i.v., and vasopressors (Caffedrine/theoadrenalin, etilefrine, or norepinephrine).

Degree 4 is a failure of vital organs resulting in cardiorespiratory arrest. Immediate basic and advanced life support must be initiated. In addition to the measures taken in degree 3 anaphylaxis, fluid resuscitation exceeding the amount of 2,000 – 3,000 ml and norepinephrine in boluses of 10 – 50 μg i.v. must be given (Heck and Fresenius 2004).

3.4 Sepsis

3.4.1 Definitions

3.4.1.1 Systemic Inflammatory Response Syndrome

If a patient presents with at least two of the criteria listed in Table 3.5, but lacks evidence for infection, the conditions for a systemic inflammatory response syndrome (SIRS) are met. The SIRS is the uniform answer of the body to a variety of diseases such as pancreatitis, major operation, severe trauma, or ischemia. Additionally a drop in the platelet count and the antithrombin-III levels (AT-III) is usually seen (Fresenius and Heck 2001).

Table 3.5. Definition of the systemic inflammatory response syndrome

Temperature >38 °C or <36 °C
Tachycardia >90 beats/min
Respiratory insufficiency (at least one of the following three criteria)
Respiratory frequency >20/min
Hyperventilation p_aCO_2 <32 mm Hg (with spontaneous respiration)
p_aO_2 <70 mm Hg (during spontaneous respiration) or p_aO_2/F_IO_2 <175 (during mechanical ventilation with absence of pulmonary disease)
WBC >12,000/μl or <4,000/μl or >10 % immature bands

For the diagnosis of SIRS at least two criteria have to be met
From AACP/SCCM (1992); *WBC* white blood cell count

3.4.1.2
Sepsis

If the source of an infection can be located and the SIRS criteria are present, the definition of sepsis is met. The incidence of sepsis is five per 1,000 inpatients; the 28-day mortality varies between 25% and 35%, in severe sepsis up to 60%.

The definition for severe sepsis includes the standard sepsis criteria in conjunction with signs of organ dysfunction, hypoperfusion, or sepsis-induced hypotension, which present as lactate acidosis, oliguria, encephalopathy, or thrombocytopenia.

A septic shock is the combination of sepsis with arterial hypotension, defined as arterial blood pressure below 90 mm Hg (or a decrease of more than 40 mm Hg from the baseline value for more than 1 h) despite adequate fluid resuscitation. It is accompanied by decreased perfusion or dysfunction of the organs.

3.4.2
Standard Therapy for Sepsis

The standard therapy for sepsis consists of the following:

- Identification and verification of the origin of the sepsis and removal of this focus (surgery and/or anti-infectious therapy)
- Accompanying antimicrobiologic treatment, initially as broad calculated antibiotic therapy using a combination of two or more antibiotics according to the CID (Centre of Infectious Disease) guidelines, after antibiogram testing-specific deescalating antibiotic treatment
- Optimization of organ perfusion and oxygen delivery with catecholamines
- Early mechanical ventilation
- Transfusion of red blood cells until the hematocrit reaches 30%
- Volume resuscitation with crystalloid or colloid solutions
- Decreasing peripheral oxygen consumption by lowering of body temperature, analgesia, and sedation
- Early enteral nutrition

3.4.3
Early Goal-Directed Therapy for Sepsis

In 2001 Rivers et al. (2001) presented a new treatment strategy for sepsis that reduced the in-hospital mortality from 46.5% to 30.5% when compared to standard treatment with the so called early goal-directed therapy (EGDT). Patients were included in this study if they met the SIRS criteria and showed signs of global tissue hypoxia, which was defined by a systolic pressure of 90 mm Hg or below or a lactate level of 4 mmol/l or higher.

After assessment and consent, the patients were randomized either to the standard therapy group or the EGDT group. In both groups, treatment was commenced in the emergency room; after at least 6 h the patients were transferred to an intensive care unit, where the consecutive treatment did not differ between groups and where the intensivists were blinded to the initial treatment group assignments. In both groups, the central venous pressure (CVP) was kept at or above 8–12 mm Hg with boluses of 500 ml crystalloid solutions every 30 min, the mean arterial pressure (MAP) monitored with an arterial cannula was kept at or above 65 mm Hg with vasoactive agents and the urine output was kept at or above 0.5 ml/kg/h.

The particular feature of the EGDT was to install continuous central venous oxygen saturation monitoring ($ScvO_2$), which was achieved by inserting a specialized central venous catheter and monitoring system (Edwards Lifesciences, Irvine, CA, USA). $ScvO_2$ has been shown to be a surrogate for the cardiac index as a target for hemodynamic therapy. If $ScvO_2$ was below 70%, transfusion of red cells was begun until the hematocrit reached 30%. If $ScvO_2$ was still below 70% infusion of dobutamine began. Dobutamine was started at a dose of 2.5 μg/kg/min that was increased by 2.5 μg/kg/min every 30 min until $ScvO_2$ reached 70% or a maximum dose of 20 μg/kg/min was given. Dobutamine was decreased in dose or discontinued if the mean arterial pressure was less than 65 mm Hg or if the heart rate was above 120 beats per minute. To decrease oxygen consumption, patients in whom hemodynamic optimization could not be achieved received mechanical ventilation and sedatives (see Fig. 3.5).

3.4.4
Heidelberg Sepsis Pathway

See Fig. 3.6 for the Heidelberg sepsis pathway.

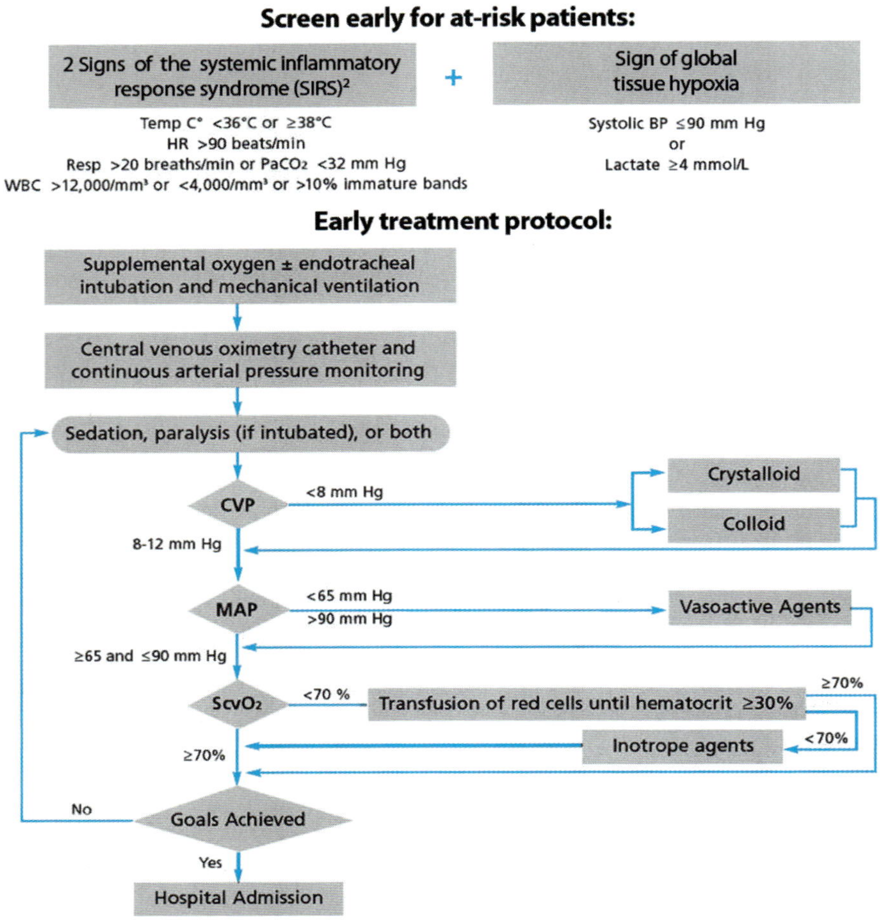

Fig. 3.5. Protocol for early goal directed therapy for sepsis. *CVP* central venous pressure, *MAP* mean arterial pressure, *ScvO₂* central venous oxygen saturation. From Edwards Lifesciences (2006)

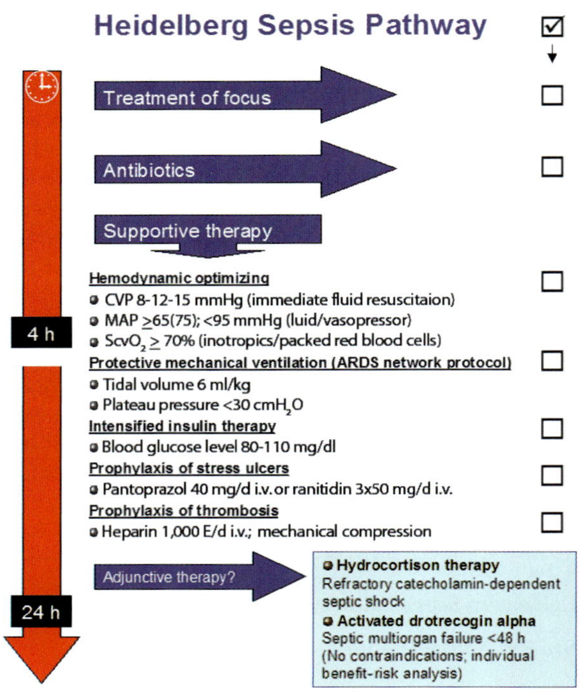

◁ **Fig. 3.6.** Heidelberg sepsis pathway. *CVP* central venous pressure, *MAP* mean arterial pressure, *ScvO₂* central venous oxygen saturation. Modified from Nieminen et al. (2005)

3.5 Intensive Care Procedures

3.5.1 Analgosedation

The use of analgetics and sedatives for the treatment of pain, anxiety, and agitation is a daily challenge in the intensive care environment. It is usually needed for the mechanically ventilated patient. To achieve a sufficient level of patient shielding while minimizing side effects and a short and cost-effective weaning period, the algorithm for analgosedation (AS) is an important task for the clinician. Emphasis should be placed on the consequent and correct implementation of a concept while the details of the concept are not as important. Another key aspect is the regular documentation of the indication for continuing AS, the definition of a therapeutic goal, the assessment of the patient's degree of agitation and pain, and finally the adjustments in the drug therapy. If the underlying diseases permit, a regular daily suspension of the AS is advisable to evaluate the patient neurologically and discover a prolonged effect of the AS (Martin et al. 2005).

There are manifold causes of pain in the intensive care environment: preexisting disease, invasive procedures, trauma, monitoring and therapeutic devices (such as catheters, drains, noninvasive ventilating devices, endotracheal tubes), routine nursing care (airway suctioning, physical therapy, dressing changes, patient mobilization), and prolonged immobility. Unrelieved pain leads to inadequate sleep, causing exhaustion, disorientation, agitation, stress response (tachycardia, increased myocardial oxygen consumption, hypercoagulability, immunosuppression, persistent catabolism), pulmonary dysfunction through localized guarding of muscles around the area of pain and a generalized muscle rigidity or spasm that restricts movement of the chest wall and diaphragm.

The causes for anxiety in the intensive care unit can be secondary to an inability to communicate due to continuous noise (alarms, personnel, and equipment), continuous ambiguous lighting, excessive stimulation (inadequate analgesia, frequent measurements of vital signs, repositioning, lack of mobility, room temperature, sleep deprivation, and the underlying disease that led to ICU admission. Causes for agitation include extreme anxiety, delirium, adverse drug effects, and pain. If agitation is present, it is important to identify and treat any underlying physiological disturbances: hypoxemia, hypoglycemia, hypotension, pain, withdrawal from alcohol, and other drug effects. Special attention should be paid to the treatment of agitation, because it can pose a serious threat to patients by contributing to ventilator dyssynchrony, increase in oxygen consumption, or inadvertent removal of devices and catheters (Jacobi et al. 2002).

3.5.1.1 Algorithm

Before the start of analgosedation, it is important to assess the indication and define a therapeutic goal. Today the patients in the intensive care unit should react adequately to verbal stimulation, perceive their environment, communicate their needs, and tolerate the diagnostic and therapeutic measures.

The next step is to assess the degree of agitation and pain. A good approach is the concept by Martin and Messelken (1998), which implements the Richmond Agitation-Sedation Scale (RASS) (Sessler et al. 2002) at the outset and continues depending on the RASS score with an adequate pain score. For the unresponsive to lightly sedated patient, the behavioral pain scale (BPS) by Payen et al. (2001) is applicable, for the sleepy to

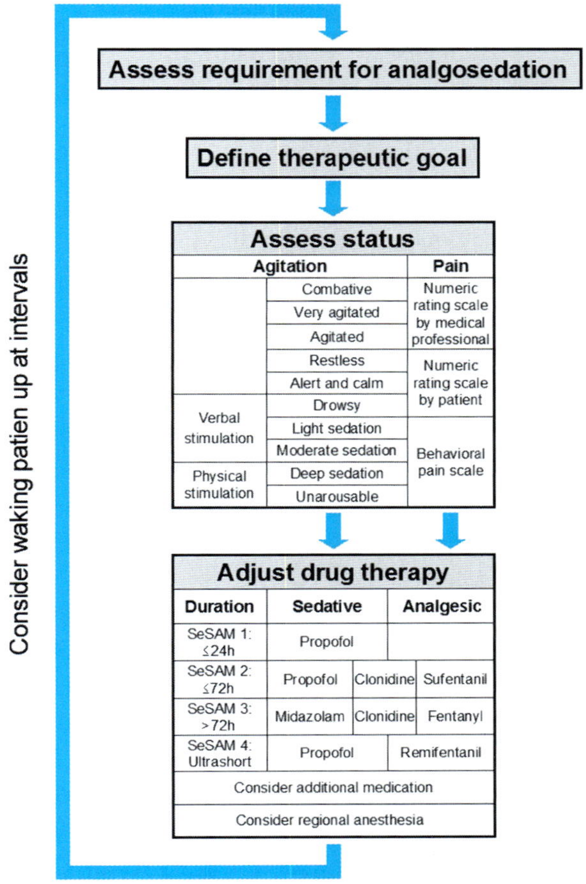

Fig. 3.7. Algorithm of analgosedation. Assembled from Jacobi et al. (2002); Martin et al. (2005); Martin and Messelken (1998)

restless patient the numeric rating scale (NRS: 0 = no pain to 10 = highest pain possible) assessed by the patient himself is applicable, and for the agitated to fighting patient the NRS rated by a medical professional (physician or nurse) is applicable. For details of the assessment of agitation and pain, please refer to Tables 3.6 and 3.7.

The last step is to schedule the duration of the AS and choose the appropriate drug accordingly. The SeSAM concept (Martin and Messelken 1998) provides four duration categories: up to 24 h, up to 72 h, more than 72 h, and ultrashort analgosedation (e.g., for short painful diagnostic procedures). The drugs were chosen such that the length of the context-sensitive half-life meets the requirements of the duration of AS needed and prolonged action is unlikely. For dosages of the drugs, please refer to Tables 3.8 and 3.9. Co-medication such as nonopioids should be considered to support the AS in an additive way, but strict adherence to the contraindications of these drugs is mandatory. Another therapeutic option is continuous regional anesthetic techniques such as epidural catheter analgesia

Table 3.6. Richmond agitation-sedation scale (RASS)

Score	Term	Description	Procedure
+4	Combative	Overtly combative or violent; immediate danger to staff	1. Observe patient. Is patient alert and calm (score 0)? Does patient have behavior that is consistent with restlessness or agitation (score +1 to +4 using the criteria listed above, under "description")?
+3	Very agitated	Pulls on or removes tube(s) or catheter(s) or has aggressive behavior toward staff	
+2	Agitated	Frequent nonpurposeful movement or patient–ventilator dyssynchrony	2. If patient is not alert, in a loud speaking voice state patient's name and direct patient to open eyes and look at speaker. Repeat once if necessary. Can prompt patient to continue looking at speaker. Patient has eye opening and eye contact, which is sustained for more than 10 s (score –1). Patient has eye opening and eye contact, but this is not sustained for 10 seconds (score –2). Patient has any movement in response to voice, excluding eye contact (score –3).
+1	Restless	Anxious or apprehensive but movements not aggressive or vigorous	
0	Alert and calm		
–1	Drowsy	Not fully awake, but has sustained (more than 10 s) awakening, with eye contact, to voice	
–2	Light sedation	Briefly (less than 10 s) awakens with eye contact to voice	3. If patient does not respond to voice, physically stimulate patient by shaking shoulder and then rubbing sternum if there is no response to shaking shoulder. Patient has any movement to physical stimulation (score –4). Patient has no response to voice or physical stimulation (score –5).
–3	Moderate sedation	Any movement (but not eye contact) to voice	
–4	Deep sedation	No response to voice, but any movement to physical stimulation	
–5	Unarousable	No response to voice or physical stimulation	

From Sessler et al. (2002)

Table 3.7. Behavioral pain scale (BPS)

Item	Description	Score
Facial expression	Relaxed	1
	Partially tightened (e.g., brow lowering)	2
	Fully tightened (e.g., eyelid closing)	3
	Grimacing	4
Upper limbs	No movement	1
	Partially bent	2
	Fully bent with finger flexion	3
	Permanently retracted	4
Compliance with ventilation	Tolerating movement	1
	Coughing but tolerating ventilation most of the time	2
	Fighting ventilator	3
	Unable to control ventilation	4

From Payen et al. (2001)

or continuous femoral nerve block. With the use of regional anesthesia techniques, a dose reduction of opioids and their side effects can be achieved. Spinal-applied local anesthetics provide sympathicolysis with improved bowel function and less postoperative ileus. A drawback of the continuous regional anesthesia techniques is the risk of infection at the puncture site and the risk of spinal hematoma formation, when a hypocoagulatory state is caused by disease or treatment with antithrombotic agents (therapeutic anticoagulation).

Table 3.8. Drugs for analgesia, sedation and vegetative attenuation. On usage of Ketamin-S cut dosages in half. All dosages refer to a middle aged adult of 60–80 kg.

Drug	Loading (mg/50 ml)	Dosage [mg(µg)/kg/h] Low	Dosage [mg(µg)/kg/h] High	Application speed (ml/h) Low	Application speed (ml/h) High	Metabolism	Active metabolites	Daily costs (Germany)
Propofol 2%	1,000	0.8 mg	4 mg	3.0	14	Oxidation	No	+++
Midazolam	90	0.01 mg	0.18 mg	0.5	6.9	Oxidation	Yes (prolonged sedation)	++
Remifentanil	5	1.5 µg	18 µg	1	12	Serum esterase	No	+++
Fentanyl	1.5	0.9 µg	3.5 µg	2.0	8.0	Oxidation	No Accumulation	+
Sufentanil	0.5	0.15 µg	0.7 µg	2.0	10.0	Oxidation	No	++
Ketamine	2,500	0.4 mg	3.0 mg	0.6	4.0	Glucuronidized	Yes	+++
Clonidine	2.25	0.32 µg	1.3 µg	0.6	2.0	Hydroxylized	No	+

Modified from Martin et al. (2005)

Table 3.9. Co-medication to analgosedation.

Drug	Dosage	Terminal half-life	Metabolism	Active metabolites	Cost per application
Piritramide	3.75 – 15 mg i.v.	4 – 10h	Oxidation	No	++
Pethidine	12.5 – 50 mg i.v.	3 – 12h	Demethyl.	No	++
Paracetamol	4 × 1 g i.v./day	2.7 – 3.5h	Conjugation	No	++
Metamizol	1.0 – 2.5 g short infusion, max 5 g/day	2.7 – 11.5h	Hydroxyliz.	Yes	++
Diclofenac	50 – 100 mg supp, max 150 – 200 mg/day	1 – 2h	Hydroxyliz.+Conjugation	No	+
CEA	Ropivacaine 0.2 % 10 – 20 mg/h, or in combination with an opioid (sufentanil or fentanyl)	3h	Hydroxyliz	No	+++
	Or 15 ml bupivacaine 0.25 % 3 – 4/day	1.5 – 5.5h			+
Block of femoral nerve	Ropivacaine 0.2 % 20 – 30 ml Or bupivacaine 0.25 % 20 – 30 ml				

Please be aware of contraindications
Modified from Martin et al. (2005)
CEA continuous epidural anesthesia

3.5.1.2 Assessment of Agitation and Pain

See Tables 3.6 and 3.7 for the assessment of agitation and pain.

At regular intervals (e.g., once every 8-h shift), the algorithm for assessing sedation, pain, and agitation should be followed again.

3.5.1.3 Drug Adjustment

See Tables 3.8 and 3.9.

3.5.2 Monitoring

3.5.2.1 Transesophageal Echocardiography

Transesophageal echocardiography (TEE) enables the experienced examiner to evaluate online the morphology of the anatomic structures of the heart and the large vessels, contractility of the ventricles, and blood flow.

The ACC/AHA/ASE 2003 guidelines (Cheitlin et al. 2003) state the following indication for an intraoperative TEE. Only the indications that apply to the urologic environment are stated:

- Class I (evidence or general agreement that a given procedure or treatment is useful and effective): evaluation of acute, persistent, and life-threatening hemodynamic disturbances in which ventricular function and its determinants are uncertain and have not responded to treatment.
- Class IIa (weight of evidence/opinion is in favor of usefulness/efficacy): surgical procedures in patients at increased risk of myocardial ischemia, myocardial infarction, or hemodynamic disturbances.

3.5.2.2 PiCCO

With the PiCCO-system, cardiac output, the stroke volume index, the heart rate, the mean arterial pressure, the systemic vascular resistance, stroke volume variation (indicator of volume deficit), and left ventricular contractility can be measured continuously with a relatively noninvasive device. First a special arterial catheter must be placed in a large arteria (e.g., the femoral artery). This catheter has two functions: it has a transducer to measure the arterial pressure and a thermistor for the registration of changes in blood temperature for calibration. Second, a regular central venous catheter is needed to calibrate the system. After the setup, it should be calibrated at regular intervals (e.g., every 8 h), and changes in central venous pressure should be entered into the monitor to allow calculation of additional parameters. Please refer to Fig. 3.8 for the configuration of the PiCCO-system, to Table 3.10 for the overview of the complete parameters of the PiCCO-system, and to Fig. 3.9 for the decision tree and the therapeutic suggestions.

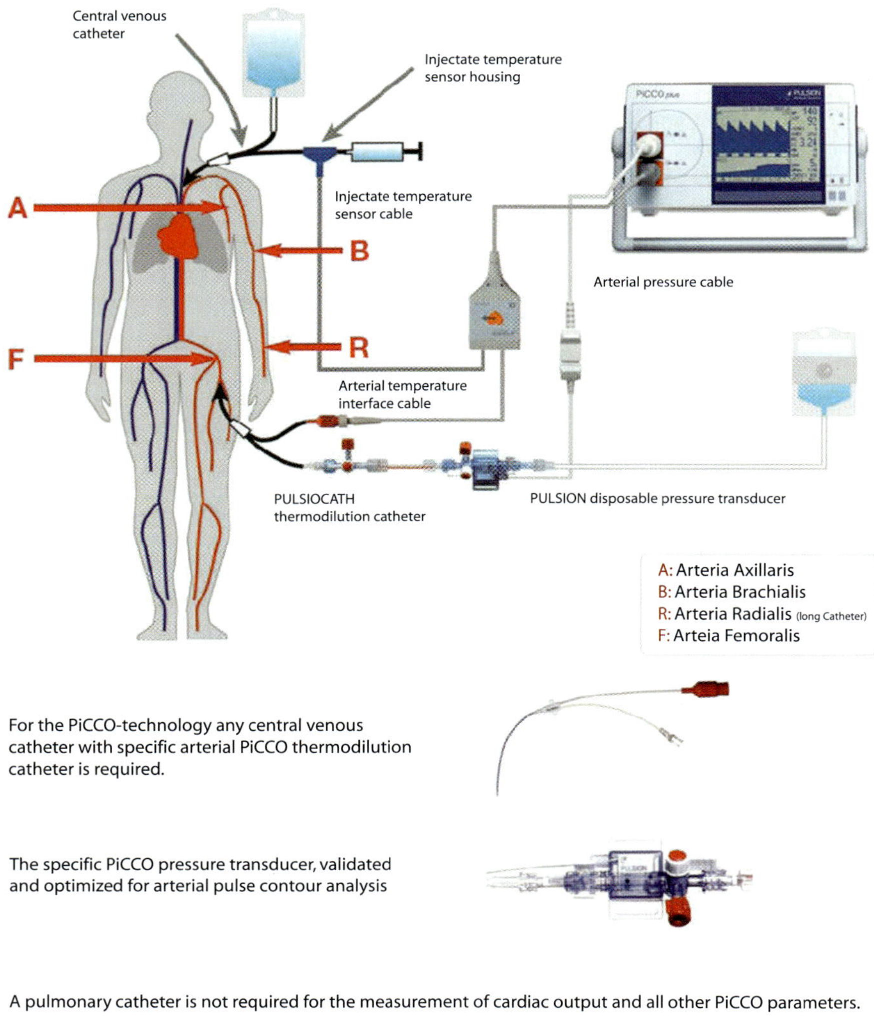

Fig. 3.8. Configuration of the PiCCO-System (Pulsion Technology 2006)

Table 3.10. Parameters and normal values of the PiCCO system

Category	Parameter	Abbr.	Value	Unit
Flow/afterload	Cardiac Index	CI	3.0–5.0	l/min/m²
	Stroke Volume Index	SVI	40–60	ml/m²
	Heart rate	HR	60–100	1/min
	Mean arterial pressure	MAP	70–90	mm Hg
	Systemic Vascular Resistance Index	SVRI	1700–2,400	dyn*s*cm^{-5}m^2
Volume management	Global End-Diastolic Volume Index	GEDI	680–800	ml/m²
	Intrathoracic Blood Volume Index	ITBI	850–1,000	ml/m²
	Stroke volume variation	SVV	≤10	%
	Pulse pressure variation	PPV	≤10	%
Lungs	Extravascular Lung Water Index	ELWI	3.0–7.0	ml/kg
	Pulmonary Vascular Permeability Index	PVPI	1.0–3.0	
Contractility	Global ejection fraction	GEF	25–35	%
	Cardiac Function Index	CFI	4.5–6.5	1/min
	Left ventricular contractility	dP/mx		

Continuous parameters/discontinuous parameters
Modified from Pulsion Technology (2006)

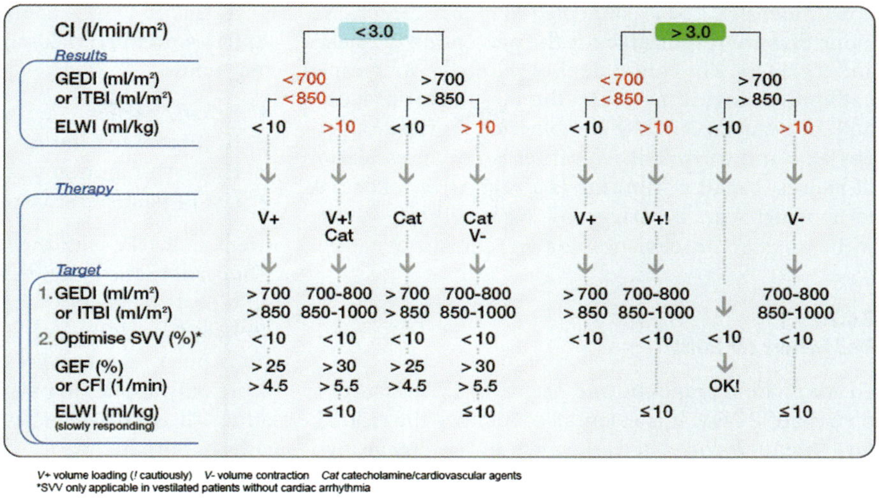

Fig. 3.9. PiCCO Decision Tree (Pulsion Technology 2006)

3.6 Intraoperative and Postoperative Procedures

3.6.1 TUR Syndrome

Many endoscopic procedures such as the transurethral resection of the prostate or bladder, operative hysteroscopies, cystoscopy, arthroscopy, rectal tumor surgery, vesical ultrasonic lithotripsy, or percutaneous nephrolithotripsy require the use of an irrigation fluid. If monopolar electrocauterization is necessary, the irrigation fluid must not contain any electrolytes. Accidental resorption of the irrigation fluid can therefore cause the so-called TUR syndrome, which poses a serious threat to the patient. The consequences for the patient depend on the rate, volume, and nature of the absorbed fluid. Possible symptoms are chest pain, bradycardia, hypertension, hypotension with drops over 50 mm Hg, poor urine output up to anuria despite diuretics, blurred vision to transient blindness, nausea, vomiting, uneasiness, confusion, tiredness, unconsciousness needing ventilatory support, and headache.

Traditional countermeasures to prevent TUR syndrome are limitation of the resection time, limiting the height of the bag containing the irrigating fluid to the maximum of 1 m above the patient, and inserting a suprapubic catheter. Early discovery of TUR syndrome is possible in patients under regional anesthesia by recognizing the symptoms described above. To quantify the amount of absorbed irrigation fluid, the latter must be mixed with a known quantity of ethanol. By measuring the exhaled ethanol concentration with an apparatus called Alcotest, absorption of irrigation fluid is detected and quantified.

Modern strategies to prevent TUR syndrome exchange the electrolyte-free irrigation solutions causing a hypotonic hyperhydration, hemolysis, hyponatremia, and specific symptoms of the other ingredients of the irrigation fluid (glycine, mannitol, sorbitol) for a normal saline solution. Closing vessels opened during resection when using electrolyte-containing irrigation solution is possible with bipolar cauterization or laser-evaporation or other techniques. In this case, absorption of irrigating fluid causes a normotonic hyperhydration, which is less dangerous (Hahn 2006).

3.6.2 Prevention of Postoperative Nausea and Vomiting

Postoperative nausea and vomiting (PONV) is the second most common postanesthetic complication after pain, the most distressing for the patient. The overall incidence of PONV for all surgeries and patient populations varies between 25 % and 30 %, in high-risk groups PONV occurs in up to 70 % of all cases (Ho and Chiu 2005).

PONV is usually self-limiting and not associated with severe consecutive complications, but the patients' assessment classifies the prevention and treatment of PONV as important as pain (Apfel and Roewer 2004). Complications of PONV such as tension on suture lines, wound bleeding and dehiscence, increased intracranial pressure, pulmonary aspiration, dehydration, and electrolyte imbalance pose a threat to the patient and result in consecutive costs.

The pathophysiology of PONV still remains unclear, with the exception of the chemotherapy- or opioid-induced vomiting despite the identification of many anatomical and histological structures and the interconnections involved in the PONV process. The vomiting center in the brainstem receives stimuli from vagal afferents of the gastrointestinal tract (particularly serotoninergic), the vestibular system (particularly histaminergic), the chemoreceptor trigger zone (particularly dopaminergic), and is connected to higher cerebral regions that are responsible for the perception of nausea and dizziness. The conclusions of the above-mentioned pathophysiological facts are: the multifactorial nature of PONV may necessitate combination therapy for prophylaxis and treatment. Vomiting is not an escalation of nausea, because vomiting is a vegetative reflex pattern, which can be triggered even without nausea, while cortical consciousness is a prerequisite of nausea.

3.6.2.1 Risk Factors for PONV

To adapt the therapeutic and prophylactic measures to the risk of PONV, it is essential to identify the risk factors with their correlated relevance and deduct an algorithm for the optimal and cost-effective measures to be taken. The clinically relevant patient-specific risk factors are:

- Female gender increases the risk of PONV threefold.
- Non-smoking increases the risk twofold.
- A history of former PONV or motion-sickness increases the risk.
- An age older than 5 years increases the risk.

The validated and clinically relevant anesthesiologic risk factors are:

- Use of volatile anesthetics (dependent on dosage) increases the risk of PONV compared to total intravenous anesthesia (TIVA).
- The use of nitrous oxide.
- The administration of postoperative opioids.
- The use of antagonists of nondepolarizing muscle relaxants (e.g., more than 2.5 mg neostigmine) also increases the risk.

There exists controversy over whether the type of surgery influences the rate of PONV in adults, because some studies have shown significant results, while others demonstrated no significance on the same type of surgeries. There is one study from Stadler et al. (2003) where the type of surgery was correlated with the incidence of nausea but not with the incidence of vomiting. In children, it was proved that the surgical technique can be related to the risk of PONV, e.g., in strabismus operations (Ruesch et al. 1999). Obesity, menstruation cycle, anxiety, or personality can definitely be ruled out as risk factors. Table 3.11 summarizes the degree of relevance and certainty of risk factors for PONV.

3.6.2.2 Antiemetic Strategy

A number of complicated scores and strategies taking the type of surgery into account exist to adapt the prophylaxis for PONV to the needs of the patient, while Apfel's simplified risk score (Apfel et al. 1999) with the four items

- Female gender
- Non-smoking status
- History of motion sickness or PONV
- Use of postoperative opioids

predicts PONV with the same reliability of about 70%. Concerning the latter, the number of risk factors (0, 1, 2, 3, or 4) correlates with a PONV risk of 10%, 20%, 40%, 60%, or 80% (see Fig. 3.10). The following limitations must be taken into account: The simplified risk score only applies to balanced anesthesia techniques in adults. It is unclear whether it yields reproducible results in outpatients.

Table 3.11. Risk factors for PONV, classified by evidence and clinical relevance

Evidence demonstrated and clinically relevant	●●● Female gender ●● Non-smoking status ●● Medical history for PONV or motion sickness ●●● General anesthesia ●● Volatile anesthetics ●● Duration of anesthesia ●● Postoperative opioids
Evidence demonstrated, but not as clinically significant	● Young age and ASA status 1 or 2 ● Nitrous oxide ● Neostigmine, Pyridostigmine
Controversial data	Type of surgery Experience of anesthesiologist Routine use of gastric tube
Insufficient data	Pain Movements
Refuted	Obese patients (body mass index) Menstruation cycle Anxiety and personality

Modified from Apfel and Roewer (2004)
● Moderate, ●● strong, ●●● very strong

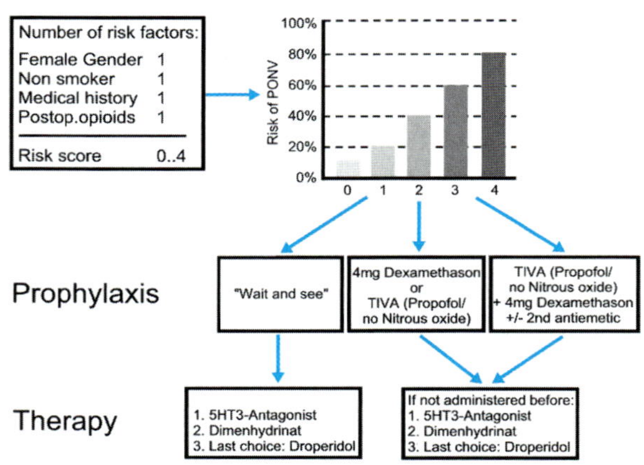

Fig. 3.10. Risk-adapted strategy for prophylaxis and therapy of PONV. modified from Apfel and Rozwer (2004)

In patients with none or only one risk factor, no prophylactic PONV therapy is required. If there are two risk factors, it is advisable to administer dexamethasone 4 mg i.v. or use total-intravenous anesthesia (TIVA) prophylactically. In TIVA, the induction and maintenance of the general anesthesia is achieved with intravenous agents, most commonly with propofol. Volatile anesthetics such as isoflurane, desflurane, sevoflurane, and nitrous oxide should be omitted. In patients with three or four risk factors for PONV, the combination of TIVA, dexamethasone prophylaxis, and optionally a second antiemetic drug is advisable.

To avoid the risk factors of volatile anesthetics and opioids, regional anesthetic techniques should be considered in patients at risk for PONV.

Every first-time vomiting or moderate nausea should be treated immediately. The dosage is approximately one-quarter of the antiemetic dosage needed for prophylaxis. Since it takes a few hours until the maximum antiemetic effect of dexamethasone is established, the use of a 5-HT_3-antagonist (e.g., ondansetron 1 mg i.v. or dolasetron 12.5 mg i.v.) or dimenhydrinate 32 mg i.v. is recommended. There is consensus on the fact that the next dose of an antiemetic drug should not be given in less than 6 h.

3.6.2.3 Antiemetic Drugs

Dexamethasone is proposed as a first-line antiemetic drug because it is effective and inexpensive, and it yields a low rate of side effects, although the antiemetic mechanism is unknown. Because of its delayed onset, dexamethasone should be given at the beginning of anesthesia.

Dimenhydrinate is an unspecific antagonist at the histamine-type 1 receptor with an antiemetic effect comparable to the other drugs mentioned. It should be used intravenously, since the amount of rectal absorption is uncertain.

Serotonin antagonists like ondansetron, tropisetron, dolasetron, or granisetron block the vagally mediated action of serotonin on the 5-hydroxytryptamin-type-3 receptor (5-HT_3). The most common side effect is a mild headache; they do not have any sedating or extrapyramidal potential. All serotonin antagonists are believed to demonstrate an equivalent antiemetic effect.

Droperidol is a highly potent neuroleptic drug acting as an antagonist at the dopamin-type-2 receptor. Because of the short duration of action, it is recommended to administer the drug at the end of surgery. The Food and Drug Administration (FDA) in the US has issued a black-box warning for the substance due to QT-interval prolongation resulting in fatal arrhythmogenic complications (prolonging of the QT interval in the electrocardiogram, torsades de points, tachycardia, bradycardia).

Metoclopramide was used by clinicians for decades, but an insufficient antiemetic effect was demonstrated by Henzi et al. (1999).

For an overview of antiemetic drugs and recommendations on dosages, please refer to Table 3.12.

3.7 Perioperative Management of Jehovah's Witnesses

Jehovah's Witnesses refuse to consent to transfusions of whole blood, red cells, plasma, platelets, white cells, and predonated autologous blood due to their religious beliefs. It is a matter of individual conscience whether Jehovah's Witnesses allow fractions derived from any primary component of blood (e.g., anti-D), medical procedures involving the use of autologous blood that do not involve storage (e.g., intraoperative cell salvage),

Table 3.12. Standard intravenous dosages of antiemetics (pediatric dosage should not exceed adult dosage), modified from (1)

Substance	Point of action	Adult prophylaxis	Adult therapy	Pediatric prophylaxis
Ondansetron	5-HT_3	4 mg	1 mg[b,c] to 4 mg[a,b]	50 µg/kg[b,c] to 100 µg/kg
Tropisetron	5-HT_3	2 mg	1 mg[c] to 2 mg[a]	100–200 µg/kg[b,c]
Dolasetron	5-HT_3	12.5 mg[a–c] to 50 mg[b,c]	12.5 mg	350 µg/kg[c]
Granisetron	5-HT_3	0.35–1 mg[b,c], 3 mg[a]	0.1–0.3 mg[c], 3 mg[a]	10–20 µg/kg[c], 40 µg/kg (>2years)[a]
Dexamethasone	Unsettled	4–5 mg early[b,c], 8–20 mg preop[a]	Not recommended[c] 8–20 mg[a]	150 µg/kg[a–c] to 500 µg/kg(>2 years)[a]
Dimenhydrinate	H_1	62[a–c] to 124 mg[a]	32 mg[c], 62–124 mg[a]	500 µg/kg[b,c] to 1.25 mg/kg[a]
Droperidol	D_2	0.625–1.25 mg[b,c]	0.625 mg[b,c]	50–75 µg/kg[b,c]
Metoclopramide	Not recommended due to insufficient antiemetic effect			

Modified from Apfel and Roewer (2004)

5-HT_3 antagonist at 5-hydroxytryptamine (serotonin)-3 receptor, *H_1* antagonist at histamin-1-receptor, *D_2* antagonist at dopamin-2 receptor

[a] Scientific information

[b] Proved by studies

[c] Expert opinion

or organ transplant. Nevertheless, Jehovah's Witnesses request all other kinds of medical treatment to save their lives.

3.7.1 Legal Issues

Patient management depends on the laws of the country; e.g., in the United States, it is the right of a competent adult to refuse transfusion even though the result of such a refusal may be death of the individual.

The perioperative strategy seems to be quite easy if the patient can express his or her wish not to receive any blood or blood products in an elective setting. The key conditions for a legal informed consent are "competency" and "adulthood". There should be a high grade of suspicion concerning competency if the patient has abnormal or unstable vital signs, altered mental status, evidence of impaired judgment as from a central nervous system injury or illness, or any sign of alcohol or drug intoxication. In regard to the definition of a minor, individuals are generally considered too young to make a decision for themselves if they are under the age of 18; however, exceptions can be made for self-sufficient minors and emancipated minors. A self-sufficient minor is one who is age 15 or older and lives separately and apart from his or her parents or legal guardian. An emancipated minor is any person under the age of 18 who has entered into a valid marriage.

Concerning minors, the courts have ordered transfusions for children in life-threatening situations despite the objections or their parents or legal guardians. The same applies to incompetent adult patients, where courts have predominantly ruled that a physician has a legally recognized right to proceed with emergency procedures such as transfusion therapy even over the objections of the relatives (Rashad Net University 2006).

3.7.2 Physiology of Anemia

To understand the physiology and compensatory measures of a reduced hemoglobin concentration and deduct possible strategies to maintain oxygen supply of the body, the following parameters should be discussed.

The oxygen delivery of the organism (DO_2) is the product of the cardiac output (CO) and the arterial oxygen content of the blood (c_aO_2).

$$DO_2 = CO \times c_aO_2 \qquad (3.1)$$

DO_2 Oxygen supply, normal range 900 – 1,200 ml/min
CO Cardiac output, normal range: 4 – 8 l/min
c_aO_2 Oxygen content of the arterial blood, normal range: 19±1 ml/dl

The content of oxygen of the arterial blood consists of the major part of 98.5 % that is stored in the hemoglobin (S_aO_2*Hb*1.39) and the minor part of 1.5 % that is physically stored (p_aO_2*0.003).

$$c_aO_2 = SaO_2 \times Hb \times 1.39 + p_aO_2 \times 0.003 \qquad (3.2)$$

S_aO_2 Oxygen saturation of the arterial blood, normal range 96 % – 100 %
Hb Hemoglobin concentration, normal range 12 – 16 g/dl in women, 14 – 18 g/dl in men
p_aO_2 Partial pressure of oxygen in arterial blood, normal range 70 – 100 mm Hg (Fresenius and Heck 2001)

Physiologic compensation of anemia (decrease in hemoglobin concentration) to maintain adequate oxygen delivery is achieved by increased cardiac output (tachycardia, increased contractility). Therapeutic measures include lowering oxygen consumption and administering high inspiratory oxygen concentrations (increase in S_aO_2 and p_aO_2) by sedation and mechanical ventilation. Oxygen consumption can also be lowered (7 % per °C) by hypothermia. When the hemoglobin concentration is very low, the oxygen content of the blood decreases dramatically, because the physically stored oxygen (p_aO_2 * 0.003) is only a minor part of oxygen transport in the blood. The physically stored oxygen can only be increased significantly in hyperbaric conditions.

Other mechanisms to improve tissue oxygenation include lowering of the hematocrit with consecutive decrease in viscosity and improvement of blood flow. The peripheral vascular resistance is lowered to additionally increase blood flow. The oxygen saturation curve, which describes the dependency of saturation on the partial pressure, shifts to the right due to acidosis, anemia, and an increase in 2,3-diphosphoglycerate and consecutively improves donation of oxygen to the tissues (Rashad Net University 2006).

3.7.3 Strategies to Avoid Blood Transfusions

Perioperative care of Jehovah's Witnesses should ideally start weeks before the surgical procedure. After a positive benefit–risk analysis by the surgeon that includes the determination of the possible blood loss, the patient should also be assessed by the anesthesiologist to determine the patient's preferences and preclusions. After all parties agree on how to proceed with medical management, the patient must sign a consent form memorializing his or her request not to transfuse under any circumstances. At this early stage of planning, an oral iron medication should be considered.

Donation and deposition of autologous blood is commonly not accepted by the patients, but the preoperative acute normovolemic hemodilution can be an option to reduce intraoperative blood loss if the collecting system "maintains in the circulatory system". Additionally a cell-saving device can be used intraoperatively, if no contraindications exist and the patient accepts its use.

Deliberate hypotension with the reduction of the systolic blood pressure to 80–90 mm Hg decreases intraoperative blood loss. Contraindications are cardiovascular disease, particularly coronary artery disease and congestive heart failure, poorly controlled hypertension, raised intracranial pressure, and coexistent central nervous system pathologies. Additional side effects of deliberate hypotension are increased alveolar dead space and decreased renal blood flow, so monitoring arterial blood gases and urinary output is advis-

Table 3.13. Perioperative management to avoid blood transfusions

Strategy	Measures	Effect
Fluids	Ringer's lactate Hydroxyethyl starch Dextran Gelatin solutions Oxygen transporting solutions	Maintain blood volume Transport of oxygen
Drugs	Erythropoietin Interleukin-11 GM-CSF, G-CSF Aprotinin, Tranexamic acid Desmopressin Vitamin K Recombinant Factor VIIa, VIII	Stimulation of red blood cells Stimulation of platelets Stimulation of white blood cells Antifibrinolytics Release of vWF Vitamin K-dependent coagulation factors Activation of extrinsic pathway
Biological hemostats	Collagen pad Cellulose woven pad Fibrin glue	Direct sealing of wounds
Blood salvage	Cell-saving machines	Recovery of red blood cells
Surgical techniques	Thorough operative planning Prompt action to stop bleeding Dividing large surgeries into smaller ones Minimally invasive procedures Endoscopic procedures Arterial embolization Applied direct pressure Ice packs Positioning of body Tourniquet	Minimizing blood loss during procedure
Surgical tools	Electrocautery or electrosurgery Laser surgery Argon beam coagulator Gamma knife radiosurgery Microwave coagulating scalpel Shaw hemostatic scalpel Ultrasonic scalpel Cryosurgery	Closing vessels
Anesthesiologic techniques	Controlled hypotension Regional anesthesia Maintaining normothermia Acute normovolemic hemodilution Pediatric microsampling equipment Multiple tests per sample	Reduced blood pressure Maintain coagulation Reduced blood loss Reduced sample volumes
Management of anemia	Stop the bleeding Oxygen support Maintain intravascular volume Iron Folic acid Vitamin B_{12} injection Hyperbaric oxygen chamber Mechanical ventilation	Basis of all efforts Increased S_aO_2 Erythropoiesis Increased p_aO_2 Reduced oxygen consumption

able. Hypotension can be achieved by inhalational anesthetics, sodium nitroprusside, nitroglycerin, and trimethaphan. Neuroaxial blocks such as spinal or epidural anesthesia also lower the blood pressure, but controlling the amount of hypotension is more difficult.

Positioning the patient so that the surgical field is at a high point may result in less blood loss.

Mild hypothermia is another possible measure to reduce oxygen demand in anemic patients, as mentioned before. A target core temperature of 30–32 °C is typically chosen to balance the reduction of oxygen consumption with the side effects of cardiac arrhythmias and the hypocoagulatory state. Desmopressin, a synthetic analog of the antidiuretic hormone, can elevate the coagulation factor VIII and von-Willebrand factor. Aminocaproic acid and other antifibrinolytics can reduce blood loss by inhibiting the physiologic or increased lysis of already formed clots. Recombinant human erythropoietin stimulates the synthesis of erythrocytes but takes a while to produce an effect and is quite expensive. The artificial substances such as perfluorocarbon that transport oxygen are not as effective as hemoglobin and still need further development.

Table 3.13 lists the possible strategies, measures, and effects to avoid blood transfusions. From this summary, the treating physician should extract the measures applicable to a specific patient.

3.7.4 Conclusion

If a hospital anticipates they might administer emergency care to Jehovah's Witnesses, it should establish a protocol for such treatment to help avoid any medical, ethical, or legal dilemmas that may arise.

All the blood-saving techniques discussed above also apply to the regular patient in order to minimize blood loss and the need for transfusions.

References

ACCP/SCCM (1992) Consensus conference of the American College of Chest Physicians/Society of Critical Care Medicine (ACCP/SCCM). Des Plains, IL, August 1991

Apfel CC, Roewer N (2004) Postoperative Nausea and Vomiting. Anaesthesist 53:377

Apfel CC, Laara F, Koivurante M et al (1999) A simplified risk score for predicting postoperative nausea and vomiting: conclusions from cross validations between two centers. Anesthesiology 91:693

Boettiger BW, Motsch J, Teschendorf P et al (2004) Postoperative 12-lead ECG predicts perioperative myocardial ischaemia associated with myocardial cell damage. Anaesthesia 59:1083

Cheitlin MD, Armstrong WF, Aurigemma GP et al (2003) ACC/AHA/Ase 2003 Guidline update for the clinical application of echocardiography: summary article. Circulation 108:1146

Cleland JG, Swedberg K, Follath F et al (2003) The Euroheart failure survey programme – a survey on the quality of care among patients with heart failure in Europe. Part 1: patient characteristics and diagnostics. Eur Heart J 24:442

Dempfle CE (2005) Perioperative coagulation diagnostics. Anaesthesist 54:167

Edwards Life Sciences (2001) Protocol for Early Goal-Directed Therapy for Sepsis. Edwards Life Sciences, Irvine, CA, USA

Fresenius M, Heck M (2001) Repetitorium of Intensive Care. Springer, Berlin Heidelberg New York

Geerts WII, Pieno GF, Heit JA et al (2004) Prevention of venous thromboembolism:the seventh ACCP conference on antithrombotic and thrombolytic therapy. Chest 126:338S

Hahn RG (2006) Fluid absorption in endoscopic surgery. Br J Anaesth 1:8

Heck M, Fresenius M (2004) Repetitorium Anaesthesiology. 4th edn. Springer, Berlin Heidelberg New York

Henzi I, Walder B, Tramer MR (1999) Metoclopramide in the prevention of postoperative nausea and vomiting: a quantitative systematic review of randomized, placebo-controlled studies. Br J Anaesth 83:761

Herold G et al (2006) Text of internal medicine. Gerd Herold, Cologne

Ho KY, Chiu JW (2005) Multimodal antiemetic therapy and emetic risk profiling. Ann Acad Med Singapore 34:196

Jacobi J, Fraser GL, Coursin DB et al (2002) Clinical practice guidelines for the sustained use of sedatives and analgetics in the critically ill adult. Crit Care Med 1:119

Larsen R (1999) Textbook of Anaesthesia, 6th edn. Urban and Schwarzenberg, Munich

Lee TH, Marcantonio ER, Mangione CM et al (1999) Derivation and prospective validation of a simple index for prediction of cardiac risk of major noncardiac surgery. Circulation 100:1043

Level 1, Inc. 160 Weymouth Street, Rockland, MA, USA. http://www.smiths-medical.com. Cited 6 November 2006

Lindenauer PK, Pekow P, Wang K et al (2005) Perioperative beta-blocker therapy and mortality after major noncardiac surgery. N Engl J Med 4:349

Larsen R, Lahme T, Wilhelm W et al. (2002) Manual of Anaesthesia, University Hospital of the Saarland, Homburg

Martin J, Messelken M (1998) Sequential management of sedation and analgesia in the intensive care medicine. W. Zuckschwerdt, Munich

Martin J, Baesell K, Buerkle H et al (2005) Analgesia and sedation in the intensive care unit. S2: guidelines of the German society of anaesthesiology and intensive care medicine. Anaesth Intensivmed 1:S1

Motsch J, Walther A, Bock M, Boettiger BW (2006) Update in the prevention and treatment of deep vein thrombosis and pulmonary embolism. Curr Opin Anaesthesiol 19:52

Murray MJ, Cowen J, DeBlock H et al (2002) Clinical practice guidelines for sustained neuromuscular blockade in the adult critically ill patient. Crit Care Med 1:142

Nieminen MS, Boehm M, Cowie MR et al (2005) Executive summary of the guidelines on the diagnosis and treatment of acute heart failure: the Task Force on Acute Heart Failure of the European Society of Cardiology. Eur Heart J 26:384

Payen JF, Bru O, Bosson JL et al (2001) Assessing pain in critically ill sedated patients by using a behavioral pain scale. Crit Care Med 12:2258

Poldermans D, Boersma E (2005) Beta-blocker therapy in noncardiac surgery. N Engl J Med 4:412

Pulsion Technology. PiCCO-System, Pulsion Technology, http://www.pulsion.com. Cited 6 Novemer 2006

Rashad Net University (2006) The Jehovah Witness Patient. Published online by the Rashad Net University, Santa Monica, California, USA. http://www.rashaduniversity.com. Cited 6 November 2006

Rivers M, Nguyen B, Havstad S et al (2001) Early goal directed therapy in the treatment of severe sepsis and septic shock. N Engl J Med 19:1368
Ruesch D, Happe W, Wulf H (1999) Is TIVA with remifentanil/propofol superior to sevoflurane/N2O regarding PONV in children undergoing strabismus surgery. Anaesthesist 48:80
Sarig G, Michaeli Y, Lanir N (2005) Mechanisms for acquired activated protein C resistance in cancer patients. J Thromb Hemost 3:589
Schouten O, Shaw L, Boersma E et al (2006) A meta-analysis of safety and effectiveness of perioperative beta-blocker use for the prevention of cardiac events in different types of non-cardiac surgery. Coron Artery Dis 2:173
Sessler CN, Gosnell MS, Grap MJ et al (2002) The Richmond Agitation-Sedation Scale – validity and reliability in adult intensive care unit patients. Am J Respir Crit Care Med 166:1338
Stadler M, Bardieu F, Seidel L et al (2003) Difference in risk factors for postoperative nausea and vomiting. Anaesthesiology 98:46
Teschendorf P (2006) Standard Operating Procedure – Perioperative Beta-Blockers. Department of Anaesthesia, University Hospital of Heidelberg, Germany
Thompson A, Balser JR (2004) Perioperative cardiac arrhythmias. Br J Anaesth 93:86
Weigand MA, Hofer S, Plachky J (2004) Heidelberg sepsis pathway – Recommendations for the therapy of sepsis. University Hospital Heidelberg, Germany

4 Anaphylaxis

P. Bader, D. Frohneberg

4.1 Definition

Anaphylaxis is a severe, life-threatening, generalized or systemic hypersensitivity reaction resulting from the sudden release of mast cell and basophil-derived mediators (Kemp and Lockey 2002).

The European Academy of Allergology and Clinical Immunology (EAACI) suggested that anaphylactic-type reactions should be reclassified as allergic and nonallergic anaphylaxis (Johansson et al. 2001). Allergic anaphylaxis is classified as IgE- or non-IgE-mediated reactions. However, these terms have not been adopted worldwide and *anaphylactoid* and *anaphylactic* remain commonly used in differentiating non-IgE-mediated and IgE-mediated reactions (Kemp and Lokkey 2002).

The incidence of anaphylaxis during general anesthesia is 1:13,000 in a French study with a mortality of 6% (Laxenaire 1999). The most frequent causes of anaphylaxis during surgical and medical procedures are muscle relaxants, natural rubber latex, antibiotics, and anesthesia induction agents (Lieberman 2002). Colloids, opioids, and (radio)contrast media account for less than 10% of all reactions. An overview of the types of reactions is listed in Table 4.1.

Table 4.1. Common agents that cause perioperative anaphylaxis

Anaphylactic (IgE-dependent)
Medications (e.g., penicillin)
Latex
Aspirin and other nonsteroidal anti-inflammatory drugs (probably)
Anaphylactoid (IgE independent): Multimediator complement activation, activation of contact system
(Radio)contrast media
Nonspecific degranulation of mast cells and basophils
Opioids
Muscle relaxants
Immune aggregates
Dextran (possibly)
Cytotoxic
Transfusion reactions to cellular elements (IgG, IgM)

4.2 Immunological Mechanism

Coombs and Gell (1975) first classified four types of hypersensitivity (immunopathologic) reactions (Table 4.2).

Type I:	Immediate (IgE-dependent)
Type II:	Cytotoxic (IgG, IgM-dependent)
Type III:	Immune complexes (IgG, IgM-dependent complex)
Type IV:	Delayed (T lymphocyte-dependent)

Table 4.2. Classification of hypersensitivity (Coombs and Gell 1975)

Type	Time to maximal reaction	Immunological components	Examples
I	30 Min and 6–12 h	IgE antibodies Mast cells Biphasic reaction	Allergic asthma
II	days	Cytotoxic reaction	Graft-versus-host reaction
III	6–8 h	Antigen–antibody complexes Complement activation	Vasculitis Glomerulonephritis Blood transfusion reactions
IV	40–72 h	Antigen-dependent T cell reaction and leukotriene production	Cutaneous contact allergy

After Coombs and Gell (1975)

4.2.1 IgE-Dependent Anaphylaxis

Classical IgE-dependent anaphylaxis is a type I immunologic reaction, which can happen when a sensitized person is re-exposed to an allergen, usually at least a few weeks after the first exposure. Allergens are usually bivalent proteins with a molecular weight between 10,000 and 70,000 D. Allergen-specific IgE antibodies – synthesized by plasma cells after the first allergen contact – reversibly bind with the F_c portion to receptors on mast cells and basophils. The antigen-binding part of the IgE antibodies (the F_{ab} portion) extends into the extracellular space. During a subsequent antigen contact, the bivalent antigen can then build a bridge between two cell-attached IgE antibodies, which will cause a release of preformed mediators, mainly histamine, from intracellular granules. It also causes the quick synthesis of other mediators such as leukotrienes C4, D4, and E4, triggered from membrane-attached phospholipids. These primary mediators cause the clinical appearance of anaphylaxis. Both mast cells and basophils additionally release chemotactic factors to attract other cells of the immune system. The eosinophils partly decrease the anaphylactic reaction by inactivating histamine and leukotrienes. Neutrophils and thrombocytes with their products are thought to be part of the delayed anaphylactic reaction 6–12 h after the initial type I reaction.

Besides this classical route of anaphylactic reaction, another type has been described: type III anaphylactic reaction. Characteristically, this type of reaction occurs in patients with a hereditary deficiency of IgA (for example, during blood transfusion) (see Sect. 4.8).

4.2.2 Non-IgE-Dependent Anaphylaxis

In non-IgE-dependent anaphylaxis, the release of the mediators can be initiated by different factors that directly interfere with the mast cells and basophils: physical (e.g., cold temperature), osmotic (e.g., contrast media), or chemical stimuli (e.g., opioids). For this type of a reaction, no sensitization is needed, and therefore this type of anaphylactic reaction may occur with the first contact to the allergen.

The main primary mediator, histamine, activates H_1 and H_2 receptors. Pruritus, rhinorrhea, tachycardia, and bronchospasm are caused by the H_1 receptors, whereas both H_1 and H_2 receptors mediate headache, flushing, and hypotension. Gastrointestinal signs and symptoms are associated with histamine more so than with tryptase levels.

The different routes of histamine release:

IgE-dependent:	Antigen	Basophils	Histamine Leukotrienes
		Mastocytes	Histamine Leukotrienes Tryptase
Nonspecific: Idiosyncratic	Chemotoxicity Physical stimuli	Basophils	Histamine

4.3 Clinical Presentation and Differential Diagnosis

The severity of the hypersensitivity reaction is classified into four grades (see Table 4.3): IgE- or non-IgE-mediated reactions and anaphylactoid or anaphylactic reactions, respectively, cannot be differentiated clinically.

The most important clinical signs are (Chiu and Kelly 2005):

- Cutaneous reactions (erythema, urticaria) and soft tissue swelling (e.g., eyelids, lips)
- Hypotension and tachycardia

Table 4.3. Severity of immediate hypersensitivity reactions

Grade	Symptoms
Grade 1	Only cutaneous signs: diffuse erythema, urticaria
Grade 2	Same as grade 1 + nausea, cough, dyspnea, tachycardia, hypotension
Grade 3	Same as grade 2 + vomiting, diarrhea, bronchospasm, cyanosis, shock
Grade 4	Cardiovascular arrest (apparent death)

After Ring and Messmer (1977)

- Respiratory symptoms (cough, dyspnea, bronchospasm, laryngeal edema, and cyanosis)
- Gastrointestinal reactions (nausea, vomiting, diarrhea)
- Neurological reaction (loss of consciousness)

Other diagnoses that might mimic anaphylaxis should be considered, since there are several conditions that can also cause abrupt and dramatic patient collapse. Acute reactions should be excluded if possible; these include vasodepressor (vasovagal) reactions, acute anxiety (e.g., panic attack or hyperventilation syndrome), myocardial dysfunction, pulmonary embolism, aspiration, and hypoglycemia.

The clinical presentation of an anaphylactic/anaphylactoid reaction can differ greatly in each patient; it is also very much dependent on the route of allergen exposure, the rate of absorption, and the grade of sensitivity to the allergen. The symptoms may appear only seconds or minutes after the contact with the allergen.

In more than 90% of all cases, cutaneous symptoms such as pruritus, flush, or erythema happen prior to systemic reaction. However, cutaneous manifestations might be delayed or absent in rapidly progressive anaphylactic shock.

Obstruction of the pulmonary system is very common and can be life threatening. The reason may be extrathoracic (caused by swelling of the larynx or pharynx) or intrathoracic (caused by obstruction of the bronchi). Most often the swelling of the larynx is the cause of death in anaphylactoid reactions and starts with hoarseness, wheeze, and stridor. As in acute shock, edema of the larynx may be the only symptom of anaphylaxis.

Gastrointestinal symptoms such as nausea, vomiting, diarrhea, abdominal pain, bowel urgency are caused by disturbance of the permeability of the gastrointestinal system and additionally by the hypermobility of the bowels due to stimulation of histamine receptors.

The exact mechanism of hemodynamic reactions is not fully understood. Leading symptoms are hypovolemia due to vasodilatation and fluid shift into the interstitium, and tachycardia as well as decreased cardiac filling pressure.

It is unknown whether cerebral signs such as dizziness, syncope, cramps, and unconsciousness are caused by cerebral lack of perfusion or a direct effect of the mediators.

4.4 Diagnostic Tests and Risk Factors

There are many different diagnostic tests, including serum tryptase, plasma histamine, specific IgE-level measurements, and skin tests. However, all of these tests have their pitfalls.

An elevated tryptase level 1–6 h after a suspected anaphylactic reaction indicates mast cell degranulation. Together with a suggestive history and clinical findings, this supports the diagnosis of anaphylaxis (Fisher and Baldo 1998). However, serum tryptase concentration may be normal even in fatal anaphylaxis.

Plasma histamine level reaches a peak within 15–30 min of the onset of anaphylaxis and returns to baseline values within 1 h. This test is therefore of very limited use and only helpful in some patients.

4.4.1 Diagnosis of Serious or Fatal Reaction to Contrast Media

During anaphylaxis/anaphylactoid reaction, histamine is released from both basophils and mast cells, while tryptase is absent from basophils but released from the granules of mast cells together with histamine. New highly reliable assays are becoming available for measuring tryptase and histamine in plasma (Laroche et al. 1998). Tryptase's half-life is about 90 min, and the best time for measuring is 1–2 h after the reaction (not later then 6 h). Only very high concentrations of serum tryptase should be regarded as specific for fatal anaphylaxis/anaphylactoid reactions (Brockow et al. 1999). Histamine has a very short half-life (approximately 2 min), and the best time for measuring its plasma level is between 10 min and 1 h after the reaction. Consequently, blood samples for histamine analysis should be drawn as soon as possible after the reaction. For tryptase, blood sampling 1–2 h after onset of the symptoms has been recommended. To enable comparison with baseline levels, new blood samples should be collected 1–2 days after the reaction (Brockow et al. 2005a).

The level of histamine release has been demonstrated to have a direct relationship to the severity of the immediate reaction to iodinated contrast media (CM) (Laroche et al. 1998). The proof of an increased histamine or tryptase level during the acute reaction can help to diagnose an anaphylactic reaction, even retrospectively.

Muscle relaxants and natural rubber latex are very significant and potent allergens in the perioperative period. In patients with a suspicious history, a search for specific IgE antibodies can be done prior to the operation to minimize the risk of a potential anaphylactic reaction (see Sects. 4.8 and 4.9). If a latex allergy is suspected, a skin prick test is recommended (see Sect. 4.9).

In suspected penicillin incompatibility, a prior skin test might be very helpful, because it has a high negative predictive value (see Sect. 4.8).

All patients with an anaphylactic reaction should undergo an consultation with an allergy and immunology specialist, and the results documented in an allergy card. After a severe reaction, the patient should be taught to do initial self-treatment in the event of contact to the allergen. In such cases, patients should therefore carry an emergency kit with them. This should include an H1-antagonist (e.g., dimetindene maleat, 2 ml = 2 mg) as a liquid and an quick effective corticosteroid in a liquid form (e.g., celestamine liquidum, 5 ml = 0.5 mg betamethasone) or for inhalation (e.g., Primatene mist epinephrine) and an adrenaline pen for self- intramuscular injection (e.g., Fastjekt or EpiPen, 0.3 ml = 0.30 mg epinephrine).

Generally, all patients with a history of asthma or atopy (including hay fever and food allergies) have an increased risk of anaphylactic/anaphylactoid reactions in the perioperative interval. Risk factors have been clearly demonstrated for two major allergens commonly found in hospital:

1. Although reactions to iodinated radiographic CM are not true allergic ones, patients with a history of a previous reaction to contrast material have a three- to fourfold greater risk of subsequent reaction than the general population (Katayama et al. 1990; Morcos and Thomsen 2001). Other important risk factors include asthma and a history of atopy, including hay fever and food allergies, increasing the risk of anaphylaxis eight- to tenfold (Morcos and Thomsen 2001; Shehadi 1982). In addition, patients treated with β-adrenergic blockers and interleukin-2 are at increased risk of acute adverse reactions to CM (Thomsen et al. 2004; Morcos 2005) (see Sect. 4.7).
2. The risk of latex hypersensitivity in patients who require chronic bladder care (e.g., individuals with bladder extrophy or meningomyelocele) has been reported to be as high as 72% (Ricci et al. 1999). The risk of anaphylaxis in the operating room is 500-fold greater in patients with spina bifida as compared with control groups (Taylor and Erkek 2004). In individuals of occupations with regular exposure to latex gloves (e.g., health care workers, hair dressers, cleaners, housekeepers) the incidence of latex sensitization is up to 12%, compared to 1%–6% in the general population (Lieberman 2002) (see Sect. 4.9).

4.5 Prevention and Treatment of Anaphylactic Reactions

Medical prevention of anaphylaxis is useful in avoiding reactions to iodinated radiographic contrast media. It is recommended in patients with a high risk for anaphylactic/anaphylactoid reaction to CM as defined earlier (Sect. 4.4). Premedication has not been proven to have any benefit in all other perioperative anaphylactic/anaphylactoid reactions, e.g., reactions to latex or muscle relaxants.

The treatment of anaphylaxis is based on a few very important factors (for details, see Table 4.4).

- Supine position, elevated legs
- Oxygen (6–10 l/min)
- Volume substitution
  - Crystalloids (saline or ringer solution) 30 ml/kg i.v.

Table 4.4. Treatment of immediate hypersensitivity reactions
HES = Hespan

Grade	Type of reaction Dermatological	Respiratory tract	Cardiovascular	Progression suspected
I	H1- (+H2-) antagonists	As needed: i.v. line Oxygen	As needed: i.v. line Oxygen	Corticoids i.v. H1-(+H2-) antagonists
II	H1- (+H2-) antagonists	Mandatory: i.v. line Oxygen β_2-Sympathicomimetica inhalation Prednisolone (250–500 mg i.v.)	Mandatory: i.v. line Oxygen Colloids, Ringer solution, HES	Corticoids i.v. H1-(+H2-) antagonists Adrenaline 0.1 mg i.v.
III	H1- (+H2-) antagonists	Mandatory: i.v. line Oxygen β_2-sympathicomimetica inhalation Prednisolone (0.5–1 g i.v.)	Mandatory: i.v. line Oxygen Colloids, Ringer solution, HES Adrenaline 0.1 mg i.v. repeated every 3 min	Corticoids i.v. H1-(+H2-) antagonists Adrenaline 0.1 mg i.v. Dopamine and/or noradrenaline as needed
IV		Cardiopulmonary Resuscitation and intubation		

From Kemp 2002

Grade of reaction	Step	What to do?
Grade I (slight to moderate general reaction)	1	Stop the cause, stop the antigen
	2	Give oxygen by mask (6–10 l/min)
	3	Place an i.v. line and apply volume (500 ml saline, Ringers solution or HES)
	4	Measure blood pressure and pulse rate
	5	Elevate patient's legs if hypotensive
	6	Inject an H1-antagonist i.v. (e.g., diphenhydramine 25–50 mg, clemastine 4 mg or dimetindene maleat 8 mg) Optionally inject an H2-antagonist (e.g., cimetidine 400 mg or ranitidine 100 mg)
Grade II (severe general reaction)	7	Call resuscitation team
	8	Give corticosteroids i.v. (e.g., prednisolone 500–1,000 mg)
	9	Give adrenaline 1:1000 i.m. (0.2–0.5 mg)
	10	In case of bronchospasm give β_2-sympathicomimetica (e.g., fenoterol inhalation 100–200 μg or terbutaline 0.25–0.5 mg SC)
Grade III (life threatening general reaction)	11	ECG monitoring
	12	Give adrenaline 1:1,000 i.v. (0.1 mg, repeated every 3 min)
	13	Cardiopulmonary resuscitation and intubation

Table 4.5. Step-by-step algorithm for the treatment of anaphylactic reactions in correlation to the grade of anaphylactic reaction

See also Table 4.4

- Antihistamines (H1 and H2)
- Corticoids
- Adrenaline (diluted 1:1,000)

A step-by-step algorithm on what to do with a patient presenting with an anaphylactic reaction is provided in Table 4.5.

Treatment for anaphylaxis is supportive and includes epinephrine/adrenaline as the first-line pharmacological agents. An incidence of 6% for a biphasic anaphylactic reaction in pediatric patients was reported. A delay in administering epinephrine was associated with increased incidence of biphasic reactions, and *unavailability of epinephrine was associated with death* (Lee and Greenes 2000; Chiu and Kelly 2005).

Therefore, patients with an anaphylactic reaction need continuous surveillance for 24 h in hospital. This is also necessary in patients with a good reaction to appropriate therapy because of the possibility of recurrence and the delayed reaction (up to 12 h after the initial reaction) with arrhythmia, myocardial ischaemia or respiratory insufficiency (Haupt 1995).

Monitoring vital functions must include continuous ECG monitoring, pulse oximetry, and blood pressure monitoring.

Management of anaphylactic shock in general is described in great detail by Kemp and Lockey (2002) and is analogous to the management of the immediate reactions to contrast media (Table 4.8).

Guidelines for the management of the cardiovascular shock are published by the American Heart Association (Cummins and Hazinski 2000), the British Resuscitation Council, and the National Guideline Clearinghouse of the United States (NGC) (for addresses of the websites, see Sect. 4.10).

4.6 The Role of Skin and Provocation Tests

The diagnostic value of skin tests has not been fully evaluated during the last decade. Reliable skin test procedures are generally lacking, and test concentrations are unknown or poorly validated for most drugs (Demoly 2005). Skin prick tests and intradermal tests are particularly important for reactive haptens in order to demonstrate an IgE-dependent mechanism. They should be performed 4–6 weeks after the reaction by specialists in an appropriate setting, since the tests themselves can induce an anaphylactic reaction, although rarely.

Depending on the drug, the sensitivity and predictive values of tests vary from excellent (penicillin, muscle relaxants) to satisfactory (opioids, thiopental) all the way to poor or unknown (local anesthetics, paracetamol, sulfonamide, contrast media, nonsteroidal anti-inflammatory drugs). For details, see Sects. 4.7 and 4.8.

The best standardized skin test exists for the β-lactam ring of penicillin. An IgE-dependent hypersensitivity can be demonstrated by a positive skin prick test and/or intradermal test after 20 min (Brockow et al. 2002).

A drug provocation test is carried out for diagnostic/therapeutic purposes and consists of the controlled administration of the drug to a patient with a history that suggests drug allergies. The European Network of Drug Allergy from the European Academy of Allergology and Clinical Immunology recommends the use of a provocation test when skin tests and biological tests are not available or not validated. This approach has elicited some controversial discussion, because with the exception of aspirin and β-lactams, results of tests are only available for very small patient groups. One of the most important reports on drug provocation tests, conducted in 1,372 patients, could show true drug hypersensitivity in only 17.6% of the patients (Demoly 2005). This is of crucial importance for the therapeutic future of these patients. Drug provocation tests should nevertheless be regarded as a serious and potentially dangerous procedure (Aberer et al. 2003).

4.7 Immediate and Nonimmediate Reactions to Contrast Media

Since their development in the 1950s tri-iodinated benzene derivates have been used for opacification of the urinary tract. The radiopacity of such compounds is produced by molecular iodine, which is attached to the benzene ring. The agents are further characterized by their ionic and nonionic side chains as well as their monomeric or dimeric ring structure.

Contrast media are used in many diagnostic and interventional procedures, including intravenous urography, CT scan, angiography, intraoperative antegrade or retrograde pyelography, urethrogram, and cystogram.

Adverse effects of contrast media are generally classified into two large groups: chemotoxic effects and idiopathic or anaphylactoid reactions. Chemotoxic effects are thought to be dose-related and have a direct toxic effect on the target organ, such as the nephrotoxicity of contrast media.

Anaphylactoid reactions simulate a true allergic reaction, but are not mediated by immunoglobulins. No antibodies to contrast material have ever been demonstrated. The diagnosis of contrast media-associated nonallergic anaphylaxis is based on clinical history alone.

Serious reactions to CM are comparable to type 1 hypersensitivity reactions (anaphylaxis), which begin within minutes after antigen exposure and are mediated by a variety of chemotactic, vasoactive, and spasmogenic compounds. Histamine seems to be the primary mediator of anaphylaxis/anaphylactoid reaction and is responsible for the intense immediate manifestations. Preformed histamine is present in basophils and mast cells and is released rapidly by degranulation of these cells in a response to a variety of stimuli. There are several other biological mediators produced by mast cells and basophils, including leukotrienes, prostaglandins, enzymes, and a variety of cytokines. These substances act in an autocrine, paracrine, and endocrine fashion, triggering a cascade of inflammatory mediators. They induce vasodilatation, an increase in vascular permeability leading to edema, contraction of smooth muscle cells precipitating bronchospasm, and an increase in airway mucous secretion. The cytokines and chemotactic factors recruit leukocytes, eosinophils, basophils, monocytes, and T cells, which release additional waves of mediators and cytokines (Morcos 2005).

The mechanisms by which CM activate basophils and mast cells to release histamine and other mediators are not completely understood. They may include direct effects of CM particles on these cells or activation of immunological mechanisms involving IgE antibodies, thymus-derived lymphocytes (T cells) or the complement system (Morcos 2005).

Hypersensitivity reactions to all classes of contrast media (CM) occur either immediately within the first hour after CM administration, or nonimmediately, more than 1 h after CM exposure.

Mild immediate reactions occur in 0.7%–3.1% of patients receiving lower-osmolar/nonionic CM (Brokkow et al. 2005a). Pruritus and mild urticaria are the most common immediate manifestations. More severe reactions involve the respiratory and cardiovascular systems.

The frequency of nonimmediate hypersensitivity reactions appears to range from 1% to 3%, and skin reactions of the maculopapular exanthematous and urticarial/angioedematous types account for the majority of them. At present, the exact pathogenesis of these delayed reactions is still unclear. There is, however, increasing evidence that a significant proportion of the reactions is T cell-mediated (Christiansen et al. 2000).

In a large study of over 330,000 patients, Katayama et al. evaluated the incidence of severe and very severe reactions following intravascular administration of CM. He found an incidence of 0.22% and 0.04%, respectively, after administration of high-osmolar contrast media (HOCM), but only 0.04% and 0.004%, respectively, after low-osmolar contrast media (LOCM) (Katayama et al. 1990; Table 4.6). The study concluded that the use of LOCM has resulted in reducing the incidence of severe and very severe reactions by a factor 10 in comparison to HOCM. However, no difference was observed in the incidence of fatal reactions to both types of CM, which were exceedingly rare (1:170,000). Nevertheless, iodinated CMs are one of the top ten drugs responsible for anaphylaxis/anaphylactoid reactions (Wang et al. 1998), with a mortality rate of 0.9 per 100,000 examinations (Pumphrey 2000; Caro 2001).

Table 4.6. Frequency of adverse reactions to contrast media (338,000 patients)

Adverse reactions	High-osmolar/ ionic contrast media	Low-osmolar/ nonionic contrast media
Total	12.66%	3.13%
Severe	0.22%	0.04%
Very severe	0.04%	0.0004%
Fatal	0.0006%	0.0006%

After Katayama et al. 1990

4.7.1 Diagnostics

4.7.1.1 Immediate Hypersensitivity Reactions

Immediate hypersensitivity reactions to CM are at least in part associated with histamine and tryptase release from basophils and mast cells (Laroche et al. 1998). The role of skin prick tests and intradermal tests (IDT) in diagnostic procedures has been evaluated for many years, but positive tests have only been reported in patients with a history of severe reactions (Brockow 2005a). Determination of plasma histamine and tryptase immediately after reactions to CM may confirm basophil or mast cell mediator release (Laroche et al. 1998). However, recent results indicate that these tests may be of limited value (Laroche 2004). Only two out of 20 patients with immediate reactions had increased levels of these mediators after CM exposure. Both patients had experienced a life-threatening reaction. Whereas tryptase levels remain relatively stable within at least 2 h, histamine is rapidly degraded, and levels have to be determined as soon as possible after the reaction.

Some investigators have reported the presence of CM-specific IgE antibodies in the serum of patients with an immediate reaction, but the frequency of positive test results varies widely between 2 % and 47 %. No commercial assay is available for routine measurement, and the relative merit of the test in diagnosing severe immediate reactions has yet to be established (Brockow 2005a).

Additionally, the role of a histamine release test and other in vitro basophil activation tests in the diagnosis of allergic reactions to CM has not yet been defined.

4.7.1.2 Skin Reactions

Skin reactions of the maculopapular exanthematous and urticarial/angioedematous types account for the majority of nonimmediate hypersensitivity reactions to CM. There is increasing evidence that a significant proportion of the reactions are T cell-mediated (Christiansen et al. 2000). Skin tests have been widely used to confirm such delayed hypersensitivity. CM have consistently tested positively as an allergen in patch tests and/or delayed intradermal tests (IDT) in reactors but not in controls (Brockow et al. 2005a). These tests may be useful in allergy diagnosis of nonimmediate skin reactions to CM, but further evaluation is needed with regard to the sensitivity and specificity as well as of the positive and negative predictive value of such tests.

More data from larger studies are needed to assess the usefulness of the skin tests and other diagnostic tests as routine tools in the follow-up of patients with either immediate or nonimmediate hypersensitivity reactions after CM exposure. *At present such tests cannot yet be recommended for routine clinical practice* (Brokkow 2005b).

4.7.2 Risk Factors

Although the majority of anaphylactoid reactions occur unpredictably, certain risk factors have been well documented. Even though these reactions are not true allergic reactions, patients with a history of a previous adverse response to contrast material have a risk of subsequent reaction that is three- to fourfold greater than the general population (Katayama et al. 1990; Morcos and Thomsen 2001). Other important risk factors include asthma and a history of atopy, including hay fever and food allergies (Morcos and Thomsen 2001; Shehadi 1982). In addition, patients treated with β-adrenergic blockers and interleukin-2 are at increased risk of acute adverse reactions to CM (Thomsen and Morcos 2004; Morcos 2005).

4.7.3 Prevention

The European Society of Urogenital Radiology (ESUR) has produced guidelines on prevention of generalized reactions to CM (Morcos et al. 2001; Table 4.7). They recommend the use of nonionic CM to decrease the risk of generalized CM reactions; they also recommend premedicating high-risk patients with prednisolone (30 mg orally) or methylprednisolone (32 mg orally) 12 and 2 h before CM exposure. However, the value of such premedication in the prevention of severe reactions to lower-osmolar CM has not been conclusively demonstrated. It has yet to be definitively decided whether antihistamines H1 and H2 are of additional benefit in premedication (Morcos et al. 2001; Morcos 2005).

In case of emergency administration of CM in patients with a high risk of severe reactions to CM, particularly those with a history of previous serious reaction to CM, pretreatment is recommended with hydrocortisone (200 mg intravenously) immediately and every 4 h until the procedure is completed, as well as with diphenhydramine (50 mg intravenously) before the procedure and the use of low-osmolar nonionic CM (Greenberger et al. 1986).

However, the best prevention of acute reactions to iodinated contrast media is to avoid its administration (Morcos 2005). Therefore in high-risk patients, imaging procedures that use other contrast media should be considered. Anaphylaxis to gadolinium-based contrast media used in magnetic resonance imaging is very rare and is a safe alternative.

Table 4.7. Prevention of generalized reactions to contrast media

A. Risk factors for reactions
- Previous generalized reaction to a contrast medium, either moderate (e.g., urticaria, bronchospasm, moderate hypotension) or severe (e.g., convulsions, severe bronchospasm, pulmonary edema, cardiovascular collapse)
- Asthma
- Allergy requiring medical treatment

B. To reduce the risk of generalized contrast medium reactions
- Use nonionic agents

C. Premedication is recommended in high-risk patients (defined in A)
- When ionic agents are used
- Opinion is divided about the value of premedication when nonionic agents are used

D. Recommended premedication
- Corticosteroids
  Prednisolone (30 mg orally) or methylprednisolone (32 mg orally) 12 and 2 h before contrast
  Medium is administered. Corticosteroids are not effective if given less than 6 h before contrast medium
- Antihistamines H1 and H2 may be used in addition to corticosteroids, but opinion is divided about the merits of this approach

Remember for all patients
- Have a trolley with resuscitation drugs in the examination room
- Observe patients for 20–30 min after contrast-medium injection

F. Extravascular administration
- When absorption or leakage into the circulation is possible, take the same precautions as for intravascular administration

After Morcos et al. (2001b); www.esur.org

4.7.4 Treatment

Severe, even life-threatening reactions may still occur in patients who receive both corticoid premedication and low-osmolar contrast media. Prompt recognition and treatment of adverse side effects to CM can be invaluable in diminishing the response and may prevent a reaction from becoming severe or even life-threatening (Morcos and Thomsen 2001). For at least 20 min after a CM injection, the patient should never be left alone, because 94%–100% of severe and fatal reactions occur in that interval. Knowledge, training, and preparation are very important for effective treatment of an adverse contrast-related reaction. Therefore, all personnel involved in intravascular application of CM should be adequately trained in cardiopulmonary resuscitation, and all equipment for resuscitation (crash cart, defibrillator, necessary drugs) should be checked regularly.

Mild reactions are usually self-limiting and do not require active treatment. However, the application of the agents must be stopped immediately, and the patient should be observed until full recovery.

Table 4.8. Simple guidelines for first-line treatment of acute reactions to CM

Nausea or vomiting
- Transient: supportive treatment
- Severe, protracted: appropriate antiemetic drugs should be considered

Urticaria
- Scattered, transient: supportive treatment including observation
- Scattered, protracted: appropriate H1-antihistamine intramuscularly or intravenously should be considered; drowsiness and/or hypotension may occur
- Profound: consider adrenaline 1:1,000, 0.1–0.3 ml (0.1–0.3 mg) intramuscularly up to 0.3 maximum in children. Repeat as needed

Bronchospasm
- Oxygen by mask (6–10 l/min)
- β-2-agonist metered dose inhaler (two to three deep inhalations)
- Adrenaline

Normal blood pressure
Intramuscular: 1:1,000, 0.1–0.3 ml (0.1–0.3 mg) (use smaller dose in a patient with coronary artery disease or elderly patient)
In pediatric patients: 0.01 mg/kg up to 0.3 mg maximum

Decreased blood pressure
Intramuscular: 1:1,000, 0.5 ml (0.5 mg), (in pediatric patients: 0.01 mg/kg intramuscularly)

Laryngeal edema
- Oxygen by mask (6–10 l/min)
- Intramuscular adrenaline (1:1,000), 0.5 ml (0.5 mg) for adults, repeat as needed

Hypotension
Isolated hypotension
- Elevate patient's legs
- Oxygen by mask (6–10 l/min)
- Intravenous fluid: rapidly, normal saline or lactated Ringer's solution
- If unresponsive: adrenaline: 1:1,000, 0.5 ml (0.5 mg) intramuscularly, repeat as needed

Vagal reaction (hypotension and bradycardia)
- Elevate patient's legs
- Oxygen by mask (6–10 l/min)
- Atropine 0.6–1.0 mg intravenously, repeat if necessary after 3–5 min, to 3 mg total (0.04 mg/kg) in adults. In pediatric patients, give 0.02 mg/kg intravenously (max. 0.6 mg per dose) repeat if necessary to 2 mg total
- Intravenous fluid: rapidly, normal saline or lactated Ringer's solution

Generalized anaphylactoid reaction
- Call for resuscitation team
- Suction airway as needed
- Elevate patient's legs if hypotensive
- Oxygen by mask (6–10 l/min)
- Intramuscular adrenaline (1:1,000), 0.5 ml (0.5 mg) in adults. Repeat as needed. In pediatric patients, 0.01 mg/kg to 0.3 mg (maximum dose)
- Intravenous fluids (e.g., normal saline, lactated Ringer's)
- H1-blocker, e.g., diphenhydramine 25–50 mg i.v.
- β-2-agonist metered dose inhaler for persistent bronchospasm: two or three inhalations

After Thomsen et al. (2004); www.esur.org

The management of acute adverse reactions to contrast media is well defined and all other anaphylactic reactions, for example to latex and drugs, are managed in the same way. This includes establishment of an adequate airway, oxygen supplementation, administration of intravascular physiological fluids, and measurement of the blood pressure and heart rate. Talking to the patient while checking the pulse rate provides useful initial information: breathing is assessed, the possibility of a vagal reaction (bradycardia) is determined, and a rough estimation of systolic pressure is obtained. H1-antihistamine and adrenaline are administered in correlation with the severity of the reaction.

Wherever an anaphylactic reaction may occur (e.g., the ward, the operating room, the examination room of the radiology department), the following basic medical equipment should be available:

- Oxygen
- Adrenalin 1:1,000 (suitable for injection)
- Antihistamine H1 (suitable for injection)
- Atropine
- β2-agonist metered-dose inhaler
- i.v. fluids: normal saline or Ringers solution
- Anticonvulsive drugs (diazepam)
- Sphygmomanometer
- One-way mouth breather apparatus

Guidelines on first-line treatment have been published by the European Society of Urogenital Radiology (ESUR) (Thomsen and Morcos 2004; Table 4.8, www.esur.org). The subsequent management of severe adverse reactions (including the administration of second-line drugs) should be handled by the resuscitation team.

H2 antihistamines and H2 receptor blockers have a limited role in treating contrast media reactions. They are used primarily to reduce symptoms from skin reactions. High-dose intravenous corticoids do not play a role in the first-line treatment of acute adverse reactions. Standard doses can be effective in reducing delayed recurrent symptoms, occurring up to 48 h after the initial reaction (intravenous prednisolone 250 mg or methylprednisolone 50 mg). However, very high doses may have an immediate stabilizing effect on the mast cell membrane and can be used in the second-line treatment (intravenous prednisolone 500–1,000 mg or methylprednisolone 100–200 mg). It can take 6 h before corticoids are fully active (Thomsen and Morcos 2004).

4.8 Reactions to Perioperative Drugs

4.8.1 General Anesthetic Agents and Neuromuscular Blocking Agents

The main agents used for induction of anesthesia are hypnotics (thiopentone, propofol, and etomidate), opioids (fentanyl), neuroleptics, and benzodiazepines (Thong and Yeow-Chan 2004). The majority of intraoperative anaphylactic reactions are caused by the neuromuscular blocking agents commonly used to induce paralysis to facilitate endotracheal intubation or to optimize surgical exposure (Birnbaum et al. 1994).

The use of intradermal skin tests for the diagnosis of IgE-mediated anaphylaxis to agents during general anesthesia is well established (Moscicki et al. 1990; Rose and Fisher 2001). Some authors have reported the usefulness of skin prick tests (Fisher and Bowey 1997). The advantage of skin prick tests is that by doing intradermal testing, potentially dangerous reactions can be prevented. However, there are no data available on the safety of subsequent anesthesia based on the results of prick testing alone, and reliability over time has not been assessed.

Skin testing is useful because alternative muscular relaxants that produce a negative skin test reaction may be used safely if skin tests show that a neuromuscular agent could cause problems (Fisher 1994). However, the true-negative predictive value for these skin tests is unknown, and false-negative skin reactions have been reported (Fisher et al. 1999).

Patients with previous reactions to an agent used during general anesthesia should have intradermal testing done for both putative agents and an alternative neuromuscular block. Low-risk agents such as pancuronium should be given preference over high-risk agents such as succinylcholine, if both yield negative skin tests. However, a negative skin test result does not eliminate the possibility of developing a reaction to one of these agents. Pretreatment for neuromuscular blocking agent allergy has been found to be ineffective.

Drug-specific IgE can be demonstrated by radioimmunoassay and radioallergosorbent testing (RAST). However, there is only one commercially available test for muscular relaxants (suxamethonium; Pharmacia, Uppsala, Sweden).

4.8.2 Local Anesthetic Agents

Adverse reactions to local anesthetics are not uncommon, but less than 1% are true allergic reactions (Schatz 1984.)

Positive skin test reactions may occur in approximately 15% of patients with no history of adverse reactions to local anesthetic agents (false positive). False-negative test results are rare but are nevertheless reported in the literature (Thong and Yeow-Chan 2004).

4.8.3 Antibiotics

The most common antibiotics given perioperatively are penicillins, cephalosporins, gentamicin, and vancomycin (in patients with methicillin-resistant *Staphylococcus aureus*) (Thong and Yeow-Chan 2004). β-Lactam antibiotics are estimated to cause 400–800 fatal anaphylactic episodes per year. The skin test is the most reliable method for evaluating suspected anaphylaxis to penicillin; 97 % of patients with a negative skin test reaction will tolerate penicillin administration. Thus the skin test has a high negative predictive value. With the presence of a positive history and a positive skin test reaction, the patient has at least a 50 % risk of an immediate reaction to penicillin (Bernstein et al. 1999). Positive drug-specific IgE test results may suggest a diagnosis of penicillin allergy; however, negative tests are unreliable. Thus, skin tests are preferred.

The cross-hypersensitivity between penicillins and cephalosporins is less than 5 %–10 %. Skin tests for cephalosporins are not standardized, and the negative predictive value is unknown.

Desensitization may be considered for patients with a positive skin test reaction to penicillin who require penicillin or cephalosporin in absence of suitable non-β-lactam alternatives (Borish et al. 1987; Kelkar and Li 2001).

Vancomycin hypersensitivity usually leads to skin flush (red man syndrome) and commonly occurs from direct mast cell histamine release. Diagnosis is made from clinical history. If the flush does not respond to a slower rate of infusion, a protocol similar to desensitization may be considered (Wazny and Daghigh 2001).

4.8.4 Opioids

Opioids are often used perioperatively for analgesia and sedation, and as adjuvants to anesthetics. Morphine, codeine, and synthetic opioids such as pethidine can cause direct mast cell degranulation without the presence of specific IgE antibodies. This explains why the skin prick test is not helpful in the diagnosis of opioid hypersensitivity (Nasser and Ewans 2001).

4.8.5 Nonsteroidal Anti-inflammatory Drugs

Nonsteroidal anti-inflammatory drugs (NSAIDs), given for pain relief in the perioperative period, may cause both anaphylactic and anaphylactoid reactions. Anaphylaxis to NSAIDs is typically drug-specific and not common to the entire group of agents.

4.8.6 Heparin

Perioperative heparin prophylaxis can cause thrombocytopenia. There are two types of heparin-induced thrombocytopenia (HIT). HIT I is characterized by a transitory, slight, and asymptomatic reduction in platelet count during the first 1–2 days of treatment. It resolves spontaneously and does not require discontinuation of the drug. The origin of HIT I is not completely understood, but may be caused by a heparin-induced platelet clumping.

The other type of heparin-induced thrombocytopenia, HIT II, has an immunological origin. It is characterized by a significant reduction in platelets (reduction >50 % or to levels $<100 \times 10^3/\mu l$), generally observed after the 5th day of treatment, and usually resolves in 5–15 days after heparin has been suspended. However, in some cases it may take months. HIT II is the most frequent and dangerous side effect of heparin. It may appear in patients who were exposed to heparin earlier. Laboratory tests confirm that the prevalence seems to be 1 %–3 % for unfractionated heparin and 0 %–0.8 % for low-molecular-weight heparin. There is a greater risk in those patients receiving heparin of bovine compared with porcine origin (Fabris et al. 2000; Menajovsky 2005).

The immunologic etiology of HIT II is largely accepted: platelet factor 4 (PF4) displaced from endothelial heparin sulphate or directly from the platelets binds to the heparin molecule to form an immunogenic complex. The IgG anti-heparin/PF4 immunocomplexes activate platelets and provoke an immunologic endothelial lesion with thrombocytopenia and/or thrombosis. Cutaneous allergic manifestation at the heparin injection sites and skin necrosis may be present as well. Interestingly, hemorrhagic events are not frequent, while the major clinical complications in at least 30 % of the patients are both arterial and venous thrombosis, with a 20 % mortality rate. The exact pathomechanism of this reaction is not clear.

During heparin therapy, platelet counts should be checked regularly, at least twice weekly. The diagnosis of HIT is based primarily on clinical criteria and in vitro demonstration of heparin-dependent antibodies. Among the different assays available, the PF4-heparin enzyme linked immunosorbent assay (ELISA) and the ^{14}C-serotonin release assay (SRA) are the most widely used tests.

If HIT II is suspected, heparin must be immediately discontinued and an alternative anticoagulation should be initiated until the resolution of the thrombocytopenia is completed. Heparinoids such as danaparoid sodium (Orgaran; no longer available in the US) or direct thrombin inhibitors such as hirudin are the safest and most effective drugs against the symptoms of HIT, significantly reducing mortality due to thrombotic complications (Fabris et al. 2000). Administration of low-molecular-weight heparin is not recommended, because there is a 60 % – 100 % cross-reactivity of the heparin-induced antibodies.

4.8.7 Colloid Infusion Products

Colloid infusion products used as a plasma expander may cause anaphylaxis during surgery (Thong and Yeow-Chan 2004). The exact pathophysiologic mechanisms are unclear. Gelatin-specific IgE and positive skin prick test as well as positive intradermal test have been demonstrated in some cases, suggesting an IgE-mediated mechanism (Laxenaire et al. 1994).

In a prospective multicenter trial, 69 cases of nonallergic anaphylaxis were observed among 200,906 infusions of colloid volume substitutes. The frequency of severe reactions such as shock, cardiac, or respiratory arrest was 0.003 % for plasma-protein solutions, 0.006 % for hydroxyethyl starch, 0.008 % for dextran, and 0.038 % for gelatin solutions (Ring and Messmer 1977).

4.8.8 Blood Products

A systemic reaction following transfusion of properly matched blood is related to a deficiency of IgA; this in turn is due to either selective IgA immunodeficiency, affecting approximately 1 in 600 individuals in the Western world, or due to common variable immunodeficiency (1 in 25,000 Caucasians) (Hammarstrom et al. 2000). A systemic anaphylactic reaction to blood transfusion is triggered by IgE and IgG antibodies to IgA in some IgA-deficient recipients (type III hypersensitivity reaction). These reactions are very rare, estimated to occur in 1 in 20,000 – 47,000 transfusions. The diagnosis is established by detecting an anti-IgA antibody in the patient's serum (Sandler et al. 1995). Nevertheless, no exact level of antibodies has been defined that will predict the risk of anaphylaxis due to blood products.

Treatment of all anaphylactic/anaphylactoid reactions to perioperative drugs and infusions is recommended according to the guidelines (see Sect. 4.5; Tables 4.4, 4.5, 4.8). There are no special recommendations beyond these.

4.9 Latex Allergy: Diagnosis and Management

Natural rubber latex is a ubiquitous component of modern life. It consists of proteins from the sap of the *Hevea brasiliensis* tree. Anaphylaxis to latex is one of the most feared and frequent anaphylactic reactions during surgery and medical procedures, and the number of reactions are increasing. In the year 2000, reactions to latex accounted for 16.6 % of anaphylactic reactions during surgery.

The populations who are at risk for anaphylaxis to latex are as follows:

- Individuals with a genetic predisposition (atopic individuals)
- Individuals with increased previous exposure to latex (e.g., anyone who requires chronic bladder care with repeated insertion of a latex catheter or chronic indwelling catheters, children with spina bifida and meningomyelocele)
- Healthcare workers who are exposed to latex mainly by inhalation
- In some cases, patients who have undergone multiple surgical procedures

The incidence of latex sensitivity in the general population ranges from 0.8 % to 6.5 %. The two main risk groups for latex allergy are physicians and nurses, with an incidence of 7 % to 18 %. The highest incidence of latex sensitivity has been reported for patients who require chronic bladder care, e.g., children with bladder exstrophy, spina bifida, or meningomyelocele, who have a risk as high as 72 % (Ricci et al. 1999; Taylor and Erkek 2004; Chiu and Kelly 2005).

There are two types of allergic reactions: The delayed hypersensitivity (type IV), which is seen usually in form of a dermatitis reaction. It is a cell-mediated reaction which develops 24 – 48 h after exposure and can be diagnosed by patch testing. Immediate hypersensitivity (type I) is the more dangerous type of allergy, and its incidence has been rapidly increasing over the last two decades. It represents a latex protein-specific IgE-mediated hypersensitivity with a clinical manifestation ranging from contact urticaria to fatal anaphylactic shock (Taylor and Erkek 2004). Exposure to latex antigen can occur by cutaneous (latex gloves), respiratory (opening latex gloves in the operating room), mucosal (gynecological examination with latex gloves), and parenteral routes (i.v. medication with latex-containing infusion sets), with the latter two having the highest risk of anaphylaxis.

There are allergic cross-reactions in patients with fruit or food sensitivities to avocado, banana, chestnut, potato, tomato, passion fruit, and kiwi (Taylor and Erkek 2004). Therefore, a preexisting fruit allergy may be an additional risk factor for clinically relevant latex allergies.

A diagnostic evaluation is recommended for high-risk patients (e.g., children with urological malformations), and for anyone with a history of urticaria or angioedema of the lips when inflating balloons or with itching or contact urticaria when donning gloves, a latex allergy should be suspected. This evaluation should become more comprehensive as needed.

Latex-specific IgE antibodies in serum can be demonstrated in vitro and quantified with RAST or ELISA. Currently, there are three FDA-approved in vitro serologic assays for the diagnosis of latex allergy available on the market (ImmunoCAP, Pharmacia-Upjohn, Sweden; AlaSTAT FEIA, Diagnostic Products Corp., Los Angeles, CA, USA; HYTEC EIA, Hycor Biomedical Inc., Garden Grove, CA, USA). All of them have a relatively high rate of false-negative results. Further disadvantages are the costs, delayed results, low sensitivity, and accessibility compared to in vivo tests. However, serology should be the initial diagnostic step for suspected latex allergy because it is safer than in vivo tests.

The skin prick test is the gold standard. It is easy to perform and provides immediate results (5–30 min). Sensitivity is highly influenced by the quality of the latex extract used, but can be as high as 87%. Additionally, at 66% the specificity of the skin prick test is higher than the in vitro tests (RAST, ELISA). There is a standardized commercial skin prick test kit available in Europe (Stallergenes SA, Antony, France), but so far no FDA-approved test is available.

The skin prick test as an in vivo test is comparable to a small-scale provocation test. Therefore it should be performed by experienced staff and with oxygen, epinephrine, and latex-free resuscitation equipment at hand. Because of rare anaphylactic reactions to the prick test, the in vitro diagnostic work-up should be performed prior to the prick test.

Another possibility is a provocation test by wearing a latex glove. This may be employed when there is a discrepancy between prick test or specific IgE results and clinical history. It begins as a one-finger test, and extended to a whole-hand test if there is no urticarial reaction after 20 min. Nonlatex vinyl gloves are used as a control. The testing staff has to be aware of the possibility of sudden anaphylactic reactions.

Corticoids and H1 and H2 antagonists can be used to pretreat patients with known latex allergy prior to medical procedures. However, *pretreatment is not very effective* in preventing reactions to latex, unlike prevention measures for reactions to contrast media. Therefore, the most important factor is avoiding exposure to the allergen. This means taking a thorough patient history, testing for latex allergy in high-risk patients, preadmission measures, and establishing a latex-free environment while the patient is hospitalized, particularly in the operating and recovery rooms (Lieberman 2002). The charts of latex allergic patients should be labeled, and surgery should be scheduled as the first case of the day to reduce exposure to the aerosolized latex allergens. Latex-free equipment should be stored separately: nonlatex gloves, glass syringes, nonlatex tape, synthetic catheters and tubes, latex-free blood pressure cuffs, and three-way stopcocks for i.v. administration of medication.

Allergic reactions to latex are treated in a manner that is analog to all other anaphylactic reactions (compare treatment recommendations in Tables 4.4, 4.5, and 4.8).

References

Aberer W, Bircher A, Romano A, Blanca M, Campi P, Fernandez J, Brockow K, Pichler WJ, Demoly P (2003) European Network for Drug Allergy (ENDA); EAACI interest group on drug hypersenitivity. Drug provocation testing in the diagnosis of drug hypersensitivity reactions:general considerations. Allergy 58:854

Bernstein IL, Gruchalla RS, Lee RE et al (1999) Executive summary of disease management of drug hypersensitivity:a practice parameter. Joint task force on practice parameters, the American Academy of Allergy, Asthma and Immunology. Ann Allergy Asthma Immunol 83:665

Birnbaum J, Porri F, Pradal M, Charpin D, Vervloet D (1994) Allergy during anaesthesia. Clin Exp Allergy 24:915

Borish L, Tamir R, Rosenwasser LJ (1987) Intravenous desensitization to beta-lactam antibiotics. J Allergy Clin Immunol 80:314

Brockow K, Vieluf D, Puschel K, Grosch J, Ring J (1999) Increased postmortem serum mast cell tryptase in a fatal anaphylactoid reaction to nonionic radiocontrast medium. J Allergy Clin Immunol 104:237

Brockow K, Romano A, Blanca M, Ring J, Pichler W, Demoly P (2002) General considerations for skin test procedures in the diagnosis of drug hypersensitivity. Allergy 57:45

Brockow K (2005) Contrast media hypersensitivity – scope of the problem. Toxicology 209:189

Brockow K, Christiansen C, Kanny G, Clément O, Barbaud A, Bircher A, DeWachter P, Guéant J-L, Guéant R-M R, Mouton-Faivre C, Ring J, Romano A, Sainte-Laudy J, Demoly P, Pichler WJ for ENDA and the EAACI interest group on drug hypersensitivity (2005) Management of hypersensitivity reactions to iodinated contrast media. Allergy 60:150

Caro JJ, Trinidade E, McGregor M (1991) The risks of death and of severe nonfatal reactions with high- vs low-osmolality contrast media: a meta-analysis. AJR Am J Roentgenol 156:825

Chiu AM, Kelly KJ (2005) Anaphylaxis: drug allergy, insect stings, and latex. Immunol Allergy Clin N Am 25:389

Christiansen C, Pichler WJ, Skotland T l (2000) Delayed allergy-like reactions to X-ray contrast media:mechanistic considerations. Eur Radio 10:1965

Coombs RRA, Gell PGH (1975) Classification of allergic reactions responsible for clinical hypersensitivity and disease. In: Gell PGH, Coombs RRA, Lachmann PJ (eds) Clinical aspects of immunology, 3rd edn. Blackwell, Oxford, pp 761

Cummins RO, Hazinski MR (2000) The most important changes in the international ECC and CPR guidelines 2000. Circulation 102 [8 Suppl]:1371

Demoly P (2005) Anaphylactic reactions – value of skin and provocation tests. Toxicology 209:221

Fabris F, Luzzatto G, Stefani PM, Girolami B, Cella G (2000) Heparin-induced thrombocytopenia. Haematologica 85:72

Fisher MM, Bowey CJ (1997) Intradermal compared with prick testing in the diagnosis of anaesthetic allergy. Br J Anaesth 79:59
Fisher MM, Baldo BA (1998) Mast cell tryptase in anaesthetic anaphylactoid reactions. Br J Anaesth 80:26
Fisher MM, Merefield D, Baldo BA (1999) Failure to prevent an anaphylactic reaction to a second neuromuscular blocking drug during anaesthesia. Br J Anaesth 82:770
Greenberger PA, Halwig JM, Patterson R, Wallemark CB (1986) Emergency administration of radio contrast media in high-risk patients. J Allergy Clin Immunol 77:630
Hammarstrom L, Vorechivsky I, Webster D. Selective IgA deficiency (SIgAD) and common variable immunodeficiency (CVID) (2000) Clin Exp Immunol 120:225
Haupt MT (1995) Anaphylaxis and anaphylactic shock. In: Parillo JE, Bone RC (eds) Critical care medicine. Mosby Year Book, St. Louis, pp 433
Johansson SG, Hourihane JO, Bousquet J, Bruijnzeel-Koomen C, Dreborg S, Haahtela T, Kowalski ML, Mygind N, Ring J, van Cauwenberge P, van Hage-Hamsten M, Wuthrich B (2001) EAACI (the European Academy of Allergology and Clinical Immunology) nomenclature task force: a revised nomenclature for allergy. An EAACI position statement from the EAACI nomenclature task force. Allergy 56:813
Katayama H, Yamaguchi K, Kozuka T, Takashima T, Seez P, Matsuura K (1990) Adverse reactions to ionic and nonionic contrast media. A report from the Japanese committee on the safety of contrast media. Radiology 175:621
Kelkar PS, Li JT (2001) Cephalosporin allergy. N Engl J Med 345:804
Kemp SF, Lockey RF (2002) Anaphylaxis: a review of causes and mechanisms. J Allergy Clin Immunol 110:341
Laroche D, Aimone-Gastin I, Dubois F, Huet H, Gerard P, Vergnaud MC, Mouton-Faivre C, Gueant JL, Laxenaire MC, Bricard H (1998) Mechanisms of severe, immediate reactions to iodinated contrast material. Radiology 209:183
Laroche D, Dewachter P, Mouton-Faivre C, Clément O (2004) Immediate reactions to iodinated contrast media :the CIRTACI study (abstract no. 56). Allergologie 27:165
Laxenaire MC, Charpentier C, Feldman L (1994) Anaphylactoid reactions to colloid plasma substitutes:incidence, risk factors, mechanisms. A French multicenter prospective study (in French). Ann Fr Anesth Reanim 13:301
Laxenaire MC (1999) Again and always allergy. Ann Fr Anesth Reanim 18:831
Lee JM, Greenes DS (2000) Biphasic anaphylactic reactions in pediatrics. Pediatrics 106:762
Lieberman P (2002) Anaphylactic reactions during surgical and medical procedures. J Allergy Clin Immunol 110:S64
Menajovsky (2005) LB Heparin-induced thrombocytopenia: clinical manifestations and management strategies. Am J Med 118:21S
Morcos SK (2005) Review article: Acute serious and fatal reactions to contrast media: our current understanding. Br J Radiol 932:686
Morcos SK, Thomsen HS (2001) Adverse reactions to iodinated contrast media. Eur Radiol 11:1267
Morcos SK, Thomsen HS, Webb JA (2001) Contrast Media Safety Committee of the European Society of Urogenital Radiology. Prevention of generalized reactions to contrast media: a consensus report and guidelines. Eur Radiol 11:1720
Moscicki RA, Sockin SM, Corsello BF, Ostro MG, Bloch KJ (1990) Anaphylaxis during induction of general anesthesia: subsequent evaluation and management. J Allergy Clin Immunol 86:325
Nasser SM, Ewans PW (2001) Opiate-sensitivity: clinical characteristics and the role of skin prick testing. Clin Exp Allergy 31:1014
Pumphrey RS (2000) Lessons for management of anaphylaxis from a study of fatal reactions. Clin Exp Allergy 30:1144
Ricci G, Gentili A, Di Lorenzo F, Righetti F, Pigna A, Masi M, DeCastro R (1999) Latex allergy in subjects who had undergone multiple surgical procedures for bladder exstrophy: relationship with clinical intervention and atopic diseases. BJU Int 84:1058
Ring J, Messmer K (1977) Incidence and severity of anaphylactoid reactions to colloid volume substitutes. Lancet 1:466–469
Rose M, Fisher M (2001) Rocuronium: high risk for anaphylaxis? Br J Anaesth 86:678
Schatz M (1984) Skin testing and incremental challenge in the evaluation of adverse reactions to local anesthetics. J Allergy Clin Immunol 74:606
Sandler SG, Mallory D, Malamut D, Eckrich R (1995) IgA anaphylactic transfusion reactions. Transfus Med Rev 9:1
Shehadi (1982) WH Contrast media adverse reactions: occurrence, recurrence, and distribution patterns. Radiology 143:11
Thomsen HS, Morcos SK (2004) Contrast Media Safety Committee of European Society of Urogenital Radiology. Management of acute adverse reactions to contrast media. Eur Radiol 14:476
Taylor JS, Erkek E (2004)Latex allergy:diagnosis and management. Dermatologic Therapy 17:289
Thong BY-H, Yeow-Chan (2004) Anaphylaxis during surgical and interventional procedures. Ann Allergy Asthma Immunol 92:619
Wang DJ, Forslund C, Persson U, Wiholm BE (1998) Drug-attributed anaphylaxis. Pharmacoepidemiol Drug Saf 7:269
Wazny LD, Daghigh B (2001) Desensitization protocols for vancomycin hypersensitivity. Ann Pharmacother 35:1458

Further Reading

Guidelines for the Management of Cardiovascular Shock

American Heart Association: www.americanheart.org. Cited 6 November 2006
Anonymous (2000) http://circ.ahajournals.org/cgi/content/full/102/suppl_1/I-1. Cited 6 November 2006
European Resuscitation Council (2000) Part 8: advanced challenges in resuscitation. Section 3: special challenges in ECC. 3D: anaphylaxis. Resuscitation 46:285
British Resuscitation Council: www.resus.org.uk. Cited 6 November 2006
National Guideline Clearinghouse of the United States (NGC) (2006) The diagnosis and management of anaphylaxis: an updated practice parameter. http://www.guideline.gov/summary/summary.aspx?doc_id=6887. Cited 6 November 2006

Urosepsis

5

H.G. Schiefer, Th. Diemer, W. Weidner

5.1 Definition

Urosepsis is caused by the invasion, from a focus in the urinary tract, of pathogenic or commensal microorganisms, or their constituents into the body, prompting a complex response by the synthesis of endogenous mediators responsible for the clinical phenomena (Dinarello 1984; Van Amersfoort et al. 2003). Progress of sepsis to severe sepsis and septic shock correlates with an increased risk of death.

5.2 Epidemiology of Sepsis

US data demonstrate an incidence of sepsis of approximately 750,000 cases/year, responsible for up to 250,000 deaths/year in the United States. In relation to the whole population, a yearly incidence of 3 cases per 1,000 persons and of 26 cases per 1,000 persons in the elderly population (older than 65 years) is reported. In approximately 50 % of cases, sepsis arises from the urinary tract (Bernard et al. 2001; Hotchkiss and Karl 2003; Russell 2006; Van Amersfoort et al. 2003).

5.3 Etiology of Urosepsis

Urosepsis is caused by Gram-negative bacteria (e.g., *Escherichia coli,* 52 %; other *Enterobacteriaceae* spp., 22 %, *Pseudomonas aeruginosa*, 4 %), Gram-positive bacteria (e.g., *Enterococcus* spp., 5 %, *Staphylococcus aureus*, 10 %), and other pathogenic bacteria in nosocomial urosepsis (1 % of all cases) (multidrug resistant bacteria, e.g., *Pseudomonas aeruginosa).*

5.4 Pathophysiology

Sepsis is caused by the invasion of intact pathogenic or commensal bacteria or bacterial cell wall constituents, especially lipopolysaccharides (LPS), in particular lipoid A = endotoxin of the outer membrane of Gram-negative bacteria, or peptidoglycan, teichoic and lipoteichoic acids of Gram-positive bacteria, or toxins, e.g., toxic-shock-syndrome-toxin 1 and *Staphylococcus aureus* toxin A. They bind to cellular receptors and co-receptors, e.g., CD14, toll-like receptors TLR2 and TLR4, CD18 (β_2 integrins), and selectins, on the surfaces of monocytes/macrophages, neutrophils, and endothelial cells. Via intracellular signaling molecules, e.g., NF-κB and protein kinase C, they activate the transcription of mediator genes to induce the synthesis and release of numerous endogenous mediators, i.e., cytokines such as interleukin (IL)-1, IL-2, IL-4, IL-6, IL-8, IL-10, tumor necrosis factor (TNF), and platelet-activating factor (PAF). These pro-inflammatory and anti-inflammatory mediators often originate in an inflammed local site. They are formed and released with various kinetics. They act in part synergistically and in part antagonistically, mainly via additional mediators (chemokines, prostaglandins, thromboxanes, leukotrienes, and endogenous vasodilators nitric oxide [NO]), on target organs, and are responsible for a plethora of local and systemic effects in the host organism (Bernard et al. 2001; Dellinger 2003; Gerard 2003; Gogos et al. 2000; Hotchkiss and Karl 2003; Russell 2006; Van Amersfoort et al. 2003; Wilson et al. 1998).

TNF-α and IL-1 are the primary pro-inflammatory cytokines and have similar biological activities (Camussi et al. 1991; Dinarello 1984). They alter the temperature regulation center in the hypothalamus, thus inducing fever. They act on the formatio reticularis in the brain stem (sleeping-waking center), the patient becomes somnolent or comatose. They stimulate the liberation of ACTH in the hypophysis. Via hematopoietic growth factors, they act on the bone marrow to stimulate the synthesis of neutrophils and liberate reserve neutrophils, causing peripheral leukocytosis and increased numbers of immature neutrophils (bands). They activate the neutrophils to rapid phagocytosis and production of bactericidal agents, i.e., proteases and oxygen radicals. They stimulate B and T lymphocytes and synthesis of antibodies and cellular immune reactions are increased; however, as sepsis persists, there is a shift to an anti-inflammatory immunosuppressive state (transient immune paralysis) because of apoptosis of B cells, CD4 helper T cells, and follicular dendritic cells (Liles 1997). In the liver, they stimulate the synthesis of acute-phase proteins, e.g., C-reactive protein (CRP), complement factors, and α_1-antitrypsin. They stimulate the decay of muscle proteins (increased protein catabolism), and liberated amino acids are used for antibody synthesis. They activate vascular endothelial cells to produce cytokines such as PAF and NO, and promote increased vascular permeability by vascular endothelial injury and endothelial detachment. They up-regulate the synthesis of cell-surface molecules that enhance neutrophil–endothelial cell adhesion. They increase pro-coagulatory activity on endothelial cells and the synthesis of plasminogen activator inhibitor, and activate the complement and blood coagulation systems, which may result in microcirculatory failure, tissue hypoxia, organ ischemia, and organ failure (Dellinger 2003; Dinarello 1984; Gogos et al. 2000; Hotchkiss and Karl 2003). On the other hand, IL-4 and IL-10 are anti-inflammatory cytokines since they inhibit the production of IL-1 and TNF (Gogos et al. 2000; Hotchkiss and Karl 2003; Russell 2006).

In summary, the pathophysiological phenomena and consequences of sepsis, severe sepsis, and septic shock result in:

- Poor perfusion of skin and internal organs with reduced arterial-venous oxygen gradient by by-passing the capillaries via multiple shunts, accumulation of lactate (metabolic acidosis), anoxia
- Activation of the complement and blood coagulation cascades
- Activation of B and T lymphocytes
- Activation of neutrophils, thus increasing their chemotaxis and adhesiveness
- Increased capillary permeability (capillary leak syndrome), hemoconcentration, decreased circulating blood volume
- Accumulation of neutrophils in the lungs where they release proteases and oxygen radicals which alter alveolar-capillary permeability to increased transudation of liquid, ions, and proteins into the interstitial space, which finally results in acute respiratory distress syndrome (ARDS, shock lung)
- Myocardial depression, hypotension
- Accelerated apoptosis of lymphocytes and gastrointestinal epithelial cells
- Disseminated intravascular coagulation (DIC)
- Impairment and finally failure of hepatic, renal, and pulmonary functions

5.5 Classification System

Identical clinical manifestations without bacterial infection are observed in patients suffering from polytrauma, ischemia, hemorrhagic shock, and acute pancreatitis, resulting in intensive care physicians proposing an expanded nomenclature and classification. The classification system that has been amended ever since is important in evaluating the prognosis of a patient suffering from sepsis and assessing of the success of new therapeutic approaches. It is based on the following criteria (Bone et al. 1992; Reinhart et al. 2004):

Criterion I: Definitive evidence of infection (positive hemoculture) or clinically suspected infection. Bacteremia may be low-grade (< 10 bacteria/ml) and transient. Multiple blood cultures may be required.

Criterion II: Systemic inflammatory response syndrome (SIRS)

1. Core temperature ≥ 38 °C or ≤ 36 °C
2. Heart rate ≥ 90 beats/min
3. Respiratory rate ≥ 20 breaths/min
4. Respiratory alkalosis $PaCO_2 \leq 32$ mm Hg
5. White cell count (≥ 12×10^9/l or ≤ 4×10^9/l)
6. Immature neutrophils (bands) > 10 %.

Criterion III: Multiple organ dysfunction syndrome (MODS)

1. Cardiovascular: arterial systolic blood pressure ≤ 90 mm Hg or > 40 mm Hg less than patient's normal blood pressure, or the mean arterial blood pressure ≤ 70 mm Hg for at least 1 h despite adequate fluid resuscitation, adequate intravascular volume status, or the use of vasopressors in an attempt to maintain a systolic blood pressure ≥ 90 mm Hg
2. Renal: urine output < 0.5 ml/kg of body weight/h for 1 h, despite adequate fluid resuscitation
3. Respiratory: $PaO_2 \leq 75$ mm Hg while breathing room air, or $PaO_2/FiO_2 \leq 250$ in the presence of

Table 5.1. Classification of sepsis stages and lethality

	Criteria	Lethality
Sepsis	Criterion I + ≥2 criteria II	2 Criteria II, 7% 3 Criteria II, 10% 4 Criteria II, 17%
Severe sepsis	Criterion I + ≥2 criteria II + ≥1 criterion III	Per afflicted organ (liver, lung, kidney), lethality is increased by 15%–20%
Septic shock	Criterion I + ≥2 criteria II + refractory hypotension (criterion III), i.e., arterial blood pressure <90 mm systolic, or 40 mm less than patient's normal blood pressure, or mean arterial blood pressure ≤70 mmHg, for ≥2 h, or need for vasopressors to maintain systolic blood pressure ≥90 mmHg or mean arterial pressure ≥70 mmHg.	>50%–80%

other dysfunctional organs or systems, or ≤200, if the lung is the only dysfunctional organ (PaO_2, partial pressure of arterial oxygen; FiO_2, fractional concentration of inspired O_2 [~0.21 when breathing room air])

4. Hematologic: platelet count $<80\times10^9$/l or 50% decrease in platelet count from highest value recorded over previous 3 days
5. Metabolic acidosis: a pH ≤7.30, or a base deficit ≥5 mm/l, a plasma level of lactate >1.5 times the upper limit of normal
6. Brain: somnolence, confusion, agitation, delirium, coma

Following these criteria, sepsis can be clinically categorized into three different stages (Table 5.1). Prognostic criteria concerning lethality are also based on the above-mentioned classification system.

In an intensive care unit (ICU), patient's illness is often categorized into grades of severity following a scoring system, e.g., the Apache II (Acute Physiology and Chronic Health Evaluation II) system, which is based upon age, type of intensive care unit admission, a chronic health problem score, and 12 physiologic variables.

5.6 Risk Factors for Urosepsis

Predisposing primary diseases such as advanced age, diabetes mellitus, malignancy, cachexia, immunodeficiency, radiotherapy, cytostatic therapy; obstructive uropathy (e.g., urethral stricture, benign prostatic hyperplasia [BPH]), carcinoma of the prostate, urolithiasis, neurogenic disturbances of micturition, inflammatory diseases (e.g., pyelonephritis, acute bacterial prostatitis, epididymitis, renal abscess, paranephritic abscess, prostatic abscess), and nosocomial infections (e.g., patients with indwelling urinary catheters, after transurethral/open surgery, endoscopy, and prostatic biopsies).

Table 5.2. Clinical stages of urosepsis

1. Hyperdynamic early stage
Precapillary sphincters shut the capillary bed, the blood rushes via precapillary arterial-venous shunts; gas exchange and removal of metabolites, e.g., lactate, cease
Hyperventilation induces respiratory alkalosis
The patient is warm
Cardiac output normal or increased (up to 10–20 l/min)
Peripheral vascular resistance and arterial-venous oxygen gradient reduced
Central venous pressure normal or increased
Patient appears as seriously ill, is pale, and sweating profusely
Pulse is frequent and soft
Hypotension
Nausea, emesis, diarrhea
Agitation, confusion, disturbance of orientation
2. Intermediate stage
Accumulation of lactate results in metabolic acidosis
Increasing myocardial depression
Due to endothelial injury and increased vascular permeability, effusion of plasma into renal, hepatic, pulmonary interstitial space, increasing organ dysfunction followed by organ failure (shock kidney, shock liver, shock lung [ARDS])
Due to activation of the complement and coagulatory cascades and increased adherence of cellular elements (neutrophils, thrombocytes, endothelial cells), disseminated intravascular coagulation (DIC) with consumption coagulopathy leading to hemorrhages, organ hypoxia, organ failure, and mostly lethal septic shock
3. Hypodynamic late stage
Patient's skin cold and cyanotic
Reduced cardiac output
Peripheral vascular resistance increased due to vasoconstriction; central venous pressure reduced

5.7 Clinical Symptoms

Premonitory symptoms are tachypnea (>20 breaths/min), tachycardia (>90 beats/min), and hyperthermia (>38°C), or hypothermia (<36°C) followed by intermittent bouts of fever with shaking chills during invasion of bacteria. The clinical course of urosepsis is differentiated in three stages (Table 5.2).

5.8 Diagnostic Procedures

Typical clinical laboratory data are provided in Table 5.3:

Table 5.3. Laboratory findings in urosepsis

Erythrocyte sedimentation rate increased (normal range: females 1–25 mm/h; males 0–17 mm/h)
C-reactive protein (CRP) increased (normal range, 0.1–≤8.2 mg/l, depends on the method used)
Leukocyte counts (>12×10⁹/l or <4×10⁹/l) with toxic granulation, and immature neutrophils (bands) >10%
Thrombocytopenia (<80×10⁹/l)
Hyperbilirubinemia (normal range, <1 mg/100 ml)
Increased creatinine level (normal range, <1.5 mg/100 ml)
Proteinuria
Initially respiratory alkalosis, later on metabolic acidosis
Hypoxemia
Biomarkers of sepsis (cytokines, procalcitonin) and of blood coagulation (D-dimer, protein C, protein S, antithrombin) may be determined and provide further hints

5.9 Microbiology

Analysis of at least two blood cultures (aerobic, anaerobic) at the same time, i.e., 2 × 10 ml of venous blood, is mandatory. Since bacteremia may be low-grade (<10 microorganisms/ml), multiple blood cultures may be required, in particular in case of negative results (>50% in cases of severe sepsis!) of the initial hemocultures. They should best be taken during the rise in body temperature, i.e., just before the fever spike. When antimicrobial therapy has already been started, blood should be drawn before repeated antibiotic administration.

5.10 Further Diagnostic Procedures

The focal source of infection must be sought carefully, and specimens for microbiological analysis such as purulent secretions, urine, and abscess pus should be taken.

5.11 Therapy

The general goals of therapy are:

1. Stabilization of hemodynamics
2. Improvement of oxygen saturation and utilization
3. Sufficient organ perfusion
4. Improved organ function (heart, lung, liver, kidney)
5. Antimicrobial treatment of sepsis
6. Sanitization of the focal source of infection
7. Essential steps of therapy (Evans 2001; Hotchkiss and Karl 2003; Rivers et al. 2001; Reinhart et al. 2004; Russel 2006) are compiled in Table 5.4

Table 5.4. Recommended therapeutic approach to patients suffering from urosepsis

Patients should immediately be transferred to the ICU 1. Volume replacement: infusion of 1–2 l of electrolyte solution over 1–2 h; goal: central venous pressure (CVP) 8–12 mmHg, mean arterial blood pressure ≥65 mmHg, but ≤90 mmHg Blood transfusion in case of central venous oxygenation <70% and of hematocrit <30; optimal: fresh erythrocyte concentrates; goal: hemoglobin value ≥7–≤10 g/100 ml whole blood, hematocrit >30 In case of hypalbuminemia (<2 g/100 ml), the additional infusion of albumin solutions has been suggested but is still controversial
2. Controlled and assisted ventilation: tidal volume, 6 ml/kg body weight; goal: arterial oxygen saturation ≥93%, central venous oxygen saturation ≥70%. If <70%, administration of dobutamine (initially 2.5 µg/kg/min, after 30 min each, increase by 2.5 µg/kg/min; maximum, 20 µg/kg/min)
3. Administration of vasopressors: if mean arterial pressure (MAP) <65 mmHg, give dopamine, 1–3 µg/kg/min, or noradrenaline (norepinephrine), 0.1–1.0 µg/kg/min, as a continuous i.v. infusion
4. Control of urine excretion; goal: >30 ml/h; if necessary, give furosemide in order to inhibit tubular re-resorption (therapeutic value not evidence-based). Tight control of blood glucose; goal: 80-110 mg/100 ml; exact stabilization with intensive insulin therapy (anti-apoptotic effect) (Evans 2001; Russell 2006; Van den Berghe et al. 2001)
5. Antimicrobial therapy: if possible, targeted (pathogen identified, sensitivity determined), otherwise calculated, or initially untargeted (wide-spectrum): reserve beta-lactam antibiotics i.v., e.g., cefotaxime, 3×2–4 g/day, or ceftazidime, 3×1–2 g/day, or ceftriaxone, 2×2 g at day 1, then 1×2 g/day, plus aminoglycoside i.v., e.g., gentamicin, 1×240–320 mg/day, by infusion. Monitor blood levels of aminoglycoside, trough concentration should be <1–2 µg/ml, and creatinine levels, three to seven times/week (Bodmann and Vogel 2001; Gilbert et al. 2006)
6. After stabilization of cardiovascular function and start of antimicrobial therapy, removal of the infectious focus is mandatory. Abscesses have to be drained, and pyonephrosis has to be treated either by intraureteral JJ catheters or percutaneous nephrostomy. A Foley catheter should be inserted in any case
7. Supportive measures: for patients in septic shock and/or those with proved adrenocortical insufficiency (serum cortisol level <15 µg/100 ml; corticotropin test: within 30–60 min after i.m. or i.v. injection of 250 µg of adrenocorticotropin hormone, increase of serum cortisol level <9 µg/100 ml), the i.v./i.m. administration of hydrocortisone (4×50 mg/day), or equivalent, is indicated (Cooper and Stewart 2003; Hamrahian et al. 2004; Rhen and Cidlowski 2005; Russell 2006)
8. In order to inhibit imminent disseminated intravascular coagulation (reduced levels of plasma protein C) in cases of severe sepsis, recombinant human activated protein C (drotrecogin alpha-activated) with a dose of 24 µg/kg/h as a continuous i.v. infusion for 96 h is recommended (Bernard et al. 2001; Dellinger 2003; Matthay 2001; Opal et al. 2003). The drug is approved for patients with an Apache II score of ≥25, but should not be used in patients with severe sepsis who are at low risk for death, such as those with single-organ failure or an Apache II score <25 (Abraham et al. 2005; Parrillo 2005; Russell 2006). The substance has antithrombotic, anti-apoptotic, antiinflammatory, and pro-fibrinolytic properties. Potential adverse effect is hemorrhagic diathesis

References

Abraham E, Laterre PF, Garg R et al (2005) Drotrecogin alfa (activated) for adults with severe sepsis and a low risk of death. N Engl J Med 353:1322

Bernard GR, Vincent JL, Laterre PF et al (2001) Efficacy and safety of recombinant human activated protein C for severe sepsis. N Engl J Med 344:699

Bodmann KF, Vogel F (2001) Antimikrobielle Therapie der Sepsis. Chemother J 10:43

Bone RC, Balk RA, Cerra FB et al (1992) Definitions for sepsis and organ failure and guidelines for the use of innovative therapies in sepsis. Chest 101:1644

Camussi G, Albano E, Tetta C et al (1991) The molecular action of tumor necrosis factor-α. Eur J Biochem 202:3

Cooper MS, Stewart PM (2003) Current concepts: Corticosteroid insufficiency in acutely ill patients. N Engl J Med 348: 727

Dellinger RP (2003) Inflammation and coagulation: implications for the septic patient. Clin Infect Dis 36:1259

Dinarello CA (1984) Interleukin-1 and the pathogenesis of the acute-phase response. N Engl J Med 311:1413

Evans TW (2001) Hemodynamic and metabolic therapy in critically ill patients. N Engl J Med 345:1417

Gerard C (2003) Complement C5a in the sepsis syndrome – too much of a good thing? N Engl J Med 348:167

Gilbert DN, Moellering RC, Eliopoulos GM, Sande MA (2006) The Sanford guide to antimicrobial therapy 2006, 36th edn. Antimicrobial Therapy Inc., Sperryville, VA, USA, p 44

Gogos CA, Drosou E, Bassaris HP et al (2000) Pro-versus anti-inflammatory cytokine profile in patients with severe sepsis: a marker for prognosis and future therapeutic options. J Infect Dis 181:176

Hamrahian AH, Oseni TS, Arafah BM (2004) Measurement of serum free cortisol in critically ill patients. N Engl J Med 350:1629

Hotchkiss RS, Karl IE (2003) The pathophysiology and treatment of sepsis. N Engl J Med 348:138

Liles WC (1997) Apoptosis – role in infection and inflammation. Curr Opin Infect Dis 10:165

Matthay MA (2001) Severe sepsis – a new treatment with both anticoagulant and anti-inflammatory properties. N Engl J Med 344:759

Opal SM, Garber GE, La Rosa SP et al (2003) Systemic host responses in severe sepsis analyzed by causative microorganism and treatment effects of drotrecogin alfa (activated). Clin Infect Dis 37:50

Parrillo JE (2005) Severe sepsis and therapy with activated protein C. N Engl J Med 353:1398

Reinhart K, Hüttemann E, Meier-Hellmann A (2004) Sepsis. In: Burchardi H, Larsen R, Schuster H-P, Suter PM (eds) Die Intensivmedizin. Springer Berlin Heidelberg New York, p 851

Rhen T, Cidlowski JA (2005) Anti-inflammatory action of glucocorticoids – new mechanisms for old drugs. N Engl J Med 353:1711

Rivers E, Nguyen B, Havstad S et al (2001) Early goal-directed therapy in the treatment of severe sepsis and septic shock. N Engl J Med 345:1368

Russel JA (2006) Management of sepsis. N Engl J Med 355:1699

Van Amersfoort ES, Van Berkel TJC, Kuiper J (2003) Receptors, mediators, and mechanisms involved in bacterial sepsis and septic shock. Clin Microbiol Rev 16:379

Van den Berghe G, Wouters P, Weekers F et al (2001) Intensive insulin therapy in critically ill patients. N Engl J Med 345:1359

Wilson M, Seymour R, Henderson B (1998) Bacterial perturbation of cytokine networks. Infect Immun 66:2401

6 Fournier's Gangrene

C.F. Heyns, P.D. Theron

6.1 Definition and Historical Perspective

Fournier's gangrene is a synergistic polymicrobial necrotizing fasciitis of the perineum and genitalia. It can progress to a fulminant soft tissue infection that spreads rapidly along the fascial planes, causing necrosis of the skin, subcutaneous soft tissue, and fascia, with associated systemic sepsis. If it is not diagnosed early and treated promptly, significant morbidity with prolonged hospital stay and even mortality will ensue.

In 1764, Baurienne described a fulminant gangrene of the male perineum. However, Jean Alfred Fournier, a French dermatologist and venereologist, became famous for this notorious condition when, in 1883, he described a series of five young men in whom gangrene of the genitalia occurred without any apparent etiologic factor. As knowledge of the condition increased over the years, it became clear that Fournier's gangrene is most common in older men (peak incidence in the 5th and 6th decades) and that most cases have an identifiable cause.

Fortunately, it is a rare condition, with a reported incidence of 1/7,500, and accounting for only 1 % – 2 % of urologic hospital admissions (Bejanga 1979; Bahlmann et al. 1983; Hejase et al. 1996). However, the incidence is rising, most likely due to an increase in the mean age of the population, as well as increased numbers of patients on immunosuppressive therapy or suffering from human immunodeficiency virus (HIV) infection, especially in Africa (McKay and Waters 1994; Elem and Ranjan 1995; Merino et al. 2001; Heyns and Fisher 2005).

6.2 Etiology

An etiological factor or factors can be identified in more than 90 % of cases and should be actively sought, because it may determine the treatment and prognosis (Smith et al. 1998; Santora and Rukstalis 2001). In apparently idiopathic cases, the cause may have been overlooked or obscured by the necrotizing disease process.

Any process where a virulent, synergistic infection gains access to the subcutaneous tissue of the perineum may serve as the point of origin. The cause of infection may be from a urogenital, anorectal, cutaneous, or retroperitoneal origin. The urogenital area is the most common etiologic site, where urethral stricture disease is at the top of the list (Edino et al. 2005). Knowledge of the anatomy of the perineum, urogenital area, and lower abdomen is necessary to understand the etiology and pathogenesis of this fulminant infection.

The possible causes of Fournier's gangrene are listed in Table 6.1. Infection may originate in any of the listed areas, with extension to the fascial planes leading to a proliferating fasciitis (Jones et al. 1979; Karim 1984; Walker et al. 1984; Walther et al. 1987; Baskin et al. 1990; Sengoku et al. 1990; Gaeta et al. 1991; Attah 1992; Paty and Smith 1992; Theiss et al. 1995; Benizri et al. 1996; Hejase et al. 1996; Fialkov et al. 1998; Corman et al. 1999; Eke 2000; Kilic et al. 2001; Ali 2004; Jeong 2004; Yeniyol et al. 2004; Edino et al. 2005).

Although Fournier's gangrene is predominantly a condition of the older male, it may occur at any age, and approximately 10 % of cases occur in females (Kilic et al. 2001; Quatan and Kirby 2004). Specific causes in women include pudendal nerve block or episiotomy for

Table 6.1. Causes of Fournier's gangrene

Urogenital
Urethral stricture
Indwelling transurethral catheter
Prolonged or neglected use of condom catheter
Urethral calculi
Urethritis
Transurethral surgery
Infection of periurethral glands and paraurethral abscess
Urogenital tuberculosis
Urethral cancer
Prostate biopsy
Prostatic massage
Prostate abscess
Insertion of penile prosthesis
Constriction ring device for management of ED
Iatrogenic trauma
Cauterization of genital warts
Circumcision
Manipulation of longstanding paraphimosis
Noniatrogenic trauma
Animal, insect, or human bite
Scrotal abscess
Infected hydrocele
Hydrocelectomy
Vasectomy
Balanitis
Phimosis
Anorectal
Ischiorectal or perianal or intersphincteric abscess
Rectal mucosal biopsy
Banding of hemorrhoids
Anal dilatation
Cancer of sigmoid or rectum
Diverticulitis
Rectal perforation by foreign body
Ischemic colitis
Anal stenosis
Cutaneous
Hidradenitis suppurativa
Folliculitis
Scrotal pressure sore
Post-scrotal surgery wound infection
Cellulitis of scrotum
Pyoderma gangrenosum
Femoral access for intravenous drug users
Retroperitoneal causes
Psoas abscess
Perinephric abscess
Appendicitis and appendix abscess
Pancreatitis with retroperitoneal fat necrosis
Other
Inguinal hernia repair
Filariasis in endemic areas
Strangulated Richter hernia

vaginal delivery, septic abortion, hysterectomy, and Bartholin and vulval abscess (Roberts and Hester 1972; Addison et al. 1984).

A prominent feature of patients with Fournier's gangrene is that most of them have an underlying systemic disorder causing vascular disease or suppressed immunity, which increases their susceptibility to polymicrobial infection (Table 6.2). Fournier's gangrene is often a marker of an underlying disease such as diabetes mellitus, urogenital tuberculosis, syphilis, or HIV.

Table 6.2. Underlying disorders in patients with Fournier's gangrene

Diabetes mellitus
Chronic alcoholism
Malnutrition
Obesity
Liver cirrhosis
Poor personal hygiene
Immunosuppression:
Chronic steroid use
Organ transplantation
Chemotherapy for malignancy
HIV/AIDS
Tuberculosis
Syphilis

Diabetes mellitus is the most common associated underlying systemic disease, affecting two-thirds of patients with Fournier's gangrene. Diabetic patients have a higher incidence of urinary tract infections, due to cystopathy with urinary stasis (Baskin et al. 1990). Hyperglycemia decreases cellular immunity by decreasing phagocytic function. It retards chemotaxis of leukocytes to the site of inflammation, neutrophil adhesion, and intracellular oxidative destruction of pathogens. Wound healing is also retarded due to defective epithelialization and collagen deposition (Hejase et al. 1996; Nisbet and Thompson 2002). Apart from hyperglycemia, diabetic patients also have microvascular disease, which contributes significantly to the pathogenesis. Although diabetes mellitus increases the risk for development of Fournier's gangrene, it does not increase the mortality (Baskin et al. 1990; Benizri et al. 1996; Hejase et al. 1996; Yeniyol et al. 2004).

Chronic alcoholism, malnutrition, liver cirrhosis, poor personal hygiene, and personal neglect are quite common in patients with Fournier's gangrene (Benizri et al. 1996; Hejase et al. 1996; Yeniyol et al. 2004). Other conditions causing depressed immunity that may predispose to the development of Fournier's gangrene include chronic steroid use, organ transplantation, chemotherapy for malignancies such as leukemia, as well as HIV infection (Paty and Smith 1992; Elem and Ranjan 1995; Heyns and Fisher 2005).

The rising incidence of HIV is paralleled by a rising incidence of Fournier's gangrene, especially in Africa. Fournier's gangrene may be the first presenting condition in patients with HIV infection (McKay and Waters 1994; Elem and Ranjan 1995; Roca et al. 1998; Heyns and Fisher 2005). Risk factors include a CD4 count under 400, chemotherapy for Kaposi's sarcoma, and femoral access for the administration of intravenous drugs. HIV-positive patients with Fournier's gangrene present at a younger age and have a wider spectrum of causative bacteria (McKay and Waters 1994).

6.3 Anatomy

The pelvic outlet can be divided into anterior and posterior triangles by drawing a line between the ischial tuberosities with the symphysis pubis and coccyx being the apices (Fig. 6.1). Urogenital causes of Fournier's gangrene lead to initial involvement of the anterior triangle, whereas anorectal causes primarily involve the posterior triangle.

The five fascial planes that can be affected are: Colles' fascia, dartos fascia, Buck's fascia, Scarpa's fascia, and Camper's fascia.

Colles' fascia is the fascia of the anterior triangle of the perineum. Laterally it is attached to the pubic rami and fascia lata, posteriorly it fuses with the perineal membrane and perineal body, and anterosuperiorly it is continuous with Scarpa's fascia (Smith et al. 1998). It prevents the spread of infection in a posterior or lateral direction, but provides no resistance to spread in an anterosuperior direction towards the abdominal wall.

The dartos fascia is the continuation of Colles' fascia over the scrotum and penis.

Buck's fascia lies deep to the dartos fascia, covering the penile corpora. It fuses distally with the corona of the glans and proximally with the suspensory ligament and crura of the penis.

Camper's fascia is the loose areolar fascial layer deep to the skin of the abdominal wall, but superficial to Scarpa's fascia. Together with Scarpa's fascia it is continuous with Colles' fascia inferomedially.

Scarpa's fascia lies deep to Camper's fascia, covering the muscles of the anterior abdominal wall and thorax. It terminates at the level of the clavicles.

The perineal membrane lies deep to Colles' fascia. It is triangular in shape and lies between the pubic rami from the symphysis pubis to the ischial tuberosities. It has a distinct posterior border, with the central perineal tendon in the midline. Colles' fascia terminates in this posterior border.

The central perineal tendon (or perineal body) lies between the anus and bulbar urethra. It serves as an attachment for the various perineal muscles and helps to maintain the integrity of the pelvic floor.

Via the internal and external fascial layers of the spermatic cord, the perineal fascia is continuous with the retroperitoneal fascia. This is a potential path for the spread of infection from the perineum to the perivesical and retroperitoneal areas, and vice versa (Paty and Smith 1992; Fialkov et al. 1998).

Spread of infection along the fascial planes will follow the path of least resistance (Jones et al. 1979). Infection in the anterior perineal triangle will spread preferentially in an anterosuperior direction along Scarpa's

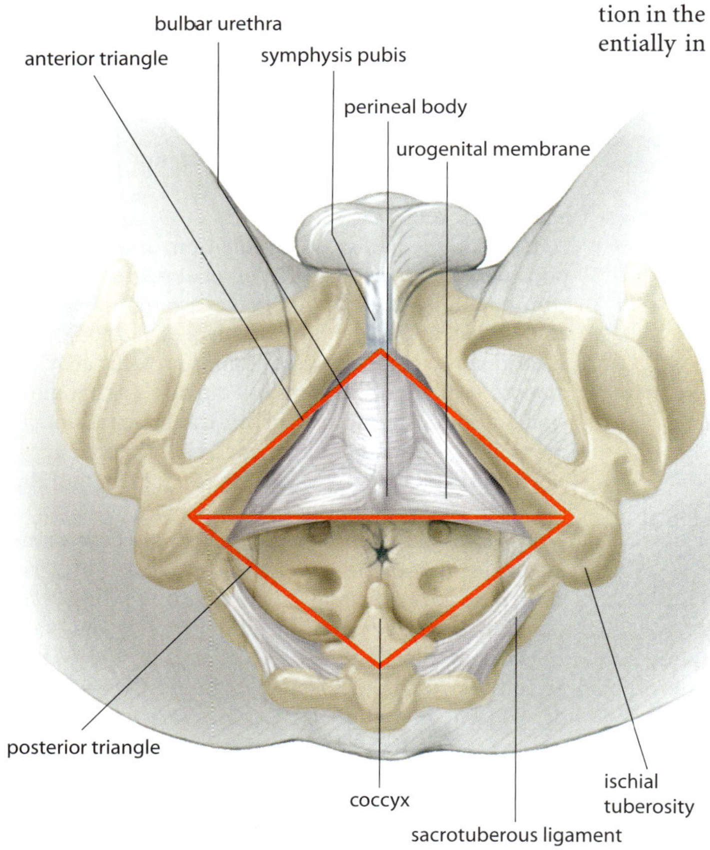

Fig. 6.1. The pelvic outlet can be divided into anterior and posterior triangles by drawing a line between the ischial tuberosities with the symphysis pubis and coccyx being the apices (© Hohenfellner 2007)

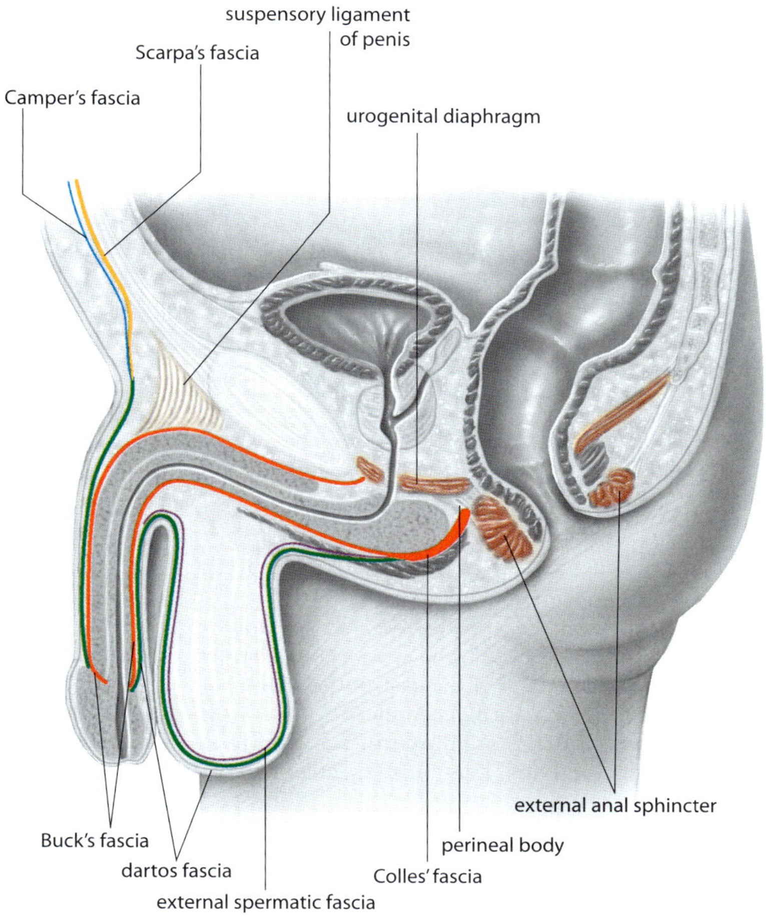

Fig. 6.2. Diagram of a sagittal section showing the fascial planes of the male external genitalia, perineum, and lower abdomen (© Hohenfellner 2007)

fascia, whereas lateral spread will be limited by fusion of Colles' fascia to the ischiopubic rami, and posterior spread to the anal region will be limited by the termination of Colles' fascia in the posterior edge of the perineal membrane (Fig. 6.2).

Infection from the perianal region may sometimes penetrate Colles' fascia, which is fenestrated at the level of the bulbocavernosus muscle, leading to spread of infection to the anterior triangle (Tobin and Benjamin 1949). Thus, while anterior triangle infection rarely spreads to the posterior triangle, it is possible for infection to spread from the posterior to the anterior triangle and then to the anterior abdominal wall (Jones et al. 1979; Walker et al. 1984; Laucks 1994).

In the perineum, the vascular supply to the cutaneous and subcutaneous tissues is mainly derived from the perineal branches of the internal pudendal artery. The deep circumflex iliac artery and superficial inferior epigastric artery supply blood to the lower abdominal wall. These arteries traverse the various fascial planes, supplying nutrients and oxygen to the skin and subcutaneous tissues. With the fascial planes infected, these vessels become thrombosed, facilitating the proliferation of anaerobic bacteria.

Blood supply to the testis, bladder, and rectum originates directly from the aorta and not from the perineal vasculature, and for this reason they are rarely affected in Fournier's gangrene. If the testes are affected, it may be from specific testicular pathology such as epididymo-orchitis, or from a retroperitoneal infection spreading along the spermatic fascia, causing thrombosis of the testicular arteries.

6.4 Microbiology

One of the characteristics of Fournier's gangrene is that it is a polymicrobial infection, with a mean of four different organisms usually cultured (Bahlmann et al. 1983; Baskin et al. 1990).

Aerobic, anaerobic, Gram-positive and Gram-negative bacteria, yeasts, and even mycobacteria can be found (Table 6.3). The most commonly cultured organ-

Table 6.3. Most common causative organisms

Gram-negative
E. coli
Klebsiella pneumoniae
Pseudomonas aeruginosa
Proteus mirabilis
Enterobacteria
Gram-positive
Staphylococcus aureus
Beta-hemolytic streptococci
Streptococcus faecalis
Staphylococcus epidermidis
Anaerobes
Bacteroides fragilis
Peptococcus
Fusobacterium
Clostridium perfringens
Mycobacteria
Mycobacterium tuberculosis
Yeasts
Candida albicans

isms are *Escherichia coli*, *Bacteroides*, beta-hemolytic streptococci, *Staphylococcus* spp., and *Proteus*. Besides being found in the lumen of the gastrointestinal tract, these bacteria are also normal commensal flora of the skin folds and hair follicles of the perineum (Benizri et al. 1996; Smith et al. 1998). This mixed spectrum of bacteria acts in a synergistic fashion to produce and promote a fulminant necrotizing fasciitis.

Anaerobic organisms are responsible for the formation of subcutaneous gas, which leads to the characteristic crepitus often found on palpation. Clostridial infection, classically associated with gas formation, is not commonly encountered, but should be suspected when there is a colorectal origin (Spirnak et al. 1984; Baskin et al. 1990).

It is extremely important to obtain cultures in order to identify the causative organism(s), because this determines the correct choice of antibiotic treatment. Because of the difficulty of culturing anaerobic organisms, a subcutaneous aspirate should be obtained, and at initial debridement a piece of infected tissue should also be sent for anaerobic culture. Microbiological studies should include acid fast staining for *Mycobacterium tuberculosis* and culture for fungal infection.

6.5 Pathogenesis

The pathogenesis of Fournier's gangrene is characterized by polymicrobial aerobic and anaerobic infection with subsequent vascular thrombosis and tissue necrosis, aggravated by poor host defense due to one or more underlying systemic disorders.

Aerobic organisms cause intravascular coagulation by inducing platelet aggregation and complement fixation, while anaerobes produce heparinase. Vascular thrombosis causes necrosis of tissue and decreased clearance of toxic bacterial metabolites, with subsequent proliferation of anaerobic bacteria (Paty and Smith 1992; Hejase et al. 1996).

Hypoxic tissue leads to the formation of oxygen free radicals (superoxide anions, hydrogen peroxide, hydroxyl radicals), which play an important role in the pathogenesis. The effects of free radicals include cell membrane disruption leading to cell death, decreased ATP production leading to decreased energy delivery, and DNA damage, which leads to decreased protein production (Anderson and Vaslef 1997).

Anaerobic organisms secrete various enzymes and toxins. Lecithinase, collagenase, and hyaluronidase cause digestion of the fascial planes (Baskin et al. 1990). They produce insoluble hydrogen and nitrogen, leading to the formation of gas in the subcutaneous tissues, clinically palpable as crepitus. Aerobic bacteria produce CO_2, which is soluble and rarely leads to subcutaneous gas accumulation.

Endotoxins are released from the cell walls of Gram-negative bacteria. Macrophage activation and subsequent complement activation ensues with release of pro-inflammatory cytokines and eventual development of septic shock (Anderson and Vaslef 1997).

Depending on the origin of the infection, the various paths of spread can be explained with reference to the anatomy of the fascial planes and adhesions.

Infection from a urogenital cause, e.g., a patient with a urethral stricture and urinary tract infection leading to a paraurethral abscess, will spread from the corpus spongiosum by penetrating the tunica albuginea and Buck's fascia, and will then spread under the dartos fascia and Colles' fascia to Scarpa's fascia, thereby involving the anterior abdominal wall.

Infection from an anorectal cause, e.g., an ischiorectal abscess, will spread from the perirectal tissues to Colles' fascia. Because Colles' fascia is fenestrated, it allows spread from the perirectal area to the dartos fascia of the scrotum and penis, and from there the infection can spread to Scarpa's fascia and the anterior abdominal wall. Because Colles' fascia terminates in the perineal membrane, infection from the anterior triangle of the perineum, which contains the bulbar urethra and scrotum, cannot spread to the perirectal area, but because Colles' fascia is fenestrated, the opposite is possible, i.e., posterior triangle infections may sometimes spread to the anterior triangle and from there to the anterior abdominal wall. This is important in trying to localize the origin of the initial infection.

Retroperitoneal infection, e.g., from a perinephric or psoas abscess, may spread along the inguinal canal and spermatic fascia, which connects to Colles' fascia deep to the bulbocavernosus muscle. Retroperitoneal infection should be considered as a cause of Fournier's gangrene if no obvious point of origin can be found.

6.6 Clinical Presentation

The diagnosis of Fournier's gangrene is made on clinical grounds. It is usually preceded by prodromal symptoms such as fever, prostration, nausea and vomiting, perineal discomfort, and poor glucose control in diabetics, for a period ranging from 2 to 9 days (Bahlmann et al. 1983; Paty and Smith 1992; Benizri et al. 1996; Edino et al. 2005).

Genital and perineal discomfort worsens, leading to pain, itching, burning sensation, erythema, swelling, and eventual skin necrosis. There may be a purulent discharge with a feculent odor. The pain may subside as neural damage develops (Corman et al. 1999). Crepitus may be difficult to elicit, due to pain on palpation, but is present in up to 50%–60% of cases (Corman et al. 1999; Benizri et al. 1996).

Clinical signs such as an elevated temperature, tachycardia, tachypnea, ileus, poor glucose control, and vascular collapse may be found, but are not very consistent, especially with underlying immunosuppressive disorders.

The diagnosis is sometimes delayed due to morbid obesity, poor communication (stroke, dementia), or inadequate physical examination. In Africa, patients may first seek help from a traditional healer, thereby delaying proper medical attention (Attah 1992).

Once there is necrosis of the skin, the underlying fascia has already undergone extensive necrosis. This explains the frequent finding of systemic symptoms, which are out of proportion to the visible pathology.

Other symptoms and signs depend on the origin of the infection. A history of lower urinary tract symptoms may indicate a urethral stricture. Preceding anorectal symptoms such as pain, fissures, or hemorrhoids may indicate an anorectal origin of Fournier's gangrene.

It is essential that the attending doctor have a high index of suspicion in patients presenting with perineal discomfort accompanied by systemic symptoms. A missed or delayed diagnosis may have catastrophic effects.

6.7 Special Investigations

Special investigations to be done include a full blood count, clotting profile, urea, creatinine and electrolytes, liver function tests, blood glucose, blood gases, group and screen, HIV and VDRL.

Abnormal findings include anemia, thrombocytopenia, coagulopathy, hyponatremia, and raised urea and creatinine. Hypocalcemia may occur in some cases, subsequent to the chelation of ionized calcium by triglycerides liberated by bacterial lipases.

Leukocytosis with a white cell count above 15,000 mm^3 and a left shift is found in more than 90% of cases. Neutrophilia indicates overwhelming bacterial infection. It is noteworthy that leukocytosis may not be present in immunosuppressed patients (Baskin et al. 1990; Laucks 1994). Anemia may be present as part of the septic profile. Coagulopathy may be indicated by a raised prothrombin time (PT) and partial thromboplastin time (PTT), and thrombocytopenia. Raised fibrinogen levels and positive D-dimers may herald the onset of disseminated intravascular coagulation (DIC).

Blood and urine cultures, together with wound swabs and tissue specimens for bacterial culture are very important. The HIV status should be determined in all patients, as Fournier's gangrene may be the presenting condition in patients with HIV.

Radiologic imaging may be useful if the diagnosis is in doubt, but it should not delay the surgical management. An x-ray of the abdomen and pelvis may demonstrate gas in the subcutaneous fascial layers of the perineum and abdominal wall.

Ultrasound provides superior imaging of the perineum and scrotum. The appearance of hyperacoustic shadows in the fascial planes is diagnostic of gas formation, and it may be more sensitive than clinical evaluation for crepitus (Kane et al. 1996). However, in patients with extreme tenderness on palpation, ultrasound examination may be too painful.

Computerized tomography (CT) is more sensitive in demonstrating subcutaneous and retroperitoneal gas and fluid collections, but the use of contrast should be avoided in patients with renal failure. Magnetic resonance (MR) is the most sensitive imaging modality for evaluating pathology in soft tissues, but is expensive and not readily available.

6.8 Management

The main goals in the management of Fournier's gangrene are aggressive resuscitation of the patient, administration of broad-spectrum antibiotics, and debridement of infected and necrotic tissue. Debridement is paramount, and the aim should be to get the patient to the operating room as soon as possible (Baskin et al. 1990; Smith et al. 1998; Quantan and Kirby 2004).

6.8.1 Initial and Preoperative Management

If there is doubt about the diagnosis of Fournier's gangrene, imaging and laboratory studies may be requested, but this should not delay definitive surgical management.

The cause of the infection should be established, bearing in mind that urogenital causes (urethral stricture) and anorectal infections are the most common etiological factors. Passing an F16 transurethral catheter should exclude or confirm a urethral stricture, and painful digital rectal examination may indicate an ischiorectal abscess. If rectal examination is too painful, it can be performed in the operating room with the patient under anesthesia, just before debridement.

Aggressive fluid resuscitation with crystalloid or colloid fluids is essential to optimize the hemodynamic status in these volume-depleted, septic patients.

Anemia should be corrected to a hemoglobin greater than 10 g/dl. Coagulopathy (raised international normalized ratio [INR], PT and PTT, or platelets <100,000) should be diagnosed preoperatively and platelets should be given intraoperatively if the patient is severely thrombocytopenic. Diabetic patients usually have severe hyperglycemia, which should be corrected with a glucose-insulin sliding scale. Electrolyte abnormalities must be corrected as far as possible, without incurring unnecessary delay of surgical debridement.

Antibiotic therapy must be initiated promptly, after appropriate specimens have been obtained for bacteriological culture. High-dose, broad-spectrum parenteral antibiotics covering Gram-positive and Gram-negative aerobe as well as anaerobe organisms should be used (Baskin et al. 1990; Paty and Smith 1992; Hejase et al. 1996; Smith et al. 1998). Aminoglycosides and third- or fourth-generation cephalosporins are effective against Gram-negative bacteria, metronidazole against anaerobic infection, and penicillins against Gram-positive bacteria. Usually combined use of three antibiotics, one from each of these groups, is clinically effective. However, to ensure adequate cover against enterococci, some groups advocate the combined use of the ureidopenicillin piperacillin with the beta-lactamase inhibitor tazobactam. It is important to note that antibiotics will not penetrate ischemic and necrotic tissues, and therefore serve only as an adjunct to definitive surgical management (Baskin et al. 1990). Tetanus toxoid should also be given to all patients (Laucks 1994).

The onset of septic shock is heralded by signs such as altered sensorium, hypotension, hypoperfusion, oliguria, and lactic acidosis. Multiorgan failure should be anticipated and prevented by aggressive fluid management and invasive vascular monitoring. A mean arterial pressure over 65 mmHg and a central venous pressure (CVP) of 8–12 cm H_2O should be maintained. The mainstay of management is to optimize oxygen delivery by striving to:

- Keep oxygen saturation above 90% using an oxygen mask, continuous positive airway pressure (CPAP) or mechanical ventilation
- Optimize cardiac output by improving the heart rate and stroke volume, using sympathomimetics and volume expansion
- Optimize oxygen transport by using packed red cells to maintain a hemoglobin above 10 g/dl

6.8.2 Surgery

Early and aggressive surgical debridement is essential, because it significantly decreases morbidity and mortality (Bahlmann et al. 1983). The procedure should be done under general anesthesia, as the true extent of the infection is usually unknown preoperatively. The patient should be placed in a dorsal lithotomy position (Paty and Smith 1992; Smith et al. 1998). The aim of debridement is to remove the origin of the infection as well as the infected tissues (Quantan and Kirby 2004). The surgeon as well as the patient should be prepared for radical debridement.

A midline perineal and scrotal incision usually gives the best initial exposure (Jones et al. 1979). Debridement is extended radially from the skin incision, keeping the anatomy of the fascial planes in mind. Only skin that is clearly necrotic should be excised. Viable skin should be mobilized so that all the underlying necrotic subcutaneous tissue and fascia can be excised.

A good indication of the extent of the infection is where the affected fascia fails to separate from the deep fascia and muscle on blunt dissection (Jones et al. 1979; Smith et al. 1998; Santora and Rukstalis 2001). The wound edges should bleed like normal tissue, indicating patent nutrient vessels.

If no purulent discharge can be milked from the urethra, and an F16 catheter can be passed into the bladder, it is reasonable to assume that the urethra is not the origin of the infection. However, if it is not possible to pass a transurethral catheter easily, a suprapubic catheter should be inserted (Benizri et al. 1996). Catheterization of the bladder is essential for monitoring fluid management and for adequate wound care (Laucks 1994).

Colostomy is indicated if the anal sphincter is involved, if rectal or colon perforation is present, in immunocompromised patients with fecal incontinence, and if there is extensive involvement of the posterior perineal triangle (Fig. 6.3). Colostomy allows for better wound care (Paty and Smith 1992; Laucks 1994, Benizri et al. 1996). Some authors feel that doing a diverting co-

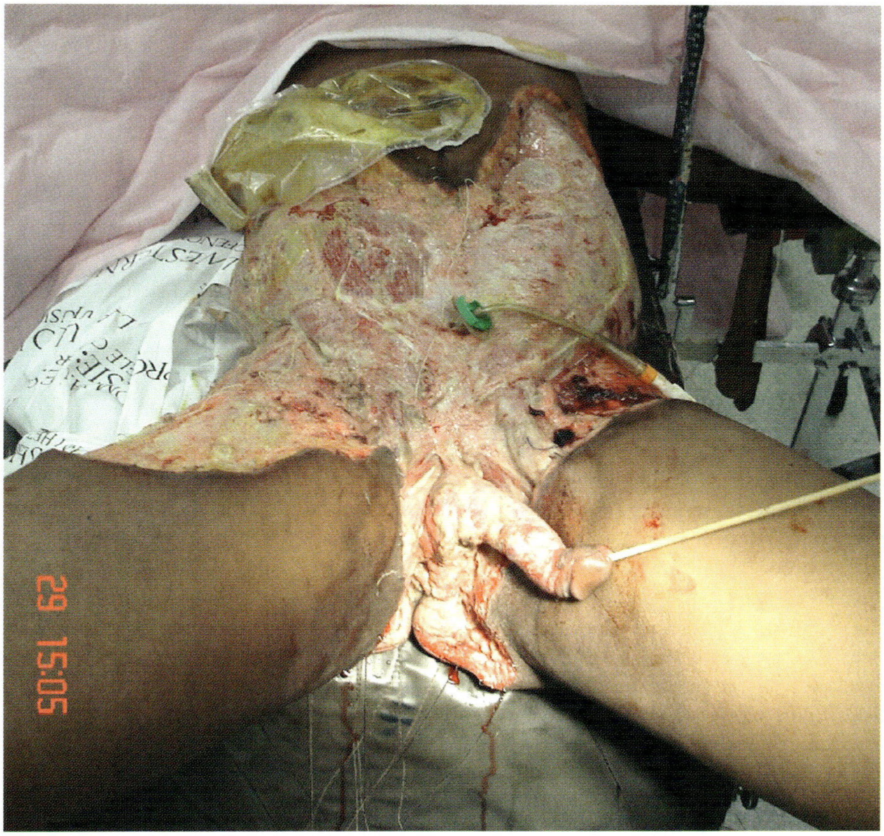

Fig. 6.3. Extensive debridement for necrotizing fasciitis arising from ischio-rectal area (note transurethral as well as suprapubic catheters, and stoma bag for transverse colostomy)

lostomy can be delayed until the second-look debridement when the patient is better resuscitated and more stable, because most acutely ill patients have an ileus for at least 48 h after admission (Bronder et al. 2004).

The testes, because of their nonperineal blood supply, are rarely affected, and orchidectomy is required in only 10%–20% of cases, if there is extensive involvement or a testicular cause for the infection (Baskin et al. 1990; Okeke 2000).

During scrotectomy, all necrotic tissues except the testes and spermatic cords should be debrided. The testis can be buried in a lateral thigh pouch or in a subcutaneous abdominal pouch, depending on the extent of the debridement. This should not be done during the initial debridement, but during one of the subsequent procedures, because this decreases the risk of a thigh abscess and extension of the infection. If the testes are buried in thigh pouches, they should be placed at different levels, eliminating the risk of the testes rubbing against each other with the patient walking (Laucks 1994). Removal of the testes from the pouches and scrotal reconstruction can be considered later.

6.8.3 Postoperative Management

The wound should be inspected daily, and the surgeon should have a low threshold for redebridement. A mean of 2.5 debridements per patient is reported in the literature (Baskin et al. 1990; Corman et al. 1999). Bacterial culture results should be checked to make sure that appropriate antibiotic therapy is given. If the patient is in renal failure, aminoglycosides should be avoided and a third- or fourth-generation cephalosporin should be given.

Nosocomial infections should be prevented as far as possible. Pulmonary complications (e.g., atelectasis) should be prevented. If postoperative fever persists or the patient does not improve clinically, a persistent source of infection should be suspected. CT or MR imaging may demonstrate an intraabdominal or retroperitoneal infective cause. However, even if these studies are negative, there should be a low threshold for reexploration and redebridement of the patient under anesthesia.

Maintaining a blood glucose level of 4–6 mmol/l (74–110 mg/dl) optimizes cellular immunity and reduces morbidity and mortality in the septic patient, regardless of whether there was preexisting diabetes or not (Van den Berghe et al. 2001; Fourie 2003).

In the acutely ill patient, the development of ileus, stress ulcers, and translocation of gut flora are common complications. Stress ulcers can be prevented by giving sucralfate (1 g every 6–8 h). Gut integrity can be maintained by starting early with gastrointestinal feeding and by using enteral rather than parenteral nutrition (Anderson and Vaslef 1997). The caloric needs of 25–35 kcal/kg per day and protein of 1.5–2 g/kg per day should be met, especially in patients with large wounds, malnutrition, and those on ventilation (Baskin et al. 1990; Anderson and Vaslef 1997).

6.8.4 Hyperbaric Oxygen

Hyperbaric oxygen (HBO) has been used as an adjunct in the treatment of Fournier's gangrene. The usual protocol is multiple sessions at 2.5 atm for 90 min with 100 % oxygen inhalation every 20 min (Pizzorno et al. 1997).

HBO increases oxygen tension levels in the tissues and has various beneficial effects on wound healing. Oxygen free radicals are liberated from hypoxic tissues, which are directly toxic to anaerobic bacteria. Fibroblast activity increases, with subsequent angiogenesis leading to accelerated wound healing.

However, HBO is expensive and logistically cumbersome. It is contraindicated where closed air spaces in the body can cause damage due to expansion upon returning to normal atmospheric pressure, such as sinusitis, otitis media, asthma, and bullous pulmonary disease. Care should be taken with diabetic patients, as hypoglycemia may be exacerbated by HBO.

Some authors question the efficacy of empirical HBO, suggesting that patients should be selected only if there is large body surface area involvement or poorly responding anaerobic infection. It is important to note that HBO is only an adjunct and should not delay prompt antibiotic therapy and surgical debridement (Paty and Smith 1992; Laucks 1994; Benizri et al. 1996; Pizzorno et al. 1997; Mindrup et al. 2005).

6.8.5 Wound Care

Care of the debrided wounds should allow for additional chemical debridement, prevent reinfection and promote natural healing and granulation.

Hydrogen peroxide, Eusol, povidone iodine, and sodium hypochlorite (Dakin solution) are the agents most often used (Jones et al. 1979; Paty and Smith 1992; Hejase et al. 1996; Edino et al. 2005). Eusol (Edinburgh University solution) is a chlorinated disinfectant included in the World Health Organization's "essential therapeutic group" of agents. It consists of calcium hypochlorite 1.25 g and boric acid 1.25 g in 100 ml sterile water. Even if not commercially available, it can be easily prepared by the hospital dispensary, and is an inexpensive and effective agent for use in developing countries. Simple irrigation with sterile saline solution to keep dressings moist can be very effective in cleansing large open wounds. Honey has also been used, because its high osmolarity and low pH make it a good desloughing agent, while it increases local oxygen concentration and helps with wound epithelialization (Hejase et al. 1996). Pseudomonas wound infection, characterized by its distinctive odor and green residue on the dressings, can be effectively treated with 5 % acetic acid dressings.

Once the patient is stable and in an anabolic state with granulating wounds, reconstruction of the denuded areas can be done (Fig. 6.4). Skin grafting should on-

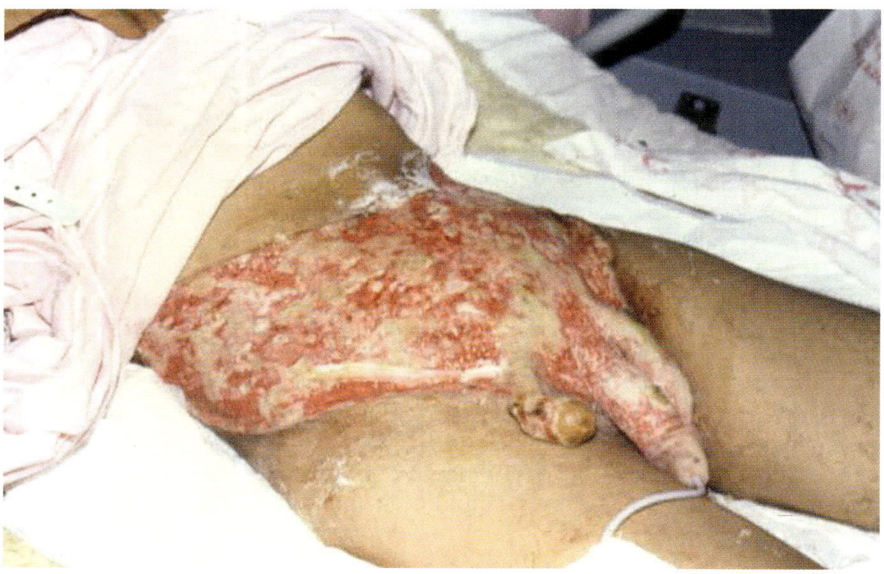

Fig. 6.4. Well granulated areas ready for skin transplantation

ly be performed if the wounds are clean and healthy, with a negative bacterial swab culture.

6.8.6 Reconstructive Surgery

Depending on the extent of skin defects, the options in reconstruction are suturing, split thickness skin grafting, or myocutaneous vascularized pedicle flaps.

Small defects can be closed by primary suturing, especially where only the pliable scrotal skin is involved. Split thickness skin grafting is most often used and yields acceptable results, even in large defects (Hesselfeldt-Nielsen et al. 1986). Healthy skin from the legs, buttocks, and arms can be used, in a single or multiple settings. Skin defects on the penile shaft should be liberally grafted so as to prevent fibrotic scar formation with future erectile problems.

In extensive defects, especially where tendons are exposed, myocutaneous vascularized flaps should be used. Medial thigh flaps, e.g., the gracilis myocutaneous pedicle flap, give the best results, because of their close proximity to the perineum, good mobility, and hidden donor site scars (Banks et al. 1986; Paty and Smith 1992; Kayikcioglu 2003). Other flaps using the inferior epigastric arteries can also be considered.

In men with underlying urethral stricture disease, urethroplasty may be extremely difficult or impossible due to extensive loss of penoscrotal skin and even of the urethra itself. Buccal mucosa may be used to reconstruct the urethra, but in some cases with extensive tissue loss, a permanent perineal urethrostomy may be the best solution.

6.9 Complications

Nonresolving sepsis may be due to incomplete debridement, a persisting occult source of infection, or a poor patient immune response. Multiple organ failure is a feared consequence of unresolved sepsis and most commonly involves the cardiovascular, pulmonary, and renal systems. Coagulopathy, acalculous cholecystitis, and cerebrovascular accidents have also been reported (Baskin et al. 1990). Myositis and myonecrosis of the upper thigh may occur as a result of sepsis from subcutaneous testicular pouches made during the first rather than secondary debridement (Choe et al. 2001).

Late complications include the following:

- Chordee, painful erections, and erectile dysfunction
- Infertility as a result of burying the testes in thigh pouches (high temperature)
- Squamous cell carcinoma in the scar tissue (Chintamani et al. 2004)
- Contractures due to prolonged immobilization
- Depression secondary to dysmorphic body changes
- Loss of income and disruption of family life due to prolonged hospitalization
- Lymphodema of the legs secondary to pelvic debridement and subsequent thrombophlebitis.

6.10 Prognosis

The reported mortality of Fournier's gangrene ranges from 0% to 70%, with an average of 20%–30%. The factors associated with an adverse outcome are physical disability, extent of the infection, delayed treatment, poor immune status, diabetes mellitus, old age, and multiorgan failure (Akgun and Yilmaz 2005). Laboratory values associated with an increased mortality are leukocytosis, elevated urea, creatinine, alkaline phosphatase (ALP) and lactate dehydrogenase (LD), and a decrease in the hemoglobin, albumin, bicarbonate, sodium, and potassium (Laor et al. 1995).

References

Addison WA, Livengood CH 3rd, Hill GB, Sutton GP, Fortier KJ (1984) Necrotizing fasciitis of vulval origin in diabetic patients. Obstet Gynecol 63:473

Akgun Y, Yilmaz G (2005) Factors affecting mortality in Fournier's gangrene (in Turkish). Ulus Travma Derg 11:49

Ali MZ (2004) Fournier's gangrene – a rare complication of hydrocele aspiration. J Coll Physicians Surg Pak 14:304

Anderson RW, Vaslef SN (1997) Shock. Causes and management of circulatory collapse. In: Sabiston DC, Lyerly HK (eds) Sabiston textbook of surgery – the biological basis of modern surgical practice, 15th edn. WB Saunders Company, Philadelphia, p 68

Attah CA (1992) New approach to the management of Fournier's gangrene. Br J Urol 70:78

Bahlmann JC, Fourie IJ, Arndt TC (1983) Fournier's gangrene: necrotising fasciitis of the male genitalia. Br J Urol 55:85

Banks DW, O'Brien DP 3rd, Amerson JR, Hester TR Jr (1986) Gracilis musculocutaneous flap reconstruction after Fournier gangrene. Urology 28:275

Baskin LS, Carroll PR, Cattolica EV, McAninch JW (1990) Necrotising soft tissue infections of the perineum and genitalia. Br J Urol 65:524

Bejanga BL (1979) Fournier's gangrene. Br J Urol 51:312

Benizri E, Fabiani P, Migliori G, Chevallier D, Peyrottes A, Raucoules M, Amiel J, Mouiel J, Toubol J (1996) Gangrene of the perineum. Urology 47:935

Bronder CS, Cowey A, Hill J (2004) Delayed stoma formation in Fournier's gangrene. Colorectal Dis 6:518

Chintamani, Shankar M, Singhal V, Singh JP, Bansal A, Saxena S (2004) Squamous cell carcinoma developing in the scar of Fournier's gangrene – case report. BMC Cancer 4:16

Choe JM, Battino BS, Benedict J, Bell TE (2001) Myositis and myonecrosis of the thigh: an unusual complication of a testicular thigh pouch. J Urol 165:1217

Corman JM, Moody JA, Aronson WJ (1999) Fournier's gangrene in a modern surgical setting: improved survival with aggressive management. Br J Urol 84:85
Edino ST, Yakubu AA, Obidiaso A (2005) Fournier's gangrene in a tertiary health facility in Nigeria. Afr J Urol 11:1
Eke N (2000) Fournier's gangrene: a review of 1726 cases. Br J Surg 87:718
Elem B, Ranjan P (1995) Impact of immunodeficiency virus (HIV) on Fournier's gangrene: observations in Zambia. Ann R Coll Surg Engl 77:283
Fialkov JM, Watkins K, Fallon B Kealey GP (1998) Fournier's gangrene with an unusual urologic etiology. Urology 52:324
Fourie CE (2003) The role of glycaemic control in preventing complications in the critically ill. South Afr J Crit Care 19:46
Gaeta M, Volta S, Minutoli A, Bartiromo A, Pandolfo I (1991) Fournier's gangrene caused by perforated retroperitoneal appendix. AJR Am J Roentgenol 156:341
Hejase MJ, Simonin JE, Bihrle R, Coogan CL (1996) Genital Fournier's gangrene: experience with 38 patients. Urology 47:734
Hesselfeldt-Nielsen J, Bang-Jensen E, Riegels-Nielsen P (1986) Scrotal reconstruction after Fournier's gangrene. Ann Plast Surg 17:310
Heyns CF, Fisher M (2005) The urological management of the patient with acquired immunodeficiency syndrome. BJU Int 95:709
Jeong HJ (2004) Fournier's gangrene associated with sparganosis in the scrotum. Urology 63:176
Jones RB, Hirschmann JV, Brown GS, Tremann JA (1979) Fournier's syndrome: Necrotising subcutaneous infection of the male genitalia. J Urol 122:279
Kane CJ, Nash P, McAninch JW (1996) Ultrasonographic appearance of necrotizing gangrene: aid in early diagnosis. Urology 48:142
Karim MS (1984) Fournier gangrene following urethral necrosis by indwelling catheter. Urology 23:173
Kayikcioglu A (2003) A new technique in scrotal reconstruction: short gracilis flap. Urology 61:1254
Kilic A, Aksoy Y, Kilic L (2001) Fournier's gangrene: etiology, treatment, and complications. Ann Plast Surg 47:523
Laor E, Palmer LS, Tolia BM, Reid RE, Winter HI (1995) Outcome prediction in patients with Fournier's gangrene. J Urol 154:89
Laucks SS 2nd (1994) Fournier's gangrene. Surg Clin North Am 74:1339
McKay TC, Waters WB (1994) Fournier's gangrene as the presenting sign of an undiagnosed human immunodeficiency virus infection. J Urol 152:1552
Merino E, Boix V, Portilla J, Reus S, Priego M (2001) Fournier's gangrene in HIV-infected patients. Eur J Clin Microbiol Infect Dis 20:910
Mindrup SR, Kealey GP, Fallon B (2005) Hyperbaric oxygen for the treatment of Fournier's gangrene. J Urol 173:1975
Nisbet AA, Thompson IM (2002) Impact of diabetes mellitus on the presentation and outcomes of Fournier's gangrene. Urology 60:775
Okeke LI (2000) Fournier's gangrene in Ibadan. Afr J Med Sci 29:323
Paty R, Smith AD (1992) Gangrene and Fournier's gangrene. Urol Clin North Am 19:149
Pizzorno R, Bonini F, Donelli A, Stubinski R, Medica M, Carmignani G (1997) Hyperbaric oxygen therapy in the treatment of Fournier's disease in 11 male patients. J Urol 158:837
Quatan N, Kirby RS (2004) Improving outcomes in Fournier's gangrene. BJU Int 93:691
Roberts DB, Hester LL Jr (1972) Progressive synergistic bacterial gangrene arising from an abscess of the vulva and Bartholin's gland duct. Am J Obstet Gynecol 114:285
Roca B, Cunat E, Simon E (1998) HIV infection presenting with Fournier's gangrene. Neth J Med 53:168
Santora T, Rukstalis DB (2001) Fournier's gangrene. www.emedicine.com/med/UROLOGY.htm. Cited 6 November 2006
Sengoku A, Yamashita M, Umezu K (1990) A case of Fournier's gangrene: was it triggered by prostatic massage (in Japanese)? Hinyokika Kiyo 36:1097
Smith GL, Bunker CB, Dinneen MD (1998) Fournier's gangrene. Br J Urol 81:347
Spirnak JP, Resnick MI, Hampel N, Persky L (1984) Fournier's gangrene: report of 20 patients. J Urol 131:289
Theiss M, Hofmockel G, Frohmuller HG (1995) Fournier's gangrene in a patient with erectile dysfunction following use of a mechanical erection aid device. J Urol 153:1921
Tobin CE, Benjamin JA (1949) Anatomic and clinical re-evaluation of scrotum. Surg Gynec Obstet 88:545
Van den Berghe G, Wouters P, Weekers F, Verwaest C, Bruyninckx F, Schetz M, Vlasselaers D, Ferdinande P, Lauwers P, Bouillon R (2001) Intensive insulin therapy in critically ill patients. N Engl J Med 345:1359
Walker L, Cassidy MT, Hutchison AG, Abel BJ, Lewi HJ (1984) Fournier's gangrene and urethral problems. Br J Urol 56:509
Walther PJ, Andriani RT, Maggio MI, Carson CC 3rd (1987) Fournier's gangrene: a complication of penile prosthetic implantation in a renal transplant patient. J Urol 137:299
Yeniyol CO, Suelozgen T, Arslan M, Ayder AR (2004) Fournier's gangrene: experience with 25 patients and use of Fournier's gangrene severity index score. Urology 64:218

Urologic Emergencies in Pregnant Women: Special Considerations

7

J.F. Hermieu, L. Boccon-Gibod

7.1 Introduction

In view of anatomical, physiological, and functional modifications, pregnancy can be responsible for many urological disorders, some of which may be life-threatening for the mother and fetus, requiring emergency treatment. Pregnancy often makes diagnosis difficult because many investigative procedures are inadvisable in pregnant women. The therapeutic possibilities are also limited, and many drugs and certain surgical procedures are contraindicated, present a risk of inducing labor, or are harmful to the fetus. Therefore, finding a compromise between the patient's comfort and the normal development of the fetus is sometimes necessary. The risk–benefit ratio should be particularly well analyzed, which requires perfect knowledge of the particularities of urological disorders in pregnant women.

7.2 Anatomical and Physiological Modifications During Pregnancy

During pregnancy, an increase in vascular volume, renal output (+60 %), and glomerular filtration rate (+40 %) is noted. Other than a 1-cm increase in the size of the kidneys, these changes result in an increase in the rate of filtered creatinine, urea, sodium, calcium, and uric acid (Biyani and Joyce 2002a). Hypercalciuria is induced by the decrease in the production of parathormone and by an increase in the 1-25 OH-D3 produced by the placenta, which is responsible for an increase in the intestinal absorption of calcium. Despite hypercalciuria and physiological hyperuricuria, the incidence of calculi does not rise during pregnancy, since the rate of factors inhibitory crystallization (citrate, magnesium, glycoproteins) is also higher (Biyani and Joyce 2002a; Meria et al. 1995). Urine, more alkaline because of respiratory alkalosis, opposes the formation of uric acid stones despite hyperuricuria.

Physiological dilatation of the upper urinary tract is found in more than 90 % of pregnant women. This dilatation occurs between the 6th and 10th weeks and disappears 4–6 weeks after delivery (McAleer and Loughlin 2004). For anatomical reasons, it predominates on the right side. Different theories seek to explain this dilatation:

- The hormonal theory involves the inhibiting role of progesterone on the ureteral smooth musculature (Biyani and Joyce 2002a; Saidi et al. 2005). This theory is supported by experimental studies that have shown that administering progesterone to the female rat increases ureteral dilatation. This has not been confirmed by other authors. The hormonal theory does not explain the predominance of ureteral dilatation on the right side. It undoubtedly plays an accessory role in the first months of pregnancy (Biyani and Joyce 2002a; McAleer and Loughlin 2004).
- The mechanical theory involves the compressive role of the uterus, with this effect predominating on the right because of the uterus's dextrorotation. Ureteral compression by the ovarian vein and by the dilated uterine veins has also been suggested. The protection of the left ureter by the sigmoid reinforces the asymmetric character of the dilatation (Chaliha and Stanton 2002; Gorton and Whitfieldd 1997; Grenier et al. 2000). The absence of ureteral dilatation in cases of pelvic kidney, after ileal conduit urinary derivation, or in the quadruped confirms the involvement of mechanical phenomena in this dilatation (Biyani and Joyce 2002a).

Physiological dilatation during pregnancy is sometimes the cause of painful symptoms that usually regress with the use of mild analgesics. The persistence of pain or the appearance of infectious signs require urine drainage by a ureteral drainage stent or a percutaneous nephrostomy (Puskar et al. 2001).

7.3 Diagnostic Procedures in the Pregnant Patient

7.3.1 Doppler Ultrasound

Doppler ultrasound is the first-line examination to perform when there is suspicion of renal colic in the pregnant woman. However, it does not differentiate physiological dilatation of pregnancy from pathological dilatation related, for example, to a kidney calculus. Since it only explores the high lumbar ureter or pelvic ureter, it misjudges many cases of calculi. With a sensitivity of 34% and a specificity of 86% (Mauroy et al. 1996; Stothers and Lee 1992), this exam is often flawed as a diagnostic procedure. Different devices have been developed in an attempt to improve its performance:

7.3.1.1 Evaluating the Dilatation of the Urinary Tract

Muller-Suur and Tyden (1985) defined the pathological limit for renal pelvis as a diameter greater than 17 mm. Erickson et al. (1979), beginning with the 2nd trimester, suggest a limit of 27 mm on the right and 18 mm on the left. Brandt and Desroches (1985) retained the same references for the 2nd and 3rd trimesters, with the pathological limits of 18 mm on the right and 15 mm on the left for the 1st trimester. Finally, discovery of ureter dilatation extending to the pelvic ureter most often indicates pathological dilatation (Saidi et al. 2005).

7.3.1.2 The Study of Ureteral Jets

The ultrasound study of ureteral jets in real-time or color echo-Doppler can be a diagnostic aid. Deyoe (1995) considered that the unilateral absence of a ureteral jet demonstrates a complete obstruction, with 100% sensitivity and 91% specificity. Unfortunately, this measure is sometimes flawed. Wachsberg (1998) advised carrying out this test in the lateral decubitus position to prevent errors related to physiological mechanical compression. Burke and Washowich (1998) reported the complete absence of unilateral jet in asymptomatic pregnant women. The search for ureteral jets must therefore be interpreted cautiously, particularly in cases of partial obstruction (Biyani and Joyce 2002a; Evans and Wollin 2001).

7.3.1.3 Vaginal Ultrasound

The vaginal route first allows a reliable study of the lower ureter and can identify lithiasis when necessary (Laing et al. 1994).

7.3.1.4 Measuring the Resistivity Index

Renal vascular resistance increases during acute obstruction, particularly during the first 6–48 h (Ulrich et al. 1995). This increase is related to vasoconstriction mediated by different factors such as prostaglandins. Using these parameters, Shokeir et al. (2000) indicated that a resistivity index of at least 0.7 diagnoses obstruction, with a sensitivity of 77% and a specificity of 83%, with 88% sensitivity and 98% specificity if the resistivity index's variation is greater than 0.06. This measurement's performance is flawed, however, when the measurement is taken before 6 h or after 48 h, in cases of single kidney, of pathological kidney, or when nonsteroidal anti-inflammatory drug (NSAID) treatment interfering with the metabolism of prostaglandins is used (Shokeir et al. 2000; Ulrich et al. 1995).

7.3.2 Irradiation and Pregnancy

Studies on animals or human fetuses and embryos irradiated in utero at Hiroshima or Nagasaki have evaluated the three risks of irradiation during pregnancy: risk of fetal malformation, risk of induced tumor, and risk of transmissible chromosome malformation. These risks are proportional to the dose delivered and the period of irradiation, with the first weeks of pregnancy the most critical (Doll 1995).

7.3.2.1 Risk of Fetal Malformation

Fetal malformation, developmental delay, growth delay, or in utero death are the usual consequences reported. There is a linear relation between the radiation dose and the risk of delays in mental development (Biyani and Joyce 2002a). Several experimental studies in animals show that the risk of irradiation during the first weeks of pregnancy often obeys the all-or-nothing law: miscarriage or absence of malformation (Gorton and Whitfield 1997). Below 50 mGy, the risk of malformation seems negligible even if minimal biochemical modifications are possible. This threshold value is well under the dose delivered by radiological diagnostic tests (plain abdomen = 1 mGy/radiograph, 1 min of image intensifier = 2 mGy) (Denstedt and Razvi 1992).

7.3.2.2 Risk of Radiation-Induced Tumors

Stewart estimated that an in utero irradiation of 10 - 20 mGy increases the risk of cancer in the child by 1.5 - 2 (Stewart 1973). Harvey et al. (1985), who studied twin pregnancies subjected or not subjected to diagnostic radiation averaging 1 cGy, evaluated the relative risk at 2.4. However, this risk continues to be debated. It is surprising to note that the risk of radiation-induced cancer is higher when the radiation is received at the end of pregnancy rather than just after birth (Miller 1995). In addition, the tumors observed in children are more of the embryonic type, which does not correspond to tumors known to be radiation-induced.

7.3.2.3 Mutagenic Risk

A dose of 0.5 - 1 Gy is necessary to double the spontaneous rate of genetic mutation (Hall 1991). This level of radiation is never reached by the common radiographic diagnostic tests.

In conclusion, even if the consequences of diagnostic irradiation during pregnancy are low, particularly in the second and third trimesters, the risk–benefit ratio of radiological exploration should always be evaluated and compared to the risk of an unrecognized urinary tract obstruction treated late (Gorton and Whitfield 1997).

7.3.3 Intravenous Urography

While intravenous urography (IVU) was considered the gold standard of radiological workup for urinary lithiasis, its utility has greatly diminished since the advent of unenhanced helical CT. It is superior to ultrasound in diagnosis but IVU requires an injection of contrast solution and leads to a low but not inconsiderable dose of radiation, especially during the first trimester. Different examination protocols have been proposed aiming to limit the radiation exposure as much as possible to three or four radiographs: plain abdomen, 30 s, 20 min (McAleer and Loughlin 2004; Stothers and Lee 1992) plus or minus one late x-ray (Dore 2004); plain abdomen, 20 min, late x-ray (Klein 1984). It is important to use high-sensitivity films, reduce the aperture as much as possible, have large radiology rooms available, choose digital radiology, and use a lead apron for the side of the healthy kidney (Biyani and Joyce 2002a; McAleer and Loughlin 2004). Given bony superposition and the voluminous uterus, identifying small stones is sometimes difficult (Biyani and Joyce 2002a; Dore 2004; Evans and Wollin 2001). The exam does not always differentiate physiological and pathological dilatations (Biyani and Joyce 2002a; Evans and Wollin 2001).

7.3.4 Computerized Tomography

The advantage of unenhanced helical computerized tomography (CT) to evidence a kidney stone and the resulting dilatation no longer needs to be demonstrated in terms of both sensitivity and specificity when compared to plain abdomen, ultrasound, or the plain abdomen–ultrasound combination. However, this exam requires high-dose radiation that is incompatible with pregnancy. It should be avoided in the pregnant patient.

7.3.5 Retrograde Ureteropyelography

Retrograde ureteropyelography (RUP) results in radiation that is not inconsiderable and results in a risk of sepsis when infection is present. Its advantages are limited to a few patients for whom diagnosis remains uncertain, during an operation, and immediately before double-J stenting.

7.3.6 Magnetic Resonance Imaging

The recent progress in magnetic resonance imaging (MRI), providing reduced acquisition time, makes reliable exploration of the urinary tract feasible. To the sequences without injection of contrast medium can be added sequences with injection of gadolinium for a uro-MRI with no iodine injection or irradiation. The exam provides reconstitutions in the different spatial planes (frontal, sagittal, etc.).

Although the MRI has no known native implication for the fetus, for reasons of caution this examination is not advised in the course of the first trimester during the organogenesis phase (Louca 1999; Murthy 1997; Spencer 2000). MRI does not display small stones well (Roy et al. 1995) and has the disadvantage of high cost and reduced accessibility to the patient during the study. Although MRI is infrequently used in standard urinary lithiasis workups, it can be useful in difficult cases involving pregnant patients (Roy et al. 1995).

7.4 Treatment

7.4.1 Oral Treatment

7.4.1.1 Analgesics

Paracetamol, acetaminophen and dextropropoxyphene can be used with no risk (Biyani and Joyce 2002a). Codeine is contraindicated during the first trimester because of its potential teratogenic side effects but can be used episodically during the second and third trimesters (Pedersen and Finster 1979). In cases of intense pain, morphine can be necessary. The prescription should be of short duration to prevent any risk of maternofetal dependence, growth delay, or prematurely induced labor (Barron 1985). Morphine should not be used at the beginning of or during labor.

7.4.1.2 Nonsteroidal Anti-inflammatory Drugs

Given their blocking action of the synthesis of prostaglandins, NSAIDs should be avoided during pregnancy because of the risk of premature closing of the ductus arteriosus (Rasanen and Jouppila 1995) and of fetal pulmonary hypertension (Van Marter et al. 1996). Aspirin can delay or prolong labor. Also, through its effect on platelet aggregation, it also induces a hemorrhagic risk at delivery.

7.4.1.3 Alpha 1 Adrenergic Blockers

Recent studies show the advantages of alpha 1 blocker, used as a spasmolytic drug, for the spontaneous expulsion of distal ureteral stones (Dellabella et al. 2003). The side effects in pregnant women and the possibility of teratogenicity are not currently known. Further evaluations are necessary before using this class of substances in pregnancy.

7.4.1.4 Antibiotic Therapy

Aminopenicillins (Ampicillin, Amoxicillin)

Antibiotics of the penicillin group, aminopenicillins have low toxicity and generate few side effects other than a risk of allergy. Forty to 50 % of enterobacteria are resistant to these antibiotics (Goldstein 2000). Adding clavulanic acid-inhibiting beta-lactamases has increased the efficacy, but 30 % – 40 % of bacteria are currently resistant to it (Goldstein 2000). The aminopenicillins are very effective on streptococci. This group of antibiotics can be used without risk in pregnant women but after having verified the sensitivity of the bacterium on the antibiogram.

Third-Generation Cephalosporins

Belonging to the beta-lactam group, third-generation cephalosporins have low toxicity and generate few side effects. They can be administered orally or by intramuscular or intravenous routes. Because of their efficacy, their pharmacological properties, and a low rate of enterobacterial resistance, third-generation cephalosporins are the first-line antibiotic therapy for treating acute pyelonephritis in pregnant women while waiting for the result of the antibiogram.

Aminoglycosides

Aminoglycosides have a synergetic action with betalactamines and a wide spectrum of activity on enterobacteria. They have a risk of nephrotoxicity and ototoxicity. While aminoglycosides have been said by some authors to potentially cause neuromuscular blockade in humans, and have experimentally caused it in animals, there has never been a reported case of human neuromuscular blockade after aminoglycosides administration (Santucci and Krieger 2000; Wong and Brown 1996) Administrable parenterally, they cross the placental barrier. Because of their risk to the fetus, in pregnant patients they can only be used for short periods for severe acute pyelonephritis threatening maternal–fetal prognosis.

Fluoroquinolones

Fluoroquinolones are very effective on enterobacteria but also on certain negative-coagulase staphylococci. They are ineffective against enterococci. *Escherichia coli* has a low resistance rate to ciprofloxacin (1%–2%) (Goldstein 2000). They are classically contraindicated in the pregnant patient because of the risk of toxicity to fetal cartilage and joints. Nevertheless, in cases of severe acute pyelonephritis presenting a life-threatening risk to mother and fetus or of multiresistant bacteria, they can be used for a short period of time.

Quinolones (Nalidixic Acid, Pipemidic Acid)

Quinolones are active on enterobacteria, but they are contraindicated for patients with G6PD deficit and should be avoided during pregnancy. Their main side effects are digestive problems, photosensitization, and neurosensory phenomena (disturbed vision, somnolence, dizziness, headaches, and more rarely hallucinations and convulsions).

Nitrofurantoin

Active on enterobacteria, nitrofurantoin only slightly modifies the fecal flora and induces little resistance. It is contraindicated in patients with G6PD deficit. It can be responsible for digestive problems, allergic reactions, and more rarely pulmonary fibrosis, hepatitis, and optical or peripheral neuritis during prolonged use. It can be used during pregnancy except in the last trimester when it can result in hemolytic anemia.

Fosfomycin-Trometamol

Fosfomycin-trometamol is active on enterobacteria, has low toxicity, and generates few side effects. It modifies fecal flora only slightly. It can be used with no risk during pregnancy (Patel et al. 1997).

Trimethoprim-Sulfamethoxazole

The association of trimethoprim and sulfamethoxazole is very active on enterobacteria. Resistance rates of 20%–40% have been reported, however (Goldstein 2000). It is contraindicated during the first trimester of pregnancy because of a potential teratogenic risk (antifolic property) and during the third trimester because of a risk of neonatal jaundice. However, it can be used during the second trimester except in cases of G6PD deficiency suspect in Mediterranean patients or with first-degree relatives affected.

Other Antibiotics

Chloramphenicol and tetracyclines are contraindicated during pregnancy. Erythromycin have no fetal morbidity, although erythromycin estolate salt compounds can cause cholestatic jaundice and should not be used (Biyani and Joyce 2002b; Dorosz 2003).

7.4.1.5 Other Medications

The thiazide diuretics decrease urinary excretion of calcium in an attempt to lower the incidence of urinary calculus formation. They have been suspected of inducing fetal thrombocytopenia. Even if this effect is uncertain (Collins et al. 1985), they should be avoided during pregnancy. The same holds true for xanthine oxydase inhibitors such as allopurinol or D-penicillamine, for which fetal malformations have been described in animals (Maikranz 1994).

Beta-1-blockers (Hettenbach et al. 1988) have been suggested in the treatment of hydronephrosis during pregnancy. They act by stimulating the contractile activity of the renal pelvis and the ureter. Limited experience with these treatments does not allow confirmation of their efficacy (Zwergel et al. 1996).

7.4.2 Surgical Treatment

7.4.2.1 Ureteral Stents

When a urinary calculus requires surgery during pregnancy, the classical attitude is to ensure urine flow, with the definitive treatment undertaken after the child is born (Denstedt and Razvi 1992). Placing a double-J ureteral stent easily removes the obstruction. In very septic patients, the stent can be placed without sedation. When urine is thick, it is preferable to first position an open ureteral stent, which can be replaced after a few days with a double-J stent when the sepsis is under control and the urine more liquid (Dore 2004). The double-J stent presents several advantages. It can be placed under local anesthesia and presents no radiation to the patient, as the procedure is guided by ultrasound (Jarrard et al. 1993). It allows the patient to return to normal activities rapidly and permits vaginal delivery. It is not always easy to place, especially during the 3rd trimester, when the bladder is pushed back by the uterus, the trigone deformed, and the mucous membrane of the bladder rendered hyperemic by pelvic hypervascularization. In addition, the stent carries a certain number of disadvantages: bladder irritation by the lower J that may cause urinary frequency, increased micturition urge or hematuria, risk of displacement due to dilatation of the excretory tract, and vesicorenal reflux, which can cause lower back pain or acute pyelonephritis (Zwergel et al. 1996).

Many authors have reported the risk of incrustation secondary to hypercalciuria of pregnancy (Borboroglu and Kane 2000; Goldfarb et al. 1989; Loughlin 1994). This risk is reduced by increasing fluid intake, controlling calcium intake, and treatment of UTI if necessary (Biyani and Joyce 2002b). To avoid incrustations, some authors advise changing the double-J stent every 4–8 weeks (Denstedt and Razvi 1992; Loughlin and Bailey 1986), thus multiplying hospitalizations and the risks related to endoscopic procedures. Other authors prefer to avoid the double-J stent at the beginning of pregnancy and reserve its use for after the 22nd week (Denstedt and Razvi 1992; Goldfarb et al. 1989; Loughlin and Bailey 1986; Stothers and Lee 1992).

7.4.2.2 Percutaneous Nephrostomy

An alternative to placing a ureteral stent is percutaneous nephrostomy (Biyani and Joyce 2002b). Dilatation of the urinary tract during pregnancy facilitates its placement. Denstedt preferred this procedure before the 22nd week of pregnancy (Denstedt and Razvi 1992). It can be done under local anesthesia, ultrasound localization, and in the three-quarter position (Kavoussi et al. 1992). It may result in discomfort of an external derivation, exposes the patient to the risks of stent displacement, cutaneous infection at the site of entry, and bacterial colonization following prolonged use of the stent (Biyani and Joyce 2002b; Kavoussi et al. 1992; Loughlin and Lindsey 2002; Zwergel et al. 1996). The risk of incrustation is identical to that of the ureteral stent, requiring that the stent be changed every 4–8 weeks (Kavoussi et al. 1992). In very septic patients, who rarely cannot tolerate intravenous sedation, percutaneous nephrostomy should be a good choice even if the three-quarter position is not always possible in such patients.

7.4.2.3 Ureteroscopy

Ureteroscopy during pregnancy is contraindicated by most experts, as it exposes the patient to radiation, a risk of ureteral perforation, or a vascular injury in a cramped hypervascularized pelvis. However, a few authors, considering the discomfort of prolonged use of a double-J stent or of a nephrostomy until delivery and the risk of incrustations, have successfully performed ureteroscopies in pregnant women (Rittenberg and Bagley 1988; Shokeir and Mutabagani 1998; Ulvik et al. 1995). The ureteroscopy can be done under locoregional anesthesia (Carringer et al. 1996; Rittenberg and Bagley 1988; Scarpa et al. 1996; Shokeir and Mutabagani 1998; Ulvik et al. 1995). Progesterone absorption and dilatation of the urinary track provide problem-free scope advancement without dilating the ureteral meatus beforehand (Shokeir and Mutabagani 1998; Ulvik et al. 1995; Watterson et al. 2002), which is further facilitated by continual technical improvements in equipment (such as 7.5-F rigid ureteroscopes and flexible ureteroscopes) (Scarpa et al. 1996; Shokeir and Mutabagani 1998). Scope progression can be observed visually, without radiological guidance and with no radiation, provided that a confirmed and experienced endoscopist does the procedure. Although some experts do not recommend ureteroscopy during the 3rd trimester (Vest and Warden 1990), others consider this procedure possible at any time during the pregnancy (Carringer et al. 1996; Rittenberg and Bagley 1988; Watterson et al. 2002). The calculus is ideally extracted with a Dormia basket (Ulvik et al. 1995). When the calculus must be fragmented, electrohydraulic shock is not advised because it risks inducing labor (Evans and Wollin 2001; Zheng and Denstedt 2000). Ultrasonic lithotriptors present a risk for the fetal auditory system (Ulvik et al. 1995). Using the Holmium laser on uric acid calculi presents the theoretical risk of producing cyanide ions (Teichman et al. 1998a) whose harmful effect has never been proven (Teichman et al. 1998b), probably because the majority of these ions are eliminated by the irrigating fluid (Evans and Wollin 2001; Mauroy et al. 1996). Carringer et al. (1996) consider that laser can be used with no risk in pregnant women. The promotors of the technique refer to a few contraindications to ureteroscopy during pregnancy: inexperienced operator, calculi larger than 1 cm, multiple calculi, transplanted kidney, and sepsis (Biyani and Joyce 2002b).

7.4.2.4 Extracorporal Shock-Wave Lithotripsy

Pregnancy is one of the common contraindications for extracorporal shock-wave lithotripsy (ESWL) because of the potential risk of the shock waves on the fetus (Chaussy and Fuchs 1989). Smith et al. (1992) reported fetal growth delay in the pregnant rat treated with ESWL. The risk of irradiation when the calculus is located by imaging and premature induction of labor (Vieweg et al. 1992) have also been reported. However, seven patients have undergone this treatment during their pregnancy, either because the pregnancy had not been diagnosed at the time of treatment or after informed consent (Asgari et al. 1999; Frankenschmidt and Sommerkamp 1998). These women continued their pregnancy to term and delivered a perfectly healthy child. Despite these encouraging reports, most learned societies contraindicate ESWL during pregnancy.

7.4.2.5
Percutaneous Nephrolithotomy

Although some authors have successfully performed percutaneous nephrolithotomy (PCNL) in women at the end of pregnancy (Holman et al. 1992), this technique is classically contraindicated in pregnant patients. It requires a ventral decubitus position that is problematic, as well as prolonged anesthesia. It carries high irradiation and can induce labor (Biyani and Joyce 2002b; Loughlin 1994; McAleer and Loughlin 2004).

7.4.2.6
Open Surgery

With the improvements in treatment methods, recourse to surgery to treat a urinary tract calculus remains exceptional. In pregnant women, placing a double-J stent or a nephrostomy makes it possible to reach the pregnancy's term so that lithotripsy or endoscopic treatment of the stone can be undertaken at that time. Even if surgery in the pregnant patient presents a risk of hemorrhage because of the hypervascularization of the pelvic area, and a nearly 10 % risk of premature delivery (Shnider and Webster 1965), there remain a few exceptional cases where open surgery is the last recourse to removing calculus formation that causes of life-threatening complications. Exceptionally, in pregnant women in a state of urinary sepsis that cannot be controlled by antibiotics and urinary diversion via a ureteral catheter or a nephrostomy, emergency nephrectomy is indicated after preparation including vasoactive drugs, platelets, or coagulating factor transfusions if necessary. A three-quarter operating position and a retroperitoneal approach and an experienced surgeon are required to execute quickly the procedure and limit morbidity and mortality.

7.5
Particular Treatments of Certain Urological Emergencies in Pregnant Women

7.5.1
Urinary Tract Calculi

The incidence of urinary lithiasis during pregnancy is on the order of 1:200 to 1:1,500 (Evans and Wollin 2001; Gorton and Whitfield 1997; Loughlin 1997; McAller and Loughlin 2004; Meria et al. 1993; Stothers and Lee 1992), with the mean figure of 1:1,500 cited most often. This incidence is identical in women who are not pregnant (Biyani and Joyce 2002a; McAleer and Loughlin 2004; Saidi et al. 2005). Onset occurs eight or nine times out of ten during the 2nd or 3rd trimester (Leaphart et al. 1997; McAleer and Loughlin 2004; Meria et al. 1993; Stothers and Lee 1992). It is more frequent in multiparous women (Kroovand 1992; Stothers and Lee 1992). The calculi are essentially composed of calcium carbonitee and more rarely of struvite (Meria et al. 1993; Saidi et al. 2005; Stothers and Lee 1992). The revealing symptom is most often lower back pain (89 %) followed by microscopic hematuria, sometimes macroscopic hematuria (95 %) (Leaphart et al. 1997; McAleer and Loughlin 2004; Stothers and Lee 1992). Symptoms can be deceptive, bringing to mind cholecystitis or right-sided appendicitis, left-sided sigmoiditis, an occlusion, adnexal pathology, or placental detachment (Biyani and Joyce 2002a; Evans and Wollin 2001; McAleer and Loughlin 2004). Elsewhere, the calculus is discovered by signs in the lower urinary structures, abortion, the threat of premature delivery (Biyani and Joyce 2002a; Loughlin 1994), atypical abdominal pain, or nausea or vomiting (Evans and Wollin 2001). More rarely, lithiasis presents as an infectious complication or anuria (Carringer et al. 1996; Meria et al. 1993; Stothers and Lee 1992).

While seven or eight urinary calculi out of ten are eliminated spontaneously, medical treatment should be proposed initially. Rest and sufficient hydration (2 – 3 l/24 h) are prescribed. When pain is present, fluid restriction is routine. The proper procedure is summarized in Fig. 7.1.

7.5.2
Urinary Tract Infections

Because of anatomic, functional, and hormonal modifications, urinary tract infection is frequent during pregnancy. It can present as three different entities: asymptomatic bacteriuria, acute cystitis, or acute pyelonephritis (Ovalle and Levancini 2001).

Different risk factors have been discussed: maternal age, socioeconomic status, antecedents of UTI, sexual intercourse, hemoglobinopathies, diabetes, immunodepression of HIV infection, multiparity, and race (Connolly and Thorpe 1999; Ovalle and Levancini 2001; Pastore et al. 1999a, b).

The most frequently encountered bacteria are enterobacteria, with *E. coli* ranked first (65 % – 90 %), although streptococci are found more and more often (Hill et al. 2005).

Although many authors have established a relation between asymptomatic bacteruria and the risk of prematurity and low birth weight, today this relation is disputed. However, it is clear that untreated bacteruria induces a 20 % – 50 % risk of acute pyelonephritis, with this risk dropping to 1 % – 2 % if the bacteriuria is treated (Connolly and Thorpe 1999; Naber et al. 2001; Ovalle and Levancini 2001; Santos et al. 2002).

Although nitrite test strips and leukotests are useful in screening and monitoring, with a negative predictive value of 97.5 %, cytobacteriological urine analysis

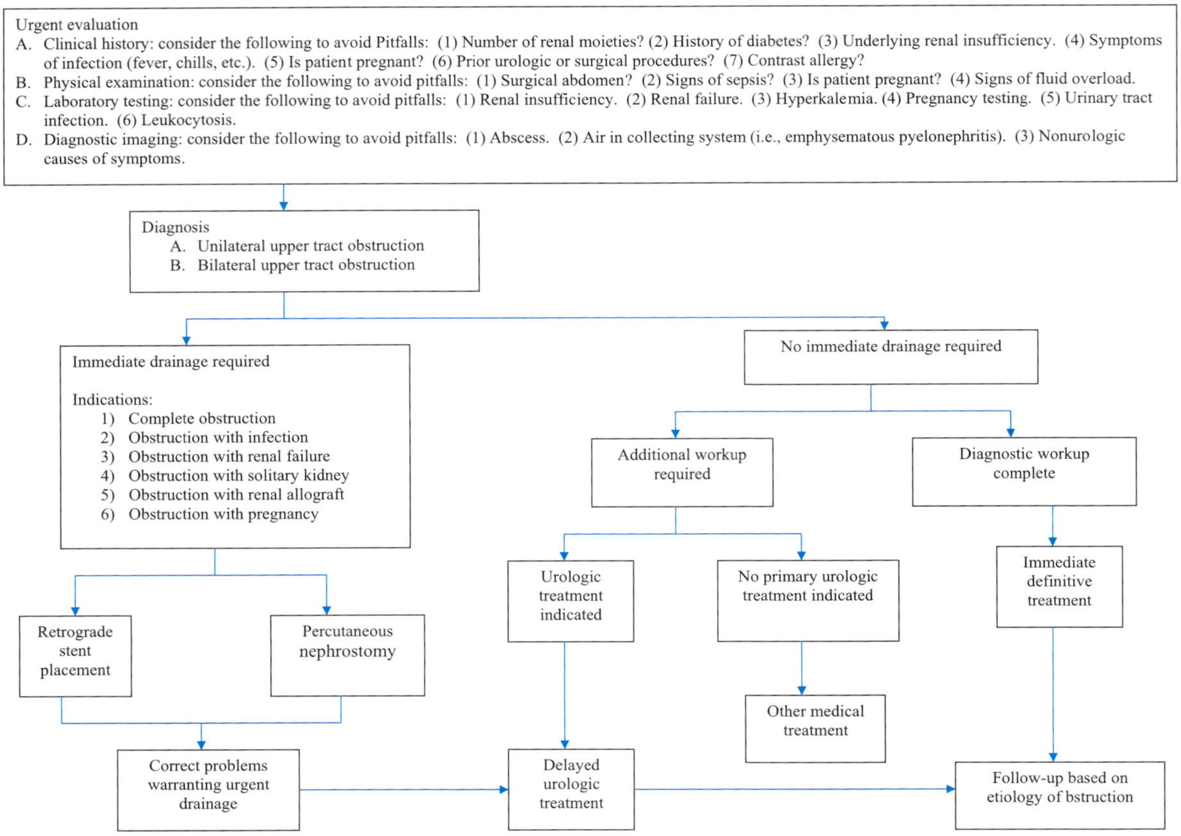

Fig. 7.1. Treatment of urinary tract calculi in pregnant patients

should be systematic to establish the diagnosis and have an antibiogram done. The upper limit of 10^5 bacteria/ml for the cytobacteriological urine analysis established by Kass to confirm the diagnosis of UTI has been questioned. The association of clinical signs with 10^2 of a single pathogenic bacterium per milliliter provides the diagnosis (Delcroix et al. 1994).

The treatment of asymptomatic bacteriuria can be based on a single-dose treatment, as effective as classical antibiotic treatment lasting 1 week (Dafnis and Sabatini 1992; Gerstner et al. 1978; Jakobi et al. 1987; McNeely 1987). On the other hand, there is no consensus on the duration of the optimal treatment of acute cystitis (Delcroix et al. 1994). The risk of recurrence (18%) requires monthly monitoring of urine and, in case of recurrence, antibiotic prophylaxis until delivery. Sometimes postcoital antibiotic prophylaxis is sufficient (Connolly and Thorpe 1999; Delcroix et al. 1994; Naber et al. 2001). Hygiene and diet advice is always useful: high fluid intake, voiding every 4 h, postcoital voiding, and perineal hygiene (Santos et al. 2002). The prescription of cranberry juice or extract can be proposed but is much debated (Connolly and Thorpe 1999).

Acute pyelonephritis in a pregnant woman often requires hospitalization (Ovalle and Levancini 2001) to make the diagnosis, begin treatment, and provide the initial monitoring. For some authors, however, this hospitalization is not always necessary (Wing et al. 1999). Parenteral antibiotic therapy, often a third-generation cephalosporin, is the preferred treatment, and can be started presumptively, then change subsequently to the antibiogram results to an appropriate oral antibiotic treatment for a total duration of 10–14 days (Connolly and Thorpe 1999; Mauroy et al. 1996). Severe forms often require prescription of an aminoglycoside during the first 48 h of treatment. Ultrasound to look for pyelocaliceal dilatation is particularly useful. When infectious or severe local signs do not respond to antibiotics or when there is substantial dilatation of the urinary tract with suspicion of obstruction, urine diversion using a ureteral stent or percutaneous nephrostomy is necessary (Naber et al. 2001). In all cases, noninvasive obstetric monitoring is indispensable (Delcroix et al. 1994).

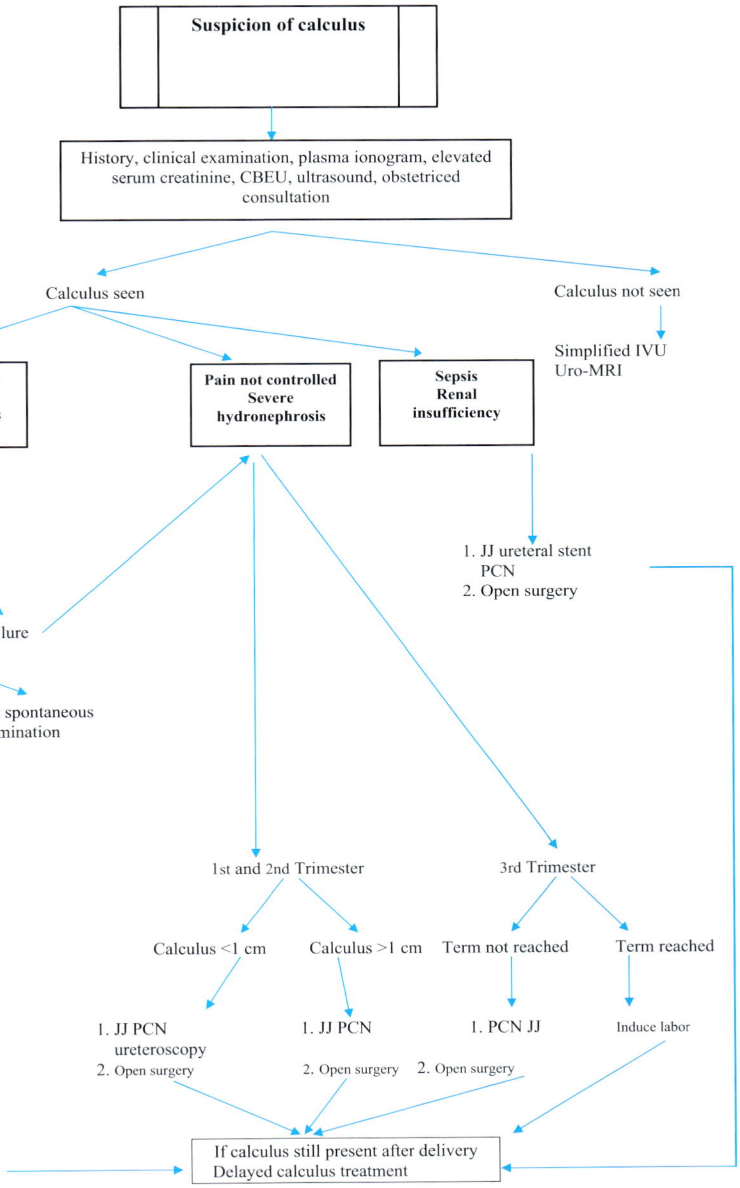

Fig. 7.2. Suspicion of calculus

7.5.3 Spontaneous Renal Rupture

Spontaneous renal rupture is a rare complication during pregnancy. It can occur in three circumstances (Middleton et al. 1980): spontaneous rupture with no cause, rupture of the excretory tract related to an obstruction, and renal rupture secondary to a tumor, most often an angiomyolipoma. Clinically, the spontaneous rupture is manifested by lumbar or abdominal pain with thickening of the lumbar fossa and sometimes hemorrhagic shock. Ultrasound is a diagnostic aide that shows an effusion of urine around the kidney or a retroperitoneal hematoma. When there is rupture of the excretory tract related to obstruction, placing a double-J stent to remove the obstruction is the best approach (Oesterling et al. 1988). If this is not possible, percutaneous nephrostomy can be undertaken. Percutaneous drainage of a collection is sometimes necessary. When there is renal parenchyma rupture, strict monitoring is indispensable. Bleeding can stop spontaneously because of the pressure exerted on the retroperitoneum. When bleeding cannot be controlled and hemodynamics are unstable, open surgery is sometimes the only choice possible, with a nephrectomy often necessary.

7.5.4 Placenta Percreta Involving Urinary Bladder

The incidence of placenta accreta is estimated from one in 540 to one in 93,000 deliveries (Smith and Ferrara 1992). Placenta percreta is a variant of placenta accreta in which chorionic villi penetrate the entire thickness of the myometrium and may involve adjacent structures. Placenta percreta involving the bladder is extremely rare (less than 60 published cases) (Washecka and Behling 2002) and is encouraged by uterine scars and cesarean section.

This potentially catastrophic condition may remain undiagnosed or underappreciated until delivery (Leaphart et al. 1997) and diagnosis is often made only at the time of operation in a life-threatening bleeding. In 31 % of cases, hematuria is present during pregnancy and a preoperative diagnosis established by ultrasound (presence of multiple linear irregular vascular spaces within the placenta) (Comstock et al. 2004) or MRI (Washecka and Behling 2002).

Cystoscopy is not always useful. If placenta percreta is suspected, transurethral biopsy should be avoided because of severe hemorrhage (Teo et al. 1996). The goal of the surgical treatment must be to control bleeding, which usually requires hysterectomy, resection of all tissue involved by the infiltrating placenta, and eventually partial cystectomy or ureteral reimplantation (Price et al. 1991). The tissue planes are often very much indurated and extremely difficult to dissect. Teo et al. (1996) and Bakri et al. (1993) prefer to leave the invasive portion in situ associated, if necessary, with bilateral hypogastric arterial ligation and pressure packing. Methotrexate adjuvant therapy may be helpful in expediting absorption of the remaining placental tissue.

7.6 Conclusion

Urologic emergencies during pregnancy are far from exceptional. Some can be life-threatening to the mother or endanger the development or viability of the fetus. Good knowledge of the diagnostic and therapeutic particularities in the pregnant patient and close collaboration between the urologist and the obstetrician make for optimal care that limits maternal and fetal risks to the greatest degree.

References

Asgari MA, Safarinejad MA, Hosseini SY, Dadhkah F (1999) Extracorporeal shock wave lithotripsy of renal calculi during early pregnancy. BJU Int 84:615

Bakri YN et al (1993) Placenta percreta with bladder invasion: report of three cases. Am J Perinatol 10:468

Barron WM (1985) Medical evaluation of the pregnant patient requiring non-obstetric surgery. Clin Perinatol 12:481

Biyani CS, Joyce AD (2002a) Urolithiasis in pregnancy. I: pathophysiology, fetal considerations and diagnosis. BJU Int 89:811

Biyani CS, Joyce AD (2002b) Urolithiasis in pregnancy. II: management. BJU Int 89:819

Borboroglu PG, Kane CJ (2000) Current management of severely encrusted ureteral stents with a large associated stone burden. J Urol 164:648

Brandt B, Desroches A (1985) Echographie rénale chez la femme enceinte. In: Chatelain C et al (eds) Urologie : pathologie infectieuse et parasitaire, Masson, Paris, pp 400

Burke BJ, Washowich TL (1998) Ureteral jets in normal second and third trimester pregnancy. J Clin Ultrasound 26:423

Carringer M et al (1996) Management of ureteric calculi during pregnancy by ureteroscopy and laser lithotripsy. Br J Urol 77:17

Chaliha C, Stanton SL (2002) Urological problems in pregnancy. BJU 89:469

Chaussy CG, Fuchs GJ (1989) Current state and future developments of noninvasive treatment of human urinary stones with extracorporeal shock wave lithotripsy. J Urol 141:782

Collins R, Yusuf S, Peto R (1985) Overview of randomised trials of diuretics in pregnancy. BMJ 290:17

Comstock CH et al (2004) Sonographic detection of placenta accreta in the second and third trimesters of pregnancy. Am J Obstet Gynecol 190:1135

Connolly A, Thorpe JM Jr (1999) Urinary tract infections in pregnancy. Urol Clin North Am 26:779

Dafnis E, Sabatini S (1992) The effect of pregnancy on renal function: physiology and pathophysiology. Am J Med Sci 303:184

Dellabella M et al (2003) Efficacy of tamsulosine in the medical management of juxta vesical ureteral stones. J Urol 170:2202

Delcroix M, Zone V, Cheront C et al (1994) L'infection urinaire de la femme enceinte. Rev Fr Gynécol Obstet 89:277

Denstedt JD, Razvi H (1992) Management of urinary calculi during pregnancy. J Urol 148:1072

Deyoe LA (1995) New techniques of ultrasound and color Doppler in the prospective evaluation of acute renal obstruction: do they replace the intravenous urogram ? Abdom Imaging 20:58

Doll R (1995) Hazards of ionising radiation: 100 years of observations on man. Br J Cancer 72:1339

Dore B (2004) La lithiase urinaire de la femme enceinte. In: Dore B (ed) Les lithiases rénales. Springer Berlin Heidelberg New York, pp 353

Dorosz P (2003) Guide pratique des médicaments. Maloine, Paris, pp 1460

Erickson LM, Nicholson SF, Lewel DB et al (1979) Ultrasound evaluation of hydronephrosis of pregnancy. J Clin Ultrasound 7:128

Evans HJ, Wollin TA (2001) The management of urinary calculi in pregnancy. Curr Opin Urol 11:379

Frankenschmidt A, Sommerkamp H (1998) Shock wave lithotripsy during pregnancy: a successful clinical experiment. J Urol 159:501

Gerstner GJ et al (1978) Amoxicillin in the treatment of asymptomatic bacteriura in pregnancy: a single dose of 3 g amoxicillin versus a 4-days of 3 doses 750 mg amoxicillin. Gynecol Obstet Invst 27:84

Goldfarb RA, Neerhut GJ, Lederer E (1989) Management of acute hydronephrosis of pregnancy by ureteral stenting: risk of stone formation. J Urol 141:921

Goldstein FW (2000) Histoire naturelle, évolution de la sensibilité, participation à la résistance bactérienne. In: Choutet

P, Goldstein FW (eds) Escherichia coli. Phase 5. Editions Médicales, Paris, p 7
Gorton E, Whitfield HN (1997) Renal calculi in pregnancy. Br J Urol 80 [Suppl 1]:4
Grenier N, Pariente JL, Trillaud H et al (2000) Dilatation of the collecting system during pregnancy: physiologic vs obstructive dilatation. Eur Radiol 10:271
Hall EJ (1991) Scientific view of low level radiation risks. Radiographics 11:509
Harvey EB, Boice JD Jr, Honeyman M, Flanner JT (1985) Prenatal x-ray exposure and childhood cancer in twins. N Engl J Med 312:541
Hettenbach A, Tschada R, Hiltmann WD, Zimmermann T (1988) Untersuchungen zum Einfluss von beta-Stimulation and beta-1-Blockade auf die Motilitatt des oberen Harntraktes. Z Geburtshilfe Perinatol 192:273
Hill JB, Sheffield JS, McIntire DD, Wendel GD Jr (2005) Acute pyelonephritis in pregnancy. Obstet Gynecol 105:18
Holman E et al (1992) Percutaneous nephrolithotomy in late pregnancy. J Endourol 6:421
Jakobi P, Neiger R, Merzbach D, Paldi E (1987) Single-dose antimicrobial therapy in the treatment of asymptomatic bacteriuria in pregnancy. Am J Obstet Gynecol 156:1148
Jarrard DJ, Gerber GS, Lyon ES (1993) Management of acute ureteral obstruction in pregnancy utilizing ultrasound-guided placement of ureteral stents. Urology 42:263
Kavoussi LR, Albala DM, Basler JW et al (1992) Percutaneous management of urolithiasis during pregnancy. J Urol 148: 1069
Klein EA (1984) Urologic problems of pregnancy. Obst Gynec Surv 39:605
Kroovand RL (1992) Stones in pregnancy and children. J Urol 148:1076
Laing FC, Benson CB, DiSalvo DN et al (1994) Distal ureteral calculi: detection with vaginal US. Radiology 192:545
Leaphart WL et al (1997) Placenta previa percreta with bladder invasion. Obstet Gynecol 89:834
Louca G (1999) MR urography in the diagnosis of urinary tract obstruction. Eur Urol 35:102
Loughlin KR (1994) Management of urologic problems during pregnancy. Urology 44:159
Loughlin KR (1997) Management of urologic problems in the pregnant patient. AUA Update Series 16:10
Loughlin K, Bailey R (1986) Internal ureteral stent for conservative management of ureteral calculi during pregnancy. N Engl J Med 315:1647
Loughlin KR, Lindsey AK (2002) The current management of urolithiasis during pregnancy. Urol Clin N Am 29:701
Maikranz P (1994) Nephrolithiasis in pregnancy. Balliere's Clin Obstet Gynaecol 8:375
Mauroy B, Beuscart C, Biserte J et al (1996) L'infection urinaire chez la femme enceinte. Prog Urol 6:607
McAleer SJ, Loughlin KR (2004) Nephrolithiasis and pregnancy. Curr Opin Urol 14:123
McNeely SG Jr (1987) Treatment of urinary tract infections during pregnancy. Clin Obstet Gynecol 13:480
Meria P, Anidjar M, Hermieu JF, Boccon-Gibod L (1993) Lithiase urinaire et grossesse. Prog Urol, 3:937
Middleton AW Jr, Middleton GW, Dean LK (1980) Spontaneous renal rupture in pregnancy. Urology 15:60
Miller RW (1995) Delayed effects of external radiation exposure: a brief history. Radiat Res 144:160
Muller-Suur R, Tyden O (1985) Evaluation of hydronephrosis in pregnancy using ultrasound and renography. Scand J Urol 19:267
Murthy LNS (1997) Urinary tract obstruction during pregnancy: recent developments in imaging. Br J Urol 80 [Suppl 1]:1
Naber KG, Bergman B, Bishop MC et al (2001) EAU guidelines for the management of urinary and male genital tract infections. Eur Urol 40:576
Oesterling JE, Besinger RE, Brendler CB (1988) Spontaneous rupture of the renal collecting system during pregnancy: successful management with a temporary ureteral catheter. J Urol 140:588
Ovalle A, Levancini M (2001) Urinary tract infections in pregnancy. Curr Opin Urol 11:55
Pastore LM, Savitz DA, Thorp JM Jr et al (1999a) Predictors of symptomatic urinary tract infection after 20 weeks' gestation. J Perinatol 19:488
Pastore LM, Savitz DA, Thorp JM Jr (1999b) Predictors of urinary tract infection at the first prenatal visit. Epidemiology 10:282
Patel SS, Balfour JA, Bryson HM (1997) Fosfomycin tromethamine: a review of its antibacterial activity, pharmacokinetic properties and therapeutic efficacy as single-dose oral treatment for acute uncomplicated lower urinary tract infection. Drugs 53:637
Pedersen H, Finster M (1979) Anaesthetic risk in the pregnant surgical patient. Anaethesiology 51:439
Price FV, Resnik E, Heller KA et al (1991) Placenta previa percreta involving the urinary bladder: a report of two cases and review of the literature. Obstet Gynecol 78:508
Puskar D, Balagovic I, Filipovic A et al (2001) Symptomatic physiologic hydronephrosis in pregnancy: incidence, complications, and treatment. Eur Urol 39:260
Rasanen J, Jouppila P (1995) Fetal cardiac function and ductus arteriosus during indomethacin and sulindac therapy for threatened preterm labor: a randomised study. Am J Obstet Gynecol 173:20
Rittenberg M, Bagley D (1988) Ureteroscopic diagnosis and treatment of urinary calculi during pregnancy. Urology 32:427
Roy C, Saussine A, Jahn C et al (1995) Fast imaging MR assessment of ureterohydronephrosis during pregnancy. Magn Reson Imaging 13:767
Saidi A, Delaporte V, Lechevallier E (2005) Problèmes urologiques rencontrés au cours de la grossesse. Prog Urol 15:1
Santos JFM et al (2002) Urinary tract infections in pregnant women. Int Urogynecol J 13:204
Santucci RA, Krieger JN (2000) Gentamicin for the praticing urologist: review of efficacy, singne daily dosing and "switch therapy". J Urol 163:1076
Scarpa RM, De Lisa A, Usai E (1996) Diagnosis and treatment of ureteral calculi during pregnancy with rigid ureteroscopes. J Urol 155:875
Shnider SM, Webster GM (1965) Maternal and fetal hazards of surgery during pregnancy. Am J Obstet Gynecol 92:891
Shokeir AA, Mutabagani H (1998) Rigid ureteroscopy in pregnant women. Br J Urol 81:678
Shokeir AA, Mahran MR, Abdulmaamoud A (2000) Renal colic in pregnant women: role of renal resistive index. Urology 55:344
Smith CS, Ferrara LP (1992) Placenta previa percreta with bladder invasion presenting as incarcerated hernia. Urology 29:371
Smith D, Graham JB, Prystowski JB et al (1992) The effects of ultrasound-guided shock waves early in pregnancy in Sprague-Dawley rats. J Urol 147:1197
Spencer JA (2000) Early report: comparison of breath-hold MR excretory urography, Doppler ultrasound and isotope renography in evaluation of symptomatic hydronephrosis in pregnancy. Clin Radiol 55:446
Stewart A (1973) The carcinogenic effects of low-level radiation: a reappraisal of epidemiologists, methods and observations. Health Phys 24:223
Stothers L, Lee LM (1992) Renal colic in pregnancy. J Urol 148:1383

Teichman JM, Champion PC, Wollin TA, Denstedt JD (1998a) Holmium: YAG lithotripsy of uric acid calculi. J Urol 160:2130

Teichman JM, Vassar GJ, Glickman RD et al (1998b) Holmium: YAG lithotripsy: photothermal mechanism converts uric acid calculi to cyanide. J Urol 160:320

Teo REC et al (1996) Placenta percreta involving urinary bladder. BJU 78:140

Ulrich J, York JP, Koff SA (1995) The renal vascular response to acutely elevated intrapelvic pressure: resistive index measurements in experimental urinary obstruction. J Urol 154:1202

Ulvik NM, Bakke A, Hoisaeter PA (1995) Ureteroscopy in pregnancy. J Urol 154:1660

Van Marter LJ, Leviton A, Allred EN et al (1996) Persistent pulmonary hypertension of the newborn and smoking and aspirin and nonsteroidal anti-inflammatory drug consumption during pregnancy. Pediatrics 97:658

Vest JM, Warden SS (1990) Ureteroscopic stone manipulation during pregnancy. Urology 35:250

Vieweg J, Weber HM, Miller K, Hautmann R (1992) Female fertility following extracorporeal shock wave lithotripsy of distal ureteral calculi. J Urol 148:1007

Wachsberg R (1998) Unilateral absence of ureteral jets in the third trimester of pregnancy: pitfall in color Doppler US diagnosis of urinary obstruction. Radiology 209:279

Washecka R, Behling A (2002) Urologic complications of placenta percreta invading the urinary bladder: a case report and review of the literature. Hawaii Med J 61:66

Watterson J et al (2002) Ureteroscopy and holmium: YAG laser lithotripsy: an emerging definitive management strategy for symptomatic ureteral calculi in pregnancy. Urology 60:683

Whitfield HN (1999) The management of ureteric stones. Part II: therapy. BJU Int 84:916

Wing DA, Hendershott CM, Dubuque L, Miller LK (1999) Outpatient treatment of acute pyelonephritis in pregnancy after 24 weeks. Obstet Gynecol 94:683

Wong J, Brown G (1996) Does once-daily dosing of aminoglycosides affect neuromuscular function? J Clin Pharm Ther 21:407

Zheng W, Denstedt J (2000) Intracorporeal lithotripsy. Urol Clin North Am 27:301

Zwergel T, Lindenmeyer T, Wullich B (1996) Management of acute hydronephrosis in pregnancy by ureteral stenting. Eur Urol 29:292

Urologic Emergencies in Children: Special Considerations

8

A. Cook, A.E. Koury

8.1 Introduction

Pediatric urologic emergencies fortunately remain rare occurrences within the emergency department of a hospital or ambulatory care center. More commonly, congenital anomalies noted at birth, or benign lesions that prompt significant parental anxiety (such as benign scrotal conditions), often result in a visit to the emergency department for evaluation. These urgencies nonetheless require both the appropriate investigations and management in order to allay patient and parental concern. The objective of this chapter is to therefore cover common emergent and urgent pediatric urologic consultations encountered from birth through childhood. Prenatal diagnoses and their respective management options (such as fetal obstructive uropathy) will not be considered, as they are beyond the scope of this chapter and do not necessarily reflect the typical urologic conditions encountered in the emergency department. The chapter will progress via an anatomical top-down approach, emphasizing various conditions from adrenal disorders to scrotal and testicular pathology.

8.2 Adrenal

8.2.1 CAH and Intersex

Although sexual ambiguity in the newborn can be a very distressing condition for the new parents of an affected child, investigations attempting to elucidate the underlying etiology for ambiguity must be undertaken rapidly in order to avoid potentially fatal complications. Intersexuality results from either the genital masculinization of a female fetus or the arrest thereof in a male during development. This usually occurs be-

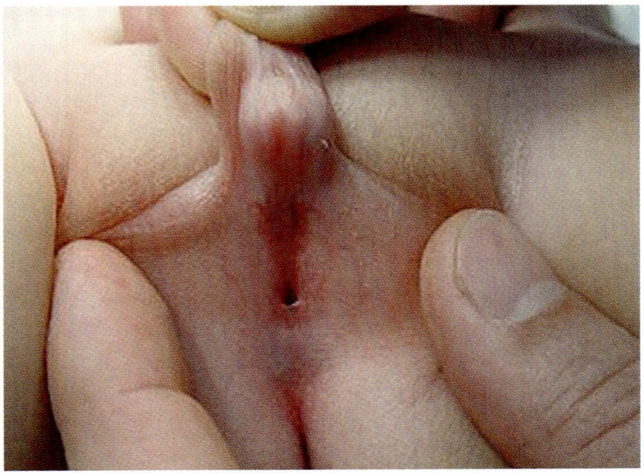

Fig. 8.1. Phenotypic appearance of a newborn 46, XX female with moderate virilization secondary to CAH

Table 8.1. Classification of intersex disorders

Category	Gonadal histology	Genotype	Phenotype
Female pseudohermaphroditism	Histologically normal ovaries	46, XX	Variable degrees of virilization
True hermaphroditism	Ovarian and testicular tissue	Variable, most commonly mosaic 46,XX/46,XY or 47,XXX/46XY	Variable appearance, depending on amount of viable testicular tissue
Male pseudohermaphroditism	Histologically normal testes	46, XY	Partial or complete failure of masculinization
Pure or mixed gonadal dysgenesis	Dysplastic gonads with abundant fibrous stroma	Usually both XY and XO cell lines	Variable appearance, depending on amount of viable testicular tissue

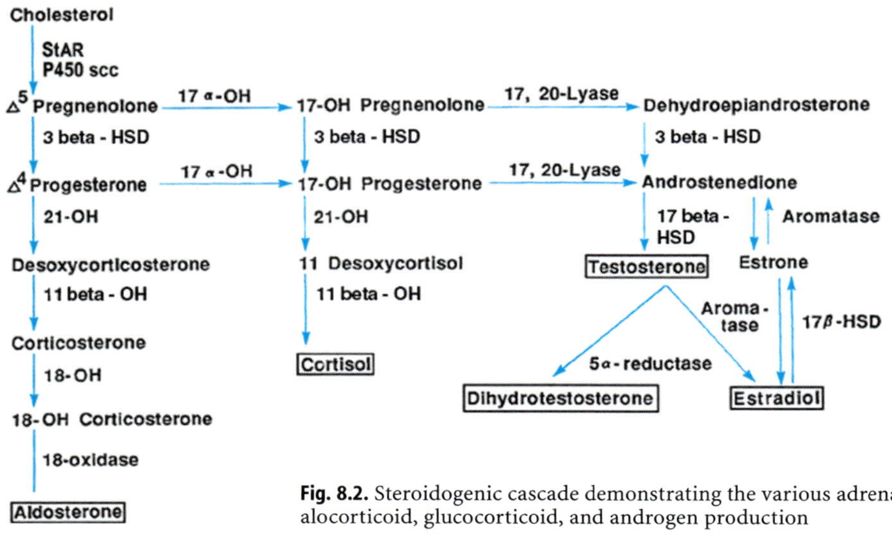

Fig. 8.2. Steroidogenic cascade demonstrating the various adrenal enzymes involved in mineralocorticoid, glucocorticoid, and androgen production

tween the 7th and 14th weeks of gestation and, depending on the underlying etiology, may have profound effects on the ultimate phenotypic appearance of the genitalia (Fig. 8.1).

Intersexuality is most conveniently classified according to gonadal histology. Four main categories have been identified that effectively enable the appropriate diagnosis and prognosis of these children with respect to sexual assignment, potential fertility as well as future gender identity (Table 8.1).

Congenital adrenal hyperplasia (CAH) is the most common underlying cause of sexual ambiguity and, if not recognized, may lead to death in the neonatal period. Although other causes of intersexuality, such as mixed gonadal dysgenesis or true hermaphroditism, may cause distress to the family in the newborn period secondary to inability to assign appropriate gender, only patients with CAH affected by the salt-wasting form represent a true urologic emergency. Consequently, the scope of this section will concentrate on the management of the infant with CAH, bearing in mind that the initial evaluation is similar for all infants with ambiguous genitalia.

CAH is caused by an inherited defect in cortisol metabolism occurring in 1 in 10,000 to 1 in 15,000 live births (Perry et al. 2005) (Fig. 8.2). Although numerous enzymatic defects have been identified, deficiencies in 21-hydroxylase account for more than 90% of cases (Forest 2004). Deficient 21-hydroxylase activity leads to an overproduction of the weak adrenal androgens, androstenedione and dehydroepiandrosterone, while preventing appropriate mineralocorticoid and glucocorticoid production. These weak androgens are subsequently converted to testosterone and dihydrotestosterone, resulting in virilization in the female fetus. The salt-wasting form affects two-thirds of CAH patients, where mineralocorticoid and glucocorticoid deficiencies lead to severe dehydration, hyponatremia, and hyperkalemia. This in turn can lead to fatal cardiac arrhythmias and hypovolemic shock (Lee and Donahoe 1997). If not recognized immediately postpartum, patients with the salt-wasting form typically present 7–10 days following birth with lethargy, poor feeding, vomiting, or even subsequent to near-miss SIDS episodes (Gassner et al. 2004).

Other potential causes of female pseudohermaphroditism include maternal ingestion of androgenic medications during pregnancy, placental aromatase deficiency, or, rarely, hormonally active maternal ovarian

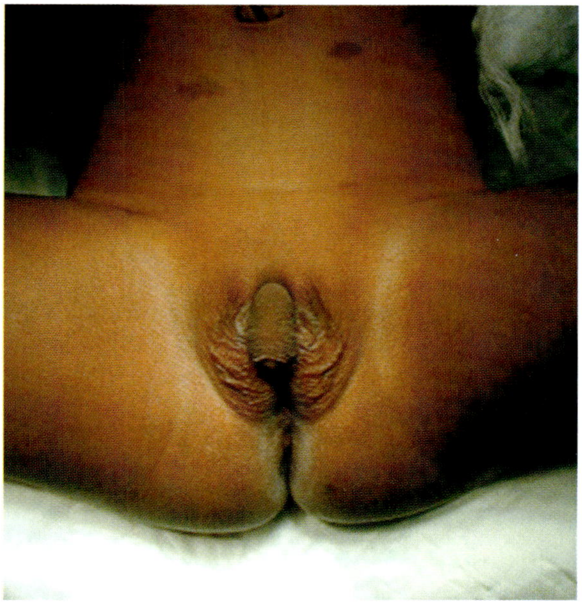

Fig. 8.3. Severe virilization of a 46, XX female with 21-hydroxylase deficiency. As do most CAH patients with significant virilization, this patient presented with the salt-wasting variety

or adrenal tumors (Ludwig et al. 1998; McClamrock and Adashi 1992). Therefore, a careful history, particularly ascertaining potential maternal drug exposure, is important for elucidating the potential underlying etiology for virilization. A family history of neonatal death or sexual ambiguity may also identify potential cases.

Acute resuscitative measures are obviously indicated for those infants presenting with signs of shock and dehydration. Physical examination will reveal various degrees of virilization, from mild clitoral hypertrophy, to a fully developed phallus, rugated scrotum and impalpable gonads (Fig. 8.3). In general, patients with salt-wasting tend to present with more severe virilization. Laboratory investigations are directed toward determining the underlying cause and typically include serum electrolytes, glucose, gonadotropin, testosterone, dihydrotestosterone, androstenedione, dehydroepiandrosterone, as well as chromosomal analysis. As the vast majority of females with CAH will harbor a defect in the 21-hydroxylase enzyme, they will demonstrate significantly elevated levels of that enzyme's substrate, namely 17-hydroxyprogesterone. If 17-hydroxyprogesterone levels are not elevated, other rare enzymatic defects may be present such as 11-betahydroxylase, 20,22-desmolase, or 3B-hydroxysteroid dehydrogenase (Dacou-Vouteakis et al. 2001).

Abdominal and pelvic ultrasound (US) is important to document the presence of a uterus and ovaries as well as rule-out any upper urinary tract anomalies. Furthermore, fluoroscopic genitography will demonstrate the confluence of the urogenital sinus, urethra,

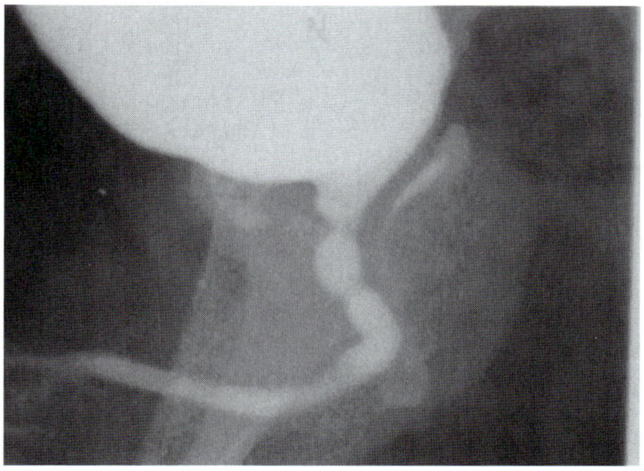

Fig. 8.4. Urogenital sinogram demonstrating the confluence of the vagina posteriorly and the anteriorly oriented urethra, bladder neck, and bladder

and vagina as well as assess for vesicoureteral reflux (Fig. 8.4).

These patients require lifelong mineralocorticoid and glucocorticoid replacement and their optimal management involves a multidisciplinary health care team consisting of pediatric urology, gynecology, endocrinology, genetics, as well as psychiatry and social work. As the vast majority with CAH can appropriately be reared as females (46, XX) with potential fertility, lifelong follow-up of these unique patients is imperative in order to address not only medical, but psychosocial issues as well, which may arise during growth into adulthood.

8.2.2 Adrenal Hemorrhage

Adrenal hemorrhage uncommonly presents as an adrenal mass. Most are incidentally discovered on imaging and are associated with birth trauma, neonatal asphyxia, septicemia, or coagulopathies. Expectant management and serial US are usually all that are required; however, pathologic jaundice may necessitate a course of phototherapy or even transfusion (Sherer et al. 1994). Subsequent adrenal insufficiency very rarely occurs and usually necessitates temporary steroid replacement only (Velaphi and Perlman 2001).

8.3 Kidney

8.3.1 Anomalies and Masses

A number of lesions (both of GU and non-GU origin) may present as a palpable abdominal mass in the infant or young child and require assessment in the emergen-

Table 8.2. Classification of palpable abdominal masses

Cystic renal lesions	Solid renal/ juxtarenal lesions	Midline lesions	Nongenitourinary lesions
Hydro-nephrosis	CMN	Urinary retention	Gastrointestinal duplications
Dilated upper-pole duplex	Neuro-blastoma	Renal ectopia	Hepatic lesions
MCDK	Wilms tumor	Urachal cyst	Pyloric stenosis
ADPKD	RCC	Ovarian cyst	Intestinal lymphatic malformations
ARPKD	Renal vein thrombosis	Hydrome-trocolpos	Omphalomesenteric remnants
Cystic nephroma	Adrenal hemorrhage	Teratoma	Mid-abdominal wall defects

MCDK multicystic dysplastic kidney, *ARPKD* autosomal recessive polycystic kidney disease, *ADPKD* autosomal dominant polycystic kidney disease, *CMN* congenital mesoblastic nephroma, *RCC* renal cell carcinoma

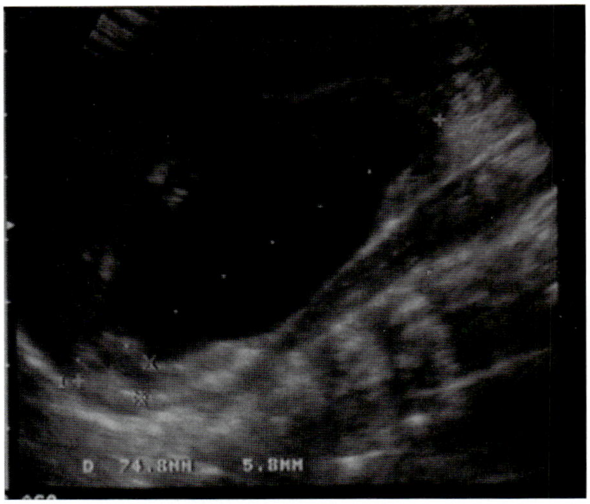

Fig. 8.5. Postnatal US demonstrating severe grade 4 hydronephrosis with parenchymal thinning. This patient underwent pyeloplasty at 6 weeks of age

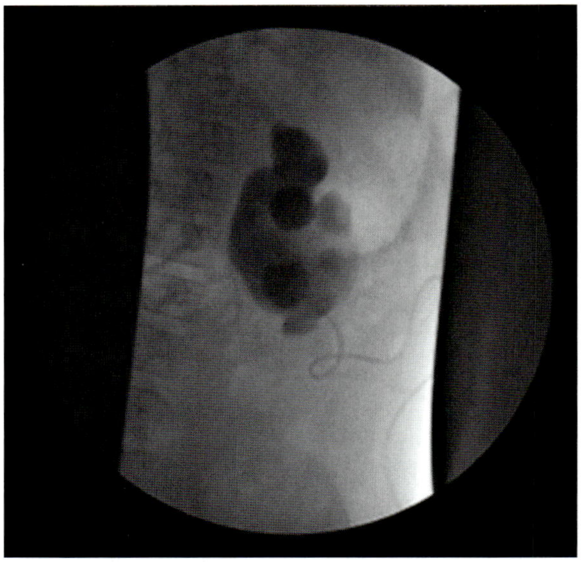

Fig. 8.6. Newborn male who presented with obstructive renal failure secondary to UPJ obstruction of a solitary kidney. Percutaneous nephrostomy was utilized as a temporizing measure and the patient subsequently underwent pyeloplasty at 3 weeks of age

cy department. Table 8.2 lists a broad spectrum of possible etiologies, categorized depending on their ultrasonographic appearance and location within the abdomen.

8.3.2 Cystic Renal Lesions

With the advent of antenatal ultrasonography, congenital anomalies, particularly of genitourinary (GU) origin, have become frequently identified during the prenatal period (Kim and Song 1996). Unilateral hydronephrosis secondary to UPJ obstruction and pelviectasis are the most common prenatally detected GU lesions, while severe hydronephrosis remains the most common cause of an abdominal mass in the neonate (Griscom et al. 1977) (Fig. 8.5). The vast majority can be managed conservatively and evaluated as outpatients in the urology clinic; however, infants with bilaterality (in up to 20%–40%) or obstruction in a functionally solitary kidney, may present with oliguria or even overt renal failure (Murphy et al. 1984). Occasionally, these infants require temporary urinary diversion (usually in the form of a percutaneous nephrostomy) in order to relieve the obstruction and to allow for the appropriate nephrourological evaluation (Fig. 8.6).

Nuclear medicine renography and voiding cystourethrography are necessary investigations to document differential renal function and assess the degree of obstruction as well as rule out lower urinary tract anomalies such as vesicoureteral reflux (VUR) or posterior urethral valves (PUV). Antibiotic prophylaxis (trimethoprim 2 mg/kg once daily) is continued until VUR or obstruction is excluded. Early pyeloplasty for those with documented obstruction and preserved function has been shown to be safe and effective even in the very young (King et al. 1984). Controversy persists regarding potential recovery in poorly functioning kidneys, with some authors documenting improved function following pyeloplasty (particularly in patients less than 6 months of age) and others showing little or even no improvement (Shokeir et al. 2005; MacNeily et al. 1993).

Multicystic dysplastic kidney (MCDK) is the second most common cause of a palpable abdominal mass in infants (Pathak and Williams 1964). It consists of multi-

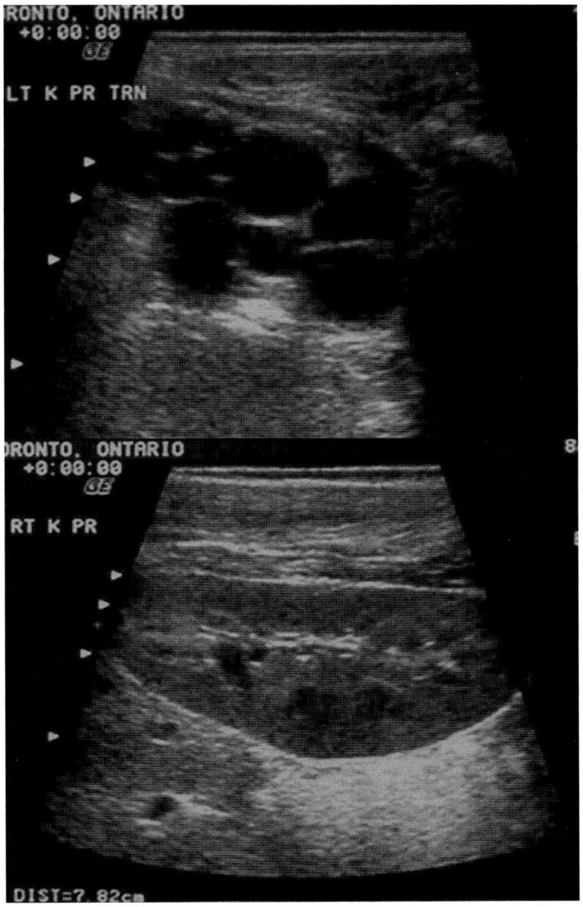

Fig. 8.7. US demonstrating typical cluster-of-grapes appearance of left-sided MCDK consisting of a number of noncommunicating cysts separated by sparse, dysplastic parenchyma. The contralateral normal kidney demonstrates compensatory hypertrophy

ple cysts of varying sizes separated by scant dysplastic parenchyma. It is usually secondary to ureteral atresia and can be visualized as a number of noncommunicating cysts or "cluster of grapes" on US (Fig. 8.7). Occasionally an infant with a very large MCDK may present with either respiratory or gastrointestinal compromise due to diaphragmatic or gastric compression, respectively. The diagnosis of MCDK mandates a complete GU evaluation because of the high incidence of contralateral abnormalities, including UPJ obstruction and VUR. Dimercaptosuccinic acid (DMSA) scanning will document no function on the affected side and VCUG will demonstrate VUR in up to 26% (Miller et al. 2004).

Contemporary management of children with MCDK consists of serial ultrasonography, physical examination, and blood pressure determinations. Over 50% of MCDK involute over the first 5 years of life, although it may take up to 20 years for others to completely regress (Rabelo et al. 2004). The remainder usually remain stable on follow-up; however, a minority increase in size (Oliveira et al. 2001). Both hypertension and malignant deterioration have shown very weak associations with MCDK; most investigators currently believe that these weak associations should not prompt the use of routine prophylactic nephrectomy for MCDK in an otherwise healthy child. However, nephrectomy is warranted for children who present with symptoms secondary to mass effect, enlargement suspicious for cancer, pain, infection, or documented renin-mediated hypertension (Kuwertz-Broeking et al. 2004).

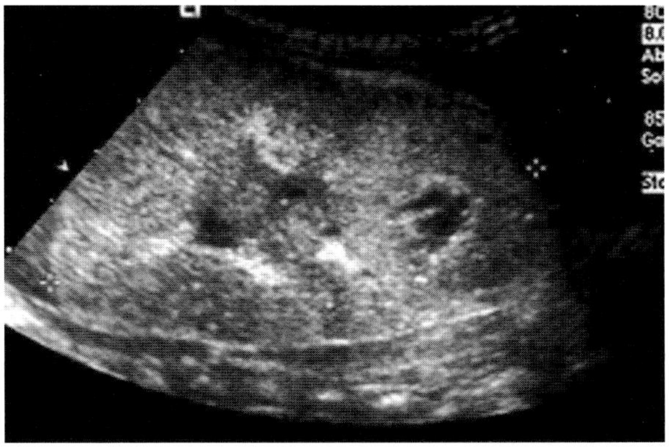

Fig. 8.8. Postnatal US of a newborn boy with ARPKD. Note the enlarged, hyperechoic kidney secondary to innumerable microscopic cysts. This patient died within the 1st week of life due to pulmonary hypoplasia

Although bilateral renal enlargement in the neonatal period is most commonly caused by bilateral UPJ obstruction, renal cystic disease is also responsible for a number of children presenting with massive abdominal distension. Autosomal recessive polycystic kidney disease (ARPKD) is a rare disorder with an overall incidence of 1 in 40,000; children typically present with massively enlarged hyperechoic kidneys on prenatal and postnatal US (Zerres et al. 1998) (Fig. 8.8). Oligohydramnios leads to significant morbidity such as pulmonary hypoplasia, limb defects, and even Potter's facies. Hepatic fibrosis has also been associated with ARPKD and was previously thought to be inversely proportional to the degree of renal impairment (Landing et al. 1980). However, it has since been realized that both hepatic and renal involvement occur essentially independently of each other (Gagnadoux et al. 1989). The prognosis is generally poor, children surviving beyond the neonatal period universally require some form of renal replacement therapy (Cole et al. 1987).

Although autosomal dominant polycystic kidney disease (ADPK) has a much higher incidence in the general population (1 in 500–1,000), it is usually first identified in older individuals on screening US (resulting from family history) or in those with hypertension, impaired renal function, proteinuria, or hematuria (Papadopoulou et al. 1999). However, when affected, infants usually present with massive renomegaly similar to ARPKD. Severely affected infants have poor prognoses; although associated anomalies, such as hepatic and pancreatic cysts, mitral valve prolapse and cerebral aneurysms, may manifest at any time throughout childhood (Ivy et al. 1995). Gradual replacement and destruction of renal parenchyma by growing cysts eventually leads to renal failure in the majority by the 6th–7th decades of life (Badani et al. 2004).

8.3.3 Solid Renal and Juxtarenal Lesions

The majority of solid renal or juxtarenal lesions present either prenatally or as a palpable abdominal mass in childhood. The most common renal tumor in the neonate remains congenital mesoblastic nephroma (CMN). More than 80% are diagnosed in the 1st month of life and essentially all are identified by 1 year of age (Geller et al. 1997). CMN usually presents as an asymptomatic abdominal mass; however, prenatal US has also demonstrated polyhydramnios, fetal hydrops, and premature delivery in affected fetuses (Lowe et al. 2000). CMN is believed to consist of a proliferation in metanephric mesenchyme and appears leiomyomatous on gross pathological analysis. Cross-sectional imaging is mandatory and demonstrates a solid intrarenal mass that may contain cystic, hemorrhagic, and necrotic regions (Fig. 8.9). Although benign in greater than 95% of cases, complete surgical excision is necessary as local recurrence, and even metastases, have been reported (Heidelberger et al. 1993). Significant hemorrhage or spontaneous tumor rupture may mandate urgent nephrectomy (Matsumura et al. 1993; Arensman and Belman 1980).

Neuroblastoma is the most common solid extracranial malignancy in childhood. It arises from primitive sympathetic nerve cells and may occur anywhere sympathetic tissue is found. However, over 75% are intraabdominal, with 65% of these arising from the adrenal glands (Chandler and Gauderer 2004). Neuroblastoma is an unusual tumor characterized by its variability in presentation. Well-advanced lesions may regress spontaneously, whereas others may progress despite aggressive therapy.

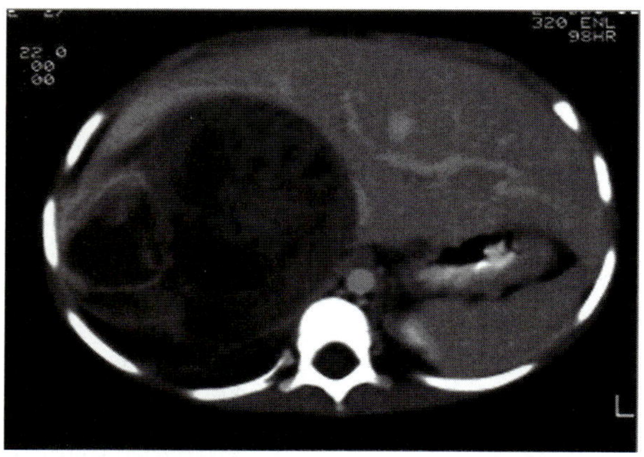

Fig. 8.9. CT of a large right palpable renal mass found in a newborn female. Nephrectomy was carried out and the tumor was identified as congenital mesoblastic nephroma (CMN)

Because of their biologically active nature, neuroblastomas may secrete a significant amount of catecholamines and hence, patients may present with palpitations, tachycardia, hypertension, flushing, and sweating. Intractable diarrhea may result from the secretion of vasoactive intestinal peptide (VIP) (Gesundheit et al. 2004). Another unusual symptom is cerebellar ataxia and opsomyoclonus (dancing feet, dancing eyes; myoclonic encephalopathy of infants). This syndrome is rare, of unknown etiology, and is usually associated with thoracic lesions (Bousvaros et al. 1986). Malaise, pain, and anemia may be the presenting complaint in up to 60% secondary to metastatic disease.

Physical examination classically reveals a firm, fixed lesion that is nodular to palpation and may cross the midline (Fig. 8.10). Children with neuroblastoma typically look unwell, are pale and cachectic compared to their rather robust appearing counterparts with Wilms tumor. Other differentiating features are summarized in Table 8.3. Investigations include cross-sectional imaging, complete blood work, serum and urine catecholamine levels including vanillylmandelic acid (VMA) and metanephrines, and bone marrow cytopathology. Surgical resection is the primary treatment for those with localized disease. Adjuvant chemotherapy and radiotherapy is added depending on disease stage and patient age. Overall, the prognosis is good; however, those with advanced disease tend to do poorly despite aggressive multimodal therapy (Haase et al. 1999).

Wilms tumor is the most common pediatric malignancy of renal origin, accounting for nearly 90% of renal masses (Lowe et al. 2000). It typically presents between the 3rd and 4th year of life and over 80% are diag-

Table 8.3. Characteristics of Wilms tumor and neuroblastoma

	Wilms Tumor	Neuroblastoma
Typical age at presentation	3–4 years of age	50% less than 1 year
Clinical appearance	Robust, healthy	Pale, anemic, cachectic, signs/symptoms of metastatic disease
Physical examination	Smooth mass does not cross midline	Nodular, craggy mass, crosses midline
Imaging	Intrarenal, compresses adjacent parenchyma, stippled calcification in 50%	Extrarenal, displaces kidney

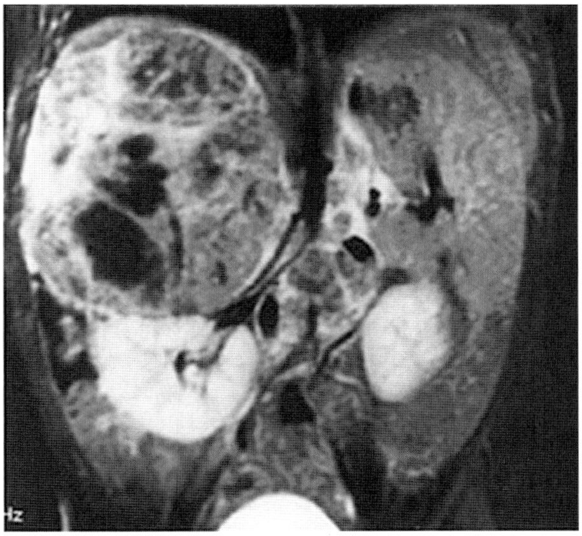

Fig. 8.10. MRI of a large right adrenal neuroblastoma found in a 2-year-old boy who presented with malaise, lethargy, and a large palpable abdominal mass

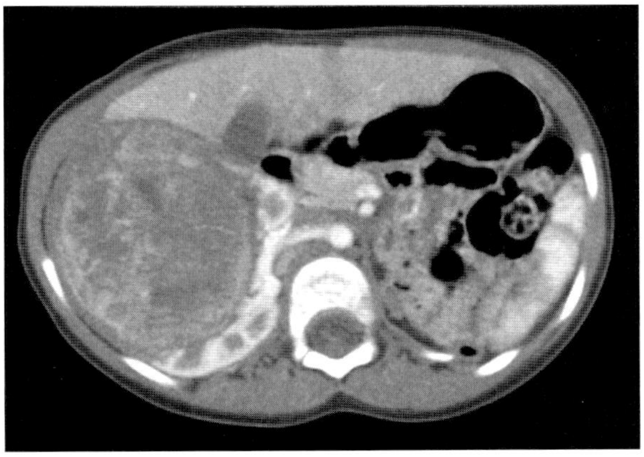

Fig. 8.11. CT of a large right intrarenal mass found to be Wilms tumor on pathological analysis in a 3-year-old female. Note the compression and distortion of the surrounding normal parenchyma by the tumor

nosed prior to 5 years of age (Lonergan et al. 1998). Synchronous or metachronous bilaterality occurs in 4%–13% (Lonergan et al. 1998). A number of associated conditions have been identified, including cryptorchidism, hemihypertrophy, hypospadias, and sporadic aniridia (White and Grossman 1991). Other congenital disorders have also been implicated such as WAGR syndrome, Beckwith-Wiedemann syndrome, Denys-Drash syndrome, and neurofibromatosis (Bove 1999). These syndromes primarily result in somatic overgrowth and it is believed that abnormalities at two genetic loci, WT1 at *11p13* and WT2 at *11p15*, are responsible for Wilms tumor development in these syndromes (Coppes et al. 1994; Ping et al. 1989).

Wilms tumor most commonly initially manifests as an asymptomatic abdominal mass; however, associated coincidental trauma is present in up to 10% (Lonergan et al. 1998). Other signs and symptoms include abdominal pain, gross hematuria and fever. Tumor rupture causing severe abdominal pain and hemodynamic instability secondary to intraperitoneal hemorrhage has been reported in up to 3% (Godzinski et al. 2001). Atypical presentations such as varicocele, hepatomegaly, ascites, and congestive heart failure can occur in 10% secondary to renal vein and inferior vena cava tumor extension (Ritchey et al. 1988). Acquired von Willebrand disease has been identified in 8% of cases (Coppes et al. 1992).

Appropriate metastatic evaluation includes complete blood work as well as cross-sectional imaging including the thorax. CT or MRI usually reveals a large intrarenal mass with a pseudocapsule and distortion of the renal parenchyma and collecting system (Fig. 8.11). The majority of children with unilateral disease can safely undergo radical nephrectomy; subsequent adjuvant therapy is based on specific tumor stage and subtype. Bilaterality or tumor in a solitary kidney is initially treated by needle biopsy and neoadjuvant chemotherapy (Fig. 8.12 a, b). This usually results in signifi-

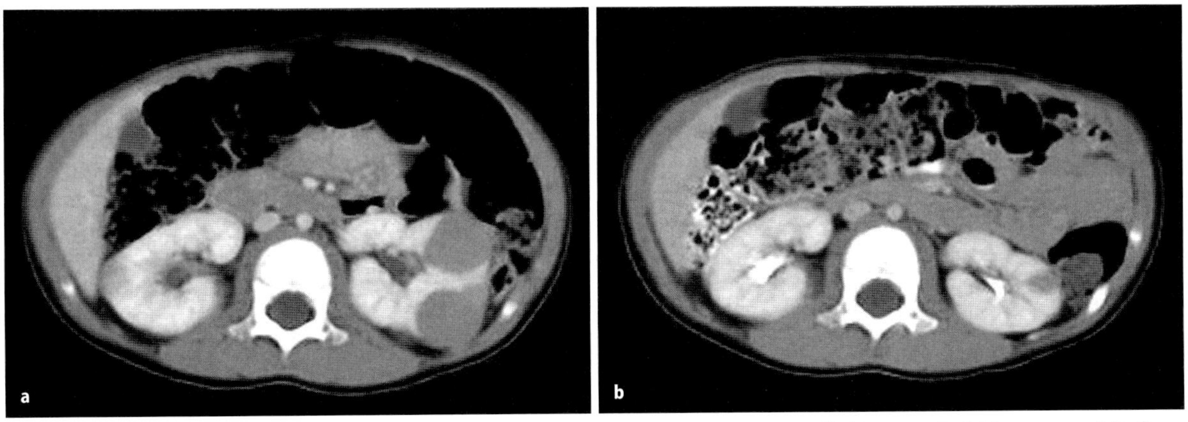

Fig. 8.12. a CT demonstrating multiple bilateral renal masses found on percutaneous needle biopsy to be Wilms tumor. **b** Follow-up CT in same patient after three courses of actinomycin-, vincristine-, and doxorubicin-based chemotherapy

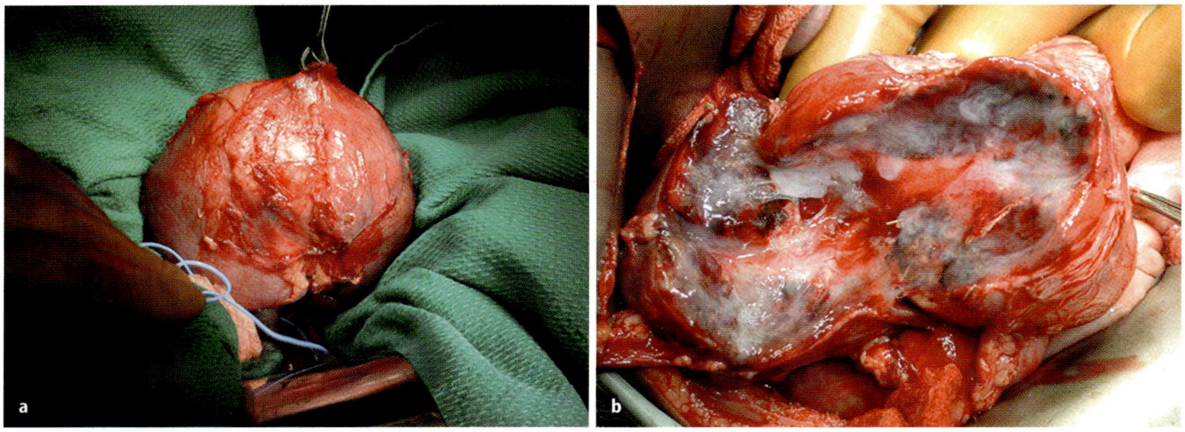

Fig. 8.13. a Intraoperative photograph of a large central Wilms tumor in a 4-year-old girl with a solitary right kidney. **b** Intraoperative photograph in the same patient following tumor resection prior to reconstruction of the renal parenchyma. Note the tumor bed with Tissel gel to aid in hemostasis

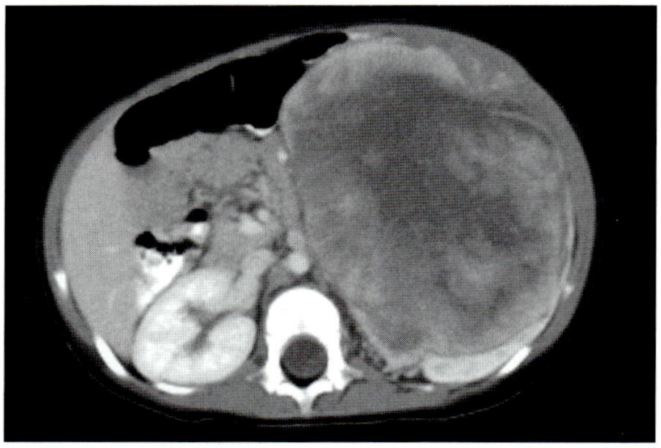

Fig. 8.14. CT of a very large left renal mass in a 9-year-old boy. The patient underwent radical nephrectomy; pathological analysis demonstrated clear cell renal cell carcinoma (RCC)

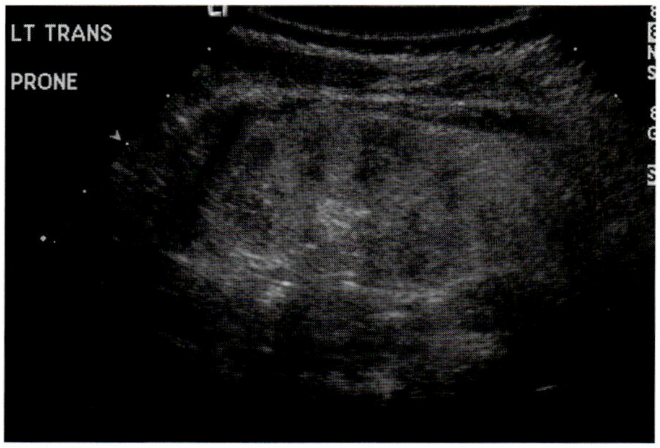

Fig. 8.15. US of a newborn female who presented with gross hematuria showing left RVT. Note the hyperechoic clot in the renal vein located in the renal sinus

cant tumor shrinkage, enabling a subsequent nephron-sparing approach in the majority (Fig. 8.13 a, b).

Renal cell carcinoma (RCC) is rare in the pediatric population, accounting for only 7% of all primary renal tumors in the first 2 decades of life (Lack et al. 1985). It is associated with von Hippel-Lindau syndrome and this disease must be ruled-out in patients presenting with RCC in the pediatric age group. Children with RCC tend to present later in life and are more apt to manifest signs and symptoms of disease. At the Hospital for Sick Children in Toronto, Canada, review of 15 patients treated over a 25-year period revealed the mean age at presentation to be over 7 years and that nearly 75% presented with signs or symptoms of disease such as gross hematuria, abdominal pain, or polycythemia. CT demonstrates a typical enhancing renal mass (Fig. 8.14). Treatment is similar to adults, with radical extirpative surgery providing the best outcomes.

Renal vein thrombosis is rarely responsible for a palpable abdominal mass in the neonate. Venous thrombosis leads to vascular congestion and enlargement of the kidney and is marked clinically by hematuria, proteinuria, hypertension, and consumptive thrombocytopenia. It is associated with dehydration, sepsis, maternal diabetes, birth asphyxia, and coagulopathies (Lowe et al. 2000). Doppler US is the best imaging modality, as it can demonstrate renal vein and vena cava extension (Fig. 8.15). Unilateral disease is best treated conservatively, with rehydration and correction of predisposing factors; however, bilateral thrombosis requires more aggressive treatment such as systemic anticoagulation or thrombolysis and is associated with a worse prognosis (Nuss et al. 1994).

8.3.4 Pyelonephritis and Pyonephrosis

Urinary tract infection (UTI) occurs in approximately 8% of girls and 6% of boys during their first 6 years of life (Marild and Jodal 1998). Although older patients

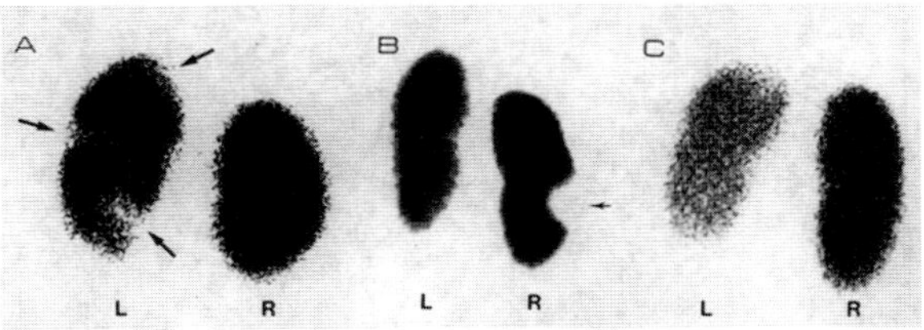

Fig. 8.16a–c. DMSA scan showing multiple photopenic areas consistent with renal scars (Courtesy H.G. Rushton)

may complain of irritative voiding symptoms and thus direct clinical suspicion to the urinary tract, infants and neonates may present with only nonspecific symptoms such as poor feeding, irritability, and failure to thrive. Therefore, urinalysis and urine culture are necessary investigations during the septic workup of all infants presenting with fever of unknown origin.

Although VCUG and renal US are necessary investigations that must be performed following the diagnosis and treatment of UTI in children, controversy persists regarding the utility of nuclear medicine renography to diagnose acute pyelonephritis. In general, most investigators believe that dimercaptosuccinic acid (DMSA) scanning could be safely omitted in children with mild to moderate infection; however, patients with signs of upper urinary tract infection, including high fever (>38.5 °C), flank pain, or abnormalities detected on US, should undergo renography (Naber et al. 2001; Deshpande and Jones 2001) (Fig. 8.16). Not only will this act as a baseline, but also acute photopenic areas detected on DMSA can be subsequently reevaluated in order to determine if renal scarring has occurred.

Uncomplicated lower-tract infection may be treated with trimethoprim-sulfamethoxazole, nitrofurantoin, or oral cephalosporins. Physicians, in general, are most comfortable with a 7-day course; however, studies demonstrating equipoise with as little as 3 days of therapy have been reported (Ruberto et al. 1989). Older children with acute pyelonephritis may also be treated as outpatients with oral antimicrobial therapy as long as they do not demonstrate signs of sepsis and can tolerate PO fluids. However, young children and those with signs of systemic illness require aggressive rehydration and parenteral broad-spectrum antibiotic therapy. Until the results of both urine and blood cultures are available to help direct specific antibiotic therapy, intravenous ampicillin and an aminoglycoside are commonly utilized synergistic antibiotics. Third-generation cephalosporins are also used; however, they are more expensive and tend to have more limited Gram-positive bactericidal coverage. Out-patient oral therapy can be instituted following 24–48 h of remaining afebrile; however, a full 10- to 14-day course of therapy is recommended (Bloomfield et al. 2005).

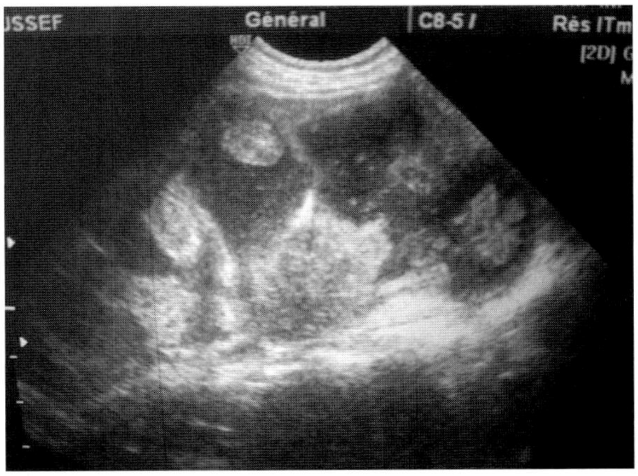

Fig. 8.17. US demonstrating right pyonephrosis in a patient who initially presented with symptoms of a lower urinary tract infection. The patient become acutely septic 5 days following antibiotic treatment and complained of abdominal and flank pain associated with a high fever

Children who remain febrile or appear toxic despite appropriate antibiotic therapy should undergo renal US as a first-line test in order to rule out renal abscess or obstructive uropathy. If necessary, CT can then be utilized in order to more accurately visualize the upper tracts as well as other abdominal viscera. Review of urine and blood culture results is important to document the presence of resistant organisms. Temporary percutaneous nephrostomy drainage is indicated in patients with ongoing signs of septicemia and evidence of pyonephrosis on US (Fig. 8.17).

Fungus (particularly *Candida* species) is a common cause of UTI among neonates in an intensive care unit (Philipps et al. 1997). It can range from simple isolated candiduria to pyonephrosis and obstructive uropathy secondary to fungus balls. Risk factors for candidal UTI include low birth weight, prematurity, indwelling central venous catheters, concomitant broad-spectrum antibiotic therapy, intravenous lipids, corticosteroids, and parenteral nutrition (Benjamin et al. 1999). Diagnosis is usually made following fungal culture of urine and renal US, which typically demonstrates hyperechoic debris in the collecting system (Fig. 8.18). Most recommend a course of amphotericin B as first-line treatment of candidal UTI; uncomplicated fungal UTI may be treated with a 7-day course, while renal candidiasis requires long-term therapy (up to 60 days) (Rowen and Tate 1998). Prompt diagnosis and aggressive systemic antifungal therapy has resulted in not only improved outcomes, but also a significant decrease in the incidence of obstructive uropathy secondary to fungus balls (Bryant et al. 1999). However, infants with evidence of obstruction and abscess formation associated with renal candidiasis require prompt percutaneous drainage in order to decrease morbidity and mortality from systemic candidiasis.

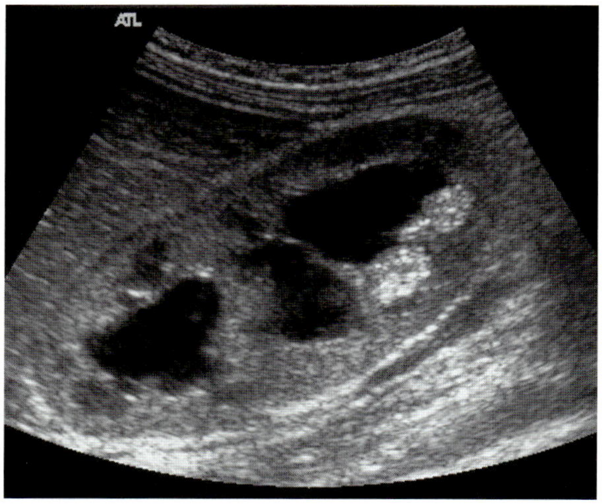

Fig. 8.18. US showing hyperechoic fungal debris in the collecting system of the lower pole of the right kidney

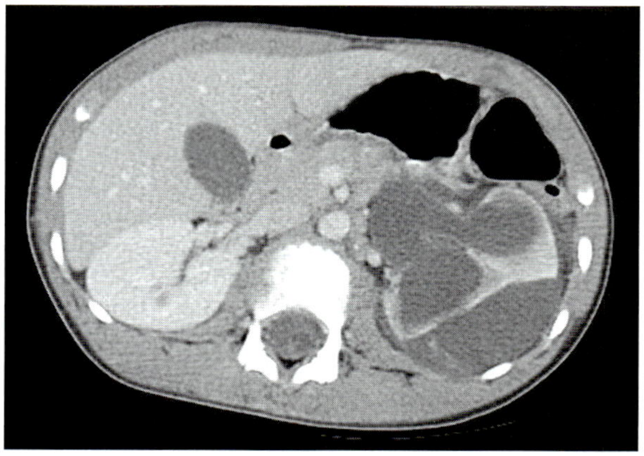

Fig. 8.19. Delayed CT with intravenous contrast demonstrating a large perinephric urinoma in an 8-year-old boy who presented to hospital with gross hematuria following a fall. Note the thinned parenchyma and severe hydronephrosis consistent with chronic obstruction

8.3.5 Trauma

The kidney is the most commonly injured organ following abdominal trauma. Children in particular are at an increased risk of renal injury due to several unique anatomical features of the pediatric axial skeleton and surrounding soft tissue. These include the less well-developed and ossified ribcage as well as decreased perirenal fat and smaller paraspinal and abdominal muscles. These features all contribute to the increased susceptibility to renal trauma in the pediatric patient (McAleer et al. 2002b). Furthermore, preexisting congenital renal anomalies can also predispose to injury (Miller et al. 1966; McAleer et al. 2002a). Approximately 10%–12% of renal injuries in children are associated with some preexisting renal anomaly (Chopra et al. 2002). All children who present with a clinical suspicion of a renal injury following seemingly trivial trauma should be suspected of harboring some underlying abnormality. Ureteropelvic junction (UPJ) disruption is also rather unique in children. The UPJ is particularly vulnerable in children secondary to increased flexion of the spine and mobility of the kidney associated with rapid deceleration (Fig. 8.19).

The vast majority of renal injuries in children are due to blunt trauma secondary to motor-vehicle collisions, falls, or sports-related injuries. The most popular grading system utilized in pediatric renal trauma is that proposed by the American Association for the Surgery of Trauma (Table 8.4). It is also used in adults and has been validated to have good prognostic value (Kansas et al. 2004). Radiological evaluation typically involves contrast-enhanced CT scanning, which enables a rapid assessment of the upper urinary tract as well as intraabdominal viscera to rule out associated injuries (Fig. 8.20).

Table 8.4. American Association for the Surgery of Trauma Renal Injury Grading System

Grade[a]	Renal injury
1	No laceration, contusion or nonexpanding subcapsular hematoma
2	Cortical laceration <1 cm without evidence of urinary extravasation
	Nonexpanding perirenal hematoma
3	Cortical laceration >1 cm without evidence of urinary extravasation
4	Laceration extending through corticomedullary junction into collecting system
	Segmental renal vascular injury with contained hematoma
5	Shattered kidney Renal pedicle injury or avulsion

[a] Advance one grade for bilateral injuries up to grade III

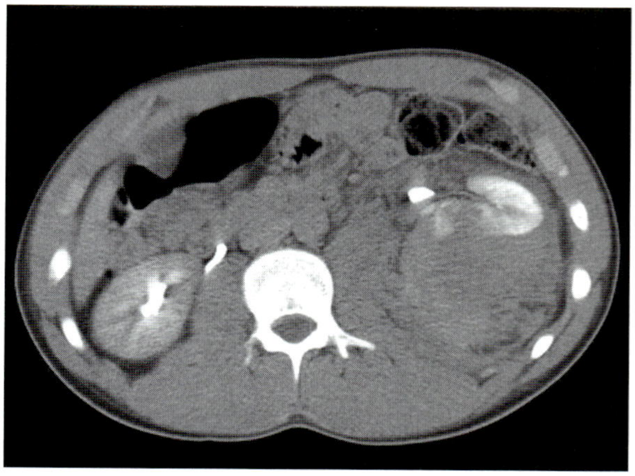

Fig. 8.20. Abdominal CT scan demonstrating grade 4 left blunt renal injury secondary to a snowboarding fall in a 12-year-old boy. This patient was successfully managed conservatively

The initial assessment of children presenting with renal trauma involves the rapid ascertainment of hemodynamic stability and evaluation to determine those who require emergent operative exploration. The indications for surgery are similar to that in adults, that is, ongoing hemodynamic instability, a pulsatile or expanding retroperitoneal hematoma, or, with rare exceptions, penetrating trauma. Relative indications include urinary extravasation, nonviable tissue, arterial injury, or incomplete staging.

Classically, all hemodynamically stable patients with a clinical suspicion of renal trauma underwent cross-sectional imaging. However, large outcome series have recently demonstrated that, depending on the degree of microhematuria and the nature of the injury, not all children with renal trauma require imaging (Buckley and McAninch 2004) Buckley and McAninch, in an expansive series of pediatric renal injuries, only recommend imaging if the urinalysis shows more than 50 red blood cells (RBC) per high power field (HPF) for those with a history of blunt trauma, or more than 5 RBC/HPF in those with penetrating renal trauma (Fig. 8.21). In their series, the majority of significant renal injuries (i.e., grade 2) were identified using these RBC/HPF values and no adverse sequelae occurred in patients for whom imaging was omitted (Buckley and McAninch 2004).

A nonoperative approach is also indicated for select patients with high-grade renal injuries. Recent reports have concluded that the majority of hemodynamically stable patients with grade IV injuries will not experience adverse outcomes nor suffer significant renal functional deterioration following a conservative management approach (Keller et al. 2004; Nance et al. 2004). An initial trial of bedrest, urethral catheter drainage, and serial hematology is thus warranted in most stable patients with high-grade injuries. Ambulation is subsequently undertaken following resolution of hematuria and documentation of stable hemoglobin levels. Patients with complete renal fracture or significant contrast extravasation may benefit from temporary upper tract urinary diversion in order to prevent urinoma formation (Rogers et al. 2004). Patients who fail conservative management usually present with ongoing hemorrhage secondary to an expanding hematoma requiring transfusion, persistent urinary extravasation despite upper tract diversion, or abdominal and flank pain.

Occasionally, controversy occurs when a pediatric patient presents following trauma whose parents are members of Jehovah's Witnesses and therefore refuse all blood products. Although this is fortunately a rare occurrence, the situation must be recognized early, and the appropriate safeguards obtained, so as not to compromise patient care. One must be cognizant and respectful of that patient's family's choice that the use of blood products is absolutely condemned within their religious belief system. Therefore, all possible attempts must be made by medical staff in order to prevent the need for transfusion. The early involvement of an expert hematologist will aid in the decision to use hemoglobin substitutes and various colloid and crystalloid fluid expanders, as necessary. However, in the event that a pediatric patient requires blood or blood products as the only life-saving alternative, a court injunction may be granted in order to temporarily award custody of the child to the state. Most hospitals and jurisdictions will have a senior administrator and judiciary official on call in order to facilitate this process in the event of such an emergency.

8.3.6 Calculi

Children with urinary tract calculi present for evaluation with similar signs and symptoms as do their adult counterparts. It was previously thought that pediatric urolithiasis was unique and distinct from adult urolithiasis; however, it has become clear that the two entities share many basic characteristics. One important dis-

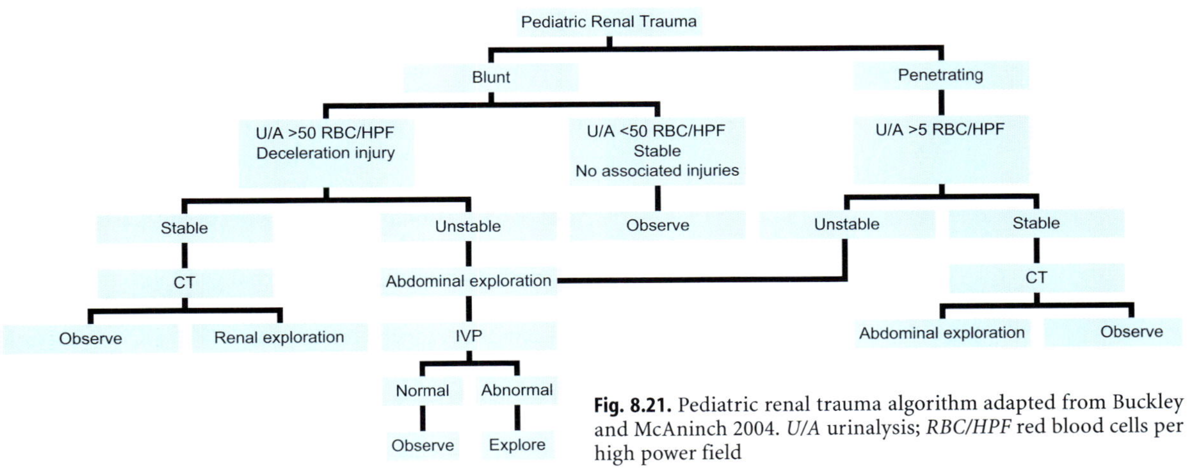

Fig. 8.21. Pediatric renal trauma algorithm adapted from Buckley and McAninch 2004. *U/A* urinalysis; *RBC/HPF* red blood cells per high power field

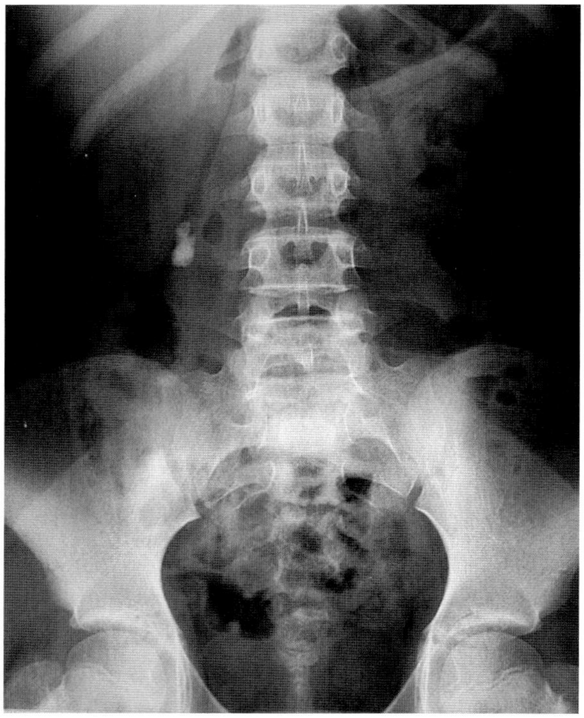

Fig. 8.22. Plain film radiograph of a 12-year-old male cystinuric patient with a history of gross hematuria and intermittent right flank pain

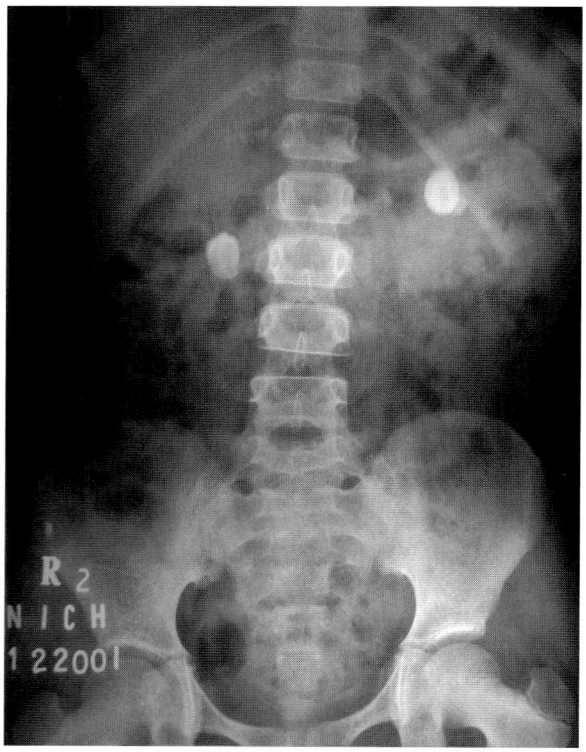

Fig. 8.23. Plain film radiograph demonstrating large, bilateral renal pelvic calculi. This patient successfully underwent staged bilateral ESWL

tinction between the two is that children are much more likely to harbor some underlying metabolic or enzymatic defect as the etiology for their stone disease (Milliner and Murphy 1993) (Fig. 8.22). Therefore, all children who present with urinary calculi require a complete metabolic evaluation following the resolution and treatment of the acute stone episode. The surgical treatment of pediatric urolithiasis consists of the same endourological practices and techniques that originated in adults. ESWL is very effective for even larger intrarenal and proximal ureteral calculi (Pearle 2003) (Fig. 8.23). With advancements in technology and miniaturization of endoscopes, when indicated, virtually every child can undergo ureteroscopic evaluation and intracorporeal laser lithotripsy (Tan et al. 2005).

8.4 Bladder

8.4.1 Exstrophy

Bladder exstrophy represents one of the most significant neonatal urologic anomalies a family may face. It has an overall incidence of 1 in 50,000 births and occurs in a 3–6:1 male to female ratio (Engel 1974; Ives et al. 1980). Cloacal exstrophy occurs even more rarely, with a reported incidence of up to 1 in 400,000(Engel 1974). However, the incidence appears to be decreasing as more and more patients are being diagnosed prenatally with subsequent parental termination of pregnancy. A number of prenatal ultrasonographic features have been found that correlate with exstrophy in the newborn, including an absent bladder, lower abdominal protrusion, an anteriorly displaced scrotum and small phallus in males, a low-set umbilicus, and pubic diastasis and iliac crest widening (Gearhart et al. 1995). Nonetheless, the majority of infants born with bladder exstrophy are not identified prenatally and still only present in the newborn period (Skari et al. 1998). Therefore it is incumbent on the physician to recognize this rare anomaly and treat these unique patients in an efficient and effective manner.

Typically, infants with classic bladder exstrophy present following birth and, apart from the exstrophic bladder, are usually healthy and robust. The abdominal wall defect and exstrophic bladder are obvious, as is the epispadiac penis and pubic diastasis (Fig. 8.24). Females look similar to their male counterparts with respect to the abdominal wall defect and boney pelvic anomalies; however, the external genitalia characteristically demonstrate a bifid clitoris and anterior displacement of the vaginal introitus (Fig. 8.25). Although infants with classic bladder exstrophy rarely have any other underlying congenital anomalies, in contrast, most children with cloacal exstrophy harbor a number of other associated abnormalities (Diamond and Jeffs

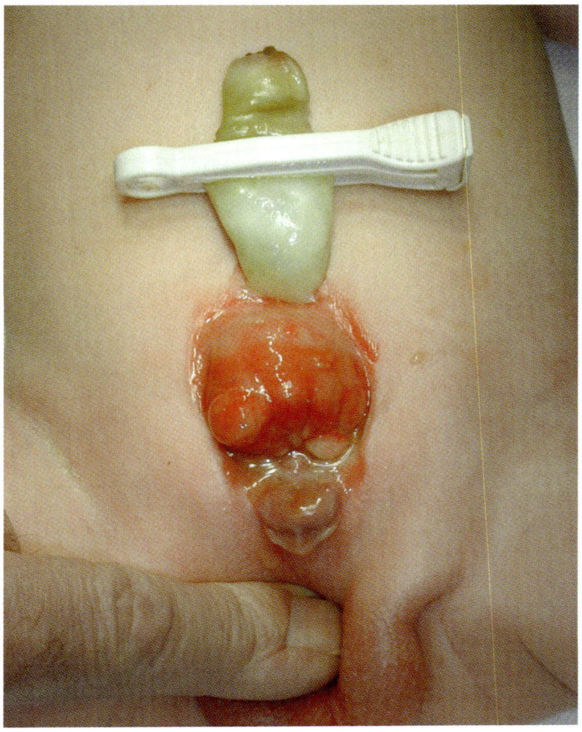

Fig. 8.24. Newborn male with classic bladder exstrophy. The exstrophic bladder, epispadiac penis, and pubic diastasis are clearly visible

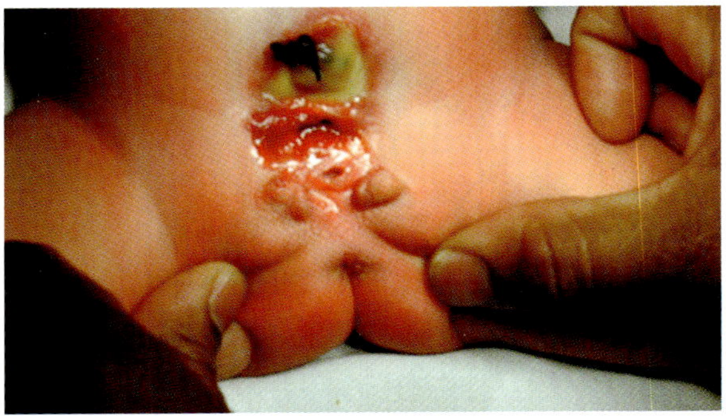

Fig. 8.25. Newborn female with classic bladder exstrophy. Note the bifid clitoris and anteriorly displaced vaginal introitus

1985) (Fig. 8.26). Appropriate screening investigations, such as echocardiography, abdominal and spinal US, as well as complete blood work, will aid in the identification of concomitant congenital defects.

Parental psychosocial support is paramount in the management of exstrophy patients. Detailed explanations regarding the disease process and surgical plan for closure as well as allaying any feelings of blame or guilt parents routinely harbor for having a child with exstrophy, are very important to maximize the initial and long-term health outcomes of the child and family. Initially, the umbilical stump is suture-ligated at the level of the abdominal wall and the plastic umbilical

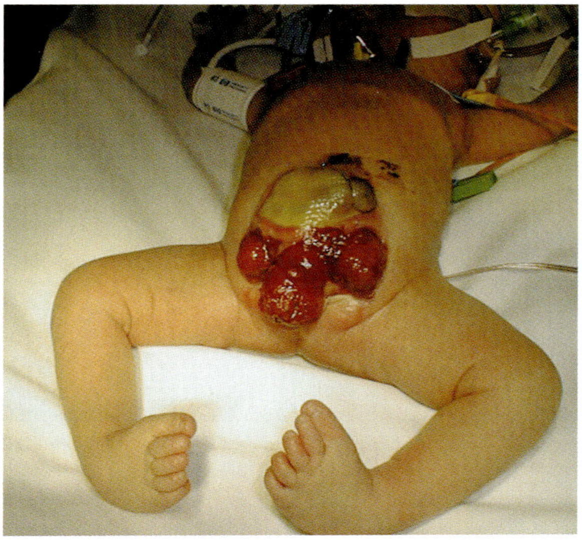

Fig. 8.26. Newborn with cloacal exstrophy. The lower limb orthopedic anomalies are obvious

clamp and redundant umbilical tissue excised. The friable bladder mucosa must be protected and remain moist until definitive operative closure. A nonadherent cellophane dressing and frequent saline soaks will protect the bladder mucosa; alternatively, a modified humidifier tent may be utilized in order to protect the fragile bladder plate. Patients should be managed in a qualified exstrophy-closure center where both technical expertise and ancillary support services exist to provide the best possible care for these complex infants.

Most patients can safely undergo reconstructive surgery in the first few days of life. Two techniques have emerged which, depending on the surgeon's preference, are most commonly utilized for exstrophy repair. The modern staged approach consists of initial abdominal wall and bladder closure in the newborn period with or without iliac osteotomy followed by epispadias repair at 6 – 18 months of age, and finally, bladder neck reconstruction in order to gain urinary continence around 4 – 6 years of age (Baker and G earhart 1998. In contrast, the complete primary repair of bladder exstrophy (CPRE) advocates incorporating the epispadias repair at the same time as abdominal wall and bladder closure in the newborn period (Grady and Mitchell 1999). Modifications of this technique are emerging and some authors have even performed both a mini-bladder neck reconstruction as well as ureteroneocystostomy for VUR at the time of neonatal CPRE (Borer et al. 2005). Regardless of the technique employed, the goals of exstrophy surgery include a secure abdominal wall and bladder closure, protection of the upper urinary tracts, urinary continence, and cosmetically and functionally acceptable external genitalia (Cook et al. 2005) (Fig. 8.27).

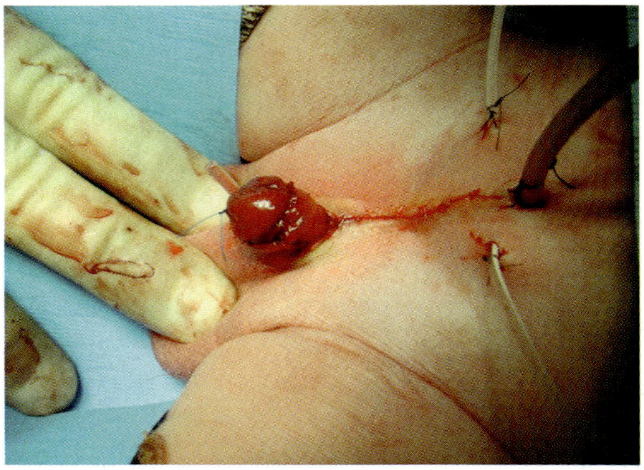

Fig. 8.27. Appearance of abdominal wall and external genitalia following complete primary reconstruction

8.4.2 Bladder Trauma

Although the bladder is an abdominal organ in children, bladder trauma is a relatively rare event, occurring in approximately 5 % – 7 % of pediatric patients assessed for trauma (McAleer et al. 1993). Pelvic fracture, and other concomitant injuries, is associated with bladder rupture in more than 95 % of cases. Blunt trauma, secondary to motor vehicle collisions, is the most common cause of bladder rupture in both the pediatric and adult trauma populations (Hochberg and Stone 1993). Depending on the nature of the trauma, bladder rupture can occur either in an intraperitoneal or extraperitoneal fashion and, similar to the management in adults, treatment in children is dictated by differentiating these two types of underlying injuries.

Intraperitoneal rupture is usually secondary to direct lower abdominal trauma at the level of the bladder dome. Children typically present with severe lower abdominal pain and an inability to void. Blood at the meatus or gross hematuria is present in more than 95 % – 100 % of cases (Carroll and McAninch 1984). Extraperitoneal rupture must be considered in those presenting with hematuria and concomitant pelvic fractures. The bladder injury may be secondary to shearing forces created from disruption of the pelvic ring or direct laceration of the bladder due to the displacement of bony fragments (Cass and Luxenberg 1989).

Presently, the diagnostic test of choice is an abdominopelvic CT scan with the retrograde instillation of contrast. It is at least as accurate as conventional retrograde cystography, but also allows the accurate visualization of other intraabdominal viscera (Deck et al. 2001). Adequate bladder distension is necessary in order to minimize the potential of a false-negative study and therefore the bladder should be filled to capacity during the contrast-phase of the examination using the

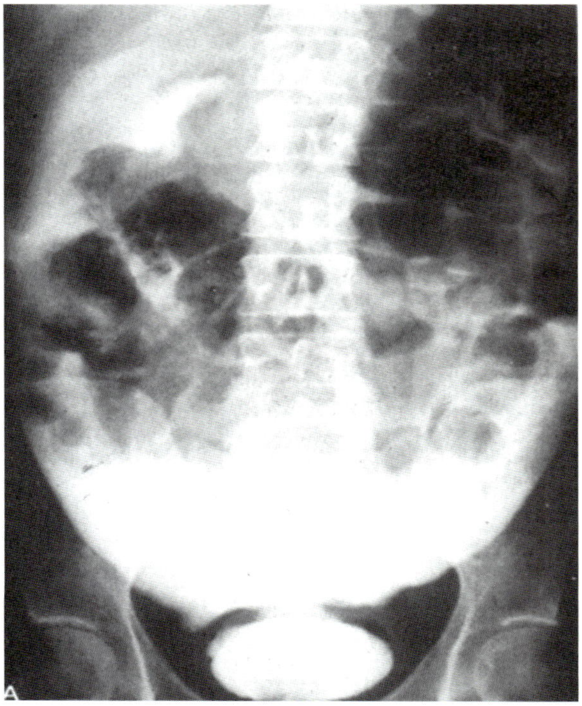

Fig. 8.28. Retrograde cystography demonstrating large intraperitoneal bladder perforation following blunt trauma secondary to a motor vehicle collision

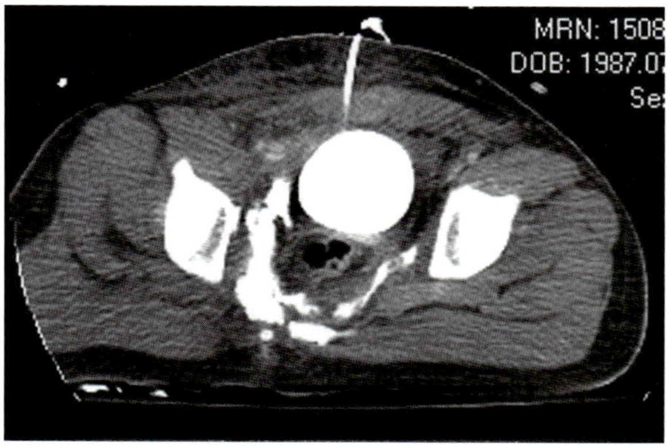

Fig. 8.29. CT scan demonstrating flame-shaped contrast extravasation typically seen in extraperitoneal bladder rupture

formula (age +2) × 30 ml, as a guide. Indirect cystography should not be performed, as it is an unreliable technique for the evaluation of bladder rupture (Haas et al. 1999). Intraperitoneal bladder rupture will easily be identified by the presence of contrast outlining loops of bowel within the peritoneal cavity (Fig. 8.28). Extraperitoneal lacerations are typically identified by flame-shaped collections of contrast in the space of Retzius and pelvis (Fig. 8.29).

As previously mentioned, the management of bladder rupture in the pediatric patient is similar to that in adults. Intraperitoneal injury is best treated by laparotomy and repair of the laceration using multiple layers of absorbable suture. Urinary diversion and antibiotic prophylaxis are continued for at least 10–14 days. Postoperative cystography will determine adequacy of the repair and dictate at which point the catheters may be removed and trials of voiding ensue. Most extraperitoneal lacerations respond well to catheter drainage and a trial of observational therapy. Antibiotic prophylaxis has been shown to reduce potential infective complications for the duration of urinary diversion (usually 10–14 days) (Kotkin and Koch 1995). Indications for repair of an extraperitoneal injury include clot retention, injury involving the bladder neck, the presence of an intravesical bony fragment, concomitant rectal or vaginal lacerations, and any patient presenting with penetrating trauma.

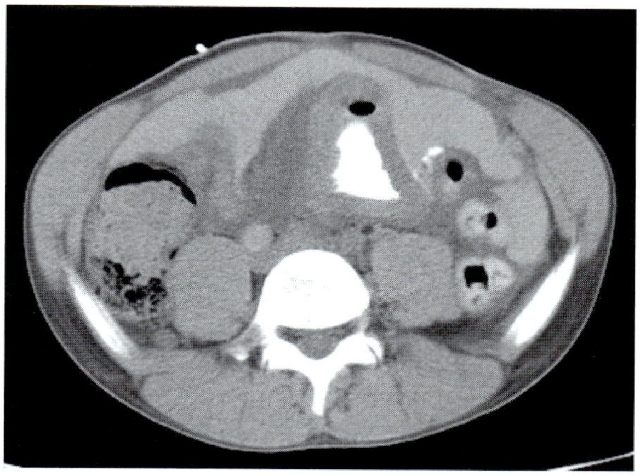

Fig. 8.30. CT showing contrast extravasation in a 15-year-old boy with a history of bladder augmentation and appendicovesicostomy and noncompliant intermittent catheterization

8.4.3 Bladder Rupture Postaugmentation

Enterocystoplasty is a commonly utilized technique within pediatric urology as a method of both increasing vesical storage capacity and decreasing pressure transmission to the upper urinary tracts in children with inadequate bladder volumes and abnormal bladder wall dynamics. The most frequent indications for augmentation include a poorly compliant, high-pressure, low-capacity bladder secondary to spina bifida (or other spinal cord anomaly or insult), posterior urethral valves (PUV), or bladder exstrophy. Augmentation is inherently associated with significant risks and therefore should only be recommended in select patients following an exhaustive trial of medical therapy. Only those with ongoing risk of renal deterioration or socially unacceptable urinary incontinence, despite maximal medical treatment and clean intermittent catheterization (CIC), should be considered for augmentation. Furthermore, vigilance and selection of patients and their families in whom compliance with CIC is assured, is important to reduce potentially catastrophic complications. Unfortunately, despite these precautions, a small number of patients present to the emergency department with an acute abdomen secondary to spontaneous bladder rupture postaugmentation. A high index of suspicion must be maintained in these patients, as this condition is frequently associated with a delay in diagnosis with potentially lethal results (Couillard et al. 1993).

Although the exact etiology of bladder perforation is unknown, traumatic catheterization, noncompliance with CIC leading to chronic bladder overdistension, and blunt trauma have all been implicated (Elder et al. 1988; Jayanthi et al. 1995; Rushton et al. 1988). The diagnosis must be suspected, and the condition ruled out, in any patient who presents with abdominal pain and a history of augmentation. The majority of children who undergo augmentation are neurologically impaired; therefore, lower abdominal sensation is diminished and signs and symptoms may be nonspecific. Patients may complain of nausea, vomiting, fever, obstipation, gross hematuria, and oliguria; physical examination demonstrates a distended rigid abdomen with positive peritoneal signs.

If suspected, a CT cystogram must be performed immediately and is the most sensitive test to rule out perforation in these patients. The bladder must be filled to capacity with the retrograde instillation of contrast and both pre- and post-contrast images taken in order to accurately determine the diagnosis (Fig. 8.30). Complete blood work, including blood and urine cultures, should be taken and fluid resuscitation, catheter drainage, and parenteral broad-spectrum antibiotics initiated immediately. Stable patients without signs of sepsis and in whom a small perforation is suspected, may be managed nonoperatively. Serial blood work and physical examinations are paramount to this approach, as any sign of clinical deterioration mandates immediate operative intervention. The majority of patients with bladder rupture, however, will require immediate exploratory laparotomy, closure of the perforation and irrigation of the peritoneal cavity. Broad-spectrum parenteral antibiotics are continued and patients are monitored closely for signs of postoperative intraperitoneal abscess formation during convalescence.

8.4.4 Urinary Retention

The majority of newborns will void within the first 8 h of life, though some may void up to 24 h following birth (Mesrobian et al. 2004). If more than 24 h elapses, obstruction must be considered and investigated accordingly. Furthermore, a complete newborn physical ex-

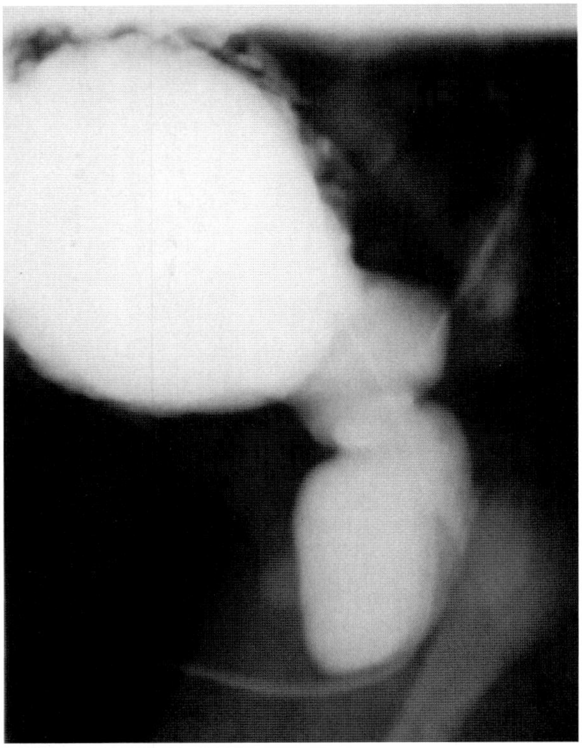

Fig. 8.31. VCUG demonstrating posterior urethral valves in a newborn male with a known prenatal history of bilateral hydroureteronephrosis and bladder wall thickening.

amination is important as even an apparently normal void does not rule out the presence of lower urinary tract obstruction due to the bladder's potential for compensation in the face of obstruction. The presence of a lower midline abdominal mass in a male infant is suspicious for posterior urethral valves (PUVs) despite normal micturition. If suspected, passage of a small feeding tube or Foley catheter will decompress the urinary tract and allow subsequent investigations to be carried out in a timely manner. PUVs occur in approximately 1 in 5,000 boys and are the most common cause of lower urinary tract obstruction in male infants (Mesrobian et al. 2004). Both US and VCUG are mandatory to visualize the upper tracts and definitively diagnose the presence of PUV (Fig. 8.31). Five signs of PUV on cystography are:

1. The presence of VUR
2. A thick-walled trabeculated bladder ± diverticula
3. Bladder neck hypertrophy
4. A dilated posterior urethra ± visualization of the PUV
5. Significant caliber change in the urethra distal to the PUV

Boys with stable renal function can usually undergo primary valve ablation in the 1st week of life. However, vesicostomy may be necessary to decompress and temporize the upper urinary tracts in those who cannot undergo cystoscopy such as preterm or small infants. Vesicostomy closure and valve ablation are then usually performed at 6–12 months of age following interval growth of the child. Overall, early prognosis is usually dependent on oligohydramnios and its consequent ramifications on pulmonary development in utero. Subsequently, the degree of renal impairment, secondary to dysplasia, will contribute to early postnatal morbidity and mortality.

Females may also present in the neonatal period with urinary retention and a palpable lower midline abdominal mass. Urogenital sinus anomalies, ectopic ureteroceles, and hydrometrocolpos may all lead to outlet obstruction and urinary tract dilatation. The diagnosis of a prolapsing ureterocele or imperforate hymen may not initially be obvious on physical examination. Both appear as cystic interlabial masses; however, careful inspection of the introitus will differentiate the two lesions (Fig. 8.32 a, b). Hydrometrocolpos due to an imperforate hymen results from the accumulation of uterine and vaginal secretions secondary to prenatal maternal estrogen stimulation (Hahn-Pederssen et al. 1984). Incision and drainage results in resolution of the vaginal, uterine, and urinary tract dilatation. Ectopic ureteroceles can also cause outlet obstruction in the newborn; however, they may also present later in childhood with a history of a protruding "bubble" or mass when voiding or recurrent UTIs (Fig. 8.33). Incision of the ureterocele will relieve the outlet obstruction and temporize the newborn while a complete evaluation of the upper urinary tracts is undertaken. Older children with an intermittently prolapsing ureterocele may be evaluated on a more elective basis with US, VCUG, and DMSA renal scan. The majority of girls with a ureterocele will have a duplicated collecting system; definitive reconstruction will largely depend on the function of the renal moiety subtended by the ureterocele, although it should be directed at the prevention of UTI.

Occasionally urogenital sinus or anorectal anomalies will cause outlet obstruction and urinary retention in newborn females. The abnormal Mullerian duct structures penetrate the urogenital sinus and form a valve mechanism that leads to the prenatal accumulation of urine in the vagina and uterus. Newborns can present with a massively distended abdomen secondary to the urometrocolpos that causes both gastrointestinal and respiratory compromise (Fig. 8.34). It is important to thoroughly evaluate these infants, as congenital adrenal hyperplasia and a salt-wasting nephropathy can be associated with persistent urogenital sinus anomalies (Hamza et al. 2001). Careful inspection of the perineum will reveal a single orifice (in the case of a persistent cloaca) or two orifices when a urogenital sinus malformation is present. The treating physician

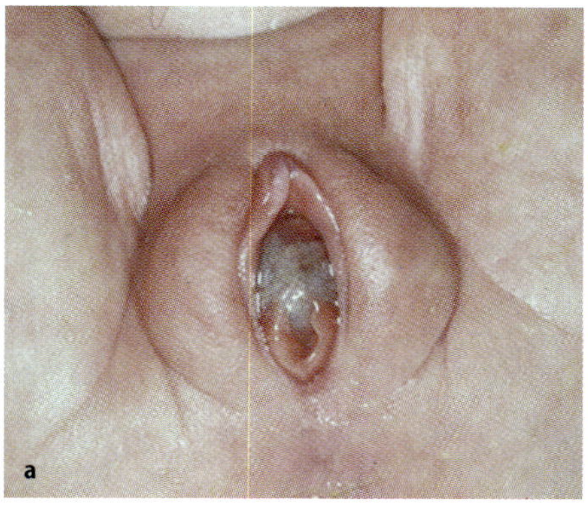

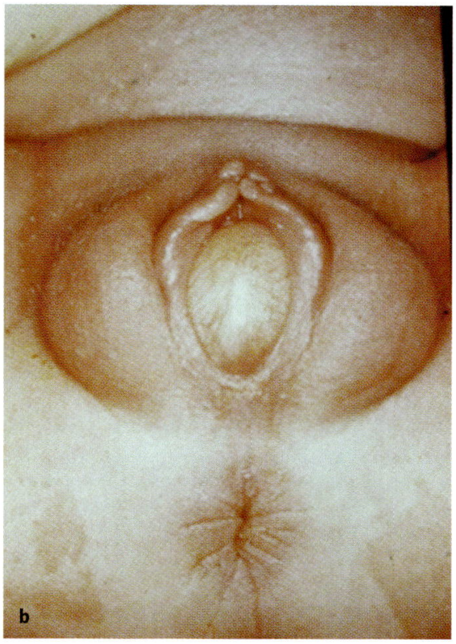

Fig. 8.32. a Interlabial mass in a newborn female subsequently found to be a prolapsing ectopic ureterocele. Note the hymenal remnant inferiorly which aids in the differentiation between Fig. 8.32b. **b** Interlabial mass in a different newborn female. This mass was secondary to an imperforate hymen. Hydrometrocolpos was drained following simple vertical incision of the hymen

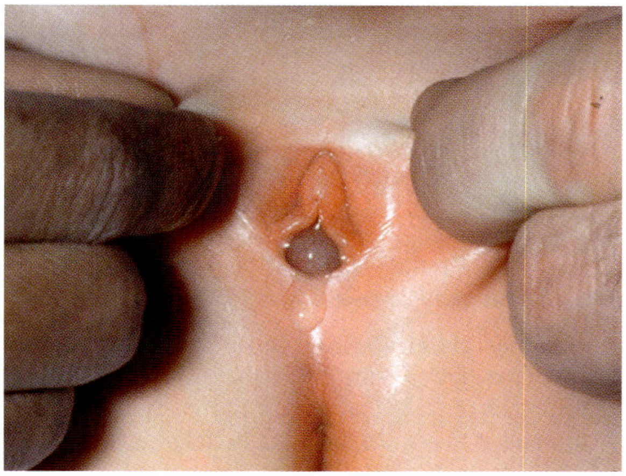

Fig. 8.33. Photograph of an intermittently prolapsing ectopic ureterocele in a 6-year-old female with a history of "passing a bubble" while micturating

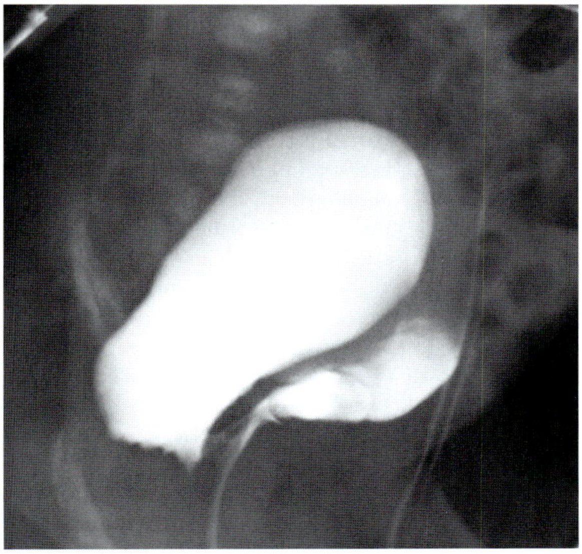

Fig. 8.34. Urogenital sinogram in a newborn female with an isolated urogenital sinus anomaly and massive abdominal distension. The patient was subsequently found to have severe urometrocolpos requiring acute decompression

must be willing to undertake prompt decompression and diversion of both urine and feces (depending on the underlying anomaly) to allow interval growth and elective planning of the reconstructive surgery. Girls with isolated urogenital sinus anomalies and urinary retention may be managed initially by intermittent catheterization of the urogenital sinus followed by total urogenital mobilization (TUM) around 1 year of age (Gosalbez et al. 2005). Anorectal and cloacal anomalies are best treated by the cloacal disassembly technique advocated by Pena utilizing a posterior-sagittal approach for anorectal, vaginal, and urethral reconstruction (Pena et al. 2004).

8.5 External Genitalia

8.5.1 Penis

8.5.1.1 Circumcision Injuries

Newborn circumcision is the most common surgical procedure performed in the United States. Over 61 % of newborn boys underwent circumcision in 2000 and the incidence continues to increase (Nelson et al. 2005). Although some lay people and professionals alike still question the need for circumcision, it has become apparent that it does afford a number of recognized medical benefits. Firstly, the risk of UTI in male infants is reduced in those who undergo circumcision, from 1 % to 0.1 % (Singh-Grewal et al. 2005). Furthermore, boys with recurrent UTIs or identified genitourinary pathol-

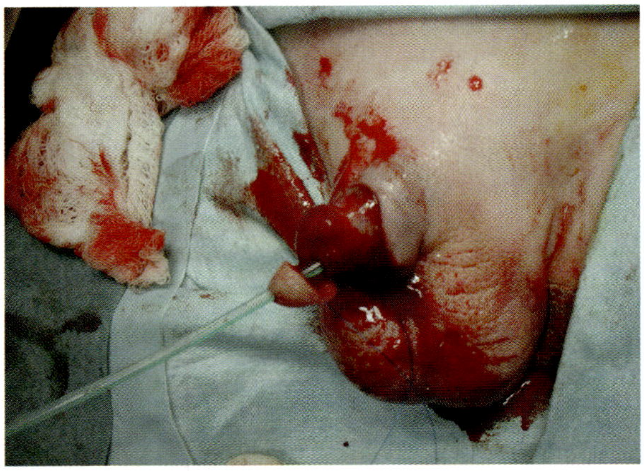

Fig. 8.35. Intraoperative photograph of an 8-day-old the day following partial glans amputation at the time of ritual circumcision. This was successfully reattached and healed without meatal stenosis or urethral fistula

ogy such as PUV, high-grade VUR or hydronephrosis, are at an even greater likelihood of risk reduction (Singh-Grewal et al. 2005; Herndon et al. 1999). Sexually transmitted diseases and HIV transmission are also greatly reduced in circumcised men (Baeten et al. 2005). Finally, early circumcision prevents conditions and diseases associated with an intact prepuce such as phimosis, paraphimosis, penile cancer, and recurrent balanitis (Busby and Pettaway 2005; Daling et al. 2005). However, it should not be considered lightly, as increased complications have been noted in children who undergo circumcision by untrained vs licensed practitioners (Aitkeler et al. 2005).

Although the majority of complications are minor, significant morbidity and even death has been reported following circumcision (Sullivan 2002). Strict adherence to technique including sterility, hemostasis, protection of the glans, removal of appropriate amounts of penile and preputial skin, and early recognition of complications will decrease potentially adverse outcomes (Davenport 1996). Complications are best managed by the immediate evaluation and treatment under subspecialist supervision. Bleeding is usually controlled by hematoma evacuation and suture ligation while partial or complete glans amputation requires emergent repair using fine absorbable suture and urinary diversion, if necessary (Fig. 8.35).

Finally, prevention is obviously the best tool to avoid potential complications. Circumcision should be delayed in premature infants or those with severe comorbid disease or coagulopathy. Additionally, boys with an underlying congenital anomaly of the phallus, such as hypospadias or buried penis, should not undergo circumcision until thoroughly evaluated by a pediatric urologist. Table 8.5 lists acute complications and their respective treatments.

Table 8.5. Potential complications following circumcision

Complication	Treatment	Prevention
Bleeding	Temporary pressure dressing, suture ligation	Careful use of Plastibell devices
Infection	Broad-spectrum antibiotics	Sterile technique, use of antibiotic ointment after circumcision
Amputation	Emergent reattachment	Careful placement of clamp at time of circumcision
Excessive skin loss	Wound care, gradual re-epithelization	Careful placement of clamp, appropriate marking of coronal sulcus
Penile necrosis	Conservative treatment, debridement if necessary	Judicious use of cautery
Buried penis	Operative phalloplasty	Recognition of the abnormality, circumcision at time of phalloplasty

8.5.1.2
Paraphimosis and Phimosis

Paraphimosis is a frequently encountered condition in the pediatric emergency department. Because of their age and lack of understanding, children have a tendency to neglect to reduce their foreskin following retraction at the time of micturition. Occasionally medical personnel will cause an iatrogenic paraphimosis by inadvertently leaving the foreskin retracted following insertion of an indwelling urethral catheter. Subsequent edema and venous congestion proximally could lead to decreased blood flow to the foreskin and glans (Fig. 8.36). It is imperative that the foreskin be reduced immediately to avoid further swelling. The best technique to treat a paraphimosis involves the use of sustained gradual pressure on the glans by both thumbs while the first and second digits reduce the edematous foreskin (Fig. 8.37). Wrapping the penis in gauze and applying a hypertonic solution (such as 3% saline) for 20–30 min before will cause a dramatic reduction in the amount of edema and facilitate manual decompression. If unsuccessful, a dorsal slit may be necessary to incise the tight preputial ring in order to reduce the foreskin and relieve the venous congestion. Formal circumcision can be performed at a later date, if necessary. Children should not retract their foreskin for at least 2 weeks following reduction of a paraphimosis.

Although rarely a true urologic emergency, phimosis nonetheless causes significant parental concern and frequently results in an emergency department consultation. It is important to differentiate physiologic phimosis from true or pathologic phimosis. Physiologic phimosis is a natural adherence of the inner prepuce to

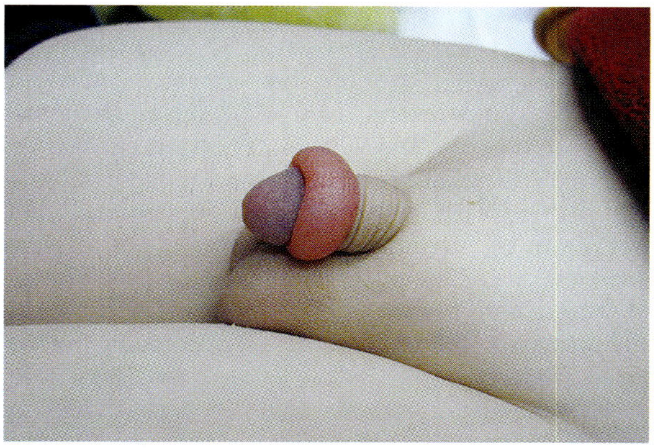

Fig. 8.36. Typical appearance of a boy with paraphimosis. Venous return from the glans is impaired and the prepuce is edematous and engorged distal to the phimotic ring

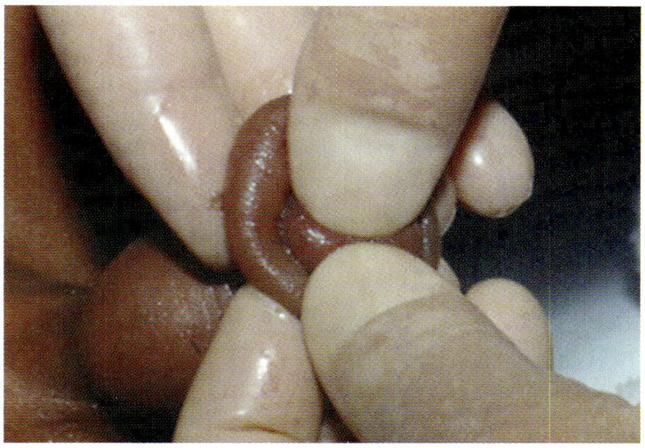

Fig. 8.37. The proper technique to manually reduce paraphimosis. Sustained gentle pressure is required in order to reduce the edematous foreskin over the glans

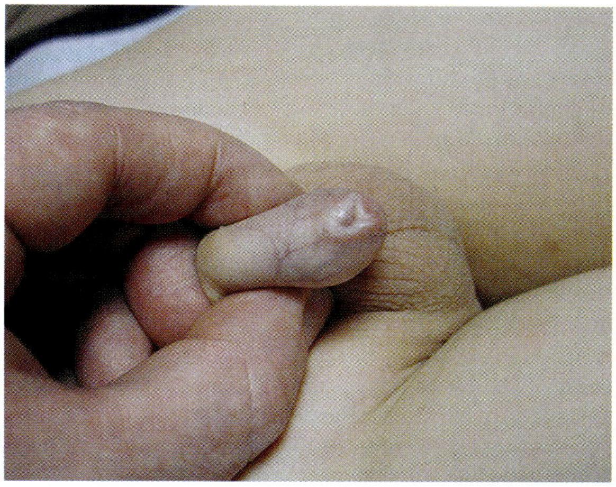

Fig. 8.38. Pathological phimosis showing a thickened indurated phimotic band. This patient failed a course of topical steroid therapy and required circumcision

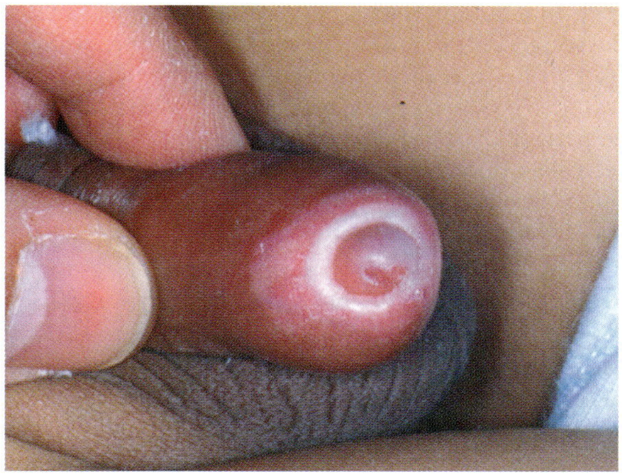

Fig. 8.39. Pathological phimosis secondary to BXO. Note the whitish discoloration similar to the patient in Fig. 8.38. Both patients were found to have BXO on pathological analysis

the glans and, with interval growth, usually resolves spontaneously. Desuamation of epithelial cells and build-up of smegma aid in this process of preputial separation. On examination, the phimotic prepuce appears quite supple and there is no evidence of an indurated, thickened phimotic band, as visualized in true pathologic phimosis (Fig. 8.38). Although a course of topical mid-potency steroid cream, applied two to three times a day for 6 weeks, is effective for separating physiologic adhesions, circumcision is usually required for indurated, pathologically phimotic conditions (Yang et al. 2005). Occasionally, children with previously retractile foreskins may present with a history of progressive difficulty retracting the foreskin associated with significant induration and fibrosis. It is imperative to rule out (via circumcision or biopsy) balanitis xerotica obliterans (BXO), also known as lichen sclerosis et atrophicus, in this patient population, as progressive meatal stenosis and ongoing obstructive voiding has been reported following circumcision (Gargollo et al. 2005). BXO has a characteristic whitish discoloration of the prepuce and can involve both the glans and distal urethra (Fig. 8.39).

8.5.1.3
Urethral Trauma

The majority of posterior urethral injuries are associated with blunt trauma and shearing forces secondary to pelvic fracture. Complete evaluation of the urinary tract is necessary, as 10 % – 30 % of boys with posterior urethral injuries will also have an associated bladder perforation (Baskin and McAninch 1993). Urethral and bladder neck injuries in females, although quite rare, are typically associated with pelvic fractures and anterior vaginal wall lacerations.

Any patient presenting with a history of pelvic trauma and blood at the level of the meatus requires retrograde urethrography prior to urethral catheter insertion. Careful inspection of the vaginal introitus, and even examination under anesthesia, may be necessary in female patients. If there is no evidence of contrast extravasation, a urethral catheter may be passed gently and left in situ for 5–7 days to allow healing of the urethral contusion. Partial disruptions may also be amenable to retrograde catheter insertion; however, the use of flexible cystoscopy and insertion of a catheter under direct vision is a safer technique to ensure proper catheter placement. In general, a retrograde periurethrogram or VCUG is performed 7–10 days following the injury and the catheter removed if no evidence of extravasation exists. Occasionally, prolonged drainage (up to 3 weeks) is required in order to allow complete healing of the injury.

Management of complete posterior urethral disruptions remains controversial; however, two approaches are presently most commonly utilized in pediatric urology, that is, suprapubic cystostomy insertion and delayed reconstruction, or primary endoscopic realignment. Choice of either technique will depend largely on severity of associated injuries as well as the surgeon's experience. Open cystostomy and suprapubic tube placement can be performed quickly in the unstable, multi-injured patient. Delayed reconstruction of the resultant posterior urethral stricture can be safely undertaken via a perineal approach at least 3 months after the injury (Hafez et al. 2005).

Primary realignment may be performed acutely, or within the first several days following injury. Combined retrograde and antegrade cystourethroscopy, with the utilization of endoscopic techniques, will usually enable placement of a urethral catheter and allow healing of the urethral defect. The resultant urethral stricture is usually shorter and more amenable to visual internal urethrotomy or one-stage urethroplasty than in those who undergo urinary diversion and delayed reconstruction (Balkan et al. 2005) (Figs. 8.40, 8.41). Immediate sutured repair in boys should be avoided; however, urethral injury in females should be treated by early repair and reconstruction of the urethra in order to avoid potentially devastating complications such as complete urethral obliteration and urethrovaginal fistulae (Huang et al. 2003).

Anterior urethral injuries are usually blunt and secondary to straddle injuries to the perineum. The bulbar urethra is the most commonly affected segment. Children typically present with an inability to void and blood at the meatus. Retrograde urethrography will identify the degree of injury. Furthermore, the extent of penile and perineal hematoma will help identify injury to associated tissue planes. If Buck's fascia is intact, the hematoma will be isolated along the penile shaft only;

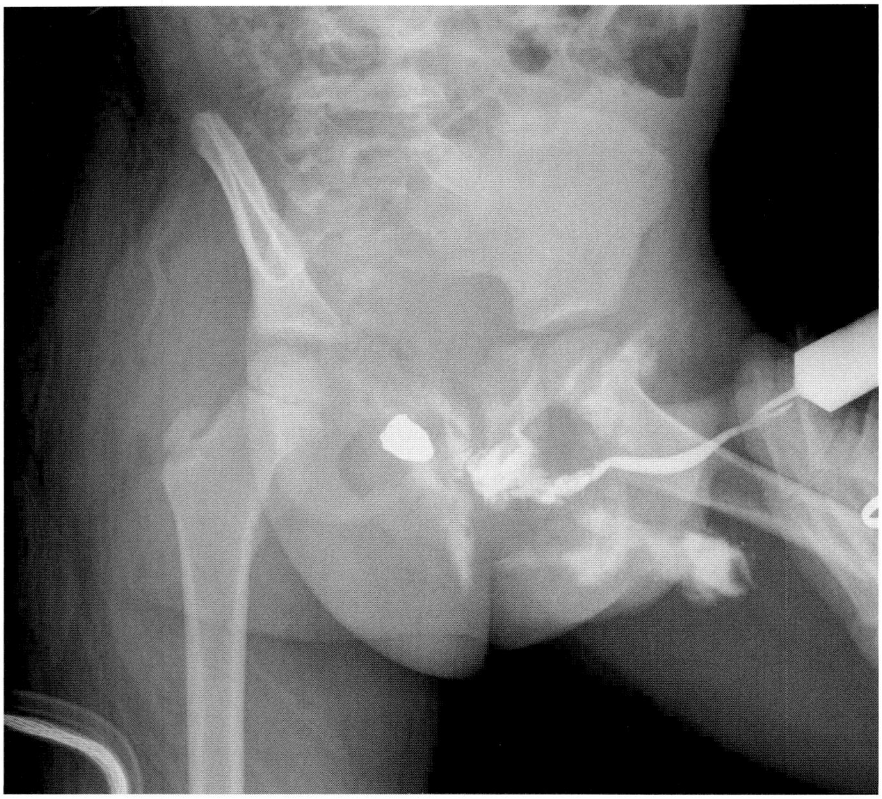

Fig. 8.40. Retrograde urethrogram in a 4-year-old boy demonstrating contrast extravasation at the level of the proximal urethra following penetrating trauma. Note the bullet fragment lodged in the right pelvis

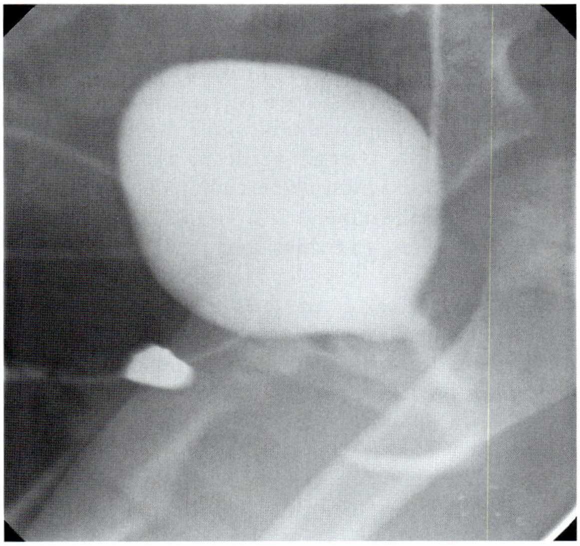

Fig. 8.41. Antegrade urethrogram in the same patient following primary endoscopic realignment and suprapubic diversion. A relatively short bulbar urethral stricture was found on subsequent cystoscopy

however, extension of the hematoma to the scrotum and perineum will signify rupture of Buck's fascia. In this case, the hematoma and urinary extravasation will only be limited by Colles fascia.

Incomplete disruptions may be managed by temporary catheter drainage and appropriate antibiotic prophylaxis. However, children with complete disruptions should not undergo further instrumentation, and a suprapubic cystostomy inserted for urinary diversion. Subsequent delayed repair of the urethral stricture is carried out following resolution of the inflammatory process. In contrast, penetrating urethral injuries require immediate surgical debridement and reconstruction using fine absorbable suture over an indwelling urethral catheter.

8.5.2 Scrotum

8.5.2.1 The Acute Scrotum

The presentation of a child with a scrotal mass is frequently accompanied by significant distress regarding the potential medicolegal implications of the misdiagnosis of an acute surgically correctible lesion, namely testicular torsion. However, a rational, thoughtful approach to the child with an acutely symptomatic scrotum will aid in the rapid diagnosis and treatment of this commonly encountered entity. The history will determine the age of the patient, associated symptoms, and the presence or absence of pain. Pertinent physical findings and appropriate investigations will help clarify the diagnosis and enable treatment in a timely fashion.

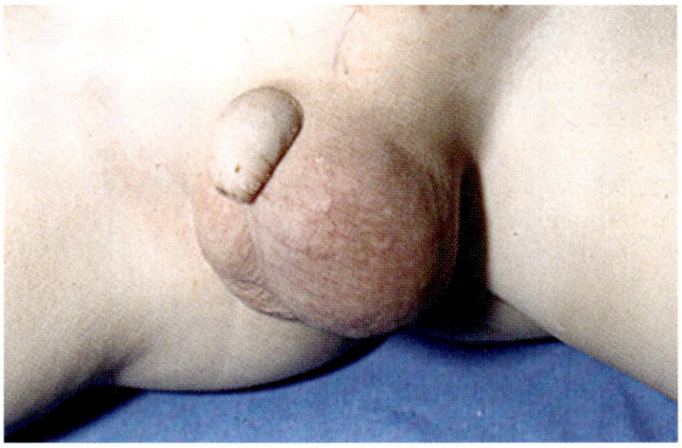

Fig. 8.42. Newborn boy with an enlarged, nontender, discolored left hemiscrotum at the time of newborn examination. Neonatal torsion was diagnosed and the patient underwent orchidectomy and contralateral orchiopexy at 2 weeks of age

8.5.2.2 Testicular Torsion

Testicular torsion is a true urologic emergency and must remain a diagnosis of exclusion in any boy presenting with a painful scrotum. A bimodal age distribution has been identified that corresponds to specific inherent anatomic abnormalities at the level of the testis that present either perinatally or around puberty (Melekos 1988).

8.5.2.3 Neonatal Torsion

Perinatal torsion, also referred to as neonatal or prenatal torsion, is usually secondary to lack of gubernacular adherence to the scrotal wall and results in extravaginal torsion, involving the entire spermatic cord and its associated tunica layers. It may occur prior to, or around delivery, and patients typically present with an enlarged, discolored, nontender hemiscrotum (Fig. 8.42). Some believe that prenatal torsion can occur very early in gestation and results in the majority of cases of unilateral testicular agenesis (Gong et al. 1996). Contemporary high-frequency Doppler US is generally accurate in confirming the diagnosis.

Controversy persists regarding the optimal management of neonatal torsion: some advocate early exploration in order to avoid potentially synchronous or metachronous bilaterality while others feel that, because the torsion occurs prenatally, operative exploration is redundant and simple observation is all that is required (Yerkes et al. 2005; Dewan and Walton 1987). However, since the gubernaculum dehydrates and fixates to the scrotal wall over the first 6–8 weeks postnatally, patients are at a theoretically increased risk of metachronous bilateral torsion during that time; therefore, urgent exploration and contralateral orchiopexy is not an unreasonable treatment option. Beyond this timeframe, the risk of contralateral torsion appears to decrease, and conservative observational therapy alone is warranted thereafter.

8.5.2.4
Pediatric Torsion

The history, including the onset and severity of pain as well as associated symptoms, is vital in the assessment of the older child with suspected testicular torsion. Patients typically present with sudden-onset severe pain associated with nausea, vomiting, and scrotal swelling. There is no history of fever, irritative voiding symptoms, or urethral discharge. Physical examination demonstrates an enlarged hemiscrotum containing a high-riding tender, swollen testicle with no evidence of spermatic cord swelling or inguinal adenopathy. The epididymis may be palpable in an abnormal location due to the testicle's transverse lie. The cremasteric reflex is usually absent and urinalysis is routinely normal. Surgical exploration usually reveals torsion in these cases and should not be delayed by radiologic confirmation (Fig. 8.43). Doppler US should be reserved for those cases in which the diagnosis is questionable.

Pediatric torsion is usually secondary to the bell-clapper deformity and occurs intravaginally. Prompt recognition and surgical detorsion will prevent atrophy and testicular nonfunction. Orchidopexy within 4 h will result in almost certain complete testicular viability; however, some germ and Leydig cell function can still be preserved after 12 h of untreated torsion. Beyond 24 h, nearly complete testicular atrophy occurs despite detorsion and orchidopexy (Rampaul and Hosking 1998). As the bell-clapper deformity affects both testes, contralateral orchidopexy should be performed at the time of exploration of the involved testis.

Frequently, torsion of a testicular appendage will present in a similar fashion; however, careful examination will reveal a normal, vertically oriented testicle with an intact cremasteric reflex and pain on palpation limited only to the upper pole of the testicle. Occasionally, the blue-dot sign (which consists of a small bluish discoloration of the overlying scrotal skin) is appreciated as the congested, torted appendix is identified at the level of the upper pole. Doppler US should be performed and can easily diagnose appendix testis or appendix epididymis torsion and rule out testicular torsion proper. Supportive therapy and NSAIDS are the mainstays of treatment.

8.5.2.5
Epididymitis

Epididymitis must also be considered in boys presenting with acute scrotal pain. However, it is usually of a more insidious onset and may be accompanied with urinary symptoms and progressive scrotal swelling. Physical examination demonstrates a swollen erythematous hemiscrotum associated with epididymal engorgement and tenderness (Fig. 8.44). In contrast to torsion, the cremasteric reflex is usually intact and elevation of the testis improves pain (Prehn's sign) (Kadish and Bolte 1998). Doppler US should be performed; it typically reveals an enlarged hyperemic epididymis, a thickened scrotal wall and normal or increased blood flow to the testis (Munden and Trautwein 2000). Although a bacterial etiology must be considered, the majority of episodes of epididymitis in prepubertal children is secondary to a postinfectious viral etiology (Somekh et al. 2004). Symptoms usually resolve within

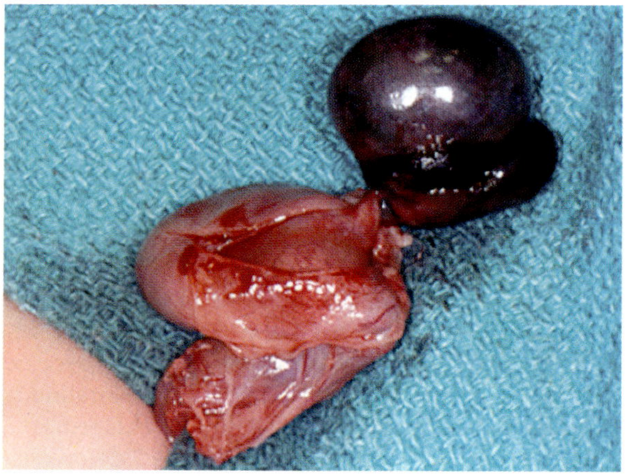

Fig. 8.43. Intraoperative photograph demonstrating testicular and epididymal ischemia secondary to spermatic cord torsion

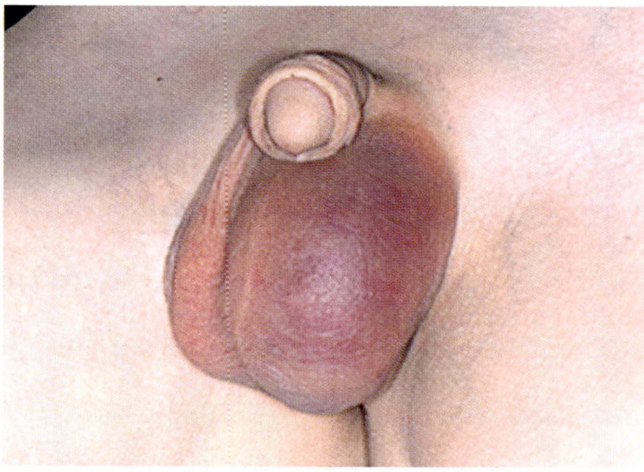

Fig. 8.44. Left epididimo-orchitis in a 5-year-old boy. The left hemiscrotum is red, indurated, and edematous; the underlying left epididymis and testis were diffusely tender

1–3 days following a course of reassurance, scrotal elevation, and nonsteroidal anti-inflammatories. There is usually no role for antibiotics; however, if the urine is positive for bacteruria, an appropriate course of antimicrobial therapy is obviously warranted. The most common underlying bacterium in prepubertal children is *Escherichia coli*; however, *Chlamydia trachomatis* must also be considered in sexually active postpubertal boys.

In the past, any boy presenting with epididymitis underwent a complete evaluation of the upper urinary tract in order to rule out potentially contributing urinary tract pathology such as an ectopic ureter or PUV. However, as most cases of epididymitis are postinfectious and nonbacterial in origin, renal US has been shown to be unnecessary in the majority. In general, only boys under the age of 4, those with documented bacterial infection, evidence of sepsis, and those with urinary tract symptoms are more likely to harbor some underlying urogenital anomaly, and would thus benefit from antibiotic therapy and radiologic evaluation.

8.5.2.6 Idiopathic Scrotal Edema

Acute idiopathic scrotal edema (AISE) is a fairly common, yet underreported cause of the acute scrotum in children, accounting for as many as 30% of patients who undergo assessment (Najmaldin and Burge 1987). It is characterized by the rapid onset of nontender, frequently unilateral scrotal and penile erythema and edema. The patient is usually afebrile and is otherwise asymptomatic, apart from the distressing appearance of the genitalia. It is usually found in prepubertal children from 5 to 11 years of age. As the name implies, the cause of AISE is unknown; however, some children present with a history of asthma or allergic conditions such as eczema or dermatitis (Klin et al. 2002). Laboratory investigations are usually normal, with occasional patients demonstrating mild peripheral eosinophilia. This has led many to believe the underlying cause of AISE is atopic in origin; other possible etiologies include insect bites, scrotal trauma, and parasitic infection (Hanstead and John 1964).

Physical examination reveals an edematous, erythematous, hyperthermic scrotal wall without underlying testicular tenderness. The penile shaft skin may be involved; however, there is no history of irritative or obstructive voiding symptoms. Lower abdominal, inguinal, and perineal involvement is also frequently encountered. Urine and blood work is usually normal, apart from the previously mentioned occasional eosinophilia. Scrotal US should be performed to rule out surgically correctible conditions such as testicular torsion, infection, or abscess formation. US consistently demonstrates thickening and increased echogenicity of the scrotal wall with increased peritesticular and scrotal blood flow (Herman et al. 1994).

AISE is a self-limiting phenomenon and therefore reassurance, scrotal support, and close observation are the mainstays of therapy. Antibiotics and anti-inflammatory medications are usually redundant; however, the use of antihistamines is a reasonable option, as an underlying allergic etiology is likely responsible for this condition.

Other scrotal masses, which may mimic testicular torsion, include hydroceles, hernias, tumors, and lesions secondary to a patent processus vaginalis. History, physical examination, and scrotal US will usually determine the underlying etiology and dictate further management. Communicating hydroceles are common in infancy; patients typically present with an otherwise asymptomatic intermittently swollen hemiscrotum. If the child is older, the swelling may enlarge with ambulation and subsequently decrease in size upon recumbence. Physical examination will reveal a fluid filled mass, which easily transilluminates and can be reduced with gentle pressure (Fig. 8.45a, b). The underlying tes-

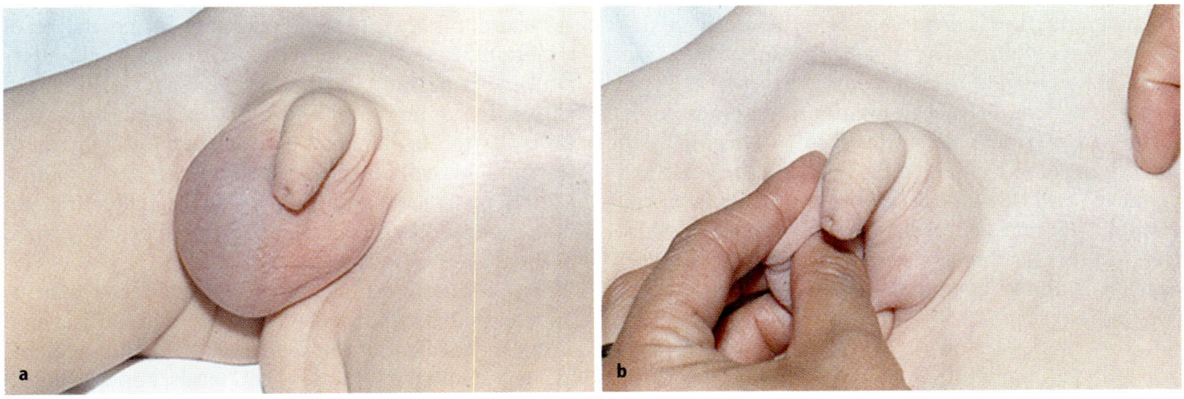

Fig. 8.45. a Typical appearance of a communicating hydrocele in a 1-year-old boy. **b** Decompression of the hydrocele and verifying the presence of a patent processus vaginalis

tis is usually normal. Treatment consists of conservative therapy, as most resolve by 12–18 months of age. Thereafter, inguinal hydrocele repair is the treatment of choice.

8.5.2.7
Henoch-Schönlein Purpura

Henoch-Schönlein purpura (HSP) is a small vessel vasculitis characterized by arthritis, nonthrombocytopenic purpura, abdominal pain and renal disease (Mills et al. 1990). It typically presents in patients less than 20 years of age and is the one of the most common vasculitides of childhood. One of the hallmarks of the disease is the presence of palpable purpura; raised hemorrhagic purple-blue skin lesions unrelated to thrombocytopenia (Mills et al. 1990). GU manifestations include hematuria, acute scrotal pain, bluish discoloration of the glans, penile shaft purpura, and priapism (Lind et al. 2002; Sandell et al. 2002). Boys may present with acute scrotal pain mimicking torsion, thought to be secondary to transient ischemia similar to the bowel angina commonly identified in HSP patients (Ballinger 2003). Therefore, any patient with a history of scrotal pain in the presence of the typical signs and symptoms of HSP should undergo urgent hematological consultation as well as scrotal Doppler ultrasonography in order to rule out both HSP and testicular torsion, respectively. Treatment for HSP is largely supportive, consisting of steroids and other immunomodulating medications such as azathioprine (Singh et al. 2002). The majority of patients with HSP will not suffer significant long-term sequelae; however, those with renal involvement may require lifelong treatment (Ronkainen et al. 2002).

8.5.2.8
Scrotal Masses

Inguinal hernias may also present acutely and, if incarcerated, do represent a true surgical emergency. If manual reduction is unsuccessful, ischemic necrosis of the contents of the hernia is a significant concern, and therefore, emergent hernia repair is necessary. Examination will demonstrate an inguinoscrotal mass with a thickened spermatic cord (Fig. 8.46). Occasionally the underlying blood supply to the testis may become compromised and US will not be able to distinguish if concomitant torsion is present with the hernia. Exploration will reveal compression of the spermatic vessels by the hernia and its contents.

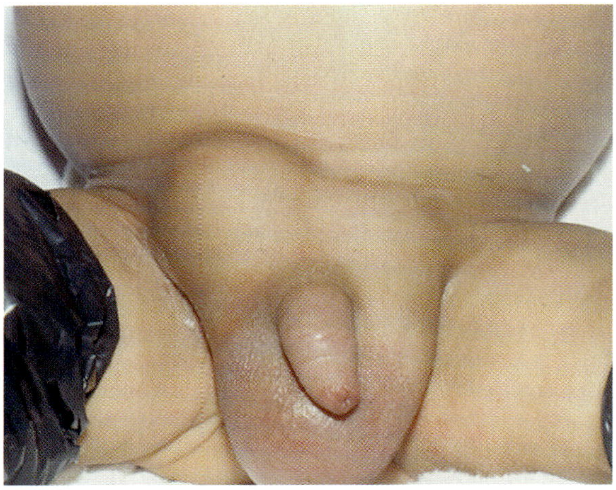

Fig. 8.46. Large bilateral inguinal hernias in a 3-month-old boy. The right hernia became incarcerated, which required emergent inguinal repair

8.5.2.9
Testis Tumors

Neonatal and pediatric testicular tumors are rarely initially seen in the emergency department. The majority are first recognized by a parent/caregiver or by primary care physicians during routine well-child examinations. Although yolk sac tumors, gonadal stromal tumors, and teratomas are most commonly encountered in the neonatal period, recent reviews have identified teratoma as the most common underlying pathologic diagnosis of a solid testicular mass in pediatric patients (Levy et al. 1994; Pohl et al. 2004). History is often consistent with a gradually enlarging, painless, scrotal mass and physical examination will identify a nontender firm mass involving or replacing the ipsilateral testis (Fig. 8.47). Blood work for testicular tumor markers including alpha-fetal protein (AFP) and beta-human chorionic gonadotropin (B-HCG) as well as scrotal US should be performed as soon as possible. Newborn and infant AFP levels may be normally elevated in the 1st year of life and, therefore, cautious interpretation of a seemingly elevated AFP level in an infant with a testicular tumor must be undertaken and rationalized within the context of the entire clinical scenario. Scrotal US is key to the diagnosis and will demonstrate an intraparenchymal mass compressing the surrounding normal testicular tissue. Intralesional calcification and cystic spaces may be seen and are more likely identified in those with teratoma (Fig. 8.48).

Any pediatric patient with a suspected testicular tumor should be approached via an inguinal incision with early control of the spermatic cord and, depending on the initial AFP and B-HCG levels, undergo either radical or partial orchidectomy. Those with clearly elevated AFP and/or B-HCG levels consistent with a germ

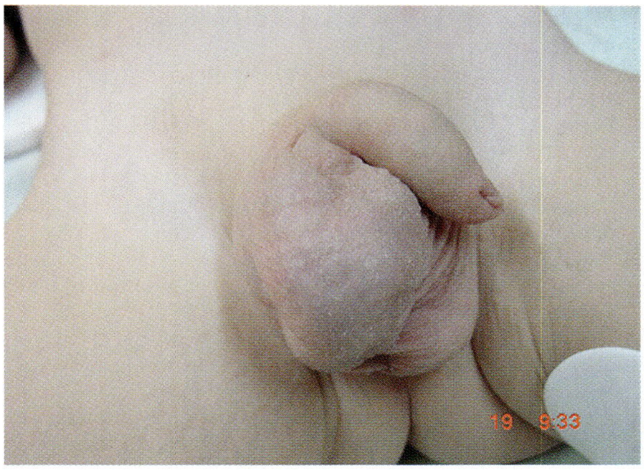

Fig. 8.47. Clinical appearance of a large right testicular mass. Pathological analysis was consistent with mature teratoma following partial orchidectomy

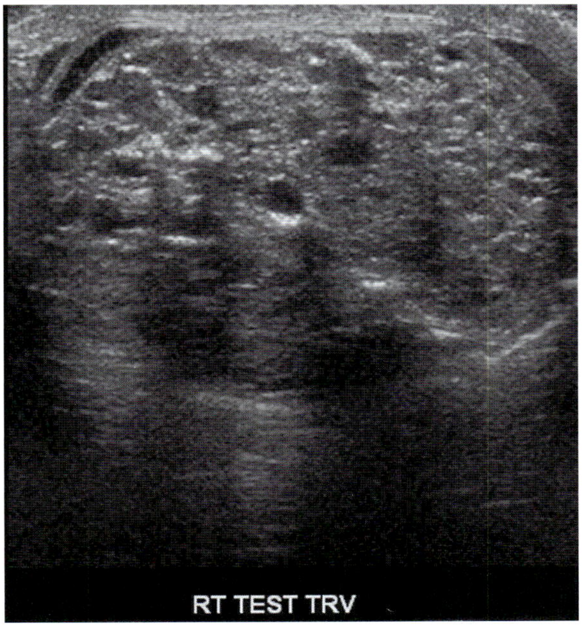

Fig. 8.48. US of same patient as Fig. 8.47. Note the cystic spaces and focal areas of calcification consistent with teratoma. The patient underwent partial orchidectomy and remains recurrence-free

cell malignancy should be treated by radical orchidectomy. CT scan should be performed preoperatively in order to avoid potentially false-positive retroperitoneal adenopathy secondary to surgery. However, patients with normal AFP and B-HCG levels can initially undergo resection of the tumor and frozen-section pathological analysis. If teratoma is identified, reconstruction of the remaining testicle is undertaken and orchiopexy performed, as it has been clearly demonstrated that prepubertal pediatric teratoma is a uniformly benign disease process(Shukla et al. 2004). However, if malignancy is identified, the remaining testicular tissue is resected and high ligation of the spermatic cord carried out. Follow-up studies have demonstrated good long-term outcomes utilizing this approach (Shukla et al. 2004; Gupta et al. 1999; Ciftci et al. 2001).

References

Arensman RM, Belman AB (1980) Ruptured congenital mesoblastic nephroma: chemotherapy and irradiation as adjuvants to nephrectomy. Urology 15:394

Atikeler MK, Gecit I, Yuzgec V, Yalcin O (2005) Complications of circumcision performed within and outside the hospital. Int Urol Nephrol 37:97

Badani KK, Hemal AK, Menon M (2004) Autosomal dominant polycystic kidney disease and pain – a review of the disease from aetiology, evaluation, past surgical treatment options to current practice. J Postgrad Med 50:222

Baeten JM, Richardson BA, Lavreys L, Rakwar JP, Mandaliya K, Bwayo JJ et al (2005) Female-to-male infectivity of HIV-1 among circumcised and uncircumcised Kenyan men. J Infect Dis 191:546

Baker LA, Gearhart JP (1998) The staged approach to bladder exstrophy closure and the role of osteotomies. World J Urol 16:205

Balkan E, Kilic N, Dogruyol H (2005) The effectiveness of early primary realignment in children with posterior urethral injury. Int J Urol 12:62

Ballinger S (2003) Henoch-Schonlein purpura. Curr Opin Rheumatol 15:591

Baskin LS, McAninch JW (1993) Childhood urethral injuries: perspectives on outcome and treatment. Br J Urol 72:241

Benjamin DK Jr, Fisher RG, McKinney RE Jr, Benjamin DK (1999) Candidal mycetoma in the neonatal kidney. Pediatrics 104:1126

Bloomfield P, Hodson EM, Craig JC (2005) Antibiotics for acute pyelonephritis in children. Cochrane Database Syst Rev: CD003772

Borer JG, Gargollo PC, Hendren WH, Diamond DA, Peters CA, Atala A et al (2005) Early outcome following complete primary repair of bladder exstrophy in the newborn. J Urol 174:1674

Bousvaros A, Kirks DR, Grossman H (1986) Imaging of neuroblastoma: an overview. Pediatr Radiol 16:89

Bove KE (1999) Wilms' tumor and related abnormalities in the fetus and newborn. Semin Perinatol 23:310

Bryant K, Maxfield C, Rabalais G (1999) Renal candidiasis in neonates with candiduria. Pediatr Infect Dis J 18:959

Buckley JC, McAninch JW (2004) Pediatric renal injuries: management guidelines from a 25-year experience. J Urol 172:687

Busby JE, Pettaway CA (2005) What's new in the management of penile cancer? Curr Opin Urol 15:350

Carroll PR, McAninch JW (1984) Major bladder trauma: mechanisms of injury and a unified method of diagnosis and repair. J Urol 132:254

Cass AS, Luxenberg M (1989) Management of extraperitoneal ruptures of bladder caused by external trauma. Urology 33:179

Chandler JC, Gauderer MW (2004) The neonate with an abdominal mass. Pediatr Clin North Am 51:979

Chopra P, St-Vil D, Yazbeck S (2002) Blunt renal trauma–blessing in disguise? J Pediatr Surg 37:779

Ciftci AO, Bingol-Kologlu M, Senocak ME, Tanyel FC, Buyukpamukcu M, Buyukpamukcu N (2001) Testicular tumors in children. J Pediatr Surg, 36:1796

Cole BR, Conley SB, Stapleton FB (1987) Polycystic kidney disease in the first year of life. J Pediatr 111:693
Cook AJ, Farhat WA, Cartwright LM, Khoury AE, Pippi Salle JL (2005) Simplified mons plasty: a new technique to improve cosmesis in females with the exstrophy-epispadias complex. J Urol 173:2117
Coppes MJ, Zandvoort SW, Sparling CR, Poon AO, Weitzman S, Blanchette VS (1992) Acquired von Willebrand disease in Wilms' tumor patients. J Clin Oncol 10:422
Coppes MJ, Haber DA, Grundy PE (1994) Genetic events in the development of Wilms' tumor. N Engl J Med 331:586
Couillard DR, Vapnek JM, Rentzepis MJ, Stone AR (1993) Fatal perforation of augmentation cystoplasty in an adult. Urology 42:585
Dacou-Voutetakis C, Maniati-Christidi M, Dracopoulou-Vabouli M (2001) Genetic aspects of congenital adrenal hyperplasia. J Pediatr Endocrinol Metab 14 [Suppl 5]:1303
Daling JR, Madeleine MM, Johnson LG, Schwartz SM, Shera KA, Wurscher MA et al (2005) Penile cancer: importance of circumcision, human papillomavirus and smoking in in situ and invasive disease. Int J Cancer 116:606
Davenport M (1996) ABC of general surgery in children. Problems with the penis and prepuce. BMJ 312:299
Deck AJ, Shaves S, Talner L, Porter JR (2001) Current experience with computed tomographic cystography and blunt trauma. World J Surg 25:1592
Deshpande PV, Jones KV (2001) An audit of RCP guidelines on DMSA scanning after urinary tract infection. Arch Dis Child 84:324
Dewan PA, Walton JK (1987) Spermatic cord torsion in the neonate. Aust N Z J Surg 57:331
Diamond DA, Jeffs RD (1985) Cloacal exstrophy: a 22-year experience. J Urol 133:779
Elder JS, Snyder HM, Hulbert WC, Duckett JW (1988) Perforation of the augmented bladder in patients undergoing clean intermittent catheterization. J Urol 140:1159
Engel RM (1974) Exstrophy of the bladder and associated anomalies. Birth Defects Orig Artic Ser 10:146
Forest MG (2004) Recent advances in the diagnosis and management of congenital adrenal hyperplasia due to 21-hydroxylase deficiency. Hum Reprod Update 10:469
Gagnadoux MF, Habib R, Levy M, Brunelle F, Broyer M (1989) Cystic renal diseases in children. Adv Nephrol Necker Hosp 18:33
Gargollo PC, Kozakewich HP, Bauer SB, Borer JG, Peters CA, Retik AB et al (2005) Balanitis xerotica obliterans in boys. J Urol 174:1409
Gassner HL, Toppari J, Quinteiro Gonzalez S, Miller WL (2004) Near-miss apparent SIDS from adrenal crisis. J Pediatr 145:178
Gearhart JP, Ben-Chaim J, Jeffs RD, Sanders RC (1995) Criteria for the prenatal diagnosis of classic bladder exstrophy. Obstet Gynecol 85:961
Geller E, Smergel EM, Lowry PA (1997) Renal neoplasms of childhood. Radiol Clin North Am 35:1391
Gesundheit B, Smith CR, Gerstle JT, Weitzman SS, Chan HS (2004) Ataxia and secretory diarrhea: two unusual paraneoplastic syndromes occurring concurrently in the same patient with ganglioneuroblastoma. J Pediatr Hematol Oncol 26:549
Godzinski J, Weirich A, Tournade MF, Gauthier F, Buerger D, Moorman-Voestermans CG et al (2001) Primary nephrectomy for emergency: a rare event in the International Society of Paediatric Oncology Nephroblastoma Trial and Study no 9. Eur J Pediatr Surg 11:36
Gong M, Geary ES, Shortliffe LM (1996) Testicular torsion with contralateral vanishing testis. Urology 48:306
Gosalbez R, Castellan M, Ibrahim E, DiSandro M, Labbie A (2005) New concepts in feminizing genitoplasty–is the Fortunoff flap obsolete? J Urol 174:2350
Grady RW, Mitchell ME (1999) Complete primary repair of exstrophy. J Urol 162:1415
Griscom NT, Colodny AH, Rosenberg HK, Fliegel CP, Hardy BE (1977) Diagnostic aspects of neonatal ascites: report of 27 cases. AJR Am J Roentgenol 128:961
Gupta DK, Kataria R, Sharma MC (1999) Prepubertal testicular teratomas. Eur J Pediatr Surg 9:173
Haas CA, Brown SL, Spirnak JP (1999) Limitations of routine spiral computerized tomography in the evaluation of bladder trauma. J Urol 162:51
Haase GM, Perez C, Atkinson JB (1999) Current aspects of biology, risk assessment, and treatment of neuroblastoma. Semin Surg Oncol 16:91
Hafez AT, El-Assmy A, Sarhan O, El-Hefnawy AS, Ghoneim MA (2005) Perineal anastomotic urethroplasty for managing post-traumatic urethral strictures in children: the long-term outcome. BJU Int 95:403
Hahn-Pedersen J, Kvist N, Nielsen OH (1984) Hydrometrocolpos: current views on pathogenesis and management. J Urol 132:537
Hamza AF, Soliman HA, Abdel Hay SA, Kabesh AA, Elbehery MM (2001) Total urogenital sinus mobilization in the repair of cloacal anomalies and congenital adrenal hyperplasia. J Pediatr Surg 36:1656
Hanstead B, John HT (1964) Idiopathic scrotal oedema of children. Br J Urol 36:110
Heidelberger KP, Ritchey ML, Dauser RC, McKeever PE, Beckwith JB (1993) Congenital mesoblastic nephroma metastatic to the brain. Cancer 72:2499
Herman TE, Shackelford GD, McAlister WH (1994) Acute idiopathic scrotal edema: role of scrotal sonography. J Ultrasound Med 13:53
Herndon CD, McKenna PH, Kolon TF, Gonzales ET, Baker LA, Docimo SG (1999) A multicenter outcomes analysis of patients with neonatal reflux presenting with prenatal hydronephrosis. J Urol 162:1203
Hochberg E, Stone NN (1993) Bladder rupture associated with pelvic fracture due to blunt trauma. Urology 41:531
Huang CR, Sun N, Wei P, Xie HW, Hwang AH, Hardy BE (2003) The management of old urethral injury in young girls: analysis of 44 cases. J Pediatr Surg 38:1329
Ives E, Coffey R, Carter CO (1980) A family study of bladder exstrophy. J Med Genet 17:139
Ivy DD, Shaffer EM, Johnson AM, Kimberling WJ, Dobin A, Gabow PA (1995) Cardiovascular abnormalities in children with autosomal dominant polycystic kidney disease. J Am Soc Nephrol 5:2032
Jayanthi VR, Churchill BM, McLorie GA, Khoury AE (1995) Concomitant bladder neck closure and Mitrofanoff diversion for the management of intractable urinary incontinence. J Urol 154:886
Kadish HA, Bolte RG (1998) A retrospective review of pediatric patients with epididymitis, testicular torsion, and torsion of testicular appendages. Pediatrics 102:73
Kansas BT, Eddy MJ, Mydlo JH, Uzzo RG (2004) Incidence and management of penetrating renal trauma in patients with multiorgan injury: extended experience at an inner city trauma center. J Urol 172:1355
Keller MS, Eric Coln C, Garza JJ, Sartorelli KH, Christine Green M, Weber TR (2004) Functional outcome of nonoperatively managed renal injuries in children. J Trauma 57:108
Kim EK, Song TB (1996) A study on fetal urinary tract anomaly: antenatal ultrasonographic diagnosis and postnatal follow-up. J Obstet Gynaecol Res 22:569
King LR, Coughlin PW, Bloch EC, Bowie JD, Ansong K, Hanna MK (1984) The case for immediate pyeloplasty in the neonate with ureteropelvic junction obstruction. J Urol 132:725

Klin B, Lotan G, Efrati Y, Zlotkevich L, Strauss S (2002) Acute idiopathic scrotal edema in children–revisited. J Pediatr Surg 37:1200

Kotkin L, Koch MO (1995) Morbidity associated with nonoperative management of extraperitoneal bladder injuries. J Trauma 38:895

Kuwertz-Broeking E, Brinkmann OA, Von Lengerke HJ, Sciuk J, Fruend S, Bulla M et al (2004) Unilateral multicystic dysplastic kidney: experience in children. BJU Int 93:388

Lack EE, Cassady JR, Sallan SE (1985) Renal cell carcinoma in childhood and adolescence: a clinical and pathological study of 17 cases. J Urol 133:822

Landing BH, Wells TR, Claireaux AE (1980) Morphometric analysis of liver lesions in cystic diseases of childhood. Hum Pathol 11:549

Lee MM, Donahoe PK (1997) The infant with ambiguous genitalia. Curr Ther Endocrinol Metab 6:216

Levy DA, Kay R, Elder JS (1994) Neonatal testis tumors: a review of the Prepubertal Testis Tumor Registry. J Urol 151:715

Lind J, Mackay A, Withers SJ (2002) Henoch-Schönlein purpura and priapism. J Paediatr Child Health 38:526

Lonergan GJ, Martinez-Leon MI, Agrons GA, Montemarano H, Suarez ES (1998) Nephrogenic rests, nephroblastomatosis, and associated lesions of the kidney. Radiographics 18:947

Lowe LH, Isuani BH, Heller RM, Stein SM, Johnson JE, Navarro OM et al (2000) Pediatric renal masses: Wilms tumor and beyond. Radiographics 20:1585

Ludwig M, Beck A, Wickert L, Bolkenius U, Tittel B, Hinkel K et al (1998) Female pseudohermaphroditism associated with a novel homozygous G-to-A (V370-to-M) substitution in the P-450 aromatase gene. J Pediatr Endocrinol Metab 11:657

MacNeily AE, Maizels M, Kaplan WE, Firlit CF, Conway JJ (1993) Does early pyeloplasty really avert loss of renal function? A retrospective review. J Urol 150:769

Marild S, Jodal U (1998) Incidence rate of first-time symptomatic urinary tract infection in children under 6 years of age. Acta Paediatr 87:549

Matsumura M, Nishi T, Sasaki Y, Yamada R, Yamamoto H, Ohhama Y et al (1993) Prenatal diagnosis and treatment strategy for congenital mesoblastic nephroma. J Pediatr Surg 28:1607

McAleer IM, Kaplan GW, Scherz HC, Packer MG, Lynch FP (1993) Genitourinary trauma in the pediatric patient. Urology 42:563

McAleer IM, Kaplan GW, LoSasso BE (2002a) Congenital urinary tract anomalies in pediatric renal trauma patients. J Urol 168:1808

McAleer IM, Kaplan GW, LoSasso BE (2002b) Renal and testis injuries in team sports. J Urol 168:1805

McClamrock HD, Adashi EY: Gestational hyperandrogenism. Fertil Steril 57:257

Melekos MD (1988) Re: testicular torsion in a 62-year-old man. J Urol 140:387

Mesrobian HG, Balcom AH, Durkee CT (2004) Urologic problems of the neonate. Pediatr Clin North Am 51:1051

Miller DC, Rumohr JA, Dunn RL, Bloom DA, Park JM (2004) What is the fate of the refluxing contralateral kidney in children with multicystic dysplastic kidney? J Urol 172:1630

Miller RC, Sterioff S Jr, Drucker WR, Persky L, Wright HK, Davis JH (1966) The incidental discovery of occult abdominal tumors in children following blunt abdominal trauma. J Trauma 6:99

Milliner DS, Murphy ME (1993) Urolithiasis in pediatric patients. Mayo Clin Proc 68:241

Mills JA, Michel BA, Bloch DA, Calabrese LH, Hunder GG, Arend WP et al (1990) The American College of Rheumatology: 1990 criteria for the classification of Henoch-Schönlein purpura. Arthritis Rheum 33:1114

Munden MM, Trautwein LM (2000) Scrotal pathology in pediatrics with sonographic imaging. Curr Probl Diagn Radiol 29:185

Murphy JP, Holder TM, Ashcraft KW, Sharp RJ, Goodwin CD, Amoury RA (1984) Ureteropelvic junction obstruction in the newborn. J Pediatr Surg 19:642

Naber KG, Bergman B, Bishop MC, Bjerklund-Johansen TE, Botto H, Lobel B et al (2001) EAU guidelines for the management of urinary and male genital tract infections. Urinary Tract Infection (UTI) Working Group of the Health Care Office (HCO) of the European Association of Urology (EAU) Eur Urol 40:576

Najmaldin A, Burge DM (1987) Acute idiopathic scrotal oedema: incidence, manifestations and aetiology. Br J Surg 74:634

Nance ML, Lutz N, Carr MC, Canning DA, Stafford PW (2004) Blunt renal injuries in children can be managed nonoperatively: outcome in a consecutive series of patients. J Trauma 57:474

Nelson CP, Dunn R, Wan J, Wei JT (2005) The increasing incidence of newborn circumcision: data from the nationwide inpatient sample. J Urol 173:978

Nuss R, Hays T, Manco-Johnson M (1994) Efficacy and safety of heparin anticoagulation for neonatal renal vein thrombosis. Am J Pediatr Hematol Oncol 16:127

Oliveira EA, Diniz JS, Vilasboas AS, Rabelo EA, Silva JM, Filgueiras MT (2001) Multicystic dysplastic kidney detected by fetal sonography: conservative management and follow-up. Pediatr Surg Int 17:54

Papadopoulou D, Tsakiris D, Papadimitriou M (1999) The use of ultrasonography and linkage studies for early diagnosis of autosomal dominant polycystic kidney disease (ADPKD) Ren Fail 21:67

Pathak IG, Williams DI (1964) Multicystic and cystic dysplastic kidneys. Br J Urol 36:318

Pearle MS (2003) Pediatric staghorn calculi: the role of extracorporeal shock wave lithotripsy monotherapy with special reference to ureteral stenting. Int Braz J Urol 29:168

Pena A, Levitt MA, Hong A, Midulla P (2004) Surgical management of cloacal malformations: a review of 339 patients. J Pediatr Surg 39:470

Perry R, Kecha O, Paquette J, Huot C, Van Vliet G, Deal C (2005) Primary adrenal insufficiency in children: twenty years experience at the Sainte-Justine Hospital Montreal. J Clin Endocrinol Metab 90:3243

Phillips JR, Karlowicz MG (1997) Prevalence of Candida species in hospital-acquired urinary tract infections in a neonatal intensive care unit. Pediatr Infect Dis J 16:190

Ping AJ, Reeve AE, Law DJ, Young MR, Boehnke M, Feinberg AP (1989) Genetic linkage of Beckwith-Wiedemann syndrome to 11p. Am J Hum Genet, 44:720

Pohl HG, Shukla AR, Metcalf PD, Cilento BG, Retik AB, Bagli DJ et al (2004) Prepubertal testis tumors: actual prevalence rate of histological types. J Urol 172:2370

Rabelo EA, Oliveira EA, Diniz JS, Silva JM, Filgueiras MT, Pezzuti IL et al (2004) Natural history of multicystic kidney conservatively managed: a prospective study. Pediatr Nephrol 19:1102

Rampaul MS, Hosking SW (1998) Testicular torsion: most delay occurs outside hospital. Ann R Coll Surg Engl 80:169

Ritchey ML, Kelalis PP, Breslow N, Offord KP, Shochat SJ, D'Angio GJ (1988) Intracaval and atrial involvement with nephroblastoma: review of National Wilms Tumor Study-3. J Urol, 140:1113

Rogers CG, Knight V, MacUra KJ, Ziegfeld S, Paidas CN, Mathews RI (2004) High-grade renal injuries in children–is conservative management possible? Urology 64:574

Ronkainen J, Nuutinen M, Koskimies O (2002) The adult kid-

ney 24 years after childhood Henoch-Schönlein purpura: a retrospective cohort study. Lancet 360:666
Rowen JL, Tate JM (1998) Management of neonatal candidiasis. Neonatal Candidiasis Study Group. Pediatr Infect Dis J 17:1007
Ruberto U, D'Eufemia P, Martino F, Giardini O (1989) Amoxycillin and clavulanic acid in the treatment of urinary tract infections in children. J Int Med Res 17:168
Rushton HG, Woodard JR, Parrott TS, Jeffs RD, Gearhart JP (1988) Delayed bladder rupture after augmentation enterocystoplasty. J Urol 140:344
Sandell J, Ramanan R, Shah D (2002) Penile involvement in Henoch-Schönlein purpura. Indian J Pediatr 69:529
Sherer DM, Kendig JW, Sickel JZ, Salafia CM, Donahue ML (1994) In utero adrenal hemorrhage associated with fetal distress, subsequent transient neonatal hypertension, and a nonfunctioning ipsilateral kidney. Am J Perinatol 11:302
Shokeir AA, El-Sherbiny MT, Gad HM, Dawaba M, Hafez AT, Taha MA et al (2005) Postnatal unilateral pelviureteral junction obstruction: impact of pyeloplasty and conservative management on renal function. Urology 65:980
Shukla AR, Woodard C, Carr MC, Huff DS, Canning DA, Zderic SA et al (1999) Experience with testis sparing surgery for testicular teratoma. J Urol 171:161
Singh S, Devidayal Kumar L, Joshi K, Minz RW, Datta U (2002) Severe Henoch-Schönlein nephritis: resolution with azathioprine and steroids. Rheumatol Int 22:133
Singh-Grewal D, Macdessi J, Craig J (2005) Circumcision for the prevention of urinary tract infection in boys: a systematic review of randomised trials and observational studies. Arch Dis Child 90:853
Skari H, Bjornland K, Bjornstad-Ostensen A, Haugen G, Emblem R (1998) Consequences of prenatal ultrasound diagnosis: a preliminary report on neonates with congenital malformations. Acta Obstet Gynecol Scand 77:635
Somekh E, Gorenstein A, Serour F (2004) Acute epididymitis in boys: evidence of a post-infectious etiology. J Urol 171:391
Sullivan P (2002) Infant's death: another nail in circumcision's coffin, group says. CMAJ, 167:789
Tan AH, Al-Omar M, Denstedt JD, Razvi H (2005) Ureteroscopy for pediatric urolithiasis: an evolving first-line therapy. Urology 65:153
Velaphi SC, Perlman JM (2001) Neonatal adrenal hemorrhage: clinical and abdominal sonographic findings. Clin Pediatr (Phila) 40:545
White KS, Grossman H (1991) Wilms' and associated renal tumors of childhood. Pediatr Radiol 21:81
Yang SS, Tsai YC, Wu CC, Liu SP, Wang CC (2005) Highly potent and moderately potent topical steroids are effective in treating phimosis: a prospective randomized study. J Urol 173:1361
Yerkes EB, Robertson FM, Gitlin J, Kaefer M, Cain MP, Rink RC (2005) Management of perinatal torsion: today, tomorrow or never? J Urol 174:1579
Zerres K, Rudnik-Schoneborn S, Steinkamm C, Becker J, Mucher G (1998) Autosomal recessive polycystic kidney disease. J Mol Med 76:303

Autonomic Dysreflexia and Emergencies in Neurogenic Bladder

B. Wefer, K.-P. Jünemann

9.1 Autonomic Dysreflexia

Autonomic dysreflexia is an acute syndrome characterized by abrupt onset of excessively high blood pressure caused by uncontrolled sympathetic nervous system discharge in patients with spinal cord injury (SCI). Autonomic dysreflexia is potentially life-threatening.

The syndrome was first described by Head and Riddoch in 1917 (Head and Riddoch 1917). In 1947, Guttmann and Whitteridge showed the effects of bladder distensions on the cardiovascular system (Guttmann and Whitteridge 1947). Autonomic dysreflexia is also known as autonomic hyperreflexia, paroxysmal neurogenic hypertension, sympathetic hyperreflexia, and neurovegetative syndrome.

9.1.1 Epidemiology, Pathophysiology, and Clinical Features

The frequency of autonomic dysreflexia varies widely, but appears to be relatively common in spinal cord-injured patients with a lesion at or above the sixth thoracic neurologic level (T6). Sometimes autonomic dysreflexia is also seen in paraplegic patients with lesions below T6, but usually the clinical presentation is milder. Lifetime frequency of autonomic dysreflexia is between 19% and 85% (Snow et al. 1978; Braddom and Rocco 1991; Shergill et al. 2004). In particular, patients with cervical lesions (60%) show autonomic dysreflexia compared to patients with thoracic lesions (20%).

In healthy persons, an afferent stimulus enters the spinal cord and then ascends to the brain. Some interneurons are reflexively connected with preganglionic sympathetic neurons and excite them, resulting in vasoconstriction below the neurologic lesion and causing a rise in blood pressure. In neurologically intact persons, higher centers inhibit these sympathetic effects by a compensatory vasodilatation of the splanchnic bed, resulting in normalized blood pressure.

In SCI patients, these higher inhibitory pathways are not intact and cannot reach the splanchnic bed, resulting in high blood pressure. As a parasympathetic reflex, the heart beat is also reduced (bradycardia).

Typical clinical signs and symptoms are:

- Sudden severe hypertension
- Bradycardia (tachycardia is also possible)
- Severe pounding headache
- Flushed (reddened) face
- Paresthesia neck, shoulder, and arms
- Nasal congestion
- Blurred vision
- Tightness in chest
- Nausea
- Feeling of anxiety and agitation
- Arrhythmia
- Bladder and bowel contraction
- Penile erection
- Sweating and red blotches *above* the level of spinal cord injury
- Piloerection (goose bumps) and cold, clammy skin *below* the level of spinal cord injury

It is important to note that the resting blood pressure decreases after a spinal cord injury. Often a blood pressure of 90/60 mm Hg is normal for SCI patients and this means that even a normal blood pressure of 120/80 mm Hg might be considered increased. If possible, SCI patients should be asked for their normal resting blood pressure.

9.1.2 Etiology

Almost any precipitant below the neurologic lesion can trigger autonomic dysreflexia. Important to the urologist, a genitourinary cause is responsible in 81%–87% of cases (Shergill et al. 2004). The commonest reason for autonomic dysreflexia is bladder distension, accounting for 75%–85% of cases (Blackmer 2003). Bladder distension can be a consequence of a kinked or obstructed catheter as well as an insufficient intermittent catheterization frequency. Other urinary triggers are infection, instrumentation, stones, and urethral distension.

As almost 90% of cases have a genitourinary cause, it is particularly important for the urologist to prevent autonomic dysreflexia. When treating patients with SCI, the urologist should be aware of the possibility of autonomic dysreflexia. When performing instrumentation of the lower urinary tract, for example changing a catheter, local anesthetic jelly and an aseptic technique (to avoid urinary tract infection as a precipitant of autonomic dysreflexia) should be used. If the instrumentation takes more than a few minutes (cystoscopy, urodynamic investigation) sufficient blood pressure monitoring should also be provided. It should also be noted that even sexual intercourse can effect autonomic dysreflexia. Therefore the andrologist should keep in mind this risk when applying vibroejaculation to a SCI patient.

The second most common precipitant for autonomic dysreflexia is bowel distension (13%–19% of cases).

Table 9.1 displays precipitants for autonomic dysreflexia.

Table 9.1. Precipitants for autonomic dysreflexia

Urological	Bladder distension (kinked/obstructed catheter) Infection Urethral distension Instrumentation (indwelling catheter, cystoscopy, urodynamics) Stones Ejaculation (vibro- or electroejaculation) Sexual intercourse
Gastrointestinal	Bowel distension (fecal impaction) Instrumentation Infection or inflammation (colitis, peritonitis) Gastric ulcer Reflux Hemorrhoids Anal fissure
Dermatologic	Pressure sore Ingrown toenail Burns (sunburns, burns from hot water) Tight clothing or pressure to skin
Skeletal	Heterotopic ossification Fracture Joint dislocation
Reproductive	Labor and delivery Menstruation Testicular torsion
Hematologic	Deep vein thrombosis Pulmonary embolism

9.1.3 Treatment

Acute management of autonomic dysreflexia is important to prevent complications. If untreated autonomic dysreflexia can lead to convulsions, subarachnoid hemorrhage, intracerebral bleeding, hypertensive encephalopathy, cardiac arrhythmias, neurogenic pulmonary edema and death (Shergill et al. 2004).

The acute management aims to relieve the precipitant cause and management of symptoms to prevent potential complications. The long-term goal is to prevent recurrence of autonomic dysreflexia.

Immediately the precipitant should be identified and treated.

To prevent a further increase in blood pressure, the patient should be seated upright with the head raised to induce an orthostatic drop in blood pressure. Tight clothing should be removed and during treatment the blood pressure should be monitored carefully (every 2–5 min).

Then the trigger for autonomic dysreflexia should be identified and eliminated. In most cases, a genitourinary problem is the precipitant. Therefore, if the patient has an indwelling catheter the catheter should be checked for kinks and obstructions. In addition, a full urinary bag can cause bladder distension leading to autonomic dysreflexia. If necessary, the catheter should be carefully flushed with saline solution. Irrigation should be limited to 5–10 ml in children under 2 years and 10–15 ml in children older than 2 years and adults.

If no indwelling catheter is placed but bladder distension is the suspected trigger, a catheter should be inserted. Before inserting the catheter, the urethra should be instilled with lidocaine jelly to avoid further triggers for autonomic dysreflexia. In many cases, draining the bladder alleviates the symptoms of autonomic dysreflexia.

If afferent stimulation of bladder wall receptors (infection, stones) is supporting the autonomic dysreflexia, local anesthetic (lidocaine) instillation of the bladder might be effective (Dietz 1996).

High-dose antibiotics are delivered if urinary tract infection is suspected to be the cause. If symptoms persist other triggers must be sought.

The next step is a rectal examination for fecal impaction and a gentle manual evacuation if necessary.

If the precipitant for autonomic dysreflexia is not found within the first few minutes medical treatment is necessary when the blood pressure remains high.

There are only a few published studies on medical treatment of autonomic dysreflexia, but nifedipine and nitrates are the most commonly used drugs. The immediate release form is the preferred method of administration.

Nifedipine is given in a dose of 10 mg using the bite-and-swallow method. Adverse effects of nifedipine have been reported (reflex tachycardia and hypotension), but in these studies nifedipine was not used to treat autonomic dysreflexia (Consortium for Spinal Cord Medicine 2001).

Nitrates (glyceryl trinitrate, isosorbide dinitrate, sodium nitroprusside) are also used to treat autonomic dysreflexia. If the blood pressure remains high an intravenous drip of sodium nitroprusside could be necessary. Before using these drugs (nitrates), the patient should be questioned regarding sildenafil or other PDE-5 inhibitors. If a PDE-5 inhibitor was used in the last 24 h an alternative short-acting, rapid-onset antihypertensive drug should be used. Drugs with these characteristics are captopril and prazosin.

Other drugs that have been used to treat autonomic dysreflexia include hydralazine, phenoxybenzamine, clonidine, diazoxide, and mecamylamine (Consortium for Spinal Cord Medicine 2001; Blackmer 2003).

With recurrent episodes of autonomic dysreflexia, *prevention* is the best approach. Therefore patients with spinal cord injury and their families should be educated about proper bladder, bowel, and skin management. If a catheter is present it should be changed regularly with great care and attention to avoid autonomic dysreflexia, ideally using local anesthetic jelly. Urodynamic investigations should be done with blood pressure monitoring in SCI patients. Other colleagues should be made aware of the propensity for autonomic dysreflexia in affected patients.

9.2 Neurogenic Bladder and Spinal Shock

Directly after the spinal cord injury, all reflexes below the neurologic lesion have disappeared. This is called spinal shock. In this phase, the bladder is hypotonic. This phase takes normally 4–6 weeks, sometimes up to 6–8 months.

To prevent the bladder from overdistension (due to polyuria), it is important to drain the urine continuously. Usually indwelling catheters are used. A better approach is a suprapubic catheter, especially in men, to prevent the patient from urethral trauma and prostatic infections.

After the polyuria phase, the patient should start with an intermittent catheterization program (if possible dependent on neurologic lesion and hand function) (Dietz 1996).

When the spinal shock phase ends, bladder dysfunction will develop and a urodynamic investigation is needed to treat the dysfunction properly.

Bladder rehabilitation should be a part of the overall rehabilitation routine after spinal cord injury *and should be adjusted to the result of the urodynamic investigation.*

References

Blackmer J (2003) Rehabilitation medicine: autonomic dysreflexia. CMAJ 28:169:931

Braddom RL, RJ (1991) Autonomic dysreflexia. A survey of current treatment. Am J Phys Med Rehabil 70:234

Consortium for Spinal Cord Medicine (2001) Acute management of autonomic dysreflexia: individuals with spinal cord injury presenting to health care facilities. Washington, DC, The Consortium of Paralyzed Veterans of America

Dietz (1996) Querschnittslähmung: Physiopathologie Klinik und Therapie von Blasenfunktion Bewegung und Vegetativum. Kohlhammer, Stuttgart

Guttmann L, Whitteridge D (1947) Effects of bladder distension on automatic mechanisms after spinal cord injury. Brain 70:361

Head H, Riddoch G (1917) The autonomic bladder, excessive sweating and some other reflex conditions in gross injuries of the spinal cord. Brain 40:188

Shergill IS, Arya M, Hamid R, Khastgir J, Patel HR, Shah PJ (2004) The importance of autonomic dysreflexia to the urologist. BJU Int. 93:923

Snow JC, SH, Kripke BJ, Freed MM, Shah NK, Schlesinger RM (1978) Autonomic hyperreflexia during cystoscopy in patients with high spinal cord injuries. Paraplegia 15:327

10 Failure of Urinary Drainage: Upper Urinary

M.T. Gettman, J.W. Segura

10.1 Introduction

Failure of upper urinary drainage represents a relatively common urologic emergency. Obstruction of the upper urinary tract can be related to a variety of underlying clinical scenarios. In the current era, technologic advances have facilitated an accurate diagnosis and streamlined treatment. Nonetheless, correct management involves attention to presenting clinical signs and symptoms and an awareness of subtle nuances related to the underlying etiology. In this chapter, we describe the presenting signs and symptoms, differential diagnosis, radiographic testing, laboratory evaluation, acute management, follow-up, and pitfalls associated with failure of upper urinary tract drainage.

10.2 Presenting Signs and Symptoms

10.2.1 Patient Presentation

The patient presentation associated with upper urinary tract obstruction is varied. In addition, the differential diagnosis of upper urinary obstruction is extensive (Table 10.1). Many patients seen on an emergent basis will have classic symptoms of renal colic; however, an urgent evaluation may be requested for a totally asymptomatic patient with incidentally discovered unilateral or bilateral upper urinary tract obstruction.

The presenting signs and symptoms can be impacted by many factors related to the underlying etiology such as the interval of time in which the obstruction developed (acute vs chronic), presence of infection, nature of the obstruction (intrinsic vs extrinsic), laterality (unilateral vs bilateral), and the degree of blockage (complete obstruction vs partial obstruction) (Gulmi et al. 2002). Other important factors to consider when evaluating a patient with upper urinary obstruction are the patient's number of renal moieties, known congenital anomalies of the upper urinary tract (e.g., horseshoe kidney), and a history of renal transplantation. For example, the signs and symptoms for a patient with a blocked renal allograft would be entirely different than a patient with a blocked solitary native kidney. Specifically, pain-related symptoms of obstruction would classically be absent in the renal transplantation patient.

10.2.2 Unilateral Upper Urinary Tract Obstruction

One of the most common forms of failed drainage in the upper urinary tract is acute unilateral ureteral ob-

Table 10.1. Etiology of upper urinary tract obstruction

Intrinsic
Urothelial carcinoma
Fibroepithelial polyp
UPJ obstruction
Ureterovesical junction obstruction
Acquired stricture
Congenital stricture
Urinary stones
Tuberculosis
Papillary necrosis
Trauma
Extrinsic
Renal cell carcinoma
Wilms tumor
Cystic renal diseases
Parapelvic cysts
Renal artery aneurysm
Retroperitoneal malignancy (primary or metastatic)
Adnexal mass
Endometriosis
UPJ obstruction
Retrocaval ureter
Abscess
Appendicitis
Inflammatory bowel disease
Trauma (ureteral ligation)
Radiation therapy
Lymphocele
Urinoma
Retroperitoneal fibrosis
Pelvic lipomatosis
Aortic aneurysm
Pregnancy

struction. The underlying etiology is often urinary calculi, but the diagnostic possibilities are extensive (Kobayashi et al. 2003). In general, acute obstruction is most commonly associated with intermittent, severe flank pain that can radiate into the groin, external genitalia, and/or ipsilateral thigh (i.e., classic renal colic). Gross hematuria can also be associated with the colicky symptoms. Not uncommonly, gastrointestinal complaints including nausea and vomiting will also accompany the symptoms. In addition, patients can also experience fever and chills, especially if the obstruction is associated with infection (Nickel 2002). In some instances, patients can present with partial unilateral obstruction in the absence of flank pain. In this scenario, an urgent evaluation is often prompted by other associated symptoms including nausea and vomiting, abdominal pain, new onset of irritative voiding symptoms, or gross hematuria. In other instances, the finding of a partial obstructing stone can be an entirely incidental finding. In the setting of acute unilateral urinary obstruction, the development of gross hematuria in the presence or absence of pain also may suggest an etiology of blockage unrelated to stone disease.

The development of chronic unilateral upper urinary obstruction often occurs over extended periods of time and frequently is not associated with presenting symptoms. Unless the patient is to develop concurrent symptoms (i.e., hematuria, recurrent urinary tract infections, etc.), the obstruction is typically an incidental finding. In some instances such as unilateral ureteropelvic junction (UPJ) obstruction or ureterovesical obstruction, pain-related symptoms may occur only after increased fluid intake. A classic example of this would be the development of flank pain following the ingestion of alcohol in a patient with UPJ obstruction. More commonly, chronic unilateral obstruction is related to an extrinsic process that has developed slowly over time. In most cases, the obstruction will be evaluated as an incidental finding in the ambulatory care setting.

10.2.3 Bilateral Upper Urinary Tract Obstruction

The classic presentation of bilateral upper urinary tract obstruction often differs clinically when compared to unilateral obstruction. Bilateral upper urinary obstruction most commonly occurs on a more chronic basis, related to an extrinsic process that progresses slowly over time. In this scenario, signs and symptoms directly related to the extrinsic process often prompt the workup which ultimately leads to the diagnosis of bilateral obstruction. When bilateral chronic upper urinary tract obstruction progresses to the point of causing symptoms, manifestations of renal failure are also commonplace. A common presentation for acute bilateral upper urinary obstruction is related to bilateral obstructing ureteral or UPJ stones. The tip-off to this diagnosis can be the development of bilateral flank pain in the setting of anuria; however, more commonly the bilateral stones will be only partially obstructing and the patient will maintain an adequate urine output. Urgent management of chronic bilateral upper urinary obstruction is frequently not related to pain or hematuria, but rather the development of renal failure or the sequelae of fluid overload. For example, patients with chronic bilateral upper urinary obstruction may report nonspecific symptoms including pedal edema, weight gain, fatigue, shortness of breath, increased waist size, and vague gastrointestinal complaints (Gulmi et al. 2002). In the urgent setting, ultimately the development of these signs or the frank symptoms of uremia may prompt the initial evaluation and treatment.

10.3 Diagnostic Evaluation

10.3.1 Patient History

Many clues to the pathogenesis of upper urinary tract obstruction can be obtained from the initial patient encounter. It is important to take a complete history and do a physical examination when urgently evaluating a patient with upper urinary tract obstruction (Fig. 10.1). In addition to the duration and type of symptoms experienced, the patient's past medical and surgical history, current medications, and allergies should be thoroughly reviewed. Particular emphasis should be placed on the patient's prior urologic history including prior episodes and treatments of urinary calculi, current voiding patterns, prior urologic surgeries, prior history with urinary tract infections, and the presence of gross hematuria. The patient's prior history of urothelial carcinoma should be well documented as well as a history of other urologic and nonurologic malignancies. Pregnant females and patients with urinary diversion, renal transplantation, or history of urethral/ureteral strictures can pose additional diagnostic and therapeutic challenges. A patient's smoking history should also be noted as well as familial factors that could be contributing to the underlying etiology (e.g., familial stone disease, hereditary nonpolyposis colorectal cancer syndrome associated with urothelial carcinoma).

10.3.2 Physical Examination

The general appearance of the patient is one of the most important factors to consider when examining the patient. The diagnostic possibilities for a patient with cachexia are different than a well-nourished patient complaining of flank pain. Patients with classic colic will appear uncomfortable; however, the diagnosis is not always stone disease. A similar appearance can be seen in patients with other urologic problems such as UPJ obstruction or less commonly ureteral tumors. Completely nonurologic problems such as acute appendicitis, gynecologic disorders, or dissecting aortic aneurysms can also present with symptoms of renal colic (Rucker et al. 2004). In all patients, vital signs should be documented. In addition to blood pressure, heart rate, and respirations, the presence of fever is a very important finding. Fever suggests the presence of renal parenchymal infection or abscess and overall increases the urgency of the diagnostic evaluation, especially among diabetic patients or those with significant comorbidity (Nickel 2002). Indeed, the presence of upper urinary obstruction in a patient with urinary infection war-

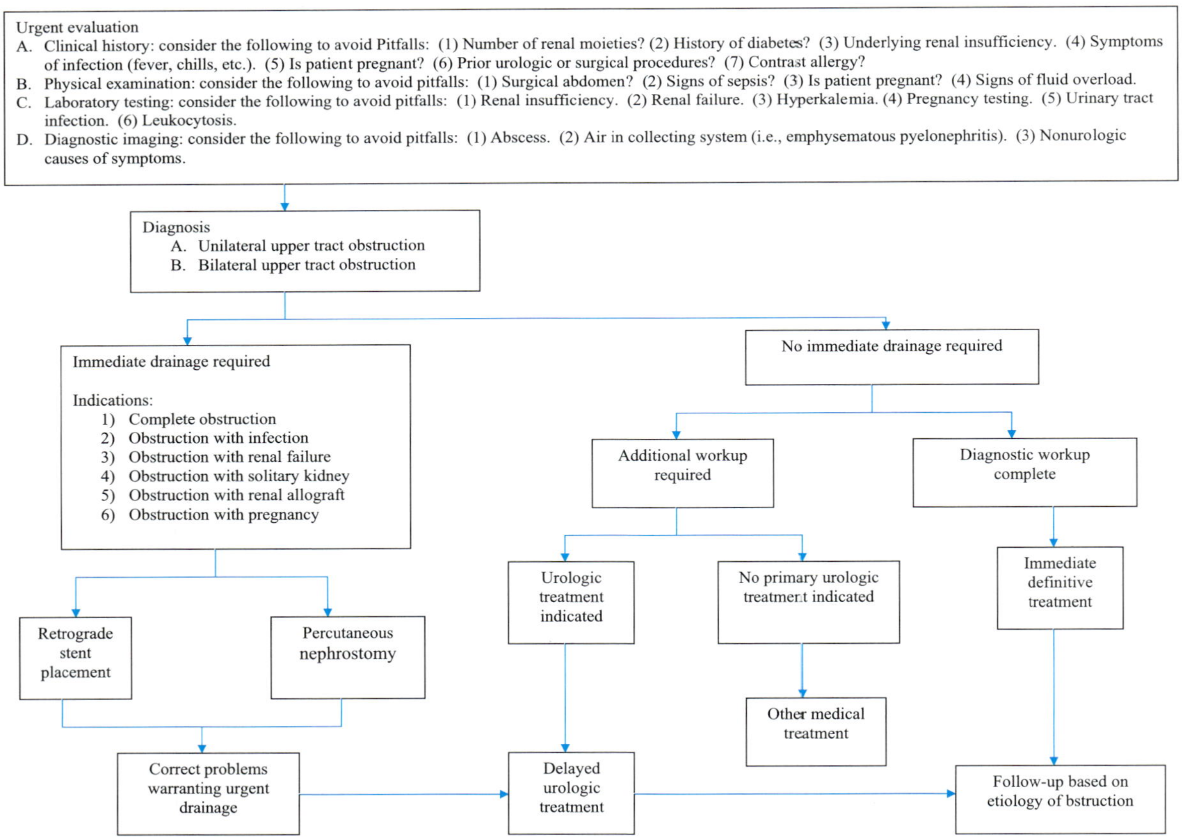

Fig. 10.1. Treatment algorithm for patients with failed upper urinary tract drainage

rants a prompt urinary drainage procedure and is considered a true urologic emergency. During the physical examination, symptoms suggestive of fluid overload or uremia should also be documented. The abdomen should also be palpated for the presence of an abdominal mass or associated abnormality, yet a clinically recognized mass aside from UPJ obstruction is a relatively uncommon presentation for upper urinary obstruction related to urologic causes. The examination should also rule out the presence of peritoneal signs (i.e., guarding, rebound tenderness, etc.), which that suggest a surgical abdomen. The presence of a surgical abdomen would frequently imply that the etiology of the patient's presenting symptomatology is entirely unrelated to urinary obstruction and it is likely that the etiology is nonurologic. Costovertebral angle tenderness may also be present among patients with upper urinary obstruction; however, this is also a nonspecific finding. For pregnant females requiring an urgent evaluation of suspected upper urinary obstruction, the welfare of the fetus should also be documented as part of the initial evaluation. In addition, appropriate safeguards should be undertaken to protect and monitor the fetus throughout diagnostic evaluations and therapeutic interventions at a minimum with documentation of fetal heart tones.

10.3.3 Concurrent Medical Evaluations

Before any required therapeutic procedures, all patients should undergo a preoperative medical examination by colleagues in primary care medicine and/or anesthesiology. Patients with renal failure should also be evaluated by nephrology. In relatively rare instances, a patient's overall medical condition may require optimization before proceeding with the required therapeutic interventions. In rare instances, this may include the use of hemodialysis before proceeding with relief of upper urinary obstruction. Acutely ill patients should be appropriately monitored in the hospital setting. In fact, those patients deemed too unstable for therapeutic intervention should have their clinical situation optimized in the intensive care unit setting.

10.3.4 Analgesia

In the urgent care setting, pain control is another consideration when evaluating a patient with upper urinary tract obstruction. The cornerstone of pain control for patients with renal colic and upper urinary tract function has traditionally been parenteral narcotics (Gulmi et al. 2002). Nonsteroidal anti-inflammatory drugs (NSAIDs) have recently gained popularity in the urgent care setting (Larkin et al. 1999). NSAIDs provide effective analgesia in the absence of significant sedation or exacerbation of associated nausea and vomiting. In a prospective, randomized, double-blind trial, Larkin and colleagues compared efficacy of the NSAID, ketorolac, to meperidine among 70 patients evaluated for acute renal colic. They noted that ketorolac provided superior analgesia and facilitated quicker discharges from the emergency room setting (Larkin et al. 1999). Despite the analgesic benefits of NSAIDs, associated physiologic effects in the kidney can be detrimental especially for patients with renal obstruction. In fact, the use of NSAIDS in the absence of renal obstruction has led to case reports of acute renal failure (Kim et al. 1999; Simckes et al. 1999). Despite these reports, other groups have noted safety in clinical use of ketorolac (Diblasio et al. 2004; Lee et al. 2004). For patients with upper urinary tract obstruction, NSAIDS should be administered with caution. Prior to the administration of analgesics in the urgent care setting, assessment of renal function should be documented. For patients with renal insufficiency or patients with bilateral obstruction, selection of narcotic-based analgesics may be preferred.

10.3.5 Laboratory-Based Evaluation

Laboratory testing is necessary when urgently evaluating any patient with presumed upper urinary tract obstruction. Standard tests include a complete blood count, serum chemistry testing, complete urinalysis with evaluation of the urinary sediment, urine Gram stain, and urine culture. In addition, for patients with fever or findings of pyelonephritis on radiographic imaging, multiple blood cultures should also be obtained. Ideally, cultures would be obtained before antibiotics are started. A complete blood count is obtained predominantly to exclude leukocytosis, which could suggest presence of infection concurrent with the obstruction. Depending on the etiology and duration of the obstruction, the following laboratory findings can be observed with chemistry testing: elevated serum creatinine, elevated blood urea nitrogen, hyperkalemia, and/or acidosis. Normally, elevated creatinine, acidosis, and hyperkalemia will accompany bilateral upper tract obstruction or patients with an obstructed solitary functioning kidney (i.e., previous nephrectomy patient, contralateral nonfunctioning kidney, renal transplantation patient). Typically, the patients with the most dramatic chemistry abnormalities are likely to have a rather longstanding or chronic source of underlying obstruction in all renal moieties (Gulmi et al. 2002). Even for patients with complete unilateral obstruction (acute or chronic), serum chemistry findings would commonly be normal or just slightly elevated (serum creatinine 1.2 – 1.6 mEq/l) unless the patient had preexisting renal insufficiency. A serum creatinine above 2.0 would be considered pathologic and possibly suggest a prerenal component of renal dysfunction or preexisting medical renal disease. Microscopic evaluation of the urine can show a variety of findings in the setting of obstruction including hematuria, pyuria, proteinuria, cast formation, and/or crystal formation. The urinalysis can also show changes in concentrating ability based on the duration of the obstruction and overall condition of the kidneys. In patients with obstruction related to a chronic condition affecting both kidneys, urine electrolytes may provide additional diagnostic value. In this setting, decreased urine to plasma creatinine ratios and elevated urinary sodium concentrations are typically noted in addition to poor concentrating ability. For the patient with acute unilateral obstruction, concentrating ability is less commonly affected and urine testing will typically show increased urine osmolality values and relatively low urine sodium concentrations (Gulmi et al. 2002). For patients with hyperkalemia, an emergent electrocardiogram should be performed and appropriate medical management is required to address the elevated serum potassium levels prior to treating the obstruction. In situations where obstructing is thought to be related to urothelial carcinoma, a voided urine cytology can help assist with the correct diagnosis. Lastly, all child-bearing females should have a pregnancy test performed before undergoing any diagnostic radiologic evaluations or treatment, if pregnancy is a possibility.

10.3.6 Radiographic Evaluation

10.3.6.1 Traditional Diagnostic Imaging

Technologic advances in radiographic imaging have radically changed the diagnostic approach to upper urinary obstruction (Smith et al. 1999; Kawashima et al. 2004). For years, the radiographic gold standard in the diagnosis of acute urinary obstruction was plain radiographs (KUB) with or without tomography and excretory urography (EXU) (Hattery et al. 1988; Heidenreich et al. 2002). The KUB would provide important evidence on the presence of radiopaque stone disease. EXU provided both functional and anatomic detail regarding upper tract obstruction. Classic findings of upper urinary obstruction on EXU include a delayed nephrogram, persistent nephrogram, delayed excretion of contrast into the collecting system, and/or failure of contrast to enter the bladder on delayed films. In the setting of upper urinary tract obstruction, other associated findings can include contrast extravasation secondary to forniceal rupture or rarely pyelovenous/pyelolymphatic backflow (Hattery et al. 1988). EXU can provide excellent detail of the calices, renal pelvis, and ureter, but anatomic detail of the renal parenchyma and surrounding soft tissues is poor in comparison to cross-sectional imaging techniques (Kawashima et al. 2004). EXU is also more time-consuming and labor-intensive than other imaging modalities. In addition, nonurologic causes of urinary obstruction and flank pain are less optimally evaluated with EXU (Rucker et al. 2004). Performing EXU on patients with renal colic can also be problematic in the setting of ureteral obstruction. In the setting of ureteral obstruction, the osmotic effect of the contrast may result in a forced diuresis and subsequent fornix rupture and resultant urinoma. In the current era, emphasis has been placed on more advanced imaging techniques including ultrasonography (US), magnetic resonance imaging (MRI), and particularly computerized tomography (CT).

10.3.6.2 Noncontrast Helical Abdominal/Pelvic CT

In the emergency room setting, noncontrast helical abdominal/pelvic CT has become the examination of choice in the evaluation of flank pain and obstructive anuria (Niall et al. 2002; Shokeir et al. 2002, 2004; Colistro et al. 2002). Introduced by Smith and colleagues in 1995, noncontrast CT is quick, relatively easy to interpret, and obviates risks associated with the use of contrast media (Smith et al. 1999). Noncontrast CT is the gold standard in the detection of urinary calculi with an associated sensitivity of more than 95% and an associated specificity greater than 98% (Fig. 10.2) (Rukker et al. 2004). When upper urinary tract obstruction is related to stone disease, CT can provide a wealth of diagnostic information. In addition, when stone disease does not exist, noncontrast CT can provide an accurate first glance to the underlying etiology of upper urinary obstruction (Rucker et al. 2004). In comparison to KUB with abdominal US, Shokeir and co-workers noted that noncontrast CT had a superior sensitivity (94% vs 58%) and diagnostic accuracy (95% vs 77%) for patients with obstructive anuria, respectively (Shokeir et al. 2002). Also, noncontrast CT can provide incidentally discovered findings and nonurologic sources of flank pain. Indeed, up to one-third of unenhanced CT scans performed for flank pain may reveal unsuspected findings unrelated to stone disease that are contributing to the patient's symptomatology (Rukker et al. 2004; Ather et al. 2005). When flank pain is unrelated to stone disease, the most common alternative diagnoses with unenhanced CT include adnexal masses, pyelonephritis, appendicitis, and diverticulitis. In cases where additional diagnostic information is needed on the basis of the noncontrast examination, additional CT phases can be easily performed after the administration of contrast. For instance, CT is the imaging modality of choice to evaluate associated inflam-

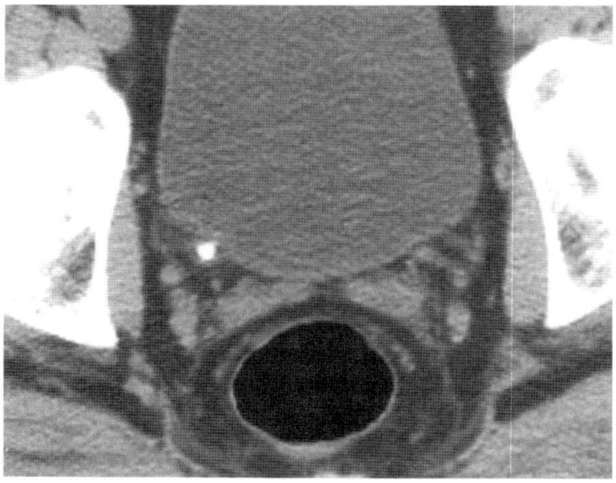

Fig. 10.2. Appearance of obstructing ureteral stone on noncontrast CT scan

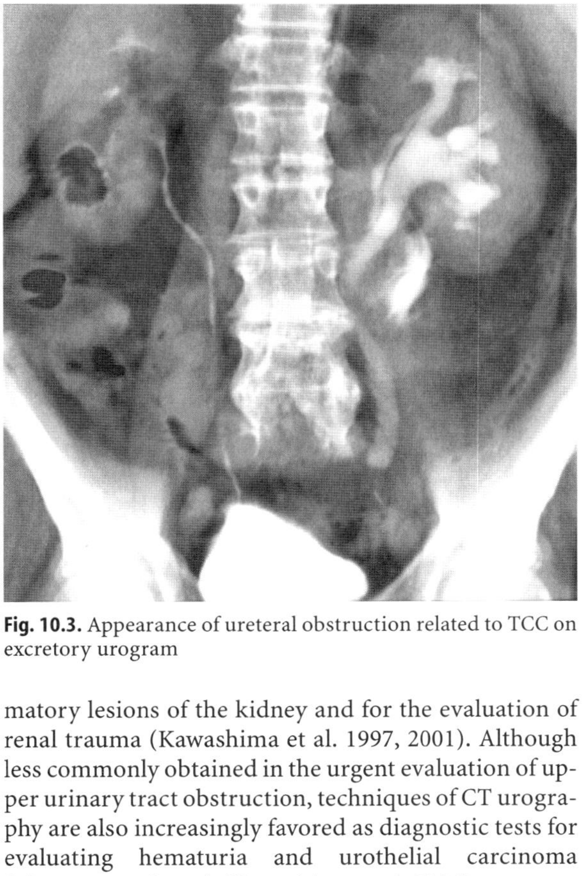

Fig. 10.3. Appearance of ureteral obstruction related to TCC on excretory urogram

matory lesions of the kidney and for the evaluation of renal trauma (Kawashima et al. 1997, 2001). Although less commonly obtained in the urgent evaluation of upper urinary tract obstruction, techniques of CT urography are also increasingly favored as diagnostic tests for evaluating hematuria and urothelial carcinoma (Figs. 10.3 and 10.4) (Kawashima et al. 2004).

Both noncontrast and contrast-enhanced CT can reveal characteristic signs associated with the diagnosis of upper urinary tract obstruction. Stone disease, essentially regardless of composition, is easily recognized on noncontrast CT because the attenuation of stones is higher than that of soft tissue. The possible exception to this rule would be human immunodeficiency virus

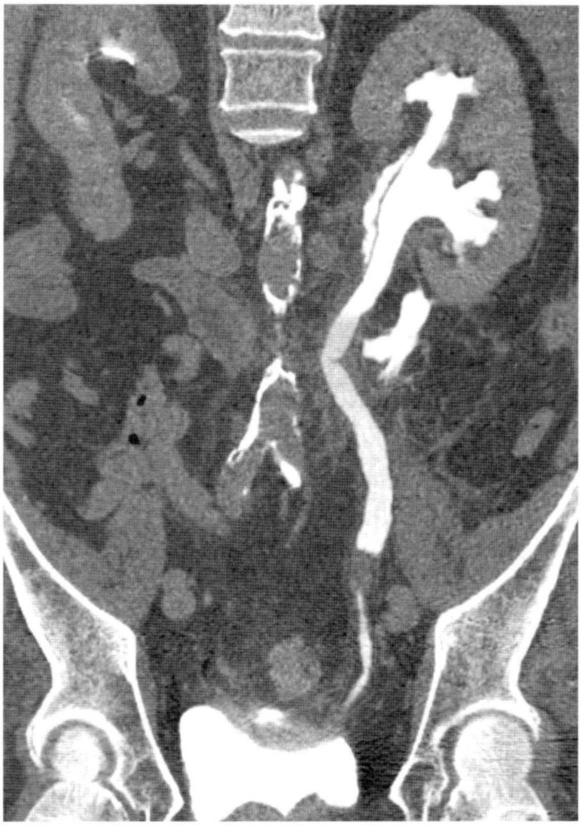

Fig. 10.4. Corresponding appearance of obstructive urothelial carcinoma of the ureter on contrast-enhanced CT urogram

patients with indinavir stones and select patients with completely uncalcified matrix stones. The diagnosis of stone disease on noncontrast CT is simplified by the appearance of proximal ureteral dilation, hydronephrosis, and the possibility of stranding in the perinephric fat (Colistro et al. 2002). Another secondary sign of acute obstruction recently described by Özer and associates is the difference in renal parenchyma density on noncontrast CT. In a study of 49 patients with obstructing ureteral stones, a Hounsfield unit (HU) decrease in the ipsilateral kidney was observed in all cases. When a parenchyma decrease of more than 5 HU was observed on the obstructed side, the sensitivity, specificity, positive predictive value, and accuracy of acute obstructing stone on the ipsilateral side were 89.1%, 100%, 100%, and 93.4%, respectively (Özer et al. 2004).

Concurrent findings of pyelonephritis or abscess can also be suggested on noncontrast CT by nephromegaly and changes in the renal parenchyma. It is especially important to recognize the presence of air in the collecting system or renal parenchyma, as this may suggest a diagnosis of emphysematous pyelonephritis. With advanced transaxial imaging, our ability to diagnose air in the urinary tract has increased. On computerized tomography, some gas in the collecting system can be observed after instrumentation or among patients that have had a ureterosigmoidostomy urinary diversion, and this is not worrisome. On the other hand, gas in the renal parenchyma on computerized tomography or gas in the collecting system on a less advanced imaging test (i.e., plain abdominal radiograph) can represent the more serious problem of emphysematous pyelonephritis. It is important to correlate finding of gas in the collecting system to other clinical findings for the patient. In some instances, pelvic phleboliths may cloud the accurate diagnosis of upper urinary tract obstruction. A soft-tissue rim sign (i.e., soft tissue ring around the calcification) favors the diagnosis of stone on noncontrast CT (Colistro et al. 2002). Upper tract obstruction related to UPJ obstruction can often show associated hydronephrosis on noncontrast CT. Clues to a diagnosis of upper tract obstruction related to a retroperitoneal process (e.g., retroperitoneal fibrosis, adenopathy, primary retroperitoneal malignancy, metastatic retroperitoneal malignancy, aneurysm, etc.) are also initially deciphered or frequently diagnosed on noncontrast CT.

When the noncontrast CT shows associated abnormalities without presence of stone disease or when unrelated abnormalities are encountered that require further characterization, contrast administration should be strongly considered in patients with acceptable renal function. Use of contrast-enhanced CT in the setting of upper urinary tract obstruction provides the same diagnostic signs as seen on EXU; however, the anatomic details of the parenchyma and the ability to diagnose associated findings such as forniceal rupture are superior. Contrast-enhanced CT can provide superior diagnostic information when obstruction is related to urothelial carcinoma (Kawashima et al. 2004). Nonetheless, the presence of obstruction related to urothelial carcinoma is relatively rare in the kidney and UPJ. Among five presentation patterns described by Lowe and Roylance, the presence of urothelial carcinoma associated with long-standing UPJ obstruction and atrophy was relatively uncommon (13% incidence), as was the presence of urothelial carcinoma in the setting of hydronephrosis, renal enlargement, and acute UPJ obstruction (6% incidence). More commonly, urothelial carcinoma located at or above the UPJ will be associated with irregular filling defects of the renal pelvis or calices (61% incidence) or infundibular amputations (20% incidence) (Lowe and Roylance 1976). Upper urinary tract obstruction related to urothelial carcinoma is more commonly associated with tumors in a ureteral location. Among the presentations of ureteral tumors, the presence of concurrent nonfunctioning kidneys with high-grade obstruction was seen in 46% and hydronephrosis with or without hydroureter was the presenting finding in 34% of cases. In the remaining 20% of cases, ureteral tumors were observed on standard urographic or cross-sectional imaging as ureteral filling defects or as irregular narrowed segments of the ureteral lumen, respectively (Kawashima et al. 2004).

10.3.6.3 Ultrasonography

While CT is the favored imaging modality in the evaluation of upper urinary tract obstruction, other radiographic tests also have indications in the acute setting. For pregnant patients, abdominal and/or transvaginal US or less commonly MRI remain important tests for evaluation of urinary obstruction. Renal US, in particular, is also more commonly ordered as a first-line test in the pediatric population. While US does not provide the anatomic detail of CT or MRI, parenchymal abnormalities such as pyelonephritis, hydronephrosis, and stone disease can be detected quickly and fairly reliably without concerns about radiation exposure or contrast-related complications (Gulmi et al. 2002). Furthermore, US does further evaluate the character of urine in the obstructed upper urinary tract. Sedimentation, for example, may be visualized with US and this can provide additional evidence for pyonephrosis and would lead to more urgent need for drainage. In addition, findings noted on US can often help determine the duration of the obstruction. Long-standing obstruction can frequently be associated with thinning of the renal parenchyma. A common scenario is the presence of chronic obstruction related to stone disease or stricture with the appearance of a kidney that has extremely thinned renal parenchyma. The degree of observed hydronephrosis on US, however, is not as reliable when evaluating for duration of renal obstruction. Completely unobstructed upper urinary tract systems can show pyelocaliectasis, ureterectasis, or hydronephrosis that can be related to congenital variation (e.g., prune belly syndrome, megacystis/megaureter syndrome), lower urinary tract obstruction (e.g., urinary retention secondary to benign prostatic hyperplasia or urethral stricture), or reflux. In cases of dehydration, very early obstruction, or intrarenal collecting systems, US may also miss a diagnosis of upper urinary tract obstruction (Gulmi et al. 2002). To increase the sensitivity of US, a renal resistive index (RI) may provide important diagnostic information (Oktar et al. 2004). As initially described, a RI above 0.7 is defined as obstruction, yet underlying medical renal disease can be associated with RI values over 0.7 in the absence of renal obstruction. Because of this finding as well as the finding that renal obstruction can occur with RI below 0.7, use of RI in the diagnosis of failed upper urinary tract drainage is controversial (Gulmi et al. 2004).

Indeed, US findings should be considered in context with other presenting clinical factors to arrive at the diagnosis of obstruction. Shokeir and co-workers recently reported, for instance, that renal RI measurements correlate positively with serum creatinine values in the setting of obstructive anuria (Shokeir et al. 2002). In addition, the group found that RI significantly improves after obstruction is drained and that rapid improvement in RI can predict early recoverability of renal function. At 3 days following drainage, however, the mean renal RI among the 48 treated patients remained at 0.70, a value classically associated with obstruction (Shokeir et al. 2002). Given such reported inconsistencies in the use of renal RI measurements and the concern with false-negative US findings for obstruction, a lower threshold should be made for obtaining additional diagnostic testing to evaluate for obstruction.

10.3.6.4
Magnetic Resonance Imaging

For all practical purposes, MRI is not routinely used in the urgent evaluation of upper tract obstruction. In comparison to the other imaging modalities, MRI is less available, more costly, and frequently less sensitive in the accurate diagnosis of upper tract obstruction, especially related to stone disease. For example, urinary calcifications are poorly visualized with MRI, making this a less valuable test in instances of obstruction related to stones. For select patients including pregnant females in whom more anatomic detail is required than that available with US, however, MRI may be considered as a confirmatory imaging test. The use of MRI may also have a role in the evaluation of patients with upper urinary tract obstruction and compromised renal function (serum creatinine >2.5 mg/dl). In a study by Shokeir and colleagues, 149 patients with upper tract obstruction were evaluated with not only KUB and US but also MRI urography (MRU) and noncontrast CT (Shokeir et al. 2004). While noncontrast CT was superior for detecting obstructing stones (100% sensitivity), MRU was superior in detecting the 113 cases in which obstruction unrelated to stone disease (sensitivity of 89%) compared to noncontrast CT (sensitivity of 40%) or combined KUB and US (sensitivity of 18%).

10.3.6.5
Diuretic Renography

Another confirmatory test, used extensively in the office setting to confirm the diagnosis of upper urinary obstruction but rarely in the emergency room setting, is diuretic renography. Like EXU, diuretic renography is a dynamic test providing functional data for the kidneys. Not only can diuretic renography help with the diagnosis of obstruction, the test can also provide data on split renal function. In contrast to EXU, diuretic renography is associated with minimal risk of contrast-related side effects (i.e., allergic reactions are unlikely), minimal risk of contrast-related nephrotoxicity, and can be performed with a lower amount of radiation exposure. The most commonly used radiotracer for diuretic renography is technetium 99m mercaptoacetyltriglycine (99mTc-MAG3). When information regarding renal function is preferentially required, the favored radiotracer is dimercaptosuccinic acid (DMSA). Because DMSA accumulates in the kidneys over a period of several hours, the role of this test is limited in the urgent evaluation and management of upper urinary tract obstruction (Croft et al. 1996). Before the introduction of diuretic renography, the Whitaker test was routinely used to confirm the diagnosis of upper urinary tract obstruction. In the urgent evaluation of a patient with presumed upper urinary tract obstruction nowadays, the role for this test is even less justified than that of diuretic renography.

10.4
Acute Urologic Management

The acute treatment of upper urinary tract obstruction is to re-establish urinary drainage. The timing (immediate vs delayed), approach (endoscopic, percutaneous, open, laparoscopic), and goals of treatment (temporizing vs definitive) depend heavily on the diagnostic workup. When safe and possible, an effort should be made to provide definitive treatment at the same time as urinary drainage is established. In cases of renal failure, concurrent infection, or complete obstruction, however, the only goal of treatment should be urgent decompression of the blocked upper tract.

10.4.1
Temporary Interventions

Despite the multitude of diagnoses and associated problems contributing to the etiology of upper urinary tract obstruction, urgent temporary decompression, when warranted, is performed either with retrograde placement of ureteral stents or percutaneous nephrostomy tube placement. The retrograde technique also provides the option that drainage be performed with an external ureteral catheter or an internal double pigtail stent. Both procedures have an established track record with high success rates and low complication rates. The following clinical scenarios would typically warrant a temporary drainage procedure (i.e., stenting or percutaneous nephrostomy):

1. Complete ureteral obstruction (unilateral or bilateral)
2. Obstruction with infection

3. Obstruction with acute renal failure
4. Obstruction in a solitary native kidney
5. Obstruction in a renal allograft
6. Obstruction in a pregnant female

Individualized clinical circumstances may also dictate use of temporizing interventions for other patient populations such as uncontrollable flank pain, fever, or uncontrollable gastrointestinal complaints. Indeed, when a decision is being made regarding the use of a temporary drainage procedure vs definitive therapy for initial relief of upper tract urinary obstruction, it is advisable to err on the side of conservative temporizing therapy rather than immediate definitive treatment. Not uncommonly, patients requiring an acute drainage procedure can have significant morbidity and can be acutely ill.

In a recent report by Yoshimura and co-workers, the need for temporizing interventions related to upper urinary tract obstruction appears to be increasing in older, more debilitated patients (Yoshimura et al. 2005). Among 424 patients with 473 upper tract stones treated in Japan, emergency drainage events in 59 renal units were performed for associated urosepsis by either ureteral stenting (35/59 events, 59%) or percutaneous nephrostomy tube placement (24/59 events, 41%). In 24% of the emergency drainage cases, intensive care management with the use of vasopressors and anticoagulants was required. In addition, one death was reported related to sepsis. As would be expected, emergency drainage was associated with a significantly prolonged hospitalization in comparison to nonseptic patients (25.2 days vs 14.8 days, $p<0.001$). In univariate and multivariate modeling, the need for a temporizing drainage procedure was related to age over 75 years (odds ratio, 2.1; $p=0.038$), poor performance status (odds ratio, 2.9; $p=0.003$), or female gender (odds ratio, 1.9; $p=0.046$). Based on the increasing life span in developed countries, the authors suggested that the issue of emergency drainage procedures in the elderly patient population with significant comorbidity is likely to become more commonplace.

10.4.1.1
Temporary Drainage Procedures: Recommendations

For patients with a normal urinary tract, we have favored an attempt at cystoscopy with retrograde ureteral catheterization before trying percutaneous drainage techniques. When turbid urine is encountered at the time of retrograde catheterization, not uncommonly we will initially place an external ureteral catheter rather than immediately placing an indwelling double pigtail stent. This provides an opportunity to directly monitor the character of the drainage and can provide an option for flushing the catheter to maintain adequate drainage. We typically use an open ended 6-F angiographic catheter for a patient requiring external drainage, but a variety of other open-ended ureteral catheters are also available for this purpose. The external catheter is fixed to the Foley catheter with suture and drained separately into an external collection device. This permits evaluation of the amount and nature of the drainage. When turbid urine is encountered, the fluid should be sent for culture. In addition, the presence of infection with obstruction also mandates urgent antibiotics. Typically, intravenous therapy is initiated with aminoglycosides with ampicillin, a fluoroquinolone, or a third-generation cephalosporin. Antibiotics are started before any manipulation of the obstructed upper urinary tract. While patients are in the hospital, we do aggressively hydrate our patients to induce a water diuresis. This can facilitate a mechanical washout of the upper tract. Based on culture results, antibiotic therapy is modified with a typical duration of therapy of 7–14 days (Nickel 2002; Kalyanakrishnan and Scheid 2005). When the patient's clinical picture improves, internalization of drainage is then performed by placing a double pigtail stent. For pregnant females needing urgent decompression, we traditionally have favored retrograde stent placement. For patients with a urinary diversion, renal allograft, or significant anatomic variation, urgent decompression at our institution is most commonly performed immediately with percutaneous drainage. After temporary drainage, individual clinical circumstances dictate the follow-up plan for further diagnostic or therapeutic intervention. When urgent drainage is performed for obstructing stones, a minimum of 2–3 weeks is allowed for complete treatment of concurrent infections and to permit resolution of obstruction-induced inflammation of the upper tract.

10.4.1.2
Temporary Drainage Procedures in Pregnancy

Temporizing drainage procedures in pregnant females pose additional treatment-related concerns warranting comment. Because of physiologic changes in renal function during pregnancy resulting in hypercalcuria and hyperuricosuria, encrustation of stents and percutaneous nephrostomy tubes can occur (McAleer and Loughlin 2004; Evans and Wollin 2001). Pregnant women with stents are therefore recommended to have stent exchanges approximately every 4–6 weeks to prevent this problem. For a woman in the first or second trimester, the need for multiple stent exchanges is a disadvantage and could potentially be associated with complications putting the fetus at risk. In addition, the impact of typical stent-related irritations such as pain, hematuria, infection, and lower urinary tract voiding symptoms may be greater in the pregnant female.

Nephrostomy tubes are likewise associated with similar irritations and because of encrustation or blockage must also be frequently exchanged. With nephrostomy tubes, other disadvantages include the risk of traumatic removal and the need for wearing an external collection bag potentially for the duration of the pregnancy. Despite the disadvantages, the traditional treatment of pregnant females requiring a temporizing treatment is unchanged from other patient populations.

10.4.1.3 Comparison of Temporary Drainage Techniques

Despite limited options, the method for urgent decompression of the obstructed urinary tract is controversial. Proponents of percutaneous nephrostomy suggest that drainage is improved with the larger sized nephrostomy tube and that complications related to manipulation of a stent across the area of blockage are eliminated (i.e., ureteral perforation). In addition, percutaneous nephrostomy can be performed under local anesthesia, which is a true benefit for many patients. In some institutions where percutaneous nephrostomy tubes are placed by interventional radiologists, a time delay can be associated with use of this drainage technique. To facilitate expeditious treatment, advocates of retrograde stent placement suggest that this drainage technique can be performed more quickly and is less invasive (Pearle et al. 1998).

For patients with normal upper urinary tracts, Pearle and colleagues compared the efficacy of percutaneous nephrostomy vs retrograde catheterization in cases of obstruction and infection associated with ureteral stones (Pearle et al. 1998). Among 42 consecutive patients with obstructing ureteral stones, patients were randomized into percutaneous or retrograde drainage. Mean operative time (32.7 min vs 49.2 min) and fluoroscopy time (5.1 min vs 7.7 min) were significantly lower among the patients drained via retrograde catheter placement. One patient failed drainage in the percutaneous treatment group and was salvaged with retrograde stent placement. When comparing percutaneous nephrostomy tube placement to retrograde stenting, no significant differences were observed in time to treatment, time to normal temperature (2.3 days vs 2.6 days), time to normal white blood cell count (2 days vs 1.7 days), or length of hospitalization (4.5 days vs 3.2 days). Nonetheless, a twofold cost advantage was realized for percutaneous nephrostomy tube placement in comparison to retrograde stent placement. The authors concluded that neither technique was superior. They recommended that selection of the drainage modality must be made on the basis of the surgeon's preference, logistic factors, and stone characteristics.

On the other hand, Mokhmalji and co-workers reported a prospective randomized comparison of percutaneous nephrostomy tube placement vs ureteral stent placement for obstructing stones (Mokhmalji et al. 2001). In this evaluation of 40 stone patients, percutaneous nephrostomy tube placement was successful in 100 % of cases, while ureteral stent placement was successful in 80 % of cases. In contrast to the report by Pearle and colleagues, the authors noted that analgesic use was more common and quality of life reduced in patients undergoing stent placement. In addition, the reduction in quality of life was most pronounced in men and younger patients within the retrograde stent placement group. Based on their data, the authors recommended percutaneous nephrostomy tube placement as the drainage procedure of choice with obstructed stones.

In another attempt to optimize choice of emergent drainage procedures, Yossepowitch and associates evaluated risk factors for retrograde stent placement in a group of 92 consecutive patients with ureteral obstruction (Yossepowitch et al. 2001). Among patients with intrinsic and extrinsic ureteral obstructions, stenting was initially successful in 94 % and 73 % of patients, respectively. At 3-month follow-up, however, the success rate was constant in all intrinsic obstruction patients but decreased to 56 % in the extrinsic obstruction patients. In a multivariate analysis of failure, extrinsic ureteral obstructions with more significant hydronephrosis and a more distal level of obstruction were more common to fail retrograde stent placement regardless of stent diameter. The authors suggested based on their analysis that percutaneous nephrostomy tube placement may be superior in this subset of patients.

Among 101 patients with extrinsic ureteral obstruction, Chung and colleagues evaluated their 15-year experience with retrograde ureteral stenting (Chung et al. 2004). The etiology of extrinsic obstruction was metastatic cancer in 89 % (90/101 patients) and at a mean followup of 5.8 months after stenting, 32.2 % of these patients had died. Overall, stent failure occurred in 58 renal units. For 40 renal units, salvage percutaneous nephrostomy tubes were placed at a mean follow-up of 40 days. In 18 of the 40 renal units, a nephrostomy tube was placed as salvage therapy less than 1 week from retrograde stenting. In the remaining renal units not salvaged by nephrostomy tube placement, the mean time to failure was 52.4 days. In a multivariate analysis model, the following factors were suggestive of retrograde stent failure: diagnosis of cancer, baseline renal insufficiency, and metastatic disease requiring chemotherapy or radiation therapy.

10.4.1.4 Summary

In summary, the indications for temporary drainage in the setting of upper urinary tract obstruction are clearly established. Either drainage technique can be highly effective with minimal risk of treatment-related complications. Since no clear consensus regarding optimal treatment can be gleaned from published series, the choice of drainage should be selected on the basis of individualized patient characteristics, the planned duration of stenting, available institutional resources, and the surgeon's preference.

10.4.2 Immediate Definitive Interventions

If no indications exist for temporary drainage procedures, immediate definitive therapy can be considered. Use of immediate definitive therapy is more common when the cause of flank pain is urinary calculi and only considered when partial upper tract obstruction is present. In this scenario, the size, number, and location of the stones impact the choice of endourologic treatment. Immediate management of partially obstructing stones in the kidney and ureter should follow the recommendations set forth in the AUA nephrolithiasis treatment guidelines (Preminger et al. 2005; Segura et al. 1997). In reality, advances in endoscope design and instrumentation make ureteroscopic approaches to these problems much more appealing than ever before. An additional benefit of ureteroscopic treatment in the setting of acute management with partial obstruction is the ability to assess intraoperatively for unrecognized infection or contributing abnormalities such as ureteral stricture. Also, if circumstances are encountered that make ureteroscopy less optimal in the acute setting, the threshold should be low for stenting the patient and returning at a later date for definitive treatment.

In the setting of life-threatening urinary tract infections such as emphysematous pyelonephritis with obstruction, temporary drainage procedures may provide suboptimal treatment. Nickel has noted that relief of obstruction and antibiotics are usually sufficient treatment, but that nephrectomy should be considered in non-responders (Nickel 2002). Since the contemporary mortality rate remains approximately 75% for the typical diabetic patient that develops emphysematous pyelonephritis (Nickel 2002), we favor immediate traditional treatment with nephrectomy rather than an initial trial of temporary drainage.

10.4.2.1 Immediate Shock Wave Lithotripsy

In the setting of partially obstructing stones, shock wave lithotripsy (SWL) has also been performed as immediate treatment (Kravchick et al. 2005; Doublet et al. 1997; Tligui et al. 2003; Joshi et al. 1999). While SWL in this situation would be less invasive, one theoretical concern would be treating a stone with SWL in the setting of unrecognized infection. SWL would provide little opportunity to diagnose an unsuspected infection and thereby alter treatment plans. Nonetheless, in the absence of indications for urgent upper tract decompression, some authors have acutely utilized SWL. In a recent report, Kravchick and colleagues reported a prospective randomized trial of emergent SWL vs scheduled SWL (treatment within 30 days of diagnosis) for upper urinary tract stones associated with acute renal colic (Kravchick et al. 2005). None of the patients had presenting indications that warranted a temporary drainage procedure. Emergent SWL was associated with a higher success rate (72%) than delayed treatment (64%). In addition, scheduled (delayed) treatment was associated with significantly prolonged hospitalizations and recovery at home. Other groups have noted favorable experiences with emergency SWL. For instance, Doublet and associates found a significant relationship between stone location and stone-free rates after emergent SWL (Doublet et al. 1997). In their report, proximal stone treatment was associated with a 65% success rate.

More controversial is the use of emergency shock wave lithotripsy (SWL) for immediate definitive management of completely obstructing stones (Joshi et al. 1999). Among 82 consecutive patients with completely obstructing stones treated by Joshi and co-workers, 26 patients underwent percutaneous nephrostomy tube placement followed by scheduled SWL, 40 patients underwent retrograde stent placement followed by scheduled SWL, and 16 patients underwent urgent in situ SWL alone without prior drainage procedures (Joshi et al. 1999). All SWL procedures were performed on a Siemens Lithostar Multiline or Lithostar Plus lithotripter. The mean stone size was 8.98 mm (range, 4–25 mm) and stone size was not significantly different among treatment groups. Infectious complications related to urgent in situ SWL were not observed. Urgent in situ SWL was associated with an overall success rate of 81% compared to a 70% success rate in the stent + SWL group and 54% success rate in the nephrostomy tube + SWL group. Success rates were highest for in situ SWL performed on proximal ureteral stones. While Joshi and colleagues report favorable results, additional clinical evaluation appears warranted before urgent SWL can be recommended for emergent treatment of completely obstructed stones. Indeed, the presence of completely obstructing stones would traditionally mandate the use of a temporary drainage technique prior to delayed definitive treatment.

10.4.2.2 Immediate Definitive Treatment in Pregnancy

Definitive management of pregnant females with obstructing stones is also controversial. Traditional treatment has been temporizing with placement of a stent or percutaneous nephrostomy until the postpartum period in which definitive endourologic management is performed. With advances in intracorporeal lithotripsy and ureteroscope design, ureteroscopic stone fragmentation and extraction has been successfully performed in pregnancy as an alternative to temporary drainage techniques. Despite the gravid uterus, small-caliber semirigid ureteroscopes can typically be placed without difficulty (Watterson et al. 2002). In part, physiologic dilation of the ureter during pregnancy facilitates ureteroscope passage. Since ureteroscope passage is relatively straightforward in pregnancy, the need for intraoperative fluoroscopy is typically minimized, if needed at all. In fact, if imaging is needed, this can alternatively be accomplished with US monitoring (Watterson et al. 2002).

Watterson and colleagues reported use of ureteroscopy and holmium:yttrium-aluminum-garnet (YAG) laser lithotripsy in eight patients with ten symptomatic ureteral stones and two encrusted stents (Watterson et al. 2002). Treatment was performed at a mean gestational age of 22 weeks (range, 10–35 weeks) and the mean stone diameter was 8.1 mm (range, 4–15 mm). The mean operative time was 39 min (range, 20–70) and an overall success rate of 91% was achieved without obstetric or urologic complications. The authors concluded that modern ureteroscopic techniques in pregnant females were safe and obviated the disadvantages associated with long-term stenting or nephrostomy tube placement. Favorable results with ureteroscopy have also been suggested by Lifshitz and Lingeman. Among ten patients with ureteral calculi in pregnancy, six patients underwent first-line ureteroscopic evaluation without complication (Lifshitz and Lingeman 2002).

10.4.2.3
Postobstructive Diuresis

After urgent relief of upper urinary tract blockage, patients with bilateral obstruction or obstruction of a solitary kidney are at risk for postobstructive diuresis. The chronically obstructed patient with signs and symptoms of fluid overload including pedal edema, congestive heart failure, increased abdominal girth, weight gain, and azotemia is more likely to have this problem (Gulmi et al. 2002). Postobstructive diuresis is classified as physiologic, pathologic, or iatrogenic. In the physiologic form, the diuresis is caused by retained free water, sodium, and urea. The pathologic form is associated with impairment in renal concentrating ability or sodium reabsorption. When patients are given high volumes of intravenous fluid containing dextrose, glucose reabsorption in the proximal tubule can be exceeded, leading to the iatrogenic type of postobstructive diuresis. While postobstructive diuresis can be thought of as these three types, the reality is that many patients experience mixed patterns. In addition, the development of postobstructive diuresis after relief of upper tract obstruction is relatively rare. Furthermore, most patients that develop the problem have a physiologic-type diuresis that rapidly returns to normal. In fact, providing the patient access to free water and avoiding the use of intravenous fluids usually is enough to remedy the situation (Gulmi et al. 2002).

Nonetheless, it is important to identify patients at risk for postobstructive diuresis after relief of upper tract obstruction. Following the drainage procedure, urine output should be carefully monitored, especially for patients with evidence of chronic obstruction and fluid overload. When urine outputs are higher than 200 ml/h for 2 consecutive hours, urine and plasma osmolality should be obtained to determine the type of diuresis. In the presence of low or iso-osmolar urine, the alert patient with access to water will typically normalize the serum creatinine and blood urea nitrogen within 1 or 2 days. Until the diuresis is corrected, urine output should be carefully monitored (every 2 h), the patient should be weighed daily, and serum electrolytes should be checked twice daily (Gulmi et al. 2002). Furthermore, it is important to assess the adequacy of hydration while the postobstructive diuresis is being treated. To achieve this goal, postural vital sign assessments should be utilized at a minimum of every 8 h as the patient is being treated for the postobstructive diuresis.

In situations where the diuresis continues for more than 2 days and the urine persists with a low osmolarity, concern for a pathologic type of diuresis is increased. The alert patient continues with oral intake, but if serum electrolytes show unchanged elevations in creatinine and blood urea nitrogen, intravenous fluid (0.45% sodium chloride with 5% dextrose) should additionally be started. In most instances, urine output is replaced with the intravenous fluid as a ratio 0.5 cc of saline to 1.0 cc of urine output and this treatment is continued with frequent monitoring until the diuresis stops. This type of pathologic diuresis is related to a water diuresis secondary to damage in the distal tubules. In the rarest form of pathologic postobstructive diuresis, significant sodium loss also occurs secondary to distal tubule damage. Correction of this diuresis involves 1:1 replacement of urinary sodium with intravenous saline. In this form of diuresis, patients are at risk of volume depletion and vascular collapse (Gulmi et al. 2002). Faced with issues of postobstructive diuresis in a patient with fluid overload and uremia, nephrologic consultation is advised.

10.4.2.4 Summary

In summary, patients without indications for temporary drainage procedures can be definitively treated at presentation. In the majority of cases, this urgent management is comparable to management of symptomatic stone patients with partial obstructing stones who are not candidates for conservative treatment protocols. In this setting, all endourologic treatments have been used to treat stone disease. With improvements in ureteroscope design and instrumentation, however, we have increased utilization of ureteroscopy for these stones. Favorable results can be expected with ureteroscopy. In addition, direct stone manipulation provides an opportunity to alter treatment in the setting of an unrecognized infection. Despite favorable early results with the use of ureteroscopic treatment of stones in pregnancy, we have continued to favor retrograde stenting in symptomatic patients failing conservative treatment.

10.5 Delayed Definitive Interventions

Delayed definitive interventions for patients with upper urinary tract obstruction are performed for patients who have responded appropriately to temporary drainage. Most commonly this is the stone patient that for one reason or another required a temporary drainage procedure. After resolution of the underlying treatment concerns (i.e., infection, inflammation, etc.), definitive stone treatment can be given with endourologic techniques catering to the size, location, and laterality of the stones. In most instances, a minimum delay of 2–3 weeks is needed before definitive treatment is performed.

For upper urinary tract obstruction unrelated to stone disease, delayed definitive interventions are also undertaken once the additional diagnostic workup has been completed to recommend optimal treatment. The complete diagnostic workup and must be tailored to the individual patient. When obstruction is unrelated to stone disease and the patient presents urgently, emphasis is typically first made on temporizing interventions. Once the patient's obstruction has been temporarily relieved and once the urgent presenting signs and symptoms have been stabilized, additional diagnostic and therapeutic intervention is based predominantly on the radiographic evaluation. Not uncommonly, the diagnostic workup can be completed on an outpatient basis after the patient has been released from the acute care setting. A discussion of definitive treatment options for the variety of problems associated with upper urinary tract obstruction is beyond the scope of this chapter.

10.6 Conclusion

Failure of upper urinary tract drainage is an emergent urologic condition. In many cases, a thorough history and physical examination can facilitate an accurate diagnosis. Advances in radiographic imaging have also improved the ability to differentiate both intrinsic and extrinsic causes of obstruction occurring in one or both kidneys. On the basis of the presenting signs and symptoms and with the radiographic information, a safe treatment plan can be instituted, providing necessary temporizing therapy or immediate definitive treatment. After the urgent problem is addressed, further diagnostic evaluation can be performed to ultimately treat underlying factors contributing to the initial presentation.

References

Ather MH, Memon W, Rees JR (2005) Clinical impact of incidental diagnosis of disease on non-contrast-enhanced helical CT for acute ureteral colic. Semin Ultrasound CT MRI 26:20

Chung SY, Stein RJ, Landsittel D et al (2004) 15-year experience with the management of extrinsic ureteral obstruction with indwelling ureteral stents. J Urol 172:592

Colistro R, Torreggiani WC, Lyburn ID et al (2002) Unenhanced helical CT in the investigation of acute flank pain. Clin Radiol 57:435

Croft BY, Joyce JM, Parekh J et al (1996) Nuclide studies. In: Gillenwater et al (eds) Adult and pediatric urology, 3rd edn. Mosby, St Louis, pp 193

Evans HJ, Wollin TA (2001) The management of urinary calculi in pregnancy. Cur Opin Urol 11:379

Diblasio CJ, Snyder ME, Kattan MW et al (2004) Ketorolac: safe and effective analgesia for the management of renal cortical tumors with partial nephrectomy. J Urol 171:1062

Doublet JD, Tchala K, Tligui M et al (1997) In situ extracorporeal shock wave lithotripsy for acute colic due to obstructing ureteral stones. Scand J Urol Nephrol 31:137

Gulmi FA, Felsen D, Vaughan ED Jr (2002) Pathophysiology of upper tract obstruction. In: Walsh PC et al (eds) Campbell's urology, 8th edn. Saunders, Philadelphia, pp 411

Hattery RR, Williamson B Jr, Hartman GW et al (1988) Intravenous urographic technique. Radiology 167:593

Heidenreich A, Desgrandschamps F, Terrier F (2002) Modern approach of diagnosis and management of acute flank pain: review of all imaging modalities. Eur Urol 41:351

Joshi HB, Obadeyi OO, Rao PN (1999) A comparative analysis of nephrostomy JJ stent and urgent in situ extracorporeal shock wave lithotripsy for obstructing ureteric stones. BJU Int 84:264

Kalyanakrishnan K, Scheid DC (2005) Diagnosis and management of acute pyelonephritis in adults. Am Fam Physician 71:933

Kawashima A, Sandler CM, Goldman SM et al (1997) CT of renal inflammatory disease. Radiographics 17:851

Kawashima A, Sandler CM, Corl FM et al (2001) Imaging of renal trauma: comprehensive review. Radiographics 21:557

Kawashima A, Vrtiska T, LeRoy AJ et al (2004) CT Urography. RadioGraphics 24:S35

Kim H, Xu M, Lin Y et al (1999) Renal dysfunction associated with the perioperative use of diclofenac. Anesth Analg 89:999

Kobayashi T, Nishizawa K, Watanabe J et al (2003) Clinical characteristics of ureteral calculi detected by nonenhanced computerized tomography after unclear results of plain radiography and ultrasonography. J Urol 170:799

Kravchick S, Bunkin I, Stepnov E et al (2005) Emergency extracorporeal shockwave lithotripsy for acute renal colic caused by upper urinary tract stone. J Endourol 19:1

Larkin GL, Peacock WF 4th, Pearl SM et al (1999) Efficacy of ketorolac tromethamine versus meperidine in the ED treatment of acute renal colic. Am J Emerg Med 17:6

Lee A, Cooper MC, Craig JC et al (2004) Effects of nonsteroidal anti-inflammatory drugs on post-operative renal function in adults with normal renal function. Cochrane Database Syst Rev 2:CD002765

Lifshitz DA, Lingeman JE (2002) Ureteroscopy as a first-line intervention for ureteral calculi in pregnancy. J Endourol 16:19

Lowe PP, Roylance J (1976) Transitional cell carcinoma of the kidney. Clin Radiol 27:503

McAleer SJ, Loughlin KR (2004) Nephrolithiasis and pregnancy. Cur Opin Urol 14:123

Mokhmalji H, Braun PM, Martinez Portillo FJ et al (2001) Percutaneous nephrostomy versus ureteral stents for diversion of hydronephrosis caused by stones: a prospective, randomized clinical trial. J Urol 165:1088

Niall O, Russell J, MacGregor R et al (1999) A comparison of noncontrast computerized tomography with excretory urography in the assessment of acute flank pain. J Urol 161:534

Nickel JC (2002) Acute pyelonephritis in adults. AUA Updates 21:306

Oktar SÖ, Yucel C, Özdemir H, Karaosmanoglu D (2004) Doppler sonography of renal obstruction: value of venous impedance index measurements. J Ultrasound Med 23:929

Özer C, Yencilek E, Apaydin FD et al (2004) Diagnostic value of renal parenchyma density difference on unenhanced helical computed tomography scan in acutely obstructing ureteral stone disease. Urology 64:223

Pearle MS, Pierce HL, Miller GL et al (1998) Optimal method of urgent decompression of the collecting system for obstruction and infection due to ureteral calculi. J Urol 160:1260

Preminger GM, Assimos DG, Lingeman JE et al (2005) Chapter 1: AUA guideline on management of staghorn calculi: diagnosis and treatment recommendations. J Urol 173:1991

Rucker CM, Menias CO, Bhalla S (2004) Mimics of renal colic: alternative diagnoses at unenhanced helical CT. Radiographics 24:S11

Segura JW, Preminger GM, Assimos DG et al (1997) Ureteral stones clinical guidelines panel summary report on the management of ureteral calculi. The American Urological Association. J Urol 158:1915

Smith RC, Levine J, Dalrymple NC et al (1999) Acute flank pain: a modern approach to diagnosis and management. Semin Ultrasound CT MR 20:108

Shokeir AA, Shoma AM, Essam A et al (2002) Recoverability of renal function after relief of acute complete ureteral obstruction: clinical prospective study of the role of renal resistive index. Urology 59:506

Shokeir AA, Shoma AM, Mosbah A et al (2002) Noncontrast computed tomography in obstructive anuria: a prospective study. Urology 59:861

Shokeir AA, El-Diasty T, Eassa W et al (2004) Diagnosis of ureteral obstruction in patients with compromised renal function: the role of noninvasive imaging modalities. J Urol 171:2303

Simckes AM, Chen SS, Osorio AV et al (1999) Ketorolac-induced irreversible renal failure in sickle cell disease: a case report. Pediatr Nephrol 13:63

Tligui M, Khadime MR, Tchala K et al (2003) Emergency extracorporeal shock wave lithotripsy (ESWL) for obstructing ureteral stones. Eur Urol 43:552

Watterson JD, Girvan AR, Beiko DT et al (2002) Ureteroscopy and holmium:YAG laser lithotripsy: an emerging definitive management strategy for symptomatic ureteral calculi in pregnancy. Urology 60:383

Yoshimura K, Utsunomiya N, Ichioka K et al (2005) Emergency drainage for urosepsis associated with upper urinary tract calculi. J Urol 173:458

Yossepowitch O, Lifshitz DA, Dekel et al (2001) Predicting the success of retrograde stenting for managing ureteral obstruction. J Urol 166:1746

11 Failure of Urinary Drainage: Lower Tract

J.M. Patterson, C.R. Chapple

11.1 Introduction

Failure of the lower urinary tract to drain adequately is one of the most common presenting emergencies seen by the practicing urologist. The wide variety of pathologies that can cause this problem needs to be taken into account when assessing the patient, as it is important not to subject the patient to undue risks.

In the emergency situation, the most common presenting symptom is that of urinary retention (UR), which itself can present in varied forms. It is often associated with pain and an intense desire to pass urine, most commonly termed acute urinary retention (AUR) (Fitzpatrick and Kirby 2006; Emberton and Anson 1999; Weiss et al. 2001), but it can also be a painless entity, sometimes noted by a report of not passing urine for several hours or even days, termed chronic urinary retention (CUR) (Kurasawa et al. 2005; Chooong and Emberton 2000). In some circumstances, presentation is not associated with a full urinary bladder but with a sensation of needing to void when the bladder is empty or near-empty. In some cases this can itself cause significant distress, and along with the discomfort felt by those in AUR, exemplifies the rapidity needed in the assessment and treatment of these patients.

Because of the variety of conditions causing UR, it is difficult to design a simple, single algorithm for their management. If the advice in this chapter is followed, however, we hope that the reader will be able to manage effectively the majority of problems seen in everyday practice.

11.2 The Male Patient

11.2.1 Introduction

The vast majority of patients with failure of lower urinary tract drainage seen as emergencies are male. Of these, the largest proportion will present with AUR, either to emergency departments or to primary care physicians. While many patients will have been complaining for some time of lower urinary tract symptoms (LUTS) (Abrams and et al. 2002), in some, the emergency presentation is the first indication that they had any functional abnormality of their lower urinary tract.

11.2.2 Benign Prostatic Hyperplasia

11.2.2.1 Pathophysiology

Benign prostatic hyperplasia (BPH) is the commonest benign adenoma in the male and develops almost exclusively in the transitional zone of the prostate gland. The growth and development of the prostate is under the influence of testosterone, specifically its active metabolite dihydrotestosterone (DHT). After conversion by the enzyme 5-α reductase, DHT stimulates androgen receptors in the prostate, which results in the production of growth factors such as epidermal growth factor (EGF). These factors then promote the hyperplasia seen in BPH. It has been postulated that a reduction in apoptosis is also involved in the development of BPH, by causing an imbalance in the ratio of proliferation and apoptosis and hence leading to glandular hyperplasia. The process also involves an increase in the amount of stromal and smooth muscle tissue of the transitional zone. Histologically, initially small stromal nodules are seen in the transitional zone around the urethra, followed by hyperplasia of the glandular structures. These changes are seen in prostates of men as young as 40, and are increasingly prevalent as the population ages. The size of the gland also tends to increase with age, which is in part responsible for the fact that aging male patients experience an increasing incidence of bladder outflow obstruction (BOO), and although there is no statistically significant link between size of prostate and degree of BOO, there is a correlation between size of prostate and the risk of complications of BPH, including AUR and the need for surgical intervention (Anderson et al. 2001; Chute et al. 1991; Fitzpatrick 2006; Jacobsen et al. 2005; Kirby 2000; Masumori et al. 2003; Thomas et al. 2004).

The smooth muscle of the prostate is under sympathetic nervous control, with synaptic release of norepinephrine from nerve terminal granules diffusing across the synaptic gap to stimulate large numbers of α_1-adrenoceptors. These are predominantly of the α_{1A}-adrenoceptor subtype, compared with α_{1B}-subtype and α_{1D}-subtype, which are found on blood vessels (causing vasodilatation) and viscera, respectively, and hence antagonists of these receptors are therapeutic targets of interest in the management of BPH. It has been shown that in AUR secondary to BPH, excess α-adrenergic receptor stimulation may be causative (Caine et al. 1975; Chapple 2001).

Histological BPH tends to progress gradually. Initially, the enlarging transitional zone tissue compresses the surrounding normal prostate tissue, and in time also begins to compress the prostatic urethra. It is this compression that causes a diminishing peak urine flow rate and progressive LUTS. As the caliber of the prostatic urethra is reduced by the hyperplastic prostate, it becomes less distensible, and the hyperplastic gland is also less able to relax to allow normal voiding function. Population studies have shown that the prostate increases by an average of 1–2 cm^3 per year, and in the same series, peak urine flow rates were also seen to diminish by 0.2 ml/s per year. However, individuals show considerable variety, and although in general patients with larger prostate glands tend toward faster rates of growth, the symptoms these patients describe fluctuate greatly. Patients also often find ways of managing their disease so that despite enlarging gland size, their symptoms remain stable (Girman et al. 1999; Roehrborn et al. 2002).

Associated with the increasing obstruction caused by the enlarging prostate, several associated morphological changes in the bladder are commonly seen. The detrusor muscle tends to hypertrophy as a consequence of increasing voiding pressures and associated collagenous infiltration of smooth muscle, which leads to reduced bladder compliance during filling. In a significant proportion of patients, there is evidence of detrusor overactivity causing involuntary bladder contractions, although at present it is unclear whether this is directly related to the BOO or is an unrelated age-dependent phenomenon. LUTS therefore seen in patients with BPH causing a degree of BOO (Weiss et al. 2001; Fitzpatrick 2006; Roehrborn et al. 2002; Fong et al. 2005) comprise a combination of *storage* (frequency, urgency, nocturia) and *voiding* (hesitancy, intermittency, reduced stream, incomplete emptying) and *postmicturition* symptoms (postmicturition and terminal dribbling).

With increased age, the problems with bladder emptying tend to progress. Some patients may develop problems fully emptying their bladder, with the development of increased residuals due to an encroaching prostate and worsening obstruction whereby the failing or tiring detrusor is unable to adequately compensate for the obstruction. This can culminate in acute-on-chronic UR, where the patient is unable to void despite a volume often in excess of 1.5 l in the bladder. These patients also often have enuresis (so-called overflow incontinence), and in some cases the volumes retained may preclude full recovery of detrusor function (Chapple and Smith 1994). Others may have an episode of AUR, which typically presents as described in Sects. 11.2.2.2 and 11.2.2.4, and requires emergency treatment by catheterization (see Chap. 19, "Surgical Techniques and Percutaneous Procedures"). In some cases, prolonged BOO and the development of residuals will predispose to the formation of bladder stone(s), recurrent urinary tract infections (UTIs; see Sect. 11.2.5.2), and in some cases deterioration of renal function, when the intravesical pressure exceeds the ureteric pressure, hence exerting a back-pressure on the kidneys that can lead to renal failure if left untreated.

11.2.2.2
Epidemiology and Diagnosis

It is important to remember that BPH is a pathological diagnosis, and most of the patients seen in practice have clinically enlarged prostate glands but no histological confirmation of BPH. Hence the term "benign prostatic enlargement" (BPE) is more appropriate in those in whom tissue diagnosis is not confirmed. BPH is one of the most prevalent conditions affecting men aged 40 and above. Histological studies have shown features of BPH to be present in the prostate of approximately 60% of men aged 60, and closer to 100% of men aged 80 and above. The only clear risk factors for the development of BPH are increasing age and the presence of circulating androgens. Clearly there are specific genetic patterns since histological BPH has been shown to be more prevalent in Afro-Caribbean than Caucasian populations. Asians tend to have a lower incidence still, but this is not maintained in migratory populations, also implying environmental factors in the development of BPH. Clinical BPH seems to run in families, although the genes responsible are yet to be identified.

There are three components to the clinical picture of BPH. It has been shown that there is considerable overlap between BPH and LUTS, and again between BPH and BOO, but they are by no means the same entities. LUTS may or may not be due to BPH, and BOO may or may not be present with BPH and/or LUTS (see Fig. 11.1). What can be said with certainty is that patients with BPH, LUTS, and BOO are at greatest risk of disease progression, including episodes of AUR (Weiss et al. 2001; Choong and Emberton 2000; Anderson et al. 2001; Abrams 1997; Kirby and McConnell 2005).

Diagnosis is based on clinical history and examination, including an assessment of LUTS and digital rectal examination (DRE). Although the International Prostate Symptom Score (IPSS) (the American Urology Association [AUA] Symptom Score Index) is advocated for the office assessment of LUTS and it is widely used in clinical trials to assess response to treatments (Weiss et al. 1991), in the emergency situation it is of limited applicability.

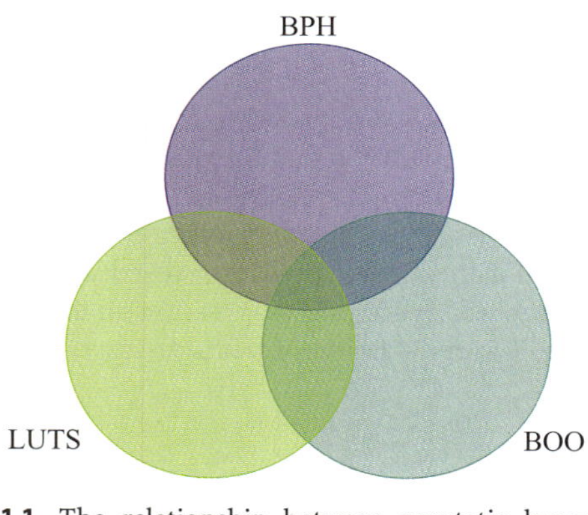

Fig. 11.1. The relationship between prostatic hypertrophy, symptoms and obstruction. Each may exist independently or in combination in each individual patient

Acutely, patients presenting with AUR will typically complain of both an intense desire to void and a degree of suprapubic pain (Fitzpatrick and Kirby 2006). They may give a history of preceding LUTS, with a reduced urine flow rate and a sensation of incomplete bladder emptying correlating best with subsequent progression to AUR. Those with chronic retention will not typically have pain. Some may describe a feeling of fullness, and some may even notice a suprapubic swelling. Usually, however, they present simply with an inability to pass urine, often having not voided for over 24 h. Some of these patients will, however, present *in extremis* with acute renal failure. These patients are often uremic, and some may have life-threatening electrolyte imbalances including hyperkalemia. Typically, on catheterization, they will have very large residual volumes and subsequently may have a significant diuresis, which needs careful observation and management with appropriate fluid replacement. In the presence of disturbed renal function, investigations into the state of the upper urinary tracts (typically ultrasound) should also be carried out (see Sect. 11.2.2.5).

In the history it is important, as well as asking about LUTS, to exclude any other co-morbidities that could be contributing to the presentation. It is important to exclude neurological disorders, including cerebrovascular events, multiple sclerosis (MS), spinal cord injury (SCI), pelvic or perineal trauma, Parkinson's disease, multisystem atrophy (MSA), and motor neuron disease (MND), and consider if they are taking any drugs that could contribute to dysfunctional voiding (anticholinergics, antidepressants, anesthetic agents, analgesics). Also, it is important to assess the patient's general medical state to ensure that they are not going to come to any harm as a result of any therapy instigated.

Physical examination is performed as a matter of routine. It should include a full cardiorespiratory assessment, neurological examination including cognitive state (specifically examining the low lumbar and sacral dermatomes and myotomes to rule out cauda equina syndrome), and examination of the abdomen, paying special attention to the kidneys and the presence or absence of a palpable urinary bladder. Examination of the external genitalia is important to ensure urethral catheterization is not going to be impossible and to identify phimosis or meatal stenosis, as well as to rule out associated infective complications such as epididymitis. If suprapubic catheterization is to be considered, then inspection of the lower abdomen to look for lower midline scars is essential (see Chap. 19, "Surgical Techniques and Percutaneous Procedures").

DRE is performed to both give an estimation of prostate size and to exclude malignancy and prostatitis as alternative causes of UR (see also Sects. 11.2.3 and 11.2.5.2). As such it is possibly the most important part of the examination in male patients presenting with failure to empty their bladder. The normal male prostate is less than 20 cm^3 in volume, so BPE can be diagnosed by the experienced clinician based on DRE alone, although the accuracy of size estimation tends to be very subjective and is certainly reduced in glands bigger than 50 cm^3. The gland should be symmetrical. Any nodules or irregularity, or a gland that is diffusely firm or asymmetrical could represent malignancy. It is important to note that inflammatory conditions such as prostatitis can also feel firm and irregular, but the difference is that in the acute phase, these will be tender to palpation.

In the acute setting, especially in cases presenting with UR, testing for prostate-specific antigen (PSA) is deferred. Although PSA correlates well with both gland size in BPH and tumor size in prostate cancer, it is also usually significantly raised in episodes of retention or infection and after instrumentation or examination. (In the nonacute office setting, with patients presenting with LUTS and BPE, it is entirely reasonable to perform PSA testing as long as the implications are understood by the patient. Important information can also be obtained in this setting by assessment of peak urine flow and concurrent assessment of postvoid residual urine volume.)

Urinalysis should be performed on the urine obtained immediately after catheterization (if the patient is completely unable to void) and if anything abnormal is seen, the urine should be sent for formal microscopy and culture, and if sexually transmitted infection is suspected, particularly in younger sexually active patients, urine should also be sent for gonorrhea and chlamydia PCR testing (see also Sect. 11.2.5.2).

In some cases, patients may present with symptoms suggestive of both AUR and UTI, for example, a few days history of dysuria and offensive smelling urine, with an acute history of inability to pass urine. In these patients, to avoid instrumenting the urinary tract unnecessarily and in the presence of infection, a measurement of residual urine volume can be helpful. This is typically carried out using a bedside portable ultrasound bladder scanner (Bladderscan BVI 3000, Verathon Inc., Bothel, WA, USA). If the residual volume is very low (less than 150 ml) then the patient should not be catheterized. A course of antibiotics should be commenced and the patient should only be catheterized if he is unable to void with a more significant urine volume in the bladder.

11.2.2.3
Lower Urinary Tract Symptoms

LUTS is a relatively new term coined to lessen the confusion caused by terms such as prostatism, symptomatic obstructive uropathy, etc. They comprise three groups of symptoms: storage, voiding, and postmicturition symptoms (Abrams et al. 2002). Storage symptoms include frequency, nocturia, urgency, and urgency incontinence. It is important to differentiate a normal urge to void and urgency, and similarly nocturia from nocturnal polyuria. Voiding symptoms include hesitancy, poor stream, intermittency, straining to void, incomplete bladder emptying, and UR. A case can be made for considering enuresis secondary to chronic retention – overflow incontinence – as both a storage and a voiding disorder. Postmicturition symptoms include terminal and postmicturition dribbling.

Clearly these symptoms are not disease-specific and a wide range of other disease states can cause LUTS. These include neurological conditions such as those mentioned above, malignancy (including prostate cancer and urothelial tumors), inflammatory conditions (including UTI, bladder stones, interstitial cystitis), polyuria (diabetes, congestive cardiac failure), and other causes of BOO, including bladder neck or external sphincter dyssynergia, urethral stricture (see Sect. 11.2.4) and severe phimosis. Some symptoms such as a poor urine stream are also found in conditions such as detrusor underactivity or detrusor failure, which do not necessarily have an obstructive component.

The role of inflammation within the prostate has also been investigated recently, with several series showing that in tissue samples from prostates of patients in AUR, there is more inflammation than in prostates with BPH/BOO, which in turn have more inflammation than normal prostates (Anjum et al. 1998; Roehrborn 2006b; Tuncel et al. 2005).

11.2.2.4
Bladder Outflow Obstruction

BOO is a clearly defined urodynamic diagnosis. The most widely accepted diagnosis of obstruction is by the use of the Abrams-Griffiths (AG) number and its associated nomogram. The AG number can be derived from conventional cystometry by the following equation:

$$\text{AG number} = \text{pDet.}Q_{max} - 2\ (Q_{max})$$

If the AG number is less than 20, the patient is unobstructed. If the result is between 20 and 40, the result is said to be equivocal, whereas if it is over 40, the patient has BOO (Abrams 1997; Chapple and MacDiarmid 2000).

In male patients above the age of 40, BOO is typically caused by BPE, although other causes exist, as outlined above (other causes of BOO are also discussed in Sect. 11.2.5). In most examples, it tends to be a progressive problem, and serial cystometry in these patients will show progressive increases in voiding pressures with an associated reduction in maximum urine flow rates.

In cases caused by BPE, there may be a critical point beyond which the patient is unable to generate a sustained detrusor contraction sufficient to overcome the outlet resistance, and it is at this point that they may present in AUR. In many cases presenting acutely, however, this information is unknown, and cannot easily be derived in the acute setting.

11.2.2.5 Management

Immediate Management

The immediate management of any patient presenting with failure to empty their bladder, history and examination aside, is directed to draining the bladder. This is discussed in detail in Chap. 19, "Surgical Techniques and Percutaneous Procedures". In most cases, the passage of a Foley urethral catheter (under aseptic conditions) is sufficient to bypass the obstruction and establish drainage of the bladder. Typically, the catheter stays in place for at least 24–48 h while long-term management is decided and instigated. In some cases, however, it is not possible to pass a Foley catheter due to the nature of the obstruction. This can be overcome in some patients by using alternative catheters, such as those with a Coudé tip, which are often able to navigate the obstruction as described in Chap. 19, "Surgical Techniques and Percutaneous Procedures". If no urethral access is available, then the next option is to proceed to suprapubic cystostomy. In some patients, specifically those with prior lower abdominal surgery, this may need to be carried out under ultrasound guidance. Finally, if this is not possible, then there is no option other than open surgical cystostomy, but this should be regarded as a last resort.

If catheterization is successful, and there are no features suggestive of high risk of recurrent UR, and the patient has normal renal function, i.e., a diagnosis of "typical" uncomplicated UR secondary to BPE (which should make up approximately 70% patients with AUR), then typically we would proceed to institute pharmacological therapy to aid chances of a successful trial without catheter (TWOC).

However, in patients not meeting the above criteria, further investigations are required. In cases where renal function is disturbed, it is appropriate to perform ultrasonographic examination of the upper tracts to both diagnose obstructive uropathy and exclude any coexisting renal abnormality. In patients with true high-pressure CUR, there may be a degree of hydronephrosis, but this should resolve promptly (within 48 h) of catheterization. These patients will typically need definitive bladder drainage, usually via long-term urethral or suprapubic drainage, with surgical intervention as deemed appropriate by TURP. If definitive bladder drainage is not ensured, then the high-pressure CUR will almost invariably recur.

Cases of CUR with no hydronephrosis or renal impairment are termed low-pressure CUR and are usually associated with a low-pressure low-flow voiding pattern. These patients fare badly with TURP, and are best managed with clean intermittent self-catheterization (CISC), as the detrusor muscle tends not to recover from its chronically distensible hypercompliant state. CISC is an alternative long-term method of bladder drainage in those patients with BOO who are unfit for surgery, but some patients encounter difficulties with large obstructing prostate glands actually passing the catheters into the bladder. Also, the technique needs to be closely observed prior to discharge to the community, as some patients find it much harder than others.

Pharmacotherapy

α-Antagonists. The receptors responsible for maintaining smooth muscle tone in the prostate are α_{1A}-adrenoceptors, and it is in part due to failure of the prostatic smooth muscle to relax effectively that voiding is obstructed in BOO caused by BPH, leading in some to AUR, possibly as a result of excess stimulation of the α-adrenoceptors as a precipitative event.

There has been a large shift in recent years in the management of uncomplicated AUR. Previously, the majority of patients would have undergone transurethral resection of the prostate (TURP) either in the acute setting or several weeks from initial presentation. The advent of α-adrenoceptor antagonists has meant that a lot of patients who previously would have undergone surgery can be managed conservatively for a period of time. Standard policy has become starting α-antagonists at presentation, at least 24 h prior to TWOC, with very good outcomes. In patients presenting routinely with LUTS suggestive of BPH and BOO, significant symptomatic improvements are seen within 24–48 h of commencing α-antagonist therapy (Fitzpatrick and Kirby 2006; Chapple 2001; Andersson et al. 2002; Chapple 2004; Djavan et al. 2004; Elhilali et al. 2006).

Commonly used examples include doxazosin, prazosin, terazosin, indoramin (used less than previously), alfuzosin, and tamsulosin. The latter two are associated with fewer systemic side effects. Alfuzosin is to date the only member of this class of drugs to have statistically proven benefits in aiding TWOC in patients with episodes of AUR (Elhilali et al. 2006; Roehrborn 2006a; McNeill et al. 1999), although it is likely that similar efficacy would be expected to be present for the other agents in the class.

Several studies have shown benefits in terms of prolonging time to retention or surgery, and recent studies have compounded these benefits by using combination therapy with 5α-reductase inhibitors (McConnell et al. 2003).

5α-Reductase Inhibitors. The 5α-reductase inhibitors work by inhibiting the enzyme responsible for converting testosterone into the more active form DHT. There are two commercially available examples, finasteride and dutasteride. The method of action is to reduce the effect of circulating androgens on the prostate. They effectively reduce growth of the prostate, and have been shown to shrink the glandular component of histological BPH. They are most effective in large prostate glands, but unfortunately the beneficial effects take approximately 4–6 months to appear, so their use in the short term is of limited value. However, if a patient presents with a large volume gland causing BPE and AUR, then adding in a 5α-reductase inhibitor to α-antagonist therapy will prolong the time to further episodes of AUR and the need for surgical intervention (McConnell et al. 2003; Andriole et al. 2004; Kaplan et al. 2006).

11.2.2.6 *Pitfalls*

It is important when managing patients with UR associated with BPH that the following points are carefully taken into consideration.

1. Perform DRE to make or confirm diagnosis and exclude malignancy and infection.
2. Measure residual urine prior to catheterization if UTI is suspected.
3. Measure serum creatinine to ensure high-pressure chronic retention is not overlooked, and if present monitor, treat diuresis appropriately, and ensure definitive bladder drainage is in place either via surgery or catheterization.
4. TURP is still appropriate as first-line management of AUR for between 20% and 40% of patients, either acutely or electively.
5. Many patients failing TWOC are not suitable for surgical treatment due to high-risk co-morbidity, and many of these can safely be managed with long-term catheterization, either urethral or suprapubic according to choice and suitability

11.2.3 Malignant Prostatic Disease

11.2.3.1 *Pathophysiology*

Although prostate cancer is increasingly common, the incidence of AUR secondary to malignant disease is very low, probably less than 1% of cases of AUR seen in practice. Having said that, there may be a significant proportion of men, especially those over the age of 70, who present in AUR who have both BPH and undiagnosed prostate cancer, and most men with prostate cancer will have BPH to a certain extent. Therefore, the mechanisms of BOO are similar to those in BPH, and prepresentation LUTS will also tend to be similar. In some cases, however, the obstruction to voiding will be directly related to local tumor burden causing either compression of the prostatic urethra, or in some cases local invasion into the urethra, seminal vesicles, or ejaculatory ducts, causing mechanical obstruction or stricturing of the prostatic urethra (Anson et al. 1993; Sandhu et al. 1992). The effects on the detrusor are similar to those seen in BPH.

11.2.3.2 *Epidemiology and Diagnosis*

The population incidence of prostate cancer has dramatically increased since the advent of PSA testing. It now represents the most common cancer in males, although this includes many cancers not requiring intervention other than monitoring, and is among the leading causes of cancer death in men. This does not mean that the true incidence of prostate cancer is higher, but that more cases are being diagnosed than previously. Most men presenting acutely with symptoms of UR of any cause will most likely have BPH, but several large population studies have shown that a significant proportion of these will have clinically undetectable foci of prostate cancer. This proportion increases dramatically with age (Johansson et al. 2004; Kessler and Albertsen 2003).

The patient may present in exactly the same manner as the patient with BPH, i.e., in AUR or less commonly CUR. On initial assessment, it may be evident that they are under investigation for, or being treated for, prostate cancer. DRE may reveal an overtly malignant-feeling prostate, or more commonly a benign-feeling gland. If there is no history of prostate cancer, and the DRE is benign, then one should proceed as per AUR secondary to BPH, and PSA should be checked once voiding is re-established. There is little use in checking PSA acutely, as it will be raised secondary to the episode of AUR. If there is a history of prostate cancer or investigation into the same, or the DRE is suspicious for malignancy, then a different approach should be taken; see Sect. 11.2.3.3.

If the patient is known to have prostate cancer that is being monitored for presumed small-volume organ-confined disease, then episodes of AUR can represent local disease progression, which should alter management, unless this is contrary to the patient's wishes.

11.2.3.3 *Management*

Management depends on the etiology of the episode of UR. If likely related to BPH rather than prostate cancer, then manage as per BPH above. If the patient is known to have prostate cancer, or the diagnosis is clinically very likely, then the management should be as follows. Initially, the important step is to establish bladder drainage, as before, including any appropriate investigations that should be performed.

Once bladder drainage has been established, TWOC is unlikely to be successful if AUR has been caused by local disease progression. Similarly, the addition of α-adrenoceptor antagonists is unlikely to be beneficial, as the tissue causing the obstruction is not predominantly smooth muscle. In some cases, TURP (often referred to as channel TURP to differentiate between operations for benign and malignant disease) can be performed, either acutely (within 2–3 days) or electively (after 4–6 weeks). This will provide symptomatic relief of voiding LUTS, but clearly is not intended as curative surgery for the prostate cancer. Alternative treatments have included prostatic stents (Anson et al. 1993), although these have largely gone out of favor. In select patients unsuitable for TURP, however, they may still have a role (Parikh and Milroy 1995; Wilson et al. 2002).

If the diagnosis of prostate cancer is not yet confirmed, then prostate biopsies should be obtained, usually via transrectal ultrasound. Once the diagnosis has been confirmed, then an alternative first-line treatment would be to instigate androgen deprivation treatment. This will shrink the prostate gland and potentially allow the patient to void normally again. Many centers would advocate the use of androgen deprivation therapy synchronously with TURP or stenting. Some patients, however, will have androgen-resistant disease, and in these cases any palliative treatment to improve LUTS is the most appropriate course of action, as outcome in this group tends to be very poor (Weiss et al. 2001; Gnanapragasam et al. 2006).

11.2.3.4 Pitfalls

The pitfalls of managing AUR in patients with prostate malignancy are the same as those for BPH. In addition, it is important to consider the following factors:

1. Is the episode of retention secondary to a known prostate cancer and if so, is BOO caused by local disease progression?
2. If the patient is known to have prostate cancer, ensure current status is known with respect to stage, grade, and any previous therapy.
3. PSA will be elevated secondary to both AUR and CUR, so this does not necessarily represent disease progression.
4. Is the patient on androgen deprivation therapy already; if not, is this appropriate?
5. In some circumstances, specifically hormone refractory prostate cancer, palliative measures are the most appropriate.

11.2.4 Urethral Stricture Disease

11.2.4.1 Pathophysiology

Urethral strictures are essentially urethral scars, of varying etiology. Historically they were most commonly caused by gonococcal urethritis (Singh and Blandy 1976), but in recent years they are typically the result of trauma, either external or iatrogenic. Some are still caused by inflammatory conditions such as balanitis xerotica obliterans (BXO) and a large percentage are of unknown etiology, presumed secondary to infection or inflammation in the paraurethral glands. One of the known causative agents is extravasation of urine following urothelial damage (Singh and Blandy 1976), but a common feature is the progressive nature of the majority of these scars to cause circumferential urethral lumen narrowing (Weiss et al. 2001).

11.2.4.2 Epidemiology and Diagnosis

Urethral stricture disease rarely presents for the first time acutely outside of the trauma setting; however, there is always a group of patients who present late with retention of urine consequent to an undiagnosed stricture. Most patients with urethral strictures describe a typical progressive deterioration in urine flow rate and loss of flow caliber, eventually describing storage, voiding, and postmicturition LUTS. Some have recurrent UTI and a proportion will describe bleeding per urethra that is not always associated with voiding. If symptoms progress without intervention, patients may in time present with AUR. Some patients with meatal stenosis and/or phimosis may also present in AUR, although the majority of these patients will also usually have had deteriorating voiding symptoms for some time.

Traumatic disruption of the male urethra, causing failure of bladder drainage, is a well-described feature of many types of injuries; most commonly pelvic fractures, fall-astride injuries, foreign bodies, etc.; these are covered in Sect. 11.2.5.5.

In patients presenting acutely with UR who are known to have urethral stricture, the diagnosis is simple. If it is the first presentation, then a comprehensive history of deteriorating LUTS can raise the suspicion of stricture disease. This is especially true in patients younger than 40, or those with a history of urinary tract instrumentation, injuries, or foreign bodies. The examination may be unremarkable, but in some cases, as previously, a bladder will be palpable above the symphysis pubis. DRE should be normal; however, some patients may have coexisting BPE. In some cases, an area of thickening of the corpus spongiosum is palpable in the penile urethra or in the bulbar urethra, felt at the perineum; this suggests severe stricturing that will almost certainly necessitate surgical intervention (Weiss et al. 2001). There may be features of UTI, including epididymitis, and these would be corroborated by a history of dysuria and cloudy, offensive urine.

Definitive diagnosis is sometimes not made until attempts at urethral catheterization are made, which will invariably fail in patients with AUR secondary to stricture(s). Alternatively, if stricture is suspected, retrograde urethrography can be performed to identify the site and extent of the stricture(s). This also helps to guide future management.

11.2.4.3
Management

The patient in AUR caused by stricture disease has the same requirement for bladder drainage as the patient with obstruction caused by BPH. However, urethral access is almost invariably not available. In these cases, insertion of a suprapubic catheter is often the only option available. This is discussed further in Chap. 19, "Surgical Techniques and Percutaneous Procedures". Rarely, suprapubic catheterization may be contraindicated (e.g., urothelial malignancy, although this is a relative contraindication in the acute setting) or technically impossible (e.g., morbid obesity, presence of abdominal viscera between abdominal wall on ultrasonographic examination). In these cases, the only two options available both involve surgical intervention. Open surgical cystostomy is one option, with the attending risks of an abdominal incision (although the peritoneum need not be opened in most cases). The other option would be to attempt direct inline visual urethrotomy (DIVU) after passing a guidewire across the stricture and incising it, although very dense strictures are usually not successfully by-passed in this manner. A last-resort option would be to consider acute-setting formal urethroplasty, but this is so rarely carried out that it should not be considered unless everything else has failed.

It is very rare for suprapubic drainage to be impossible, and once established, the patient can safely be managed with a suprapubic catheter until definitive treatment for their stricture can be planned.

In cases of AUR due purely to phimosis, acute circumcision or a dorsal slit procedure of the prepuce can be performed to allow the patient to void, or if necessary allow access to the urethral meatus for catheterization. Similarly, meatal dilatation under local anesthetic can relieve meatal stenosis sufficiently to allow the patient to void (or a urethral catheter to be passed as indicated) if this is the cause of the AUR. Meatal dilatation is usually performed with urethral sounds, graduated female urethral dilators, or bougies, depending on local availability. Some patients will need definitive treatment at a later date for these conditions; others can be managed conservatively.

11.2.4.4
Pitfalls

Some strictures are associated with other conditions, and elements of the history may be unclear; however, the acute management remains the same. It is important to consider the following when a diagnosis of stricture is made as the cause for AUR.

1. When attempting urethral catheterization and encountering resistance at the level of a stricture, it is imperative not to attempt to force a catheter through a stricture, as false passages can be easily created, which can cause problems when it comes to definitive management procedures.
2. Some patients may have undergone previous surgery to the bladder neck, such as TURP, radical prostatectomy, or bladder neck incision, which are known to cause stenosis and obstruction in some cases. The acute management is the same, however, as indicated above.
3. It is essential in these patients that a full sexual health history is taken to exclude sexually transmitted infection as a cause, and also to allow formal contact tracing if indicated.

11.2.5
Other Causes of Failure of Lower Urinary Tract Drainage

11.2.5.1
Postoperative Urinary Retention

One of the most common presentations of AUR is postoperative UR. This is surprisingly common and can occur associated with up to 23% of anesthetic procedures, with an especially high prevalence in those undergoing epidural or spinal anesthetic (Dolin and Cashman 2005; Kim et al. 2006). It is more likely to occur in patients undergoing major abdominal, pelvic, or lower limb surgery, and is also more likely in those patients receiving opiate analgesia. The precise mechanism of postoperative UR is unclear, although the most widely believed theory is that detrusor contractility is suppressed, combined with activation of stress-mediated inhibitory sympathetic pathways (Kim et al. 2006). This is often as a side effect of anesthetic agents, but it is thought to be potentiated by opiates. Lesser effects have been seen with the opioids alfentanil and sufentanil, especially relating to epidural use, than with conventional opiates (Kim et al. 2006). Epidural-related detrusor dysfunction is clearly recognized as a cause for litigation in pregnant patients undergoing labor with an epidural in situ, where there is a failure to drain the bladder that then becomes overdistended, with resultant detrusor dysfunction that can lead both acute and chronic retention. In some patients, especially those undergoing pelvic surgery, there is a risk of direct neurological damage as a cause of abnormal detrusor function. Other causes of postoperative UR include immobility, constipation, pain, local edema and preexisting BOO.

The mainstay of management is again to drain the bladder by urethral or suprapubic catheterization. In motivated and able patients, CISC can be taught as acute management of postoperative UR. Usually, after a period of either in-dwelling catheterization or institution of CISC, normal voiding function returns. This is typically within 6 weeks of surgery, although it can take up to 12 months in cases where neuropraxia is implicated. In patients with postoperative UR, BOO is rarely demonstrated on urodynamic testing, although it may coexist in many patients incidentally (Leveckis et al. 1995; Anderson and Grant 1991). If BOO is demonstrated in male patients and return to normal voiding function has not occurred within 6 weeks, then TURP is usually beneficial. In patients who fail to return to normal, including those in whom neurological damage is suspected, a regime of CISC is the best acute management strategy (Weiss et al. 2001).

11.2.5.2 Urinary Tract Infection

Urinary tract infections are relatively rare in male patients, but they do represent a proportion of men attending with AUR. Many of these patients will have a degree of BOO and/or LUTS, and some will be known to have incomplete bladder emptying. They are also commonly seen in BOO caused by stricture disease. The patient will typically give a history of LUTS, but associated with a short-term history of dysuria, offensive-smelling or dark/cloudy urine, and suprapubic pain. Some patients may describe passing debris and others may have frank hematuria. They may have perineal pain if the prostate is infected, with associated pain on defecation. In some cases, one or both epididymides and testes may be affected also. The patient will usually volunteer this information, although it tends to be obvious on examination. On examination, the patient will typically complain of suprapubic discomfort on palpation, and in cases with prostatic involvement, the prostate will be exquisitely tender on DRE. It may also be grossly abnormal to palpation, and if so it is important that the patient be re-examined once the infective episode has resolved, typically at 6 – 8 weeks.

The history of the episode of AUR is similar to patients with uncomplicated AUR, but in some cases the patient will have been passing small volumes of urine intermittently. In view of this, it is always worth assessing the residual urine volume using an ultrasound bladder scanner prior to catheterization. Often the patient will have a very small residual volume and the risks of systemic sepsis associated with catheterizing him can therefore be avoided. In these cases, treatment with systemic antibiotics and α-antagonist is often sufficient to overcome the obstructed voiding. However, patients will also often have a full bladder, in which case the AUR should be managed as normal, with broad-spectrum antibiotic cover with systemic antibiotics or quinolones for at least 24 h prior to TWOC. As any episode of UTI causing AUR is by definition a complicated UTI; it should be treated with at least 7 days of antibiotics, and if prostate involvement or epididymoorchitis is suspected, then this course should be extended to 2 – 3 full weeks.

If acute prostatitis is thought to be the sole cause of the episode of AUR, or there is a prostatic abscess palpable on DRE, then urinary tract instrumentation is contraindicated due to the risk of spreading the infection to the soft tissues (possibly culminating in necrotizing fasciitis or Fournier's gangrene). In these cases, it is best to drain the bladder by suprapubic catheterization. The choice of antibiotic is important, as some have better prostatic penetration than others. Currently, quinolones offer the best penetration into the tissues and should be used as first-line treatment, although if the patient is showing signs of systemic infection, then broad spectrum intravenous antibiotics such as ampicillin, gentamicin, and metronidazole in combination should be used until the patient is consistently apyrexial and cultures return to normal. If abscess or evidence to suggest spreading soft tissue infection is present, then surgical debridement is the first-line treatment as well as the above management (Weiss et al. 2001).

Any patient with prostatitis and/or epididymoorchitis should be evaluated with a full sexual health history to rule out gonococcal and chlamydial urinary tract infections, as these may require slightly different treatment as well as formal contact tracing to limit the community impact of these potentially sexually transmitted infections.

11.2.5.3 Urothelial Malignancy

The most common cause of failure of drainage of the lower urinary tract associated with urothelial malignancy is related to hematuria and AUR caused by the mechanical obstruction of the bladder outflow tract with clot. The patient will present with a variable history: they may be known to have an urothelial tumor, or rarely a renal tumor, or this may be their first episode of hematuria. Typically, they describe hematuria for a period of time, often associated with severe bladder spasms (as blood is highly irritant to the trigone) culminating in a complete inability to void, which is almost invariably painful. Some patients may have coexisting LUTS, BOO, or BPH, and others may have coexisting detrusor failure or CUR. Examination findings will rarely be different from patients with uncomplicated AUR, but it is important to examine the kidneys to identify any large masses suggestive of renal tumor. If the patient has advanced malignancy, they may be cachectic or show features of secondary disease such as jaundice. DRE may reveal a fixed bladder base mass or evidence of prostatic infiltration or may be normal.

It is important to realize that not all episodes of AUR with clot are caused by malignancy, with common alternative reasons being infection, iatrogenic (instrumentation), bladder calculi, and upper tract urolithiasis.

Acute management is also directed at establishing and maintaining effective bladder drainage. In cases of clot retention, however, it is usually not sufficient to pass a standard two-way catheter, as this will in turn block with clot, even with diligent washouts. The most straightforward means of establishing bladder drainage is via a large 24-F or larger three-way catheter. Irrigating the bladder typically breaks up clots to allow them to be drained more efficiently, and in time all clot debris will be removed from the bladder. In some situations, operative bladder washouts are necessary. Once the urine is clear, the bladder can be inspected and the cause of the bleeding identified and treated, if appropriate, or diagnosed to allow longer-term management to be planned.

Bladder neoplasms themselves are rare causes of AUR. Large pedunculated tumors can act in a similar fashion to ball-valves, causing mechanical obstruction of the bladder neck, but this is very unusual. More commonly, a bladder tumor may invade the base of the bladder or the prostate, causing progressive stenosis of either the bladder neck or the prostatic urethra in the same way as prostatic malignancy can lead to BOO.

11.2.5.4 Neurological Abnormalities

Patients with neurological causes of AUR tend to present either acutely, at the same time as their neurological insult, e.g., cerebrovascular event (CVE) or with AUR as a new component of a progressive neurological condition such as multiple sklerosis (MS). In either case, the initial management is the same as previously, namely urethral or suprapubic catheterization.

The majority of neurological causes of UR relate to loss of detrusor function rather than excess sympathetic activity, and because of this the UR may not always be painful, especially on a background of progressive LUTS or difficulty voiding. The most commonly associated neurological abnormalities associated with voiding dysfunction include CVEs, cauda equina syndrome or spinal cord compression, Parkinson's disease, Shy-Drager syndrome (multisystem atrophy), multiple sclerosis (MS), and motor neuron disease (MND). Spinal cord injury also causes long-term voiding dysfunction, but rarely AUR. Most patients are, however, managed with an in-dwelling catheter after the initial injury, until the period of spinal shock has passed when a better idea of long-term bladder function can be ascertained.

On presentation of patients in UR with neurological disease, it is important to ascertain not only the diagnosis of the neurological impairment, but how this is likely to affect their urinary tract function. Some patients with acute conditions such as CVE may fully recover normal urinary tract function, so may only need catheterization for a short period of time. Others are more likely to need definitive longer-term management to be in place once the initial event is treated.

On examination of these patients, it is imperative to perform a full neurological examination paying specific attention to the sacral dermatomes and myotomes and their associated reflexes. Assessment of anal tone and sensation can be performed at the same time as DRE. In patients with symptoms suggestive of cauda equina compression, such as back pain and saddle anesthesia, urgent magnetic resonance imaging (MRI) scanning should be performed with a view to urgent neurosurgical intervention where appropriate. Some patients in this group may have known metastatic bone disease, in which case MRI followed by urgent radiotherapy may be required. Both of these events will not effect the immediate management of AUR, i.e., catheterization. If treated early, normal neurological function should return after a period of time, but any delays to treatment are associated with worse long-term recovery.

In cases caused by progression of chronic neurological disease, those patients with reasonable motor function, specifically with reference to the hands and upper limbs, and normal cognitive function, CISC is the best option for long-term bladder management. Some patients, however, may not be able to manage this independently, and long-term management of these individuals needs to be decided on a case-by-case basis to ensure all parties involved in the patient's on-going care are informed and capable of whatever is needed. Some patients may require long-term suprapubic catheterization as a less intensive method of long-term bladder management.

11.2.5.5 Trauma

Trauma is a rare cause of failure of drainage of the lower urinary tract. The most common mechanism is that of urethral disruption, although rarely foreign bodies can cause complete obstruction to voiding. The most common injuries associated with urethral injury are fall-astride injuries, pelvic fractures, penetrating or blunt trauma to the perineum, and fracture injuries of the corpora. Also, bladder injuries, such as intraperitoneal rupture, can cause failure to void. Most bladder injuries have a typical history of falling onto the lower abdomen while the bladder was full, or of obvious blunt or penetrating trauma.

The management of all trauma patients should adhere to Advanced Trauma Life Support (ATLS) protocols (American College of Surgeons 1997), especially as a large proportion of these patients may have multiple injuries. Urethral injuries may not immediately be apparent on primary survey, although presence of blood at the urethral meatus should give a high incidence of suspicion. The patient may not be in AUR, as the trauma may have occurred when the bladder was empty, but the presence or absence of urethral trauma needs to be excluded if there is any suspicion of its presence.

Prior to insertion of a urethral catheter, a retrograde urethrogram should be performed. If any extravasation of contrast is seen, then a urethral catheter should not be inserted, and the drainage of the bladder should be established by suprapubic catheterization. If the patient is undergoing any abdominal or pelvic surgery then this can be performed synchronously; otherwise one needs to either wait until the bladder is full enough for percutaneous suprapubic cystostomy, or perform the procedure using ultrasound to show the position of the bladder (Morey et al. 1999; McAninch et al. 1996). Once bladder drainage is established, cystography can be performed to exclude concomitant bladder injuries.

If the patient is suspected of having a bladder injury, and urethral injury is either unlikely given the mechanism of injury or has been ruled out on urethrography, then the first-line investigation should usually be computed tomography (CT) scanning with synchronous cystography. If this is unavailable, then plain x-ray cystography is usually sufficient to diagnose the need for surgical repair. Generally speaking, extraperitoneal bladder rupture with insignificant contrast extravasation can be managed effectively with prolonged urethral catheterization, typically for 10 days, with cystography prior to removal of catheter to ensure no ongoing leak. If intraperitoneal bladder rupture is seen, then surgical repair is needed. This should be carried out acutely, and postoperatively the bladder should be drained for at least 10 days, with some surgeons advocating both urethral and suprapubic catheters to ensure drainage and reduce the risk of complications.

A summarizing algorithm for the management of (male) patients presenting with AUR is presented in Fig. 11.2.

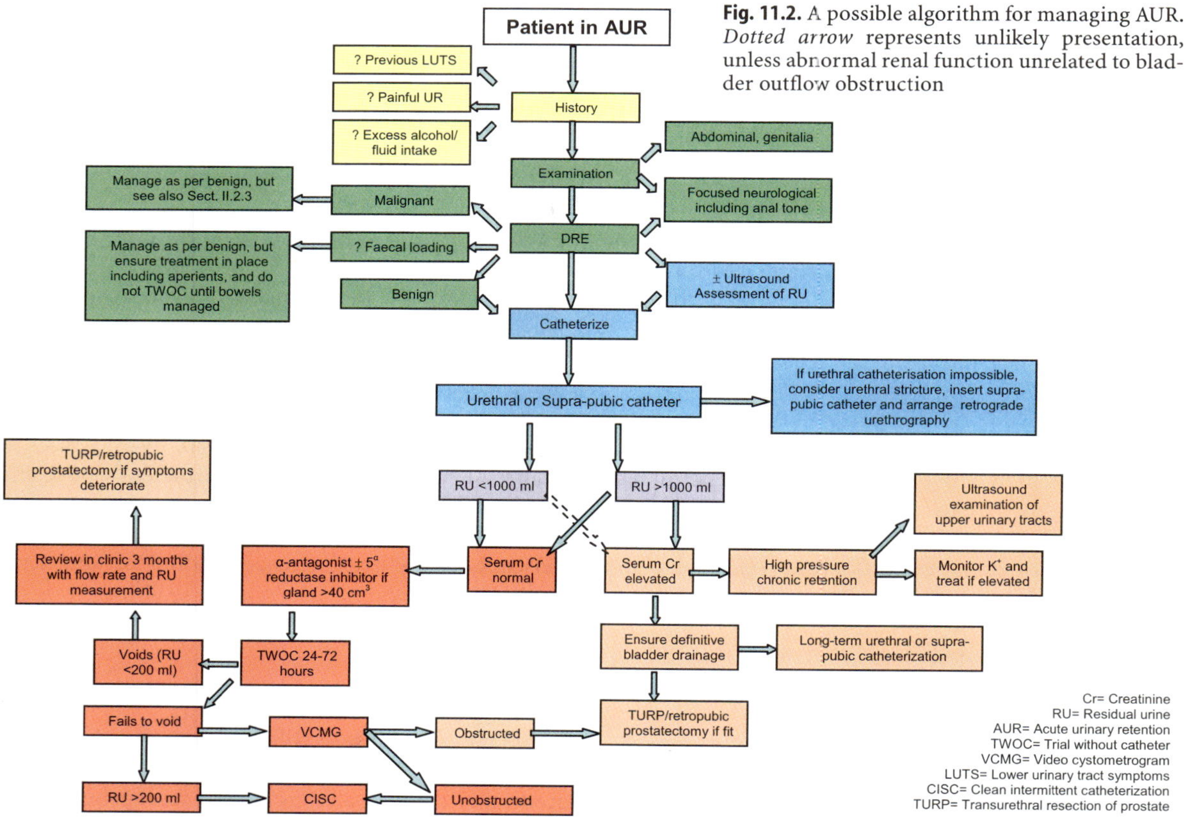

Fig. 11.2. A possible algorithm for managing AUR. *Dotted arrow* represents unlikely presentation, unless abnormal renal function unrelated to bladder outflow obstruction

11.3 The Female Patient

11.3.1 Introduction

Although female patients make up a small percentage or those in AUR, they are not as uncommon as one might think. Many of the conditions causing AUR or CUR in women are the same as in men, and these shall therefore not be covered again. However, due to obvious anatomical differences, the causes of AUR can be very different.

Largely speaking, the management is the same as in men in the acute phase. If the bladder is failing to drain, then drainage needs to be re-established. In some cases, as with men, this is achieved by the passage of a urethral catheter, and in others suprapubic catheterization is required. Also, long-term management is often the same, although the teaching of CISC involves explaining to many women the location of the urethral meatus, since it is not as obviously sited as it is in male patients.

A few women may have disturbed renal function and chronic outflow tract obstruction, but this is extremely rare and much more commonly related to another cause of renal impairment. The assessment of the female patient should be no different from assessment in the male, with thorough history taking and examination being the cornerstone of diagnosis.

11.3.2 Urinary Tract Infection

UTI is extremely common in women, although it is rarely complicated and usually managed in primary care. It is, however, the one of the most common causes of voiding dysfunction in female patients. It frequently causes symptoms of AUR, but the patient may be able to void small volumes but associated with significant discomfort. The cause of the retention is most likely the patient preventing herself from voiding to prevent these symptoms, and the patient rarely needs catheterization, with most settling with a course of antibiotics. Very occasionally, patients have high residual volumes and a complete inability to void, in which cases catheterization is needed, but again the majority of these settle quickly with antibiotic therapy and need no further treatment.

There is an argument for investigating women with recurrent UTIs to exclude other causes of BOO, such as pelvic prolapse, urethral stricture, meatal stenosis, urethral diverticulum, Skene's gland cysts or abscesses, bladder stones, or tumor of the urethra or bladder (Goldman and Simmern 2006). Clinical examination coupled with out-patient flexible urethrocystoscopy is usually sufficient to rule out most lesions, although if urethral diverticulum is suspected MRI is the gold standard (Patel and Chapple 2006).

11.3.3 Neurological Abnormalities

All the abnormalities mentioned above have similar presentation and management in women, in fact some conditions such as MS are far more prevalent in the female population.

Generally, women with voiding dysfunction in the absence of structural abnormalities of the lower urinary tract are very difficult to manage. A small group of female patients with obstructed voiding, and in some cases AUR, have been shown to have a specific electromyographic abnormality of the striated urethral sphincter, explaining their symptoms. When associated with features of polycystic ovary syndrome (PCOS), these patients are said to have Fowler's syndrome (Kavia et al. 2006; Fowler and Kirby 1984, 1985). They characteristically present at age 20–30, with episodes of AUR, and are often intolerant of urethral catheterization. Acutely, they can be managed with urethral catheterization, if tolerated, or CISC, although this is often tolerated even less well. Some patients will require suprapubic bladder drainage for this reason.

On initial presentation, any other neurological cause of AUR must be excluded, as well as any other structural abnormalities, before a diagnosis of Fowler's syndrome is made.

Long-term management is also a problem, with the only effective treatment that can restore normal voiding function (to date) being sacral nerve stimulation (Kavia et al. 2006).

11.3.4 Postsurgery for Stress Incontinence

The aims of stress incontinence surgery is to increase the outlet resistance of the urethra by either injection of bulking agents into the urethral musculature, by elevating the bladder base by colposuspension or by inserting tapes or slings to support the urethra under circumstances of raised abdominal pressures, thereby preventing leakage. Unfortunately, in some cases, this is too effective and many women undergoing surgery for stress incontinence develop BOO, which their bladder is unable to cope with in the acute setting, consequent to their surgery, and develop AUR.

The majority of these cases are diagnosed at the point of removing the urethral catheter for a trial of voiding after their surgery, but a degree of BOO that is not clinically evident may have potential to progress insidiously, culminating in AUR.

If the patient is unable to void after surgery, a urethral catheter is typically replaced for a further 2-week period to allow any edema and inflammation around a sling or tape to subside, which is sometimes sufficient to restore normal voiding. However, some patients are still unable to void after this and will go into AUR. For this reason, it is part of good practice to ensure any patient undergoing surgery for stress urinary incontinence is counseled on the possible need for CISC preoperatively, and has the technique demonstrated so that she is able to perform it should the need arise. Consequently, most patients presenting in AUR after this sort of surgery should be able to perform CISC.

Occasionally, tapes and slings can cause problems related to fibrosis and scarring around the tape or sling. This can in turn cause BOO and ultimately AUR, but the management should initially be the same. In the long-term, the patient may need her sling or tape incised to relieve obstructed voiding.

11.3.5 Other Causes of Failure of Lower Urinary Tract Drainage

Most other causes of failure of lower tract drainage in women are mentioned above (Sect. 11.3.2) as causes of BOO progressing to AUR. In addition, traumatic urethral disruption can occur in female patients, although less commonly than in males. The management is the same, with diagnosis being the key as well as managing a potentially multiply injured patient (American College of Surgeons 1997).

Luminal lesions such as urethral caruncles, which can be seen protruding from the external urethral meatus as a fleshy mass, can thrombose and cause obstruction, and these can usually be managed by transurethral resection prior to catheterization. Urethral diverticula, if they become infected, can lead to AUR, but this is an uncommon mode of presentation.

Other lesions of the urethra and bladder base, as mentioned above, can usually be diagnosed from history and examination in correlation with urethrocystoscopy, and if they are causing obstruction or AUR, can then be managed appropriately.

References

Abrams P (1997) Urodynamics. Springer, Berlin New York Heidelberg

Abrams P, Cardozo L, Fall M et al (2002) The standardisation of terminology of lower urinary tract function: report from the Standardisation Sub-committee of the International Continence Society. Neurourol Urodyn 21:167

American College of Surgeons. Committee on T (1997) Advanced trauma life support program for doctors: ATLS. American College of Surgeons, Chicago

Anderson JB, Grant JB (1991) Postoperative retention of urine: a prospective urodynamic study. BMJ 302:894

Anderson JB, Roehrborn CG, Schalken JA et al (2001) The progression of benign prostatic hyperplasia: examining the evidence and determining the risk. Eur Urol 39:390

Andersson KE, Chapple CR, Hofner K (2002) Future drugs for the treatment of benign prostatic hyperplasia. World J Urol 19:436

Andriole G, Bruchovsky N, Chung LW et al (2004) Dihydrotestosterone and the prostate: the scientific rationale for 5-alpha-reductase inhibitors in the treatment of benign prostatic hyperplasia. J Urol 172:1399

Anjum I, Ahmed M, Azzopardi A et al (1998) Prostatic infarction/infection in acute urinary retention secondary to benign prostatic hyperplasia. J Urol 160:792

Anson KM, Barnes DG, Briggs TP et al (1993) Temporary prostatic stenting and androgen suppression: a new minimally invasive approach to malignant prostatic retention. J R Soc Med 86:634

Caine M, Raz S, Zeigler M (1975) Adrenergic and cholinergic receptors in the human prostate, prostatic capsule and bladder neck. Br J Urol 47:193

Chapple CR (2001) Alpha adrenoceptor antagonists in the year 2000: is there anything new? Curr Opin Urol 11:9

Chapple CR (2004) Pharmacological therapy of benign prostatic hyperplasia/lower urinary tract symptoms: an overview for the practising clinician. BJU Int 94:738

Chapple CR, MacDiarmid SA (2000) Urodynamics made easy. Churchill Livingstone, Edinburgh

Chapple CR, Smith D (1994) The pathophysiological changes in the bladder obstructed by benign prostatic hyperplasia. Br J Urol 73:117

Choong S, Emberton M (2000) Acute urinary retention. BJU Int 85:186

Chute CG, Stephenson WP, Guess HA et al (1991) Benign prostatic hyperplasia: a population-based study. Eur Urol 20 [Suppl 1]:11

Djavan B, Chapple C, Milani S et al (2004) State of the art on the efficacy and tolerability of alpha1-adrenoceptor antagonists in patients with lower urinary tract symptoms suggestive of benign prostatic hyperplasia. Urology 64:1081

Dolin SJ, Cashman JN (2005) Tolerability of acute postoperative pain management: nausea, vomiting, sedation, pruritus, and urinary retention. Evidence from published data. Br J Anaesth 95:584

Elhilali M, Emberton M, Matzkin H et al (2006) Long-term efficacy and safety of alfuzosin 10 mg once daily: a 2-year experience in 'real-life' practice. BJU Int 97:513

Emberton M, Anson K (1999) Acute urinary retention in men: an age old problem. BMJ 318:921

Fitzpatrick JM (2006) The natural history of benign prostatic hyperplasia. BJU Int 97:3

Fitzpatrick JM, Kirby RS (2006) Management of acute urinary retention. BJU Int 97:16

Fong YK, Milani S, Djavan B (2005) Natural history and clinical predictors of clinical progression in benign prostatic hyperplasia. Curr Opin Urol 15:35

Fowler CJ, Kirby RS (1985) Abnormal electromyographic activity (decelerating burst and complex repetitive discharges) in the striated muscle of the urethral sphincter in 5 women with persisting urinary retention. Br J Urol 57:67

Fowler CJ, Kirby RS, Harrison MJ et al (1984) Individual motor unit analysis in the diagnosis of disorders of urethral sphincter innervation. J Neurol Neurosurg Psychiatry 47:637

Fowler CJ, Kirby RS, Harrison MJ (1985) Decelerating burst and complex repetitive discharges in the striated muscle of the urethral sphincter, associated with urinary retention in women. J Neurol Neurosurg Psychiatry 48:1004

Girman CJ, Jacobsen SJ, Rhodes T et al (1999) Association of health-related quality of life and benign prostatic enlargement. Eur Urol 35:277

Gnanapragasam VJ, Kumar V, Langton D et al (2006) Outcome of transurethral prostatectomy for the palliative management of lower urinary tract symptoms in men with prostate cancer. Int J Urol 13:711

Goldman HB, Zimmern PE (2006) The treatment of female bladder outlet obstruction. BJU Int 98 [Suppl 1]:17

Jacobsen SJ, Girman CJ, Lieber MM (2001) Natural history of benign prostatic hyperplasia. Urology 58:5

Johansson JE, Andren O, Andersson SO et al (2004) Natural history of early, localized prostate cancer. JAMA 291:2713

Kaplan SA, McConnell JD, Roehrborn CG et al (2006) Combination therapy with doxazosin and finasteride for benign prostatic hyperplasia in patients with lower urinary tract symptoms and a baseline total prostate volume of 25 ml or greater. J Urol 175:217

Kavia RB, Datta SN, Dasgupta R et al (2006) Urinary retention in women: its causes and management. BJU Int 97:281

Kessler B, Albertsen P (2003) The natural history of prostate cancer. Urol Clin North Am 30:219

Kim JY, Lee SJ, Koo BN et al (2006) The effect of epidural sufentanil in ropivacaine on urinary retention in patients undergoing gastrectomy. Br J Anaesth 97:414

Kirby RS (2000) The natural history of benign prostatic hyperplasia: what have we learned in the last decade? Urology 56:3

Kirby RS, McConnell JD (2005) Fast facts: benign prostatic hyperplasia. Health Press, Oxford

Kurasawa G, Kotani K, Kurasawa M et al (2005) Causes of chronic retention of urine in the primary care setting. Intern Med 44:761

Leveckis J, Boucher NR, Parys BT et al (1995) Bladder and erectile dysfunction before and after rectal surgery for cancer. Br J Urol 76:752

Masumori N, Tsukamoto T, Rhodes T et al (2003) Natural history of lower urinary tract symptoms in men–result of a longitudinal community-based study in Japan. Urology 61:956

McAninch JW, Carroll PR, Jordan GH (1996) Traumatic and reconstructive urology. WB Saunders, Philadelphia

McConnell JD, Roehrborn CG, Bautista OM et al (2003) The long-term effect of doxazosin, finasteride, and combination therapy on the clinical progression of benign prostatic hyperplasia. N Engl J Med 349:2387

McNeill SA, Daruwala PD, Mitchell ID et al (1999) Sustained-release alfuzosin and trial without catheter after acute urinary retention: a prospective, placebo-controlled. BJU Int 84:622

Morey AF, Hernandez J, McAninch JW (1999) Reconstructive surgery for trauma of the lower urinary tract. Urol Clin North Am 26:49

Parikh AM, Milroy EJ (1995) Precautions and complications in the use of the UroLume wall stent. Eur Urol 27:1

Patel AK, Chapple CR (2006) Female urethral diverticula. Curr Opin Urol 16:248

Roehrborn CG (2006a) Alfuzosin 10 mg once daily prevents overall clinical progression of benign prostatic hyperplasia but not acute urinary retention: results of a 2-year placebo-controlled study. BJU Int 97:734

Roehrborn CG (2006b) Definition of at-risk patients: baseline variables. BJU Int 97 [Suppl 2]:7

Roehrborn CG, McConnell JD, Saltzman B et al (2002) Storage (irritative) and voiding (obstructive) symptoms as predictors of benign prostatic hyperplasia progression and related outcomes. Eur Urol 42:1

Sandhu DP, Mayor PE, Sambrook PA et al (1992) Outcome and prognostic factors in patients with advanced prostate cancer and obstructive uropathy. Br J Urol 70:412

Singh M, Blandy JP (1976) The pathology of urethral stricture. J Urol 115:673

Thomas K, Chow K, Kirby RS (2004) Acute urinary retention: a review of the aetiology and management. Prostate Cancer Prostatic Dis 7:32

Tuncel A, Uzun B, Eruyar T et al (2005) Do prostatic infarction, prostatic inflammation and prostate morphology play a role in acute urinary retention? Eur Urol 48:277

Weiss RM, George NJR, O'Reilly PH (2001) Comprehensive urology. Mosby, London

Wilson TS, Lemack GE, Dmochowski RR (2002) UroLume stents: lessons learned. J Urol 167:2477

12 Scrotal Emergencies

V. Master

12.1 Introduction

Scrotal emergencies frequently result in a call to the urologist. It is important to remember that emergencies that involve the scrotum may be confined to scrotal structures or referred from other sources. There are a number of differential diagnoses to consider (Table 12.1), as the scrotum itself contains numerous structures: the testicles, epididymis, spermatic cord, and the scrotal tissue itself, comprised of several muscular and fascial layers. Without a thorough differential diagnosis of intrinsic and extrinsic causes of scrotal pain, a diagnosis may be missed. Careful history tak-

Table 1. Differential diagnosis of scrotal pathology

Painless scrotal masses
Inguinal hernia (nonstrangulated, nonincacerated)
Testicular tumors (these may also be painful)
Hydrocele
Spermatocele
Varicocele
Paratesticular tumors/masses
Scrotal edema
Epididymal caput distension from bilateral congenital absence of the vas
Painful scrotal masses
Inguinal hernia (incarcated or strangulated)
Testicular tumors
Testicular torsion
Appendicial torsion (of testicular appendages)
Epididymitis
Epididymo-orchitis
Trauma
Dermatological lesions
Inflammatory vasculitis
Hematocele
Miscellaneous
Empty scrotum (cryptorchidism)

Table 2. Findings on evaluation for common scrotal emergencies

Pathology	Pain	Illumination	Urinalysis	Ultrasound	Doppler
Epididymitis	Yes	No	Abnormal	Heterogenous testis echotexture	Increased flow
Inguinal hernia	Maybe	Maybe	Normal	Hernia sac	Normal
Hydrocele	No	Yes	Normal	Fluid without echos	Normal
Spermatocele	No	Maybe	Normal	Fluid usually with echos	Normal
Testicular rupture	Yes	No	Normal	Heterogeneous testicle Possible incomplete tunica	Usually abnormal
Testicular tumor	Maybe	No	Normal	Heterogeneous echotexture	Normal
Testicular torsion	No	No	Yes	Normal	Decreased Flow

ing, directed physical exam, and urinalysis with the occasional use of Doppler ultrasound can discriminate between processes quite effectively (Table 12.2). In the hierarchy of concern when dealing with scrotal emergencies, the testicle assumes the position of importance, as loss of a testicle from torsion or failure to diagnose a testicular tumor carry disastrous consequences. Scrotal examination therefore absolutely must document the presence and characteristics of the testicles.

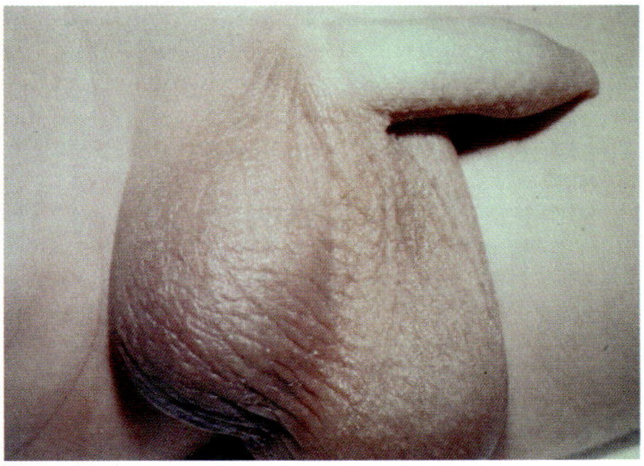

12.1. Physical examination of extravaginal torsion. Note the lie of the affected testicle

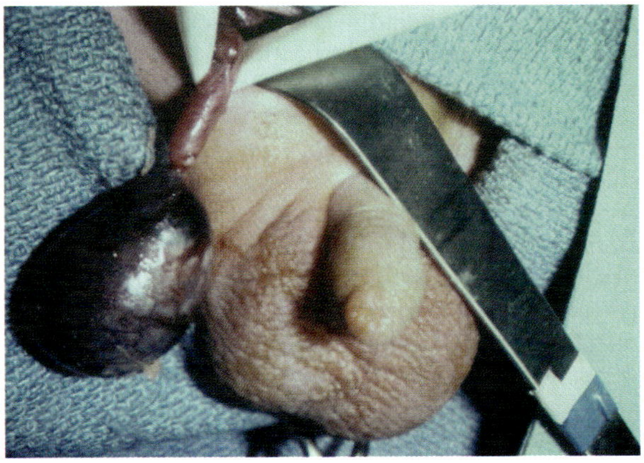

12.2. Intraoperative photograph of extravaginal testicular torsion

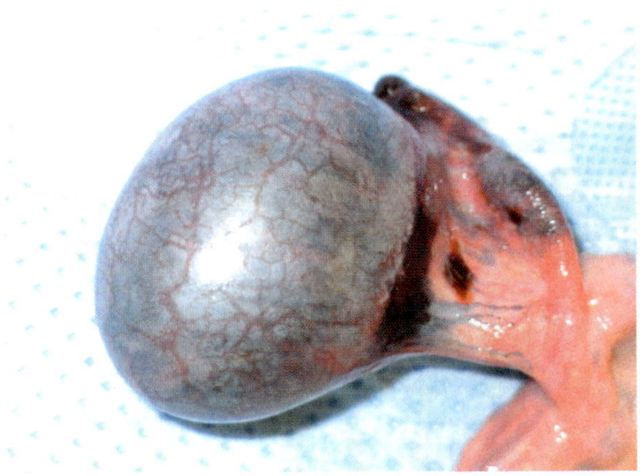

12.3. Intraoperative photograph of intravaginal torsion

12.2 Testis

12.2.1 Torsion

Torsion is defined by Webster's dictionary as a noun which means "the action of being twisted, or the state of being twisted, especially one end of an object relative to another." Torsion of the testicle is the disease process whereby there is cessation of blood flow to the testicle because of an occlusion of arterial blood supply due to twisting of the artery (and associated structures), which can lead to testicular loss unless there is timely intervention. Anatomically defined, torsion can either be intravaginal or extravaginal. The entity of intermittent or minimal torsion, is created by a short-lived torsion process in which venous obstruction occurs first. This causes tissue congestion and edema, which then impairs arterial inflow into the testicle, causing acute pain.

12.2.2 Extravaginal

This type of torsion can occur in utero (incidence unknown) and in neonates. In this type of torsion, there is lack of fixation of the gubernaculum and testicular tunica to the scrotal wall, which allows for the entire testis, spermatic cord, and tunica vaginalis to twist, often to the level of the internal inguinal ring (Figs. 12.1, 12.2). A risk factor for extravaginal torsion is cryptorchidism. Generally, salvage rates are low for this variant of torsion.

12.2.3 Intravaginal

In this type of torsion, the spermatic cord twists inside the tunica vaginalis. This is thought to occur because of an abnormal attachment of the spermatic cord to the testis, which allows the testis to turn easily within the scrotum. This anatomic relationship, in which the testicle has a transverse lie, is termed the bell-clapper deformity (Fig. 12.3). This horizontal lie is a risk factor for torsion. Generally, intravaginal torsion occurs in children as well as adults, but usually in adolescents.

12.2.4 Presentation

The most common age for the development of torsion is early puberty, while the newborn period is the second most common. The vascular compromise results in the rapid onset of swelling because of venous outflow obstruction in the face of continued arterial inflow. The testicle can be completely salvaged with up to 6 h of torsion, but is unlikely to be salvaged beyond 12 h, so expedient diagnosis and surgical detorsion should be pursued.

Patients generally present with acute testicular pain, often being awoken from sleep with pain. If the patient has mild pain, which has increased over a few days, a torsion of a testicular appendage should be suspected, rather than testicular torsion. If the patient complains of intermittent acute pain, which completely resolves, a diagnosis of intermittent testicular torsion should be suspected (Eaton et al. 2005). In classic testicular torsion, there tends to be nausea and vomiting, along with referred abdominal pain. On inspection, the typical torsion patient is lying quite still on the exam table. A patient who is ambulating easily without pain is unlikely to have torsion. Close inspection of the scrotum may show asymmetric positioning of the testicles with the torsed testicle occupying a high position in the scrotum, which is termed a high-riding testicle. A cremasteric reflex should be elicited next, before palpation, as absence of a cremasteric reflex is associated with torsion. This sign is not fully specific, as a cremasteric reflex can sometimes be elicited with torsion. Next, palpation should occur. When palpating the scrotum, the normal testicle must be palpated first. It should be in a vertical position. Next the spermatic cord of the affected testis is palpated. If painful and swollen, the suspicion of torsion is raised. Finally, the affected testis is palpated. This is often difficult for the patient. Sometimes the epididymis faces anteriorly. Pain at the lower pole of the testis is more likely to signify torsion than pain at the upper pole of the testis, which is where many of the testicular appendages are located. If a hydrocele is present, preventing testicular palpation, and the diagnosis is mostly equivocal, an imaging modality can be obtained to examine the testicle and its flow characteristics, if it can be obtained in a timely manner. Scrotal ultrasound with color Doppler is widely used (Fig. 12.4), although some institutions have expertise in rapid nuclear medicine imaging with technicium-99m radionuclide scanning looking for blood flow to the testicle, which is equally sensitive (Nussbaum Blask et al. 2002). Occasionally, MRI has been used to evaluate for torsion. However, if the imaging modality cannot be obtained in a timely manner, and the index of suspicion is high, then intraoperative exploration is mandatory.

12.2.5 Torsion Treatment

Surgical treatment is identical for both intravaginal and extravaginal torsion and consists of scrotal exploration. If the testicle is necrotic it should be removed. If the testis appears nonviable initially, it should be placed in a warm gauze pad. Appropriate color and turgor may return, in which case orchidopexy should be performed; otherwise orchiectomy is recommended. For the viable testicle, orchidopexy with creation of a three-point nonabsorbable suture fixation of the testicle should be performed. Some authors also advocate placement of the testicle in to a subdartos pouch to fix the testicle by tissue as well as by suture.

The single most important point about testicular torsion is quite simply keeping torsion firmly near the top of the differential diagnosis when evaluating a scrotal emergency. Even if the patient has symptoms of epi-

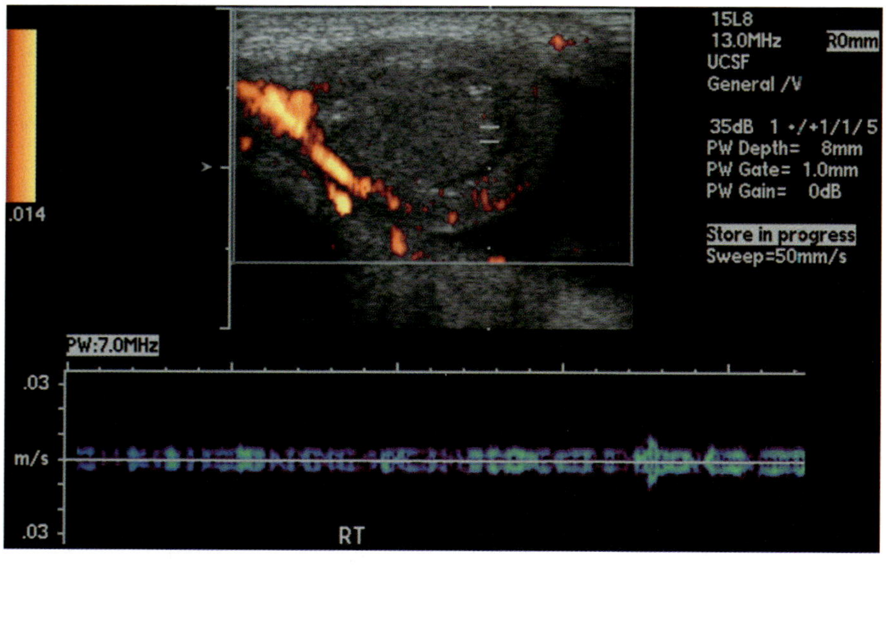

12.4. Color Doppler ultrasound image of testicular torsion. Note the absence of flow to the testicle didymitis, torsion may still occur. A patient may claim testicular trauma, but torsion may actually be the reason that patient is in the emergency room. Finally, paradoxically, even if a patient had a previous orchidopexy, they may (rarely) develop torsion again (Mor et al. 2006)!

If a testicular torsion is not repaired and testicular loss occurs, the dead testicle should be removed because of the possibility of the development of significant orchalgia, as well as the theoretical risk of the production of antisperm antibodies as the blood–testis barrier breaks down (Anderson and Williamson 1988). However, some authorities advocate leaving the testicle in place so as to maintain Leydig cell function (testosterone production). Contralateral orchidopexy is often performed, but this approach continues to generate controversy. Manual detorsion has been reported by one group.

12.2.6 Torsion of Testicular Appendages

The most common testicular appendage susceptible to torsion is the appendix testis, which is a remnant of the Mullerian duct. Presentation is usually the same as that for testicular torsion. Patients are most often adolescents and present with the sudden onset of orchalgia. Occasionally, early in the course of the process, before edema has developed, it is possible to palpate the twisted appendage as a small (3- to 5-mm) tender area or mass close to the upper pole of the testis. Also, rarely, a blue dot sign may be seen through the skin of the scrotum, corresponding to a torsed, ischemic testicular appendage. As time passes, edema develops, thus making physical examination impossible, which usually requires an ultrasound examination to evaluate whether testicular torsion is present.

Management, if the diagnosis is certain, consists of supportive care, with the liberal use of analgesic, in the form of anti-inflammatory medications. If diagnosis is uncertain, meaning that testicular torsion is suspected, then exploration is mandatory (Fig. 12.5).

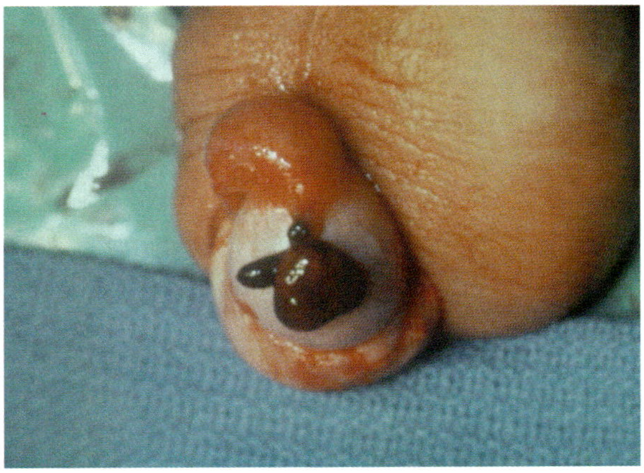

12.5. Torsion of the appendix of testis

12.2.7 Tumors

Any mass originating from the testicle must be presumed to be testicular cancer until otherwise proven, because of the explosive growth and metastatic potential of germ cell testicular cancers. While rare, testis cancers are the most common solid tumor of young adult males. Germ cell tumors make up approximately 95% of all testis tumors and are seminoma, yolk sac, choriocarcinoma, embryonal, and teratoma. Stromal testis tumors are rare and are found almost exclusively in prepubertal individuals. These mostly exhibit benign behavior but undifferentiated stromal tumors may exhibit metastatic behavior. Men with a testis mass in their 50s are more likely to have a testicular lymphoma. Benign tumors of the testis are rare, less than 1%. These include an intratesticular cyst, tunica cyst, dermoid cyst, and epidermoid cyst (different from epidermoid tumor of the epididymis, which is also benign.

Testis cancers usually present as an incidental finding of a painless lump, nodule, swelling, or abnormality in the scrotum in men in their 20s to 40s. A feeling of dull aching or heaviness may also be present. A hydrocele may co-exist on physical exam, which may make testicular palpation difficult. Exceedingly rapidly growing testis cancers, which are hemorrhaging, may cause the patient to present with a painful scrotal mass (see Table 12.1). Palpation will usually reveal a hard testis mass and very often a significant size discrepancy. Metastatic adenopathy is rarely palpable, but huge retroperitoneal adenopathy may cause nausea, vomiting, or early satiety. Rarely, supraclavicular lymphadenopathy will be palpable with massive supradiaphragmatic disease. Scrotal ultrasound will show a heterogeneous testis mass (Fig. 12.6).

Treatment is standard and should invariably be an inguinal radical orchiectomy (Fig. 12.7). Tumor markers consisting of alpha fetoprotein (AFP), beta human chorionic gonadotropin (B-HCG), and lactate dehydrogenase (LDH) should be sent prior to orchiectomy. Chest x-ray and contrast CT scan of the abdomen and pelvis should be obtained. Patients should be risk-stratified and counseled for the need for repeating tumor markers after orchiectomy, as well as the fact that testis cancer represents the most curable solid organ malignancy presently.

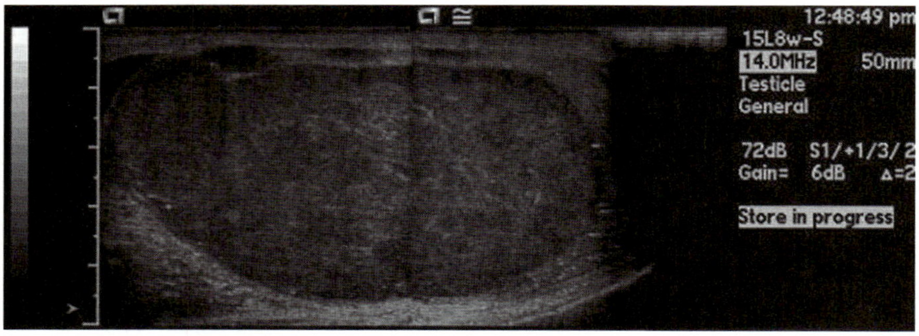

12.6. Ultrasound showing heterogenous echotexture of a testis cancer

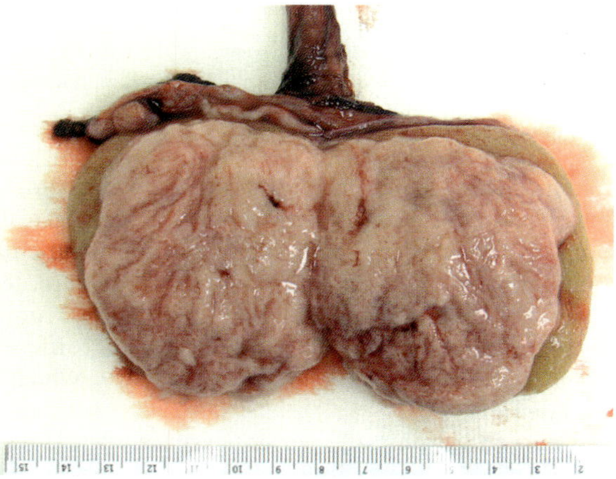

12.7. Intraoperative picture of bivalved specimen from a radical orchiectomy. Note the thin rim of normal tissue seen on the ultrasound of the same patient in Fig. 12.6

12.3 Paratesticular Emergencies

12.3.1 Epididymitis

Epididymitis is an inflammatory reaction of the epididymis to one of several infectious agents or to local trauma. Acute epididymitis may present at any age, with a sudden onset of pain and swelling of the epididymis in the scrotum. Epididymitis can present in a sexually transmitted form or one associated with urinary tract infections and prostatitis. Thus, eliciting a specific history of sexual exposure or of prior genitourinary tract disease is crucial for diagnosis and appropriate treatment. Much less frequently, epididymitis may also be caused by a reflux of sterile urine into the epididymis, causing a local sterile chemical inflammation.

The patient's age suggests the most likely etiology of epididymitis. Within each age group, the cause appears to be the same as the most common cause of genitourinary infection in that group. In heterosexual men younger than 35, urethritis caused by *Neisseria gonorrhoeae* or *Chlamydia trachomatis* is more common than bacteriuria. Thus, in this patient population, epididymitis is most commonly caused by these same organisms, with *C. trachomatis* causing about two-thirds of the cases of noncoliform, nongonococcal epididymitis in these patients. By contrast, in men older than 35, sexually transmitted urethritis is uncommon; thus, a nonsexually transmitted form of epididymitis is more likely, most commonly caused by Enterobacteriaceae or *Pseudomonas*. Epididymitis that develops in children, which is rare, is most commonly caused by the coliform organisms that cause bacteriuria. It is important, however, to rule out anatomic abnormalities in children with epididymitis. In infants, epididymitis is more likely to result from genitourinary abnormalities. In immunosuppressed males, a very small percentage may have epididymitis resulting from systemic disease such as tuberculosis, cryptococcus, or brucella.

While some men may have only a nonspecific finding of fever or other signs of infection, patients with acute epididymitis usually complain of sudden-onset, severely painful swelling of the scrotum. Pain may radiate along the spermatic cord and reach the abdomen, or possibly even the flank. The onset may be acute over 1 or 2 days, or sometimes more gradual; it is often accompanied by dysuria or irritative lower urinary tract symptoms. Erythema of the scrotum may develop, and the epididymis may double in size in as little as 3–4 h. Many patients also have urethral discharge. In acute epididymitis, inflammation and swelling usually begin in the tail of the epididymis and may spread to involve the rest of the epididymis and testicle. The spermatic cord is usually tender and swollen. Epididymitis is frequently accompanied by erythema, which is generally unilateral and primarily in the posterior aspect of the scrotum. If the patient is examined early in the course of the disease, the swelling may be localized to one portion of the epididymis. Later, the ipsilateral testis is often involved, producing epididymo-orchitis and making it difficult to distinguish the testicle from the epididymis within the inflammatory mass. Scrotal examination often reveals the presence of a hydrocele, caused by the secretion of inflammatory fluid between the layers of the tunica vaginalis testis. Urinalysis usually shows leukocytes and often bacteria. Usually, the microbial etiology of epididymitis can be determined by examining a Gram-stained urethral smear and Gram stain of a midstream urine specimen for Gram-negative bacteriuria. The presence of intracellular Gram-negative diplococci on the smear correlates with the presence of *N. gonorrhoeae*, whereas the presence of only white blood cells on the urethral smear indicates the presence of nongonococcal urethritis. *C. trachomatis* will be isolated in approximately two-thirds of these patients. In older men, the presence of coliform bacteria often leads to diagnosis. Treatment for patients with bacterial epididymitis depends on the age and history of the patient, and underlying co-morbidities. Infirm individuals with a fever and in severe cases, leukocytosis, should be admitted for intravenous antibiotics. In young, sexually active men, suspected sexually transmitted epididymitis should be treated with a single dose of ceftriaxone (250 mg i.m.) followed by tetracycline (500 mg p.o. q.i.d.) or doxycycline (100 mg p.o. b.i.d.) for 21 days. This regimen covers both *C. trachomatis* and *N. gonorrhoeae*. In older patients, empiric treatment with agents appropriate for both Gram-negative rods and Gram-positive cocci should be initiated, pending urine culture and sensitivity results. Usually, treatment with a fluoroquinolone (levofloxacin 500 mg/d p.o. or ciprofloxacin 500 mg p.o. bid for at least 3 weeks) and an anti-inflammatory medication should be started. Bed rest, scrotal elevation, analgesics, and local ice packs are exceedingly helpful. Surgery may be necessary to manage complications of acute epididymal infections such as a testicular abscess. Making the differential diagnosis between epididymitis and testicular torsion at the beginning of the patient encounter is imperative, particularly in men younger than 35. Delayed diagnosis of torsion can result in testicular infarction and loss of a testicle. Generally, Prehn's sign, which is elevation of the scrotum upward toward the abdomen, manifests as relief of testicular discomfort in the patient with epididymitis, and worsening discomfort in the patient with torsion. While Prehn's sign is useful, it is not always accurate. If the clinician is trying to differentiate between torsion and epididymitis ultrasonography of the scrotum, preferably with color flow Doppler imaging, should be performed to evaluate blood flow to the testicle, in which epididymitis has increased blood flow to the testicle (Fig. 12.8). Finally, tuberculous epididymitis must be considered. Although this condition is more likely to be confused with a malignancy than a cause of an acute scrotal mass, it can be an important cause of epididymitis in patients from areas where tuberculosis is endemic. Testicular malignancy must also be suspected, since as many as 10 % of patients with testicular cancer may present with epididymitis.

12.4 Spermatocele

Spermatocele is defined as a painless, sperm-containing mass in the caput of the epididymis. They generally occur in middle-aged men and are never seen in children. This lesion is generally not painful and is palpable above the testicle, which is usually palpable. They

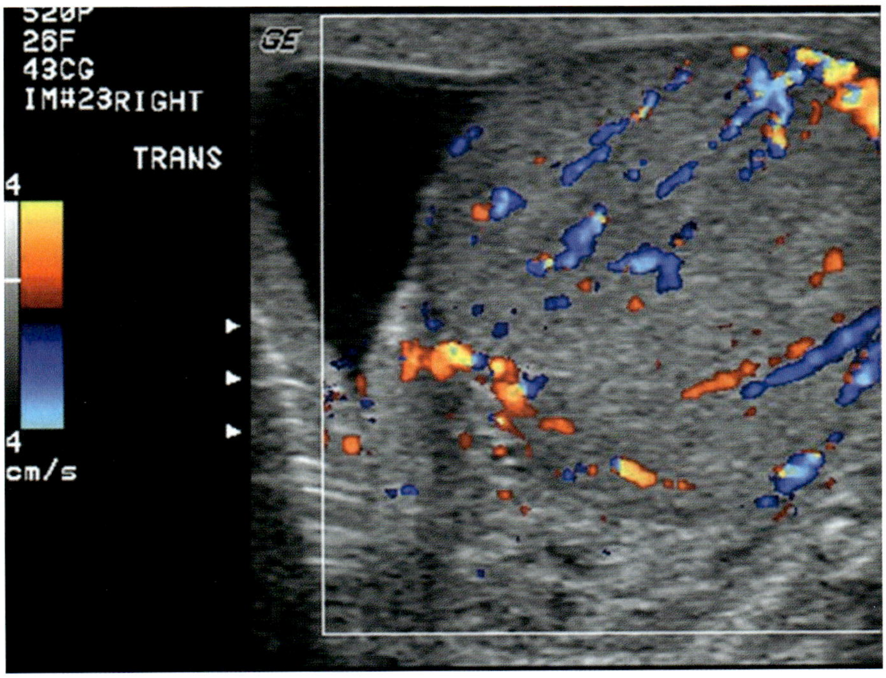

12.8. Ultrasound of epididymo-orchitis. Note the increased vascularity to the testicle

can reach a massive size and extend up to the external ring. A not uncommon presentation is to have the patient come to the office complaining of the feeling of having a third testicle. Spermatoceles can be thought of diverticula of the epididymal tubules. The can be uni- or multiloculated and contain a mixture of sperm and sloughed epithelium. Importantly, these do not obstruct sperm transport. Most spermatoceles are idiopathic but some have a history of trauma. There appears to be no relation to vasectomy.

On questioning, patients will report a painless scrotal mass that was discovered during self-examination. On exam, the mass does not change in size with position or Valsalva. Ultrasound is diagnostic if the physical exam is equivocal and should certainly be done if any testicular pathology is suspected.

Treatment of the spermatocele should be based upon symptoms as well as patient age. A risk factor for spermatocelectomy in patients who wish to father children is that there may be complete epididymal obstruction if the delicate epididymal tubule is damaged. However, if patients are significantly bothered by the spermatocele, then repair should be offered. A microsurgical approach has the best chance of avoiding epididymal damage. Additionally, small cysts can be seen with the microscope. Huge spermatoceles can sometimes obscure the vas deferens and the testicular artery. Both of these structures should be dissected and preserved by directing attention to the area cephalad to the lesion.

12.5 Varicocele

Varicocele is defined as a dilation of the pampiniform plexus of the veins within and surrounding the spermatic cord secondary to absent or incompetent venous values, which are congenital or acquired, respectively. Varicoceles may be visible, nonvisible but palpable (the classic sign is the so-called scrotal "bag of worms", referring to vermiform appearance of the dilated veins), or nonvisible and nonpalpable. Both adults and children present as a scrotal emergency with a varicocele. Varicoceles are more common on the left, which is thought to be due to increased venous pressure. The classic teaching is that an isolated right varicoceles should prompt a search for abdominal pathology such as renal tumors with vena caval thrombus, retroperitoneal fibrosis, renal vein thrombosis and retroperitoneal cancers. Multiple teleological arguments have been invoked, including of a longer drainage path of the left gonadal vein, a right angle entry into the left renal vein, erect posture of humans (four-legged animals do not get varicoceles), compression of the left renal vein by the superior mesenteric artery, and a lack of venous valves in the proximal testicular vein.

Table 3. Grades of varicoceles. Traditional grading is on the basis of physical examination, but many are now seen on ultrasound (grade 0)

Grade	Description
0	Not detected on physical exam, but on ultrasound with: Dilated pampiniform plexus veins to >2mm and/or Blood flow reversal during Valsalva maneuver seen on Doppler
1	Palpable on Valsalva
2	Palpable without need for Valsalva
3	visible on scrotal inspection alone

Varicoceles can be seen in 15% of adult males, depending on the definition of varicocele. Most times varicoceles present because of symptoms, but the bulk of men with varicoceles are asymptomatic. Interestingly, infertile males do have 40% incidence of varicoceles. If patients do have symptomatic varicoceles, symptoms are usually a pulling sensation or a dull ache that does not radiate. These symptoms are relieved by achieving a recumbent position. The pain is never present on awakening from sleep, but increases over the day, especially with exertion. In a pediatric population, there may be ipsilateral testicular growth retardation from the varicocele.

Examination for a varicocele should be conducted in a warm room with the patient in a standing position for 5–10 min before the examination starts, so that the pampiniform plexus veins fill and demonstrate the varicocele. A varicocele is felt as a mass separate from the testicle. There are usually three grades of varicocele on examination, although with the adjunctive use of ultrasound, there are essentially four grades of varicoceles (see Table 12.3). Varicoceles should get larger with Valsalva maneuvers.

Treatment should be offered for multiple indications. Primarily, treatment is given for patients with complaints of signs or symptoms of the varicocele. Adolescents are offered varicocele repair if there is testicular growth retardation secondary to the varicocele. Finally, patients with male factor infertility due to abnormal semen analysis with a varicocele are offered repair (Cayan et al. 2002). Surgical approaches to repair are either suprainguinal (Palomo repair), inguinal, or subinguinal. Magnification is very helpful to avoid inadvertent ligation of the testicular artery and lymphatics. Ligation of lymphatics is likely to cause a hydrocele and ligation of the testicular artery is likely to result in some degree of testicular atrophy. Microsurgical approaches are believed to decrease morbidity and recurrences to approximately 1% (Grober et al. 2004). Interventional radiology approaches have also been used, but are reported to have a higher rate of recurrence, approximately 20% (Feneley et al. 1997).

12.6 Trauma

Testicular, spermatic cord and scrotal wall trauma is covered in Chap. 15.7, “Genital Trauma.”

12.7 Paratesticular Masses

12.7.1 Hernia

An inguinal hernia may present as a scrotal mass secondary to loops of bowel within the scrotum. Exam will reveal peristalsis of the scrotum and auscultation will reveal bowel sounds. Direct inguinal hernias result from an acquired weakness in the transversalis fascia at Hesselbach’s triangle, bounded by the inguinal ligament, the exterior border of the rectus muscle, and the inferior epigastric vessels, and the peritoneum rarely outpouches beyond the area of the external ring; thus scrotal involvement is rare. Indirect inguinal hernias may occur secondary to a patent processus vaginalis, which is mostly found in a pediatric population. Indirect hernias in the adult are mostly protrusions of a new peritoneal process following the same path as the spermatic cord into the scrotum.

Management is dictated by the characteristic of the hernia. Strangulated hernias will require urgent surgical exploration. Incarcerated hernias will require open surgical management or closed reduction under anesthesia. The accuracy of ultrasound in making this diagnosis is operator-dependent, and thus, operative repair should not be delayed if incarceration or strangulation of an inguinal hernia is suspected. Reducible hernias can be repaired on an elective basis.

12.7.2 Hydrocele

A hydrocele is a collection of fluid within the tunica vaginalis, which surrounds the testicle. During homeostasis, there is a small amount of fluid with the tunica vaginalis, the so-called physiologic hydrocele. When there is a profound increase in this amount of fluid, it is termed a clinical hydrocele. On presentation, it is most often a painless swelling of the scrotum which transilluminates and may prevent testicular palpation.

12.7.3 Acquired

Acquired, or adult, hydroceles are usually idiopathic, but may also be present as a consequence of a primary process such as a tumor, infection, or systemic disease. The visceral and parietal layers of the tunica vaginalis appear to have an imbalance between fluid production and fluid reabsorption.

Treatment is generally indicated for symptomatic relief. Needle aspiration is very effective for temporary relief, but the hydrocele will often recur. Aspiration, accompanied by a sclerosing solution, may sometimes be effective. There are many sclerosing agents. Historically, tetracycline mixed with local anesthetic such as lidocaine was used, but modern authors report using sodium tetradecylsulfate (STDS), phenol, Betadine, and fibrin glue. More definitive treatment is surgical, either via a Lord or Jabouley-type repair, which are a plication or excision of the redundant tunica vaginalis, respectively.

12.7.4 Infant

Infant hydroceles are usually the result of peritoneal fluid that accumulates in the scrotum. This can be either via a patent processus vaginalis (communicating hydrocele), or by a nonpatent processus that has trapped a significant amount of peritoneal fluid, causing a scrotal bulge. The most important differential between the two is that the size of the scrotal mass changes with recumbency, or with crying, in the case of communicating hydroceles. Most communicating hydroceles tend to close within the 1st year of life, so surgical repair should be delayed to 1 year of life. An inguinal approach to surgical ligation should be used. In the case of premature infants, however, surgical repair should be performed before discharge from the hospital because of the risk of bowel herniation (Benjamin 2002).

12.8 Scrotal Wall Problems

12.8.1 Fournier’s Gangrene

Necrotizing ascending infection of the scrotal wall, or Fournier’s gangrene, is a urologic emergency requiring immediate diagnosis and expedient treatment, as delayed diagnosis and treatment can result in a 50 % mortality in high-risk patients such as older diabetic patients. It involves the skin, subcutaneous fat, and superficial fascia of the external genitalia and perineum. This disease process is characterized by a polymicrobial fasciitis involving the perineum and external genitalia. This infective process was first reported by Baurienne in 1764, and later by Fournier in 1883, whose name is eponymous with the disease. Although initially thought to be a fulminant disease restricted to young men, it has now been found to involve all ages and genders, and in some cases, to follow an indolent course.

The origin is most often from a genitourinary source, such as a periurethral abscess, or from a colorectal source, such as a perirectal abscess. Additionally, surgery or local trauma to the genitalia are additional risk factors. In presentation of the patient in the classic form, there is an acute onset of spreading cellulitis adjacent to the site of injury and very often frank necrosis (Fig. 12.9). Genital and scrotal pain out of proportion to the exam, swelling, and erythema are the most common symptoms. Interval examination usually shows rapid progression of the disease. Radiographic studies may be valuable when the physical examination is in doubt. While CT scans may be most sensitive at determining the presence of subcutaneous gas, bedside ultrasound may be more rapid, depending on the institutional capabilities (Morrison et al. 2005). Occasionally, subcutaneous and deep tissue gas can be observed on a KUB by an observant radiographer. The identification of subcutaneous gas should prompt immediate surgery. Incidentally, if a urethral source is suspected, retrograde urethrography will be helpful in determining whether the patient needs a suprapubic tube to drain the bladder.

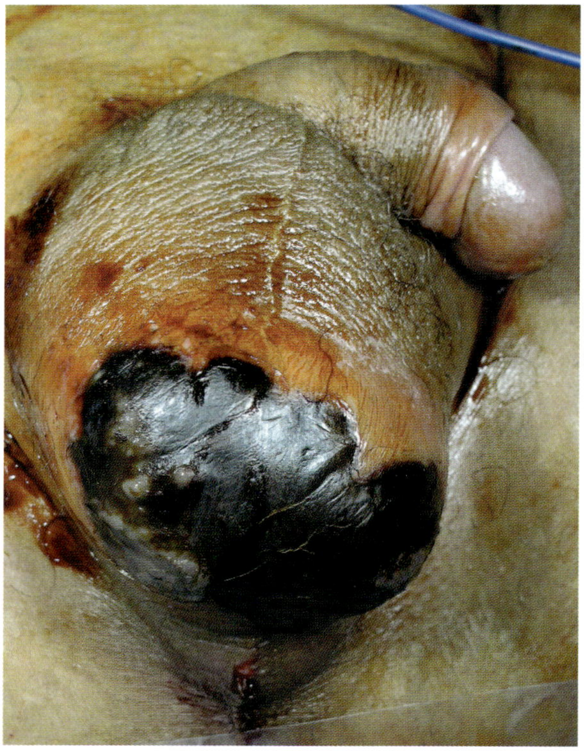

12.9. Fournier's Gangrene. This patient, a diabetic male aged 65, sustained minor trauma to his scrotum while zipping his trousers 21 h prior to presentation. Note the necrotic, large amount of scrotum that is affected. A large amount of purulent material was also found in the perineum, which can be seen to be swollen in the picture

Management is emergent (Baskin et al. 1990). Rapid recognition, speedy resuscitation with fluids and oxygen, administration of broad-spectrum antibiotics, and wide debridement of all necrotic tissue are the cornerstones of treatment, along with the recognized need for a second trip to the operating room for a second look within 24 h. Many times additional surgery is required beyond the second surgery. Support in an intensive care unit may be required, including a large amount of fluid resuscitation, ventilatory support, and vasopressor support. Antibiotic coverage should include metronidazole or clindamycin for anaerobes, a third-generation cephalosporin or aminoglycoside for Gram-negative infections and penicillin for Gram-positive bacteria. Debridement should extend to fresh, vital tissue at every surgical margin. The glans, corpus spongiosum, corpora cavernosa and testes are almost always uninfected and preserved because of their deep blood supply. However, if the tunica vaginalis is violated during the course of debridement, the testis may become superinfected and require orchiectomy at a later time. Primary removal of the testicle should be performed at the time of surgical debridement if the etiology of the necrotizing infection is epididymo-orchitis. Cystoscopy and rigid sigmoidoscopy should be performed to find the primary source of infection. Fecal diversion via end colostomy is rarely required unless there is massive contamination of the wound by feces or simultaneous colorectal and urinary tract involvement. Testicles can be places in subcutaneous thigh pouches.

After the patient is stabilized in the operating room, debrided wounds are managed with moist gauze dressings and repeat debridement. Secondary coverage takes place via split thickness skin grafting only after the primary infective process has been eradicated.

12.8.2 Edema of Scrotal Wall

Scrotal wall edema is a very frequent consultation request to the inpatient urology service. Many patients tend to have congestive heart failure, but the majority of cases are idiopathic in origin (Brandes et al. 1994). It is important for the physician to examine the scrotum and perineum and ascertain that there are no areas of skin breakdown, or referred swelling from a perineal abscess. Equally importantly, patient and careful squeezing of the edematous fluid out of the scrotum and away from the testes will allow for careful testicular palpation, so that epididymo-orchitis or other testicular abnormalities can be ruled out.

Management of scrotal edema is purely supportive. The scrotum should be elevated with towels and the patient kept in a supine position, if possible.

12.8.3 Cancer of Scrotum

Cancer of the scrotum is not an acute problem in terms of the time of the disease's course of development. However, it is a true emergency because of the virulent nature of scrotal wall cancers. The largest and most immediate factor is to properly stage the malignancy after the tissue diagnosis is obtained.

12.9 Miscellaneous

12.9.1 Henoch-Schönlein Purpura

Henoch-Schönlein purpura (HSP) is a disease that manifests symptoms of purple spots on the skin, joint pain, gastrointestinal symptoms, and glomerulonephritis. HSP is a type of hypersensitivity vasculitis and inflammatory response within the blood vessel. It is caused by an abnormal response of the immune system. The exact cause for this disorder is unknown. The syndrome is usually seen in children, but people of any age may be affected. It is more common in boys than in girls. Many people with HSP had an upper respiratory illness in the previous weeks. Purpuric lesions are usually over the buttocks, lower legs, and elbows. Besides purpuric lesions, nephritis, angioedema, joint pains, abdominal pain, nausea, vomiting, diarrhea, and hematochezia can be seen. The scrotum can also be affected in 13%–35% of cases (Ioannides and Turnock 2001). While the testis and/or scrotum can rarely be involved, usually the scrotum is diffusely tender with erythema distributed all over the scrotum. Involvement of the scrotum by HSP is self-limiting and therefore treatment is primarily expectant. The exquisite pain experienced by boys with this syndrome can mislead the surgical team to suspect torsion; in HSP cases, this can be ruled out with a Doppler ultrasound (Ioannides and Turnock 2001).

12.9.2 Other

Finally, there can be referred pain to the scrotum from a variety of etiologies (McGee 1993). The most common would be pain from the impaction, or passage, of a distal ureteral stone. More rarely, pain from appendicitis when the appendix is in a retrocecal position can cause scrotal pain (Friedman and Sheynkin 1995). The rarest are patients with a ruptured abdominal aortic aneurysm can present with scrotal pain (Crausman and Bravo 1997).

12.10 Summary of Diagnostic Workup

1. History and careful physical examination of the scrotum, genitals, and perineum. Transillumination of the scrotum is valuable.
2. Urinalysis
3. Scrotal Ultrasound with Doppler

References

Anderson JB, Williamson RC (1988) Testicular torsion in Bristol: a 25-year review. Br J Surg 75:988

Baskin LS, Carroll PR, Cattolica EV, McAninch JW (1990) Necrotising soft tissue infections of the perineum and genitalia. Bacteriology, treatment and risk assessment. Br J Urol 65: 524

Benjamin K (2002) Scrotal and inguinal masses in the newborn period. Adv Neonatal Care 2:140

Brandes SB, Chelsky MJ, Hanno PM (1994) Adult acute idiopathic scrotal edema. Urology 44:602

Cayan S, Erdemir F, Ozbey I, Turek PJ, Kadioglu A, Tellaloglu S (2002) Can varicocelectomy significantly change the way couples use assisted reproductive technologies? J Urol 167:1749

Crausman RS, Bravo K (1997) Ruptured abdominal aortic aneurysm masquerading as testicular pain. Am J Emerg Med 15:445

Eaton SH, Cendron MA, Estrada CR, Bauer SB, Borer JG, Cilento BG et al (2005) Intermittent testicular torsion: diagnostic features and management outcomes. J Urol 174:1532

Feneley MR, Pal MK, Nockler IB, Hendry WF (1997) Retrograde embolization and causes of failure in the primary treatment of varicocele. Br J Urol 80:642

Friedman SC, Sheynkin YR (1995) Acute scrotal symptoms due to perforated appendix in children: case report and review of literature. Pediatr Emerg Care 11:181

Grober ED, Chan PT, Zini A, Goldstein M (2004) Microsurgical treatment of persistent or recurrent varicocele. Fertil Steril 82:718

Ioannides AS, Turnock R (2001) An audit of the management of the acute scrotum in children with Henoch-Schonlein Purpura. J R Coll Surg Edinb 46:98

McGee SR (1993) Referred scrotal pain: case reports and review. J Gen Intern Med 8:694

Mor Y, Pinthus JH, Nadu A, Raviv G, Golomb J, Winkler H et al (2006) Testicular fixation following torsion of the spermatic cord–does it guarantee prevention of recurrent torsion events? J Urol 175:171

Morrison D, Blaivas M, Lyon M (2005) Emergency diagnosis of Fournier's gangrene with bedside ultrasound. Am J Emerg Med 23:544

Nussbaum Blask AR, Bulas D, Shalaby-Rana E, Rushton G, Shao C, Majd M (2002) Color Doppler sonography and scintigraphy of the testis: a prospective, comparative analysis in children with acute scrotal pain. Pediatr Emerg Care 18:67

13 Oncologic Emergencies

N.-E.B. Jacobsen, S.D.W. Beck, R.S. Foster

13.1 Introduction

It has been estimated that genitourinary malignancies will account for 25% of new cancer diagnoses in the United States in 2005 (Jemal et al. 2005). While the incidence of many of these malignancies has increased over the past two decades, the mortality rates appear to be decreasing. Early cancer detection combined with improvements in surgical and nonsurgical oncologic therapy account for these trends. Although not common, newly diagnosed cancer patients occasionally present in an emergent, life-threatening manner that warrants immediate medical or surgical intervention. As the prevalence of genitourinary malignancies continues to expand, additional patients can be expected to develop disease or treatment-related complications. This chapter will serve to review the diagnosis and management of oncologic emergencies as they pertain to the urologist.

13.2 Spontaneous Perinephric Hemorrhage

Renal cell carcinoma (RCC) is the fourth most common genitourinary malignancy in the United States, with an estimated 36,000 new cases expected in 2005 (Jemal et al. 2005). In contrast to years past, the majority of cases are now diagnosed incidentally due to the widespread availability and performance of abdominal imaging. While presentation with the classic triad of flank pain, gross hematuria, and a palpable abdominal mass is now rare (Jayson and Sanders 1998), a small proportion of cases complicated by a spontaneous perinephric hemorrhage (SPH) will demonstrate one or all of these findings. It is difficult to estimate the true incidence of spontaneous tumor hemorrhage since SPH is not specific to RCC and most descriptions of SPH amount to case reports only. Nonetheless, this would appear to be an uncommon mode of presentation for RCC. Neovascularity and propensity for necrosis are possible explanations for tumor rupture and hemorrhage (Hora et al. 2004).

13.2.1 Background

Spontaneous perinephric hemorrhage represents a diagnostic and therapeutic challenge. Appropriate treatment depends on the hemodynamic stability of the patient and a correct determination of its cause. In light of its infrequent occurrence, management guidelines for SPH are based on data acquired through meta-analyses of case reports. Since 1933, four available meta-analyses have reviewed 448 cases of SPH, 165 of which took place after 1985 (Polkey and Vynalek 1933; McDougal et al. 1975; Cinman et al. 1985; Zhang et al. 2002). It appears that SPH occurs with equal frequency in males and females as well as in right and left kidneys. Flank or abdominal pain of acute onset is the most common presenting symptom (83% – 100%) (Zhang et al. 2002; Pereverzev et al. 2005). Interestingly, only a minority of SPH cases demonstrate gross or microscopic hematuria (0% – 19%). Up to 11% present with signs and symptoms of hypovolemic shock indicative of a severe retroperitoneal hemorrhage. Numerous etiologies exist, the most common of which is neoplasm (57% – 66%), benign or malignant, followed by vascular disease (17% – 26%), idiopathic hemorrhage (6.7%), and infection (2.4%). Angiomyolipoma (AML) and RCC represent the most common benign and malignant neoplastic causes of SPH, accounting for 24% – 33% and 30% – 33% of all cases, respectively. With such disparate etiologic possibilities, accurate diagnosis is of the utmost importance to ensure appropriate treatment is provided.

Computed tomography (CT) with intravenous (i.v.) contrast is the imaging study of choice for SPH (Fig. 13.1). The diagnostic accuracy of CT for a perinephric hematoma approaches 100%, and the reported sensitivity and specificity for identification of an underlying mass is 57% and 82%, respectively (Zhang et al. 2002). Contemporary series employing state-of-the-art CT imaging technology report up to 92% diagnostic accuracy for determination of the underlying cause of SPH (Sebastia et al. 1997). In contrast, the sensitivity and specificity of ultrasound (US) is 11% and 33%, respectively. Magnetic resonance imaging (MRI) is an appropriate substitute in cases where contraindications to i.v. contrast exist or CT is unavailable. Diagnostic arteriography is indicated if CT or MRI does not demonstrate a mass or if a vascular etiology is suspected (Zagoria et al. 1991). Bilateral SPH, reported in 3% of cases, suggests a vascular diagnosis such as polyarteritis nodosa (Zhang et al. 2002).

Identification of fat content (< 10 Hounsfield Units) within a renal mass on CT, although not sensitive, is a highly specific finding for AML (Fig. 13.2) (Bosniak et

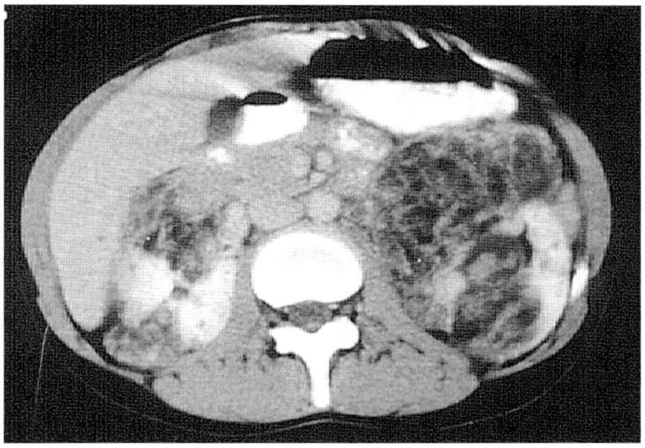

Fig. 13.2. Angiomyolipoma. CT demonstrating bilateral angiomyolipomas with characteristic fat attenuation

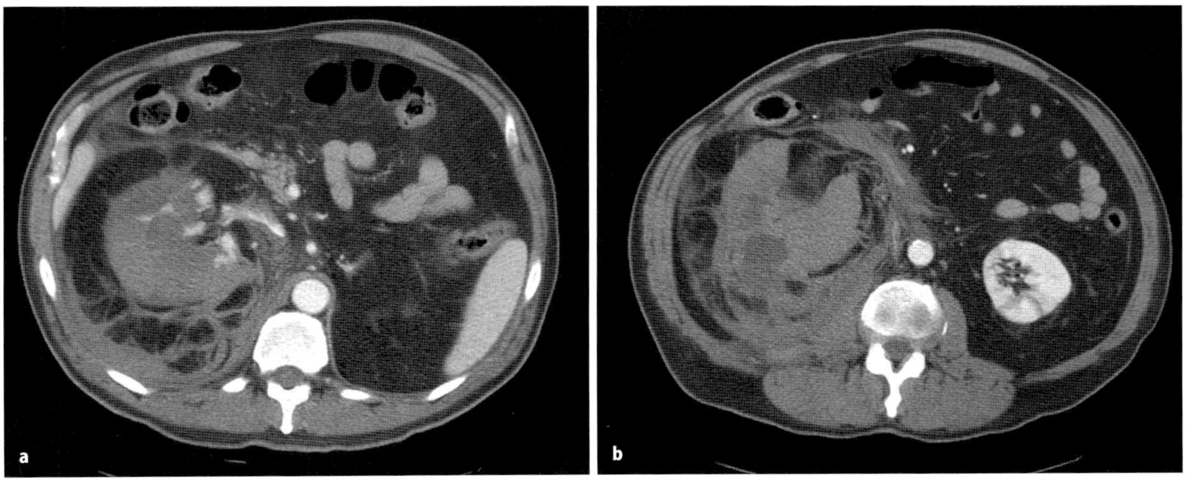

Fig. 13.1a, b. Spontaneous right hemorrhage. **a, b** Contrast-enhanced CT demonstrating right renal hemorrhage into perinephric space. No mass lesion is discernible. Patient was subsequently diagnosed with renovascular disease

al. 1988; Lemaitre et al. 1997). In contrast, any heterogenous solid or cystic mass without fat should be regarded as RCC until proven otherwise. Of note, tumor size does correlate with risk of hemorrhage for AML; however, no such correlation has been shown for RCC (Zhang et al. 2002).

13.2.2 Evaluation

At the time of presentation, a thorough history, physical examination, and determination of hemodynamic stability should ensue. Given that flank pain arising from SPH is commonly confused with renal colic, a noncontrast CT of the abdomen and pelvis is often performed. In fact, a contrast-enhanced CT is the first-line study and should be obtained in the event that a noncontrast CT or US suggests the presence of a retroperitoneal hematoma. Laboratory studies should include a complete blood count (CBC), electrolytes, blood urea nitrogen (BUN), creatinine, and a coagulation profile.

13.2.3 Treatment

The management of SPH is similar to that of renal trauma wherein conservative measures are first-line and nephrectomy is reserved as an option of last resort (Santucci and Fisher 2005). Initial steps are directed toward maintaining hemodynamic support through i.v. hydration and blood and blood product replacement as necessary. Bed rest is instituted along with periodic monitoring of vital statistics and serum hemoglobin in those patients who are hemodynamically stable. Unstable patients or those in whom the hemoglobin continues to decrease despite repeated transfusions require diagnostic arteriography and selective embolization. Only patients who remain unstable or continue to bleed despite embolization need undergo open nephrectomy. Partial nephrectomy remains an option in the early period but should be restricted to patients with a solitary kidney or those with a small (<4 cm), easily identifiable exophytic mass whose hemodynamic parameters do not prohibit an extended procedure. Seven percent of patients with a renal mass in available series have undergone early partial nephrectomy in the setting of SPH (Zhang et al. 2002). Unfortunately, no data on local recurrence is available at this time.

Patients with hemodynamic stability including those responding to conservative measures, including embolization, require inpatient monitoring and symptomatic treatment only. Ambulation and subsequent hospital discharge can be initiated when vital signs and hemoglobin remain stable for 24 h and gross hematuria, if present, has resolved. Given the 25% risk of underlying malignancy, repeat abdominal imaging with CT scan should be performed in 1–3 months (Zhang et al. 2002; Yip et al. 1998). If a mass suggestive of RCC is identified at presentation or in follow-up, definitive treatment can be performed on an elective basis.

13.3 Hypercalcemia of Malignancy

Hypercalcemia is the most common paraneoplastic syndrome of malignancy (Fojo 2005). Among genitourinary malignancies, it is most frequently identified in association with RCC (3%–25%) (Zekri et al. 2001; Walther et al. 1997; Papac and Poo-Hwu 1999; Skinner et al. 1971). In comparison, hypercalcemia is an uncommon manifestation of prostate cancer and transitional cell carcinoma (Coleman 1997). The incidence of hypercalcemia in RCC correlates with the stage of the primary tumor as well as with the presence or absence of bone metastases (Fahn et al. 1991). Hypercalcemia typically occurs late in the course of disease and has demonstrated independent significance as a poor prognostic factor in patients with advanced RCC (Motzer et al. 1999).

13.3.1 Pathophysiology

Two pathogenic mechanisms are involved in the generation of hypercalcemia: (1) focal osteolytic bone destruction secondary to bone metastases and (2) uncoupling of bone turnover secondary to tumor-secreted humoral factors. Focal bone destruction by metastases involves the paracrine secretion of various cytokines that stimulate local osteoclasts and inhibit osteoblasts. Although this mechanism certainly contributes to hypercalcemia, it appears that systemic factors play a more important role. Malignant hypercalcemia caused by the production of humoral factors is often referred to as humoral hypercalcemia of malignancy (HHM). The humoral factor most commonly associated with HHM, including that of RCC, is parathyroid hormone-related protein (PTHrP) (Burtis et al. 1990; Mundy 1990). PTHrP causes hypercalcemia through bone resorption, as well as through renal calcium reabsorption (Rosol and Capen 1992). Partial sequence homology between PTHrP and parathyroid hormone (PTH) helps to explain the mechanisms by which this occurs. Unlike primary hyperparathyroidism, PTH levels are often normal or suppressed in cases of HHM (Walther et al. 1997; Flombaum 2000). Interleukin-6 (IL-6) and prostaglandin (PG), both of which stimulate osteoclast activity, represent additional humoral factors involved in HHM (Papac and Poo-Hwu 1999).

13.3.2
Presentation

The most common presenting symptoms of hypercalcemia are nonspecific and include fatigue, anorexia, nausea, and constipation. Through the induction of an osmotic diuresis and inhibition of antidiuretic hormone activity, hypercalcemia also causes polyuria and progressive dehydration. Not uncommonly, patients are found to have acute or chronic renal insufficiency at the time of presentation. Neurologic symptoms such as weakness, lethargy, and disorientation may progress into seizures, coma, and even death if treatment is delayed. Symptom severity depends upon the degree of hypercalcemia and the rate at which it develops.

13.3.3
Evaluation

Appropriate treatment of hypercalcemia depends upon the symptom severity, serum calcium level, renal function, and overall health status of the patient. Tumor stage and oncologic prognosis are also important and must be taken into consideration when formulating a management plan. Laboratory investigations include a CBC, serum electrolytes, ionized and total serum calcium, albumin, BUN, and serum creatinine. Serum magnesium should also be measured since hypercalcemia commonly induces renal magnesium wasting through actions exerted at the loop of Henle. Assays for PTHrP are available; however, the utility of this test is questionable at present. Perhaps in cases without a definitive diagnosis of malignancy, PTHrP and PTH levels should both be evaluated.

13.3.4
Treatment

Asymptomatic patients with mild to moderately elevated serum calcium ($\leq$3.25 mmol/l, $\leq$14 mg/dl) do not require immediate treatment as an inpatient (Fojo 2005). Rather, medical therapy may be instituted on an outpatient basis with periodic monitoring of serum calcium and renal function. Symptomatic patients, or those with a serum calcium level above 3.25 mmol/l (>14 mg/dl) indicating severe hypercalcemia require hospital admission and immediate intervention. The traditional and most basic treatment for hypercalcemia is i.v. hydration with isotonic saline. By increasing urine calcium excretion, hydration results in a rapid, yet modest (0.5 mmol/l) reduction in serum calcium levels. Renal function can also be expected to improve as the prerenal component of dysfunction is corrected. Hydration is generally begun with the infusion of 1–2 l of isotonic saline over 1–4 h (Flombaum 2000). Total volumes and rate of delivery will depend on the hydration and cardiovascular status of the patient. Furosemide, a loop diuretic that inhibits calcium reabsorption at the loop of Henle, can be used to augment renal calcium excretion. Loop diuretics should only be used when rehydration has been completed.

Table 13.1. Treatment options for hypercalcemia of malignancy

Treatment	Dose	Route	Frequency
Normal saline hydration	1–2 l	IV	As necessary
Furosemide	20–40 mg	IV	As necessary
Zoledronate	4–8 mg over 5–15 min	IV	Every 4–6 weeks
Calcitonin	4–8 IU/kg	IM/SC	Every 6–8 h
Gallium nitrate	100–200 mg/m^2/day × 5 days	IV	
Dialysis Nephrectomy			

Rehydration alone is often inadequate (Hosking et al. 1981). The majority of patients with hypercalcemia of malignancy will require additional medical therapy as outlined in Table 13.1. The cornerstone of such therapy is the bisphosphonate group of medications. As pyrophosphate analogs with a high affinity for hydroxyapatite, bisphosphonates concentrate in areas of high bone turnover where they become internalized into osteoclasts and inhibit bone resorption (Fleisch 1991; Lin 1996; Sato et al. 1991; Fojo 2005). Three generations of bisphosphonates are now available, each providing an incremental improvement in potency, response duration, and toxicity profile. Etidronate, the original bisphosphonate, corrects hypercalcemia in 50% of patients; however, this is achieved at the expense of significant demineralization (Singer and Minoofar 1995). The success rate of second- and third-generation bisphosphonates exceeds 80% (Purohit et al. 1995; Nussbaum et al. 1993). The current drug of choice is zoledronate, a third-generation bisphosphonate that achieves normocalcemia in more than 90% of patients (Major et al. 2001). As with all bisphosphonates, this agent must be given intravenously because of poor oral absorption. Zoledronate usually corrects hypercalcemia within 4–10 days for a duration of 4–6 weeks. Bisphosphonates are more effective against hypercalcemia arising from focal bone destruction secondary to metastases than against HHM. Despite potent inhibition of focal and systemic bone resorption, bisphosphonates have no effect on renal calcium reabsorption, which plays a prominent role in HHM. Animal studies suggest that bisphosphonates may cause or exacerbate renal failure; therefore, these agents should be used with caution if the serum creatinine exceeds 3.0 mg/dl (Stewart 2005).

Calcitonin is another treatment option for hypercalcemia. Reduction in serum calcium occurs primarily through the inhibition of osteoclast-mediated bone resorption. However, supraphysiologic doses have also been shown to improve renal calcium excretion (Lin 1996; Sato et al. 1991). Tachyphylaxis occurs within 2–3 days of repeated calcitonin dosing; therefore long-term efficacy is not possible. The primary utility of calcitonin lies in the rapidity of its onset (2–6 h) (Warrell et al. 1988). As such, calcitonin is ideally used in combination with longer-acting medications with delayed-onset such as bisphosphonates. With the exception of rare allergic reactions, calcitonin is considered safe and nontoxic.

Gallium nitrate, originally developed as an anticancer drug, is a potent inhibitor of bone resorption (Warrell et al. 1991). In addition to osteoclast inhibition, gallium nitrate reduces serum calcium through the inhibition of both renal calcium reabsorption and PTH secretion (Warrell et al. 1984; Warrell 1997). A continuous 5-day i.v. infusion corrects hypercalcemia in approximately 80% of patients for a median duration of 8 days (Warrell et al. 1991). Serum calcium begins to normalize within hours but maximal effect takes place after the infusion is complete. Ten percent of treated patients experience an elevation in serum creatinine; therefore, gallium nitrate should be used with caution in patients with baseline renal dysfunction (Zojer et al. 1999). Based on its lengthy administration protocol and potential for nephrotoxicity, gallium nitrate is rarely used today. It does, however, remain an important treatment option in cases of hypercalcemia refractory to bisphosphonate therapy.

Dialysis is indicated in patients with severe hypercalcemia complicated by significant mental changes. Patients with chronic renal failure or congestive heart failure often cannot tolerate i.v. hydration therapy; therefore, hemodialysis is frequently necessary in these cases as well.

Depending on the extent of disease and the oncologic prognosis, nephrectomy may also be a consideration. Hypercalcemia typically normalizes after nephrectomy in cases of localized RCC (Gold and Fefer 1996; Fahn et al. 1991). Persistence or relapse of hypercalcemia is often an indication of local recurrence or occult metastatic disease. Cytoreductive nephrectomy has been shown to correct hypercalcemia in two-thirds of patients with metastatic RCC; however, this effect is only temporary (Walther et al. 1997).

13.4 Complications of Bacille Calmette-Guérin Therapy

Bacille Calmette-Guérin (BCG) is the most effective intravesical agent available for the treatment of high-risk superficial transitional cell carcinoma (TCC) of the bladder. A live attenuated strain of the bovine tuberculous mycobacterium, BCG exerts its antineoplastic effect through the stimulation of a nonspecific inflammatory reaction at the bladder level. Intravesical treatment is generally safe with fewer than 10% of patients experiencing complications that require treatment beyond symptomatic palliation (Lamm et al. 1992, Rischmann et al. 2000). Side effects can be categorized into local and systemic subtypes. The most common local toxicity is cystitis, with 80% of patients describing varying degrees of irritative voiding symptoms (Resel Folkersma et al. 1999). Low-grade fever (<38.5°C), which occurs in many as one-third of patients soon after intravesical therapy, is the most frequent systemic effect reported (Rischmann et al. 2000). The most serious toxic effects of BCG treatment include BCG-osis, manifested as pulmonary or hepatic infection, and BCG sepsis. Since both present with fever as an early sign, the difficulty lies in differentiating benign, transient fever from that which heralds serious systemic illness. Fortunately, BCG-osis and BCG sepsis each affect less than 1% of patients (Lamm et al. 1992).

In the setting of serious systemic illness following BCG therapy, suspicion for hematogenous dissemination of mycobacteria or other urinary tract pathogens should be high. Although BCG virulence and host immunocompetence play a role, trauma to the lower urinary tract is the most common predisposing factor (Lamm et al. 1992). This is reflected in the list of contraindications to intravesical BCG therapy, which include traumatic catheterization and gross or microscopic hematuria (Table 13.2) (Malkowicz 2002; Lamm et al. 1992). While the literature is sparse, small series have demonstrated no significant morbidity with the use of intravesical BCG in renal transplant patients (Palou et al. 2003). Apart from a lower rate of fever with the Pasteur strain, the relative rates of fever, BCG-osis and

Table 13.2. Contraindications to intravesical BCG therapy

Absolute	Relative
Traumatic catheterization	Microscopic hematuria
Gross hematuria	Poor performance status
Immunocompromised	Advanced age
Acquired immunodeficiency syndrome	Prior history of tuberculosis
Seropositive human immunodeficiency virus	
Leukemia	
Hodgkin's disease	
Transplant recipients	
Prior BCG sepsis	
Prior BCG-osis (pulmonary, hepatic)	
Intractable urinary tract infection	
Pregnancy	
Lactation	

BCG sepsis among the five commercially available strains of BCG are quite similar (Lamm et al. 1992). Prior febrile responses to BCG therapy and positive skin reactivity to purified protein derivative have both been shown to be predictive of an increased risk of fever and a trend toward an increased risk of systemic side effects (Lamm 1992; Bilen et al. 2003). Interestingly, patients who develop systemic side effects to BCG demonstrate longer disease-free and progression-free survival from an oncologic standpoint (Bilen et al. 2003; Suzuki et al. 2002). This implies that patients who mount an augmented systemic reaction toward BCG may also mount a more effective inflammatory response against the bladder tumor.

13.4.1 BCG-Related Fever

Low-grade fever (<38.5°C) in the absence of hemodynamic instability is a benign immune response to mycobacterial exposure in most cases. Outpatient symptomatic treatment with oral antipyretics is typically all that is necessary. Resolution should be expected within 24–48 h of treatment (Rischmann et al. 2000). High-grade fever (>39.5°C), which develops in 3%–4% of patients, or persistent low-grade fever are more worrisome (Lamm et al. 1992; Resel Folkersma et al. 1999). Current recommendations are to evaluate all patients with fevers above 38.5°C or 39.5°C lasting longer than 24 or 12 h, respectively, and to initiate single-agent antitubercular treatment on an empiric basis (Malkowicz 2002). The evaluation of BCG-related fever includes a CBC as well as serum electrolytes, creatinine, liver function studies, and mycobacterial blood cultures. Gram-negative sepsis is not an uncommon cause of fever in this patient population; therefore standard blood and urine cultures should also be obtained in order to rule out infection by common urinary pathogens. Respiratory symptoms suspicious for pulmonary infection warrant a plain radiograph of the chest. Isoniazid (INH) (300 mg once a day by mouth) is the antitubercular agent of choice for BCG-related fever. The most common adverse effect of INH is transient hepatitis manifest as elevated serum transaminase levels. This occurs in 10%–20% of patients and should normalize despite the continuation of treatment (Lamm et al. 1992). Isoniazid is continued for 3 months and need only be discontinued if transaminases rise above three times the upper limit of normal. Prophylactic INH has not been shown to reduce the incidence of fever or systemic infection (Durek et al. 2000). Moreover, prophylactic INH diminishes the immune response and impairs antitumor activity (de Boer et al. 1992).

13.4.2 BCG Sepsis

The most serious complication of BCG therapy is generalized sepsis secondary to intravascular absorption of mycobacteria or other urinary pathogens. Traumatic catheterization, identified in more than two-thirds of such cases, is the most common etiologic factor (Lamm 1992). Severe cystitis and recent transurethral surgery (within 1 week) are other potential routes for dissemination. Fever is the most common presenting sign and typically occurs within 12 h of BCG instillation (Paterson and Patel 1998). High-grade fever within 2 h of BCG instillation is especially worrisome, as is hemodynamic instability and other signs of multisystem organ failure (Dalbagni and O'Donnell 2006). Blood and urine cultures are typically negative. The mortality rate of BCG sepsis approaches 50%; therefore empiric triple-drug therapy is indicated in any patient with persistent fever and evidence of sepsis in temporal association with BCG administration (Malkowicz 2002; Paterson and Patel 1998). A 6-month course of INH, rifampin, and ethambutol is the current standard of care (Table 13.3). Ethambutol may be discontinued after 2 months depending upon organism susceptibility and clinical resolution (Blumberg et al. 2003). Since the treatment response to antitubercular medications is delayed by 2–7 days, traditional guidelines recommended concurrent therapy with cycloserine, an antibiotic capable of controlling mycobacteria within 24 h (Lamm et al. 1992; Lotte et al. 1984). Recent susceptibility studies, however, have demonstrated that commercially available BCG strains are highly resistant to cycloserine. In contrast, fluoroquinolones, gentamicin, and all antitubercular drugs, except pyrazinamide, retain activity against BCG (Durek et al. 2000). As such, contemporary guidelines recommend the addition of a fluoroquinolone or ampicillin plus gentamicin combination to standard antitubercular therapy in cases of BCG sepsis (Durek et al. 2000; Paterson and Patel 1998). This allows rapid inhibition of mycobacterial growth while also providing adequate empiric coverage for possible Gram-negative sepsis. The duration of treatment with supplementary antibiotics, determined by the results of

Table 13.3. Treatment of BCG sepsis

Medication	Dosage	Duration
Isoniazid plus	300 mg p.o. daily	6 Months
Rifampin plus	600 mg p.o. daily	6 Months
Ethambutol plus	1,200 mg p.o. daily	2–6 Months
Ampicillin plus	1 g i.v. every 6 h	Await culture results
Gentamicin[a]	7 mg/kg i.v. every 24 h	
Or ciprofloxacin	500 mg p.o. twice daily or 400 mg i.v. every 12 h	

[a] Based on potential nephrotoxicity, gentamicin dosing requires assessment of renal function

standard blood and urine cultures, need only be short-term in true BCG sepsis. One caveat is the development of intolerance or systemic complication to any of the standard antitubercular drugs, in which case a fluoroquinolone may be used in substitution.

The use of corticosteroids in BCG sepsis is somewhat controversial. Severe type IV hypersensitivity is an important diagnosis to consider in any patient with suspected BCG sepsis. Since the two diagnoses are often difficult to differentiate, most authorities recommend the addition of corticosteroids (prednisolone 40 mg p.o. daily) or hydrocortisone 100 mg i.v. four times daily (Lamm 1992; Paterson and Patel 1998) to standard treatment in the short term. Animal studies have shown that prednisolone in combination with standard antitubercular therapy is more effective than standard therapy alone (DeHaven et al. 1992). Exacerbation of true BCG sepsis secondary to immunosuppression remains a concern; therefore the decision to continue steroid therapy should be made relatively soon, based on clinical and laboratory parameters.

13.4.3 BCG-osis

BCG-osis is a variant of systemic infection wherein the lungs, liver, or both are primarily affected (Malkowicz 2002). The clinical picture is similar to that of BCG sepsis; however, patients with BCG-osis are generally hemodynamically stable and present with signs and symptoms indicating pulmonary or hepatic disease. Although an abnormal chest radiograph or elevated liver enzymes suggest the diagnosis, only bronchoalveolar aspiration or biopsy of the lungs or liver are conclusive (Rischmann et al. 2000). Not uncommonly, these biopsies are negative, indicating that many such cases represent a hypersensitivity reaction rather than a true mycobacterial infection. Regardless, a 6-month course of INH and rifampin is indicated if clinical suspicion is high (refer to Table 13.3) (Lamm et al. 1992). Ethambutol is added if the patient is acutely ill, as are corticosteroids in cases unresponsive to standard treatment. A prior history of BCG sepsis or BCG-osis precludes future treatment with intravesical BCG.

13.5 Malignant Spinal Cord Compression

Spinal cord compression is a debilitating complication of metastatic cancer identified in 5%–14% of cancer patients (Patchell et al. 2005). Among urologic malignancies, it is most commonly seen with prostate cancer (PCa), which accounts for 9%–24% of cases overall (van der Linden et al. 2005; Flynn and Shipley 1991). In fact, PCa is the second most common cause of malignant spinal cord compression, with a cumulative incidence of 7% (Manglani et al. 2000; Rosenthal et al. 1992; Sorenson et al. 1990). Although RCC and TCC account for 6% and 2% of cases, respectively, PCa, by virtue of its higher incidence and preponderance for vertebral metastases, warrants the bulk of discussion. However, despite a few minor variances, the treatment principles are the same regardless of malignant etiology.

Prostate cancer is the most commonly diagnosed noncutaneous malignancy in American men today and the second most common cause of cancer death (Jemal et al. 2005). Screening through the use of serum prostate-specific antigen (PSA) has led to both stage and risk migration such that the proportion of patients presenting with metastatic disease has fallen from 14.1% in 1988 to 3.3% in 1998 (Paquette et al. 2002). While distant metastatic disease is now uncommon at presentation, an additional 70% of patients with locally advanced PCa can be expected to develop metastases in follow-up (Coleman 1997). Skeletal metastases are the most common form of extralymphatic disease, and based on venous drainage patterns the bony pelvis and spine often represent the first sites involved.

In addition to significant pain and the potential for pathologic fracture, metastases to the vertebral column may cause spinal cord compression through local growth into the epidural space (Byrne 1992). Direct compression of the spinal cord causes edema, venous congestion, and demyelination, all of which impair neurologic function (Patchell et al. 2005). Prolonged compression eventually leads to infarction of the spinal cord. Without prompt diagnosis and treatment, progressive and irreversible loss of neurologic function will occur. All too often, however, presentation and diagnosis are delayed.

13.5.1 Presentation

Midline back pain is the most common presenting symptom (90%) (Gilbert et al. 1978; Sundaresan et al. 1985; Harrington 1988; Maranzano and Latini 1995). It is typically localized to the level of cord compression and, unlike degenerative disc disease, it is exacerbated by recumbency and improved by upright posture (Dodge et al. 1951). Radicular pain secondary to nerve root compression is less frequent but highly localizing. Symptom progression is usually slow with pain predating further neurologic changes by a median of 7 weeks (Quinn and DeAngelis 2000). Progression of neurologic dysfunction can, on occasion, take place over a matter of hours or days; therefore, new onset back pain in a cancer patient requires urgent evaluation.

Motor weakness is the second most common feature of cord compression. As a result of delays in both presentation and diagnosis, more than three-quarters of patients present with objective motor deficits (Gilbert et al. 1978; Harrington 1988). Regardless of the compression site, weakness begins in the legs and affects proximal muscle groups first (Quinn and DeAngelis 2000). Progression to paraplegia is typically a late event. Sensory changes are also common (50%) and occur soon after the onset of muscle weakness (Tazi et al. 2003). Symptoms include hyperesthesia at the level of compression or paresthesias and sensory loss in the toes with proximal ascent. Urinary retention, fecal incontinence, and impotence are usually late signs indicating autonomic dysfunction. An exception is cauda equina syndrome in which lumbar metastases cause compression of the conus medullaris. Autonomic dysfunction can occur early in this setting and sensory loss often assumes a saddle-like distribution.

13.5.2 Evaluation

Any cancer patient with new-onset back pain or neurologic change requires a thorough evaluation to rule out cord compression. A meticulous neurologic exam is performed to determine the initial spinal level and severity of compression. Interval changes are documented through periodic repeat examinations. A normal neurologic exam does not exclude the presence of impending cord compression. Up to 36% of patients with back pain and no neurologic deficits will have epidural metastases demonstrated on imaging (Rodichok et al. 1981). MRI is the imaging modality of choice in cases of suspected spinal cord compression (Fig. 13.3) (Manglani et al. 2000; Quinn and DeAngelis 2000). While plain radiography allows a quick assessment of vertebral collapse and deformity, MRI provides an accurate determination of both the degree of compression and the number of cord levels affected. A total of 10%–38% of cases involve multiple noncontiguous levels; therefore, the entire spine must be imaged (Byrne 1992; Helweg-Larsen et al. 1995). The thoracic spine is the most common site of cord compression, and accounts for approximately two-thirds of cases involving PCa (Flynn and Shipley 1991). CT with or without myelography may be used in cases where MRI is contraindicated or unavailable. Serum PSA and testosterone levels should be measured in cases of PCa to determine the androgen sensitivity of the malignancy.

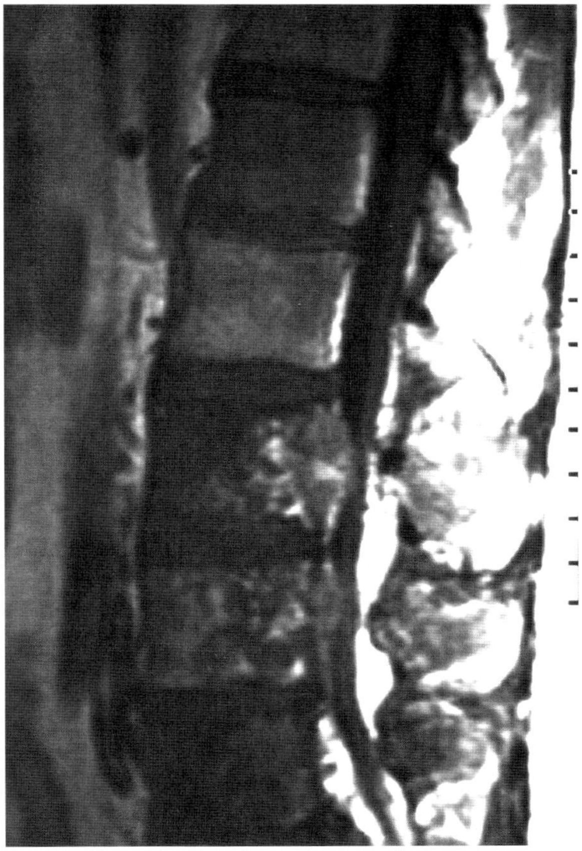

Fig. 13.3. Spinal cord compression. MRI demonstrating neoplastic replacement of L3 and L4 vertebrae and epidural compression of spinal cord in patient with metastatic prostate cancer

13.5.3 Treatment

As a late manifestation of advanced disease, the treatment of malignant spinal cord compression is palliative. The primary objectives are pain relief and neurologic preservation while reduction of tumor bulk remains a secondary goal only. Available treatment options include medical, radiation, and surgical therapies, which are typically delivered in a multidisciplinary fashion. Historically, intravenous corticosteroids in combination with external beam radiotherapy (EBRT) were the treatment of choice. Recent advances in spinal instrumentation and surgical techniques have led to a renewed interest in the use of surgery as primary therapy. Since there are no large-scale studies of urologic or PCa-related spinal cord compression, current guidelines are based upon the results of studies incorporating numerous tumor types. Although oncologic prognosis, presence of co-morbidities, and overall performance status are important, ambulatory status and spinal stability at presentation are the primary considerations when formulating a treatment plan. Numerous studies have demonstrated the prognostic significance of baseline ambulatory status with regard to treatment outcome. The majority of ambulatory patients can expect to remain ambulatory with early treatment, whereas only 50% of nonambulatory patients, at best, can expect the same (Ok et al. 2005).

Table 13.4. Steroid protocols for malignant spinal cord compression

Dexamethasone	Bolus	Maintenance
High dose	100 mg i.v.	24 mg i.v./p.o. every 6 hs for 3 days then taper
Moderate dose	10 mg i.v.	4 mg p.o./i.v. every 6 h for 3 days then taper

Regardless of ambulatory status and spinal stability, corticosteroids are the first treatment administered in cases of suspected or confirmed spinal cord compression. Through a rapid reduction in vasogenic edema, corticosteroids decrease mechanical compression on the spinal cord until more definitive therapy can be provided. Additional steroid actions include pain relief, reduction in inflammation, and a direct oncolytic effect (Ok et al. 2005). Corticosteroids can be given in both high-dose and moderate-dose schedules (Table 13.4) (Manglani et al. 2000). The two dosing schedules appear to provide similar rates of neurologic and ambulatory preservation; however, high-dose corticosteroids are associated with superior analgesia at the expense of a greater risk of steroid-related complications (gastroduodenal ulceration, psychosis, *Pneumocystis carinii* pneumonia) (Heimdal et al. 1992; Delattre et al. 1988). Since no randomized controlled trials have directly compared these two schedules, it is difficult to make firm recommendations for steroid dosing. To minimize the potential for steroid-related morbidity, it has been suggested that corticosteroid therapy begin with the moderate dose schedule. If neurologic improvement does not occur within 6–12 h, the high-dose schedule can be implemented at that time (Manglani et al. 2000). Maintenance dosing is continued until the neurologic status remains stable for 48 h, after which steroids are tapered over 2–3 weeks.

Androgen deprivation therapy maintains an important role in the treatment of metastatic spinal cord compression involving hormonally naïve PCa. Unfortunately, most patients with PCa who develop spinal cord compression have exhausted hormonal therapy and are resistant to such therapy. Nevertheless, all PCa patients require an evaluation of serum PSA and testosterone to determine the level of androgen sensitivity that remains. Hormonally naïve cases demonstrate improved ambulatory rates (80 % vs 42 %) and overall survival (16 vs 6 months) relative to hormone-resistant cases when androgen deprivation is incorporated into the overall management plan (Iacovou et al. 1985; Flynn and Shipley 1991). Methods available for hormonal therapy include both surgical (bilateral orchiectomy) and chemical (ketoconazole) castration. Orchiectomy and ketoconazole allow the most immediate reduction in serum testosterone levels. Ketoconazole, an oral synthetic imidazole antifungal agent, reduces gonadal and adrenal testosterone synthesis through the inhibition of cytochrome P450 enzyme-dependent 14-demethylation of lanosterol to cholesterol. At a dose of 400 mg three times daily, ketoconazole suppresses serum testosterone to castrate levels within 48 h (Trachtenberg 1984). Prostate cancer-related spinal cord compression with neurologic compromise is a relative contraindication to the use of luteinizing hormone-releasing hormone (LHRH) agonists. These agents induce a temporary rise in serum testosterone, termed the flare phenomenon, which begins within 2–3 days and lasts approximately 1 week from the initiation of therapy (Bubley 2001). Such a rise in serum testosterone may lead to symptomatic disease progression, which, in the context of documented spinal cord compression, can involve a further deterioration in neurologic function. Patients in whom spinal cord compression is impending rather than proven may be candidates for LHRH agonist therapy; however, pretreatment with a steroidal or nonsteroidal antiandrogen is recommended. Antiandrogen therapy is preferably begun 1 week before the initiation of LHRH agonist treatment and continued for 1 month. Luteinizing hormone-releasing hormone antagonists, such as abarelix, represent an acceptable alternative to LHRH agonists since they rapidly achieve castrate serum testosterone levels (68 %–78 % within 7 days, 96 % within 1 month) and avoid the testosterone surge altogether (Trachtenberg et al. 2002; Koch et al. 2003). Abarelix has demonstrated safe and effective provision of medical castration in men with symptomatic PCa, including those with impending spinal cord compression (Koch et al. 2003).

Ambulatory patients with spinal stability are usually managed nonoperatively. For this group, the gold standard treatment is corticosteroids in combination with EBRT. Radiotherapy is begun soon after the initiation of corticosteroids with dosages of 2,000–4,000 cGy administered over a 2- to 4-week period (Manglani et al. 2000). For optimal results, the radiation portal includes a margin of one or two vertebral bodies above and below the site of compression (Quinn and DeAngelis 2000). Radiotherapy decreases cord compression through a reduction in tumor mass and bone turgor. Paradoxically, this may lead to weakening of the vertebral body and subsequent collapse; therefore, patients often require 6–10 weeks of external bracing while bone healing takes place. Preservation of ambulation can be expected in 70 %–100 % of patients treated in this manner (Sundaresan et al. 1985; Maranzano and Latini 1995; Katagiri et al. 1998; Helweg-Larsen 1996; Tomita et al. 1983). Radiotherapy and corticosteroids together are more effective than EBRT alone with ambulatory rates of 81 % and 61 %, respectively, demonstrated in a randomized controlled trial (Sundaresan et al. 1985).

Nonambulatory, nonparaplegic patients with stable spines are more difficult to manage. Significant motor deficit is a sign of severe and longstanding spinal cord compression and only a minority of treated patients can be expected to regain the ability to walk. Corticosteroids plus EBRT provide post-treatment ambulatory rates of 6%–60% and likely favor the lower end of this spectrum (Maranzano and Latini 1995; Tomita et al. 1983; Turner et al. 1993; Sorensen et al. 1994; Leviov et al. 1993). Based on a clear inferiority to EBRT and a lack of proven benefit in combination with EBRT, surgery has not had a prominent role in this subgroup. However, this practice was based upon the results of decompressive laminectomy, a historical procedure with inferior outcomes. Although most vertebral metastases are located anterior to the spinal cord, laminectomy typically removes only posterior elements and does not remove the bulk of the compressive tumor. Furthermore, laminectomy may actually destabilize the spine, thereby worsening postoperative ambulatory rates. Over the past two decades, vertebrectomy and spinal stabilization have gained popularity based on the successful results of several nonrandomized studies (Siegel et al. 1982, 1985; Harrington 1984; Sundaresan et al. 1984; Overby and Rothman 1985; Klimo et al. 2005). This procedure, which takes an anterior approach, seeks to decompress the spinal cord through the resection of all gross disease. Concurrent spinal instrumentation provides immediate spinal stabilization even in cases of near-total vertebral body excision.

A recent randomized trial comparing vertebrectomy plus spinal stabilization in combination with EBRT vs EBRT alone has confirmed the utility of primary surgery in cases of metastatic spinal cord compression (Patchell et al. 2005). Postoperative ambulatory rates (84% vs 57% overall) and duration of ambulation (median, 122 days vs 13 days) were both superior with direct decompressive surgery, regardless of baseline ambulatory status. In fact, 62% of nonambulatory patients regained the ability to walk after surgery compared to 19% with radiation alone. Although this study did not include patients with paraplegia persisting longer than 48 h, older series suggest that immediate surgery is also advantageous in this group (Barcena et al. 1984). Unfortunately, only a minority of paraplegic patients (<30%) can expect to regain ambulation with such treatment. The superior functional results of surgery likely reflect the provision of immediate decompression before irreversible spinal infarction takes place as well as the removal of maximal tumor bulk, which minimizes the possibility of malignant regrowth and secondary compression. Of importance, no excess morbidity or mortality could be ascribed to surgery and the mean duration of hospitalization was only 10 days in both groups. Although this randomized study demonstrated a superior functional outcome with surgery for both ambulatory and nonambulatory patients, vertebrectomy and spinal stabilization is not yet considered a panacea. Commonly accepted indications for surgical decompression are outlined in Table 13.5 (Baehring 2005).

Table 13.5. Indications for surgical management of spinal cord compression secondary to prostate cancer metastases

Surgical indications
Spinal instability or vertebral body collapse
Nonambulatory patients who fail to respond to radiotherapy
Progressive neurologic deterioration during radiotherapy
Bone extending into spinal canal causing thecal compression
Radiculopathy with progressive or uncontrolled symptoms
Spinal cord compression in a previously irradiated area
Paraplegic or severely paraparetic patients with recent neurologic deterioration

13.6 Neutropenia

Neutropenia, defined as an absolute neutrophil count of less than 500 cells/μl, occurs frequently in cancer patients undergoing systemic chemotherapy. Among patients with genitourinary malignancies, this scenario is most common in patients with advanced TCC of the bladder. In this setting, the administration of MVAC (methotrexate, vinblastine, doxorubicin, cisplatin) or GC (gemcitabine, cisplatin) chemotherapy leads to the development of grade 3 or 4 neutropenia (World Health Organization classification) in 80% and 43%–71% of patients, respectively (von der Masse et al. 2000). Although less frequent, neutropenia may also occur with conventional (bleomycin, etoposide, cisplatin) and salvage (ifosfamide-based) chemotherapy during the treatment of metastatic germ cell cancer (Bosl et al. 2005).

Neutrophils represent the first cellular component of the inflammatory response. As such, neutropenia poses significant risk for the development of infection. Both the degree and duration of neutropenia have been shown to correlate strongly with the incidence of serious infection (Bodey et al. 1966). Numerous risk factors have been identified for the development of neutropenia and subsequent infection. Patient-specific risk factors include hematologic malignancy, advanced tumor stage, significant co-morbidities, poor performance status, and advanced age, while treatment-specific risk factors include chemotherapy type and dose intensity (Crawford et al. 2004). Incorporation of these risk factors into predictive models serves to guide prophylaxis and treatment recommendations against neutropenia (Lyman et al. 2005).

The inflammatory response to infection is severely weakened in the setting of neutropenia. Not only does this predispose to the development and rapid progression of infection, but it also lessens the associated signs and symptoms thereof. To prevent the development of infection and infection-related complications, it is essential that neutropenic cancer patients receive prompt evaluation and appropriate management. Antimicrobial prophylaxis for the prevention of infection is controversial. While clinicians are divided on its use, current guidelines recommend against the use of prophylactic antibiotics in neutropenic patients without fever, citing a lack of consistent reduction in mortality rates as well as concern over the emergence and propagation of drug-resistant bacteria and fungi (Hughes et al. 2002). An exception to this rule is found in patients considered to be at high risk for the development of *Pneumocystis carinii* pneumonitis. In these patients, prophylactic trimethoprim-sulfamethoxazole is recommended. Hematopoietic growth factors such as granulocyte colony-stimulating factor (filgrastim) or granulocyte-macrophage colony-stimulating factor (sargramostim) represent additional potential treatment options. When given as primary prophylaxis, these agents can reduce the incidence of febrile neutropenia by as much as 50% (Ozer et al. 2000). However, the American Society of Clinical Oncology (ASCO) does not recommend the routine use of prophylactic colony-stimulating factors in patients undergoing chemotherapy since no improvements in survival or response rate have been demonstrated with such practice (Ozer et al. 2000). Likewise, therapeutic colony-stimulating factor is not recommended as routine treatment for afebrile neutropenic patients based on a demonstrated lack of clinical benefit. Finally, adjustments to the chemotherapy regimen may become necessary in some neutropenic patients. Although this allows for bone marrow recovery, it should be considered an option of last resort since lower cancer-specific survival is well documented among patients receiving less than full-dose chemotherapy (Lepage et al. 1993; Budman et al. 1998).

13.6.1 Febrile Neutropenia

Febrile neutropenia is defined as: (1) a single oral temperature above 38.3°C or a temperature of 38.0°C or higher lasting longer than 1 h, and (2) an absolute neutrophil count below 500 cells/µl (Hughes et al. 2002). Of bladder cancer patients undergoing CMV or MVAC chemotherapy regimens, 10%–14% meet these established criteria (Gilligan et al. 2003). The importance of febrile neutropenia lies in the fact that infection is the most common cause of fever in the neutropenic setting (50%) and, in turn, the leading cause of chemotherapy-related death (Schimpff 1986). As such, fever in the context of neutropenia is considered to reflect active infection until proven otherwise.

13.6.1.1 Evaluation

Patients that meet the criteria for febrile neutropenia require urgent evaluation. The purpose of initial evaluation is twofold: (1) assess for the presence and site of infection and (2) determine the risk of significant infection-related complications. Evaluation begins with a thorough history and meticulous physical examination. Among immunocompromised patients, the classic signs and symptoms of infection are unreliable. A complete head-to-toe examination should be undertaken wherein every minor finding suspicious as a site or route of infection is investigated further. The gastrointestinal tract, lungs, skin, mouth, and pharynx deserve special consideration since endogenous flora originating from these sites account for the majority of neutropenic infections (Marchetti and Calandra 2004; Crawford et al. 2004). Careful evaluation of surgical scars, biopsy sites and venous catheter sites, if present, should also be made. The perineum and perianal region are often overlooked sites of infection that require careful inspection and palpation.

The initial laboratory evaluation includes a CBC and differential, electrolytes, BUN, creatinine, liver function studies, as well as cultures of blood (two sites) and urine. Sputum, cerebral spinal fluid, skin lesions, and stool should also be cultured if there is clinical suspicion of infection involving these sites. Most recommend obtaining a plain chest radiograph in all patients regardless of clinical findings. Ambulatory patients without clinical signs of pulmonary infection do not routinely require imaging of the chest because it is often of low diagnostic yield (Oude Nijhuis 2003; Sipsas et al. 2005). Laboratory and radiologic examinations may be insensitive markers of infection in the setting of neutropenia. As an example, up to 89% of febrile neutropenic patients with urinary tract infection lack pyuria and 40% of patients with pneumonia will have no abnormal findings on chest radiography.

13.6.1.2 Treatment

Empiric antibiotic therapy forms the cornerstone of treatment for febrile neutropenia and should be started immediately upon diagnosis. With such treatment, reductions in infection-related mortality have been observed over the past three decades. However, a mortality rate of 8% among contemporary hospitalized cancer patients with febrile neutropenia would seem to indicate that this condition remains a serious threat to life (Crawford et al. 2004). It has become clear that patients with febrile neutropenia are not all alike, and treatment regimens may be individualized. The Infectious Diseases Society of America (IDSA) has published guide-

Table 13.6. Infectious Diseases Society of America (IDSA) recommended antibiotic regimens for empiric treatment of febrile neutropenia

Setting	Regimen
Low risk	Ciprofloxacin plus amoxicillin-clavulanate
High risk	
Monotherapy	Cefepime or Ceftazidime or Imipenem or Meropenem
Combination	Aminoglycoside plus Antipseudomonal penicillin or Cephalosporin (cefepime or ceftazidime) or Carbapenem
Combination with vancomycin	Cefepime or ceftazidime ± aminoglycoside or Carbapenem ± aminoglycoside or Antipseudomonal penicillin + aminoglycoside

lines to facilitate the treatment of cancer patients with neutropenic fever (Table 13.6) (Hughes et al. 2002). A complete review of this complex topic is beyond the scope of this chapter; however, the treatment principles deserve discussion.

The IDSA treatment guidelines are based upon an individualized assessment of risk as determined by prognostic models. One such model, the Multinational Association of Supportive Care in Cancer (MASCC) Scoring Index, accurately predicts the risk of infection-related complications in neutropenic patients based upon seven clinical variables each with independent prognostic significance (Klastersky et al. 2000) (Table 13.7). Patients are generally divided into two groups: (1) low-risk (<5% risk of developing serious infection-related complications) and (2) high-risk (all other patients). Low-risk, compliant patients may be treated on an outpatient basis with oral antibiotics, the preferred agents being ciprofloxacin in combination with amoxicillin-clavulanate. In contrast, high-risk patients require hospitalization for i.v. antibiotics and close monitoring. The antibiotic of choice in high-risk patients is controversial and depends upon patient, cancer, and pathogen-related factors. Gram-negative bacilli and Gram-positive cocci are the predominant organisms involved and account for one-third and two-thirds of all cases, respectively (Table 13.8) (Hughes et al. 2002). Not only should the selected antibiotic regimen provide broad coverage of both groups, but it should also reflect the prevalence and susceptibility profiles of the individual institution. Historically, all patients received aminoglycoside-containing combination antibiotic therapy. The results of numerous contemporary studies have found that empiric antibiotic monotherapy provides similar efficacy to combination therapy in cases of uncomplicated neutropenic fever,

Table 13.7. The Multinational Association of Supportive Care in Cancer (MASCC) Risk Scoring Index for identification of low-risk febrile neutropenic patients at presentation

Characteristic	Score[a]
Extent of illness[b]	
No symptoms	5
Mild symptoms	5
Moderate symptoms	3
No hypotension	5
No chronic obstructive pulmonary disease	4
Solid tumor or no fungal infection	4
No dehydration	3
Outpatient at onset of fever	3
Age <60 years[c]	2

[a] Highest theoretical score is 26. A risk index score of ≥21 indicates that the patient is likely to be at low risk for complications and morbidity
[b] Choose one item only
[c] Does not apply to patients ≤16 years of age

Table 13.8. Most common bacterial causes of febrile neutropenia

Gram-positive cocci	Gram-negative bacilli
***Staphylococcus* species**	*Escherichia coli*
Coagulase-positive (*S. aureus*)	*Klebsiella* species
Coagulase-negative (*S. epidermidis* and others)	*Pseudomonas aeruginosa*
***Streptococcus* species**	
S. pneumoniae	
S. pyogenes	
Viridans group	
Enterococcus faecalis, E. faecium	
Corynebacterium species	

but with a lower rate of adverse reactions (De Pauw et al. 1994; Furno et al. 2002). This has led to a paradigm shift in treatment such that empiric antibiotic monotherapy is now considered appropriate for the majority of patients. The IDSA currently recommends four antibiotics as appropriate empiric monotherapy: ceftazidime, cefepime, imipenem, and meropenem (Hughes et al. 2002). Piperacillin-tazobactam represents a fifth monotherapy option with proven efficacy (Bow et al. 2003). Combination antibiotic therapy remains the standard of care for low-risk cases treated with oral therapy, high-risk cases involving hemodynamic instability, and cases arising from institutions with a high-frequency of multidrug-resistant pathogens. Recommended combination regimens include an aminoglycoside with an antipseudomonal β-lactam or cephalosporin (Table 13.6). The decision to add vancomycin is based upon a presumed risk of Gram-positive infection rather than routine practice. Indications for its empiric use include (1) apparent catheter-related infection; (2) positive blood culture for a Gram-positive bacterium; (3) colonization with methicillin-resistant *Staphylococcus aureus*; and (4) hemodynamic instability without an identifiable organism (Segal et al. 2005).

The response to treatment is evaluated after 2–3 days of therapy. If the causative organism is identified, antibiotics may be tailored accordingly. Unfortunately, the causative organism is confirmed in only one-third of patients (Bodey et al. 1978). In the event that the culture results are inconclusive, low-risk patients who remain afebrile and clinically stable may be switched to, or continued on, oral ciprofloxacin plus amoxicillin-clavulanate. Patients who demonstrate persistent fever after 3–5 days of empiric therapy are at risk for cryptic foci (e.g., abscess, endocarditis), resistant organisms, as well as fungal or viral infections (Sipsas et al. 2005). These patients require repeat evaluation and, most likely, modification of empiric antibiotic therapy. This should be done in consultation with an infectious disease specialist knowledgeable in the care of cancer patients. The recommended duration of antibiotic therapy for febrile neutropenia depends upon the absolute neutrophil count, presence or absence of fever on day 3, culture results, clinical course, and overall risk strata. The reader is referred to the 2002 IDSA guidelines in this regard (Hughes et al. 2002).

Antifungal therapy deserves appropriate consideration in cases of persistent neutropenic fever. Fungal infections account for 2%–10% of neutropenic infections overall, and up to 30% of infections in patients with persistent neutropenic fever (Wisplinghoff et al. 2003; de Pauw et al. 1994). Furthermore, fungal septicemia carries with it a high mortality rate, which approaches 90% in certain subgroups of patients (Sipsas et al. 2005). Based on the high prevalence and significant mortality of fungal infections, the IDSA recommends the empiric initiation of systemic antifungal therapy in neutropenic patients with fever persisting 5 days despite appropriate empiric antibiotic therapy (Hughes et al. 2002). *Candida* and *Aspergillus* species constitute the most common fungi identified. The drug of choice is amphotericin B, although fluconazole is an acceptable alternative. In contrast, there is no indication for empiric antiviral therapy in febrile neutropenic patients, nor are colony-stimulating factors routinely recommended. The use of antiviral agents is generally limited to cases of documented viral respiratory tract infection or documented herpes simplex or varicella-zoster cutaneous infection. Cutaneous viral infections, even if not the source of fever, require treatment since they are potential portals of entry for bacteria and fungi. Acyclovir, valacyclovir, or famciclovir are all appropriate antiviral treatment options.

13.7 Intractable Bladder Hemorrhage

Gross hematuria is not uncommon among patients with genitourinary malignancies. It can be the presenting sign of cancer involving the urinary tract or it may arise as a direct complication of cancer treatment. In most cases, the hematuria is of mild to moderate severity and resolves with conservative measures. Some cases, however, involve intractable hemorrhage that can be life-threatening without prompt and effective treatment. Intractable gross hematuria usually arises from the bladder secondary to advanced urothelial carcinoma, severe infection, chemotherapy-induced hemorrhagic cystitis, and radiation cystitis. Not only are these disease processes the most common causes of severe bladder hemorrhage, but they are also among the most difficult to treat. The optimal management of intractable bladder hemorrhage rests upon a determination of its cause and the institution of specific treatment at that time. Commonalities do exist, however, and they form the basis for management guidelines with broad application to all patients with severe bladder hemorrhage.

13.7.1 Transitional Cell Carcinoma

Transitional cell carcinoma (TCC) of the bladder is the fourth and ninth most common cancer in men and women, respectively (Jemal et al. 2005). Gross or microscopic hematuria is the typical manner of presentation (>80%). Seventy-five percent of patients are found to have superficial TCC while the remaining 25% are diagnosed with muscle-invasive disease. Treatment is primarily surgical with transurethral resection and radical cystectomy representing the standard options for superficial and invasive TCC, respectively. Since hematuria arises from the tumor itself, isolated or recurrent episodes of bleeding can be expected to resolve upon resection of the primary tumor. Exceptions do exist, however. These include: (1) large or locally advanced tumors deemed unresectable by cystectomy and (2) invasive tumors diagnosed in patients whose health status precludes cystectomy. Transurethral resection alone is inadequate in these cases and patients often develop troublesome hematuria as a consequence of inevitable tumor progression. Patients with advanced bladder cancer who fail conservative measures, as outlined below, may receive benefit from the addition of external beam radiotherapy. Radiotherapy for this purpose is generally well tolerated and may lead to resolution of hematuria in up to 59% of patients (Srinivasan et al. 1994).

13.7.2 Hemorrhagic Cystitis

Hemorrhagic cystitis is defined as gross hematuria secondary to diffuse inflammation of the bladder. Viral infection, radiation-induced inflammation, and chemotherapy-induced inflammation account for the majority of cases among cancer patients. While relatively uncommon in patients with genitourinary malignancies, viral-mediated hemorrhagic cystitis occurs in as many as 50 % of patients undergoing bone marrow transplantation (Bedi et al. 1995). The principle etiologic factor involved is the BK polyomavirus. Viral-mediated hemorrhagic cystitis often occurs several weeks after transplantation and is usually self-limited. The role of antiviral therapy is unclear at present; therefore, no specific treatment recommendations beyond standard hematuria management can be made for viral hemorrhagic cystitis.

The association between hemorrhagic cystitis and the oxazaphosphorine alkylating agents, cyclophosphamide and ifosfamide, has been well documented (Philips et al. 1961; Burkert 1983; Klastersky 2003). These chemotherapeutic drugs are used frequently in the treatment of breast cancer, lymphoma, and sarcoma but also have application in poor-risk and chemotherapy-resistant germ cell tumors. Cyclophosphamide is associated with a 24 % incidence of irritative voiding symptoms, 7 % – 53 % incidence of microscopic hematuria, and 1 % – 15 % incidence of gross hematuria (Talar-Williams et al. 1996). Older series report hemorrhagic cystitis in as many as 68 % of patients treated with cyclophosphamide (Burkert 1983). The causative agent of urothelial toxicity is acrolein, a hepatic metabolite eliminated primarily through urinary excretion (Cox 1979). Peak urine levels occur approximately 5 h after the start of chemotherapy infusion (Takamoto et al. 2004). Early pathologic changes include transmural edema, mucosal ulceration, and urothelial necrosis all of which may occur within 24 h of a single dose (DeVries and Freiha 1990). With repeated exposure, urothelial damage is progressive and may become irreversible (Forni et al. 1964; Koss 1967). The entire urothelium is at risk; however, the bladder is most frequently affected as it receives the longest exposure. In the acute setting, cystoscopy reveals diffuse inflammatory changes, while in the delayed setting chronic changes such as edema, pale mucosa, telangiectasia, and patchy inflammation are prominent (Coleman and Walther 2005).

Contemporary studies report a lower incidence of hemorrhagic cystitis secondary to cyclophosphamide than do historical series. This is due in large part to the development and routine application of preventative measures such as hydration and prophylactic mesna (sodium 2-mercaptoethane sulfonate). Intravenous normal saline is given concurrently with cyclophosphamide infusion to reduce the urinary concentration of acrolein through an increase in urine output (Philips et al. 1961). Unfortunately, the prevention of clinically significant urothelial damage is inconsistent with hydration; therefore, hydration therapy alone cannot be recommended as adequate prophylaxis. Mesna, a non-toxic thiol compound, was specifically developed to bind and inactivate acrolein without interfering with tumor control (Brock et al. 1981). Numerous randomized trials have demonstrated the superiority of mesna relative to placebo and hydration in the prevention of gross hematuria (Araujo and Tessler 1983; Fukuoka et al. 1991; Shepherd et al. 1991). With the routine incorporation of mesna into cyclophosphamide or ifosfamide-containing chemotherapy regimens, modern rates of severe hematuria range from 0 % – 13 %. Mesna must be administered before cyclophosphamide to ensure adequate urinary levels are available when acrolein reaches peak urinary concentration. For this reason, mesna has no place in the treatment of established cyclophosphamide-induced hemorrhagic cystitis. Based on simplicity, convenience, and proven efficacy, a two-dose mesna regimen (15 min before and 4 h after cyclophosphamide) is recommended (Katz et al. 1995). There is suggestion that the addition of dexamethasone may improve the prophylactic efficacy of mesna (Vieira et al. 2003). Prior episodes of hemorrhagic cystitis do not absolutely contraindicate the repeat administration of cyclophosphamide or ifosfamide provided that mesna is given prophylactically (Andriole et al. 1987).

The management of cyclophosphamide-induced hemorrhagic cystitis can be difficult. At the present time, there is no specific therapeutic option that can be recommended ahead of standard management strategies. Intravesical prostaglandin (PGE1, PGE2, and PGF2α) therapy is one option that may hold future promise. Initial interest in the use of prostaglandins was generated by case reports of demonstrated success in cases of otherwise intractable bladder hemorrhage secondary to cyclophosphamide (Miller et al. 1994; Trigg et al. 1990; Shurafa et al. 1987). Subsequent series report 50 % complete resolution of hematuria after the administration of carboprost tromethamine (PGF2α) for a median treatment period of 6 days (Levine and Jarrard 1993). Although the exact mechanism of action is unknown, prostaglandin may improve hematuria through platelet aggregation and vasoconstriction. Bladder spasms (78 %) are a frequent occurrence with intravesical prostaglandin therapy; however, adverse effects on renal or bladder function are negligible as are systemic complications. Prostaglandins have since found application in the management of other forms of severe hemorrhagic cystitis. Hyperbaric oxygen treatment (HBO), typically reserved for cases of refractory radiation cystitis, has also been used to treat hemorrhagic cystitis resulting from cyclophosphamide. Animal models suggest that HBO may be of value as prophylaxis or treatment in this setting (Hader et al. 1993).

13.7.3 Radiation Cystitis

Radiation cystitis is a late complication of radiotherapy which, by definition, occurs at least 90 days after the initiation of radiation treatment but may be delayed up to 10 years or more (Cox et al. 1995). Most patients develop severe irritative voiding symptoms; however, gross hematuria dominates the clinical picture (Pasquier et al. 2004). While any patient receiving pelvic radiotherapy is at risk, radiation cystitis is most common among those treated for prostate or cervical cancer. Three to five percent of such patients will develop late grade 3 hematuria, the incidence of which is directly related to both the biologic dose and the volume of tissue irradiated (Perez 1998; Lawton et al. 1991; Shipley et al. 1988; Dearnaley et al. 1999). In contrast to acute changes, late radiation injuries are irreversible and often progressive. There appears to be no correlation between the development of early and late radiation injuries. The pathophysiology of late radiation damage includes cellular depletion, fibrosis, and obliterative endarteritis (Pasquier et al. 2004). All of these changes lead to tissue ischemia and, in turn, delayed wound healing. Cystoscopically, such changes give the appearance of pale, frosted mucosa, scattered telangiectasia, and ulcers (Rigaud et al. 2004).

Radiation cystitis is perhaps the most difficult form of bladder hemorrhage to treat. The reason for this lies primarily in the ischemic nature of the injury and the propensity toward poor wound healing. Based on a lack of randomized controlled trials comparing available treatment options, firm guidelines for radiation cystitis management cannot be made (Denton et al. 2002). That being said, a tremendous amount of research has been devoted to examining the role of hyperbaric oxygen therapy (HBO) in the treatment of radiation injuries. First introduced into the field of radiation oncology in 1953 as a radiosensitizer, HBO has subsequently been shown to ameliorate radiation damage among a wide range of tissues, including the bladder (Gray et al. 1953; Capelli-Schellpfeffer and Gerber 1999; Feldmeier and Hampson 2002). Hyperbaric oxygen therapy involves the inhalation of 100% oxygen pressurized to 1.4–3.0 atm in sessions of 60–120 min. Under these conditions, alveolar, arterial, and tissue oxygen levels are driven to supraphysiologic levels. By improving the oxygenation of irradiated tissue, HBO stimulates angiogenesis, fibroblast proliferation, and collagen formation (Marx et al. 1990). Not only does this promote wound healing, but the vasoconstriction induced by an abundance of oxygen may also help to control bleeding (Capelli-Schellpfeffer and Gerber 1999). Retrospective studies examining the role of HBO in severe radiation cystitis report response rates of 77%–100% (complete response, 34%–100%; partial response, 12%–45%) (Mathews et al. 1999; Neheman et al. 2005). A single prospective study of HBO demonstrated an overall response rate of 92.5% among 40 patients with radiation cystitis refractory to standard measures (Bevers et al. 1995). Patients underwent 20 treatment sessions inhaling 100% oxygen at 3 atm for 90 min each. With a mean follow-up of 23 months, the recurrence rate of severe hematuria was 12% per year. It is difficult to predict the individual treatment outcome; however, the provision of HBO within 6 months of hematuria onset appears to improve the response rate (96% vs 66%, $p=0.003$) (Chong et al. 2005). Cancer patients who do not respond to HBO require evaluation for cancer recurrence since this is a common cause of persistent hematuria (Rijkmans et al. 1989). Hyperbaric oxygen therapy is generally well tolerated, with adverse events limited to case reports of visual disturbance, spontaneous pneumothorax, oxygen toxicity seizures, hypoglycemia, and loss of respiratory drive in hypercapnic patients (Capelli-Schellpfeffer and Gerber 1999). Contraindications to the use of HBO are listed in Table 13.9 (O'Reilly et al. 2002). Concern exists over the theoretic risk of cancer stimulation through HBO-mediated neoangiogenesis, immune suppression, and free radical toxicity. A review of the world literature in 2003, however, found that available in vitro, in vivo, and clinical studies suggested no more than a neutral effect of HBO on tumor growth (Feldmeier et al. 2003). Additional studies have found no evidence that exposure to hyperbaric oxygen promotes tumor growth, including that of prostate cancer (Chong et al. 2004). As such, a history of malignancy should not be considered a contraindication to treatment with HBO. Perhaps the largest obstacle to its use is cost. The average cost per session is $ 300–$ 400, which amounts to an estimated $ 10,000–$ 15,000 per patient (Norkool et al. 1993). While there exist no formal cost-comparisons among available treatments for radiation cystitis, HBO is still regarded as a cost-effective option and should be considered for refractory cases.

WF10, the i.v. formulation of a novel wound-healing agent, tetrachlorodecaoxygen, has demonstrated benefit in patients with wound healing disorders, including that arising from radiation injury (Hinz et al. 1986; Veerasarn et al. 2004). As an immune modifier, WF10 promotes the healing process through the inhibition of the chronic inflammatory process. Two human studies, including one randomized trial have evaluated the effica-

Table 13.9. Contraindications to use of hyperbaric oxygen therapy

Absolute contraindications	Relative contraindications
Untreated pneumothorax	Upper respiratory infections
Concurrent treatment with	Seizure disorders
Cis-platinum	High fevers
Doxorubicin	History of spontaneous pneumothorax
Bleomycin	Viral infections
Disulfiram	Congenital spherocytosis
Mafenide acetate	History of optic neuritis
	History of otosclerosis

cy of this novel agent in the treatment of radiation cystitis (Veerasarn et al. 2004, 2006). Among cervical cancer patients with grade 2 or 3 radiation cystitis, WF10 provided a complete response rate of 74%–88%. Although this was not statistically superior to the standard hematuria measures employed in the control arm, patients treated with WF10 demonstrated a lower rate of hematuria recurrence (47% vs 77%, $p=0.01$) and a longer estimated time to recurrence (>300 days vs <100 days, $p=0.004$). The administration protocols in both studies involved 0.5 mg/kg WF10 in 250 ml normal saline infused over 2 h on 5 consecutive days every 3 weeks for two cycles. Transient hemoglobinemia may occur in up to one-quarter of treated patients; however, there have been no serious safety concerns with WF10 in these or any other studies to date. At this time, the role of WF10 in the management of radiation cystitis remains investigational.

13.7.4 Treatment of Intractable Bladder Hemorrhage

The approach to the patient with intractable bladder hemorrhage is fairly standard and begins with a thorough evaluation to determine its cause. Information obtained on history (e.g., prior malignancy, prior radiotherapy, prior cyclophosphamide, etc.) may suggest the etiology; however, multiple factors may be involved and assumptions should not be made. Outside of the acute setting, all cases in which the etiology has not been identified require a formal hematuria workup, including cystoscopy, urine cytology, and upper tract imaging. The chronicity and severity of the hematuria as well as any prior attempts at therapy are important to determine. This may suggest to what degree, if any, the hematuria is refractory to conservative measures. Patients with severe hematuria can develop urinary retention secondary to the accumulation of blood clot within the bladder; therefore, the ability to void should be questioned. A list of the patient's current medications should be reviewed and any anticoagulants discontinued accordingly. The primary goals of physical examination are to determine the hemodynamic stability and overall health status of the patient as well as the presence of urinary retention. Laboratory studies should include a CBC and differential, serum electrolytes, BUN, creatinine, coagulation profile, and urine culture. Initial therapy is directed toward maintaining hemodynamic support through i.v. fluids as well as through blood and blood product replacement as necessary.

Whatever the etiology, the management of gross hematuria follows the same general principles as outlined in Table 13.10. Treatment is delivered in a stepwise manner according to hemodynamic stability, hematuria severity, and treatment response. A hematuria grading system has been proposed to facilitate treatment in this regard (Table 13.11) (DeVries and Freiha 1990). The first step involves bladder decompression through the insertion of a large-bore urethral catheter for clot evacuation and saline lavage. This is a simple maneuver that may slow or stop the bleeding altogether. Continuous bladder irrigation (CBI) through a three-way Foley catheter is initiated once the effluent is clear or pink-tinged and free of clots. In some instances, bedside lavage is inadequate and formal cystoscopic clot evacuation in the operating room becomes necessary. During this time, the bladder is carefully inspected for a source of hemorrhage, and biopsies or fulguration of suspicious areas can be performed. Cases not responsive to clot evacuation and fulguration or those with cystoscopic evidence of diffuse hemorrhage

Table 13.10. Graded management options for intractable bladder hemorrhage

Clot evacuation (catheter or cystoscopic) plus
Intermittent saline irrigation or
Continuous saline irrigation
Cystoscopy ± fulguration
Oral agents
E-aminocaproic acid (Amicar) (loading 5 g p.o./i.v., then maintenance 1 g/h)[a]
Sodium pentosan polysulphate (Elmiron) (begin 100 mg p.o. three times daily)
Intravesical agents
Alum 1% (250 ml/h via continuous bladder irrigation)[b]
Prostaglandin-E1, -E2, and -F2α (see text for dosing)
Formalin (begin ≤4%, up to 10%)
Hyperbaric oxygen therapy
Embolization of internal iliac artery
Surgery (urinary diversion, with or without open bladder packing or cystectomy)

[a] Maximum daily dose of Amicar is 30 g
[b] Do not exceed 3 g/h alum in patients with renal insufficiency

Table 13.11. Hematuria grading system and suggested management

Grade	Treatment
Mild	
No acute decrease in hematocrit (Hct)	Saline irrigation Oral Amicar or Elmiron Intravesical alum
Moderate	
Drop in Hct Requires ≤6 HU of packed red blood cells to maintain hemodynamic stability Urinary clot retention	Above plus Clot evacuation Cystoscopy ± fulguration Intravesical prostaglandin or formalin
Severe	
Refractory to saline irrigation, Amicar, alum, prostaglandin Requires >6 HU of packed red blood cells to maintain hemodynamic stability	Above plus: Intravesical formalin Embolization Surgery

require supplementary therapy with systemic or intravesical agents.

E-aminocaproic acid (Amicar), given orally or parenterally, inhibits the process of fibrinolysis by preventing the activation of plasminogen to plasmin. It is used commonly in the field of cardiothoracic surgery based on demonstrated efficacy in the reduction of postoperative hemorrhage (Trinh-Duc et al. 1992). Unfortunately, there have been no comparative trials evaluating the efficacy of this agent in the context of hemorrhagic cystitis. Proponents of its use for bladder hemorrhage cite anecdotal reports of apparent success in addition to the evidence provided by disciplines outside of urology (Aroney et al. 1980; Lakhani et al. 1999; Stefanini et al. 1990). Administration involves a loading dose of 5 g followed by 1 g/h for 8 h or until bleeding stops. The maximum recommended dosage in 24 h is 30 g. As an inhibitor of fibrinolysis, E-aminocaproic acid promotes clot formation; therefore, it should be used in conjunction with CBI. Upper tract hemorrhage remains a contraindication to its use since clot formation within the ureter can lead to obstruction and acute renal failure.

Sodium pentosan polysulphate (Elmiron), given orally, is a low-molecular-weight heparinoid that replaces deficient glycosaminoglycans on the bladder surface (Parsons et al. 2002). In doing so, it removes potential triggers of hematuria by protecting the bladder wall from bacterial adherence as well as from the absorption of toxic substances within the urine. Such protection may also facilitate healing of the bladder surface. While used more commonly in the treatment of interstitial cystitis, sodium pentosan polysulphate has been shown to resolve hematuria in 50% of patients with radiation or cyclophosphamide-induced hemorrhagic cystitis when given as first-line treatment (Parsons et al. 1993; Sandhu et al. 2004). Dosing begins at 100 mg three times daily with a gradual reduction to 100 mg daily as hematuria improves. Treatment may be discontinued when the hematuria resolves completely. At this time, there is no data available regarding the rate or time to recurrence with such therapy.

Of the commonly used intravesical agents, alum and prostaglandins have the advantage of not requiring an anesthetic. Alum (aluminium ammonium sulphate or aluminium potassium sulphate) is an astringent that causes protein precipitation, vasoconstriction, and decreased capillary permeability without damaging normal urothelium (Ostroff and Chenault 1982; Arrizabalaga et al. 1987). Commonly delivered as a 1% solution (50 g alum in 5 l sterile water) via CBI at a rate of 250 ml/h, alum leads to the complete resolution of hematuria in 60%–100% of hemorrhagic cystitis patients (Ostroff and Chenault 1982; Gattegno et al. 1990; Choong et al. 2000). The median time to resolution of hematuria ranges from 3–4 days, but therapy may be required for as long as 7 days. Up to 20% of patients will develop recurrent hematuria within 5–10 months. The risk of systemic toxicity is low because urothelial permeability to aluminum is minimal and prompt renal excretion ensures elevated aluminum levels are avoided. There are case reports of aluminum encephalopathy with intravesical alum, the majority of which occurred in patients with baseline renal insufficiency (Kavoussi et al. 1986; Shoskes et al. 1992; Perazella et al. 1993). In addition to central nervous system disturbance (lethargy, confusion, seizures), aluminum toxicity can result in metabolic acidosis and coagulopathy. While renal failure is not an absolute contraindication to the use of intravesical alum, it should be used with caution and at a dose that should not exceed 3 g/h (Kennedy et al. 1984). Aluminum levels should be monitored periodically in such patients. Intravesical alum irrigation should be discontinued immediately if serum aluminum levels are elevated or systemic toxicity is suspected.

Prostaglandin-E1, -E2, and -F2α, already discussed as a treatment option for cyclophosphamide-induced hemorrhagic cystitis, may prove beneficial in cases arising from a variety of other causes as well. Numerous protocols for prostaglandin administration have been described including: (1) 50 ml of 4–10 mg/l of carboprost tromethamine left indwelling for 2 h four times per day alternating with saline CBI and (2) 8–10 mg/l of PGF2α via saline CBI at a rate of 100 ml/h for 10 h (Choong et al. 2000). Both protocols lead to a complete response in 50% of patients treated over a median period of 6 days (Levine and Jarrard 1993). A small trial comparing intravesical PGF2α and 1% alum in patients with hemorrhagic cystitis of unknown origin demonstrated similar response rates of 80% and 90%, respectively (Praveen et al. 1992). Although there was a complete lack of systemic side effects in both groups, virtually all patients developed transient bladder spasms requiring symptomatic control. Since prostaglandins are very expensive, 1% alum remains the intravesical agent of first choice.

The best known and most effective intravesical hemostatic agent is formalin, the aqueous solution of formaldehyde. When administered intravesically, formalin rapidly fixes the bladder mucosa through a process involving protein cross-linking. This prevents further necrosis and blood loss from occurring (DeVries and Freiha 1990). First introduced in 1969 for the treatment of radiation cystitis, 10% formalin led to the complete resolution of hematuria in 22 of 24 patients with no serious side effects noted (Brown 1969). Since that time, formalin has also demonstrated success in the treatment of hemorrhagic cystitis. At the same time, the potential for serious toxicity (up to 15%) with bladder formalinization is well documented. In light of the potential for significant treatment-related morbidity, formal instillation is generally reserved for cases of intractable bladder hemorrhage refractory to conservative treatment.

The results of a meta-analysis evaluating 235 cases of intractable bladder hemorrhage treated with intravesical formalin form the foundation upon which most recommendations are made (Donahue and Frank 1989). Formalin can be administered intravesically in concentrations ranging from 1%–10% (typically 1%, 5%, 10%). While there is a trend toward improved results with 10% formalin, there is no statistical difference in complete response among the three preparations (71%–83%). Hematuria typically resolves within 48 h (1–5 days) and the duration of response is 3–4 months, regardless of dose. Major complications (5%–15%) include bladder contracture, ureteral stenosis, acute renal failure, and even death. Although there appears to be a trend toward a higher rate of major complications with higher concentrations of formalin, this has never been proven. Similarly, the rate of minor complications (14%–78%), of which irritative voiding symptoms are most common, appear to correlate with dose. Given the lack of comparative studies it is difficult to make firm recommendations regarding the optimal concentration of formalin. There is some suggestion that hematuria secondary to radiation cystitis may require 5% or more formalin, while hematuria due to cyclophosphamide or bladder cancer may require less than 5% formalin; however, this is merely conjecture. Most centers advocate the initial use of 4% or less formalin since this concentration appears to optimize the treatment response (>75%) while minimizing the potential for minor and major complications (Russo 2000).

Formalin must be instilled under a spinal or general anesthetic since it is caustic to the sensory nerves of the bladder. The procedure begins with a formal cystoscopic evaluation of the entire bladder and urethra. Clot evacuation and fulguration of bleeding vessels can be performed as necessary. Vesicoureteric reflux significantly predisposes the patient to upper tract damage with intravesical formalin; therefore a cystogram must be performed prior to every instillation. Documented reflux is not a contraindication to formalin treatment but does necessitate the insertion of occlusive Fogarty balloon catheters into the affected ureteric orifice(s) (Gottesman and Ehrlich 1974). Reverse Trendelenburg positioning and the induction of a brisk diuresis can also protect against the reflux of formalin. The presence of bladder perforation, which remains an absolute contraindication to the use of formalin, can also be documented by a cystogram. Prior to beginning formalin instillation, the entire perineum should be painted with petroleum jelly and, in women, the vagina packed with petroleum jelly gauze to protect exposed skin and mucosa from the caustic effect of formalin. Through an 18-F Foley catheter, the bladder is then filled to capacity with 1%–2% formalin under gravity at a pressure kept below 15 cm H_2O (catheter level at 15 cm above pubic symphysis). Although the optimal contact time is not known, most recommend limiting the treatment session to 15 min (Choong et al. 2000).

Approximately 10%–30% of patients with severe hemorrhagic cystitis will not respond to low-dose formalin instillation. A second instillation using high-dose formalin (5%–10%) remains an option; unfortunately, repeat administration of formalin is associated with a lower complete response rate (50%) and a higher rate of major complications (40%). Treatment alternatives include hyperbaric oxygen therapy, arteriographic embolization, and urinary diversion with or without cystectomy. Hyperbaric oxygen is most appropriate for refractory radiation cystitis as described above; however, animal studies suggest that it may also be of benefit in cases of cyclophosphamide-induced hemorrhagic cystitis (Hader et al. 1993).

Therapeutic embolization of the internal iliac artery to control bladder hemorrhage was first reported in 1974 (Hald and Mygind 1974). Most studies report a response rate in excess of 80%, usually of immediate onset (McIvor et al. 1982; Rodriguez et al. 2003; Nabi et al. 2003). A common complication of embolization is severe transient gluteal pain caused by claudication of the superior gluteal artery (Choong et al. 2000). Case reports of leg ischemia and bladder necrosis also exist (Woodside et al. 1976; Braf and Koontz 1977). Improvements in both technology and technique have led to superselective embolization. With such procedures, the efficacy of embolization is maintained while patient morbidity is reduced (De Berardinis et al. 2005). Embolization is most appropriate for those patients who are refractory to conservative measures, including formalin instillation, but whose health status precludes surgical intervention.

Open surgery is an option of last resort to be used only in patients with massive intractable bladder hemorrhage who are otherwise good surgical candidates. Open cystotomy combined with bladder packing and percutaneous urinary diversion, cutaneous ureterostomy, and cystectomy with urinary diversion have all been described, each with variable outcome (Andriole et al. 1990; Pomer et al. 1983; Okaneya et al. 1993). Unfortunately, many patients with severe hemorrhagic cystitis are elderly and unfit for invasive surgery. It is in situations such as this that intractable bladder hemorrhage becomes a lethal event.

13.8 Ureteral Obstruction

Malignant ureteral obstruction is not rare among cancer patients, with a cumulative incidence of 4.4% in advanced cases (Coleman and Walther 2005). While pelvic genitourinary malignancies such as ovarian, cervical, bladder, and prostate cancer (PCa) are the most common causes of malignant ureteral obstruction (70%), retroperitoneal lymphadenopathy secondary to lymphoma, and germ cell cancer are not uncommon (Holden et al. 1979). Obstruction may result from intramural tumor growth, extramural compression, or from retroperitoneal fibrosis secondary to cancer treatment (Montana and Fowler 1989). Approximately 2.5% of women who undergo definitive radiation treatment for cervical cancer will develop ureteral obstruction (McIntyre et al. 1995).

13.8.1 Presentation

The manner of presentation of ureteral obstruction depends upon the time course over which it develops and whether or not both sides are involved. Acute unilateral obstruction presents with the symptoms typical of renal colic while chronic unilateral obstruction tends to be clinically silent and is most often identified through the incidental detection of hydronephrosis on abdominal imaging. Bilateral obstruction, acute or chronic, presents with decreased urine output and signs and symptoms of uremia.

13.8.2 Evaluation

Evaluation of the patient with suspected ureteral obstruction begins with a complete history and physical examination. Laboratory evaluation includes a CBC, serum electrolytes, BUN, creatinine, and urine culture. Since patients with ureteral obstruction may require the placement of percutaneous nephrostomy tubes, coagulation parameters should be routinely measured if obstruction is suspected. It is of the utmost importance to rule out the presence of concomitant urinary tract infection. Fever and flank pain together with leukocytosis and pyuria suggest urosepsis, a urologic emergency. Without prompt endoscopic or percutaneous decompression, obstructed urosepsis is a potentially lethal condition. Upper tract imaging should be performed in all cases of suspected ureteral obstruction. Available options include intravenous pyelography, retrograde pyelography, antegrade pyelography, renal ultrasonography, radionuclide renography, and CT or MRI of the abdomen and pelvis (Fig. 13.4). These studies can confirm the presence and site of obstruction and may also provide clues as to the etiology. In this regard, CT and MRI provide the best anatomic detail of the retroperitoneum and pelvis (Fig. 13.5). Upper tract imaging can also establish the presence and severity of obstructive uropathy. The finding of small atrophic kidneys with marked cortical thinning indicates chronic obstruction (Fig. 13.6). Renal deterioration secondary to chronic obstruction is unlikely to improve with decompression; therefore, intervention is reserved for infected renal units (Logothetis et al. 2003).

13.8.3 Treatment

The management of malignant ureteral obstruction is controversial and depends upon many factors includ-

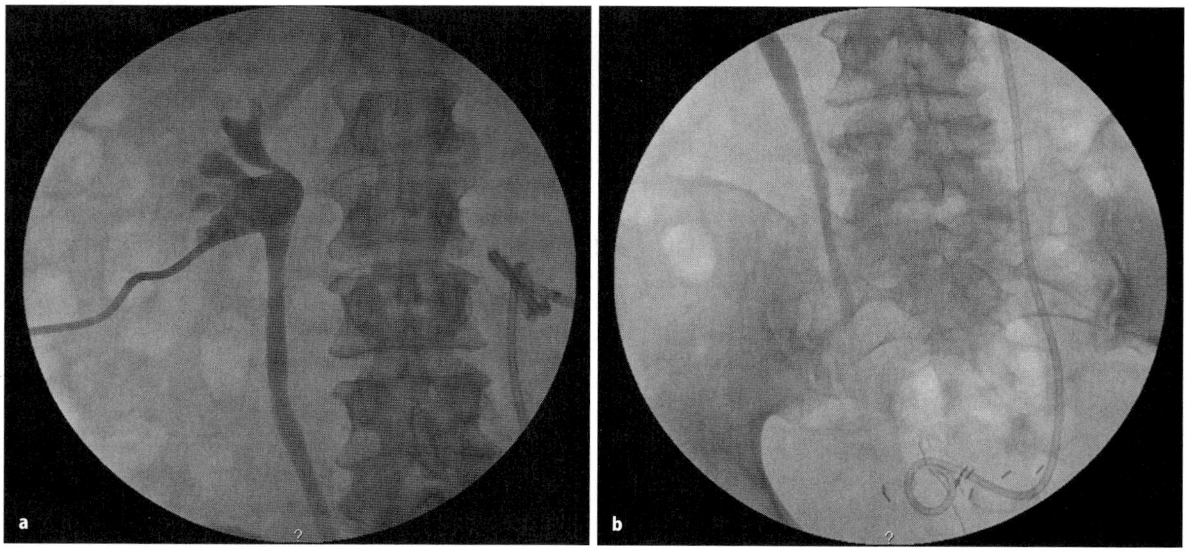

Fig. 13.4a–c. Distal ureteric obstruction in patient with locally recurrent cervical cancer. **a** Antegrade nephrostogram demonstrating left hydronephrosis and hydroureter, indwelling ureteric stent is visualized within right ureter. **b** Obstruction visualized at level of distal right ureter, no contrast within bladder.

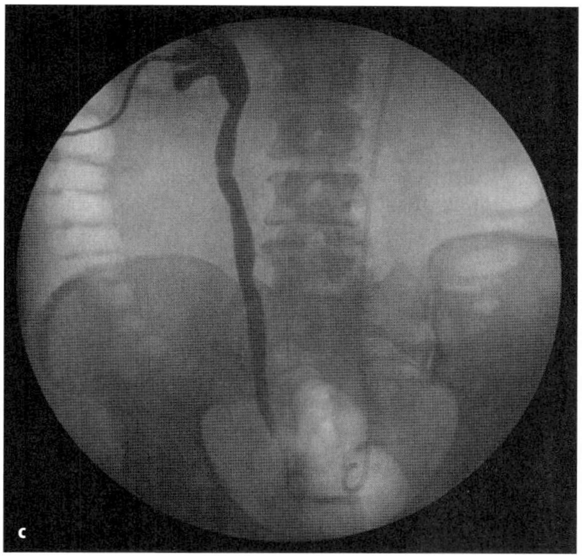

Fig. 13.4c. Ureteric stent placed beyond point of obstruction

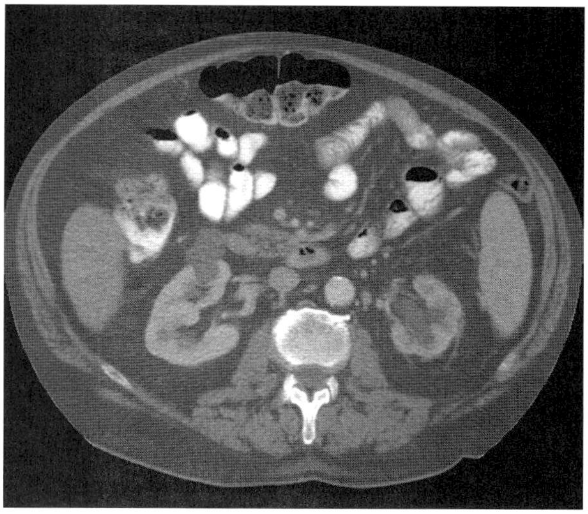

Fig. 13.6. Atrophic left kidney. Noncontrast CT demonstrating left hydronephrosis and renal atrophy in patient with distal ureteric obstruction

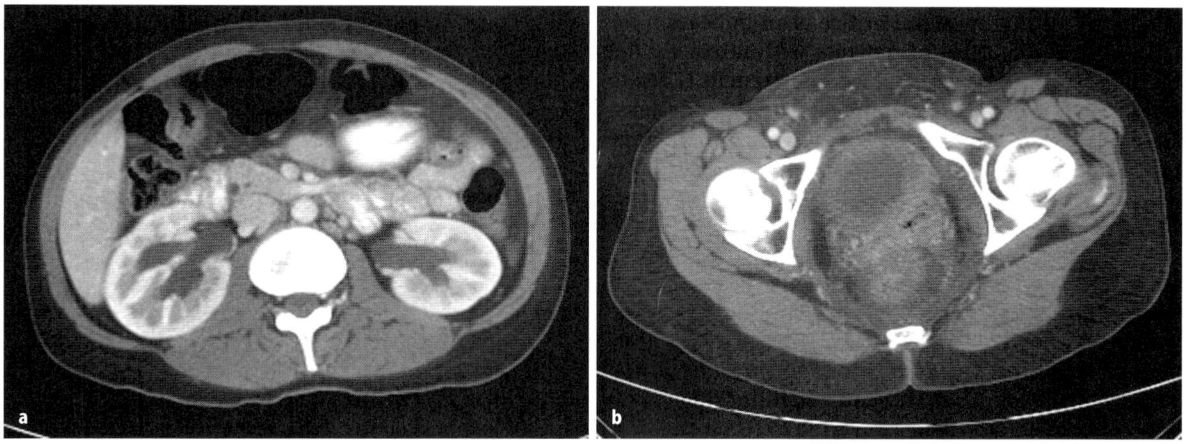

Fig. 13.5a, b. Distal ureteric obstruction in patient with locally recurrent cervical cancer. **a** CT demonstrating bilateral hydronephrosis. b Posterior pelvic mass invading and displacing posterior bladder wall

ing oncologic prognosis, quality of life, and treatment-related complications. Quite often, malignant ureteral obstruction is a late presentation of advanced, incurable malignancy and portends a poor prognosis. In this circumstance, the provision of ureteral decompression is unlikely to improve either the quality or quantity of life. The median survival of patients with active malignancy who undergo renal decompression through internal or external drainage is only 3–7 months (Wilson et al. 2005; Donat and Russo 1996; Shekarriz et al. 1999). The only situation in which ureteral decompression is uniformly recommended is in the infrequent circumstance that an improvement in renal function will facilitate the provision of therapeutic or palliative chemotherapy (Russo 2000). Lymphoma and germ cell cancer represent two such chemotherapy-sensitive malignancies wherein maximal preservation of renal function is an important determinant of chemotherapy delivery and ultimate success (Logothetis et al. 2003; Ondrus et al. 2001).

Noninvasive treatment modalities, including retrograde internal ureteral stent (IUS) insertion and radiology-guided percutaneous nephrostomy (PCN) insertion, are most appropriate for malignant ureteral obstruction. It is difficult to make a firm recommendation in either regard since the quality of life they afford appears to be similar and both options have an equally high complication rate (13%–63%) (Little et al. 2003; Ganatra and Loughlin 2005; Donat and Russo 1996; Shekarriz et al. 1999). Stent or PCN-related infection, obstruction, migration, and dislodgement are common and often necessitate prolonged hospitalization. In experienced hands, PCN drainage can be established in 98% of cases, with a major complication rate of 4% (renal hemorrhage requiring transfusion, vascular injury, sepsis, bowel injury, lung injury) and a mortality rate of 0.05%–0.3% (Dyer et al. 1997; Stables 1982). Cystoscopic IUS insertion appears to have a higher initial failure rate (15%–79%) than PCN, leading some authors to propose that PCN should be the management option of first choice in the acute setting (Ganatra and Loughlin 2005; Chitale et al. 2002; Park et al. 2002). Likewise, the accumulated incidence of recurrent obstruction may be higher with IUS (11%) than with PCN (1.3%) (Ku et al. 2004). Numerous studies have sought to determine if tumor type, degree of hydronephrosis, and level of obstruction are predictive of treatment failure; however, the results have thus far been contradictory (Ganatra and Loughlin 2005). That being said, some centers do recommend immediate PCN for ureteral obstruction secondary to advanced cervical cancer citing high failure rates with IUS in the short and long term (Ku et al. 2004). Cystoscopic evidence of tumor invasion appears to predict for IUS failure; therefore, radiographic imaging suspicious for involvement of the bladder and ureteral orifice is an indication for initial PCN. One-third of patients will ultimately fail IUS within 6 months and require long-term PCN due to repeat obstruction. Attempts to improve the long-term success rates of IUS include frequent stent exchange (every 3 months) and the ipsilateral insertion of two indwelling ureteral stents (two 7-F stents) (Ganatra and Loughlin 2005; Rotariu et al. 2001). Periodic imaging to confirm interval resolution or improvement of hydronephrosis is also warranted in patients with IUS. Despite the relatively high failure rate of IUS, most authorities recommend a trial of retrograde ureteral stents in all patients without obvious involvement of the distal ureter and bladder (Ganatra and Loughlin 2005). Likewise, PCN tubes should be converted to IUS in an antegrade fashion after a period of renal decompression. Situations in which retrograde stent insertion is advisable over PCN include those in which anatomic anomalies present a technical challenge to PCN insertion (e.g., horseshoe kidney) or cases involving a solitary kidney in which renal loss secondary to PCN-related renal hemorrhage would be disastrous (Uthappa and Cowan 2005).

Decompression of solitary or bilaterally obstructed kidneys may result in a postobstructive diuresis with urine output in excess of 200 ml/ h. Most commonly, this reflects the appropriate excretion of excess sodium, urea, and water retained during the period of obstruction. Apart from the provision of oral fluids and the periodic evaluation of serum electrolytes, this form of diuresis requires no specific intervention. Serum creatinine and blood urea nitrogen typically normalize within 48 h. On occasion, a pathologic diuresis involving water or sodium-wasting may ensue secondary to significant distal renal tubular damage. Vital statistics including postural blood pressure measurements should be performed on a frequent basis if a pathologic diuresis is suspected. These patients require careful monitoring and copious fluid replacement with 0.9% or 0.45% saline in order to avoid dehydration and electrolyte abnormalities.

In light of the significant long-term complication rate associated with mechanical drainage, patients with IUS or PCN require periodic monitoring with serum creatinine, urine culture, and upper tract imaging. Ureteral stents and percutaneous nephrostomy tubes should be exchanged every 3–4 months to prevent encrustation and obstruction. Depending on the chemotherapy or radiation-sensitivity of the etiologic malignancy, mechanical drainage may not be required indefinitely. Most cases of extrinsic obstruction secondary to germ cell or lymphomatous retroperitoneal lymphadenopathy will resolve with appropriate cytotoxic chemotherapy (Logothetis et al. 2003). Likewise, up to 70% and 85% of patients with hormonally naïve locally advanced PCa treated with androgen ablation or radiotherapy, respectively, will experience a relief of obstruction, obviating the need for mechanical drainage (Michigan and Catalona 1977; Megalli et al. 1974).

Malignant ureteral obstruction is, in most cases, a manifestation of advanced, incurable disease and portends a poor prognosis. Even with the establishment of mechanical internal or external drainage, the median survival is 3–6 months among the most common etiologic malignancies. Furthermore, treatment-related morbidity is high and patients can expect to spend a significant portion of their remaining days in hospital (18%–46%) (Little et al. 2003; Romero et al. 2005). While IUS or PCN appear to be of questionable benefit in the palliative setting, they retain utility in the treatment of chemotherapy or radiation-sensitive malignancies. Clearly, this is a situation in which treatment, however minimally invasive it may be, should be approached in a cautious mannerand only after due consideration has been given to the ultimate prognosis as well as the wishes of a fully informed patient and family.

13.9 Bladder Outlet Obstruction

Acute urinary retention is not uncommon in cancer patients, particularly those with genitourinary malignancies. Numerous etiologies exist and can be grouped into two broad categories: (1) mechanical bladder outlet obstruction (BOO) and (2) neurophysiologic dysfunction. Localized growth of PCa is a common cause of BOO. While symptomatic presentation is uncommon today, up to 82% of patients with PCa in the pre-PSA era presented with symptoms of urinary obstruction (Brawn et al. 1994). Furthermore, up to 35% of PCa patients placed on watchful waiting will eventually require transurethral prostatectomy (TURP) for symptomatic progression or urinary retention (Whitmore et al. 1991). Likewise, surgical and nonsurgical therapies directed toward prostate cancer may predispose to urinary retention. Bladder neck contracture (BNC) is reported in 1.3%–27% of patients after radical prostatectomy and 1.5%–22% of patients will develop urinary retention following prostatic brachytherapy (Anger et al. 2005; Stone and Stock 2002).

Neurophysiologic bladder dysfunction may arise secondary to medication side effects, postoperative pain and immobility, radical pelvic surgery, and chronic disease such as diabetes mellitus. Preexisting bladder dysfunction is common among elderly patients and even minor insults can trigger urinary retention. Medications with anticholinergic, sympathomimetic, and opioid activity are well known for their adverse effects on bladder function in this regard and should be discontinued or substituted if possible. Up to 50% of patients undergoing abdominoperineal resection or radical hysterectomy will develop bladder dysfunction as a result of interruption of parasympathetic innervation (Eickenberg et al. 1976). Fortunately, urinary retention secondary to radical pelvic surgery will spontaneously resolve in up to 90% of patients thus affected.

13.9.1 Evaluation

The diagnosis of urinary retention is established relatively easily. Patients typically complain of severe suprapubic pain and the inability to void. Physical examination often reveals a lower midline abdominal mass; however, dullness with percussion of the lower abdomen may be a more sensitive sign of bladder fullness. Apart from establishing urinary drainage, the next step is to differentiate mechanical obstruction from neurophysiologic dysfunction. Pelvic and rectal examination may identify a large obstructing pelvic tumor, while a focused neurologic exam demonstrating sensory or motor abnormalities may suggest a neurophysiologic cause. Further enquiry should be made into baseline voiding status, prior episodes of retention and associated treatment, overall health status, as well as the presence of medications or chronic illnesses known to undermine bladder function. Since urinary tract infection can complicate or precipitate urinary retention, the presence of irritating voiding symptoms or fever should be questioned. Renal insufficiency may complicate longstanding or severe urinary retention; therefore, azotemia and associated electrolyte abnormalities must be ruled out. Laboratory evaluation includes a CBC, serum electrolytes, BUN, and serum creatinine. Once urine becomes available, a urinalysis and urine culture should also be performed. Imaging of the upper tracts is indicated if renal dysfunction is present. Renal size and cortical thickness may suggest the degree and duration of obstruction and may also provide some measure of salvageable renal function. Ultrasound appears to be the most cost-effective imaging modality in this regard (Reisman et al. 1991).

13.9.2 Treatment

The first step in the management of urinary retention, regardless of etiology, is bladder decompression through the insertion of a urethral Foley catheter. Should this prove difficult, attempts should be made to insert a coudé-tipped catheter. Difficult catheterization often indicates the presence of an obstructing process such as urethral stricture or prostatic in-growth, benign or malignant. Situations such as this may require formal cystoscopy and possible urethral dilation for catheter insertion. In the event that all attempts at catheterization fail, the insertion of a suprapubic cystostomy tube is the most appropriate alternative. This can usually be performed percutaneously at the bedside. A history of lower abdominal or pelvic surgery is a contraindication to the percutaneous insertion of an suprapubic tube since intervening bowel may be injured. In this circumstance, suprapubic drainage should be established under radiologic guidance or in the operating room through open techniques.

Relief of longstanding bladder outlet obstruction can result in a postobstructive diuresis. This most commonly reflects the appropriate excretion of retained sodium, water and urea; however, a concentrating defect or a sodium-wasting nephropathy, both secondary to distal renal tubular damage, may also play a role. Management is similar to that arising from upper tract obstruction.

Once bladder decompression has been achieved, further management is dictated by the underlying pathologic process. Depending on the patient's health and prior voiding status, a trial of voiding is warranted in most cases. Retention secondary to neurophysiologic bladder dysfunction often resolves after a period of bladder decompression. Cases in which spontaneous voiding is slow to return require the initiation of clean intermittent catheterization every 4–6 h (Lapides et al. 1972). Intermittent catheterization has demonstrated clear superiority over chronic indwelling catheterization in terms of preserving upper tract function and minimizing urinary tract infection and stone formation. Benign prostatic hypertrophy alone or together with neurologic dysfunction warrants a trial of α-adrenergic blockade (Flomax 0.4 mg p.o. daily) and/or 5-α-reductase inhibition (Finasteride 5 mg p.o. daily) therapy.

Locally advanced prostate cancer, not uncommonly, precipitates urinary retention through compression of the prostatic urethra and bladder neck. The most appropriate initial therapy in the hormonally naïve patient is androgen deprivation therapy. This may involve either surgical (bilateral orchiectomy) or chemical castration (LHRH agonist). Although castrate levels of serum testosterone are achieved much more rapidly with bilateral orchiectomy (immediate) than with LHRH agonist therapy (3–4 weeks), the reduction in prostate and tumor volume is delayed with both, as is the ability to spontaneously void. Two-thirds of patients thus treated will ultimately regain the ability to void; however, roughly 50 % of patients will require catheterization for a period of 21–60 days in the interim (Fleischmann and Catalona 1985). Temporary drainage can be achieved through either continuous or intermittent catheterization, depending on the ease of catheterization. Up to 22 % of patients will develop urinary retention a mean of 21 months after the initiation of hormonal therapy (Sehgal et al. 2005). Prognostic factors for urinary retention in this circumstance include a high Gleason score (> 7) and urinary retention at the start of hormonal therapy. Those cases that are unresponsive to androgen deprivation or known to be resistant at baseline require TURP or intraprostatic urethral stenting. The insertion of a urethral stent is most appropriate for those patients who are poor surgical candidates and refuse an indwelling catheter. As many as 88 %–100 % of patients are able to void through a urethral stent with acceptable morbidity out to 1 year (Ok et al. 2005; Guazzoni et al. 1994). Based on concerns over the risk of infection and possible obstruction secondary to progressive tumor growth, urethral stents are only recommended in patients with a limited life expectancy.

Palliative or channel TURP is the gold standard treatment for PCa-related urinary retention unresponsive to medical therapy. Although less successful and associated with more complications than TURP performed for BPH, palliative TURP is considered a safe and efficacious procedure. Up to 79 % of patients will regain the ability to void despite the relatively high rate of failure at initial trial of voiding (42 %) (Crain et al. 2004). Morbidity is acceptable with an 8 % transfusion rate and negligible perioperative mortality rate. The reoperation rate is relatively high (22 %–29 %) and likely reflects less than complete resection (mean 12-g resection), continued local tumor growth, and the propensity of tumor to bleed (Mazur and Thompson 1991; Crain et al. 2004). Photoselective vaporization of the prostate (PVP) using high-power potassium-titanyl-phosphate (KTP) laser energy is a relatively new procedure that appears to be an acceptable alternative to standard TURP for symptomatic obstructive uropathy secondary to either PCa or BPH (Sulser et al. 2004). Although no randomized controlled trials have compared these two modalities in the setting of PCa, similar improvement in peak flow rates and urinary symptom scores have been demonstrated in patients with BPH (Shingleton et al. 1999). Perceived advantages to PVP include less bleeding, lower transfusion rate, shorter catheterization, and more rapid convalescence (Kumar 2005).

Chronic catheterization via an indwelling urethral or suprapubic catheter is an option of last resort typically reserved for terminally ill patients or those who fail medical and surgical therapies. Suprapubic catheterization may be preferable to urethral catheterization based on long-term data in spinal cord-injured patients, demonstrating lower rates of symptomatic urinary tract infection and upper tract deterioration with suprapubic drainage (Ku et al. 2005; Esclarin de Ruz et al. 2000). To minimize catheter-related morbidity, scheduled catheter changes should be conducted on a monthly basis (Russo 2000). Chronic suppressive antibiotics are not recommended in catheterized patients but short-course antibiotic therapy may be used at the time of catheter exchange.

13.9.3 Urinary Retention After Prostatectomy

Prostate cancer treatment with curative intent can also predispose to urinary retention. Although the true incidence of bladder neck contracture following radical prostatectomy is not known, 1.3 %–27 % of patients will develop symptomatic BNC requiring treatment (Anger et al. 2005). Surgical technique remains a critical determinant of BNC development; however, risk factors for microvascular disease such as smoking, hypertension, and diabetes mellitus also appear to play a role (Borboroglu et al. 2000). Simple dilation appears to be effective; however, some authors question the long-term patency rates with such treatment. Transurethral incision of the contracture using cold knife, electrocautery, or the holmium:YAG laser is the most commonly recommended treatment for severe BNC and those cases involving urinary retention (Anger et al. 2005; Salant et al. 1990). Great care must be taken when performing transurethral incision since deep incision may cause sphincteric damage and, in turn, stress urinary incontinence.

13.9.4 Urinary Retention After Brachytherapy

Urinary retention affects 1.5 %–22 % of men within a median of 2 months following prostatic brachytherapy (Stone and Stock 2002; Flam et al. 2004). Identified preimplant risk factors include an International Prostate Symptom Score above 20 and a prostate volume larger than 35 cm^3 (Terk et al. 1998; Gelblum et al. 1999). Attempts to reduce the risk of urinary retention with prophylactic α-adrenergic blockade (Flomax) have thus far been unsuccessful (Elshaikh et al. 2005).

The majority of cases respond to conservative measures such as catheter drainage plus or minus α-blockade, those that do not require TURP. According to a recent meta-analysis, up to 8.7% of brachytherapy patients undergo TURP after implantation; however, large contemporary series report a lower rate of 1.1%–2% (Stone and Stock 2002; Allen et al. 2005; Kollmeier et al. 2005). Urinary incontinence, while uncommon after TURP performed for BPH (1%–5%), is reported in up to 70% of brachytherapy patients who undergo TURP (Foote et al. 1991; Hu and Wallner 1998). The results of more recent series suggest the rate of post-TURP incontinence is 0%–18% (Stone and Stock 2002; Kollmeier et al. 2005). Radiation dose, preimplantation prostate volume, and hormonal therapy do not appear to be predictive of subsequent incontinence; however, TURP performed more than 2 years after implant does appear to be a risk factor.

13.10 Respiratory Complications

13.10.1 Pulmonary Emboli

In urologic malignancies the primary respiratory complication is fatal postoperative pulmonary emboli (PE) (Fig. 13.7). The incidence of deep venous thrombosis (DVT) and PE following urologic surgery in patients without prophylaxis has been reported to be as high as 50% and 22%, respectively (Allgood et al. 1970; Mayo et al. 1971). With the use of intermittent pneumatic compression devices, the incidence of PE has decrease to 2% (Igel et al. 1987; Leandri et al. 1992; Lepor and Kaci 2003; Soderdahl et al. 1997). Scardino and others at Baylor College of Medicine published an extensive review of published series reporting the perioperative morbidity of radical prostatectomy (Dillioglugil et al. 1997). In a combined series of nearly 1,300 patients, the mortality rate was 1.18%, with a PE incidence of 2.76%.

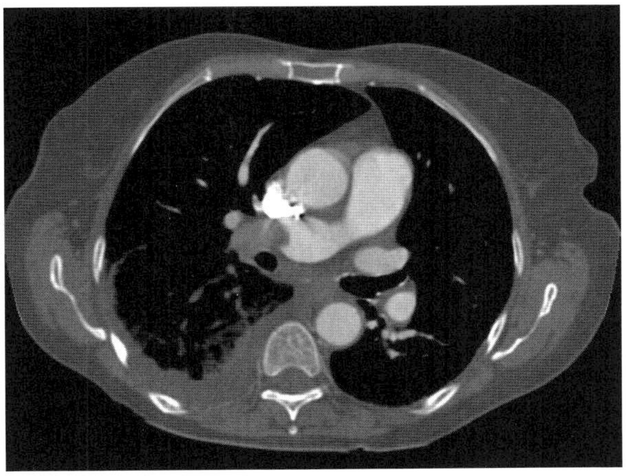

Fig. 13.7. Pulmonary embolism. Contrast-enhanced CT demonstrating pulmonary embolism as large filling defect within proximal right pulmonary artery in patient with renal cell carcinoma

Controversy exists regarding the optimal DVT prophylaxis for GU patients. The University College of Dublin forwarded questionnaires to all urology residency programs in Ireland, the United Kingdom, and the United States regarding the current practice with respect to thromboprophylaxis (Galvin et al. 2004). Among the three countries, there was no difference in the use of nonpharmacological thromboprophylaxis, with about 75% using either intermittent pneumatic compression devices or support stockings. However; just 24% of American urologists use pharmacological thromboprophylaxis, such as conventional or low-molecular-weight heparin, in contrast to 100% of British urologists.

There continues to be no consensus in regards to the optimal DVT prophylaxis, though the minimum would be the use of support stockings with either the addition of compression devices or pharmacological thromboprophylaxis.

13.10.2 Bleomycin Toxicity

Testicular cancer is unique in that cure often requires an integration of chemotherapy and surgery. Treatment of widely metastatic disease consists of cisplatin-based chemotherapy, typically with three or four courses of cisplatin, etoposide, and bleomycin. Those patients not achieving radiographic response with residual retroperitoneal disease typically undergo post-chemotherapy surgery. It is in this setting that the urologist must confront the potential postoperative pulmonary toxicity related to bleomycin use.

Bleomycin exerts its cytotoxic effect by induction of free oxygen radicals, resulting in DNA breaks and cell death, as well as the inhibition of tumor angiogenesis. Due to the lack of the bleomycin-inactivating enzyme, bleomycin hydrolase, in the lungs and skin, bleomycin-induced toxicity occurs predominately in these organs. A multi-institutional study involving 812 testis cancer patients performed serial pulmonary function testing to define pulmonary toxicity related to bleomycin administration (de Wit et al. 2001). This study found a median acute decline in carbon monoxide diffusion capacity (DCLO) of 19% in patients who received a cumulative dose of 270 units. Chronic decline in DCLO has not been shown. The toxic death rate at this dose is less than 0.2%, with no significant impairment in long-term pulmonary function. At doses of 360 units, the toxic death rate increased to 1%–2%.

Prior bleomycin exposure has been associated with an increased risk of postoperative pulmonary complications including fatal acute respiratory distress syndrome (ARDS). In the 1980s and early 1990s at our institution, the postoperative management of such patients involved the judicious administration of postoperative fluid preferring oliguria and prerenal creatinine rise to the potential of ARDS. With clinical experience, improved surgical technique with decreased blood loss and operative time, we no longer limit post-operate hydration. Massively obese patients, those who have received salvage chemotherapy, or have extensive surgical dissections are at higher risk of postoperative pulmonary complications and we would recommend judicious fluid administration with monitoring of volume status.

13.10.3 Pulmonary Metastases

On rare occasions, patients with germ cell tumors may present with respiratory compromise secondary to massive pulmonary metastases. In this circumstance, systemic chemotherapy is initiated on an emergent basis in lieu of radical orchiectomy. Although most patients would likely tolerate a primary orchiectomy, respiratory failure represents the most immediate threat to life and warrants directed therapy as such. Radical orchiectomy is generally performed within a few weeks of initiating chemotherapy.

References

Allen ZA, Merrick GS, Butler WM et al (2005) Detailed urethral dosimetry in the evaluation of prostate brachytherapy-related urinary morbidity. Int J Radiat Oncol Biol Phys 62:981

Allgood RJ, Cook JH, Weedn RJ et al (1970) Prospective analysis of pulmonary embolism in the postoperative patient. Surgery 68:116

Andriole GL, Sandlund JT, Miser JS et al (1987) The efficacy of mesna (2-mercaptoethane sodium sulfonate) as a uroprotectant in patients with hemorrhagic cystitis receiving further oxazaphosphorine chemotherapy. J Clin Oncol 5:799

Andriole GL, Yuan JJ, Catalona WJ (1990) Cystotomy, temporary urinary diversion and bladder packing in the management of severe cyclophosphamide-induced hemorrhagic cystitis. J Urol 143:1006

Anger JT, Raj GV, Delvecchio FC et al (2005) Anastomotic contracture and incontinence after radical prostatectomy: a graded approach to management. J Urol 173:1143

Araujo CE, Tessler J (1983) Treatment of ifosfamide-induced urothelial toxicity by oral administration of sodium 2-mercaptoethane sulphonate (MESNA) to patients with inoperable lung cancer. Eur J Cancer Clin Oncol 19:195

Aroney RS, Dalley DN, Levi JA (1980) Haemorrhagic cystitis treated with epsilon-aminocaproic acid. Med J Aust 2:92

Arrizabalaga M, Extramiana J, Parra JL et al (1987) Treatment of massive haematuria with aluminous salts. Br J Urol 60:223

Baehring JM, Spinal Cor Comprssion. In: DeVita VT Jr, Hellman S, Rosenberg SA (2005) Cancer principles and practice of oncology. Lippincott Williams and Wilkins, Philadelphia: 2287

Barcena A, Lobato RD, Rivas JJ (1984) Spinal metastatic disease: analysis of factors determining functional prognosis and the choice of treatment. Neurosurgery 15:820

Bedi A, Miller CB, Hanson JL et al (1995) Association of BK virus with failure of prophylaxis against hemorrhagic cystitis following bone marrow transplantation. J Clin Oncol 13: 1103

Bevers RF, Bakker DJ, Kurth KH (1995) Hyperbaric oxygen treatment for haemorrhagic radiation cystitis. Lancet 346: 803

Bilen CY, Inci K, Erkan I et al (2003) The predictive value of purified protein derivative results on complications and prognosis in patients with bladder cancer treated with bacillus Calmette-Guerin. J Urol 169:1702

Blumberg HM, Burman WJ, Chaisson RE et al (2003) American Thoracic Society/Centers for Disease Control and Prevention/Infectious Diseases Society of America: treatment of tuberculosis. Am J Respir Crit Care Med 167:603

Bodey GP, Buckley M, Sathe YS et al (1966) Quantitative relationships between circulating leukocytes and infection in patients with acute leukemia. Ann Intern Med. 64:328

Bodey GP, Rodriguez V, Chang HY et al (1978) Fever and infection in leukemic patients: a study of 494 consecutive patients. Cancer 41:1610

Borboroglu PG, Sands JP, Roberts JL et al (2000) Risk factors for vesicourethral anastomotic stricture after radical prostatectomy. Urology 56:96

Bosl GJ, Bajorin DF, Sheinfeld J et al, Cancer of the testis. In: DeVita VT Jr, Hellman S, Rosenberg SA (2005) Cancer principles and practice of oncology. Lippincott Williams and Wilkins, Philadelphia: 1269

Bosniak MA, Megibow AJ, Hulnick DH et al (1988) CT diagnosis of renal angiomyolipoma: the importance of detecting small amounts of fat. AJR Am J Roentgenol 151:497

Bow EJ, Schwarer AP, Laverdiere M et al (2003) Efficacy of piperacillin/tazobactam as initial therapy of febrile neutropenia in patients with hematologic malignancies. Paper presented at the 2003 Interscience Conference on Antimicrobial Agents and Chemotherapy, Chicago IL

Braf ZF, Koontz WW (1977) Gangrene of the bladder. Complication of hypogastric artery embolization. Urology 9:670

Brawn PN, Johnson EH, Speights VO et al (1994) Incidence, racial differences, and prognostic significance of prostate carcinomas diagnosed with obstructive symptoms. Cancer 74:1607

Brock N, Phol J, Stekar J (1981) Detoxification of urotoxic oxazaphosphorines by sulfhydryl compounds. J Cancer Res Clin Oncol 100:311

Brown RB (1969) A method of management of inoperable carcinoma of the bladder. Med J Aust 1:23

Bubley GJ (2001) Is the flare phenomenon clinically significant? Urology 58 [2 Suppl 1]:5

Budman DR, Berry DA, Cirrincione CT et al (1998) Dose and dose intensity as determinants of outcome in the adjuvant treatment of breast cancer. The Cancer and Leukemia Group B. J Natl Cancer Inst 90:1205

Burkert H (1983) Clinical overview of mesna. Cancer Treat Rev 10 [Suppl A]:175

Burtis WJ, Brady TG, Orloff JJ et al (1990) Immunochemical characterization of circulating parathyroid hormone-related protein in patients with humoral hypercalcemia of cancer. N Engl J Med 322:1106

Byrne TN (1992) Spinal cord compression from epidural metastases. N Engl J Med 327:614

Capelli-Schellpfeffer M, Gerber GS (1999) The use of hyperbaric oxygen in urology. J Urol 162:647

Chitale SV, Scott-Barrett S, Ho ET et al (2002) The management of ureteric obstruction secondary to malignant pelvic disease. Clin Radiol 57:1118

Chong KT, Hampson NB, Bostwick DG et al (2004) Hyperbaric oxygen does not accelerate latent in vivo prostate cancer: implications for the treatment of radiation-induced haemorrhagic cystitis. BJU Int 94:1275
Chong KT, Hampson NB, Corman JM (2005) Early hyperbaric oxygen therapy improves outcome for radiation-induced hemorrhagic cystitis. Urology 65:649
Choong SK, Walkden M, Kirby R (2000) The management of intractable haematuria. BJU Int 86:951
Cinman AC, Farrer J, Kaufman JJ (1985) Spontaneous perinephric hemorrhage in a 65-year-old man. J Urol 133:829
Coleman JA, Walther MM, Urologic emergencies. In: DeVita VT Jr, Hellman S, Rosenberg SA (2005) Cancer principles and practice of oncology. Lippincott Williams and Wilkins, Philadelphia: 2301
Coleman RE (1997) Skeletal complications of malignancy. Cancer 80 [Suppl 8]:1588
Cox JD, Stetz J, Pajak TF (1995) Toxicity criteria of the Radiation Therapy Oncology Group (RTOG) and the European Organization for Research and Treatment of Cancer (EORTC) Int J Radiat Oncol Biol Phys 31:1341
Cox PJ (1979) Cyclophosphamide cystitis: identification of acrolein as the causative agent. Biochem Pharmacol 28:2045
Crain DS, Amling CL, Kane CJ (2004) Palliative transurethral prostate resection for bladder outlet obstruction in patients with locally advanced prostate cancer. J Urol 171:668
Crawford J, Dale DC, Lyman GH (2004) Chemotherapy-induced neutropenia: risks, consequences, and new directions for its management. Cancer 100:228
Dalbagni G, O'Donnell M, Intravesical therapy. In: Vogelzang NJ, Scardino PT, Shipley WU, Debruyne FMJ, Linehan WM (2006) Comprehensive textbook of genitourinary oncology. Lippincott Williams and Wilkins, Philadelphia: 452
De Berardinis E, Vicini P, Salvatori F et al (2005) Superselective embolization of bladder arteries in the treatment of intractable bladder haemorrhage. Int J Urol 12:503
De Boer EC, Steerenberg PA, van der Meijden AP et al (1992) Impaired immune response by isoniazid treatment during intravesical BCG administration in the guinea pig. Prog Clin Biol Res 378:81
De Pauw BE, Deresinski SC, Feld R et al (1994) Ceftazidime compared with piperacillin and tobramycin for the empiric treatment of fever in neutropenic patients with cancer. A multicenter randomized trial. Ann Intern Med 120:834
De Vries CR, Freiha FS (1990) Hemorrhagic cystitis: a review. J Urol 143:1
De Wit R, Roberts JT, Wilkinson PM et al (2001) Equivalence of three or four cycles of bleomycin, etoposide, and cisplatin chemotherapy and of a 3- or 5-day schedule in good-prognosis germ cell cancer. J Clin Oncol 19:1629
Dearnaley D, Khoo V, Normal A et al (1999) Comparison of radiation side-effects of conformal and conventional radiotherapy in prostate cancer: a randomized trial. Lancet 353: 267
DeHaven JI, Traynellis C, Riggs DR et al (1992) Antibiotic and steroid therapy of massive systemic bacillus Calmette-Guerin toxicity. J Urol 147:738
Delattre JY, Arbit E, Rosenblum MK (1988) High dose versus low dose dexamethasone in experimental epidural spinal cord compression. Neurosurgery 22:1005
Denton AS, Clarke NW, Maher EJ (2002) Non-surgical interventions for late radiation cystitis in patients who have received radical radiotherapy to the pelvis. Cochrane Database Syst Rev (3):CD001773
Dillioglugil O, Leibman BD, Leibman NS et al (1997) Risk factors for complications and morbidity after radical retropubic prostatectomy. J Urol 157:1760
Dodge HW Jr Svien HJ, Camp JD et al (1951) Tumors of the spinal cord without neurologic manifestations, producing low back and sciatic pain. Mayo Clin Proc 26:88
Donahue LA, Frank IN (1989) Intravesical formalin for hemorrhagic cystitis: analysis of therapy. J Urol 141:809
Donat SM, Russo P (1996) Ureteral decompression in advanced nonurologic malignancies. Ann Surg Oncol 3:393
Durek C, Rusch-Gerdes S, Jocham D et al (2000) Sensitivity of BCG to modern antibiotics. Eur Urol 37 [Suppl 1]:21
Dyer RB, Assimos DG, Regan JD (1997) Update on interventional uroradiology. Urol Clin North Am 24:623
Eickenberg HU, Amin M, Klompus W et al (1976) Urologic complications following abdominoperineal resection. J Urol 115:180
Elshaikh MA, Ulchaker JC, Reddy CA et al (2005) Prophylactic tamsulosin (Flomax) in patients undergoing prostate 125I brachytherapy for prostate carcinoma: final report of a double-blind placebo-controlled randomized study. Int J Radiat Oncol Biol Phys 62:164
Esclarin de Ruz A, Leoni EG, Cabrera RH (2000) Epidemiology and risk factors for urinary tract infection in patients with spinal cord injury. J Urol 164:1285
Fahn HJ, Lee YH, Chen MT (1991) The incidence and prognostic significance of humoral hypercalcemia in renal cell carcinoma. J Urol 145:248
Feldmeier JJ, Hampson NB (2002) A systematic review of the literature reporting the application of hyperbaric oxygen prevention and treatment of delayed radiation injuries: an evidence based approach. Undersea Hyperb Med 29:4
Feldmeier J, Carl U, Hartmann K et al (2003) Hyperbaric oxygen: does it promote growth or recurrence of malignancy? Undersea Hyperb Med 30:1
Flam TA, Peyromaure M, Chauveinc L et al (2004) Post-brachytherapy transurethral resection of the prostate in patients with localized prostate cancer. J Urol 172:108
Fleisch H (1991) Bisphosphonates. Pharmacology and use in the treatment of tumour-induced hypercalcaemic and metastatic bone disease. Drugs 42:919
Fleischmann JD, Catalona WJ (1985) Endocrine therapy for bladder outlet obstruction from carcinoma of the prostate. J Urol 134:498
Flombaum CD (2000) Metabolic emergencies in the cancer patient. Semin Oncol 27:322
Flynn DF, Shipley WU (1991) Management of spinal cord compression secondary to metastatic prostatic carcinoma. Urol Clin North Am 18:145
Fojo AT, Metabolic emergencies. In: DeVita VT Jr, Hellman S, Rosenberg SA (2005) Cancer principles and practice of oncology. Lippincott Williams and Wilkins, Philadelphia: 2292
Foote J, Yun S, Leach GE (1991) Postprostatectomy incontinence. Pathophysiology, evaluation, and management. Urol Clin North Am 18:229
Forni AM, Koss LG, Geller W (1964) Cytological study of the effect of cyclophosphamide on the epithelium of the urinary bladder in man. Cancer 17:1348
Fukuoka M, Negoro S, Masuda N et al (1991) Placebo-controlled double-blind comparative study on the preventive efficacy of mesna against ifosfamide-induced urinary disorders. J Cancer Res Clin Oncol 117:473
Furno P, Bucaneve G, Del Favero A (2002) Monotherpay or aminoglycoside-containing combinations for empirical antibiotic treatment of febrile neutropenic patients: a meta-analysis. Lancet Infect Dis 2:231
Galvin DJ, Mulvin D, Quinlan DM (2004) Thromboprophylaxis for radical prostatectomy: a comparative analysis of present practice between the USA, the UK, and Ireland. Prostate 60:338
Ganatra AM, Loughlin KR (2005) The management of malignant ureteral obstruction treated with ureteral stents. J Urol 174:2125

Gattegno B, Guillemenot F, Fiatte P et al (1990) Treatment of hemorrhagic cystitis caused by cyclophosphamide using intravesical instillation of potassium alum. Apropos of 5 cases. Ann Urol (Paris) 24:190
Gelblum DY, Potters L, Ashley R et al (1999) Urinary morbidity following ultrasound-guided transperineal prostate seed implantation. Int J Radiat Oncol Biol Phys 45:59
Gilbert RW, Kim JH, Posner JB (1978) Epidural spinal cord compression from metastatic tumor: diagnosis and treatment. Ann Neurol 3:40
Gilligan TD, Steele GS, Zietman AL, Bladder cancer. In: Kufe DW, Pollock RE, Weichselbaum RR, Bast RC, Gansler TS, Holland JF, Frei E (2003) Cancer medicine. BC Decker, Hamilton: 1689
Gold PJ, Fefer A, Thompson JA (1996) Paraneoplastic manifestations of renal cell carcinoma. Semin Urol Oncol 14:216
Gottesman J, Ehrlich RM (1974) Preventing vesicoureteral reflux during intravesical formalin instillation. Urology 3:494
Gray LH, Conger AD, Ebert M et al (1953) The concentration of oxygen dissolved in tissues at the time of irradiation as a factor in radiotherapy. Br J Radiol 26:638
Guazzoni G, Montorsi F, Bergamaschi F et al (1994) Prostatic UroLume Wallstent for urinary retention due to advanced prostate cancer: a 1-year follow-up study. J Urol 152:1530
Hader JE, Marzella L, Myers RA et al (1993) Hyperbaric oxygen treatment for experimental cyclophosphamide-induced hemorrhagic cystitis. J Urol 149:1617
Hald T, Mygind T (1974) Control of life-threatening vesical hemorrhage by unilateral hypogastric artery muscle embolization. J Urol 112:60
Harrington KD (1984) Anterior cord decompression and spinal stabilization for patients with metastatic lesion of the spine. J Neurosurg 61:107
Harrington KD (1988) Anterior decompression and stabilization of the spine as a treatment for vertebral collapse and spinal cord compression from metastatic malignancy. Clin Orthop Relat Res 233:177
Heimdal K, Hirschberg H, Slettebo H et al (1992) High incidence of serious side effects of high-dose dexamethasone treatment in patients with epidural spinal cord compression. J Neurooncol 12:141
Helweg-Larsen S (1996) Clinical outcome in metastatic spinal cord compression. A prospective study of 153 patients. Acta Neurol Scand 94:269
Helweg-Larsen S, Hansen SW, Sorensen PS (1995) Second occurrence of symptomatic metastatic spinal cord compression and findings of multiple spinal epidural metastases. Int J Radiat Oncol Biol Phys 33:595
Hinz J, Hautzinger H, Stahl KW (1986) Rationale for and results from a randomised, double-blind trial of tetrachlorodecaoxygen anion complex in wound healing. Lancet 1:825
Holden S, McPhee M, Grabstald H (1979) The rationale of urinary diversion in cancer patients. J Urol 121:19
Hora M, Hes O, Klecka J et al (2004) Rupture of papillary renal cell carcinoma. Scand J Urol Nephrol 38:481
Hosking DJ, Cowley A, Bucknall CA (1981) Rehydration in the treatment of severe hypercalcemia. Q J Med 50:473
Hu K, Wallner K (1998) Urinary incontinence in patients who have a TURP/TUIP following prostate brachytherapy. Int J Radiat Oncol Biol Phys 40:783
Hughes WT, Armstrong D, Bodey GP et al (2002) 2002 guidelines for the use of antimicrobial agents in neutropenic patients with cancer. Clin Infect Dis 34:730
Iacovou JW, Marks JC, Abrams PH et al (1985) Cord compression and carcinoma of the prostate: is laminectomy justified? Br J Urol 57:733
Igel TC, Barrett DM, Segura JW et al (1987) Perioperative and postoperative complications from bilateral pelvic lymphadenectomy and radical retropubic prostatectomy. J Urol 137:1189
Jayson M, Sanders H (1998) Increased incidence of serendipitously discovered renal cell carcinoma. Urology 51:203
Jemal A, Murray T, Ward E et al (2005) Cancer statistics, 20CA. Cancer J Clin 55:10
Katagiri H, Takahashi M, Inagaki J et al (1998) Clinical results of nonsurgical treatment for spinal metastases. Int J Radiat Oncol Biol Phys 42:1127
Katz A, Epelman S, Anelli A et al (1995) A prospective randomized evaluation of three schedules of mesna administration in patients receiving an ifosfamide-containing chemotherapy regimen: sustained efficiency and simplified administration. J Cancer Res Clin Oncol 121:128
Kavoussi LR, Gelstein LD, Andriole GL (1986) Encephalopathy and an elevated serum aluminum level in a patient receiving intravesical alum irrigation for severe urinary hemorrhage. J Urol 136:665
Kennedy C, Snell ME, Witherow RO (1984) Use of alum to control intractable vesical haemorrhage. Brit J Urol 56:673
Klastersky J (2003) Side effects of ifosfamide. Oncology 65 [Suppl 2]:7
Klastersky J, Paesmans M, Rubenstein EB et al (2000) The Multinational Association for Supportive Care in Cancer risk index: a multinational scoring system for identifying low-risk febrile neutropenic cancer patients. J Clin Oncol 18:3038
Klimo P, Thompson CJ, Kestle JRW et al (2005) A meta-analysis of surgery versus conventional radiotherapy for the treatment of metastatic spinal epidural disease. Neuro-oncol 7:64
Koch M, Steidle C, Brosman S et al (2003) An open-label study of abarelix in men with symptomatic prostate cancer at risk of treatment with LHRH agonists. Urology 62:877
Kollmeier MA, Stock RG, Cesaretti J et al (2005) Urinary morbidity and incontinence following transurethral resection of the prostate after brachytherapy. J Urol 173:808
Koss LG (1967) A light and electron microscopic study of the effects of a single dose of cyclophosphamide on various organs in the rat. I. The urinary bladder. Lab Invest 16:44
Ku JH, Lee SW, Jeon HG et al (2004) Percutaneous nephrostomy versus indwelling ureteral stents in the management of extrinsic ureteral obstruction in advanced malignancies: are there differences? Urology 64:895
Ku JH, Choi WJ, Lee KY et al (2005) Complications of the upper urinary tract in patients with spinal cord injury: a long-term follow-up study. Urol Res 33:435
Kumar SM (2005) Photoselective vaporization of the prostate: a volume reduction analysis in patients with lower urinary tract symptoms secondary to benign prostatic hyperplasia and carcinoma of the prostate. J Urol 173:511
Lakhani A, Raptis A, Frame D et al (1999) Intravesicular instillation of E-aminocaproic acid for patients with adenovirus-induced hemorrhagic cystitis. Bone Marrow Transplant 24: 1259
Lamm DL (1992) Complications of bacillus Calmette-Guerin immunotherapy. Urol Clin North Am 19:565
Lamm DL, van der Meijden PM, Morales A et al (1992) Incidence and treatment of complications of bacillus Calmette-Guerin intravesical therapy in superficial bladder cancer. J Urol 147:596
Lapides J, Diokno AC, Silber SJ et al (1972) Clean, intermittent self-catheterization in the treatment of urinary tract disease. J Urol 107:458
Lawton CA, Won M, Pilepich MV et al (1991) Long-term treatment sequelae following external beam irradiation for adenocarcinoma of the prostate: analysis of RTOG studies 7506 and 77. Int J Radiat Oncol Biol Phys 21:935
Leandri P, Rossignol G, Gautier JR et al (1992) Radical retropu-

bic prostatectomy: morbidity and quality of life. Experience with 620 consecutive cases. J Urol 147:883
Lemaitre L, Claudon M, Dubrulle F et al (1997) Imaging of angiomyolipomas. Semin Ultrasound CT MR 18:100
Lepage E, Gisselbrecht C, Haioun C (1993) Prognostic significance of received relative dose intensity in non-Hodgkin's lymphoma patients: application to LNH-87 protocol. Ann Oncol 4:651
Lepor H, Kaci L (2003) Contemporary evaluation of operative parameters and complications related to open radical retropubic prostatectomy. Urology 62:702
Levine LA, Jarrard DF (1993) Treatment of cyclophosphamide-induced hemorrhagic cystitis with intravesical carboprost tromethamine. J Urol 149:719
Leviov M, Dale J, Stein M et al (1993) The management of metastatic spinal cord compression: a radiotherapeutic success ceiling. Int J Radiat Oncol Biol Phys 27:231
Lin JH (1996) Bisphosphonates: a review of their pharmacokinetic properties. Bone 18:75
Little B, Ho KJ, Gawley S et al (2003) Use of nephrostomy tubes in ureteric obstruction from incurable malignancy. Int J Clin Pract 57:180
Logothetis CJ, Assikis V, Sarriera JE, Urologic complications. In: Kufe DW, Pollock RE, Weichselbaum RR, Bast RC, Gansler TS, Holland JF, Frei E (2003) Cancer medicine. BC Decker, Hamilton: 2517
Lotte A, Wasz-Hockert O, Poisson N et al (1984) BCG complications. Estimates of the risks among vaccinated subjects and statistical analysis of their main characteristics. Adv Tuberc Res 21:107
Lyman GH, Lyman CH, Agboola O (2005) Risk models for predicting chemotherapy-induced neutropenia. Oncologist 10: 427
Major P, Lortholary A, Hon J et al (2001) Zoledronic acid is superior to pamidronate in the treatment of hypercalcemia of malignancy: a pooled analysis of two randomized, controlled clinical trials. J Clin Oncol 19:558
Malkowicz SB, Management of superficial bladder cancer. In: Walsh PC, Retik AB, Vaughan ED Jr, Wein AJ (2002) Campbell's urology. Saunders, Philadelphia: 2785
Manglani HH, Marco RA, Picciolo A et al (2000) Orthopedic emergencies in cancer patients. Semin Oncol 27:299
Maranzano E, Latini P (1995) Effectiveness of radiation therapy without surgery in metastatic spinal cord compression: final results from a prospective trial. Int J Radiat Oncol Biol Phys 32:959
Marchetti O, Calandra T, Infections in the neutropenic cancer patient. In: Cohen J, Powderly WG (2004) Infectious Diseases. Mosby, Philadelphia: 1077
Marx RE, Ehler WJ, Tayapongsak P et al (1990) Relationship of oxygen dose to angiogenesis induction in irradiated tissue. Am J Surg 160:519
Mathews R, Rajan N, Josefson L et al (1999) Hyperbaric oxygen therapy for radiation induced hemorrhagic cystitis. J Urol 161:435
Mayo ME, Halil T, Browse NL et al (1971) The incidence of deep vein thrombosis after prostatectomy. Br J Urol 43:738
Mazur AW, Thompson IM (1991) Efficacy and morbidity of "channel" TURP. Urology 38:526
McDougal WS, Kursh ED, Persky L (1975) Spontaneous rupture of the kidney with perirenal hematoma. J Urol 114:181
McIntyre JF, Eifel PJ, Levenmack C et al (1995) Ureteral stricture as a late complication of radiotherapy for stage IB carcinoma of the uterine cervix. Cancer 75:836
McIvor J, Williams G, Greswick Southcott RD (1982) Control of severe vesical haemorrhage by therapeutic embolisation. Clin Radiol 33:561
Megalli MR, Gursel EO, Demirag H et al (1974) External radiotherapy in ureteral obstruction secondary to locally invasive prostatic cancer. Urology 3:562
Michigan S, Catalona WJ (1977) Ureteral obstruction from prostatic carcinoma: response to endocrine and radiation therapy. J Urol 118:733
Miller LJ, Chandler SW, Ippoliti CM (1994) Treatment of cyclophosphamide-induced hemorrhagic cystitis with prostaglandins. Ann Pharmacother 28:590
Montana GS, Fowler WC (1989) Carcinoma of the cervix: analysis of bladder and rectal radiation dose and complications. Int J Radiat Oncol Biol Phys 16:95
Motzer RJ, Mazumdar M, Bacik J et al (1999) Survival and prognostic stratification of 670 patients with advanced renal cell carcinoma. J Clin Oncol 17:2530
Mundy GR (1990) Pathophysiology of cancer-associated hypercalcemia. Semin Oncol 17 [2 Suppl 5]:10
Nabi G, Sheikh N, Greene D et al (2003) Therapeutic transcatheter arterial embolization in the management of intractable haemorrhage from pelvic urological malignancies: preliminary experience and long-term follow-up. BJU Int 92:245
Neheman A, Nativ O, Moskovitz B et al (2005) Hyperbaric oxygen therapy for radiation-induced haemorrhagic cystitis. BJU Int 96:107
Norkool DM, Hampson NB, Gibbons RP et al (1993) Hyperbaric oxygen therapy for radiation-induced hemorrhagic cystitis. J Urol 150:332
Nussbaum SR, Younger J, Vandepol CJ et al (1993) Single-dose intravenous therapy with pamidronate for the treatment of hypercalcemia of malignancy: comparison of 30-, 60-, and 90-mg dosages. Am J Med 95:297
O'Reilly KJ, Hampson NB, Corman JM (2002) Hyperbaric oxygen in urology. AUA Update Series 21:26
Ok JH, Meyers FJ, Evans CP (2005) Medical and surgical palliative care of patients with urological malignancies. J Urol 174:1177
Okaneya T, Kontani K, Komiyama I et al (1993) Severe cyclophosphamide-induced hemorrhagic cystitis successfully treated by total cystectomy with ileal neobladder substitution: a case report. J Urol 150:1909
Ondrus D, Hornak M, Breza J et al (2001) Delayed orchiectomy after chemotherapy in patients with advanced testicular cancer. Int Urol Nephrol 32:665
Ostroff EB, Chenault Ow Jr (1982) Alum irrigation for the control of massive bladder hemorrhage. J Urol 128:929
Oude Nijhuis CS, Gietema JA, Vellenga et al (2003) Routine radiography does not have a role in the diagnostic evaluation of ambulatory adult febrile neutropenic cancer patients. Eur J Cancer 39:2495
Overby MC, Rothman AS (1985) Anterolateral decompression for metastatic epidural spinal cord tumors. J Neurosurg 62:344
Ozer H, Armitage JO, Bennett CL et al (2000) 2000 update of recommendations for the use of hematopoietic colony-stimulating factors: evidence-based, clinical practice guidelines. J Clin Oncol 18:3558
Palou J, Angerri O, Segarra J et al (2003) Intravesical bacillus Calmette-Guerin for the treatment of superficial bladder cancer in renal transplant patients. Transplantation 76:1514
Papac RJ, Poo-Hwu WJ (1999) Renal cell carcinoma: a paradigm of lanthanic disease. Am J Clin Oncol 22:223
Paquette EL, Sun L, Paquette LR et al (2002) Improved prostate cancer-specific survival and other disease parameters: impact of prostate-specific antigen testing. Urology 60:756
Park DS, Park JH, Lee YT (2002) Percutaneous nephrostomy versus indwelling ureteral stents in patients with bilateral nongenitourinary malignant extrinsic obstruction. J Endourol 16:153
Parsons CL, Benson G, Childs SJ et al (1993) A quantitatively

controlled method to study prospectively interstitial cystitis and demonstrate the efficacy of pentosan polysulfate. J Urol 150:845
Parsons CL, Forrest J, Nickel JC et al (2002) Effect of pentosan polysulfate therapy on intravesical potassium sensitivity. Urology 59:329
Pasquier D, Hoelscher T, Schmutz J et al (2004) Hyperbaric oxygen therapy in the treatment of radio-induced lesions in normal tissues: a literature review. Radiother Oncol 72:1
Patchell RA, Tibbs PA, Regine WF (2005) Direct decompressive surgical resection in the treatment of spinal cord compression caused by metastatic cancer: a randomised trial. Lancet 366:643
Paterson DL, Patel A (1998) Bacillus Calmette-Guerin (BCG) immunotherapy for bladder cancer: review of complications and their treatment. Aust N Z J Surg 68:340
Perazella M, Brown E (1993) Acute aluminum toxicity and alum bladder irrigation in patients with renal failure. Am J Kidney Dis 21:44
Pereverzev AS, Shchukin DV, Iliukhin IA et al (2005) Spontaneous ruptures of renal tumors. Urologiia 2:21
Perez CA, Uterine cervix. In: Perez CA, Brady LW (1998) Principles and practice of radiation oncology. Lippincott-Raven, Philadelphia: 1733
Philips FS, Sternberg SS, Cronin AP (1961) Cyclophosphamide and urinary bladder toxicity. Cancer Res 21:1577
Polkey HJ, Vynalek WJ (1933) Spontaneous non-traumatic perirenal and renal hematomas: an experimental and clinical study. Arch Surg 26:196
Pomer S, Karcher G, Simon W (1983) Cutaneous ureterostomy as last resort treatment of intractable haemorrhagic cystitis following radiation. Br J Urol 55:392
Praveen BV, Sankaranarayanan A, Vaidyanathan S (1992) A comparative study of intravesical instillation of 15(s) 15 Me alpha and alum in the management of persistent hematuria of vesical origin. Int J Clin Pharmacol Ther Toxicol 30:7
Purohit OP, Radstone CR, Anthony C et al (1995) A randomised double-blind comparison of intravenous pamidronate and clodronate in the hypercalcaemia of malignancy. Br J Cancer 72:1289
Quinn JA, DeAngelis LM (2000) Neurologic emergencies in the cancer patient. Semin Oncol 27:311
Reisman EM, Kennedy TJ, Roehrborn CG et al (1991) A prospective study of urologist-performed sonographic evaluation of the urinary tract in patients with prostatism. J Urol 145:1186
Resel Folkersma LE, Belon Lopez Tomasetti JA, Isorna Martinez de la Riva S et al (1999) Complications of endovesical treatment with BCG in a series of 200 patients. Arch Esp Urol 52:957
Rigaud J, Hetet JF, Bouchot I (2004) Management of radiation cystitis. Prog Urol 14:568
Rijkmans BG, Bakker DJ, Dabhoiwala NF et al (1989) Successful treatment of radiation cystitis with hyperbaric oxygen. Eur Urol 16:354
Rischmann P, Desgrandchamps F, Malavaud B et al (2000) BCG intravesical instillations: recommendations for side-effects management. Eur Urol 37 [Suppl 1]:33
Rodichok LD, Harper GR, Ruckdeschel JC (1981) Early diagnosis of spinal epidural metastases. Am J Med 70:1181
Rodriguez-Patron RR, Sanz ME, Gomez GI et al (2003) Hypogastric artery embolization as a palliative treatment for bleeding secondary to intractable bladder or prostate disease. Arch Esp Urol 56:111
Romero FR, Broglio M, Pires SR et al (2005) Indications for percutaneous nephrostomy in patients with obstructive uropathy due to malignant urogenital neoplasias. Int Braz J Urol 31:117
Rosenthal MA, Rosen D, Raghavan D et al (1992) Spinal cord compression in prostate cancer. A 10-year experience. Br J Urol 69:530
Rosol TJ, Capen CC (1992) Mechanisms of cancer-induced hypercalcemia. Lab Invest 67:690
Rotariu P, Yohannes P, Alexianu M et al (2001) Management of malignant extrinsic compression of the ureter by simultaneous placement of two ipsilateral ureteral stents. J Endourol 15:979
Russo P (2000) Urologic emergencies in the cancer patient. Semin Oncol 27:284
Salant RL, Cohen MS, Warner RS (1990) Neodymium:YAG laser treatment of postoperative bladder neck contractures. Urology 35:385
Sandhu SS, Goldstraw M, Woodhouse CR (2004) The management of haemorrhagic cystitis with sodium pentosan polysulphate. BJU Int 94:845
Santucci RA, Fisher MB (2005) The literature increasingly supports expectant (conservative) management of renal trauma–a systematic review. J Trauma 59:493
Sato M, Grasser W, Endo N et al (1991) Bisphosphonate action. Alendronate localization in rat bone and effects on osteoclast ultrastructure. J Clin Invest 88:2095
Schimpff SC (1986) Empiric antibiotic therapy for granulocytopenic cancer patients. Am J Med 80:13
Sebastia MC, Perez-Molina MO, Alvarez-Castells A et al (1997) CT evaluation of underlying cause in spontaneous subcapsular and perirenal hemorrhage. Eur Radiol 7:686
Segal BH, Walsh TJ, Gea-Banacloche JC, Holland SM, Infections in the cancer patient. In: DeVita VT Jr, Hellman S, Rosenberg SA (2205) Cancer principles and practice of oncology. Lippincott Williams and Wilkins, Philadelphia: 2461
Sehgal A, Mandhani A, Gupta N et al (2005) Can the need for palliative transurethral prostatic resection in patients with advanced carcinoma of the prostate be predicted? J Endourol 19:546
Shekarriz B, Shekarriz H, Upadhyay J et al (1999) Outcome of palliative urinary diversion in the treatment of advanced malignancies. Cancer 85:998
Shepherd JD, Pringle LE, Barnett MJ et al (1991) Mesna versus hyperhydration for the prevention of cyclophosphamide-induced hemorrhagic cystitis in bone marrow transplantation. J Clin Oncol 9:2016
Shingleton WB, Terrell F, Renfroe DL et al (1999) A randomized prospective study of laser ablation of the prostate versus transurethral resection of the prostate in men with benign prostatic hyperplasia. Urology 54:1017
Shipley WU, Prout GR Jr, Coachman NM et al (1988) Radiation therapy for localized prostate carcinoma: Experience at the Massachusetts General Hospital (1973–1981) J Natl Cancer Inst Monogr 7:67
Shoskes DA, Radzinski CA, Struthers NW, Honey RJ (1992) Aluminum toxicity and death following intravesical alum irrigation in a patient with renal impairment. J Urol 147:697
Shurafa M, Shumaker E, Cronin S (1987) Prostaglandin F2-alpha bladder irrigation for control of intractable cyclophosphamide-induced hemorrhagic cystitis. J Urol 137:1230
Siegal T, Siegal T, Robin G et al (1982) Anterior decompression of the spine for metastatic epidural cord compression: a promising avenue of therapy. Ann Neurol 11:28
Siegal T, Tigva P, Siegal T et al (1985) Vertebral body resection for epidural compression by malignant tumors. J Bone Joint Surg 67:375
Singer FR, Minoofar PN (1995) Bisphosphonates in the treatment of disorders of mineral metabolism. Adv Endocrinol Metab 6:259
Sipsas NV, Bodey GP, Kontoyiannis DP (2005) Perspectives for the management of febrile neutropenic patients with cancer in the 21st century. Cancer 103:1103

Skinner DG, Calvin RB, Vermillion CD et al (1971) Diagnosis and management of renal cell carcinoma. Cancer 28:1165
Soderdahl DW, Henderson SR, Hansberry KL et al (1997) A comparison of intermittent pneumatic compression of the calf and whole leg in preventing deep venous thrombosis in urological surgery. J Urol 157:1774
Sorensen S, Borgesen SE, Rohde K et al (1990) Metastatic epidural spinal cord compression. Results of treatment and survival. Cancer 65:1502
Sorensen S, Helweg-Larsen S, Mouridsen H et al (1994) Effect of high-dose dexamethasone in carcinomatous metastatic spinal cord compression treated with radiotherapy: a randomised trial. Eur J Cancer 30A:22
Srinivasan V, Brown CH, Turner AG (1994) A comparison of two radiotherapy regimens for the treatment of symptoms from advanced bladder cancer. Clin Oncol (R Coll Radiol) 6:11
Stables DP (1982) Percutaneous nephrostomy: techniques, indications, and results. Urol Clin North Am 9:15
Stefanini M, English HA, Taylor AE (1990) Safe and effective, prolonged administration of epsilon aminocaproic acid in bleeding from the urinary tract. J Urol 143:559
Stewart AF (2005) Clinical practice. Hypercalcemia associated with cancer. N Engl J Med 352:373
Stone NN, Stock RG (2002) Complications following permanent prostate brachytherapy. Eur Urol 41:427
Sulser T, Reich O, Wyler S et al (2004) Photoselective KTP laser vaporization of the prostate: first experiences with 65 procedures. J Endourol 18:976
Sundaresan N, Galicich JH, Bains MS et al (1984) Vertebral body resection in the treatment of cancer involving the spine. Cancer 53:1393
Sundaresan N, Galicich JH, Lane JM (1985) Treatment of neoplastic epidural cord compression by vertebral body resection and stabilization. J Neurosurg 63:676
Suzuki S, Shinohara N, Harabayashi T et al (2002) Complications of bacillus Calmette-Guerin therapy in superficial urothelial cancer: clinical analysis and implications. Int J Clin Oncol 7:289
Takamoto S, Sakura N, Namera A et al (2004) Monitoring of urinary acrolein concentration in patients receiving cyclophosphamide and ifosphamide. J Chromatogr B Analyt Technol Biomed Life Sci 806:59
Talar-Williams C, Hijazi YM, Walther MM et al (1996) Cyclophosphamide-induced cystitis and bladder cancer in patients with Wegener granulomatosis. Ann Intern Med 124:477
Tazi H, Manunta A, Rodriguez A et al (2003) Spinal cord compression in metastatic prostate cancer. Eur Urol 44:527
Terk MD, Stock RG, Stone NN (1998) Identification of patients at increased risk for prolonged urinary retention following radioactive seed implantation of the prostate. J Urol 160:1379
Tomita T, Galicich JH, Sundaresan N (1983) Radiation therapy for spinal epidural metastases with complete block. Acta Radiol Oncol 22:135
Trachtenberg J (1984) Ketoconazole therapy in advanced prostatic cancer. J Urol 132:61
Trachtenberg J, Gittleman M, Steidle M et al (2002) A phase 3, multicenter, open label, randomized study of abarelix versus leuprolide plus daily antiandrogen in men with prostate cancer. J Urol 167:1670
Trigg ME, O'Reilly J, Rumelhart S et al (1990) Prostaglandin E1 bladder instillations to control severe hemorrhagic cystitis. J Urol 143:92
Trinh-Duc P, Wintrebert P, Boulfroy D et al (1992) Comparison of the effects of epsilon-aminocaproic acid and aprotinin on intra- and postoperative bleeding in heart surgery. Ann Chir 46:677
Turner S, Marosszeky B, Timms I et al (1993) Malignant spinal cord compression: a prospective evaluation. Int J Radiat Oncol Biol Phys 26:141
Uthappa MC, Cowan NC (2005) Retrograde or antegrade double-pigtail stent placement for malignant ureteric obstruction? Clin Radiol 60:608
Van der Linden YM, Dijkstra SP, Vonk EJ et al (2005) Prediction of survival in patients with metastases in the spinal column: results based on a randomized trial of radiotherapy. Cancer 103:320
Veerasarn V, Khorprasert C, Lorvidhaya V et al (2004) Reduced recurrence of late hemorrhagic radiation cystitis by WF10 therapy in cervical cancer patients: a multicenter, randomized, two-arm, open-label trial. Radiother Oncol 73:179
Veerasarn V, Boonnuch W, Kakanaporn C et al (2006) A phase II study to evaluate WF10 in patients with late hemorrhagic radiation cystitis and proctitis. Gynecol Oncol 100:179
Vieira MM, Brito GA, Belarmino-Filho JN et al (2003) Use of dexamethasone with mesna for the prevention of ifosfamide-induced hemorrhagic cystitis. Int J Urol 10:595
Von der Maase H, Hansen SW, Roberts JT et al (2000) Gemcitabine and cisplatin versus methotrexate, vinblastine, doxorubicin, and cisplatin in advanced or metastatic bladder cancer: results of a large, randomized, multinational, multicenter, phase III study. J Clin Oncol 18:3068
Walther MM, Patel B, Choyke PL et al (1997) Hypercalcemia in patients with metastatic renal cell carcinoma: effect of nephrectomy and metabolic evaluation. J Urol 158:733
Warrell RP Jr (1997) Gallium nitrate for the treatment of bone metastases. Cancer 80 [8 Suppl]:1680
Warrell RP Jr, Bockman RS, Coonley CJ et al (1984) Gallium nitrate inhibits calcium resorption from bone and is effective treatment for cancer-related hypercalcemia. J Clin Invest 73:1487
Warrell RP Jr, Israel R, Frisone M et al (1988) Gallium nitrate for acute treatment of cancer-related hypercalcemia. A randomized, double-blind comparison to calcitonin. Ann Intern Med 108:669
Warrell RP Jr, Murphy WK, Schulman P et al (1991) A randomized double-blind study of gallium nitrate compared with etidronate for acute control of cancer-related hypercalcemia. J Clin Oncol 9:1467
Whitmore WF Jr, Marner JA, Thompson IM Jr (1991) Expectant management of localized prostatic cancer. Cancer 67:1091
Wilson JR, Urwin GH, Stower MJ (2005) The role of percutaneous nephrostomy in malignant ureteric obstruction. Ann R Coll Surg Engl 87:21
Wisplinghoff H, Seifert H, Wenzel RP et al (2003) Current trends in the epidemiology of nosocomial bloodstream infections in patients with hematological malignancies and solid neoplasms in hospitals in the United States. Clin Infect Dis 36:1103
Woodside J, Schwarz H, Bergreen P (1976) Peripheral embolisation complicating bilateral renal infarction with Gelfoam. Am J Roentgenol 126:1033
Yip KH, Peh WC, Tam PC (1998) Spontaneous rupture of renal tumours: the role of imaging in diagnosis and management. Br J Radiol 71:146
Zagoria RJ, Dyer RB, Assimos DG et al (1991) Spontaneous perinephric hemorrhage: imaging and management. J Urol 145:468
Zekri J, Ahmed N, Coleman RE et al (2001) The skeletal metastatic complications of renal cell carcinoma. Int J Oncol 19:379
Zhang JQ, Fielding JR, Zou KH (2002) Etiology of spontaneous perirenal hemorrhage: a meta-analysis. J Urol 167:1593
Zojer N, Keck AV, Pecherstofer M (1999) Comparative tolerability of drug therapies for hypercalcaemia of malignancy. Drug Saf 21:389

14 Urologic Paraneoplastic Syndromes

R. Tiguert, Y. Fradet

Paraneoplastic syndromes represent a constellation of complex signs and symptoms that result from the release of various tumor-associated proteins rather than as a consequence of local or distant metastasis. Paraneoplastic syndromes have been estimated to occur in 15%–20% of all cancer patients. The syndromes may affect any of the systems of the body, may precede or follow the diagnosis of the underlying neoplasm, and may or may not parallel the course of the neoplasm in severity. The diagnosis and therapy for these syndromes can be challenging to a physician, but successful therapy may bring about worthwhile relief for the patient. These syndromes are important for many reasons. They occasionally aid in the early diagnosis of neoplasms, and they have aided in the discovery that many (and perhaps most) neoplasms produce hormones or other substances that can be used as tumor markers. These markers are of increasing use in early diagnosis, in following the course of neoplasm and targeting therapy. A better understanding of the precise mechanisms involved in neoplasm production of these remote effects may help to achieve a better understanding of the nature of the neoplastic process itself.

These peculiar paraneoplastic syndromes may be divided into endocrinologic, dermatologic, hematologic, neurologic, and osteoarticular manifestations. Among the urologic cancers, renal cell carcinoma is the most often associated with paraneoplastic syndromes. In this review, the most common paraneoplastic syndromes associated with urologic cancers will be discussed.

14.1 Renal Cell Carcinoma

The contemporary series have reported the presence of paraneoplastic manifestations associated with renal cell carcinoma (RCC) in 2%–55%. The true incidence may be higher since some biochemical and hematologic abnormalities have been overlooked in the past and other abnormalities not considered relevant. In modern series, approximately 15%–48% of paraneoplastic syndromes are present in up to 20% of patients with renal cell carcinoma (Kim et al. 2003). Two classifications have been suggested for paraneoplastic syndromes associated with renal cell carcinoma. In certain paraneoplastic syndromes, renal tumor secretion of ectopic and eutopic hormones has been demonstrated, while in others no specific etiologic substance has been identified. Classification of paraneoplastic syndromes into specific and nonspecific syndromes has been proposed in Table 14.1. Specific syndromes may be caused by eutopic factors normally produced by the kidney. Ectopic factors are substances not normally produced by the kidney. Recognition of paraneoplastic syndromes is an important component of the diagnosis and management of RCC. The most common paraneoplastic syndromes associated with renal cell carcinoma are illustrated in Table 14.2.

Table 14.1. Classification of paraneoplastic syndromes observed in renal cell carcinoma according to the factors secreted by the kidney

Nonspecific syndromes	Specific syndromes
Anemia	Hypercalcemia
Elevated sedimentation rate	Erythrocytosis
Coagulopathy	Hypertension
Hepatic dysfunction	Elevated HCG
Amyloidosis	Cushing's syndrome
Neuropathy	Hyperprolactenemia
	Ectopic insulin/glucagon

Table 14.2. Incidence of the most common paraneoplastic syndromes associated with renal cell carcinoma

Paraneoplastic syndrome	Incidence (%)
Fever	15–80
Cachexia	33
Hypertension	10–40
Anemia	10–40
Hyperglycemia	10–20
Stauffer's syndrome	3–20
Erythrocytosis	1– 8
Amyloidosis	3– 5
Hypercalcemia	5–16

Percentage of patients with paraneoplastic syndrome

14.1.1 Hypercalcemia

The first case of RCC associated with hypercalcemia was reported by Albright in 1941 (Albright 1941). Hypercalcemia has been reported to occur in as many as 16% of patients with renal cell carcinoma (Weissglas et al. 1995). Production of parathyroid hormone-related protein (PTHrP) was considered initially to be the mechanism of humoral hypercalcemia in malignancies (Fukuzumi et al. 2000). The production of PTH-like compound is detected in vivo in patients with renal cell carcinoma, as well as in the supernatant of human renal cell carcinoma cells transplanted into nude mice (Weissglas et al. 1995; Strewler et al. 1986). Recent studies have examined a possible contribution of IL-6, known to stimulate osteoclastic bone resorption, to the hypercalcemia of renal cell carcinoma (Weissglas et al. 1995). PTHrP was purified from renal cell carcinoma as a hypercalcemic factor. It has 70% homology to the first 13 amino acids of the N-terminal portion of the parathyroid hormone (PTH), binds to PTH receptors, and shares similar biologic activity to PTH. Specifically, it stimulates adenylate cyclase in renal and bone systems. PTHrP mimics many of the effects of PTH on renal tubular function by binding to and activating the PTH receptor (Fig. 14.1). This leads to alterations in normal calcium homeostasis, including increased bone resorption, decreased renal calcium clearance, increased nephrogenous cyclic adenosine monophosphate levels, and increased phosphorous excretion. Of patients with hypercalcemia, 50% had bone metastasis (Braasch 1952; Papac et al. 1977; Warrell and Bockman 1989; Chasan et al. 1989; Weissglas et al. 1995). The clinical manifestations of hypercalcemia are influenced by many factors, including the duration of hypercalcemia, performance status, age, prior chemotherapy, hepatic and or renal dysfunction, and metastatic disease. Many of the signs and symptoms, such as nausea, anorexia, fatigue, lethargy, and confusion are nonspecific, and the physician must have a high index of suspicion for the presence of hypercalcemia. This is important, because the symptoms are generally reversible with therapy. These can include muscle weakness, fatigue, volume depletion, nausea, and vomiting, and in severe cases, coma and death. Neuropsychiatric manifestations are particularly common and may include depression, confusion, or subtle deficits that are often characterized poorly and may not be noted by the patient. Increased calcium can increase gastric acid secretion, and people with hyperparathyroidism may have a higher prevalence of peptic ulcer disease. Hypercalcemia is often the immediate leading cause of death in patients with ectopic PTHrP production. These patients may rarely survive more than a few weeks or months. Bone metastases tend to cause morbidity and mortality from nerve compression and other orthopedic compli-

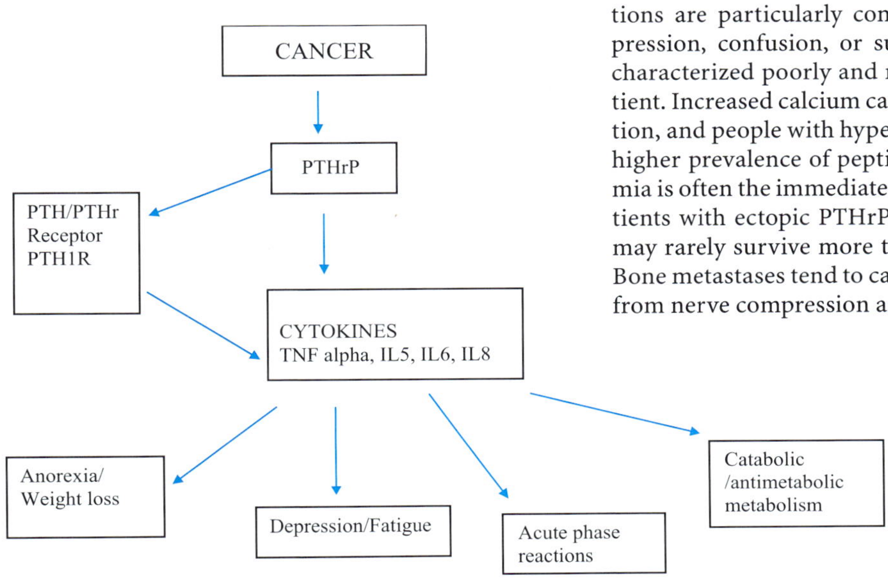

Fig. 14.1. Relationship between parathyroid hormone-related protein (PTHrP), PTH1 receptor, proinflammatory cytokines and cancer related morbidity. *TNF* tumor necrosis factor, *IL* interleukin

cations. These patients may live longer but still have a poor prognosis, especially if their serum calcium levels are very high. Ideally, treatment of the primary cancer leads to resolution of this paraneoplastic disorder. However, elevated calcium levels often require urgent, nonspecific measures, including hyperhydration therapy, diuretics, and biphosphonates.

14.1.2 Hypertension

The association between renal cell cancers and hypertension was initially based on response of blood pressure following surgical removal of the tumors (Hollifield et al. 1975). The incidence of hypertension in patients with RCC ranged from 10% to 40%. The potential mechanisms involved in the production of hypertension include hyperreninemia, arteriovenous fistula, renal artery stenosis, polycythemia, hypercalcemia, ureteral obstruction, and cerebral metastasis. It is important to keep in mind that therapeutic arterial embolization of renal cell carcinoma may cause iatrogenic hypertension. Although renin secretion generally is associated with tumors of the juxtaglomerular cells, a few patients with renin secretion from renal cell carcinoma are well documented. Unlike patients with juxtaglomerular cell tumors, the patients with renal cell carcinoma did not manifest hypokalemia or secondary aldosteronism (Hollifield et al. 1975; Lindop and Fleming 1984). In one reported patient, hypertension was associated with elevated levels of renin in the renal vein draining the tumor site and with extremely high renin levels in the tumor tissue (Hollifield et al. 1975). Following nephrectomy, blood pressure returned to normal and the assay for renin was below the limit of detection. Another study reported elevated serum levels of renin in 21 of 57 patients with renal cell carcinoma. However, tissue assays were not performed in this study (Sufrin et al. 1977). The elevated levels of renin were related to high-grade tumors and those with mixed histologic type, and there was no correlation between renin levels and hypertension. The authors suggest that renin levels could be a useful marker of the disease. Immunostaining with an antibody to renin was investigated in 19 primary and in seven metastasis renal cell carcinoma patients. Immunoreactivity was detected in seven primary cases and in two metastasis renal cell carcinoma cases, respectively. There was no correlation with hypertension and renin level. Based on these results, it was postulated that the renin secreted by the tumor may be biologically inactive. Another possible hypothesis to explain the absence of hypertension in these patients is based on the role of growth factors in renin secretion (Lindop and Fleming 1984). In animal studies, epidermal growth factor inhibits the secretion of renin, and transforming growth factor beta may enhance it (Antonipillai 1993; Antonipillai et al. 1993).

14.1.3 Hyperglycemia

There are very few reports regarding the development of diabetes or worsening of preexisting diabetes in patients with renal cell carcinoma (Elias 2005; Palgon et al. 1986; Jobe et al. 1993; Callewaert et al. 1999). In one case, the patient was diagnosed with a preexisting insulin-dependent diabetes mellitus that became uncontrollable by insulin therapy. The patient underwent partial nephrectomy because of a histological papillary type and the control of his glycemia improved immediately and insulin need became identical to the premorbid situation (Callewaert et al. 1999). The other three case reports did not have any history of diabetes mellitus and the hyperglycemia resolved following nephrectomy. The mechanism for this syndrome is unclear and none of these patients had evidence of metastatic disease or family history of diabetes. No specific etiology was found, but the possibility of ectopic glucagon production was considered. Hypothetically, diabetes could develop in patients with renal cell carcinoma if the tumor was the source of hormones that antagonized the effect of insulin or promoted neoglucogenesis. Glucagon and growth hormones are able to produce such an effect. Other potential mechanisms include ectopic ACTH production, hyperprolactinemia causing insulin resistance, and the potential for the production of an insulin receptor antagonist (Plagon et al. 1986). There are several reports of the development of diabetes mellitus in patients receiving cancer-related cytokine therapy with interleukin-2 or interferon and this may be yet another mechanism (Shiba et al. 1998).

14.1.4 Cushing's Syndrome

Ectopic production of adrenocorticotrophic hormone (ACTH) by renal cell carcinoma has been reported. However, of the 232 patients with Cushing's syndrome reported, three of them were found to have hypernephroma: one patient had an adrenal adenoma as well as a renal tumor, another had an incidental renal tumor found during adrenalectomy, and the other had a lapse of 21 years between the finding of increased ACTH production and renal cell carcinoma (Riggs and Sprague 1961). The mechanism of Cushing's syndrome is the enzymatic conversion of inactive proopiomelanocortin (POMC) to ACTH by the tumor. This leads to symptoms of cortisol excess, including weakness, muscle atrophy, fatigue, hypertension, and glucose intolerance. These symptoms resolved following nephrectomy (Watanobe et al. 1988).

14.1.5 Human Chorionic Gonadotropin

Elevation of human chorionic gonadotropin (hCG) associated with renal cell carcinoma RCC has been reported (McCloskey and O'Connor 1982; Golde et al. 1974; Fukutani et al. 1983). In males, clinical findings include gynecomastia, decreased libido, and elevated urine and serum hCG levels. Only a small number of cases have been reported, though there is no direct evidence of tumor production of these hormones. Gynecomastia and increased urinary levels gonadotropins associated with RCC have been reported with resolution of the endocrine abnormality following nephrectomy (Laski and Vugrin 1987).

14.1.6 Hematologic Syndromes

Various hematologic abnormalities have been associated with RCC. Anemia has been reported in 28%–88% of patients diagnosed with RCC, and may be the presenting symptom in 10%. The anemia is typically normochromic and normocytic, and consistent with that observed in chronic disease. Leukocytosis and thrombocytosis are also observed occasionally in patients with RCC. Some correlation of platelet levels with IL-6 levels has been shown. IL-6 is known to stimulate thrombopoiesis in murine and primate animal models. Leukocytosis could be related to tumor necrosis or could be cytokine-mediated. The presence of receptors for granulocyte-macrophage colony stimulating factor (GM-CSF) has been reported in vitro on some transformed renal cell lines. Pancytopenia has occurred occasionally in patients with RCC. It is almost always associated with disease involvement of the bone marrow (DaSilva et al. 1990; Shiramizu et al. 1994).

The occurrence of erythrocytosis in renal cell carcinoma was first reported in 1929 (Bliss 1929). However, erythropoietin production by the tumor was well documented in the early 1990s (DaSilva et al. 1990; Shiramizu et al. 1994). Erythrosis generally was considered to be a paraneoplastic phenomenon because elevated erythropoietin levels were observed in patients diagnosed with RCC. Paraneoplastic erythrocytosis is differentiated from polycythemia vera by the absence of leukocytosis, thrombocytosis, and splenomegaly, and from secondary polycythemia by the absence of low arterial oxygen saturation (Bliss 1929). Cell lines from human renal cell carcinoma have been shown to produce erythropoietin. It has been suggested that erythropoietin secreting renal tumors may be responsive to therapy IL-2 and alpha-IFN. However, this study included only five patients, which makes it difficult to draw a definitive conclusion (Janik et al. 1993).

14.1.7 Amyloidosis

Systemic amyloidosis is a collective term for a group of diseases that are characterized by the widespread extracellular deposition of insoluble amyloid protein (Callewaert et al. 1999). Amyloidosis may be primary (idiopathic) or secondary. Secondary causes include myeloma, solid malignancies and chronic inflammatory rheumatoid arthritis and tuberculosis. RCC is the most common nonlymphoid malignancy associated with systemic amyloidosis. It is detected in 3%–8% of patients with RCC. The pathogenesis of the amyloidosis is poorly understood but its disappearance following nephrectomy indicates clearly that is paraneoplastic. Amyloidosis should be suspected in patients with renal cell carcinoma who present with renal dysfunction or a nephrotic syndrome (Jobe et al. 1993; Elias 2005).

14.1.8 Hepatic Syndromes

In 1961, Stauffer described for the first time a syndrome associating abnormal liver function with RCC in the absence of metastatic disease (Stauffer 1961). The abnormalities returned to normal following nephrectomy. The incidence of Stauffer's syndrome ranged from 9% to 33%. Liver dysfunction is accompanied by hepatosplenomegaly in 50% of patients, including fever, fatigue, and weight loss. The biochemical abnormalities included elevated transaminases, elevated alkaline phosphatase, hypothrombinemia, prolonged partial thromboplastin time, elevated alpha 2 globulin levels, and hypoalbuminemia. The etiology of Stauffer's syndrome remains undefined. Some etiologic theories have been reported, including secretion of hepatotoxins or lysosomal enzymes, which might also stimulate hepatic cathepsins, phosphatase, or beta glucuronidase. Attempts to reproduce this syndrome in animals by utilizing injections of tumor extracts have been unsuccessful (Hanash et al. 1971). Liver biopsies show a nonspecific reactive hepatitis with Kupffer cell proliferation, variable hepatocellular degeneration, and portal triaditis. There is no evidence of biliary obstruction to explain the elevated alkaline phosphatase (Hannash 1982). Following nephrectomy, reversal of liver function tests to normal is usually associated with favorable prognosis; their failure to normalize implies incomplete resection or unrecognized metastasis. Furthermore, patients whose liver function became normal following radical nephrectomy and subsequently revert to abnormal have tumor recurrence locally or distant metastasis (Warren et al. 1970).

14.1.9 Constitutional Symptoms

Nonspecific symptoms, including cachexia, anorexia, weight loss, and fatigue, are common presenting features in up to one-third of patients with large RCC. The etiology is not well established, but the cancer cachexia is likely cytokine-mediated. Tumor necrosis factor alpha is the cytokine most commonly involved by altering fat metabolism and appetite regulation (Laski and Vugrin 1987). Other cytokines including interleukin-1, interleukin-6, and interferon gamma, have also been implicated in cancer cachexia (Tsukamoto et al. 1992; Walther et al. 1998). In a series of 1,046 patients treated by radical nephrectomy for renal cell carcinoma, cachexia (defined as hypoalbuminemia, weight loss, and malaise), predicts worse survival after controlling for well-established prognosticators, including TNM and Fuhrman grade (Kim and al. 2003). Fever has been associated with renal cell carcinoma in approximately 20%. In patients evaluated for fever, a renal cell carcinoma was found in up to 2% (Weinstein et al. 1961). The etiology of fever associated with renal cell carcinoma has not been clearly elucidated, but it has been postulated that the following factors may be involved: tumor necrosis with secretion of tissue pyrogens, tumor-produced toxins or pyrogens, prostaglandins, and immune mechanisms (Sufrin et al. 1989). Interleukin-6 has been incriminated in the genesis of fever. In a study evaluating 71 patients with renal cell carcinoma, 25% had higher levels of interleukin-6, 78% of whom had fever. There is no correlation of fever with necrosis or inflammatory changes in the tumor. The fever disappears after nephrectomy and may recur when metastasis develops (Tsukamoto et al. 1992).

14.1.10 Neuromuscular and Cutaneous Syndromes

Polyneuropathy, polymyositis, and myopathy are all known to occur with RCC. The myopathy is characterized by involvement of proximal muscles and association of elevated serum levels of creatine kinase and aldolase (Solon et al. 1994; Evans et al. 1990). In each condition, there are reports of resolution after nephrectomy. With the development of metastatic disease, polymyositis and polyneuromyopathy have recurred.

Myasthenia gravis is an autoimmune disorder of neural conduction in which the autoantigen is the nicotinic acetylcholine receptor at the neuromuscular junction. There are few reported cases of carcinomatous neuromyopathies associated with renal cell carcinoma. Neurological manifestations frequently manifest before discovery of the primary tumor. Effective therapy of the primary malignancy is almost always associated with resolution of the symptoms. In one case, the presenting symptom was urinary retention (Torgerson et al. 1999; Leavitt 2000).

14.2 Prostate Cancer

Prostate cancer is the second leading urological cancer after renal cell carcinoma associated with paraneoplastic syndromes. Paraneoplastic syndromes in association with prostate cancer are uncommon and include Cushing's syndrome, the inappropriate antidiuretic hormone syndrome, hypercalcemia, and hypophosphatemia (Table 14.3).

Table 14.3. Most common paraneoplastic syndromes associated with prostate cancer

Inappropriate antidiuretic hormone secretion
Cushing's syndrome
Hypercalcemia
Hypophosphatemia
HCG
Bleeding diathesis and coagulopathy
Neuromuscular
Dermatomyositis

14.2.1 Inappropriate Antidiuretic Hormone Secretion

Inappropriate antidiuretic hormone secretion (IADHS) may occur in a variety of diseases, including malignancies, acute and chronic pulmonary diseases, central nervous system and endocrine disorders, acute psychosis, and surgical stress. It can be induced by drugs such as phenothiazines, cyclophosphamide, vincristine, thiazides, morphine, carbamazepine, and cisplatin. IADHS may accompany certain malignancies, particularly small-cell lung carcinoma, head/neck carcinomas, brain tumors, and lymphomas. The symptoms of IADHS syndrome include anorexia, nausea, headache, confusion, with the possible end result being coma. Laboratory findings include serum hyponatremia, elevated urinary sodium concentrations with normal renal and adrenal homeostasis. Few cases of prostate cancer associated with IADHS syndrome have been reported, and tumors were either poorly differentiated or small cell carcinoma and were almost uniformly metastatic at the time of diagnosis. Most of the patients died a few months after the diagnosis. In one case, elevated level of antidiuretic hormone was found in the patient's serum and in the prostatic tumor. The cytoplasm of the tumor cells was positive for prostate-specific antigen and was faintly positive for antidiuretic hormone (ADH). The patient responded well to combination therapy of androgen blockade with leuprorelin acetate and flutamide and subsequently laboratory findings of SIADH and serum ADH level returned to normal. However, he died of sudden profuse bleeding caused by gastric ulcers 6 months after the therapy (Sackset al. 1975; Gasparini et al. 1993; Yamazaki et al. 2001; Kawai et al.2003; Yalcin et al. 2000).

14.2.2 Cushing's Syndrome

A small number of cases of Cushing's syndromes associated with prostate cancer has been reported. Ectopic adrenocorticotropic hormone secretion has been reported in patients with prostate cancer (Haukaas et al. 1999; Rickman et al. 2001). Tumors arising outside the lungs and secreting adrenocorticotropic hormone have histological features similar to carcinoid or small cell lung cancer.

Clinically, patients may present with a variety of signs and symptoms, including round facies, proximal muscle weakness, obesity (mainly truncal), thin skin, easy bruising, purple stria, psychiatric symptoms, hypertension, and diabetes. Although no single sign or symptom is sensitive or specific enough for the diagnosis, when a patient presents with a combination of proximal weakness, thin skin, and any of the other signs noted above, a biochemical evaluation should be pursued. (Fig. 14.2). When the ACTH value is twice the normal value, the diagnosis of ectopic ACTH syndrome is likely. Management of the ectopic ACTH syndrome involves identification of the source of its production and treatment of the underlying cause (Goldfarb 1999).

14.2.3 Hypercalcemia

Hypercalcemia is an extremely rare complication of prostatic carcinoma. It occurs mainly in patients with disseminated osseous metastases and may be corrected by bilateral orchiectomy or hormonal manipulation (Matzkin and Braf 1987; Hanazawa et al.2005). Humoral factors may be involved in its pathogenesis. Its occurrence carries an ominous prognosis.

14.2.4 Hypophosphatemia

Skeletal complications are frequently seen in prostate cancer, because the skeleton is the predilective site of metastases. These complications may respond successfully to androgen deprivation therapy, but the onset of hormone refractory status is associated with their reappearance and the resurgence in skeletal morbidity, mainly in the form of intractable bone pain (Coleman 1997; Pelger et al. 2001). A less frequent skeletal complication of prostate cancer is osteomalacia, which is resistant to various therapeutic manipulations and associated with invalidating generalized bony pain refractory to conventional analgesia. The most common pathophysiologic mechanism for osteomalacia is vitamin D deficiency, a relatively frequent finding in patients in a late stage of any malignancy. However, a severe form of osteomalacia associated with profound hypophosphatemia due to renal phosphate wasting has

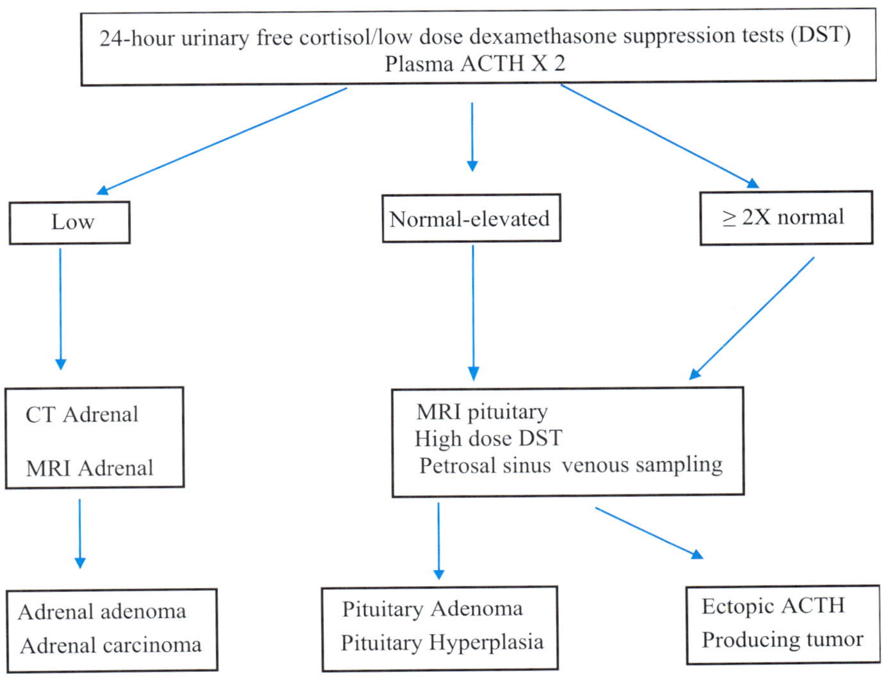

Fig. 14.2. Cushing's syndrome, diagnostic approach

been described in a number of malignancies, particularly those of mesenchymal origin. The tumor-secreted factor responsible for oncogenic hypophosphatemic osteomalacia has been identified as fibroblast growth factor 23 (FGF23) (Shimada et al. 2001). This hormone-like molecule has been recognized as playing an important role in the genesis of a number of disorders of phosphate homeostasis, having in common renal phosphate wasting and impaired mineralization of bone. Oncogenic hypophosphatemic osteomalacia presents clinically with fatigue, proximal myopathy (arthropathy, myalgia), bone pain (osteomalacia), metabolic encephalopathy (confusion, paraesthesia, seizures, coma) and gastrointestinal disturbances (anorexia, nausea, vomiting, gastric atony, ileus). It is characterized biochemically by increased urinary phosphate loss associated with low plasma phosphate and normal plasma calcium concentrations. In typical cases of oncogenic hypophosphatemic osteomalacia, low 1,25 dihydroxyvitamin D concentrations are also observed, indicating a defect in the synthetic capacity of the renal one-alpha hydroxylase enzyme, which is normally stimulated by low serum phosphate concentrations. An analysis of 18 patients with metastatic prostate cancer treated with high-dose diethylstilbestrol diphosphate and 58 patients treated with doxorubicin, doxorubicin plus cisplatinum, doxorubicin plus diethylstilbestrol diphosphate, or diethylstilbestrol diphosphate alone was conducted. A significant decrease in serum phosphate levels was seen only in patients treated with diethylstilbestrol diphosphate. In conclusion, hypophosphatemia and possibly osteomalacia in metastatic prostate cancer may be related to estrogen therapy (Citrin et al. 1984).

14.2.5 Human Chorionic Gonadotropin

The association of secretion of human chorionic gonadotropin with prostate cancer has been reported in one case. Broder et al. have analyzed prospectively 16 patients with stage D adenocarcinoma for the presence of human placental lactogen (hPL), placental alkaline phosphatase (PAP), and human chorionic gonadotropin (hCG). Ectopic production of hCG was found in one of the 16 cases. Serial serum hCG levels in that patient mirrored his course more reliably than concomitant acid phosphatase levels. Serum estradiol, testosterone, the hCG-alpha subunit, hPL, and PAP were not elevated. There was a minimal elevation of serum follicle-stimulating hormone (FSH). There were no elevations of the other placental proteins in ten evaluable cases. A retrospective evaluation of serum bank specimens from 47 patients with prostatic carcinoma revealed no elevation of the placental proteins hPL, hCG-beta, and hCG-alpha. In this peculiar case, the ectopic origin of the hormone secretion was not documented with biochemical testing on the prostate tumor for the presence of hCG (Broder et al. 1977).

14.2.6 Hematologic Syndromes

The association of bleeding diathesis and intravascular coagulopathy abnormalities in patients with prostate cancer has been reported. Bleeding problems in the prostate cancer patient may result from the effects of the tumor on hemostatic mechanisms or from the treatment of the tumor by cytotoxic and other agents. Among the tumor-related bleeding problems are disseminated intravascular coagulation, primary fibrinolysis, thrombocytopenia, acquired platelet dysfunction, and circulating inhibitors or anticoagulants. Disseminated intravascular coagulation is associated with hypercoagulability state in most solid tumors, whereas in prostate cancer tumors the most common presentation is acute promyelocytic leukemia bleeding. Treatment-related bleeding disorders include the common problem of thrombocytopenia secondary to myelosuppressive chemotherapy as well as the interesting microangiopathic hemolytic anemia syndrome associated with mitomycin C and other agents (de la Fouchardiere et al. 2003). The cornerstone of management of disseminated intravascular coagulation is treatment of the underlying condition. Unfortunately few effective therapeutic options are available in hormone refractory prostate cancer. The recent development of new active agents might reverse the situation. A case of acute disseminated intravascular coagulation (DIC) associated with hormone refractory prostate cancer was successfully treated with samarium 153 (Ruffion et al. 2000). However, systemic radiopharmaceutical treatment for bone metastases is theoretically contraindicated when disseminated intravascular coagulation occurs since the report of a death following strontium 89 therapy in 1994. Mitoxantrone chemotherapy has been reported to be effective in two patients with a survival of more than few months, but normalization of blood tests requires at least 1 week (Leong et al. 1994; Paszkowski et al. 1999).

14.2.7 Neuromuscular and Cutaneous Syndromes

The idiopathic inflammatory myopathies are systemic autoimmune diseases characterized by chronic inflammation leading to progressive weakness of the proximal muscles. In 7 % – 66 % of cases of adult dermatomyositis, different malignant tumors can promote the difficult cascade mechanisms at the cell level, leading to rapid weakness of skeletal muscles (Mooney et al. 2006). A case with all characteristic signs of acute, severe dermatomyositis associated with a low-grade, low-stage prostate cancer was reportedly cured by radical perineal prostatectomy (Tallai et al. 2006).

Only a few cases of prostate cancer associated with dermatomyositis have been reported, all of which had advanced disease (Subramonian 2000; Joseph et al. 2002). In one case, the diagnosis was made at autopsy and in the two other cases presented with bladder outflow obstruction and skin lesions.

14.3 Bladder Cancer

The association of bladder cancer and paraneoplastic syndrome is rare compared to prostate and renal malignancies.

14.3.1 Hypercalcemia

Hypercalcemia is the most common paraneoplastic syndrome encountered in bladder cancer. The proposed mechanisms are the same as for renal carcinoma and include secretion of parathyroid-like peptide and prostaglandins. The large majority of these tumors were epidermoid carcinoma with a poor prognosis. Hypercalcemia associated with bladder cancer is known to resolve with resection of the primary tumor or cystectomy and the patient should not be denied definitive local therapy (Wolchok 1998).

14.3.2 Dermatomyositis

Polymyositis is an inflammatory myopathy of unknown etiology in which the striated muscles are damaged by an inflammatory process dominated by lymphocytic infiltration. Immunohistochemical studies suggest immunologically mediated muscle damage with accumulation of B and mostly T lymphocytes. There is compelling evidence that the mechanism of paraneoplastic polymyositis relates to the activation of CD8+ T cells that become cytotoxic to a muscle antigen. However, this information is more useful for understanding pathogenesis than for making a diagnosis of the inflammatory muscle process. Polymyositis is associated with 10% of cancer-related paraneoplastic syndrome. The presence of dermatomyositis in an elderly patient may warrant a thorough search for neoplasms including a bladder tumor (Mallon et al. 1999; Apaydin et al. 2002; Rankin and Herman 2002).

14.3.3 Hematologic

It is well known that some malignant nonhematological tumors manifest leukocytosis as a paraneoplastic syndrome without any concomitant infection. This phenomenon has been suggested to be mainly due to autonomic overproduction of granulocyte colony-stimulating factor (G-CSF), which is one of the hematopoietic growth factors that stimulates the growth and proliferation and differentiation of neutrophilic granulocytes. G-CSF producing bladder cancer is associated with a poor prognosis. Of the few cases reported in the literature, only one had no evidence of recurrence at 40 months following cystectomy (Tachibana et al. 1995, 1997; Hirasawa et al. 2002).

14.4 Testicular Cancer

The two most common reported paraneoplastic syndromes associated with testicular cancer are gynecomastia and dermatomyositis

14.4.1 Gynecomastia

About 10% of choriocarcinoma of the testis and 15%–20% of gonadal/stroma sex cord testicular tumors induce gynecomastia through their autonomous synthesis and secretion of estrogens. Tumor estrogen production may also cause decreased libido and poor sperm quality. The diagnosis of these hormone producing tumors is usually clinically evident from the finding of a testicular swelling that might be painless or painful. Occasionally the sole presenting feature is gynecomastia or very rarely decreased potency and no palpable testicular lesion (Lemack et al. 1995; Haas et al. 1989). Under these circumstances the diagnosis of testicular neoplasia may be missed. The presence of such occult tumors may be suspected from the biochemical findings of raised serum estrogens and depressed testosterone hormone levels. However, this does not always apply as some clinically recognizable estrogenic tumors have been reported in patients with normal hormonal profiles. Although gynecomastia is a relatively common disorder with a benign cause in most cases, physicians should be aware that normal findings on testicular examination do not completely rule out the possibility of a testicular tumor, retroperitoneal metastasis or mediastinal germ cell tumors could be the cause. Because of the potentially high morbidity of testicular tumors and their known association with gynecomastia, early performance of testicular ultrasonography in a patient with gynecomastia of unknown cause is advised (Conway et al. 1988)

14.4.2 Dermatomyositis

A literature search revealed six cases of dermatomyositis associated with testicular germ cell tumor, including a mediastinal germ cell tumor in one case, teratoma in two, and nonseminomatous (embryonal cancer) in three. These cases illustrate the importance of palpation of the testes in young patients with dermatomyositis (Fife et al. 1984; Di Stasi et al. 2000; Yoshinaga et al. 2995).

14.5 Penile Cancer

In Western countries, carcinoma of the penis is a rare neoplasm accounting for less than 1% of all cancers in males. More than 50% of patients with squamous cell carcinoma of the penis have lymph node involvement or distant metastasis at initial presentation. Hypercalcemia is the most common life-threatening metabolic disorder associated with malignancies; it has been rarely been reported in association with primary squamous cell carcinoma of the penis. Ideally, treatment of the primary cancer leads to resolution of this paraneoplastic disorder. However, elevated calcium serum levels often require urgent, nonspecific measures including hyperhydration therapy, diuretics, and biphosphanates (Malakoff and Schmidt 1975; Videtic et al. 1997; Wolchok et al. 1998; Dorfinger et al. 1999; Akashi et al. 2002). A chemotherapy regimen of intravenous cisplatin and fluorouracil caused regression of the primary tumor and normalization of the serum calcium. A cohort of 14 men with inoperable or metastatic squamous cell carcinoma of the penis was treated with methotrexate, bleomycin, and cisplatin. In 12 patients the penis was the primary site. Two patients had tumor-related hypercalcemia. Significant responses occurred in ten patients, including both patients with hypercalcemia with correction of the hypercalcemia (Dexeus et al. 1991). Close attention should be given to hypercalcemia in patients with carcinoma of the penis, as it is a life-threatening condition, and monitoring serum calcium levels may serve as tumor marker for therapeutic effects.

14.6 Conclusion

Urologic paraneoplastic syndromes are probably less reported than before, since there is a decrease in cases of metastatic urological cancers today. Management of these syndromes involves identification of the source of the underlying cause. Sometimes it is worthwhile to look for these syndromes especially when the cancer is metastatic.

References

Akashi T, Fuse H, Muraishi Y et al (2002) Parathyroid hormone related protein producing penile cancer. J Urol 167:249

Albright F (1941) Case records of the Massachusetts general Hospital-Case 390N. Eng J Med 225:789

Antonipillai I (1993) Epidermal growth factor is a potent inhibitor of renin secretion. Hypertension 21:654

Antonipillai I, Le TH, Soceneantu L, Horton R (1993) Transforming growth factor-beta is a renin secretagogue at picomolar concentrations. Am J Physiol 265:F537

Apaydin R, Gul U, Bahadir S, Siviloglu C, Ofluoglu I (2002) Dermatomyositis without muscle weakness associated with transitional cell carcinoma of the bladder. J Eur Acad Dermatol Venereol 16:172

Braasch WF (1952) End results following nephrectomy in patients with hypertension. J Urol 68:6

Broder LE, Weintraub BD, Rosen SW, Cohen MH, Tejada F (1977) Placental proteins and their subunits as tumor markers in prostatic carcinoma. Cancer 40:211

Callewaert PR, Van Poppel H, Vanderschueren D, Baert L (1999) Uncontrollable diabetes mellitus: a rare paraneoplastic manifestation of renal cell carcinoma. Nephrol Dial Transplant 14:2263

Citrin DL, Elson P, Kies MS, Lind R (1984) Decreased serum phosphate levels after high-dose estrogens in metastatic prostate cancer. Possible implications. Am J Med 76:787

Coleman RE (1997) Skeletal complications of malignancy. Cancer 80:1588

Conway GS, MacConnell T, Wells G, Slater SD (1988) Importance of scrotal ultrasonography in gynaecomastia. BMJ 297:1176

Da Silva JL, Lacombe C, Bruneval P, Casadevall N, Leporrier M, Camilleri JP, Bariety J, Tambourin P, Varet B (1990) Tumor cells are the site of erythropoietin synthesis in human renal cancers associated with polycythemia. Blood 75:577

De la Fouchardiere C, Flechon A, Droz JP (2003) Coagulopathy in prostate cancer. Neth J Med 61:347

Dexeus FH, Logothetis CJ, Sella A et al (1991) Combination chemotherapy with methotrexate, bleomycin and cisplatin for advanced squamous cell carcinoma of the male genital tract. J Urol 146:1284

Di Stasi SM, Poggi A, Giannantoni A, Zampa G (2000) Dermatomyositis associated with testicular germ cell cancer. J Urol 163:240

Dorfinger K, Maier U, Base W (1999) Parathyroid hormone related protein and carcinoma of the penis: paraneoplastic hypercalcemia. J Urol 161:1570

Elias AN (2005) New-onset insulinopenic diabetes mellitus in a patient with an incidentally discovered renal cell carcinoma. Am J Med 118:1047

Evans BK, Fagan C, Arnold T, Dropcho EJ, Oh SJ (1990) Paraneoplastic motor neuron disease and renal cell carcinoma: improvement after nephrectomy Neurology 40:960

Fife RS, Williams S, Eyanson S (1984) Dermatomyositis associated with treated testicular carcinoma. J Rheumatol 11:397

Fukutani K, Libby JM, Panko WB, Scardino PT (1983) Human chorionic gonadotropin detected in urinary concentrates from patients with malignant tumors of the testis, prostate, bladder, ureter and kidney. J Urol 129:74

Fukuzumi M, Hamakawa H, Onishi A, Sumida T, TaniokaH (2000) Gene expression of GLUT isoforms and VHL in oral squamous cell carcinoma. Cancer Lett 161:133

Gasparini ME, Broderick GA, Narayan P (1993) The syndrome of inappropriate antidiuretic hormone secretion in a patient with adenocarcinoma of the prostate. J Urol 150:978

Golde DW, Schambelan M, Weintraub BD, Rosen SW (1974) Gonadotropin-secreting renal carcinoma. Cancer 33:1048

Goldfarb DA (1999) Contemporary evaluation and management of Cushing's syndrome. World J Urol 17:22
Haas GP, Pittaluga S, Gomella L et al (1989) Clinically occult Leydig cell tumor presenting with gynecomastia. J Urol 142:1325
Hanazawa K, Higashi N, Kawachi Y, Suzuki F, Ishi K, Fujime M (2005) Small cell carcinoma of the prostate with hypercalcemia. Int J Urol 12:108
Hanash KA (1982) The nonmetastatic hepatic dysfunction syndrome associated with renal cell carcinoma (hypernephroma): Stauffer's syndrome. Prog Clin Biol Res 100:301
Hanash KA, Utz DC, Ludwig J, Wakim KG, Ellefson RD, Kelalis PP (1971) Syndrome of reversible hepatic dysfunction associated with hypernephroma: an experimental study. Invest Urol 8:399
Haukaas SA, Halvorsen OJ, Nygaard SJ, Paus E (1999) Cushing's syndrome in prostate cancer. An aggressive course of prostatic malignancy. Urol Int 63:126
Hirasawa K, Kitamura T, Oka T, Matsushita H (2002) Bladder tumor producing granulocyte colony-stimulating factor and parathyroid hormone related protein J Urol 167:2130
Hollifield JW, Page DL, Smith C, Michelakis AM, Staab E, Rhamy R (1975) Renin-secreting clear cell carcinoma of the kidney. Arch Intern Med 135:859
Janik JE, Sznol M, Urba WJ, Figlin R, Bukowski RM, Fyfe G, Pierce WC, Belldegrun A, Sharfman WH, Smith JW 2nd et al (1993) Erythropoietin production. A potential marker for interleukin-2/interferon-responsive tumors. Cancer 72:2656
Jobe BA, Bierman MH, Mezzacappa FJ (1993) Hyperglycemia as a paraneoplastic endocrinopathy in renal cell carcinoma: a case report and review of the literature. Nebr Med J 78:349
Joseph JV, Turner KJ, Bramwell SP (2002) Dermatomyositis: a rare initial presentation of adenocarcinoma of the prostate. J Urol 168:637
Kawai S, Hiroshima K, Tsukamoto Y, Tobe T, Suzuki H, Ito H, Ohwada H, Ito H (2003) Small cell carcinoma of the prostate expressing prostate-specific antigen and showing syndrome of inappropriate secretion of antidiuretic hormone: an autopsy case report. Pathol Int 53:892
Kim HL, Belldegrun AS, Freitas DG, Bui MH, Han KR, Dorey FJ, Figlin RA (2003) Paraneoplastic signs and symptoms of renal cell carcinoma: implications for prognosis. J Urol 170:1742
Laski ME, Vugrin D (1987) Paraneoplastic syndromes in hypernephroma. Semin Nephrol 7:123
Leavitt JA (2000) Myasthenia gravis with a paraneoplastic marker. J Neuroophthalmol 20:102
Lemack GE, Poppas DP, Vaughan ED Jr (1995) Urologic causes of gynecomastia: approach to diagnosis and management. Urology 45:313
Leong C, McKenzie MR, Coupland DB, Gascoyne RD (1994) Disseminated intravascular coagulation in a patient with metastatic prostate cancer: fatal outcome following strontium-89 therapy. J Nucl Med 35:1662
Lindop GB, Fleming S (1984) Renin in renal cell carcinoma an immunocytochemical study using an antibody to pure human renin. J Clin Pathol 37:27
Malakoff AF, Schmidt JD (1975) Metastatic carcinoma of penis complicated by hypercalcemia. Urology 5:510
Mallon E, Osborne G, Dinneen M, Lane RJ, Glaser M, Bunker CB (1999) Dermatomyositis in association with transitional cell carcinoma of the bladder. Clin Exp Dermatol 24:94
Matzkin H, Braf Z (1987) Paraneoplastic syndromes associated with prostatic carcinoma J Urol 138:1129
McCloskey BG, O'Connor FA (1982) Gonadotrophin secreting carcinoma of kidney. Ir J Med Sci 151:283
Mooney CJ, Dunphy EJ, Stone B, McNeel DG (2006) Identification of autoantibodies elicited in a patient with prostate cancer presenting as dermatomyositis. Int J Urol 13:211
Palgon N, Greenstein F, Novetsky AD, Lichter SM, Rosen Y (1986) Hyperglycemia associated with renal cell carcinoma. Urology 28:516
Paszkowski AL, Hewitt DJ, Taylor A Jr (1999) Disseminated intravascular coagulation in a patient treated with strontium-89 for metastatic carcinoma of the prostate. Clin Nucl Med 24:852
Pelger RC, Soerdjbalie-Maikoe V, Hamdy NA (2001) Strategies for management of prostate cancer-related bone pain. Drugs Aging 18:899
Rankin WR, Herman JR (2002) Rapidly progressive transitional cell carcinoma associated with dermatomyositis. J Urol 167:639
Rickman T, Garmany R, Doherty T, Benson D, Okusa MD (2001) Hypokalemia, metabolic alkalosis, and hypertension: Cushing's syndrome in a patient with metastatic prostate adenocarcinoma Am J Kidney Dis 37:838
Riggs BL Jr, Sprague RG (1961) Association of Cushing's syndrome and neoplastic disease: observations in 232 cases of Cushing's syndrome and review of the literature. Arch Intern Med 108:841
Ruffion A, Manel A, Valignat C, Lopez JG, Perrin-Fayolle O, Perrin P (2000) Successful use of Samarium 153 for emergency treatment of disseminated intravascular coagulation due to metastatic hormone refractory prostate cancer. J Urol 164:782
Sacks SA, Rhodes DB, Malkasian DR, Rosenbloom AA (1975) Prostatic carcinoma producing syndrome of inappropriate secretion of antidiuretic hormone. Urology 6:489
Shiba T, Higashi N, Nishimura Y (1998) Hyperglycaemia due to insulin resistance caused by interferon-gamma. Diabet Med 15:435
Shiramizu M, Katsuoka Y, Grodberg J, Koury ST, Fletcher JA, Davis KL, Sytkowski AJ (1994) Constitutive secretion of erythropoietin by human renal adenocarcinoma cells in vivo and in vitro. Exp Cell Res 215:249
Shimada T, Mizutani S, Muto T et al (2001) Cloning and characterization of FGF23 as a causative factor of tumor-induced osteomalacia. Proc Natl Acad Sci U S A 22:6500
Solon AA, Gilbert CS, Meyer C (1994) Myopathy as a paraneoplastic manifestation of renal cell carcinoma Am J Med 97:491
Stauffer MH (1961) Nephrogenic hepatosplenomegaly (abstract). Gastroenterology 40:694
Strewler GJ, Wronski TJ, Halloran BP, Miller SC, Leung SC, Williams RD, Nissenson RA (1986) Pathogenesis of hypercalcemia in nude mice bearing a human renal carcinoma. Endocrinology 119:303
Subramonian K, Sundaram SK, MacDonald Hull SP (2000) Carcinoma of the prostate associated with dermatomyositis. BJU Int 86:401
Sufrin G, Mirand EA, Moore RH, Chu TM, Murphy GP (1977) Hormones in renal cancer. J Urol 117:433
Tachibana M, Miyakawa A, Tazaki H et al (1995) Autocrine growth of transitional cell carcinoma of the bladder induced by granulocyte-colony stimulating factor. Cancer Res 55:3438
Tachibana M, Miyakawa A, Uchida A et al (1997) Granulocyte colony-stimulating factor receptor expression on human transitional cell carcinoma of the bladder. Br J Cancer 75:1489
Tallai B, Flasko T, Gyorgy T, Ponyi A, Andras C, Toth C, Danko K (2006) Prostate cancer underlying acute, definitive dermatomyositis: successful treatment with radical perineal prostatectomy. Clin Rheumatol 25:119
Torgerson EL, Khalili R, Dobkin BH, Reiter RE (1999) Myasthenia gravis as a paraneoplastic syndrome associated with renal cell carcinoma. J Urol 162:154

Tsukamoto T, Kumamoto Y, Miyao N, Masumori N, Takahashi A, Yanase M (1992) Interleukin-6 in renal cell carcinoma. J Urol 148:1778
Videtic GM, Ago CT, Winquist EW (1997) Hypercalcemia and carcinoma of the penis. Med Pediatr Oncol 29:576
Walther MM, Johnson B, Culley D et al (1998) Serum interleukin-6 levels in metastatic renal cell carcinoma before treatment with interleukin-2 correlates with paraneoplastic syndromes but not patient survival J Urol 159:718
Watanobe H, Yoshioka M, Takebe K (1988) Ectopic ACTH syndrome due to Grawitz tumor. Horm Metab Res 20:453
Weinstein EC, Geraa JE, Greene LF (1961) Hypernephroma presenting as fever of obscure origin. Proc Mayo Clinic 36:12
Weissglas M, Schamhart D, Lowik C, Papapoulos S, Vos P, Kurth KH (1995) Hypercalcemia and cosecretion of interleukin-6 and parathyroid hormone related peptide by a human renal cell carcinoma implanted into nude mice. J Urol 153:854
Wolchok JD, Herr HW, Kelly WK (1998) Localized squamous cell carcinoma of the bladder causing hypercalcemia and inhibition of PTH secretion. Urology 51:489
Yalcin S, Erman M, Tekuzman G, Ruacan S (2000) Syndrome of inappropriate antidiuretic hormone secretion (SIADH) associated with prostatic carcinoma. Am J Clin Oncol 23:384
Yamazaki T, Suzuki H, Tobe T et al (2001) Prostate adenocarcinoma producing syndrome of inappropriate secretion of antidiuretic hormone. Int J Urol 8:513
Yoshinaga A, Hayashi T, Ishii N, Ohno R, Watanabe T, Yamada T (2005) Successful cure of dermatomyositis after treatment of nonseminomatous testicular cancer. Int J Urol 12:593

Urologic Trauma: General Considerations 15.1

S.P. Elliott, J.W. McAninch

15.1.1 Iatrogenic Injury

15.1.1.1 Background

We have all been on either the giving or receiving end of a helpful intraoperative consult. It is always remarkable how a different point of view, a different incision, or a unique approach to the operative management of a problem can turn a sour occasion into a successful one. When one is the urologist called in to repair an iatrogenic injury to the genitourinary system, it is essential that we bring that fresh perspective to the situation. This is best accomplished via two principles: (1) do your best to duplicate the operative setting with which we are all more familiar – the elective case, and (2) be flexible and change your approach as demanded by the clinical situation at hand.

15.1.1.2 Intraoperative Guidelines

When consulted for an intraoperative injury, there is often a sense of urgency to correct an iatrogenic injury immediately. However, in most cases a urologic injury is not life-threatening. One would never perform an elective operation without reviewing the patient's history and we should have the same standards when consulted for an iatrogenic injury. Depending on the situation, a brief conversation with the surgeon of record, a review of the chart, or a conversation with the patient's family may be appropriate. Knowledge about preoperative renal function or prior pelvic surgery could significantly alter one's reconstructive plans. In order to make the surgical experience as familiar and comfortable as possible, one should order special instruments or retractors early. Rather than trying to make do with what's available, optimize the surgical situation. Should bleeding be a problem, packing the wound with laparotomy pads can control the situation while preparation for repair is underway. If the incision is one with which you are not familiar, then take some time to familiarize yourself with the anatomy or extend the incision before making any moves. Since many injuries occur at the limits of a surgeon's exposure, extending the incision also helps one look for unrecognized concomitant injuries. Stage the injury completely. Assess the blood supply of the structure you are repairing. This is especially true in the case of a ureteral injury. If the ureter has been devascularized as well as transected it will alter your plan for repair. Additionally, while we recommend making the operative situation as much like an elective case as possible, this cannot always be done – one may have to modify the operative plan in light of the limitations of the operating room. For instance, whereas one may feel most comfortable staging a ureteral injury by performing cystoscopy and retrograde pyelograms, patient positioning or the orientation of the operating table may prohibit cystoscopy and/or fluoroscopy. Finally, consider the patients overall condition and the limitations of the operative setting. While it might be possible to reconstruct an injury in a single setting, it may be more judicious to temporize drainage of the urinary system until a later date if the patient is unstable.

15.1.1.3 Postoperative Guidelines

When helping a colleague with an iatrogenic injury, one should be gracious and never accusatory – in the operating room, in the operative dictation, in conversation with the family, and in casual talk with fellow urologists. One should talk with the family immediately after the case, even as a consulting surgeon. Whenever possible it is best to have the surgeon of record alongside you when talking with the family so that a uniform explanation of the circumstances surrounding the injury can be presented. Nothing is gained in the operative dictation by using words such as "error", "iatrogenic", or “mistake.” Rather, one should describe the situation in passive terms, without introducing bias, i.e., “I was called into the room to examine and repair a transected ureter” rather than “Due to the large amount of blood in the field and poor visibility the ureter had been mistakenly injured. I was asked to repair this iatrogenic injury.” The former gives the necessary information without introducing an unsolicited opinion about the factors leading to the event, whereas the latter is fodder for litigation.

15.1.2 External Trauma

Two rules should govern the management of urologic trauma. First, in the stable patient all efforts should be made to evaluate and address genitourinary injuries at presentation. Imaging of the urinary tract can be easily incorporated into computerized tomography (CT) of the abdomen by obtaining delayed images during the renal excretion phase. This allows complete staging of renal and ureteral injuries. Assessment of bladder injuries should be done with plain film or CT cystogram. Early imaging and expeditious repair of select urologic injuries is essential as delayed management can lead to increased complications (Elliott and McAninch 2003). In fact, even if an injury may eventually heal with conservative management one should consider an operative repair if the patient is being taken to the operating room for repair of another injury (Gomez et al. 2004; Santucci et al. 2004).

The first rule is illustrated by two examples. If a patient is being explored by general surgery and a gunshot wound injury of the kidney is discovered that is amenable to renorrhaphy, then a renal repair should be done, as this leads to a decreased incidence of delayed urine leak and blood transfusion (Meng et al. 1999). Likewise, if a patient with a blunt trauma is being observed for a large extraperitoneal bladder rupture and he is taken to the operating room for fixation of an unstable pelvic fracture, then the bladder rupture should be repaired, as it will decrease his recovery and catheterization time (Gomez et al. 2004).

The second rule is that in the *un*stable patient the urologic injuries must be measured alongside other, often more life-threatening, injuries; urologic injuries can often be managed without reconstruction or temporized with a drain (Elliott and McAninch 2003; Gomez et al. 2004; Santucci et al. 2004).

This rule is illustrated by the example of a patient with a gunshot wound injury to the central portion of the kidney who is hemodynamically unstable. In this case, a nephrectomy may be preferable to a complicated reconstruction. Likewise, in a patient with a ureteral injury who is unstable due to concomitant injuries, the ureteral injury may be temporized with ligation of the ureter and placement of a nephrostomy tube rather than reconstruction of the ureter.

For these reasons, it is essential that the urologist have excellent communication with the other services involved in trauma care. Our management of the urologic injuries will often need to be modified based on the management plan for concomitant injuries.

The management of iatrogenic injury and urologic trauma both demand the perfect balance of vigilance and due caution.

References

Elliott SP, McAninch JW (2003) Ureteral injuries from external violence: the 25-year experience at San Francisco General Hospital. J Urol 170:1213–1216

Gomez RG, Ceballos L, Coburn M et al (2004) Consensus statement on bladder injuries. BJU Int 94:27–32

Meng MV, Brandes SB, McAninch JW (1999) Renal trauma: indications and techniques for surgical exploration. World J Urol 17:71–77

Santucci RA, Wessells H, Bartsch G et al (2004) Evaluation and management of renal injuries: consensus statement of the renal trauma subcommittee. BJU Int 93:937–954

Modern Trauma: New Mechanisms of Injury Due to Terrorist Attacks 15.2

N.D. Kitrey, A. Nadu, Y. Mor

15.2.1 Introduction

Terrorism has increasingly become an integral part of the reality in many regions of the world. In the past few decades, there has been a surge in the number and in the intensity of terrorist attacks all over the globe, and the treatment of terror-related mass casualty incidents presents a special challenge to the medical teams involved. According to the Worldwide Incidents Tracking System (WITS) of the American National Counterterrorism Center (National Counterterrorism Center 2006), there were 3,204 terrorist incidents worldwide in the year 2004 with 6,110 fatalities and 16,257 wounded. Many of the casualties resulted from suicide bombings in Iraq, Chechnya, Uzbekistan, Israel, and Pakistan. Unfortunately, the numbers are expected to increase further and the world has realized that terrorist attacks are no longer confined to certain locations.

Consequently, management of terror-related injuries has become a global public health challenge and increased awareness of medical teams to their unique characteristics is warranted. Furthermore, the medical community should develop adequate preparedness to various nonconventional terrorist scenarios, caused by chemical, biological, and radiological weapons, in order to decrease the associated chaos and improve the probability of survival of those injured (Shemer and Shapira 2001).

The term "terrorism" itself derives from the Latin word "terrere" (to frighten), and it dates back to 1795 when it was used to describe the actions of the Jacobin Club in their rule of revolutioary France during the Reign of Terror. The modern definition of "terrorism" is emotionally and politically charged (Wikipedia 2006). However, nearly all of its definitions include certain key criteria in terms of the *unlawful* use of *violence* with political, religious or ideological *motivation*, while the *target* is civilian, and the *objective* is to demoralize and to provoke fear. According to a United Nations panel in 2004, acts of terrorism are "intended to cause death or serious bodily harm to civilians or non-combatants with the purpose of intimidating a population or compelling a government or an international organization to do or to abstain from doing any act" (Wikipedia 2006).

Bombs and explosions directed against innocents are the primary instrument of modern terrorist groups. These weapons are easily and inexpensively manufactured, often according to clear instructions that are freely distributed on the internet, and are usually very simple to activate either directly or remotely, automatically or manually, momentarily or at a deferred time using various timers (Kluger 2003; Sutphen 2005). Terrorists use explosive devices of various levels of sophistication and power, which can be military, commercial, or homemade. The common mechanism of all explosive devices is the rapid conversion of solid or liquid material into gas with associated release of energy. The explosion substances are categorized as either high- or low-order (Sutphen 2005). High-order explosives, like TNT, Semtex, and dynamite generate heat, loud noise, and a supersonic overpressurization shock wave (blast wave) that expands outward and is followed by a returning vacuum wave. Low-order explosives, like gunpowder-based bombs and Molotov cocktails, create an explosion with a relatively slow release of destructive energy without the overpressurization wave.

Suicide bombing is currently the most effective terrorist strategy since it maximizes the effect of mass casualty incidents. Suicide bombers are difficult to identify and their entrance into crowded confined places can cause an urban disaster. They may wear either an explosive belt or vest and can also use cars or trucks heavily loaded with explosives without attracting suspicion and trigger themselves with perfectly controlled timing (Sutphen 2005). The explosive device is detonated by a simple electric charge activated either remotely or more commonly by the suicide bomber himself (Kluger 2003). Occasionally, terrorists use secondary devices to detonate at a slightly delayed time, in order to harm the emergency response personnel taking care of the victims of the first act.

15.2.2 Mechanisms of Explosive Injury

Injuries inflicted by explosion have been known since the invention of gunpowder and detonation devices, although they are rarely encountered in civilian hospitals. Explosion injuries have a multidimensional pattern and complicated clinical course composed of the simultaneous combination of four distinct injury mechanisms (DePalma et al. 2005; Kluger 2003; Singer et al. 2005; Stein and Hirshberg 1999; Sutphen 2005).

15.2.2.1 Primary Mechanism (Primary Blast Injury)

The energy produced by the explosion generates a shock wave that has three components: an extremely short high-positive pressure phase, a longer but milder negative-pressure phase, and a "blast wind" – a massive movement of air. Gas-containing organs, such as the middle ear, the respiratory system, and the gastrointestinal tract, are injured by this baro-trauma with micro- and macroscopic tears of the gas–fluid interface. The common injuries consist of perforation of the eardrums, "blast lung" (alveolar capillary disruption, bronchopleural fistulas, and air emboli), and bowel perforations.

15.2.2.2 Secondary Mechanism

The secondary mechanism consists of injury caused by the impact of displaced debris and particles of the detonation device. Terrorists add nails, screws, steel pellets, and other metallic fragments to the explosive device in order to inflict as much damage as possible. These flying objects cause penetrating and blunt trauma. They have an initial velocity of 2,000 m/s but their irregular shape and unsteady course cause rapid deceleration, hence their effect is maximal at close range.

15.2.2.3 Tertiary Mechanism

These injuries occur as a result of people being thrown into fixed objects by the blast wind, especially during the deceleration phase when the body hits a stationary rigid surface. In addition, the tertiary mechanism includes extensive blunt injuries that are caused by structural collapse and fragmentation of buildings or vehicles.

15.2.2.4 Quaternary Mechanism

Other explosion-related injuries are caused by burns, smoke or toxic gas inhalation, crush injury, and exacerbation of preexisting illnesses.

15.2.3 Characteristics of Terrorist-Related Blast Injuries

The epidemiological and clinical outcomes of an explosion depend on several prognostic factors: the magnitude of explosion, the composition and amount of the explosive material, the surrounding environment, and the distance between the blast and the victim. The blast-induced injuries are considerably influenced by whether the blast occurs in an open or in a confined space. For example, in an open-air terrorist bombing in Istanbul, Turkey on November 15, 2005, there were 69 casualties that were treated in the American Hospital in Istanbul. Only four of them (5 %) had an Injury Severity Score of 16 or more and none of them had primary blast injury (Rodoplu et al. 2005). On the other hand, blast victims in confined spaces have an increased mortality rate (15.8 % vs 2.8 %), a higher mean Injury Severity Score (ISS) in survivors (11 % vs 6.8 %), a higher incidence of primary blast injury, and more extensive burn injuries (Kluger 2003; Rodoplu 2005). In ultraconfined spaces such as buses, the overpressure from the explosion is instantly magnified by reflections from the walls and has devastating consequences with an exceptionally high fatalities-to-casualties ratio and mortality rate (49 %) (Almogy et al. 2004; Kluger et al. 1997; Shaloner 2005; Sutphen 2005). Moreover, blasts that cause structural collapse are associated with an immediate mortality rate as high as 25 % (Arnold et al. 2003, 2004).

A terrorist attack can cause a unique form of severe intentional injury and it presents with a unique epidemiology and several distinctive features, differing from conventional trauma injuries. Several studies from Israel, based on the Israeli National Trauma Registry, have tried to characterize patients hospitalized as a result of terrorist injuries and to compare them to other trauma casualties (Kluger 2003; Kluger et al. 2004; Peleg et al. 2003). According to these studies, the majority of terrorist-related victims were relatively young, half of them in their 20s, since crowded public places such as malls, pubs, and buses are frequently crowded by young people (Kluger 2003; Kluger et al. 2004). It is noteworthy that children, especially adolescents, are frequently injured in terrorist attacks and the injury severity, as well as the subsequent morbidity and mortality, is exceptionally high among children injured by explosions (Aharonson-Daniel et al. 2003; Amir et al. 2005; DePalma et al. 2005).

The terrorist-related injuries were generally more severe and 29% of them had an Injury Severity Score (ISS) above 16, as compared to 10% in all other conventional trauma admissions (Kluger 2003; Kluger et al. 2004). The severity of injuries is also manifested by the state of consciousness on admission (as represented by the Glasgow Coma Scale scores), the increased frequency of hypotension on admission, and the fact that the majority of the victims sustain injuries to multiple body regions (Kluger et al. 2004). Furthermore, survivors of terrorist-related bomb explosions underwent significantly more surgical interventions (53%, especially orthopedic and abdominal surgery), they more frequently required the services of intensive care units (23%), their overall hospital stay was remarkably prolonged (20% were hospitalized for more than 14 days), and they required more rehabilitation treatment compared to casualties of other types of trauma (Kluger 2003; Kluger et al. 2004; Mintz et al. 2002; Sutphen 2005). However, despite all efforts, this group of patients eventually had an increased in-hospital mortality rate of 6.1%, as compared to 3% in motor vehicle accidents and 1.8% in other trauma, probably related to the increased injury complexity (Kluger et al. 2004). Several studies have noted that the high specific mortality rate in explosions is primarily due to abdominal injuries (19%) and severe head injuries (20–25%) (Amir et al. 2005).

15.2.4 Characteristics of Terrorist-Related Gunshot Injuries

Aside from bombs and explosions, terrorists still widely use other means of violence such as gun shooting, stabbing, and stoning. The outcomes of terrorist-related gunshot and stab wounds are similar to those seen in criminal and military scenarios. In the Israeli experience, most gunshot wounds were inflicted by sniper shootings at high velocity into passing cars or at pedestrians, though a few incidents of gunshots from automatic weapons into crowds of people were also encountered (Amir et al. 2005). Correspondingly, while explosion victims usually arrive at the hospital as a part of a mass casualty event, gunshot victims typically arrive as individuals (Peleg et al. 2004; Singer et al. 2005). Gunshot victims, compared with explosion victims, had a higher proportion of open wounds (63% vs 53%) and fractures (42% vs 31%), more frequent abdominal, spinal, and chest wounds, and overall they presented with a double incidence of moderate-severity injuries (ISS 9–14) (Mintz et al. 2002; Peleg et al. 2004; Singer et al. 2005). Explosion victims, on the other hand, had higher proportions of both minor and critical injuries (related to the distance from the focus of the explosion). The inpatient death rate is not significantly different (7.8% vs 5.3%), perhaps because the available data exclude many patients who die at the scene in an explosive incident or subsequently arrive dead at the hospital; however, a larger proportion of gunshot victims died during the first day (Peleg et al. 2004).

15.2.5 Medical Management of Terrorist-Related Injuries

Terrorist acts frequently generate mass casualty events that overwhelm the regional health care system and cause a temporary imbalance between the sudden urgent demand for large-scale resources and expertise at a specific location and the availability of such resources (Shemer and Shapira 2001). The inundation of the medical system with hundreds of victims presents two types of challenge: a medical challenge, i.e., proper medical management with accurate triage, and a logistical challenge (Hirshberg 2004; Shemer and Shapira 2001). While the management of the single patient should initially follow the guidelines of Advanced Trauma Life Support (ATLS) (Shaloner 2005), the medical team should be aware of the unique multidimensional nature of terrorist-related injuries and take this into consideration during triage, diagnosis, treatment, and hospital organization (Peleg and Aharonson-Daniel 2005). As the individual victim is often treated as part of a mass casualty scenario, prompt triage is crucial in order to utilize the hospital resources effectively, sorting the patients into urgent versus nonurgent categories and directing the efforts to a maximal number of salvageable patients (Kluger et al. 2004; Peleg et al. 2004; Stein and Hirshberg 1999; Sutphen 2005). In accordance, Israeli studies have demonstrated that only 20%–23% of the casualties present with critical injuries and require urgent care (Almogy et al. 2004; Einav et al. 2004; Frykberg 2004; Peleg et al. 2004); therefore every effort should be made to prevent treatment of unsalvageable patients and victims who do not really require immediate medical care (overtriage) from delaying the recognition and treatment of the small number of patients with urgent and salvageable life-threatening injuries (undertriage) (Frykberg 2004; Kluger 2003; Stein and Hirshberg 1999). In these circumstances, prioritization of treatment regimens is mandatory and definitive therapy should be delayed until the patient is hemodynamically stabilized: damage control principles should be applied. However, identifying those critically injured patients who are candidates for damage control maneuvers, which aims to achieve hemostasis and prevent uncontrolled spillage of bowel contents and urine, is undoubtedly a challenge. Throughout the management of the event, coordination between the primary on-scene teams responsible for the primary triage and evacuation is obligatory, followed by similar close interaction between the in-hospital teams conducting the triage, the initial treatment, the surgical interventions and the intensive care, as well as between neighboring hospitals, in order to optimize utilization of the hospitals' personnel and resources (Almogy et al. 2004; Einav et al. 2004; Hirshberg 2004). Special consideration should be given to the fact that shrapnel containing human remains might transfect hepatitis B virus (HBV) or human immunodeficiency virus (HIV); thus immunization is recommended in appropriate scenarios (Singer et al. 2005; Sutphen 2005). The psychological effects on victims and family members should not be overlooked, hence the immediate role of specialized psychological teams is critical (Kluger 2003; Rusch et al. 2002). Subsequently, during the long course of rehabilitation, one should not forget the emotional and psychological support for the trauma victims who might present posttraumatic stress disorder, depressive disorder, panic disorder, phobias, and substance abuse (Rusch et al. 2002). Similarly, the medical personnel involved should not be ignored and special sessions should be scheduled for the teams in order to minimize the individual psychological burden and alleviate the reactions (Kluger 2003).

15.2.6 Urological Aspects of Terrorist-Related Injuries

A review of the literature reveals that there is a paucity of data on terrorist-related urological injuries. Important data is available from the Israeli Trauma Registry (ITR), which records all hospitalizations for physical trauma at most of the Israeli trauma centers. Unfortunately, the accumulated experience of the Israeli medical system with terrorist-related injuries during the last two decades is exceptional in duration and intensity, out-ranging any comparable practice gained elsewhere, as only between September 2000 and December 2003, nearly 20,000 terrorist incidents were reported in Israel (Singer et al. 2005). All the patients recorded in the ITR with terrorist-related trauma to the urogenital system between 1997 and 2003 were studied retrospectively (Kitrey et al. 2005); 2% of all the terrorist attack casualties had urological injuries, one-third of them were injured by explosions, and the rest had gunshot wounds. The urological injuries were uniformly part of a multiorgan injury. The majority of the victims were young males with severe injuries, 53% of them were treated in intensive care units, and 46% were hospitalized for more than 2 weeks.

Urologic injuries during conventional wars and regional conflicts were investigated much more and seem to be comparable to terrorist-related injuries, especially the data from Northern Ireland in the 1970s and the Balkans in the 1990s. Nowadays, this comparison is increasingly accurate in view of the changing patterns of battlefield urological injuries secondary to an increased use of explosive weapons and the observation that the vast majority of urologic injuries currently sustained in war are caused by fragmentation devices (Hudak et al. 2005). This trend is evident on review of the mechanism of injury in different conflicts and wars throughout history. In the Irish conflict, 89.4% of the injuries were caused by gunshots, usually low velocity weapons (Archbold et al. 1981) and similarly in the Vietnam War, 92% of injuries were the result of penetrating missiles (Hudak et al. 2005). Later on, during the Bosnia-Herzegovina conflict, most of the urologic injuries (52.9%–75%) were inflicted by explosions of bombs, rockets, mines, mortars, and grenades, while only a minority of urologic injuries was caused by firearms (Hudolin and Hudolin 2003; Kuvezdic et al. 1996; Tucak et al. 1995; Vuckovic et al. 1995). In accordance, in the Israeli terrorist-related series, 59% of urological injuries were due to gunshots and 34% were from explosions (Kitrey et al. 2005).

Urologic war injuries are relatively infrequent and have constituted a small percentage of battlefield casualties during the past century. Review of the literature reveals that the genitourinary system is involved in 0.7%–10% of all war-related trauma cases (Table 15.2.1). Generally, the urological injuries are severe, even life-threatening, and combined with injuries to other organs in up to 76%–100% of cases (Busch et al. 1967; Hudolin and Hudolin 2003; Kuvezdic et al. 1996; Vuckovic et al. 1995). Comparably, in the Israeli experience, only 2% of all terrorist-related trauma patients had urologic injuries, uniformly as a part of a combined or a multitrauma injury (Kitrey et al. 2005), similarly to the data from the Balkans and Ireland. Since these casualties rarely suffer from injuries that are limited solely to the genitourinary system, a thorough urological evaluation is often impossible at arrival. Consequently, the genitourinary injuries are often detected during exploratory laparotomy, as the patients are hemodynamically unstable at presentation and time-consuming preoperative imaging is impossible (Hudak et

Table 15.2.1. Review of urologic injuries in recent wars

	Rate of urologic injuries	Proportion of abdominal injury (kidneys and ureters)	Proportion of pelvic and external genitalia injury
World War II[a]	0.7%–4%	14%–30%	66%–82%
Korean War[b]	1.7%		
Vietnam War (1960s)[c]	4.2%–10%	20.8%	75%
Northern Ireland (1970s)[d]	2.25%	50%	
Balkan War (1990s)[e]	2.4%–2.6%	45%–53%	47%–55%
Gulf War (1990s)[f]	<2%	17%	83%
Israel (terrorist-related)[g]	2%	67%	33%

[a] Busch et al. 1967; Hudak et al. 2005
[b] Hudak et al. 2005
[c] Busch et al. 1967; Hudak et al. 2005
[d] Archbold et al. 1981
[e] Hudolin and Hudolin 2003; Kuvezdic et al. 1996; Tucak et al. 1995; Vuckovic et al. 1995
[f] Hudak et al. 2005; Thompson et al. 1998
[g] Kitrey et al. 2005

al. 2005); consequently, damage control strategies are usually applied.

Blast injury causes injuries to the torso in 38%; only one-third of them are isolated, whereas the others are abdominal injuries combined with head, chest, or extremity injuries (Peleg et al. 2003). Gas-containing organs are the most vulnerable to primary blast effect, though injuries to solid organs such as the kidneys are also encountered as a result of acceleration and deceleration forces. At exploration, this injury usually takes the form of hemorrhage beneath the visceral peritoneum that extends into the mesentery, possibly associated with perforation of the bowel or rupture, infarction, ischemia, or hemorrhage of solid organs, including the genitourinary system (Centers for Disease Control 2006; DePalma et al. 2005; Stein and Hirshberg 1999). During warfare, the proportion of the abdominal injury with involvement of the kidneys and ureters is quite varied in different series because of the different characteristics of the conflict and the medical management. During World War II, these injuries were relatively infrequent (Table 15.2.1), perhaps because evacuation was delayed and severely wounded patients with abdominal injuries did not reach the hospital alive. Therefore, renal injury was probably underestimated then, because of high mortality rates in the combat area while awaiting evacuation and treatment (Hudak et al. 2005). On the other hand, during the Gulf war, as an example of a modern war, evacuation time was usually short, but renal and ureteral injuries were infrequent as well. This may have resulted from the fact that most of the reported wounded were American soldiers using flak jackets protecting their flank and abdomen (Thompson et al. 1998). In the same war, civilians and soldiers from the other side, not wearing flak jackets, had many more renal and ureteral injuries (Abu-Zidan et al. 1999). The urban scenarios of the Balkan and the Irish conflicts seem more comparable to terrorist attacks because both the civilian population and most of the armed forces involved did not use body armor and the evacuation was usually rapid. In these series, the kidneys and ureters were involved in half of the urologic injuries (Table 15.2.1). In accordance, in Israel, two-thirds of the terrorist-related victims with some sort of urological involvement had renal and ureteral injuries, whether injury resulted from gunshots or explosions (Kitrey et al. 2005). However, bladder injuries were more common in gunshots victims (17% vs 9%), while trauma to the external genitalia was more common following explosive injuries (26% vs 14%). Altogether, the urological injuries encountered following terrorist assaults present particularly complex and severe wounding patterns that are not typically seen in other forms of trauma, probably because they involve a combination of penetrating and blunt mechanisms (Frykberg 2004). Consequently, surgeons should be prepared to face complex renal contusions and lacerations, a high incidence of ureteral injuries, which are often overlooked, bladder ruptures, and severe injuries to the external genitalia, mostly with testicular rupture secondary to blast injury (Centers for Disease Control 2006). In view of these distinct complex urological insults associated with other multiorgan injuries, urologists should adapt their surgical approach to the situation, improvise, and often apply damage control principles in order to provide temporary stabilizing solutions. Understandably, unusual urological injuries may beget unusual original management approaches. This was previously illustrated by our colleagues (Sofer et al. 2004), by the management of a 15-year-old girl who was injured in a terrorist suicide blast. On admission, an open abdominal wound with enteral evisceration was noted and she was urgently operated on to repair a transection of the right iliac vessels. Radiological imaging performed on the following day revealed a 6-cm-long nail in the right kidney, passing through the collecting system. As the patient was asymptomatic from the urological point of view and the nail was considered to be entrapped and unlikely to migrate, conservative, nonoperative management was chosen. An intravenous urogram (Fig. 15.2.1), taken 1 year after the injury, revealed normal excretion with no migration of the nail. The patient's follow-up was uneventful for 5 years after the injury.

An early review of the published experience with terrorist bombings up to the late 1980s clearly showed that abdominal injury carries the highest specific mortality rate (19%) of any single body system injury

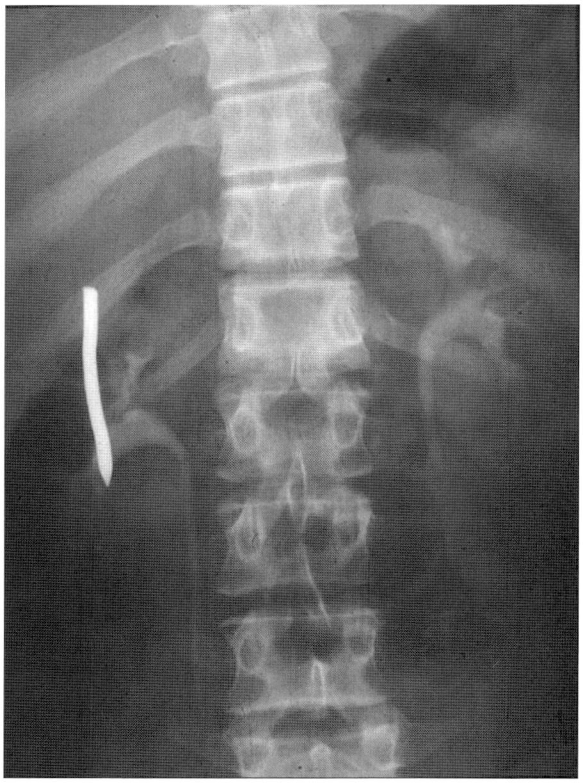

Fig. 15.2.1. Intravenous urogram showing a metallic nail in the right kidney (Sofer et al. 2001).

among the immediate survivors (Frykberg and Tepas 1988). The mortality rate among patients with urologic injuries in the Balkan war was much the same, reportedly 15.6% (Tucak et al. 1995). Similarly, in the Israeli study, 19.1% of the terrorist-related urological patients died during their hospitalization (Kitrey et al. 2005). This high mortality rate may have resulted from several factors, including the short evacuation period, which means that even very severely injured patients arrive at the hospital alive, the high prevalence of severe injuries to other organs, and the unprecedented powerful weapons.

15.2.7 Summary

Terrorist attacks have become a reality all over the world. Medical facilities and physicians alike should be prepared for terrorist-related mass casualty events with their distinctive features. Terrorist-related trauma patients tend to have severe multiorgan injuries, including some that are unique to explosions. There are no satisfactory data on urological injuries in terrorist attacks; nevertheless, it seems that these are generally combined, severe injuries that require a well-orchestrated team approach, with close cooperation between various clinical specialties and adaptation of damage control principles in urological trauma management. Undoubtedly, with the expanding role of the damage control approach, the comprehension of its principles should no longer be limited to general surgeons: urologists who are commonly involved as additional surgical specialists in severe multitrauma patients should be highly familiar with its principles.

References

Abu-Zidan FM, Al-Tawheed A, Ali YM (1999) Urologic injuries in the Gulf War. Int Urol Nephrol 31:577

Aharonson-Daniel L, Waisman Y, Dannon YL et al (2003) Epidemiology of terror-related versus non-terror-related traumatic injury in children. Pediatrics 112:280

Almogy G, Belzberg H, Mintz Y et al (2004) Suicide bombing attacks: update and modifications to the protocol. Ann Surg 239:295

Amir LD, Aharonson-Daniel L, Peleg K et al (2005) The severity of injury in children resulting from acts against civilian population. Ann Surg 241:666

Anonymous (2006) Definition of Terrorism. Wikipedia. http://en.wikipedia.org/wiki/ Definition_of_terrorism. Cited 27 January 2006

Anonymous (2006) Terrorism. Wikipedia. http://en.wikipedia.org/wiki/Terrorism. Cited 27 January 2006

Archbold JA, Barros d'sa AA, Morrison E (1981) Genito-urinary tract injuries of civil hostilities. Br J Surg 68:625

Arnold JL, Tsai MC, Halpern P et al (2003) Mass-casualty, terrorist bombings: epidemiological outcomes, resource utilization, and time course of emergency needs (part I). Prehospital Disaster Med 18:220

Arnold JL, Halpern P, Tsai MC et al (2004) Mass casualty terrorist bombings: a comparison of outcomes by bombing type. Ann Emerg Med 43:263

Busch FM, Chenault OW Jr, Clarke BG et al (1967) Urological aspects of Vietnam War injuries. J Urol 97:763

Centers for Disease Control and Prevention (2006) Explosions and blast injuries, a primer for clinicians. the Centers for Disease Control and Prevention, Atlanta. http://www.bt.cdc.gov/masstrauma/pdf/explosions-blast-injuries.pdf. Cited 27 January 2006

DePalma RG, Burris DG, Champion HR et al (2005) Blast Injuries. N Engl J Med 352:1335

Einav S, Feigenberg Z, Weissman C et al (2004) Evacuation priorities in mass casualty terror-related events: implications for contingency planning. Ann Surg 239:304

Frykberg ER (2004) Principles of Mass Casualty Management Following Terrorist Disasters. Ann Surg 239:319

Frykberg ER, Tepas JJ 3rd (1988) Terrorist bombings. Lessons learned from Belfast to Beirut. Ann Surg 208:569

Georgi BA, Massad M, Obeid M (1991) Ballistic trauma to the abdomen: shell fragments versus bullets. J Trauma 31:711

Hirshberg A (2004) Multiple casualty incidents: lessons from the front line. Ann Surg 239:322

Hudak SJ, Morey AF, Rozanski TA et al (2005) Battlefield urogenital injuries: changing patterns during the past century. Urology 65:1041

Hudolin T, Hudolin I (2003) Surgical management of urogenital injuries at a war hospital in Bosnia-Herzegovina, 1992 to 1995. J Urol 169:1357

Kitrey ND, Peleg K, Givon A et al (2005) Terror-related urological injuries in Israel between 1997 and 2003. XXth EAU congress in Istanbul, Turkey

Kluger Y (2003) Bomb explosions in acts of terrorism – detonation, wound ballistics, triage and medical concerns. Isr Med Assoc J 5:235

Kluger Y, Soffer D, Sorkine P et al (1997) Blast injury: detonation and injury pattern. Harefuah 132:591

Kluger Y, Peleg K, Daniel-Aharonson L et al (2004) The special injury pattern in terrorist bombings. J Am Coll Surg 199:875

Kuvezdic H, Tucak A, Grahovac B (1996) War injuries of the kidney. Injury 27:557

Mintz Y, Shapira SC, Pikarsky AJ et al (2002) The experience of one institution dealing with terror: the El Aqsa Intifada riots. IMAJ 4:554

National Counterterrorism Center (2006) Worldwide Incidents Tracking System (WITS) of the National Counterterrorism Center. http://www.tkb.org/NCTC/Home.jsp. Cited 28 January 2006

Peleg K, Aharonson-Daniel L (2005) Blast injuries. New Engl J Med 352:2651

Peleg K, Aharonson-Daniel L, Michael M et al (2003) Patterns of injury in hospitalized terrorist victims. Am J Emerg Med 21:258

Peleg K, Aharonson-Daniel L, Stein M et al (2004) Gunshot and explosion injuries: characteristics, outcomes, and implications for care of terror-related injuries in Israel. Ann Surg 239:311

Rodoplu U, Arnold JL, Tokyay R et al (2005) Impact of the terrorist bombings of the Neve Shalom and Beth Israel synagogues on a hospital in Istanbul, Turkey. Acad Emerg Med 12:135

Rusch MD, Gould LJ, Dzwierzynski WW et al (2002) Psychological impact of traumatic injuries: what the surgeon can do. Plast Reconstr Surg 109:18

Shaloner E (2005) Blast injury in enclosed spaces. BMJ 331:119

Shemer J, Shapira SC (2001) Terror and medicine – the challenge. Isr Med Assoc J 3:799

Singer P, Cohen JD, Stein M (2005) Conventional terrorism and critical care. Crit Care Med 33:S61

Sofer M, Kaver I, Kluger Y et al (2001) Conservative management of an uncommon renal foreign body secondary to explosion injury. J Trauma 51:594

Stein M, Hirshberg A (1999) Medical consequences of terrorism. The conventional weapon threat. Surg Clin North Am 79:1537

Sutphen SK (2005) Blast injuries: a review. http://www.medscape.com/viewarticle/516117. Cited 27 January 2006

Thompson IM, Flaherty SF, Morey AF (1998) Battlefield urologic injuries: the Gulf War experience. J Am Coll Surg 187:139

Tucak A, Lukacevic T, Kuvezdic H et al (1995) Urogenital wounds during the war in Croatia in 1991/1992. J Urol 153:121

Vuckovic I, Tucak A, Gotovac J et al (1995) Croatian experience in the treatment of 629 urogenital war injuries. J Trauma 39:733

15.3 Mass Casualties: Urologic Aspects of Triage and Definitive Management

A. Nadu, N.D. Kitrey, Y. Mor

15.3.1 Mass Casualties

15.3.1.1 Introduction

Contemporary history is unfortunately associated with pandemic civilian disasters that have made the concept of mass casualty events highly and painfully relevant for all medical and surgical specialties.

Catastrophic events resulting in mass casualties are typically associated with a number of victims that exceeds the available medical resources. Besides the sheer number of victims involved, the severity of injuries tends to be high and complex and there are usually other factors involved that further complicate the situation. These events are always unexpected and result in chaos and confusion on site and among the medical teams, with great numbers of anxious family members claiming their right for information on their loved ones and numerous patients without significant physical injuries suffering of post-traumatic reactions. In addition, the emotions of the medical personnel exposed to the results of disasters or terrorist attacks with innocent civilian victims, often children and babies, are more than likely to influence their work. Therefore, the unique characteristics of these events require a different management approach compared to day-to-day emergency room trauma care. As in sporadic complicated trauma case management, a multidisciplinary team, composed of various surgical and medical specialists, is often involved. Under these circumstances, the need for a common language and for the understanding of mass casualty treatment principles is certainly a must for all the consultants involved. Terms such as "triage" and "damage control" should not be reserved merely for the lexicon of the general surgeons in the trauma team, but should be understood and applied by all those involved in the treatment of trauma patients.

The spectrum of urogenital trauma, including life-threatening conditions (such as high-grade renal injury) or injuries that carry the potential of severe late morbidity (such as ureteral or urethral trauma), put the urologic surgeon in a position that demands thorough knowledge of the modern principles of trauma, including preparedness to catastrophic situations with mass casualty scenarios.

15.3.1.2 Definitions

A mass casualty event is defined as any event that results in a number of injured people that is sensibly higher than the number of available healthcare providers (Slater and Trunkey 1997). Although it is usually a synonym with a large number of injured people, a mass casualty disaster does not necessarily involve a large number of victims, but is actually related to the disproportion between the number of victims and the availability of a corresponding medical team. This relative paucity of medical resources dictates the application of different protocols than those existent in routine day-to-day trauma events, when the resources are greater than the casualties involved (Caro 1974; Weighlt et al. 1997).

15.3.1.3
Triage Principles

The notion of triage is somewhat problematic and debatable, as well as impregnated with difficult ethical and moral questions. During World War II, a battlefield nurse was given the responsibility of triage, i.e., dividing patients into three groups: patients with minor (non-life- or non-limb-threatening injuries) who do not need immediate attention, patients in critical condition who can mostly benefit from immediate care, and patients beyond hope who will not be treated (Frykberg 2002). Similar principles are applied in modern medicine for disaster triage, with emphasis on the fact that the essence of triage is to identify the few critically injured who can be saved by immediate intervention among the many others with non-life-threatening injuries, for whom treatment can be delayed.

The generally accepted principles of triage for mass casualty scenarios divide patients into four groups (Frykberg 2002; Jacobs et al. 1979).

1. Patients with life-threatening injuries requiring immediate and expeditious intervention in terms of the ABC care principles: airway compromise, breathing failure (tension pneumothorax, open chest wounds), and/or circulatory compromise from ongoing external hemorrhage.
2. Patients with severe but not life-threatening injuries, in whom treatment can be acceptably delayed, including fractures, vascular injuries of the limbs and soft tissue wounds.
3. Ambulatory patients with minimal injuries.
4. The most severely injured patients, for whom treatment would require allocation of resources and time that would prevent other more salvageable patients from receiving timely care. These patients are expectantly treated and reevaluated when resources become available. This group generally includes patients with severe head injuries, open skull fractures, extensive open brain wounds and patients in cardiac arrest. There is no absolute definition for the patients composing this group, who will not receive treatment initially, because triage is always to be individualized according to the existing number and severity of casualties related to the available medical resources.

The triage concept is basically in contradiction with the day-to-day principles of care, dictated by the ultimate goal of providing maximal and optimal care for any individual patient. However, in mass casualty scenarios, triage becomes legitimate as the goal changes to that of providing the minimal acceptable treatment to the maximal number of salvageable patients. Triage should therefore be implemented only in extreme situations and only as a temporary process, until further resources become available and the number of victims is clarified.

Stein and Hirshberg (1999) advocate a slightly different approach to triage by classifying victims into urgent and nonurgent groups. These authors advise against placing patients into the "expectant group" (unsalvageable patients that receive no immediate treatment) unless the victim succumbs within minutes after arrival.

Normally, immediately after a disastrous event in a civilian area, during the immediate chaos phase, family members and bystanders evacuate 5%–10% of the injured to the nearest hospital (Kluger 2003). Only subsequently, with the arrival of trained emergency medical services, is primary triage actually initiated on site with prioritized evacuation of the victims. Einav et al. (2004) described the importance of rapid primary triage, initiated within seconds or minutes after the event and conducted by experienced medical teams with minimal medical intervention and immediate evacuation to the nearest hospital. The preferred location for primary evacuation should be dictated by the condition of the patient and by the distance of each facility from the location of the event. However, there is an ongoing uncertainty in the literature regarding what is of higher priority: distance or expertise (Spira et al. 2006). While most patients will survive no matter where they are taken, there is a certain subgroup of severely injured victims who will benefit from being transferred to designated level I trauma centers (Stein 2006). Although no study showing improved outcomes in those level I centers is prospective and randomized, it seems that patients with severe head injuries and those with combined multisystem injuries will fare better there (Spira et al. 2006; Stein 2006).

The secondary and most important triage is performed at the trauma center or any other medical facility receiving the mass casualties. Almogy et al. (2004) and Kluger et al. (2004) described a model of "modern-day triage" implemented by the trauma system in Israel for terrorist bombing disasters. Accordingly, triage is performed by the most experienced trauma surgeon that does not take part in surgical or resuscitation procedures but exclusively triages patients according to the above-mentioned principles. Additionally, the same surgeon in charge is responsible for directing consultants from other specialties, urologists included, and assigning them as responsible for specific patients as dictated by their specific injuries. After all the victims have undergone triage, repeated reassessments are conducted by the senior surgeon and patients are relocated as needed. This secondary triage is intended to correct mistakes and the authors emphasize the importance of this repeated assessment in order to avoid undertriage resulting in catastrophic results, i.e., conditions such as blast lung injury that are not obvious within minutes of the explosion but eventually deteriorate to respiratory failure and death if not immediately treated by intubation and ventilation. On the other hand, overtriage, i.e., patients assigned for immediate care and eventually found not to have critical injuries, has negative and possibly disastrous implications in mass casualty events, as precious resources are misdirected and consequently the chances for survival of other critically injured casualties are eventually reduced. The early mortality of severe trauma shows a bimodal distribution with the first peak occurring within the 1st h (50%) and resulting from airway and breathing problems, while the second peak is taking place 1–6 h after admission (18%) resulting from failure to control bleeding and the consequent physiological deterioration (Spira et al. 2006).

15.3.1.4 The Concept of Damage Control

The term "damage control" is accredited to Rotondo and Schwab (Rotondo et al. 1993) who in 1993 described a prioritized three-phase approach to patients with major vascular and visceral injuries. The first phase consists of expeditious control of hemorrhage and contamination using simple and quick measures and temporary abdominal closure. This is followed by intensive care resuscitation with the goal of restoring temperature, coagulation, perfusion, and oxygenation of tissues. Only then, as a third step in a stabilized patient, is definitive surgery and abdominal wall closure considered. This concept has emerged as a life-saving strategy in multitrauma injuries. Trauma surgeons have adopted this relatively novel concept based on the observation that multitrauma patients eventually die from hypothermia, coagulopathy, and acidosis-induced irreversible physiologic insults (Feliciano et al. 2000; Hirshberg and Mattox 1993; Hirshberg and Walden 1997; Rignault 1992). In accordance, extensive and time-consuming organ-ablating and reconstructive procedures in an unstable patient might often bring the patient beyond the point of reversible physiological changes. However, identifying those critically injured patients who are candidates for damage control maneuvers, aimed to achieve hemostasis and prevent uncontrolled spillage of bowel contents and urine, is a challenge. Decisions are therefore often taken by the most senior trauma surgeon in cooperation with other specialist surgeons who should all be fully familiar with damage control principles. Increased awareness among all surgical specialists will eventually improve the communication between the members of this group, which should ultimately function as a well-orchestrated multidisciplinary team. Nowadays, damage control principles have also been successfully adopted in the context of civilian mass casualty events, military field surgery, and treatment in rural areas with long-range transfers (Holcomb et al. 2001; Rignault 1992).

15.3.2 Mechanisms of Injury and Specific Urological Injuries in Mass Casualty Events

Buildings and bridges collapses, earthquakes, floods, and tsunamis, train collisions and aircraft catastrophes tend to be associated with an inconceivably high number of victims and carry the potential of becoming mass casualty scenarios. However, such extreme situations often carry such a high fatality rate that they do not necessarily respond to the definition of a mass casualty event that can overwhelm the medical facilities available (Caro 1974; Cooper et al. 1983). Unfortunately, mass casualty events in recent history are frequently associated with civilian terrorism and are most often the result of explosions. Shootings rarely result in a large number of injuries to become a mass casualty event and other possible mechanisms, such as chemical or biological attacks, will not be discussed in the present chapter because there are no specific urological aspects of their resultant injuries.

Terrorist-related mass casualty events tend to result in a higher overall injured population and a higher mortality/injured ratio than everyday civilian trauma (Huller and Bazini 1970). The incidence of multiple penetrating injuries and the large number of multisystem and multiorgan injuries are highly associated with this type of injury mechanism. The combined effects of blast, penetrating shrapnel, and improvised projectiles (nails, screws, and bolts), burns, and gunshot wounds in those circumstances make these injuries more complex, with unpredictable damage associated with possible undertriage and unexpected subsequent deterioration.

The mechanism of injury in explosions is divided in three phases: primary blast injury caused by the powerful shock wave that spreads from the site of explosion outward. Lungs and ears (air-containing organs) are most commonly injured at this time, but any tissue can be potentially damaged by the wave passing through the body. Pneumothorax and perforated eardrums are most frequently diagnosed in survivors of primary blast (Walsh et al. 1995). Limb and earlobe amputations have been described in victims situated within a short distance of the explosion site as a result of the primary blast waves. In fatalities, the leading cause of death is believed to be air emboli in the coronary and pulmonary vessels together with severe pulmonary injuries, torn alveoli, and pulmonary bleeding (DePalma et al. 2005; Huller and Bazini 1970; Wightman and Gladish 2001). Urogenital injuries as a direct result of primary blast have not been described in survivors of blast injuries. This is probably because parenchyma and fluid-filled organs are remarkably resistant to this mechanism of injury and the rather well-protected location of the kidneys and ureters.

The secondary injury is produced by debris and projectiles set in motion by the explosion. In the recent terrorist attacks described in the literature, these secondary blasts have significantly augmented morbidity. Relatively small bombs, carried in bags or body belts by suicide bombers have inflicted disproportionately severe secondary blast injuries by being augmented with bolts, nails, and various projectiles. These projectiles behave like high- or low-velocity missiles depending on their shape and the distance of the victim from the explosion site (Almogy et al. 2004; Kluger 2003). Penetrating injuries to the urogenital system, as to any other organ, have been described as a result of these so-called upgraded killing devices (Archbold et al. 1981).

The tertiary injury occurs when the victim displaced by the blast wave hits a fixed object. An acceleration-deceleration mechanism produces severe injuries to parenchymal organs, large blood vessels, and bony structures. Blunt renal, ureteral, and bladder injuries are induced by this mechanism. (Archbold et al. 1981; Kluger 2003).

Patterns and severity of injuries caused by civilian explosions are different when the explosions are in an outdoor, open-air site, or in closed place such as a bus or a room (Almogy et al. 2004; Leibovici et al. 1996). Explosions in confined spaces are extremely devastating because of the amplification of the blast wave by reflections and structural damage with ensuing collapse of walls and concrete.

Renal vascular and parenchymal injuries can lead to significant morbidity and mortality due to severe bleeding and urine leakage. Interestingly, a review of reports of major events involving mass casualties revealed a relatively small number of reportedly major renal injuries in relation to the large number of victims and to the severity of their other injuries. The reported Irish and Balkan (Frykberg and Tepas 1988; Hudolin and Hudolin 2003) experience mentions a 2% rate of significant urogenital injuries in survivors of terrorist bombings. The overall rate is certainly higher, but these patients probably have significant associated injuries and therefore a high mortality rate. In a report describing the mass casualty event in the Oklahoma City bombing, Mallonee at al. (1996) state that in this terrorist attack that destroyed the Murrah Federal Building in 1995 and injured 759 people (168 of whom died), no specific urogenital injuries were described and urologists were not even among the list of specialists that were called to the operating room. Similarly, in the suicide bombing at the Sbarro pizzeria in Jerusalem in 2001, a suicide bomber detonated himself in a busy restaurant (Almogy et al. 2004), causing 146 casualties and 14 immediate deaths, with no specified urologic injuries.

15.3.3 The Urologic Approach in Mass Casualty Events

15.3.3.1 Urologic Aspects of Damage Control

In events involving mass casualties, the principles of triage and damage control are congruent, as both aim to diminish the mortality rates by allowing a limited number of qualified personnel treat more patients with life-saving minimal maneuvers and delayed preplanned definitive treatment.

The chances for a urologist to be involved as a trauma case manager in a mass casualty event are rather low, as this role is usually held by general surgeons. However, urologists are frequently consulted in problematic cases, as they are often involved as additional surgical specialists in severe multivisceral trauma patients. Understandably, with the expanding role of the damage control approach, the knowledge of its principles and its implications should no longer be held only by general surgeons, and surgeons from various specialties should be equally familiar with those aspects. From the urological point of view, dilemmas such as whether to explore a retroperitoneal hematoma during acute laparotomy in an unstable patient or performing time-consuming urinary reconstruction vs quick diversion for ureteral or bladder injury in the context of a multitrauma patient are to be currently addressed according to principles of the damage control approach. The thorough understanding of damage control principles that allow delayed diagnostic and reconstructive procedures in the unstable patient is thus deemed to improve the urologist's interaction with the trauma team in the emergency room or the operating room and eventually result in improved survival and diminished morbidity. Similar considerations can be applied in mass casualty events, when the number of casualties overwhelms the medical resources and every surgeon, regardless of his specialty, is expected to provide acceptable care for the maximal amount of injured patients.

In 1993, Hirshberg and Mattox (1993), in an article entitled "Damage control in trauma surgery," expressed their hope that "surgeons from all specialties involved in trauma care will adapt to the new strategy by developing appropriate surgical solutions for injuries in their respective fields." Review of the current literature, more than a decade later, reveals that their wishful prophecy is still far from being carried out in most of the surgical subspecialties. Specifically, in urology, perhaps because of the dominating elective nature of our profession, management of urological trauma has been traditionally based on temporary immediate measures and planned deferred definitive surgery, which is fortunately in line with the modern damage control principles. As previously stated, the common denominator of the already developed damage control techniques, in all kind of surgical subspecialties, is primarily increased awareness leading to creative improvisation. In Israel, as surgeons are unfortunately being exposed to urban terrorist bombings and civilian mass casualty events and are routinely trained, even in peace time, for their emergency assignment as field surgeons during war, the principles of damage control have been well implemented in various surgical specialties.

The following discussion addresses the damage control principles of management of urological injuries involving the kidney, ureter, bladder, urethra, and genital organs dictated in scenarios involving mass casualties.

15.3.3.2 The Urological Consultation in the Emergency Room During Mass Casualty Events

Initial Evaluation and Preemptive Measures

After primary assessment and triage by the surgeon in charge, urological consultations will be requested for patients triaged to group 2 (severe, nonimmediately life-threatening injuries) and group 3 (ambulatory patients with supposedly mild injuries). Gross hematuria, pelvic injuries with suspected urethral or bladder injuries, inability to insert a urethral catheter, and external genital trauma are likely scenarios that will make the patient a urologic patient in a mass casualty scenario. As discussed above, in these extreme scenarios, the luxury of a trauma surgeon who remains in charge of the patient with other specialists functioning as consultants does not exist. In mass casualty events, any available physician becomes responsible for the patients assigned by the surgeon in charge and is additionally expected to give consultations according to his or her specialty. Therefore, the consulting urologist should bear in mind that in the chaotic conditions of a mass casualty event undertriage is plausible, meaning that a complete assessment of the patient assigned should be performed and attention should not be addressed to the urogenital injury only. This assessment should be quick but comprehensive and intended to reveal any signs of life-threatening injuries that may have been missed by the primary triage. A rapid (ABCDE – airway, breathing, circulation, disability or neurological status, exposure) survey should be conducted as dictated by the ATLS principles (Weighlt et al. 1997). Only after this clearance should the specific urologic injury be approached.

Imaging

In normal conditions, evaluation of patients with penetrating and blunt abdominal or pelvic trauma routinely includes imaging procedures such as a contrast CT scan and retrograde cystourethrography (Lynch et al. 2003; McAninch and Santucci 2002). When mass casualty protocols are instituted, decisions need to be made either with or without the minimal mandatory imaging procedures. The mass casualty scenario theorists advocate a unidirectional flow of patients in order to avoid creation of bottlenecks, usually at imaging departments (Jacobs et al. 1979). The normal pattern of sending a patient for a CT scan and returning him to the emergency room for decision making is not acceptable when the protocols of mass casualties are implemented.

Planning of Definitive Treatment

In these situations when imaging facilities are impractical and need to be held to a minimum, several conceivable urologic scenarios exist:

1. Hemodynamically unstable patients with suspected intraabdominal bleeding are urgently transferred to the operating room with no preoperative imaging. At emergency laparotomy, suspicion of bleeding originating from the retroperitoneum needs to be addressed by the urologist according to principles discussed below.
2. In stable patients with suspected renal injuries (either penetrating trauma to the upper abdomen, flanks, and lower chest or blunt abdominal trauma and gross hematuria), imaging should be delayed until the protocols of mass casualty have been canceled or when resources become sufficient to restore normal management principles. These patients should be transferred to surgical departments and reevaluated by the urologist as soon as possible.
3. Patients with suspected bladder or urethral injuries (patients with pelvic fractures, high riding prostate on rectal examination, patients with blood at the urethral meatus and who are unable to void) need to undergo an evaluation of the lower urinary tract, but these injures are not considered life-threatening in themselves. Retrograde urethrocystography is generally recommended by trauma management algorithms, but in scenarios of mass casualties it should be postponed. In these cases the minimal acceptable treatment will be one gentle trial of bladder catheterization or up-front insertion of a suprapubic cystostomy followed by transfer of the patient to the surgical ward and deferred radiological evaluation. Bladder injuries, both following blunt or penetrating trauma, are usually associated with other severe injuries (McAninch and Santucci 2002) and thus deserve a prioritizing surgical approach. The patients are usually unstable, as blunt bladder injuries are often encountered with associated pelvic fractures, whereas penetrating injuries are commonly found with other major pelvic and abdominal injuries. In both

settings, the rupture should be quickly classified as either extraperitoneal or intraperitoneal injury in order to plan the management accordingly. Traditionally, the distinction between those two entities has dictated the choice between bladder drainage alone vs immediate surgical exploration and layered closure of the bladder wall (Pansadoro et al. 2002). However, it is noteworthy that the first priority in this scenario is the treatment of the associated life-threatening injuries and that despite there being no clear evidence supporting nonoperative management in penetrating bladder injury, a conservative approach seems to be equally efficient. In mass casualty scenarios, drainage of the bladder and delayed evaluation seems reasonable and concordant with the minimal acceptable treatment approach applied in these situations.

Similar principles are true for suspected urethral injuries. Injuries of the posterior urethra are commonly associated with pelvic fractures, whereas trauma of the anterior segments is usually a consequence of severe blunt trauma (Peterson 2000). The mechanism of urethral injury therefore requires significant high-energy external forces and, understandably, often creates concomitant bladder injuries (in up to 35% of patients) or other multiple organ damage (Krieger et al. 1984; Lynch et al. 2003). While urethral injury of any kind is never life-threatening per se, the associated injuries might render hemodynamic instability. Under these circumstances, the management of the associated injuries is more important and the definitive urological negotiation with the traumatized urethra is to be deferred. Moreover, even in the context of an isolated urethral injury, many urologists are reluctant to perform immediate repair because of the limited operative visibility and the adverse tissue conditions (Peterson 2000). Altogether, the standard intuitive urological approach to urethral injury dictates minimal early intervention by suprapubic catheterization, which is certainly in concordance with the principles of damage control.

4. Traumatic injuries of the external genitalia are much more common in men than in women, probably due to the anatomical differences and the different exposure to violence (Van der Horst et al. 2004). Blunt injuries of the genitalia make up 80% of the cases, but they are often isolated and can be managed conservatively. On the other hand, penetrating injuries of the genitalia, which are rather rare (11% of civilian injuries and 40%–66% of wounds during wartime), are often associated with injuries of adjacent abdominal organs and hemodynamic instability (Archbold et al. 1981; Feliciano et al. 2000). The high incidence of genital injury during military activity can be explained by the fact that military flak jackets fail to protect the external genitalia, which are particularly exposed to fragmentation injuries, especially by mines and fragments that come from below (Abu-Zidan et al. 1999).

In mass casualty scenarios, external genital injuries should be surgically addressed when resulting in major hemorrhage that needs to be expeditiously controlled either in the shock room or in the operating room, according to the available facilities. Compression dressings or clamping and ligation of bleeding vessels are highly efficient maneuvers that require a minimum of time. When severe hemorrhage is not identified, any further diagnostic steps can be postponed and the patient can be transferred to the surgical department for later reevaluation and reconstructive procedures.

In conclusion, the urologic consultation in the emergency room of a mass casualty scenario should be performed according to the following principles:

1. Rule out undertriage by the surgeon in charge and perform a rapid primary survey of every patient.
2. Stable patients with suspected renal injuries should be transferred to the surgical ward without imaging procedures. Reevaluation is warranted if there is any change in their hemodynamic status or when possible as dictated by the objective conditions of the mass casualty event. At this time every, case should be managed according to the traditional trauma management protocols.
3. Unstable patients are transferred directly to the operating room should be evaluated and treated according to the damage control principles (as discussed below, operating room management).
4. Minimal acceptable procedures should be performed in order to enable patient transfer to the surgical wards: suprapubic drainage of the bladder when bladder or urethral injuries are suspected, clamping and ligation of bleeding vessels from external genitalia wounds. Imaging procedures such as CT scans and retrograde urethrography are discouraged in those circumstances as they are time-consuming and are not intended to diagnose immediate life-threatening conditions. These imaging studies should be performed, if still needed, after repeated evaluation of patients when protocols of mass casualties have been disabled.

15.3.3.3 The Urological Consultation in the Operating Room

It needs to be reemphasized that during mass casualty events, the principle of minimum acceptable for the maximum of salvageable is applicable for the operating room as well. Procedures should be directed at expeditious control of active bleeding and control of urinary extravasation by simple diversion measures and complex, time-consuming reconstructive procedures should be delayed whenever possible.

Renal Injuries

Coexisting injuries are identified in 14% – 34% of blunt trauma and in 50% – 80% of penetrating renal trauma cases, mostly involving the liver with right-sided injury and the spleen in the left-sided cases (Krieger et al. 1984; McAninch and Santucci 2002; Peterson 2000). The urologist might therefore be involved with renal trauma as a consultant in a shared abdomen at laparotomy performed by the general surgeons for associated injuries or because of hemodynamic instability.

The ultimate goal of all renal explorations in the setting of major traumatic renal injury is to control bleeding and to preserve the maximal amount of viable renal parenchyma. In a stable patient, primary proximal vascular control, broad surgical exposure of the injured area, and the use of strict reconstructive principles have made it possible to achieve successful reconstructive outcome of the kidney in up to 87% of renal injuries (Brandes and McAninch 1999; Wessells 2002). Yet it requires temporary vascular occlusion, extensive debridement of nonviable parenchyma, meticulous hemostasis, closure of the collecting system, approximation of the parenchymal margins, and omental interposition. Altogether, these steps are time-consuming and only the reported mean arterial occlusion time exceeds 39 min (Brandes and McAninch 1999), rendering these techniques inapplicable in the context of an unstable multitrauma patient with associated injuries of other organs or in the scenario of mass casualties when the operating room cannot be and should not be saturated with time-consuming reconstructive procedures.

Whenever major active hemorrhage of renal origin can be ruled out it is probably wise not to explore the injured kidney even if a secondary delayed laparotomy will eventually be needed. The surgeon's approach should be especially selective with exploration of contained perirenal hematomas that are clinically considered unlikely to involve the renal pedicle, unless the patient is considered unstable (Brandes and McAninch 2006) or the procedure needs to be terminated as quickly as possible in order to move the patient forward and make the operating room available for the next patient in the mass casualty event. Selection of patients according to strict criteria is the key of success for this conservative approach (Wessells et al. 1997). Brandes and McAninch (1999) report an exploration rate of 77% in renal gunshot wounds and 45% in renal stab wounds. According to these authors, the only absolute indication for surgical exploration is a patient with external trauma and persistent renal bleeding. Can these recommendations be extrapolated to the operating room in the setup of an unstable, multitrauma patient or in situations of mass casualties? The answer is certainly yes. Packing the renal fossa with laparotomy pads and transferring the patient to the surgical intensive care unit until a planned second-look laparotomy becomes possible is probably a viable alternative to heroic and time-consuming nephrectomy or reconstruction (Coburn 1977).

Other techniques that were initially applied in hepatic surgery and for splenic trauma can be considered as auxiliary applicable damage control measures for controlling renal parenchymal bleeding, including application of mattress sutures, fibrin glue, absorbable mesh tamponade, and firing a stapler line over the lacerated kidney parenchyma (Chaabouni and Bittard 1996; Feliciano et al. 2000; McAninch 2003; Nadu et al., unpublished data; Shekarris and Stoller 2002).

Urinary extravasation may be ignored during the acute phase and will be drained through retroperitoneal drains, while stents or insertions of percutaneous nephrostomies are to be deferred. The abdomen is temporarily closed with towel clips or other temporizing measures (Feliciano et al. 2000). Following the urgent primary exploration, the patient is carefully monitored in an intensive care unit and only when he is sufficiently stable should radiological assessment of the injuries be undertaken in order to plan the definitive operative management accordingly (Feliciano et al. 2000; Hirshberg and Walden 1997; Hirshberg et al. 1994).

CT is advocated as the most useful imaging modality in patients who are stable enough and transportable. If the extent of renal injury has not been clearly defined at the initial laparotomy (by choosing not to explore the retroperitoneal hematoma), the CT scan performed in the interim time before the second laparotomy can provide information and help in further decision making. Data regarding existence and function of the contralateral kidney is documented, the kidney injury is graded according to traditional protocols, and therapeutic strategies are delineated concerning operative or nonoperative management of the renal trauma or whether nephrectomy or reconstruction are to be attempted.

In patients who do not stabilize after the initial acute damage control laparotomy or in patients with deteriorating hemodynamic parameters (ongoing or delayed bleeding), the management options are angiographic embolization of the bleeding kidney or reoperation. The decision should be made according to the general status of the patient and the associated injuries that have also been treated according to damage control principles (bowel injuries, packed liver, or splenic injuries) and need reoperation regardless of the renal injury. Exploration of the kidney should be approached according to the principles of renal trauma: initial control of the renal pedicle and only then opening Gerota's fascia and the perinephric space. This approach has been proved to lower the nephrectomy rates due to bleeding from the renal parenchyma. (McAninch and Santucci 2002; Peterson 2000)

Ureteral Injuries

Traumatic ureteral injuries are uncommon because the ureter is a well-protected retroperitoneal structure with a narrow diameter, accounting for only 1 % of all genitourinary injuries (Brandes et al. 2004; Elliott and McAninch 2003). Blunt ureteral trauma is rare compared to penetrating gunshot ureteral injuries, which constitute 90 % of the overall violent ureteral injuries (Peterson 2000). Yet only 2 % – 3 % of gunshot wounds of the abdomen are associated with ureteral injury, and once diagnosed, it is almost always associated with multiple intraabdominal organ injuries (Brandes et al. 2004).

The operative decisions in the presence of a ureteral injury are based on several factors: whether the tear is partial or complete, the segment of the ureter involved, the viability of the ureter and surrounding tissues, associated urological and nonurological injuries and the general condition of the patient. The options for definitive repair of a complete ureteral tear are: ureteroureterostomy, transureteroureterostomy, ureterocalicostomy, ureteroneocystostomy with Boari flap, ureterocystostomy and psoas hitch, ileal interposition graft, and autotransplantation (Lynch et al. 2003). Though excellent results can be achieved with the above-mentioned reconstructive techniques, they are all time-consuming and occupy precious operating room time and skilled personnel.

During mass casualty events, another variable is added to the equation discussed above. Diagnostic procedures such as intraoperative injection of indigo carmine, intraoperative IVP or retrograde ureteropyelography intended to confirm or rule out ureteral injuries should be discouraged. If a ureteral injury is suspected but not clearly identified, a drain may be left in place, and if urinary leak occurs a nephrostomy tube can be placed postoperatively. If a partial ureteral tear is identified (involving less than half of the circumference) and the ureter looks viable, a double-J stent may be inserted over a guidewire through the tear and the tear can be closed with interrupted absorbable stitches. This procedure takes about 10 min to perform and seems reasonable even in extreme situations of mass casualty scenarios. However, when complete ureteral injuries are identified, attempts at definitive repair should not be undertaken. Placement of a single-J or an 8-F feeding tube into the ureter, tying the distal end of the ureter over the tube, exteriorizing it (Best et al. 2005; Brandes and McAninch 1999; Coburn 1997; Elliott and McAninch 2003; McAninch and Santucci 2002) through a small stab incision of the skin and tying it to the skin has been advocated as a fast and simple procedure that produces no damage to the ureter and does not compromise delayed elective repair. The distal ureteral stump does not need to be ligated; any unnecessary manipulation should be avoided.

Tying off the injured ureteral segment and postoperative insertion of percutaneous nephrostomy (Brandes and McAninch 1999; Coburn 1997; Elliott and McAninch 2003; McAninch and Santucci 2002) is a viable alternative but should not be considered as the procedure of choice.

In rare selected cases, nephrectomy is required to treat ureteral injury with severe associated injuries of the ipsilateral kidney or other intraabdominal organs (McAninch and Santucci 2002). Though this recommendation originally refers to a situation in which ureteral injury complicates vascular procedures in which a vascular prosthesis is to be implanted, it is also relevant to the damage control situations discussed herein and should be considered in patients with ureteral injuries and high-grade renal injuries, provided documentation of a functioning contralateral kidney exists.

Hirshberg and Mattox (1994) in their report of their experience with 124 patients with multisystem trauma, describe four cases who had associated ureteral injuries; two managed by stenting, one by exteriorization, and one by ligation.

Bladder and Urethral Injuries

The approach to these injuries has been described in detail above, as they will be mainly approached in the emergency room.

Briefly, these injuries are usually not life-threatening by themselves but carry a high potential for late morbidity and tend to be associated with other significant abdominal and pelvic injuries. When discovered intraoperatively, intraperitoneal bladder tears should be addressed by rapid repair with running absorbable sutures and maximal bladder drainage by suprapubic cystostomy, urethral catheter, or both. In extreme situations when primary closure of the bladder cannot be obtained (due to lack of viable tissue), single-J ureteral catheters can be inserted and exteriorized to obtain temporary urinary drainage. Extraperitoneal tears should be treated by drainage of the bladder. Time-consuming maneuvers such as exploration of the deep pelvis and the bladder should be avoided.

High-grade urethral injuries are generally treated by cystostomy tube drainage and delayed repair, which is certainly in concordance with the minimal acceptable treatment principles.

In summary, mass casualty events involve particular treatment protocols based on principles of evacuation, triage, and damage control. A thorough knowledge of these special diagnostic and therapeutic principles by the urologist is compulsory and bound to improve communication among the other multidisciplinary trauma team members and is finally translated into improved outcome for victims.

References

Abu-Zidan FM, Al-Tawheed A, Ali YM (1999) Urologic injuries in the Gulf War. Int Urol Nephrol 31:577

Almogy G, Belzberg H, Mintz Y et al (2004) Suicide bombing attacks: update and modifications to the protocol. Ann Surg 239:295

Archbold JA, Barros d'sa AA, Morrison E (1981) Genito-urinary tract injuries of civil hostilities. Br J Surg 68:625

Best CD, Petrone P, Buscarini M et al (2005) Traumatic ureteral injuries: a single institution experience validating the American association for the surgery of trauma-organ injury scale grading scale. J Urol 173:1202

Brandes SB, McAninch JW (1999) Reconstructive surgery for trauma of the upper urinary tract. Urol Clin North Am 26:183

Brandes SB, McAninch JW. Renal trauma: a practical guide to evaluation and management. Sci World J 4[Suppl 1]:31–40

Brandes S, Coburn M, Armenakas N et al (2004) Diagnosis and management of ureteric injury: an evidence based analysis. BJU Int 94:277

Caro D (1974) Major disasters. Lancet 30:1309

Chaabouni MN, Bittard M (1996) Application of peri-renal prosthesis (vicryl mesh) in the conservative treatment of multiple ruptured kidney fragments. Ann Urol 30:61

Coburn M (1997) Damage control for urologic injuries. Surg Clin N Am 77:821

Cooper GJ, Maynard RL, Cross NL et al (1983) Casualties from terrorist bombings. J Trauma 23:955

DePalma RG, Burris DG, Champion HR et al (2005) Blast injuries. New Engl J Med 352:1335

Einav S, Feigenberg Z, Weissman C et al (2004) Evacuation priorities in mass casualty terror-related events: implications for contingency planning. Ann Surg 239:304

Elliott SP, McAninch JW (2003) Ureteral injuries from external violence: The 25-year experience at San Francisco general hospital. J Urol 170:1213

Feliciano DV, Moore EE, Mattox KL (2000) Trauma damage control. In: Mattox KL et al (eds) McGraw-Hill, New York, p 907

Frykberg ER (2002) Medical management of disasters and mass casualties from terrorist bombings: how can we cope? J Trauma 53:201

Frykberg ER, Tepas JJ 3rd (1988) Terrorist bombings. Lessons learned from Belfast to Beirut. Ann Surg 208:569

Hirshberg A, Mattox KL (1993) 'Damage control' in trauma surgery. Br J Surg 80:1501

Hirshberg A, Walden R (1997) Damage control for abdominal trauma. Surg Clin North Am 77:813

Hirshberg A, Wall MJ Jr, Mattox KL (1994) Planned reoperation for trauma: A two year experience with 124 consecutive patients. J Trauma 37:365

Holcomb JB, Helling TS, Hirshberg A (2001) Military, civilian, and rural application of the damage control philosophy. Mil Med 166:490

Hudolin T, Hudolin I (2003) Surgical management of urogenital injuries at a war hospital in Bosnia-Herzegovina, 1992 to 1995. J Urol 169:1357

Huller T, Bazini Y (1970) Blast injuries of the chest and abdomen. Arch Surg 100:24

Jacobs LM Jr, Ramp JM, Breay JM (1979) An emergency medical system approach to disaster planning. J Trauma 19:157

Kluger Y (2003) Bomb explosions in acts of terrorism – detonation, wound ballistics, triage and medical concerns. Isr Med Assoc J 5:235

Kluger Y, Mayo A, Soffer D et al (2004) Functions and principles in the management of bombing mass casualty incidents: lessons learned at the Tel-Aviv Souraski Medical Center. Eur J Emerg Med 11:329

Krieger JN, Algood CB, Mason JT et al (1984) Urological trauma in the Pacific Northwest: etiology, distribution, management and outcome. J Urol 132:70

Leibovici D, Gofrit ON, Stein M et al (1996) Blast injuries: bus versus open-air bombings – a comparative study of injuries in survivors of open-air versus confined-space explosions. J Trauma 41:1030

Lynch D, Martinez-Piñeiro L, Plas E et al (2003) European Association of Urology Guidelines on Urological Trauma. Eur Urol 47:1

McAninch JW (2003) Editorial: New technology in renal trauma. J Urol 169: 1368

McAninch JW, Santucci RA (2002) Genitourinary trauma. In: Retik AB, Vaughan ED Jr, Wein AJ (eds) Campbell's urology, 8th edn. W.B. Saunders, Philadelphia 3707

Mallonee S, Shariat S, Stennies G et al (1996) Physical injuries and fatalities resulting from the Oklahoma City bombing. JAMA 276:382

Pansadoro A, Franco G, Laurenti C, et al (2002) Conservative treatment of intraperitoneal bladder perforation during transurethral resection of bladder tumor. Urology 60:682

Peterson NE (2000) Genitourinary trauma. In: Mattox KL, Feliciano DV, Moore EE (eds) Trauma, 4th edn. McGraw-Hill, New York, p 839

Rignault DP (1992) Recent progress in surgery for the victims of disaster, terrorism, and war – Introduction. World J Surg 16:885

Rotondo MF, Schwab CW, McGonigal MD et al (1993) 'Damage control': an approach for improved survival in exsanguinating penetrating abdominal injury. Trauma 35:375

Shekarris B, Stoller ML (2002) The use of fibrin sealant in urology. J Urol 167:1218

Slater MS, Trunkey DD (1997) Terrorism in America. An evolving threat. Arch Surg. 132:1059

Spira RM, Reissman P, Goldberg S et al (2006) Evacuation of trauma patients solely to level 1 centers: Is the question patient or trauma center survival? Irs Med Assoc J 8:131

Stein M (2006) Evacuation to a trauma center or non-trauma center? Is there any doubt? Isr Med Assoc J 8: 134

Stein M, Hirshberg A (1999) Medical consequences of terrorism. The conventional weapon threat. Surg Clin North Am 79:1537

Van der Horst C, Martinez Portillo FJ, Seif C et al (2004) Male genital injury: diagnostics and treatment. BJU Int 93:927

Walsh RM, Pracy JP, Huggon AM et al (1995) Bomb blast injuries to the ear: the London Bridge incident series. J Accid Emerg Med 12:194

Weighlt JA, Krantz BE, Ali J et al (1997) Advanced Trauma Life Support Student Course Manual. American College of Surgeons Committee on Trauma, 6th edn. Chicago

Wessells H (2002) Evaluation and management of renal trauma in the 21st century. AUA Update Series, XXI, 30:234

Wessells H, McAninch JW, Meyer A et al (1997) Criteria for nonoperative treatment of significant penetrating renal lacerations. J Urol 157:24

Wightman JM, Gladish SL (2001) Explosions and blast injuries. Ann Emerg Med 37:664

Renal Trauma

15.4

E. Serafetinides

15.4.1 Anatomy

The kidneys are paired organs situated posteriorly behind the peritoneum on each side of the vertebral column and are surrounded by adipose connective tissue. Each kidney has a characteristic shape with a superior and inferior pole, a convex border placed laterally, and a concave medial border. Superiorly they are level with the upper border of the twelfth thoracic vertebra, inferiorly with the third lumbar. The right kidney is usually inferior due to the volume of the liver, while the left is a little longer and narrower and lies nearer the median plane. The long axis of each kidney is directed inferolaterally and the transverse posterolaterally.

Each kidney is about 11 cm in length, 6 cm in breadth, and 3 cm in anteroposterior dimension. Average weight is 135 – 150 g in adults. The hilum of the kidney is an anteromedial deep vertical fissure containing the renal vessels and nerves as well as the renal pelvis of the ureter. The relative positions of the main hilar structures are the vein anterior, the artery intermediate, and the pelvis posterior. Commonly, an arterial branch enters behind the renal pelvis and a renal venous tributary often leaves the hilum in the same plane

The kidney and its vessels are embedded in perirenal fat, which is thickest at the renal borders and prolonged at the hilum into the renal sinus. Fibrous connective tissue surrounding this fat is condensed as renal fascia. At the lateral renal borders, the two layers of renal fascia fuse; the anterior extends medially in front of the kidney and its vessels to merge with connective tissue enclosing the aorta and inferior vena cava, but it is thin and does not ascend above the superior mesenteric artery. The posterior layer passes medially between the kidney and the fascia on quadratus lumborum and psoas major, attaching to this fascia at the lateral and medial borders of the psoas and to the vertebrae and intervertebral discs. A deeper stratum unites the anterior and posterior layers at the medial renal border and is pierced by renal vessels. Renal fascia joins the renal capsule by numerous trabeculae traversing the perirenal fat and is strongest near the lower pole. Behind the renal fascia is a mass of fat the pararenal body. The kidney is held in position partly by renal fascia but principally by the apposition of neighboring viscera. The kidney has a thin capsule, composed of collagen--rich tissue with some elastic and non-striated muscle fibers. The organ itself has an internal medulla and external cortex.

The renal arteries are two large vessels that branch laterally from the aorta just below the inferior mesenteric; both cross the corresponding crus at right angles to the aorta. A single artery to each kidney is present in about 70 % of individuals but they vary in their level of origin (the right often being superior) and in their caliber, obliquity, and precise relations. The right renal artery is longer and often, higher, passing posterior to the inferior vena cava, right renal vein, head of the pancreas and descending part of the duodenum. The left is a little lower; it passes behind the left renal vein, the inferior mesenteric vein may cross the body of the pancreas and splenic vein anteriorly. In its extrarenal course, each renal artery gives one or more inferior suprarenal arteries and branches that supply perinephric tissue, the renal capsule, pelvis, and the proximal part of the ureter; near the renal hilum, each artery divides into an anterior and posterior division, the primary branches of which (segmental arteries) supply renal vascular segments. Accessory renal arteries are common (30% of individuals), usually arising from the aorta above or below the main renal artery and following it to the renal hilum.

The renal veins are vessels of large size and lie anterior to the renal arteries and open into the inferior vena cava almost at right angles. The left is three times the right in length (7.5 cm and 2.5 cm, respectively); it crosses the posterior abdominal wall posterior to the splenic vein and body of pancreas and, near its end, is anterior to the aorta, just below the origin of the superior mesenteric artery. The left testicular or ovarian vein enters it from below and the left suprarenal vein, usually receiving one of the left inferior phrenic veins, enters it above but nearer the midline. The left renal vein enters the inferior vena cava a little superior to the right. The right renal vein is behind the descending duodenum and sometimes the lateral part of the pancreas (Sampaio 1996).

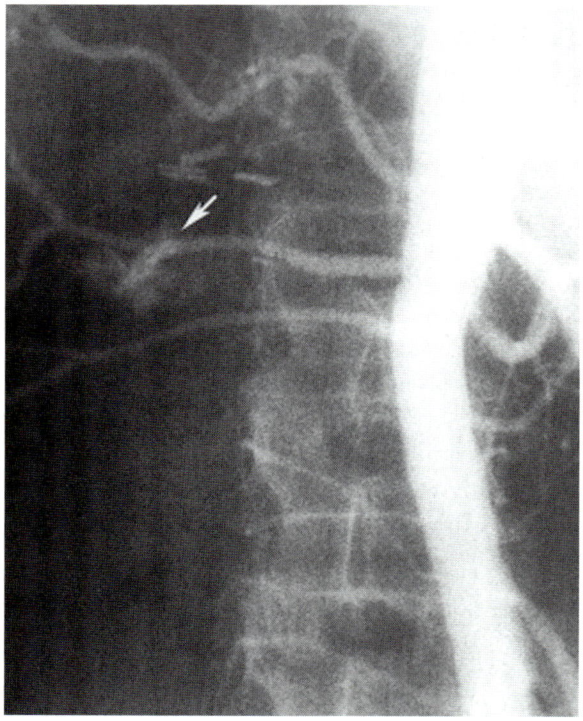

Fig. 15.4.1. Abdominal angiogram showing free contrast extravasation from the distal segment of the right main renal artery (*arrow*)

15.4.2 Iatrogenic Vascular Injuries

Iatrogenic main renal artery injuries with perforation or rupture are rare and almost exclusively reported after renal artery angioplasty or stenting with an incidence of 1.6% (Morris and Bonnevie 2001). One case of an iatrogenic renal artery perforation as a complication of cardiac catheterization has been reported (Bates et al. 2002). Since most iatrogenic renal artery lesions occur during endovascular procedures, there are no reports on the clinical symptoms, but only on the angiographic findings (Fig. 15.4.1). Arteriovenous fistulae, pseudoaneurysms, arterial dissection, or contrast extravasation are the possible radiological findings in these traumatic vascular lesions. Traditional therapy for renal perforation has been renal artery ligation followed by bypass grafting or nephrectomy, but nowadays the treatment for acute iatrogenic rupture of the main renal artery is balloon tamponade. The size of the angioplasty balloon chosen for tamponade should be 1 mm smaller in diameter than the size of the balloon or stent that caused the rupture. The balloon is fully inflated without the use of a manometer in all cases. Time of the procedure varies; a maximum of 3 min, followed by rapid deflation, and a repeat after 2 min is effective in most cases. However, in some cases inflation may need to last up to 10 min, while in other cases a single 1-min balloon inflation is enough. After the treatment of each ruptured renal artery, a selective renal digital subtraction angiogram should be performed to exclude further extravasation. However, in case of failure immediate availability of a stent graft is vital.

Patients with iatrogenic operative injuries are strikingly different from those with penetrating, blunt, or catheter-related vascular trauma. Renal vessels are vulnerable during oncologic procedures. Factors that increase technical difficulty are previous operation, tumor recurrence, radiation exposure, and chronic inflammatory changes. Renal vein injuries during elective abdominal operations are a serious complication with significant morbidity. Most patients with operative venous injuries have partial lacerations that can be managed with relatively simple techniques, such as venorraphy and patch angioplasty with autologous vein of ePTFE graft if venorraphy is not possible because of significant vessel narrowing (Oderich et al. 2004).

15.4.3 Renal Transplantation

The orthotopic kidney is protected against external force by muscles, Gerota's fascia, and perinephric fat. A renal graft is located in the lower pelvis in the iliac fossa through a retroperitoneal incision anastomosed to the iliac artery and vein and therefore is more susceptible to injury, especially from direct blows to the abdomen.

The transplanted kidney, unlike the native kidney, is fixed in position by a thick fibrosis capsule that develops after transplantation and is not really suspended by the renal vessels (Barone et al. 1997). Consequently, deceleration events that cause pedicle injury to a native kidney are less likely to affect a transplanted kidney. As transplant recipients return to more active lifestyles, including becoming a significant risk for becoming a trauma victim, a renal graft is liable to be severely affected by trauma that may not cause any injury to a native kidney.

In transplant recipients, it is very important to know the patients' baseline renal function. The knowledge of an abnormal renal baseline may prevent unnecessary extensive diagnostic evaluation. Radiographic evaluation should proceed as for the native kidney. The increased risk for contrast nephrotoxicity can be minimized with adequate hydration. A CT scan is the test of choice for a stable injured transplant recipient, as it will identify renal and associated intraabdominal injuries but it will also indirectly assess renal blood flow and function. A renal Duplex examination can be also very helpful for identifying isolated trauma to the transplanted kidney and for identifying renal blood flow. Radionuclide scans may reveal urine leaks and are good for assessing overall blood flow and renal function, while angiography can assess blood flow and identify specific arterial injuries.

The surgical management of an injured transplanted kidney is a complex procedure. A very short vascular pedicle and ureter, dense scarring, and a fibrous capsule may prevent any attempts at the direct repair of parenchymal, collecting system, and vascular pedicle injuries. Grade 1–3 injuries can be managed nonoperatively with adequate hydration and observation. Grade 4–5 injuries may require exploration with debridement and drainage or simply a subcapsular nephrectomy if associated with life-threatening bleeding. Isolated vascular injuries have a poor prognosis. Renal arteriography may be helpful with embolization of the main artery to stop bleeding or with more selective embolization to salvage part of the kidney. When renal graft injury occurs, saving the patient's life is the first priority but the saving of the graft is also very important to maintain renal function.

Obstructive uropathy in a renal graft is a serious complication caused by calculi, tumors, or ureteral strictures. Percutaneous access and antegrade intervention are regarded as the gold standard for the management of such complications. Ureteroscopy is a reliable alternative with acceptable outcomes and minimal morbidity. (Del Pizzo et al. 1998)

Iatrogenic vascular injuries of renal transplants can be managed by embolization. Angiographically successful embolization is not necessarily associated with clinical success, as nephrectomy in some cases is inevitable and the complication rate is high (Dorffner et al. 1998). On the contrary, transcatheter embolization is highly effective for biopsy-related vascular injury in the transplant kidney (Perini et al. 1998).

15.4.4 Percutaneous Renal Procedures

Percutaneous nephrostomy is achieved in nearly all patients without major complications. Hematuria is common for a few days, but massive retroperitoneal hemorrhage is rare. Small subcapsular renal hematomas resolve spontaneously, while arteriovenous–caliceal fistulas are best managed by angiographic embolization. If a nephrostomy catheter is seen to transverse the renal pelvis the possibility of injury to a large renal artery must be considered. The misplaced nephrostomy catheter should be withdrawn over a guidewire and renal artery embolization may enable rapid arrest of a life-threatening hemorrhage (Cowan et al. 1998). In more complex cases, CT may be used to detect possible catheter malposition and successfully guide catheter repositioning in the renal collecting system (Jones and McGahon 1999).

During percutaneous and renal procedures, sepsis and pelvic injuries are also reported as common complications. Sepsis can be avoided if antibiotics are administered prior to the procedure, the collecting system is not overly distended, the minimum volume of contrast medium is injected, and the attempt is not delayed. Hemorrhage can be prevented with appropriate coagulation studies, careful puncture onto target calyx and avoidance of medial punctures. A pelvic injury is less likely to occur if the dilator is not advanced further than the calyx, the peel-away sheaths are handled with care, especially when advanced around the pelvi–ureteric junction, and kinking of the guidewires is avoided (Lewis and Patel 2004).

Percutaneous renal biopsy is a relatively safe procedure. Hemorrhage, arteriovenous fistula, and renal capsular artery pseudoaneurysm may occur. Arteriovenous fistula may present with severe hypertension and is managed by embolization (Ozdemir et al. 1998). A pseudoaneurysm should be suspected if the patient presents with flank pain and decreasing hematocrit without hematuria. Arteriography and transarterial embolization is the appropriate therapy (Silberzweig et al. 1998).

Percutaneous nephrolithotomy (PCNL) is a popular procedure, wherein stones in the renal pelvis are removed via a nephroscope with forceps or by ultrasonic or electrohydraulic disruption. The complications include hemorrhage, extravasation and absorption of large volumes of irrigation fluid, fever, infection, colonic perforation, arteriovenous fistulae, and pneumothorax (Fig. 15.4.2) (Vignali et al. 2004).

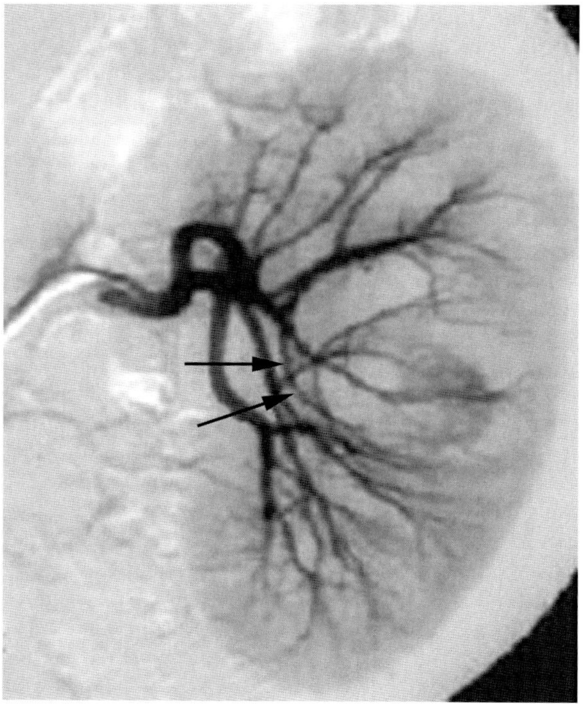

Fig. 15.4.2. Renal hematoma and pseudoaneurysm formation following percutaneous nephrolithotomy. After hyperselective catheterization, the artery is embolized with microcoils

Extravasation of fluid is often caused by a tear in the pelvicaliceal system. A close watch on irrigant fluid input and output is required for an early recognition of the complication. If the renal pelvis is torn or ruptured termination of the procedure is a safe choice. Apart from intraoperative evaluation of serum electrolytes, acid-base status and oxygenation, monitoring of airway pressure is a good indicator of this complication. Metabolic acidosis, hyponatremia, hypokalemia, peritonitis, and ileus are caused by absorption of large volumes of irrigation fluids. Management of this complication requires close monitoring, placement of an abdominal or retroperitoneal drain, correction of acidosis, and supportive measures (Ghai et al. 2003).

The diagnosis of a colon injury during or after percutaneous renal surgery can be elusive because symptoms are often variable. An unrecognized or untreated colon injury can result in abscess formation, septicemia, and/or nephrocolic or colocutaneous fistula. Surgical exploration is inevitable when the patient experiences hemorrhage, pneumoperitoneum, and peritonitis. Gerspach et al. propose an algorithm for treatment (Gerspach et al. 1997) (Fig. 15.4.3)

The majority of these cases can be successfully managed conservatively. The consistent application of proper technique, avoidance of puncturing the kidney lateral to the posterior axillary line, and puncture of the upper pole calyx when feasible will help prevent these injuries.

Vascular injuries with renal bleeding are quite frequent and can occur at any step of the percutaneous procedure, requiring transfusion in 1 % – 11 % of cases. The high number of punctures and the incorrect choice of the puncture site (access too medial or direct puncture of renal pelvis) have been incriminated in the genesis of vascular lesions after percutaneous maneuvers. Renal bleeding can arise both from venous and arterial lesions. Bleeding from venous vessels could be profuse at the end of the procedure but is generally controlled by simple maneuvers, such as placing the patient supine to reduce abdominal compression, positioning a nephrostomy catheter, forcing diuresis through hydration and parenteral administration of mannitol after clamping the nephrostomy catheter. In case of major venous trauma with massive hemorrhage, patients with concomitant renal insufficiency can be treated without open exploration or angiographic embolization using a Council balloon catheter (Gupta et al. 1997).

Arterial lesions may induce acute or late postoperative bleeding. Severe acute bleeding usually arises from the injury of the anterior or posterior segmental arteries, whereas postoperative delayed complications are usually caused by interlobar and lower pole artery lesions mainly represented by arteriovenous fistulas or post-traumatic aneurysm development. Duplex US and CT angiography can diagnose vascular injuries. Hyperselective renal embolization is considered the most appropriate technique in the treatment of iatrogenic vascular lesions. Identification of the precise site of the lesion in order to be as selective as possible and reduce the risk of renal dysfunction is essential. Hyperselective catheterization of the renal artery branches is achieved by means of both hydrophilic 5-F catheters or coaxial systems with low-profile microcatheters (2.6 F). The use of an embolic agent helps in performing a distal and irreversible occlusion with complete hemostasis. A variety of embolic materials have been used: microcoils, homologous clots, detachable balloons, polyvinyl alcohol particles, Gelfoam, silicone rubber, cotton pellets, and silk filaments. The choice of the embolic agent depends mainly on the blood flow entity at the level of the lesion, the vessel size, and the operator's preference. Complications of endopyelotomy can be classified as major (vascular injury), and minor (infection, urinoma) (Bellman 1996). Preventive steps along with proper patient selection minimize the risk for complications.

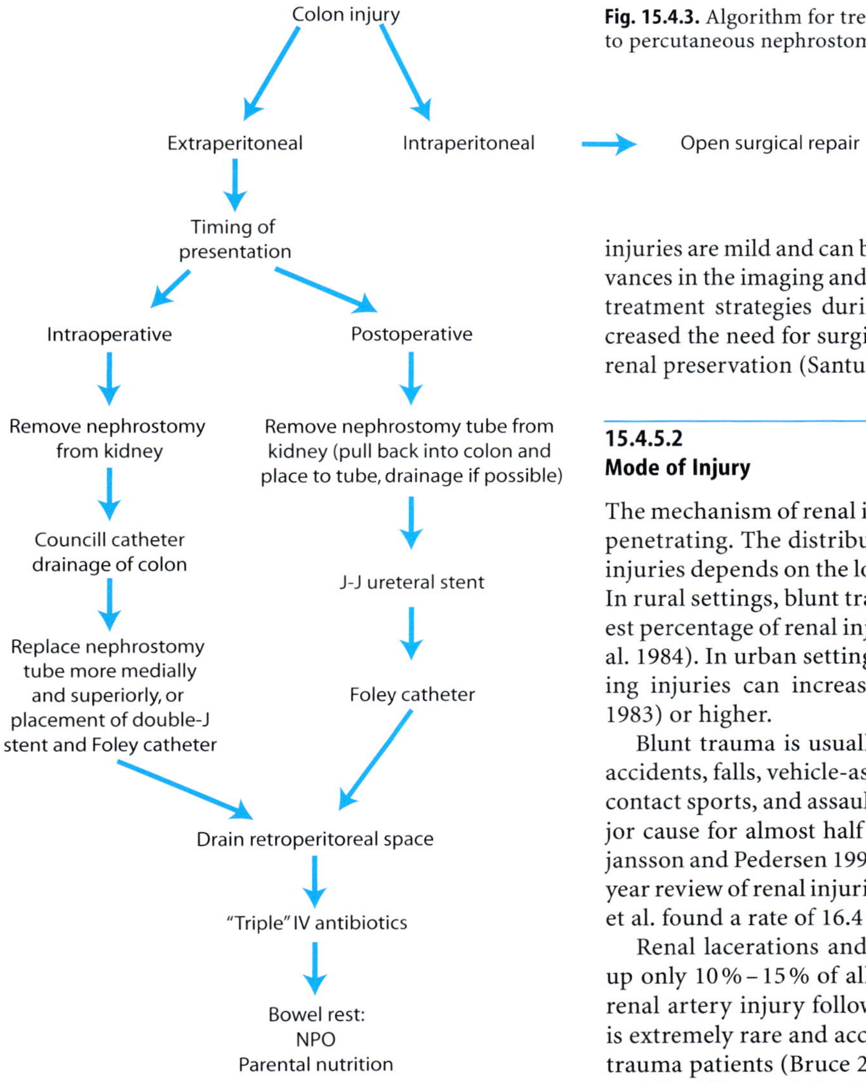

Fig. 15.4.3. Algorithm for treatment of colon injuries related to percutaneous nephrostomy injuries

15.4.5 Renal Injuries

15.4.5.1 Background

Trauma is defined as the morbid condition of the body produced by external violence. Physicians with different specialties (general surgery, urology, traumatology) evaluate and treat the trauma patient, as a high level of expertise is required to prevent mortality and reduce morbidity. Renal trauma occurs in approximately 1%–5% of all traumas (Baverstock et al. 2001; Meng et al. 1999). The kidney is the most commonly injured genitourinary and abdominal organ, with the male to female ratio being 3:1 (Herschorn et al. 1991; Kristjansson and Pedersen 1993; Danuser et al. 2001). Renal trauma can be acutely life-threatening, but the majority of renal injuries are mild and can be managed conservatively. Advances in the imaging and staging of trauma, as well as in treatment strategies during the last 20 years, have decreased the need for surgical intervention and increased renal preservation (Santucci and McAninch 2000).

15.4.5.2 Mode of Injury

The mechanism of renal injuries is classified as blunt or penetrating. The distribution of blunt and penetrating injuries depends on the location of the reference center. In rural settings, blunt trauma can account for the largest percentage of renal injuries (90%–95%) (Krieger et al. 1984). In urban settings, the percentage of penetrating injuries can increase to 18% (Sagalowsky et al. 1983) or higher.

Blunt trauma is usually secondary to motor vehicle accidents, falls, vehicle-associated pedestrian accidents, contact sports, and assault. Traffic accidents are the major cause for almost half of blunt renal injuries (Kristjansson and Pedersen 1993; Danuser et al. 2001). In a 20-year review of renal injuries following free falls, Brandes et al. found a rate of 16.4% (Brandes et al. 1999b).

Renal lacerations and renal vascular injuries make up only 10%–15% of all blunt renal injuries. Isolated renal artery injury following blunt abdominal trauma is extremely rare and accounts for less than 0.1% of all trauma patients (Bruce 2001).

Schmidlin et al. (1998b)developed an experimental model to study force transmission and stress distribution of the injured kidney and developed a hypothesis that a bending mechanism may be responsible for most blunt injuries. Maximum stress concentrations were caused by the combined effect of the applied force and the reaction generated by the liquid-filled inner renal compartment. Trauma to the injured kidney tends to concentrate at the renal periphery in this model, a finding that is often confirmed in explorations of severely damaged organs (Schmidlin et al. 1998b).

Renal artery occlusion is associated with rapid deceleration injuries. In theory, the kidney is displaced, causing renal artery traction; the resulting tear in the inelastic intima and subsequent hemorrhage into the vessel wall leads to thrombosis. Compression of the renal artery between the anterior abdominal wall and the vertebral bodies may result in thrombosis of the renal artery (Sullivan and Stables 1972). Traumatic renal vein

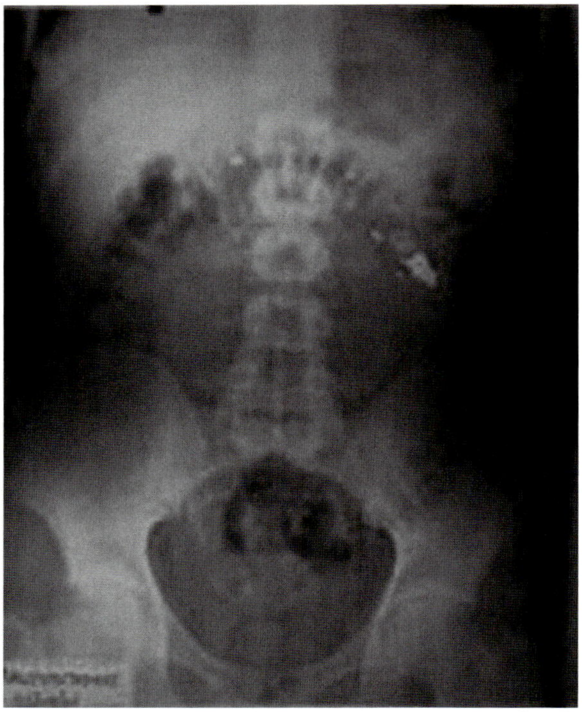

Fig. 15.4.4. Left renal injury following a gunshot wound

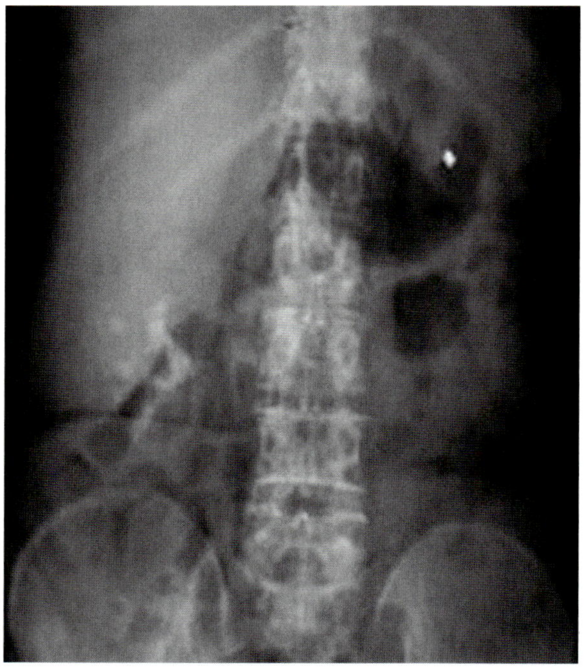

Fig. 15.4.5. Low-velocity bullet gunshot injury

thrombosis usually occurs in combination with arterial or parenchymal injury.

Gunshot and stab wounds represent the most common causes of penetrating injuries. In most cases, they result from interpersonal violence. In penetrating injuries, the retroperitoneum, and possibly the peritoneum itself, is violated depending on the path of the penetrating object. By definition, the latter leads to a nonsterile condition. In addition, the consequent bleeding and/or urine leakage that develops is an excellent media for bacterial growth. Renal injuries from penetrating trauma tend to be more severe and less predictable than those from blunt trauma (Fig. 15.4.4).

Bullets, because of their higher kinetic energy, have the potential for greater parenchymal destruction and are most often associated with multiple organ injuries (Ersay 1999). Renal injuries in recent wars are reported to be the commonest among urogenital organs. Most are found to be associated with major abdominal injuries and the rate of nephrectomies is relatively high (25% – 33%) (Abu-Zidan et al. 1999; Tucak et al. 1995) (Fig. 15.4.5).

Injury Classification

Classifying renal injuries helps to standardize different groups of patients, select appropriate therapy, and predict results. A total of 26 classifications for renal injuries have been presented in the literature in the past 50 years (Lent 1996), but the committee on organ injury scaling of the American Association for the Surgery of Trauma (AAST) has developed a renal-injury scaling system that is now widely used (Moore et al. 1989). Renal injuries are classified as Grade 1 – 5 (Table 15.4.1). Abdominal computed tomography (CT) or direct renal exploration is used to accomplish injury classification. Most recent clinical research and publications in the field of renal trauma have adopted this classification. In a retrospective review, the AAST scaling system was determined as the most important variable predicting the need for kidney repair or removal (Santucci et al. 2001) (Fig. 15.4.6).

Table 15.4.1. AAST renal injury grading scale (Moore 1989)

Grade	Description of injury
1	Contusion or nonexpanding subcapsular hematoma No laceration
2	Nonexpanding perirenal hematoma Cortical laceration < 1 cm deep without extravasation
3	Cortical laceration > 1 cm without urinary extravasation
4	Laceration: through corticomedullary junction into collecting system or Vascular: segmental renal artery or vein injury with contained hematoma or partial vessel laceration or vessel thrombosis
5	Laceration: shattered kidney or Vascular: renal pedicle or avulsion

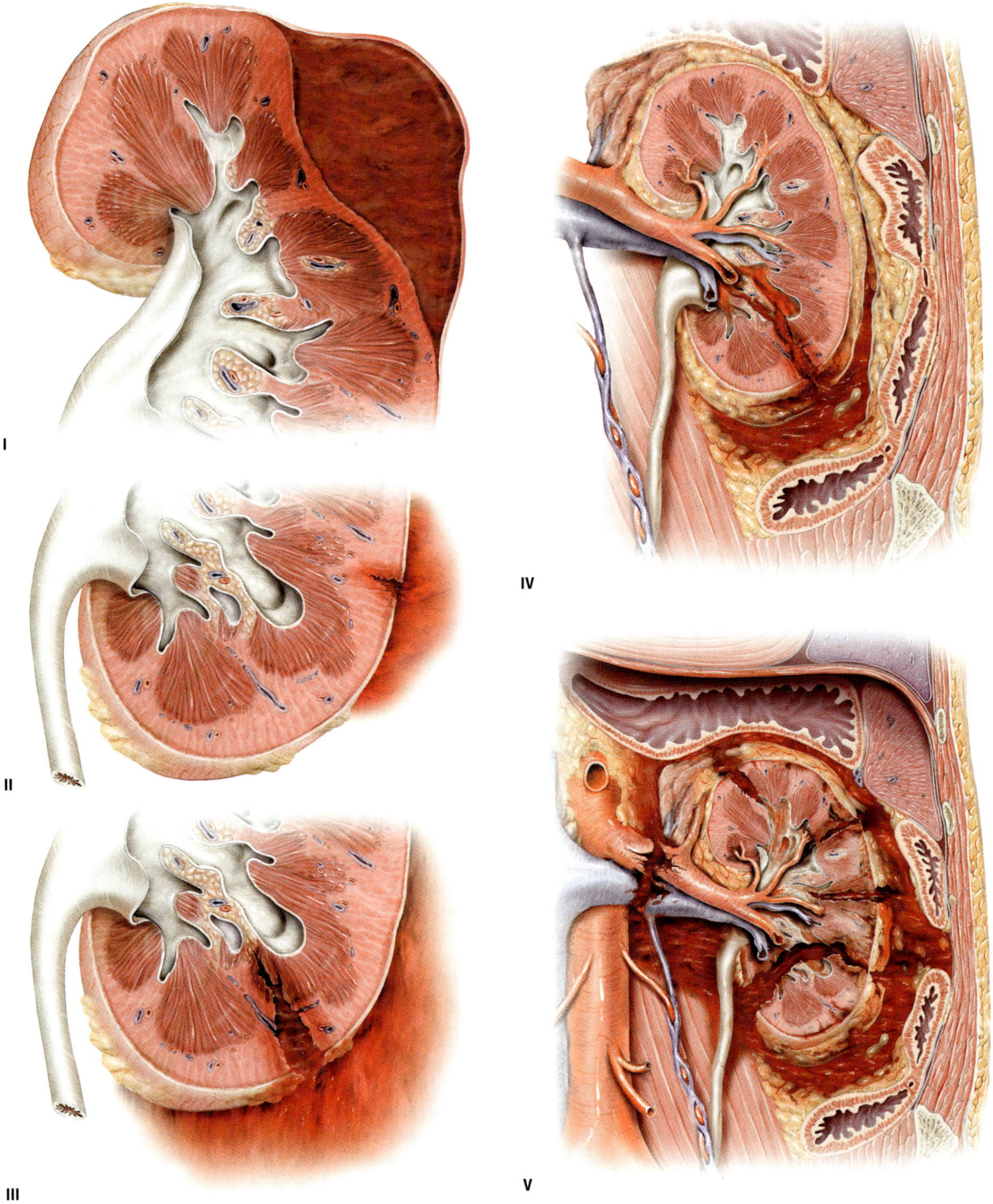

Fig. 15.4.6I–V. AAST renal injury grading scale (Moore 1989) (© Hohenfellner 2007)

15.4.5.3 Diagnosis: Initial Emergency Assessment

Initial assessment of the trauma patient should include securing the airway, controlling external bleeding, and resuscitation of shock as required. In many cases, physical examination is carried out simultaneous to stabilization of the patient. When renal injury is suspected, further evaluation is required for a prompt diagnosis.

History and Physical Examination

Direct history is obtained from conscious patients. Witnesses and emergency personnel can provide valuable information regarding unconscious or seriously injured patients. Possible indicators of major renal injury include a rapid deceleration event (fall, high-speed motor vehicle accidents) and a direct blow to the flank. In assessing trauma patients after motor vehicle accidents, the history should include the vehicle's speed and whether the patient was a passenger or pedestrian.

In penetrating injuries, important information includes the size of the weapon in stabbings and the type and caliber of the weapon used in gunshot wounds since high-velocity projectiles have the potential for more extensive damage.

The medical history should be as detailed as possible, as preexisting organ dysfunction can negatively effect on trauma patient outcome (Sacco et al. 1993). In the early resuscitation phase, special consideration should be given to preexisting renal disease (Cachecho et al. 1994). Another point of interest is the functioning renal mass of the trauma patient, as there are numerous case reports in the literature regarding renal trauma and the subsequent complications of solitary kidneys (Cozar et al. 1990).

Preexisting renal abnormality makes renal injury more likely following trauma. Any known preexisting renal pathology should be registered. Hydronephrosis due to ureteropelvic junction abnormality, renal calculi, cysts, and tumors are the most common reported entities that may complicate a minor renal injury (Sebastia et al. 1999). The overall percentage of these cases varies from 3.5% to 21.8% (Bahloul 1997; Giannopoulos et al. 1999). Trauma patients with horseshoe kidneys are at risk of losing all functioning renal tissue. In cases of severe trauma, recognition of horseshoe kidney anatomy, microvascular reconstruction, and renal autotransplantation allows the salvage of both the patient and renal function (Murphy et al. 1996).

Physical examination is the basis for the initial assessment of each trauma patient. Hemodynamic stability is the primary criterion for the management of all renal injuries. Shock is defined as a systolic blood pressure of less than 90 mm Hg found at any time during an adult patient's evaluation. Vital signs should be recorded throughout diagnostic evaluation.

Physical examination may reveal obvious penetrating trauma from a stab wound to the lower thoracic back, flanks and upper abdomen, or bullet entry or exit wounds in this area. In stab wounds, the extent of the entrance wound will not accurately reflect the depth of penetration. Blunt trauma to the back, flank, lower thorax, or upper abdomen may result in renal injury. The following findings on physical examination may indicate possible renal involvement: hematuria, flank pain, flank ecchymoses and/or abrasions, fractured ribs, abdominal distension or tenderness, and palpable mass. The clinical presentation of renal vein thrombosis depends on the balance achieved between the rapidity and degree of venous occlusion, as well as the development of collateral veins. Thus, patients may be asymptomatic, have no specific symptoms such as nausea or vomiting, or have more specific symptoms such as hematuria or flank pain (Berkovich et al. 2001).

Laboratory Evaluation

The trauma patient is evaluated by a series of laboratory tests. Urinalysis, hematocrit and baseline creatinine values are the most important tests for evaluating renal trauma. Urinalysis is considered the basic test in the evaluation of patients with suspected renal trauma. Hematuria is the presence of an abnormal quantity of red blood cells in the urine and is usually the first indicator of renal injury. Microscopic hematuria in the trauma setting may be defined as greater than 5 red blood cells per high-power field (rbc/hpf), while gross hematuria is the finding in urine that is readily visible as containing blood.

Hematuria is a hallmark sign of renal injury, but is neither sensitive nor specific enough for differentiating minor and major injuries. It does not necessarily correlate with the degree of injury (Buchberger et al. 1993). Major renal injury, such as disruption of the ureteropelvic junction, renal pedicle injuries, or segmental arterial thrombosis may occur without hematuria(Carroll et al. 1990). In a study by Eastham, 9% of patients with stab wounds and resultant proven renal injury did not manifest hematuria (Eastham et al. 1992). Hematuria out of proportion with the history of trauma may suggest preexisting renal pathology (Schmidlin et al. 1998b).

The urine dipstick is an acceptably reliable and rapid test to evaluate hematuria. Studies have shown false-negative result rates ranging from 2.5% to 10% for the dipstick test for hematuria (Chandhoke and McAninch 1988).

Serial hematocrit determination is a method of continuous evaluation of the trauma patient. Initial hematocrit in association with vital signs implies the need for emergency resuscitation. The decrease in hematocrit and the requirements for blood transfusions are indirect signs of the rate of blood loss and along with the patient's response to resuscitation are valuable in the decision-making process.

As most trauma patients are evaluated within 1 h after injury, creatinine measurement reflects renal function prior to the injury. An increased creatinine usually reflects preexisting renal pathology.

Imaging: Criteria for Radiographic Assessment in Adults

Decisions about radiographic imaging in cases of suspected renal trauma are based on the clinical findings and the mechanism of injury. Since the majority of renal injuries are not significant and resolve without any intervention, many attempts have been made to identify patients who could be spared the discomfort, radiation exposure, possible allergic reaction, and expense of a radiographic evaluation (Miller and McAninch 1995).

There is mounting evidence that following blunt renal trauma, some patients do not require radiographic evaluation. Patients with microscopic hematuria and no shock after blunt trauma have a low likelihood of concealing significant renal injury (Hardeman and Husmann 1987). The indications for radiographic evaluation are gross hematuria, microscopic hematuria and shock, or presence of major associated injuries (Miller and McAninch 1995; McAndrew and Corriere 1994). However, patients with a history of rapid deceleration injury with clinical indicators of renal trauma or associated injuries also need immediate imaging to rule out ureteral avulsion or renal pedicle injury (Brandes et al. 1999a).

Patients with penetrating trauma to the torso have a high incidence of significant renal injuries. If renal injury is clinically suspected on the basis of an entry or exit wound, renal imaging should be performed, regardless of the degree of hematuria (Miller and McAninch 1995; Mee and McAninch 1989).

Ultrasonography

Ultrasonography is a popular imaging modality in the initial evaluation of abdominal trauma. While it provides a quick, noninvasive, low-cost means of detecting peritoneal fluid collections, without exposure to radiation or contrast agents (Brown et al. 1997), the role of ultrasound in the radiographic evaluation of renal trauma has been widely questioned. Its limitations stem from the difficulty in obtaining good acoustic windows on the trauma patient who has sustained numerous associated injuries. The results are also highly dependent on the operator. Ultrasound scans can detect renal lacerations but cannot definitely assess their depth and extent and do not provide functional information about renal excretion or urine leakage. By using color Doppler, power Doppler, or ultrasound with contrast, one can usually establish the presence of blood flow to the kidney. Gray-scale techniques can determine if the kidney is intact. However, ultrasound cannot establish if renal function is present, and there is also difficulty in some cases of differentiating a shattered kidney from a congenitally absent kidney. Since adynamic ileus is often present, it can be difficult to precisely determine if the renal contour is intact (Goldman and Sandler 2004). In contrast-enhanced ultrasound, the kidneys should be covered adequately in the supine and the contralateral decubitus position. The kidney to be examined is scanned and documented longitudinally and transversely. Depending on patient size, a bolus injection of 0.3 – 1.2 ml of second-generation microbubbles is administered. The renal cortex enhances rapidly and densely, followed by the pyramids, so that the entire renal parenchyma is enhanced within approximately 40 – 50 s. There is a rapid wash-through of contrast in the kidneys, but there is adequate contrast accumulation for about 2 min, allowing reliable scanning for anechoic defects (Thorelius 2004) (Fig. 15.4.7).

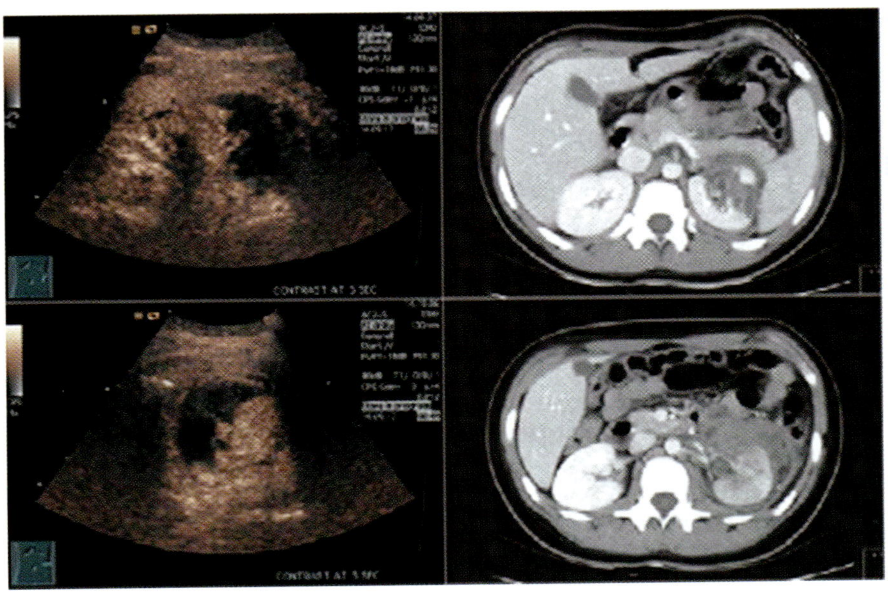

Fig. 15.4.7. *Left*, contrast-enhanced US of renal laceration; *right*, corresponding CT

Despite the drawbacks of the method, ultrasound scans can be conveniently used during the primary assessment of renal injuries (Qin and Wang 2002). During the evaluation of blunt trauma patients, ultrasound scans were more sensitive and specific than standard intravenous pyelography (IVP) in minor renal trauma (Arena 1997). In another study comparing the results of ultrasound scans and IVP, the sensitivity of ultrasound decreased as the severity of the trauma increased, while that of IVP remained high for all degrees of severity (Lopez Cubillana et al. 1998).

Another possible role for ultrasound may be for serially evaluating stable renal injuries for the resolution of urinomas and retroperitoneal hematomas (Pollack and Wein 1989). Ultrasound is considered an effective screening examination that can obviate more hazardous tests such as CT, cystography, and peritoneal lavage in most pregnant patients with trauma requiring objective evaluation of the abdomen (Brown et al. 2005) and suitable for the routine follow-up of renal parenchymal lesions or hematoma in the intensive care unit.

In conclusion, since ultrasound scans are used in the triage of patients with blunt abdominal trauma, they can be helpful in identifying which patients require a more aggressive radiological exploration to obtain a diagnosis of certainty (Buchberger et al. 1993; McGahan and Richards 1999; Rosales et al. 1992). Ultrasound findings do not provide sufficient evidence for a definite answer on the severity of renal injuries.

Standard Intravenous Pyelography

Formal IVP was the preferred imaging study for evaluating renal trauma until its replacement by CT. While standard IVP is no longer the study of choice for the evaluation of renal trauma, we acknowledge that in some centers it may be the only study available. In these situations, IVP should establish the presence or absence of one or both of the kidneys, clearly define the renal parenchyma, and outline the collecting system. In order to stage renal trauma, the IVP should include nephrotomograms, delineate the renal contour, and visualize the excretion of contrast material from both kidneys into the renal pelvis and ureter. Nonvisualization, contour deformity, or extravasation of contrast implies a major renal injury and should prompt further radiological evaluation with CT or less commonly, angiography if available.

The most significant findings on IVP are nonfunction and extravasation. Nonfunction is usually a sign of extensive trauma to the kidney, pedicle injury (vascular avulsion or thrombosis), or a severely shattered kidney. Extravasation of the contrast medium also implies a severe degree of trauma, involving the capsule, parenchyma, and collecting system. Other less reliable signs are delayed excretion, incomplete filling, calyceal distortion and obscuring of the renal shadow. The sensitivity of IVP is high (> 92 %) for all degrees of trauma severity (Lopez Cubillana et al. 1998).

One-Shot Intraoperative Intravenous Pyelography

Unstable patients selected for immediate operative intervention (and thus unable to have a CT scan) should undergo one-shot IVP in the operating suite. The technique consists of a bolus intravenous injection of 2 ml/kg radiographic contrast followed by a single plain film taken after 10 min. The study is safe, efficient, and of high quality in the majority of cases. It provides important information for decision making in the critical time of urgent laparotomy, concerning the injured kidney, as well as the presence of a normal functioning kidney on the contralateral side (Morey et al. 1999) (Fig. 15.4.8).

While the majority of experts advocate their use, not all studies have shown the one-shot IVP to be useful. In cases of penetrating abdominal trauma, Patel et al. found that the positive predictive value of the study was only 20 % (80 % of patients with normal one-shot IVP findings had renal injuries not detected by one-shot IVP (Patel and Walker 1997). The authors concluded that one-shot IVP is of no significant value in assessing penetrating abdominal trauma patients who undergo exploratory laparotomy for associated intraabdominal injuries, and should be reserved only for patients with

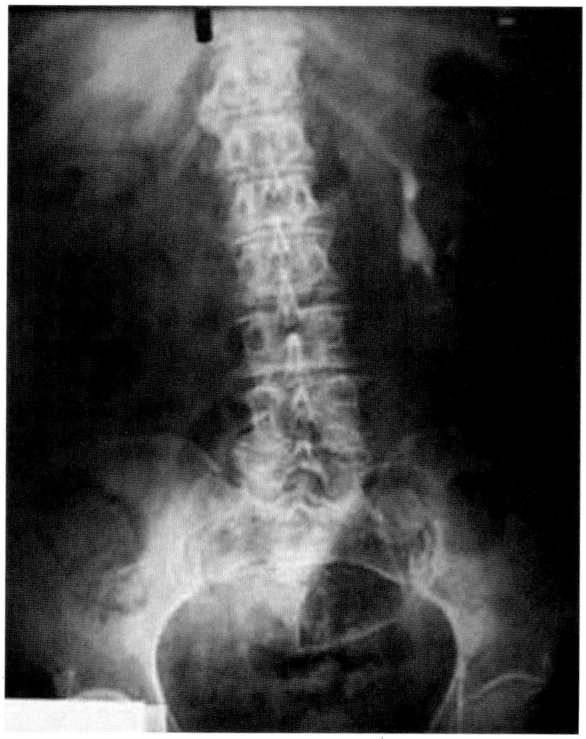

Fig. 15.4.8. One-shot IVP revealing a nonfunctioning right kidney

a flank wound or gross hematuria following penetrating trauma (Nagy et al. 1997).

Computed Tomography

Computed tomography is the gold standard method for the radiographic assessment of stable patients with renal trauma, though it may not be available in all settings, and is time-consuming. The higher cost of CT scans is a also major disadvantage, but CT is more sensitive and specific than IVP, ultrasonography, or angiography (Bretan et al. 1986). In a retrospective study, Qin et al. found that the positive rate during evaluation of 298 patients was 95.6% by CT, 90.9% by double-dose intravenous IVP, and 78.8% by ultrasound (Qin and Wang 2002).

Computed tomography more accurately defines the location of injuries, easily detects contusions and devitalized segments, visualizes the entire retroperitoneum and any associated hematomas, and simultaneously provides a view of both the abdomen and pelvis. It demonstrates superior anatomical detail, including the depth and location of renal laceration and presence of associated abdominal injuries, and establishes the presence and location of the contralateral kidney (Steinberg 1984) (Fig. 15.4.9).

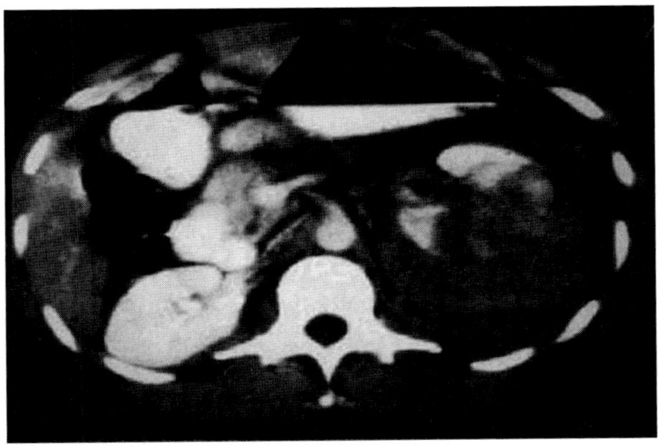

Fig. 15.4.9. CT scan of a Grade III blunt renal injury

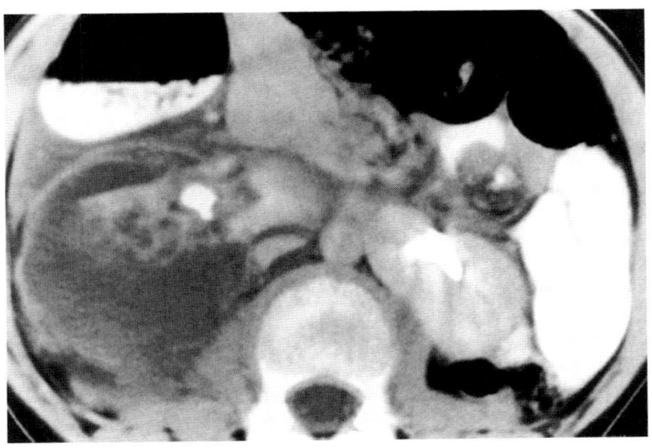

Fig. 15.4.10. Horseshoe kidney with extensive injury to the right side as evidenced by an inhomogeneous nephrogram

Computed tomography is particularly useful in evaluating traumatic injuries to kidneys with preexisting abnormalities (Sebastia et al. 1999; Kawashima et al. 2001). The ratio of hematoma area to body area on CT is very useful in evaluating blunt injuries and the change of the hematoma size is a valuable indicator for management (Ichigi et al. 1999; Goldman and Sandler 2004) (Fig. 15.4.10).

Intravenous contrast should be administered concurrently for renal evaluation. A lack of contrast enhancement of the injured kidney is a hallmark of renal pedicle injury. In cases where this typical finding is not demonstrated, central perihilar hematoma increases the possibility of renal pedicle injury. This sign should be considered even if the renal parenchyma is well-enhanced (Shima et al. 1997). Renal vein injury remains an injury that is difficult to diagnose with any type of radiographic study; however, the presence on CT of a large hematoma, medial to the kidney and displacing the renal vasculature, should raise the suspicion of venous injury.

The development and increasing availability of spiral CT has changed the diagnostic evaluation of trauma patients. Spiral CT provides shorter scanning time and thus fewer artifacts in the examinations of patients who cannot co-operate adequately (Vasile et al. 2000). Three-dimensional postprocessing modalities allow the assessment of the renal vascular pedicle by CT angiography and improve the demonstration of complex lacerations of the renal parenchyma. Contrast enhancement within a laceration or around the kidney

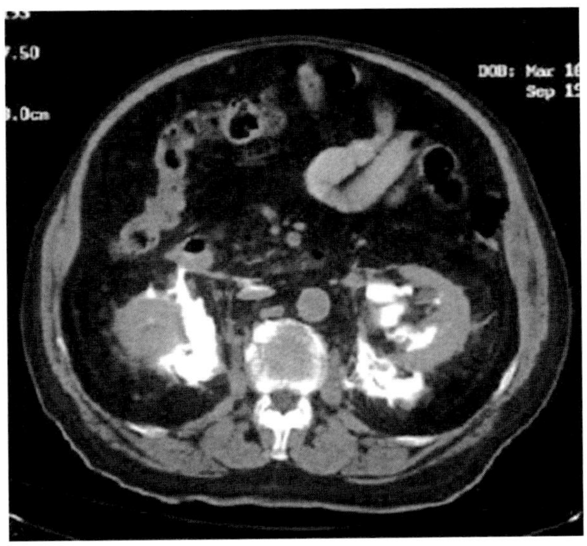

Fig. 15.4.11. Excretory phase, contrast-enhanced spiral CT performed 3 min after initial contrast administration shows bilateral extravasation of contrast medially consistent with bilateral UPJ injury

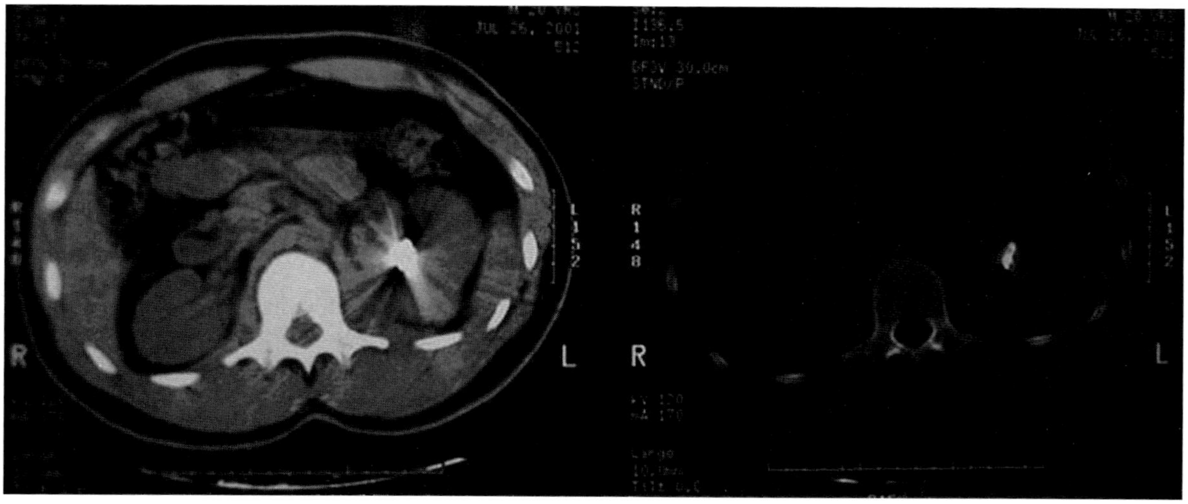

Fig. 15.4.12. Low-velocity bullet injury to the right kidney with arterial extravasation of contrast seen

during the pyelographic phase of the CT examination indicates the presence of a urine leak (Harris et al. 2001). However, injury to the renal collecting system may be missed during routine spiral CT. In all cases of suspected renal trauma evaluated with spiral CT, repeat scans of the kidneys should be performed 10–15 min after contrast injection (Brown et al. 1998b; Savage et al. 2003) (Fig. 15.4.11).

Contrast-enhanced CT can diagnose arterial extravasation in clinically stable patients. The extravasation can be used to localize anatomic sites of hemorrhage and to guide angiographic or surgical intervention. Although there is no statistical correlation between the number of patients with arterial extravasation and the need for surgical exploration (Yao et al. 2002), this finding should be considered an important indicator that a patient may be about to pass from hemodynamic stability to decompensation (Fig. 15.4.12).

Magnetic Resonance Imaging

While MRI is not used in the vast majority of renal trauma patients, Leppaniemi et al. investigated the use of high-field strength MRI (1.0 T) in the evaluation of blunt renal trauma. Magnetic resonance imaging scans were accurate in finding perirenal hematomas, assessing the viability of renal fragments, and detecting preexisting renal abnormalities, but failed to visualize urinary extravasation on initial examination. The authors concluded that MRI could replace CT in patients with iodine allergy and could be used for initial staging if CT was not available (Leppaniemi et al. 1997). The use of intravenous gadolinium-based contrast material has proved helpful in the assessment of urinary extravasation (Marcos et al. 1998). In a recent study comparing CT and MRI findings, the latter clearly revealed renal fracture with a nonviable fragment and was able to detect focal renal laceration not detected on CT due to perirenal hematoma (Ku et al. 2001).

However, MRI is not the first choice in managing the patient with trauma, because it requires longer imaging time, increases the cost, and limits access to the patient in the magnet during the examination. Thus, MRI may be useful in renal trauma only if CT is not available, in patients with iodine allergy, or in the very few cases where the findings on CT are equivocal.

Angiography

Computed tomography has largely replaced the use of angiography for staging renal injuries, since angiography is less specific, more time-consuming, and more invasive. Angiography, however, is more specific for defining the exact location and degree of vascular injuries and may be preferable when planning selective embolization for the management of persistent or delayed hemorrhage from branching renal vessels (Kawashima et al. 2001).

Angiography can define renal lacerations, extravasation, and pedicle injury. Additionally, it is the test of choice for evaluating renal venous injuries. The most common indication for arteriography is nonvisualization of a kidney on IVP after major blunt renal trauma when a CT is not available. Common causes for nonvisualization are total avulsion of the renal vessels (usually presents with life-threatening bleeding), renal artery thrombosis, or severe contusion causing major vascular spasm (Fig. 15.4.13) (Kawashima et al. 2001).

Angiography is also indicated in stable patients to assess pedicle injury, if the findings on CT are unclear, and for those who are candidates for radiological control of hemorrhage (Eastham and Bennett 1992), and in cases of persistent symptomatology as well as laborato-

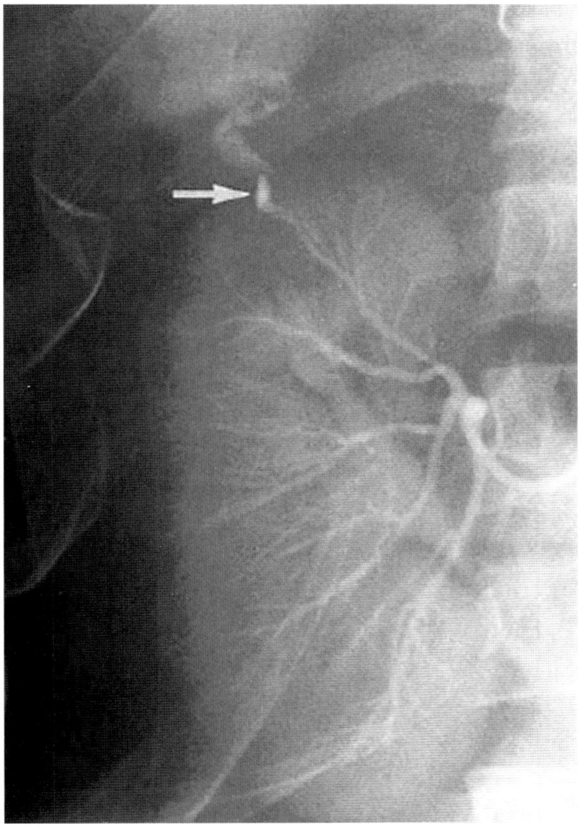

Fig. 15.4.13. Active arterial extravasation from the upper pole of the right kidney (*arrow*)

ry findings (decreasing hematocrit levels) suggestive of vascular renal injury, including prolonged hematuria (Sofocleous et al. 2005). Although complications following interventional embolization are rare, non-target vessel embolization or injury, hemodynamic compromise during or immediately after the procedure, repeated extravasation from the embolized site, pseudoaneurysm or arteriovenous fistula formation, and loss of renal function or parenchyma have been reported.

Radionuclide Scans

Radionuclide scans may be helpful to document renal blood flow in the trauma patient with severe allergy to iodinated contrast material, or in following up repair of renovascular trauma (Kawashima et al. 2001), but are not generally used or needed. Renal scintigraphy can be performed with technetium (Tc)-99m glucoheptonate, Tc-99m mercaptoacetyltriglycine, or Tc-99m diethylenetriamine pentaacetic acid.

15.4.5.4 Treatment

Indications for Renal Exploration

The goal of management of patients with renal injuries is to minimize morbidity and to preserve renal function. Thus, renal exploration should be undertaken selectively. The condition of the patient remains the absolute determinant in the decision for initial observation vs surgical intervention. However, the management of renal injury is usually influenced by the decision to explore or observe associated abdominal injuries (Kristjansson 1993; Husmann 1993). Nonoperative therapy is supported widely for the majority of blunt and penetrating injuries. The grade of renal injury, the overall injury severity of the patient, and the requirement for blood transfusions are the primary prognostic factors for nephrectomy and overall outcome (Kuo et al. 2002).

A life-threatening hemodynamic instability due to renal hemorrhage is an absolute indication for renal exploration, irrespective of the mode of injury (McAninch et al. 1991; Armenakas et al. 1999). In exsanguinated patients with severe hypovolemia, an endovascular aortic balloon catheter may control renal bleeding prior to laparotomy (Long 2004).

Other indications for exploration include an expanding or pulsatile perirenal hematoma identified at exploratory laparotomy performed for associated injuries (this finding heralds a Grade 5 vascular injury and is quite rare). A one-shot, intraoperative IVP can provide valuable information. Poor visualization or any other abnormality of the injured kidney is an indication for exploration. Grade 5 vascular renal injuries are by definition regarded as an absolute indication for exploration; however, a single report suggesting that patients who are hemodynamically stable at presentation, but with a Grade 5 parenchymal injury (shattered kidney) after blunt trauma might be safely treated conservatively (Altman et al. 2000). More research on this rare entity is required before definitive recommendations are given, and each patient must be treated individually for the best outcomes.

The management of major renal injuries with urinary extravasation and devitalized fragments is controversial. Since these injuries are very uncommon, published series report on small numbers of patients. In recent years, it seems as though it has been recognized that most major injuries heal with nonoperative treatment (Matthews et al. 1997). Moudouni et al. suggest that an initial conservative approach is feasible in stable patients with devitalized fragments (Moudouni et al. 2001a, b). These injuries, however, are associated with an increased rate of complications and late surgery (Husmann and Morris 1990). Persistent extravasation or urinoma are usually managed successfully with endourological techniques. Inconclusive renal imaging and a preexisting renal abnormality or an incidentally diagnosed tumor may require surgery even after relatively minor renal injury (Bahloul et al. 1997; Schmidlin et al. 1998b).

Operative Findings and Reconstruction

The overall exploration rate for blunt trauma is less than 10% (Baverstock et al. 2001; McAninch et al. 1991) and may be even lower in the future as more centers adopt a very conservative approach to the management of these patients (Rogers 20040; Hammer 2003). The goal of renal exploration following renal trauma is control of hemorrhage and renal salvage. Most experienced authors suggest the transperitoneal approach (McAninch et al. 1991; Robert et al. 1996; Nash et al. 1995). Access to the renal vascular pedicle is best obtained through the posterior parietal peritoneum, which is incised over the aorta, just medial to the inferior mesenteric vein.

Temporary vascular occlusion before opening of Gerota's fascia is a safe and effective method during exploration and renal reconstruction (Gonzalez 1999). It tends to lower blood loss and the nephrectomy rate, and appears not to increase postoperative azotemia or mortality (Atala et al. 1991). Renal reconstruction is feasible in most cases (Fig. 15.4.14 – 15.4.17).

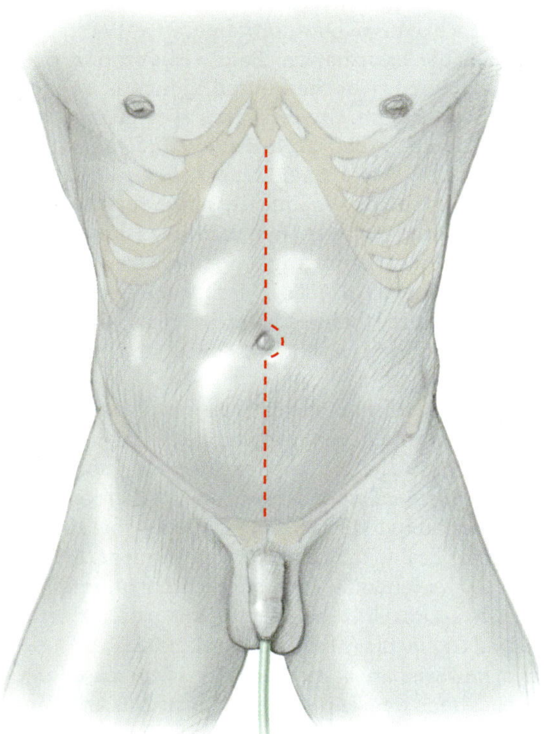

Fig. 15.4.14. Exploration and reconstruction of injured kidney. Midline incision (Fig. 15.4.14–17 © Hohenfellner 2007)

The overall rate of patients who have a nephrectomy during exploration is around 13%, usually in patients with higher rates of shock, injury severity scores, and

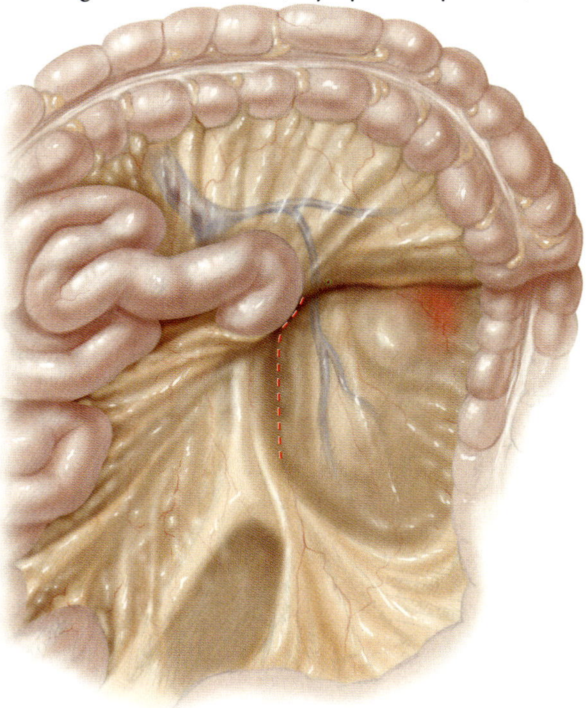

Fig. 15.4.15. Extroperitoneal incision over aorta to expose renal vessels

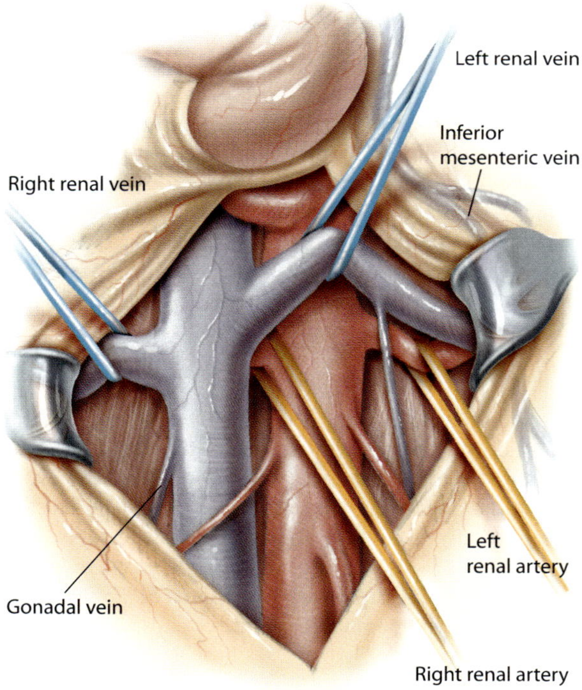

Fig. 15.4.16. Exposure and placement of vessel loops around renal vessels

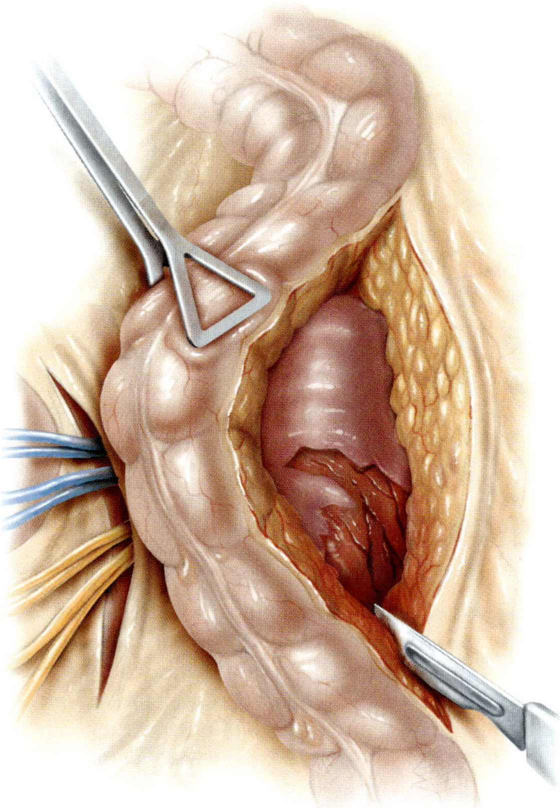

Fig. 15.4.17. Exposure of renal fossa after vascular control is achieved

mortality rates (Nash et al. 1995). The mortality in this group of patients is associated with the overall severity of the injury and is not a consequence of the renal injury itself (DiGiacomo et al. 2001). In gunshot injuries caused by a high-velocity bullet, reconstruction may be difficult and nephrectomy may be required (Ersay and Akgun 1999).

Renorrhaphy is the most common reconstructive technique. Partial nephrectomy is required when nonviable tissue is detected. Watertight closure of the collecting system if open may be desirable, although some experts merely close the parenchyma over the injured collecting system with good results. If renal capsule is not preserved, an omental pedicle flap or perirenal fat bolster may be used for coverage (McAninch et al. 1990). In a review by Shekarriz et al., the use of fibrin sealant in traumatic renal reconstruction proved to be helpful (Shekarriz et al. 2002). Newly developed hemastatic agents, which have proven useful in open and laparoscopic partial nephrectomy(Richter et al. 2003), may also be helpful but are largely unproven. In all cases, drainage of the ipsilateral retroperitoneum is recommended to provide an outlet for any temporary urinary leak. Renal wrapping with absorbable mesh is valuable in organ preservation in cases of multiple lacerations (Kluger et al. 1999).

All penetrating injuries are explored via a transabdominal approach for preserving the kidney if feasible, exploring the contralateral kidney, and controlling other abdominal injuries, since in many cases preoperative evaluation is insufficient (Kuvezdic et al. 1996). Patients with hematuria undergoing an exploration following a gunshot wound should be evaluated for the entire urinary tract. The kidney should be explored by opening Gerota's fascia in the presence of active bleeding, an expanding perirenal hematoma, or urine leak. Inspection of the hilum and proximal ureter but no incision of Gerota's fascia is mandatory in stable hematomas. Hilar control is achieved prior to renal exploration only in hemodynamically stable patients; otherwise the kidney should be immediately delivered to the laparotomy wound and active hemorrhage be controlled by manual compression. In cases of uncertainty on the adequacy of the urinary tract exploration, intravenous dye (methylene blue or indigo carmine) should be administered to unmask suspected injuries (Velmahos and Degiannis 1997).

Renovascular injuries are uncommon. They are associated with extensive associated trauma and increased peri- and postoperative mortality and morbidity. Knudson et al. (2000) found that after blunt trauma, repair of Grade 5 vascular injury was seldom if ever effective. Repair may be attempted in those very rare cases in which there is a solitary kidney or the patient has sustained bilateral injuries (Tillou et al. 2001). In all other cases, nephrectomy appears to be the treatment of choice (el Khader et al. 1998a).

Arteriography with selective renal embolization for hemorrhage control is a reasonable alternative to laparotomy, provided no other indication for immediate surgery exists (Hagiwara et al. 2001). The rate of successful hemostasis by embolization is reported to be identical in blunt and penetrating injuries (Velmahos et al. 2000; Sofocleous et al. 2005).

Nonoperative Management of Renal Injuries

As the indications for renal exploration become clearer, nonoperative management has become the treatment of choice for the majority of renal injuries. In stable patients, supportive care with bedrest, hydration, and antibiotics is the preferred initial approach. Primary conservative management is associated with a lower rate of nephrectomy, without any increase in the immediate or long-term morbidity (Schmidlin et al. 1997). The failure of conservative therapy is relatively low (5%) (Herschorn et al. 1991).

All Grade 1 and 2 renal injuries can be managed nonoperatively, whether they are due to blunt or penetrating trauma. Therapy of Grade 3 injuries has been controversial for many years. Improved results in all recent studies support expectant treatment (el Khader et al. 1998a; Thall et al. 1996; Cheng et al. 1994). The majority of patients with Grade 4 and 5 renal injuries present with major associated injuries, with resultant high exploration and nephrectomy rates (Santucci and McAninch 2001), although emerging data indicates that many of these patients can be managed safely with an expectant approach (Hammer and Santucci 2003; Rogers et al. 2004). Penetrating wounds have traditionally been approached surgically. However, stable patients should undergo complete staging to define the full extent of the injury. Renal gunshot injuries should be explored only if they involve the hilum or are accompanied by signs of continued bleeding, ureteral injuries, or renal pelvis lacerations (Velmahos et al. 1998). Low-velocity gunshot and stab wounds of minor degree may be managed conservatively with an acceptably good outcome (Baniel and Schein 1994). Meanwhile, tissue damage from high-velocity gunshot injuries may be more extensive and the majority of patients present with major associated injuries. Hemodynamic instability requiring a nephrectomy is a very common situation (Ersay and Akgun 1999).

In 1983, Bernath et al. (1983) suggested that if the site of penetration by stab wound was posterior to the anterior axillary line, 88 % of such renal injuries could be managed nonoperatively. In another study, analysis suggested that injuries to the flank were more likely to be Grade 3, whereas injuries to the abdomen were more likely to be Grade 1. A systematic approach based on clinical, laboratory, and radiological evaluation may minimize negative exploration without increasing morbidity from missed injury (Armenakas et al. 1999). Renal stab wounds producing major renal injuries (Grade 3 or higher) are more unpredictable and they are associated with a higher rate of delayed complications if treated expectantly (Wessells et al. 1997a).

Postoperative Care and Follow-up

Patients who are successfully treated conservatively carry some risk of presenting with complications. This risk correlates with increasing grade. Repeat imaging 2–4 days after trauma minimizes the risk of missed complications, especially in Grade 3–5 blunt renal injuries (Blankenship et al. 2001). However, the utility of frequent CT scanning after injury has never been satisfactorily proven. CT scans should always be performed on patients with fever, unexplained decreasing hematocrit, or significant flank pain.

Nuclear renal scans are useful for documenting and tracking functional recovery in patients following renal reconstruction before discharge from hospital (Wessells et al. 1997b). To detect many of the delayed complications, an excretory urogram is recommended within 3 months of major renal injury, although benefit to the patient has not yet been proven in the literature. Follow-up should involve physical examination, urinalysis, individualized radiological investigation, serial blood pressure measurement, and serum determination of renal function (McAninch et al. 1991; Moudouni et al. 2001a). It is recommended that follow-up examinations should continue until healing is documented and laboratory findings stabilized, although checking for latent renovascular hypertension may need to continue for years.

Literature is generally inadequate on the subject of long-term consequences of trauma on renal tissue. It appears that on histopathological evaluation, renal tissue may appear dystrophic following some cases of conservative management of minor renal injuries (Pruthi et al. 1998).

Complications

Early complications occur within the 1st month after injury and can be bleeding, arteriovenous fistulae involving the renal artery, infection, perinephric abscess, sepsis, urinary fistula, hypertension, urinary extravasation, and urinoma. Delayed complications include bleeding, hydronephrosis, calculus formation, chronic pyelonephritis, hypertension, arteriovenous fistula, hydronephrosis, and pseudoaneurysms.

Delayed retroperitoneal bleeding usually occurs within several weeks of an injury or procedure and may be life-threatening. Selective angiographic embolization is the preferred treatment (Heyns and van Vollenhoven 1992a).

Perinephric abscess formation is usually best managed by percutaneous drainage, although open drainage may sometimes be required (McAninch et al. 1991). Percutaneous management of complications may poses less risk of renal loss than reoperation, which may lead to nephrectomy when infected tissues make reconstruction difficult.

Hypertension may occur acutely as a result of external compression from perirenal hematoma (Page kidney) or chronically because of compressive scar formation. Renin-mediated hypertension may occur as a long-term complication; etiologies include renal artery thrombosis, segmental arterial thrombosis, renal artery stenosis (Goldblatt kidney), devitalized fragments, and arteriovenous fistulae. Arteriography is informative in cases of post-traumatic hypertension (Montgomery et al. 1998). Treatment is required if hypertension persists and may include medical management, excision of the ischemic parenchymal segment, vascular reconstruction, or total nephrectomy. The frequency of post-traumatic hypertension is estimated to be less than 5 % in all published series (Lebech and Strange-Vognsen 1990; Monstrey et al. 1989).

Urinary extravasation after renal reconstruction often subsides without intervention as long as ureteral obstruction and infection are not present. Ureteral, retrograde stenting may improve drainage and allow healing (Haas et al. 1998b). Persistent urinary extravasation from an otherwise viable kidney after blunt trauma often responds to stent placement and/or percutaneous drainage as necessary (Matthews et al. 1997).

Arteriovenous fistulas usually present with delayed onset of significant hematuria, hypertension, heart failure, and progressive renal failure, most often after penetrating trauma. Percutaneous embolization or stenting of the renal artery is often effective for symptomatic arteriovenous fistulas, but larger ones may require surgery (Wang et al. 1998; Kavic et al. 2002). The development of pseudoaneurysm is a rare complication following blunt renal trauma. In numerous case reports, transcatheter embolization appears to be a reliable minimally invasive solution (Franco de Castro et al. 2001; Miller et al. 2002). Acute renal colic from a retained missile has been reported and may be managed endoscopically if possible (Harrington and Kandel 1997). Other unusual late complications, such as duodenal obstruction, may result from retroperitoneal hematoma following blunt renal trauma (Park et al. 2001).

Renal Injury in the Polytrauma Patient

Approximately 8% – 10% of blunt and penetrating abdominal injuries involve the kidneys. The incidence of associated injury in penetrating renal trauma ranges from 77% to 100%. Gunshot wounds are associated with organ injury more often than stab wounds (Sagalowsky 1983; Carlton et al. 1968). The majority of patients with penetrating renal trauma have associated adjacent organ injuries that may complicate treatment. In the absence of an expanding hematoma with hemodynamic instability, associated multiorgan injuries do not increase the risk of nephrectomy (Kansas 2004).

Blunt and penetrating trauma equally contributed to combined renal and pancreatic injury, as reported by Rosen et al. (1994). Renal preservation was achieved in most patients and the complication rate of the series was 15%. A similar rate of complications (16%) was reported in patients with simultaneous colon and renal injury. In a report reviewing this combination of injuries over a period of 17 years, 58% of patients underwent an exploration, with nephrectomies performed in 16% of explorations (Wessells and McAninch 1996).

Renal injuries seem to be rather rare in patients with blunt chest trauma. In a recent study with polytrauma patients, conservative management was safely attempted in polytrauma patients without increasing morbidity (Sartorelli et al. 2000). In polytrauma patients undergoing partial or total nephrectomy, there is no increased mortality or renal failure rate (Cass et al. 1987).

Multiorgan trauma patients who need multiple operations for associated intraabdominal injuries may undergo main artery embolization for severe renal injuries. In these cases, there is a high risk for sepsis, and postembolization nephrectomy is suggested (Sofocleous et al. 2005).

15.4.6 Foreign Bodies

Renal foreign bodies are uncommon and result from penetrating injuries and retained sponges or wires during surgical or endourological procedures. There are a few case reports in the literature that suggest selective exploration of such injuries.

Penetrating injuries following blast or gunshot injuries result in multiple life-threatening injuries. Renal foreign bodies may be metallic particles, bullets, or pellets entrapped in the parenchyma or the collecting system. In stable patients, penetrating injuries are no longer absolute indications for exploration (Sofer et al. 2001). Foreign bodies may be removed endoscopically or surgically in cases of migration causing buckshot colic or infection (Harrington and Kandel 1997).

Sponges are rarely retained during surgery nowadays. The potential complications of a retained sponge are primarily related to infection and include abscess formation, fistulization to the skin or the intestinal tract, and even sepsis. Retained sponges may cause perirenal pseudotumors or appear as solid renal mass. Magnetic resonance imaging most clearly shows the characteristic features and permits preoperative diagnosis (Kuo and Wang1999; Ben Meir et al. 2003).

Absorbable hemostatic agents may also produce a foreign body giant cell reaction after partial nephrectomy for renal cell carcinoma. Imaging characteristics of this lesion are not specific and the diagnosis may be a recurrent tumor or abscess. Exploration of the lesion reveals the real nature of the lesion.

Retained stents, wires, or fractured Acucise cutting wires may also present as foreign bodies of the kidney (Johnson and Conlin 2001; Beduschi and Wolf 1997). In some cases, the foreign body may serve as nidus for stone formation. Patients are treated for calculus by endoscopy, so the true nature of the stone is revealed.

15.4.7 Spontaneous Retroperitoneal Hemorrhage

Spontaneous retroperitoneal hemorrhage is an uncommon event and the most frequent event is the rupture of a renal tumor (angiomyolipoma, sarcoma) or an adrenal mass (pheochromocytoma), severe arteriosclerosis, rupture of the renal stenotic artery in von Recklinghausen's disease (Shimizu et al. 1998), or polyarteritis nodosa (Siebels et al. 1998), spontaneous graft rupture, or rupture of the kidney after extracorporal shock wave lithotripsy. Many arguments (whether it be abdominal mechanical pressure, hormonal, or histological ones) suggest that a pregnancy could increase the risk of renal angiomyolipoma rupture. Adrenal pseudocysts may also rupture as a result of blunt injury and cause massive hemorrhage in the retroperitoneum (Favorito et al. 2004).

Rupture of the renal pelvis may result from ureteral tumor, ureteral stone, and stricture of the ureteropelvic junction. The prognosis in spontaneous urinary extravasation is usually good without drainage. Open surgery is seldom indicated. Rupture of renal pelvis during pregnancy is also uncommon. Ruptured renal neoplasms can be a catastrophic clinical presentation. Acute abdomen and severe colic pain are the common clinical manifestations.

Rupture of the kidney after extracorporal shock wave lithotripsy is an extremely rare and severe complication. Persistent flank pain with macroscopic hematuria and hemodynamic instability are the main symptoms. Emergency nephrectomy is the subsequent management of the complication (May et al. 2004) (Figs. 15.4.18 – 15.4.21).

References

Abdalati H, Bulas DI et al (1994) Blunt renal trauma in children: healing of renal injuries and recommendations for imaging follow-up. Pediatr Radiol 24:573

Abu-Zidan FM, Al-Tawheed A et al (1999) Urologic injuries in the Gulf War. Int Urol Nephrol 31:577

Acheson, AG, Graham AN et al (1998) Prospective study on factors delaying surgery in ruptured abdominal aortic aneurysms. J R Coll Surg Edinb 43:182

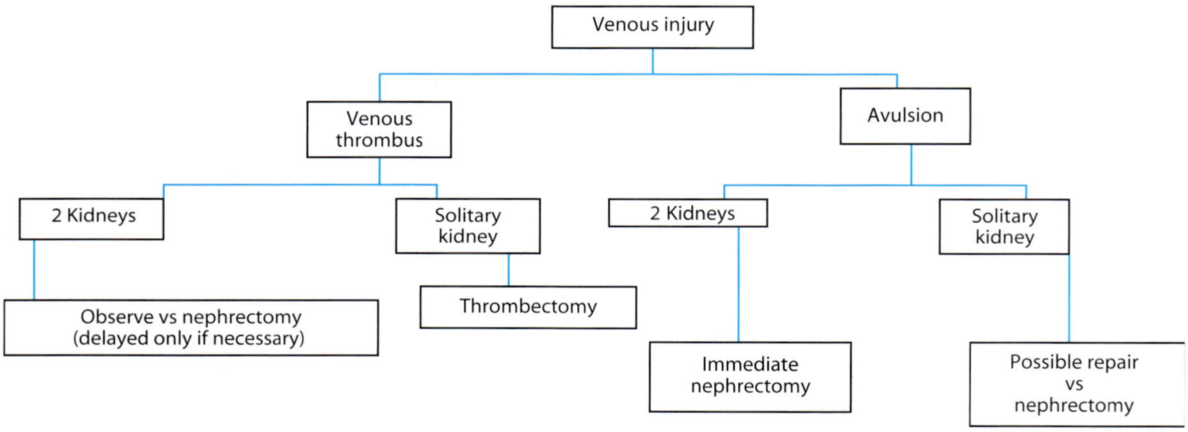

Fig. 15.4.18. Algorithm for the conservative management of venous injuries

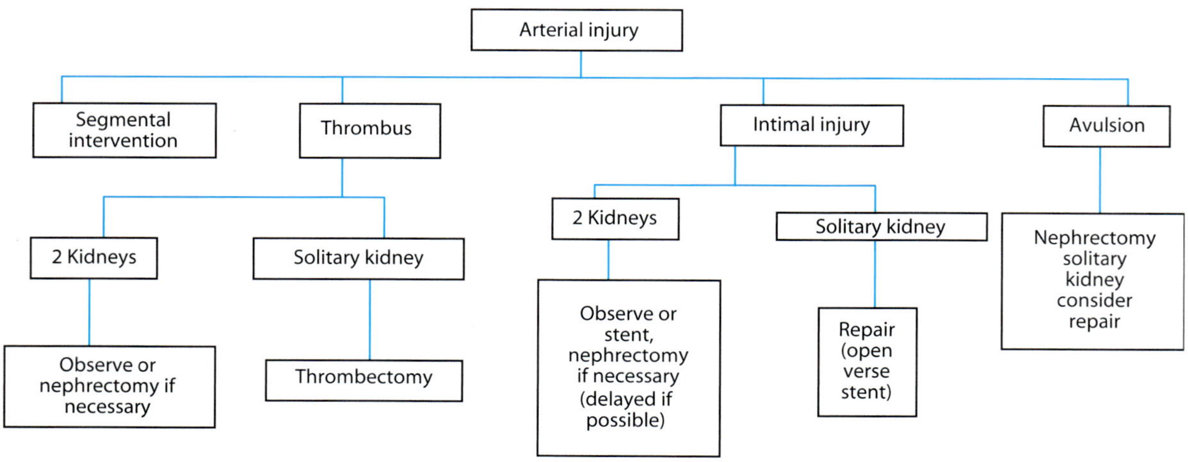

Fig. 15.4.19. Algorithm for the conservative management of arterial injuries

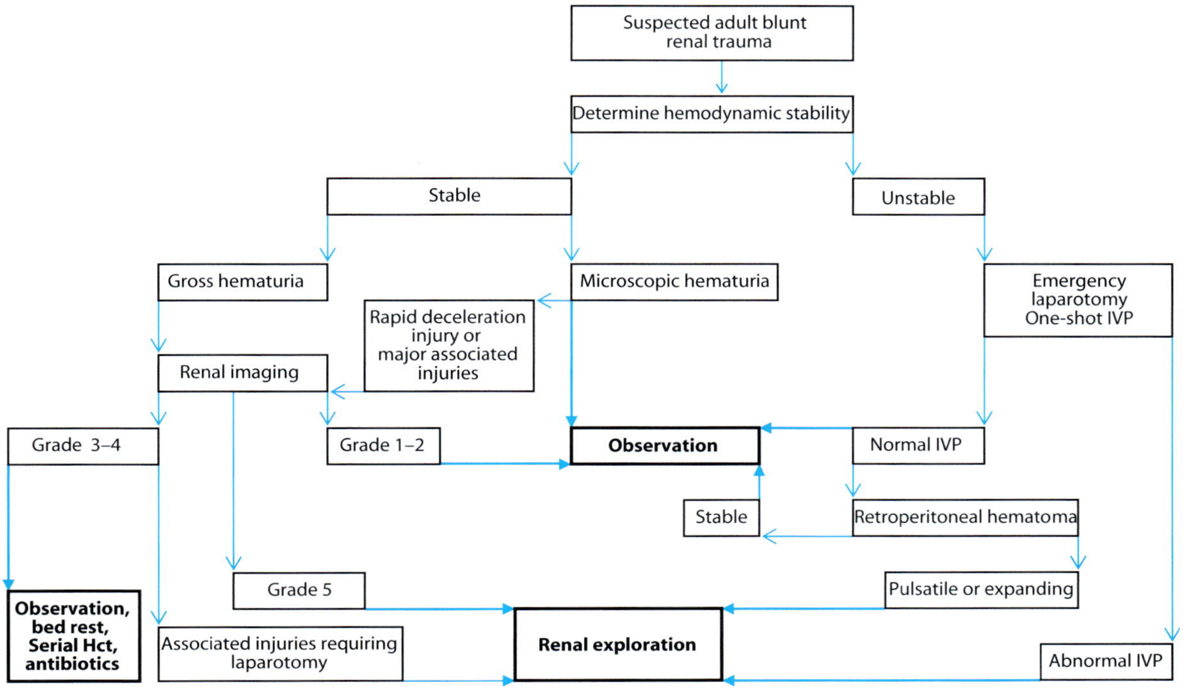

Fig. 15.4.20. Evaluation of blunt renal trauma in adults

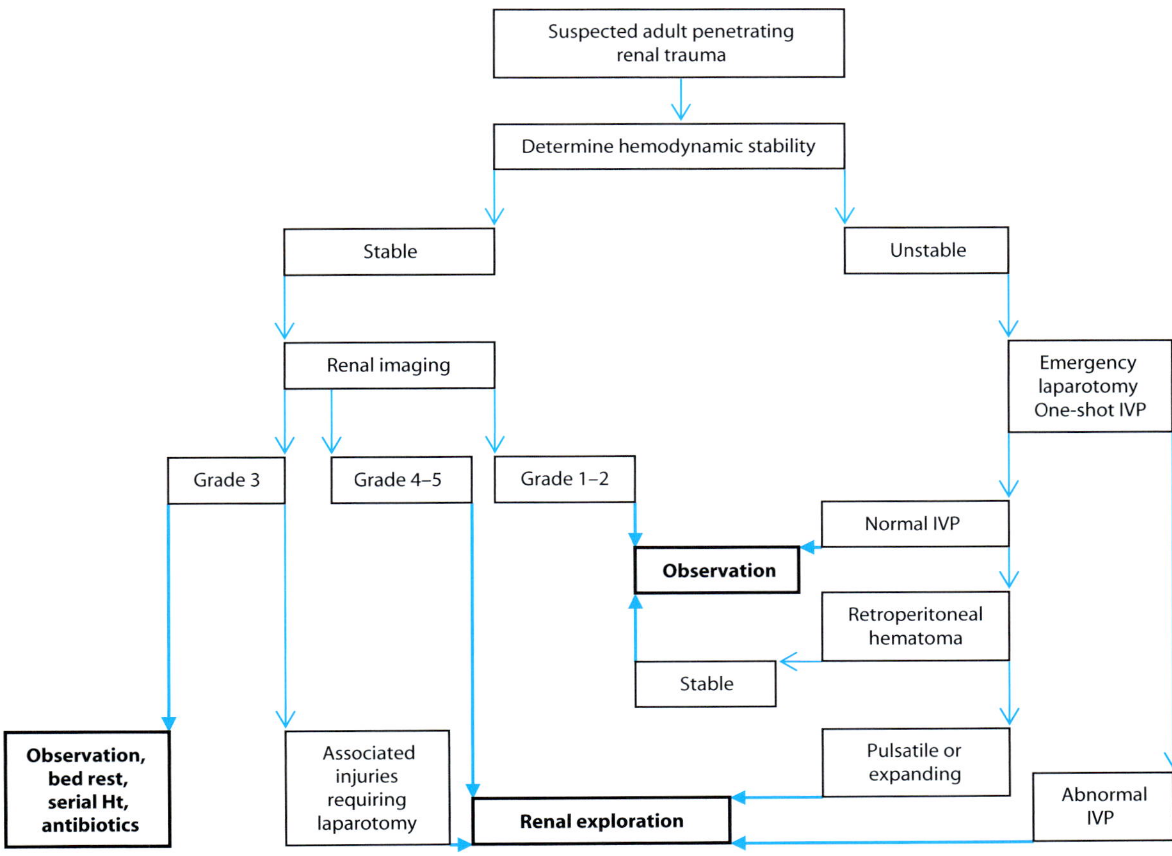

Fig. 15.4.21. Evaluation of penetrating renal trauma in adults

Adovasio R, Griselli F (2003) An unusual complication of open aortic surgery: hemorrhage due to the iatrogenic rupture of a renal cyst. Vasa 32:167
Agramunt Lerma M, Lonjedo Vicent E et al (2003) Selective embolization in the treatment of severe renal injury. Arch Esp Urol 56:83
Ahmed, S, TD Batiuk (2001) Broken kidney: traumatic fracture of a renal allograft. Am J Kidney Dis 37:e33
Akabane S, Ushiyama T et al (2001) A case of traumatic renal graft rupture with salvage of renal function. Clin Transplant 15:289
Alapont Alacreu JM, Broseta Rico E et al (2003) Complications of uretero-renoscopy. Actas Urol Esp 27:692
Aldana JP, Lee BR et al (2003) Residual air persists in the renal collecting system following percutaneous nephrolithotomy. J Laparoendosc Adv Surg Tech A 13:317
Al-Janabi MA, Ahmad R et al (1995) Case report: renal scintigraphy in the diagnosis of urinary extravasation. Br J Radiol 68:12513
Alonso-Perez M, Segura RJ et al (1999) Surgical treatment of ruptured abdominal aortic aneurysms in the elderly. Ann Vasc Surg 13:592
Altman AL, Haas C et al (2000) Selective nonoperative management of blunt grade 5 renal injury. J Urol 164:27; discussion 30
Alvi A, Doherty T et al (2003) Facial fractures and concomitant injuries in trauma patients. Laryngoscope 113:102
Amaral, JF (1997) Thoracoabdominal injuries in the athlete. Clin Sports Med 16:739
Andronikou S, Bertelsmann J (2002) CT scanning–essential for conservative management of paediatric blunt abdominal trauma. S Afr Med J 92:35
Anema JG, Morey AF et al (2001) Potential uses of absorbable fibrin adhesive bandage for genitourinary trauma. World J Surg 25:15737
Angelis M, Augenstein JS et al (2003) Ex vivo repair and renal autotransplantation after penetrating trauma: is there an upper limit of ischemic/traumatic injury beyond which a kidney is unsalvageable? J Trauma 54:606; discussion 609
Angus LD, Tachmes L et al (1993) Surgical management of pediatric renal trauma: an urban experience. Am Surg 59:388
Ansong K (1995) Re: outcome after temporary vascular occlusion for the management of renal trauma. J Urol 153:440
Anwar YA, Sullivan ED et al (1997) Abrupt, severe hypertension associated with dissection of a renal artery during selective catheterization. J Hum Hypertens 11:533
Arena F, Peracchia G et al (1997) The role of echotomography in minor renal traumatology. Acta Biomed Ateneo Parmense 68:53
Armenakas NA (1999) Current methods of diagnosis and management of ureteral injuries. World J Urol 17:78
Armenakas NA, Duckett CP et al (1999) Indications for nonoperative management of renal stab wounds. J Urol 161:768
Armstrong AL, Birch BR et al (1994) Renal arteriovenous fistula following blunt trauma. Br J Urol 73:321
Asayama K, Tsuda H et al (2005) Bilateral posterior ischemic optic neuropathy following subdural hematoma drainage. Nippon Ganka Gakkai Zasshi 109:26
Ascher E, Scheinman M et al (1999) Ruptured versus elective abdominal aortic aneurysm repair: outcome and cost. Ann Vasc Surg 13:613
Asensio JA, Chahwan S et al (2000) Operative management and outcome of 302 abdominal vascular injuries. Am J Surg 180:528; discussion 533
Ashebu SD, Dahniya MH et al (2004) Rupture of the renal pelvis of a ureteropelvic junction hydronephrosis after blunt abdominal trauma. Australas Radiol 48:256
Assenza M, Romagnoli F et al (2003) Conservative approach to IV grade renal trauma. Chir Ital 55:445
Atala A, Miller FB et al (1991) Preliminary vascular control for renal trauma. Surg Gynecol Obstet 172:386
Ather MH, Noor MA (2002) Role of imaging in the evaluation of renal trauma. J Pak Med Assoc 52:423
Aydin, MD, Akcay F et al (2005) Cerebral fat embolism: pulmonary contusion is a more important etiology than long bone fractures. Clin Neuropathol 24:86
Baba K, Yajima M et al (2001) Clinical study on renal trauma. Hinyokika Kiyo 47:159
Baeza-Herrera C, Dominguez-Perez ST et al (2002) Renal trauma in childhood. Second-level hospital experience. Gac Med Mex 138:313
Bahloul A, Krid M et al (1997) Contusions to the pathologic kidney. A retrospective study, apropos of 34 cases. Ann Urol (Paris) 31:253
Baker HW (1998) Reproductive effects of nontesticular illness. Endocrinol Metab Clin North Am 27:831
Balkan E, Kilic N et al (2005) Indirect computed tomography sign of renal artery injury: retrograde filling of the renal vein. Int J Urol 12:311
Ballesteros Sampol JJ, Alameda Quitllet F et al (2002) 3 rare cases of textiloma after renal surgery. Review of the literature. Arch Esp Urol 55:25
Ballestri M, Baraldi A et al (2001) Liver and kidney foreign bodies granulomatosis in a patient with malocclusion, bruxism, and worn dental prostheses. Gastroenterology 121: 12348
Bandhauer K, Hassler H (1990) Injuries of the urogenital system. Urologe A 29:234
Baniel J, Schein M (1994) The management of penetrating trauma to the urinary tract. J Am Coll Surg 178:417
Bar K, Klijer R et al (2002) Ureter injury as a gynecologic surgery complication–prospects for conservative treatment. Ginekol Pol 73:50
Bariol, SV, Stewart GD et al (2005) An analysis of urinary tract trauma in Scotland: imnpact on management and resource needs. Surgeon 3:27
Barone GW, Sailors DM et al (1997) Trauma management in solid organ transplant recipients. J Emerg Med 15:169
Barone R, Borson-Chazot F et al (2005) Patient-specific dosimetry in predicting renal toxicity with (90)Y-DOTATOC: relevance of kidney volume and dose rate in finding a dose-effect relationship. J Nucl Med 46 [Suppl 1]:99SS
Barsness KA, Bensard DD et al (2004) Renovascular injury: an argument for renal preservation. J Trauma 57:310
Base J, Navratilova J et al (1995) Blunt injury of the kidney–personal experience and present views on its therapy. Sb Ved Pr Lek Fak Karlovy Univerzity Hradci Kralove Suppl 38:81
Bass DH, Semple PL et al (1991) Investigation and management of blunt renal injuries in children: a review of 11 years' experience. J Pediatr Surg 26:196
Bassiri A, Ahmadnia H et al (2002) Transureteral lithotripsy in pediatric practice. J Endourol 16:257
Bates MC, Shamsham FM et al (2002) Successful treatment of iatrogenic renal artery perforation with an autologous vein-covered stent. Catheter Cardiovasc Interv 57:39
Baughman SM, Morey AF et al (2003) Percutaneous transrenal application of fibrin sealant for refractory urinary leak after gunshot wound. J Urol 170:522
Baumann L, Greenfield SP et al (1992) Nonoperative management of major blunt renal trauma in children: in- hospital morbidity and long-term followup. J Urol 148:691
Baverstock R, Simons R et al (2001) Severe blunt renal trauma: a 7-year retrospective review from a provincial trauma centre. Can J Urol 8:13726
Becker CD, Mentha G et al (1998) Blunt abdominal trauma in adults: role of CT in the diagnosis and management of visceral injuries. Part 2: gastrointestinal tract and retroperitoneal organs. Eur Radiol 8(5):772

Beduschi R, Wolf JS Jr (1997) Fragment of a catheter as a foreign body in the kidney. Tech Urol 3:222
Bellanova G, Serao A et al (2003) Hepatic and renal trauma: importance of arteriography in diagnosis and treatment. Ann Ital Chir 74:31
Bellman GC (1996) Complications of endopyelotomy. J Endourol 10:177
Ben Meir D, Lask D et al (2003) Intrarenal foreign body presenting as a solid tumor. Urology 61:1035
Benchekroun A, Lachkar A et al (1997) Kidney injuries. A propos of 30 cases. Ann Urol (Paris) 31:237
Benjamin ME, Sandager GP et al (1999) Duplex ultrasound insertion of inferior vena cava filters in multitrauma patients. Am J Surg 178:92
Bennani S, Aboutaieb R et al (1995) Evaluation and treatment of closed traumas of the kidney. J Chir (Paris) 132:142
Benson DA, Stockinger ZT et al (2005) Embolization of an acute renal arteriovenous fistula following a stab wound: case report and review of the literature. Am Surg 71:62
Berkmen F, Peker AE et al (2000) Treatment of iatrogenic ureteral injuries during various operations for malignant conditions. J Exp Clin Cancer Res 19:441
Berkovich GY, Ramchandani P et al (2001) Renal vein thrombosis after martial arts trauma. J Trauma 50:144
Bernath AS, Schutte H et al (1983) Stab wounds of the kidney: conservative management in flank penetration. J Urol 129:468
Best CD, Petrone P et al (2005) Traumatic ureteral injuries: a single institution experience validating the American Association for the Surgery of Trauma-Organ Injury Scale grading scale. J Urol 173:12025
Bhayani SB, Grubb RL 3rd et al (2002) Use of gelatin matrix to rapidly repair diaphragmatic injury during laparoscopy. Urology 60:514
Bianchi G, Lamazza A et al (1997) Diagnostic and therapeutic approach to kidney injuries. G Chir 18:308
Bilen CY, Sahin A et al (1999) Nonoliguric renal failure after transurethral resection of prostate. J Endourol 13:751
Bittard H, Chaabouni MN et al (1995) Surgery for severe traumas of the kidney. Value of initial computed tomography, problem of surgical indication and use of a perirenal resorbable prosthesis of polyglactin 910. J Urol 101:209
Biyani CS, CS Powell (1998) Guidewire fragmentation during holmium: YAG laser endopyelotomy. Tech Urol 4:51
Blake AM, Toker SI et al (2002) Trauma management in the end-stage renal disease patient. Am Surg 68:425
Blankenship B, Earls JP et al (1997) Renal vein thrombosis after vascular pedicle injuryclin conference. AJR Am J Roentgenol 168:1574
Blankenship JC, Gavant ML et al (2001) Importance of delayed imaging for blunt renal trauma. World J Surg 25:15614
Bleetman A, Dyer J (2000) Ultrasound assessment of the vulnerability of the internal organs to stabbing: determining safety standards for stab-resistant body armour. Injury 31:609
Bogdanovic J, Djozic J et al (2002) Successful surgical reconstruction of ruptured renal pelvis following blunt abdominal trauma. Urol Int 68:302
Boggi, U, R Berchiolli et al (1998) Renal hypertension due to giant perirenal haematoma: permanent resolution by percutaneous ultrasound-guided drainage. Scand J Urol Nephrol 32:64
Bozeman C, Carver B et al (2004) Selective operative management of major blunt renal trauma. J Trauma 57:305
Braams R, Vossen V et al (1999) Outcome in patients requiring renal replacement therapy after surgery for ruptured and non-ruptured aneurysm of the abdominal aorta. Eur J Vasc Endovasc Surg 18:323
Brandes SB, McAninch JW (1999a) Reconstructive surgery for trauma of the upper urinary tract. Urol Clin North Am 26:183
Brandes SB, McAninch JW (1999b) Urban free falls and patterns of renal injury: a 20-year experience with 396 cases. J Trauma 47:643; discussion 649
Breen DJ, Janzen DL et al (1997) Blunt bowel and mesenteric injury: diagnostic performance of CT signs. J Comput Assist Tomogr 21:706
Brennan PW, Everest ER et al (2002) Risk of death among cases attending South Australian major trauma services after severe trauma: the first 4 years of operation of a state trauma system. J Trauma 53:333
Bretan PN Jr, McAninch JW et al (1986) Computerized tomographic staging of renal trauma:85 consecutive cases. J Urol 136:561
Broeders IA, Blankensteijn JD et al (1999) Mid-term fixation stability of the EndoVascular Technologies endograft. EVT Investigators. Eur J Vasc Endovasc Surg 18:300
Brown DF, Rosen CL et al (1997) Renal ultrasonography. Emerg Med Clin North Am 15:877
Brown KM, Borge MA et al (2002) Pelvic lymphocele following motor vehicle collision. Ann Vasc Surg 16:121
Brown MA, Sirlin CB et al (2005) Screening sonography in pregnant patients with blunt abdominal trauma. J Ultrasound Med 24:175; quiz 183
Brown SA, Munver R et al (2000) Microdialysis assessment of shock wave lithotripsy-induced renal injury. Urology 56:364
Brown SL, Elder JS et al (1998a) Are pediatric patients more susceptible to major renal injury from blunt trauma? A comparative study. J Urol 160:138
Brown SL, Hoffman DM et al (1998b) Limitations of routine spiral computerized tomography in the evaluation of blunt renal trauma. J Urol 160:19791
Brown SL, Haas C et al (2001) Radiologic evaluation of pediatric blunt renal trauma in patients with microscopic hematuria. World J Surg 25:15570
Bruce LM, Croce MA et al (2001) Blunt renal artery injury: incidence, diagnosis, and management. Am Surg 67:550; discussion 555
Bruninx G, Wery D et al (1999) Emergency endovascular treatment of an acute traumatic rupture of the thoracic aorta complicated by a distal low-flow syndrome. Cardiovasc Intervent Radiol 22:515
Brunkwall J, Lanne T et al (1999) Acute renal impairment due to a primary aortocaval fistula is normalised after a successful operation. Eur J Vasc Endovasc Surg 17:191
Bschleipfer T, Kallieris D et al (2002) Blunt renal trauma: biomechanics and origination of renal lesions. Eur Urol 42:614
Bschleipfer T, Kallieris D et al (2003) Validity of computerized tomography in blunt renal trauma. J Urol 170:24759
Buchberger W, Penz T et al (1993) Diagnosis and staging of blunt kidney trauma. A comparison of urinalysis, i.v. urography, sonography and computed tomography. Rofo Fortschr Geb Rontgenstr Neuen Bildgeb Verfahr 158:507
Buckley JC, McAninch JW (2004) Pediatric renal injuries: management guidelines from a 25-year experience. J Urol 172:687; discussion 690
Buckman RF, AS Pathak, et al (2001) Injuries of the inferior vena cava. Surg Clin North Am 81:14317
Burbridge BE, Groot G et al (1991) Emergency excretory urography in blunt abdominal trauma. Can Assoc Radiol J 42:326
Cachecho R, Millham FH et al (1994) Management of the trauma patient with pre-existing renal disease. Crit Care Clin 10:523
Cakir B, Cevik H et al (2005) Leptin ameliorates burn-induced multiple organ damage and modulates postburn immune response in rats. Regul Pept 125:135

Cambria RP, Davison JK et al (1997) Thoracoabdominal aneurysm repair: perspectives over a decade with the clamp-and-sew technique. Ann Surg 226:294; discussion 303
Canby-Hagino ED, Morey AF et al (2000) Fibrin sealant treatment of splenic injury during open and laparoscopic left radical nephrectomy. J Urol 164:20045
Cao P, P De Rango (1999) Abdominal aortic aneurysms: current management. Cardiologia 44:711
Carcamo Valor PI, Hidalgo Togores L et al (1990) Kidney injuries in childhood: our experience in 64 cases. Arch Esp Urol 43:651; discussion 655
Carcamo Valor PI, Hidalgo Togores L et al (1991) Our experience with the diagnosis and treatment of 429 renal traumatisms. Arch Esp Urol 44:801
Carl P (1997) Diagnosis and therapy of kidney traumas. Urologe A 36:523
Carlton CE Jr, Scott R Jr, Goldman M (1968) The management of penetrating injuries of the kidney. J Trauma 8:1071
Carmona Campos EC, Prieto Castro R et al (1998) Evaluation and treatment of closed renal trauma. Actas Urol Esp 22:23
Carpio F, Morey AF (1999) Radiographic staging of renal injuries. World J Urol 17:66
Carr JA, Kralovich KA et al (2001) Primary venorraphy for traumatic inferior vena cava injuries. Am Surg 67:207; discussion 213
Carrel TP, Signer C (1999) Separate revascularization of the visceral arteries in thoracoabdominal aneurysm repair. Ann Thorac Surg 68:573
Carroll PR, McAninch JW (1985) Operative indications in penetrating renal trauma. J Trauma 25:587
Carroll PR, McAninch JW et al (1990) Renovascular trauma: risk assessment, surgical management, and outcome. J Trauma 30:547; discussion 553
Cass AS, Luxenberg M et al (1987) Deaths from urologic injury due to external trauma. J Trauma 27:319
Castrucci M, D Ghio et al (1997) Embolization of iatrogenic renal vascular lesions with coaxial catheters and microcoils. Radiol Med (Torino) 93:576
Catalano O, Lobianco R et al (1999) Contrast media extravasation in upper abdominal injuries: detection with spiral computerized tomography. Radiol Med (Torino) 97:138
Catalano O, Lobianco R et al (2004) Real-time, contrast-enhanced sonographic imaging in emergency radiology. Radiol Med (Torino) 108:454
Cetti NE (2000) Blunt renal trauma: some personal thoughts. Scand J Urol Nephrol 34:5
Ceylan H, Gunsar C et al (2003) Blunt renal injuries in Turkish children: a review of 205 cases. Pediatr Surg Int 19:710
Chaabouni MN, Bittard M (1996) Application of a peri-renal prosthesis (Vicryl mesh) in the conservative treatment of multiple ruptured kidney fragments. Ann Urol (Paris) 30:61; discussion 64
Chandhoke PS, McAninch JW (1988) Detection and significance of microscopic hematuria in patients with blunt renal trauma. J Urol 140:16
Chang SS, Koch MO (1996) The use of an extended spiral bladder flap for treatment of upper ureteral loss. J Urol 156:1981
Chatziioannou A, Brountzos E et al (2004) Effects of superselective embolization for renal vascular injuries on renal parenchyma and function. Eur J Vasc Endovasc Surg 28:201
Chazen MD, KS Miller (1997) Intrarenal pseudoaneurysm presenting 15 years after penetrating renal injury. Urology 49: 774
Chen JL, O'Shea M (1998) Extravasation injury associated with low-dose dopamine. Ann Pharmacother 32:545
Chen X, Borsa JJ et al (2002) CT of a renal artery pseudoaneurysm caused by a stab wound. AJR Am J Roentgenol 178:736
Cheng DL, D Lazan et al (1994) Conservative treatment of type III renal trauma. J Trauma 36:491
Cherniavskii AM, Marchenko AV et al (2004) A case of surgical treatment of post-traumatic false arteriovenous aneurysm of the right kidney vessels. Angiol Sosud Khir 10:130
Cherr GS, Hansen KJ (2001) Renal complications with aortic surgery. Semin Vasc Surg 14:245
Cherullo EE, Hobart MG et al (1999) Caliceal injury during laparoscopic cyst decortication in adult polycystic kidney disease. J Urol 162:1367
Chicharro Molero JA, del Rosal Samaniego JM et al (1992) Diagnostic evaluation of closed renal trauma. Actas Urol Esp 16:192
Chopra P, St-Vil D et al (2002) Blunt renal trauma-blessing in disguise? J Pediatr Surg 37:779
Chowdhary SK, Pimpalwar A et al (2000) Blunt injury of the abdomen: a plea for CT Pediatr Radiol 30:798
Christensen R (2001) Invasive radiology for pediatric trauma. Semin Pediatr Surg 10:7
Chu C, Chen K et al (2000) Delayed presentation of a posttraumatic perirenal urinoma in a 6-year-old boy. Pediatr Surg Int 16:140
Chursin VK, Stetsenko MA et al (2000) Complete abruption of kidney off vascular pedicle. Urologiia 43
Clark JY, Kearse WS Jr (1997) Extracorporeal shockwave lithotripsy for kidney stone on surgical clip. J Endourol 11:119
Clarnette TD, Beasley SW (1997) Handlebar injuries in children: patterns and prevention. Aust N Z J Surg 67:338
Cleveland RO, McAteer JA et al (1997) The effect of polypropylene vials on lithotripter shock waves. Ultrasound Med Biol 23:939
Coburn M (1997) Damage control for urologic injuries. Surg Clin North Am 77:821
Cohen M, Morales R Jr et al (2001) Staged reconstruction after gunshot wounds to the abdomen. Plast Reconstr Surg 108:83
Cohen Z, Gabriel A et al (2000) Traumatic avulsion of kidney into the chest through a ruptured diaphragm in a boy. Pediatr Emerg Care 16:180
Corriere JN Jr, McAndrew JD et al (1991) Intraoperative decision-making in renal trauma surgery. J Trauma 31:1390
Cortellini P, Ferretti S et al (1997) Major renal trauma. Therapeutic approaches and our experience. Minerva Urol Nefrol 49:183
Cowan NC, Traill ZC et al (1998) Direct percutaneous transrenal embolization for renal artery injury following percutaneous nephrostomy. Br J Radiol 71:1199
Cozar JM, Carcamo P et al (1990) Management of injury of the solitary kidney. Arch Esp Urol 43:15
Cywes S, Bass DH et al (1991) Blunt liver trauma in children. Injury 22:310
Damaraju S, Krajcer Z (1999) Successful Wallstent implantation for extensive iatrogenic renal artery dissection in a patient with fibromuscular dysplasia. J Endovasc Surg 6:297
Danuser H, Wille S et al (2001) How to treat blunt kidney ruptures: primary open surgery or conservative treatment with deferred surgery when necessary? Eur Urol 39:9
Davis PM, Gloviczki P et al (1998) Aorto-caval and ilio-iliac arteriovenous fistulae. Am J Surg 176:115
Dawson C, H Whitfield (1996) ABC of urology. Urological trauma and bladder reconstruction. BMJ 312:1352
Del Pizzo JJ, Jacobs SC et al (1998) Ureteroscopic evaluation in renal transplant recipients. J Endourol 12:135
DiGiacomo JC, Rotondo MF et al (2001) The role of nephrectomy in the acutely injured. Arch Surg 136:1045
Dorffner R, Thurnher S et al (1998) Embolization of iatrogenic vascular injuries of renal transplants: immediate and follow-up results. Cardiovasc Intervent Radiol 21:129
Eastham JA, Bennett CJ (1992) The occurrence of urologic injuries in patients with gunshot wounds to the spine. Semin Urol 10:112

Eastham JA, Wilson TG et al (1991) Radiographic assessment of blunt renal trauma. J Trauma 31:1527
Eastham JA, Wilson TG et al (1992) Angiographic embolization of renal stab wounds. J Urol 148:268
Eastham JA, Wilson TG et al (1993) Urological evaluation and management of renal-proximity stab wounds. J Urol 150: 1771
El Khader K, Bouchot O et al (1998a) Injuries of the renal pedicle: is renal revascularization justified? Prog Urol 8:995
El Khader K, A Mhidia et al (1998b) Conservative treatment of stage III kidney injuries. Acta Urol Belg 66:25
Ersay A, Akgun Y (1999) Experience with renal gunshot injuries in a rural setting. Urology 54:972
Ertekin C, Akyildiz H et al (2001) Results of conservative treatment for solid abdominal organ trauma. Ulus Travma Derg 7:224
Evan AP, Connors BA et al (1999) Renal disease potentiates the injury caused by SWLJ Endourol 13:619
Farah I, Tarabula P et al (1997) Traumatic and iatrogenic lesions of abdominal vessels. Chirurgie 122:572; discussion 578
Farid A, Sullivan TM (1996) Aortocaval fistula in ruptured inflammatory abdominal aortic aneurysm. A report of two cases and literature review. J Cardiovasc Surg (Torino) 37:561
Favorito LA, Lott FM et al (2004) Traumatic rupture of adrenal pseudocyst leading to massive hemorrhage in retroperitoneum. Int Braz J Urol 30:35
Feld LG, Waz WR et al (1997) Hematuria. An integrated medical and surgical approach. Pediatr Clin North Am 44:1191
Ferrozzi F, Bova D et al (1999) Foreign-body granuloma of the kidney: CT, MR and pathologic correlation. Eur Radiol 9:1590
Ficarra BJ (1996) Diseases and injuries in athletes. A review. J Med 27:241
Franco de Castro A, Gibanel Garanto R et al (2001) Selective embolization of post-traumatic renal pseudoaneurysm in monorenal patient. Actas Urol Esp 25:64
Frank RG, Gerard PS et al (1992) Serial sonographic evaluation of buckshot colic following a penetrating gunshot wound. Urol Radiol 14:172
Frassinelli P, Pasquale MD et al (1997) Bilateral renal artery thrombosis secondary to blunt trauma: case report and review of the literature. J Trauma 42:330
Fulford SC, Vafidis JA et al (1998) An unusual neurological complication of a staghorn renal calculus. Br J Urol 81:322
Fumi L (1997) An unexpected complication of urinary stomata. Br J Urol 79:813
Furukawa K, Ohteki H et al (1997) A case of ruptured thoracoabdominal aortic aneurysm with aortitis syndrome–operation with selective cold visceral arteries perfusion. Nippon Kyobu Geka Gakkai Zasshi 45:1747
Gabal-Shehab L, Alagiri M (2005) Traumatic adrenal injuries. J Urol 173:1330
Garner WL, Reiss M (2005) Burn care in Los Angeles, California: LAC+USC experience 1994. Burns 31 [Suppl 1]:S32
Geoghegan T, Benfayed W et al (2003) Rupture of ureteropelvic junction-obstructed kidney. AJR Am J Roentgenol 181:886
Gerspach JM, Bellman GC et al (1997) Conservative management of colon injury following percutaneous renal surgery. Urology 49:831
Gerstenbluth RE, Spirnak JP et al (2002) Sports participation and high grade renal injuries in children. J Urol 168:2575
Ghai B, Dureja GP et al (2003) Massive intra-abdominal extravasation of fluid: a life threatening complication following percutaneous nephrolithotomy. Int Urol Nephrol 35:315
Ghali AM, El Malik EM et al (1999) Ureteric injuries: diagnosis, management, and outcome. J Trauma 46:150
Giannarini G, Grossetti B et al (2004) Post-traumatic ureteropelvic junction obstruction. Arch Ital Urol Androl 76:100
Giannopoulos A, Serafetinides E et al (1999) Urogenital lesions diagnosed incidentally during evaluation for blunt renal injuries. Prog Urol 9:464
Giannopoulos A, Manousakas T et al (2004) Delayed life-threatening haematuria from a renal pseudoaneurysm caused by blunt renal trauma treated with selective embolization. Urol Int 72:352
Gintautas J, Angus LD et al (1994) Pharmacological and surgical management of pediatric renal injuries. Proc West Pharmacol Soc 37:99
Goff CD, Collin GR (1998) Management of renal trauma at a rural, level I trauma center. Am Surg 64:226
Goffette PP, Laterre PF (2002) Traumatic injuries: imaging and intervention in post-traumatic complications (delayed intervention) Eur Radiol 12:994
Goldman SM, CM Sandler (2004) Urogenital trauma: imaging upper GU trauma. Eur J Radiol 50:84
Gomes Almeida F, Reis J et al (2000) Traumatic rupture of angiomyolipoma: a case report. Arch Esp Urol 53:286
Gomez Pascual JA, Chicharro Molero JA et al (2002) Post-traumatic renal arteriovenous fistula. Conservative treatment with superselective embolization. Arch Esp Urol 55:949
Gomez Vegas A, Silmi Moyano A et al (1999) Ureteral iatrogenic disease of obstetric-gynecologic origin. Arch Esp Urol 52:923
Gonzalez RP, Falimirski M et al (1999) Surgical management of renal trauma: is vascular control necessary? J Trauma 47:1039; discussion 1042
Goodman DN, Saibil EA et al (1998) Traumatic intimal tear of the renal artery treated by insertion of a Palmaz stent. Cardiovasc Intervent Radiol 21(1:69
Gornicka G, Papierkowski A (2002) Foreign body in the kidney as a cause of erythruria in a 4-year old girl. Wiad Lek 55:338
Gorsline RT, Kaeding CC (2005) The use of NS AIDs and nutritional supplements in athletes with osteoarthritis: prevalence, benefits, and consequences. Clin Sports Med 24:71
Gosling P (1998) The cellular, immune, and metabolic response to trauma. Crit Rev Clin Lab Sci 35:59
Goswami GK, Levin DQ (2001) Traumatic renal artery thrombosis. Am J Surg 181:187
Griffet J, Bastiani-Griffet F et al (2002) Management of seat-belt syndrome in children. Gravity of 2-point seat-belt. Eur J Pediatr Surg 12:63
Griffith BC, Morey AF et al (2004) Central renal stab wounds: treatment with augmented fibrin sealant in a porcine model. J Urol 171:445
Grossman MD, Miller D et al (2002) When is an elder old? Effect of preexisting conditions on mortality in geriatric trauma. J Trauma 52:242
Gschwend JE, Sauter TW et al (1995) Renal pelvis rupture after blunt abdominal trauma. Urol Int 55:108
Guerriero WG (1989) Ureteral injury. Urol Clin North Am 16:237
Guleria S, Ahmad N et al (1998) Transplant renal artery aneurysm following venous patch repair of a traction injury to the renal artery. Nephrol Dial Transplant 13:1577
Gupta M, Bellman GC et al (1997) Massive hemorrhage from renal vein injury during percutaneous renal surgery: endourological management. J Urol 157:795
Haas CA, Dinchman KH et al (1998a) Traumatic renal artery occlusion: a 15-year review. J Trauma 45:557
Haas CA, Reigle MD et al (1998b) Use of ureteral stents in the management of major renal trauma with urinary extravasation: is there a role? J Endourol 12:545
Haas CA, Spirnak JP (1998c) Traumatic renal artery occlusion: a review of the literature. Tech Urol 4:1
Haas CA, Newman J et al (1999) Computed tomography three-

dimensional reconstruction in the diagnosis of traumatic renal artery thrombosis. Urology 54:559
Hadj-Abdelkader M, Perez N et al (1997) Post-traumatic arterial hypertension. Presse Med 26:1003
Hagiwara A, Sakaki S et al (2001) The role of interventional radiology in the management of blunt renal injury: a practical protocol. J Trauma 51:526
Hammer CC, Santucci RA (2003) Effect of an institutional policy of nonoperative treatment of grades I to IV renal injuries. J Urol 169:1751
Han Kr K, Goldstein DW et al (1998) Angiographic management of pseudoaneurysm and arteriocalyceal fistula following blunt trauma: case report and review of the literature. Can J Urol 5:654
Hani MA, Sallami S et al (2004) Trauma of an ectopic kidney. A case report. Tunis Med 82:69
Hardeman SW, Husmann DA et al (1987) Blunt urinary tract trauma: identifying those patients who require radiological diagnostic studies. J Urol 138:99
Harrington TG, Kandel LB (1997) Renal colic following a gunshot wound to the abdomen: the birdshot calculus. J Urol 157:1351
Harris AC, Zwirewich CV et al (2001) Ct findings in blunt renal trauma. Radiographics 21:S201
Hashmi A, Klassen T (1995) Correlation between urinalysis and intravenous pyelography in pediatric abdominal trauma. J Emerg Med 13:255
Hastings MK, Sinacore DR et al (2005) Bone mineral density during total contact cast immobilization for a patient with neuropathic (Charcot) arthropathy. Phys Ther 85:249
Heinz-Peer G, Helbich T (2001) Urological and nephrological emergency–value of diagnostic imaging. Wien Med Wochenschr 151:560
Hellier WP, Higgs B (1996) Severe renal laceration from blunt trauma presenting with microhaematuria and a normal intravenous urogram. Br J Urol 78:309
Henry PC, Chabannes E et al (2002) Management of severe renal trauma. Prog Urol 12:579
Herschorn S, Radomski SB et al (1991) Evaluation and treatment of blunt renal trauma. J Urol 146:274; discussion 276
Hewin DF, Campbell WB (1998) Ruptured aortic aneurysm: the decision not to operate. Ann R Coll Surg Engl 80:221
Heyns CF, van Vollenhoven P (1992a) Increasing role of angiography and segmental artery embolization in the management of renal stab wounds. J Urol 147:1231
Heyns CF, Van Vollenhoven P (1992b) Selective surgical management of renal stab wounds. Br J Urol 69:351
Hiramoto JS, Meng MV et al (2001) Successful transplantation of a donor kidney after penetrating grade 3 injury and renorrhaphy. J Urol 166:2299
Hochmuth A, Fleck M et al (2000) First experiences in using a new ultrasound mode and ultrasound contrast agent in the diagnosis of blunt renal trauma: a feasibility study in an animal model. Invest Radiol 35:205
Holmes FC, Hunt JJ et al (2003) Renal injury in sport. Curr Sports Med Rep 2:103
Holmes JF, Sokolove PE et al (2002) Identification of children with intra-abdominal injuries after blunt trauma. Ann Emerg Med 39:500
Hotker U, Rommens PM (1996) Postrenal anuria in pelvic or acetabular injury: a report of three cases. J Trauma 41:916
Huang Y, Zhu Z (1997) Massive hydronephrosis associated with traumatic rupture. Injury 28:505
Hudolin T, Hudolin I (2003) Surgical management of urogenital injuries at a war hospital in Bosnia-Hrzegovina, 1992 to 1995. J Urol 169:1357
Huerta-Alardin AL, Varon J et al (2005) Bench-to-bedside review: Rhabdomyolysis – an overview for clinicians. Crit Care 9:158
Hughes CR, Stewart PF Jr et al (1995) Renal cyst rupture following blunt abdominal trauma: case report. J Trauma 38:28
Husmann DA, Morris JS (1990) Attempted nonoperative management of blunt renal lacerations extending through the corticomedullary junction: the short-term and long-term sequelae. J Urol 143:682
Husmann DA, Gilling PJ et al (1993) Major renal lacerations with a devitalized fragment following blunt abdominal trauma: a comparison between nonoperative (expectant) versus surgical management. J Urol 150:1774
Ibanez Pradas V, Serrano Durba A et al (1999) Diagnostic attitude in a patient with kidney trauma. An Esp Pediatr 51:136
Ibarz Servio L, Perendreu Sans J et al (1997) Supraselective embolization of renal pseudoaneurysm caused by an abdominal stab wound. Arch Esp Urol 50:805
Ichigi Y, Takaki N et al (1999) Significance of hematoma size for evaluating the grade of blunt renal trauma. Int J Urol 6:502
Igun GO, Nwadiaro HC et al (2001) Surgical experience with management of vascular injuries. West Afr J Med 20:102
Inenaga T, Takishita TS (2000) Hypertension following renal trauma. Nippon Rinsho 58 [Suppl 2]:483
Inoue S, Koizumi J et al (2004) Self-expanding metallic stent placement for renal artery dissection due to blunt trauma. J Urol 171:347
Inoue S, Sugitani A et al (2005) Effect of synthetic protease inhibitor gabexate mesilate on the attenuation of ischemia/reperfusion injury in canine kidney autotransplantation. Surgery 137:216
Iqbal N, Chughtai MN (2004) Management of blunt renal trauma: a profile of 65 patients. J Pak Med Assoc 54:516
Issa MM, McNamara DE et al (1998) Surgical challenge of massive bilateral staghorn renal calculi in a spinal cord injury patient. Urol Int 61:247
Izumi M, Yokoyama K et al (1997) A young man with acute renal failure and severe loin pain. Nephron 76:215
Jackson MR, Taher MM et al (1998) Hemostatic efficacy of a fibrin sealant dressing in an animal model of kidney injury. J Trauma 45:662
Jan WA, Samad A et al (2004) Mortality and morbidity of abdominal inferior vena-caval injuries. J Coll Physicians Surg Pak 14:622
Jebara VA, El Rassi I et al (1998) Renal artery pseudoaneurysm after blunt abdominal trauma. J Vasc Surg 27:362
Johnson JE, Conlin M (2001) Calculus formation on a retained Acucise wire. Urology 57:168
Johnston WK 3rd, Patel BN et al (2005) Wireless teleradiology for renal colic and renal trauma. J Endourol 19:32
Jones CD, McGahan JP (1999) Computed tomographic evaluation and guided correction of malpositioned nephrostomy catheters. Abdom Imaging 24:422
Jones J, Shah J et al (1999) An unusual renal mass after partial nephrectomy for renal cell carcinoma. J Urol 161:913
Jordan GH, Jezior JR et al (2001) Injury to the genitourinary tract and functional reconstruction of the urethra. Curr Opin Urol 11:257
Kamel IR, Berkowitz JF (1996) Assessment of the cortical rim sign in posttraumatic renal infarction. J Comput Assist Tomogr 20:803
Kansas BT, Eddy MJ et al (2004) Incidence and management of penetrating renal trauma in patients with multiorgan injury: extended experience at an inner city trauma center. J Urol 172:1355
Kao LS, Bulger EM et al (2003) Predictors of morbidity after traumatic pancreatic injury. J Trauma 55:898
Kaplan GW (1994) Major renal trauma in children. Urology 43:131

Karabulut Z, Bostanoglu S et al (2002) Pancreatic injuries: analysis of 20 cases. Ulus Travma Derg 8:237
Karpenko LN, Driuk NF et al (2004) Surgical treatment of injured persons with the main blood vessels damage. Klin Khir:32
Kase H, Nagashima H et al (1995) Clinical analysis of 62 patients with blunt renal trauma. Hinyokika Kiyo 41:855
Kastelan Z, Derezic D et al (2004) Renal autotransplantation in management of bilateral ureteral mortar shell injuries: a case report. Mil Med 169:894
Katz R, Meretyk S et al (1997) Abdominal compartment syndrome due to delayed identification of a ureteral perforation following abdomino-perineal resection for rectal carcinoma. Int J Urol 4:615
Kau E, Patel R et al (2004) Isolated renal vein thrombosis after blunt trauma. Urology 64:807
Kavic SM, Atweh N et al (2002) Renal artery to inferior vena cava fistula following gunshot wound to the abdomen. Ann Vasc Surg 16:666
Kawashima A, Sandler CM et al (1997) Ureteropelvic junction injuries secondary to blunt abdominal trauma. Radiology 205:487
Kawashima A, Sandler CM et al (2001) Imaging of renal trauma: a comprehensive review. Radiographics 21:557
Kawashima A, Sandler CM et al (2002) Imaging evaluation of posttraumatic renal injuries. Abdom Imaging 27:199
Keller MS, Eric Coln C et al (2004) Functional outcome of nonoperatively managed renal injuries in children. J Trauma 57:108; discussion 110
Kern EO, Newman LN et al (2002) Abdominal catastrophe revisited: the risk and outcome of enteric peritoneal contamination. Perit Dial Int 22:323
Khan AB, Reid AW (1994) Management of renal stab wounds by arteriographic embolisation. Scand J Urol Nephrol 28:109
Khriakov AS, Esetov AK et al (2005) Perforating shotgun wound of the abdomen with injuries multiple visceral. Khirurgiia (Mosk) 1:65
Kiberd B, Panek R et al (1999) The morbidity of prolonged wound drainage after kidney transplantation. J Urol 161: 1467
Kirton OC, Jacobs JP et al (1994) Incidental finding of occult hydronephrosis after blunt abdominal trauma. Eur J Emerg Med 1:139
Klaric Custovic R, Krolo I et al (2004) Retained surgical textilomas occur more often during war. Croat Med J 45:422
Klein AJ, Kozar RA et al (1999) Traumatic hematuria in patients with polycystic kidney disease. Am Surg 65:464
Klochkov ND, Sidorin VS (1998) Pathology of traumatic disease in wounded people. Arkh Patol 60:43
Kluger Y, Makarin V et al (1999) Absorbable mesh wrapping of injured kidney: a renal salvage technique. Harefuah 136:647
Knight CG, Omert L (2004) Chylous ascites after nephrectomy for trauma. Am Surg 70:1083
Knudson MM, McAninch JW et al (1992) Hematuria as a predictor of abdominal injury after blunt trauma. Am J Surg 164:482; discussion 485
Knudson MM, Maull KI (1999) Nonoperative management of solid organ injuries. Past, present, and future. Surg Clin North Am 79:1357
Knudson MM, Harrison PB et al (2000) Outcome after major renovascular injuries: a Western trauma association multicenter report. J Trauma 49:1116
Kos X, Fanchamps JM et al (1999) Radiologic damage control: evaluation of a combined CT and angiography suite with a pivoting table. Cardiovasc Intervent Radiol 22:124
Kovacevic Z, Skataric V et al (1999) Complications of percutaneous transluminal renal angioplasty–case report. Vojnosanit Pregl 56:431
Kracun MD, Wooten CL (1998) Crush injuries: a case of entrapment. Crit Care Nurs Q 21:81
Kramer SC, Gorich J et al (1998) The percutaneous transarterial embolization therapy of traumatic kidney hemorrhages. ROFO 169:297
Krid M, Bahloul A et al (1997) Kidney injuries in children. Apropos of 65 cases. Ann Urol 31:259
Krieger JN, Algood CB et al (1984) Urological trauma in the Pacific Northwest: etiology, distribution, management and outcome. J Urol 132:70
Kristjansson A, Pedersen J (1993) Management of blunt renal trauma. Br J Urol 72:692
Ku JH, Jeon YS et al (2001) Is there a role for magnetic resonance imaging in renal trauma? Int J Urol 8:261
Kumar M, Aron M et al (1999) Stenturia: An unusual manifestation of spontaneous ureteral stent fragmentation. Urol Int 62:114
Kuo YT, Wang CK et al (1999) Imaging features of simultaneous occurrence of renal and pancreatic foreign body granuloma due to chronically retained gauze: a case report. Kaohsiung J Med Sci 15:104
Kuo RL, Eachempati SR et al (2002) Factors affecting management and outcome in blunt renal injury. World J Surg 26:416
Kuvezdic H, Tucak A et al (1996) War injuries of the kidney. Injury 27:557
Lambert AW, Nathan M et al (2001) A case of fatal tumor embolus following trauma in a patient with undiagnosed Wilms' tumor. Pediatr Emerg Care 17:356
Langer JE (2001) Computed tomography and ultrasonography of acute renal abnormalities. Semin Roentgenol 36:99
Lanoix R, Leak LV et al (2000) A preliminary evaluation of emergency ultrasound in the setting of an emergency medicine training program. Am J Emerg Med 18:41
Lawrentschuk N, Bolton DM (2005) Occult renal segmental arterial injury after trauma. Urology 65:386
Lazarides MK, Tsoupanos SS et al (1998) Incidence and patterns of iatrogenic arterial injuries. A decade's experience. J Cardiovasc Surg (Torino) 39:281
Lebech A, HH Strange-Vognsen (1990) Hypertension following blunt kidney injury. Ugeskr Laeger 152:994
Lee JT, White RA (2002) Endovascular management of blunt traumatic renal artery dissection. J Endovasc Ther 9:354
Lee S, Thavaseelan J et al (2004) Renal trauma in Australian rules football: an institutional experience. Aust N Z J Surg 74:766
Legg EA, Herbert FB et al (1998) Super-selective arterial embolization for blunt trauma in the horseshoe kidney. Urology 51:320
Lemaitre L, Gaillandre L et al (1996) Spiral scanners: the key to imaging of kidney injuries. Chirurgie 121:355
Lent V (1995) What treatment in kidney trauma? A critical evaluation treatment reports up to now based on a new classification. Chirurg 66:708
Lent V (1996) What classification is appropriate in renal trauma? Eur Urol 30:327
Leppaniemi A, Lamminen A et al (1995) Comparison of high-field magnetic resonance imaging with computed tomography in the evaluation of blunt renal trauma. J Trauma 38:420
Leppaniemi A, Lamminen A et al (1997) MRI and CT in blunt renal trauma: an update. Semin Ultrasound CT MR 18:129
Leppaniemi AK, Kivisaari AO et al (1991) Role of magnetic resonance imaging in blunt renal parenchymal trauma. Br J Urol 68:355
Levy JB, Baskin LS et al (1993) Nonoperative management of blunt pediatric major renal trauma. Urology 42:418
Lewis S, Patel U (2004) Major complications after percutaneous nephrostomy-lessons from a department audit. Clin Radiol 59:171
Lim JH, Kim B et al (1998) Anatomical communications of the

perirenal space. Br J Radiol 71:450
Lojanapiwat B, Sripralakit S et al (1999) Ureteric obstruction by shotgun pellet pellet colic. J Med Assoc Thai 82:1048
Long JA, Descotes JL et al (2004) Endovascular aortic balloon catheter occlusion for severe renal trauma. Prog Urol 14:394; discussion 397
Lont AP, Lamme B et al (2005) The aortocaval fistula, a rare complication of an aneurysm of the abdominal aorta. Ned Tijdschr Geneeskd 149:325
Lopez Cubillana P, Rigabert Montiel M, Nicolas Torralba JA, Banon Perez V, Valdelvira Nadal P, Prieto Gonzalez A, Server Pastor G, Gomez Gomez G, Aguayo Albasino JA, Perez Albacete YM (1998) Ultrasonography and intravenous urography in the diagnosis of blunt renal trauma. Arch Esp Urol 51:669
Lorelli DR, Kralovich KA et al (2001) The impact of pre-existing end-stage renal disease on survival in acutely injured trauma patients. Am Surg 67:693
Lozen Y (1999) Intraabdominal hypertension and abdominal compartment syndrome in trauma: pathophysiology and interventions. AACN Clin Issues 10:104; quiz 135
Lu CY, Penfield JG et al (1999) Hypothesis: is renal allograft rejection initiated by the response to injury sustained during the transplant process? Kidney Int 55:2157
Luks FI, Lemire A et al (1993) Blunt abdominal trauma in children: the practical value of ultrasonography. J Trauma 34:607; discussion 610
Luther B, Sandmann W et al (1997) Aortic aneurysm in horseshoe kidney–special diagnosis and therapy. Chirurg 68:403
Machida T, Hanazaki K et al (1999) Snowboarding injuries of the abdomen: comparison with skiing injuries. Injury 30:47
Madhavan P, Sproule J et al (1999) Aorta–left renal vein fistula: an unusual complication of an abdominal aortic aneurysm. Eur J Vasc Endovasc Surg 17:87
Madiba TE, Haffejee AA et al (2002) Renal trauma secondary to stab, blunt and firearm injuries–a 5-year study. S Afr J Surg 40:5; discussion 9
Mali V, Liu B et al (2005) Blunt renal trauma in occult congenital hydronephrosis. Singapore Med J 46:28
Mansi MK, Alkhudair WK (1997) Conservative management with percutaneous intervention of major blunt renal injuries. Am J Emerg Med 15:633
Marcos HB, Noone TC et al (1998) MRI evaluation of acute renal trauma. J Magn Reson Imaging 8:989
Margenthaler JA, Weber TR et al (2002) Blunt renal trauma in children: experience with conservative management at a pediatric trauma center. J Trauma 52:928
Marzocco S, Di Paola R et al (2005) The cyclopentenone prostaglandin 15-deoxyDelta(12,14)-prostaglandin J(2) attenuates the development of zymosan-induced shock. Intensive Care Med 31:693
Master VA, Franks J et al (2002) Grade V renal injury: avulsion of the renal pedicle. J Am Coll Surg 195:425
Mateo E, Marin JP et al (1999) Perioperative morbidity and mortality in surgery for dissecting aneurysm of the ascending aorta. Rev Esp Anestesiol Reanim 46:333
Mathews R, Marshall FF (1997) Versatility of the adult psoas hitch ureteral reimplantation. J Urol 158:2078
Matsuura T, Nose K et al (2002) Evaluation of the management of blunt renal trauma and indication for surgery. Nippon Hinyokika Gakkai Zasshi 93:511
Matthews LA, JP Spirnak (1995) The nonoperative approach to major blunt renal trauma. Semin Urol 13:77
Matthews LA, Smith EM et al (1997) Nonoperative treatment of major blunt renal lacerations with urinary extravasation. J Urol 157:2056
Mattila A, S Lundstedt et al (1999) Ureteropelvic rupture caused by a fall. Duodecim 115:1850
Maudgil DD, McHugh K (2002) The role of computed tomography in modern paediatric uroradiology. Eur J Radiol 43:129
May M, Gunia S et al (2004) An unusual complication of extracorporeal shock wave lithotripsy: rupture of the kidney with consecutive nephrectomy. Aktuelle Urol 35:316
Mayor B, Gudinchet F et al (1995) Imaging evaluation of blunt renal trauma in children: diagnostic accuracy of intravenous pyelography and ultrasonography. Pediatr Radiol 25:214
McAndrew JD, Corriere JN Jr (1994) Radiographic evaluation of renal trauma: evaluation of 1103 consecutive patients. Br J Urol 73:352
McAninch JW, Carroll PR et al (1993) Renal gunshot wounds: methods of salvage and reconstruction. J Trauma 35:279; discussion 283
McAninch JW, Dixon CM et al (1990) The surgical treatment of renal trauma. Vestn Khir Im II Grek 145:64
McAninch JW, Carroll PR et al (1991) Renal reconstruction after injury. J Urol 145:932
McGahan JP, Richards JR et al (1999) Use of ultrasonography in the patient with acute renal trauma. J Ultrasound Med 18:207; quiz 215
Medica J, Caldamone A (1995) Pediatric renal trauma: special considerations. Semin Urol 13:73
Mee SL, McAninch JW (1989) Indications for radiographic assessment in suspected renal trauma. Urol Clin North Am 16:187
Mee SL, McAninch JW et al (1989) Radiographic assessment of renal trauma: a 10-year prospective study of patient selection. J Urol 141:1095
Mejean A, Vogt B et al (1999) Mortality and morbidity after nephrectomy for renal cell carcinoma using a transperitoneal anterior subcostal incision. Eur Urol 36:298
Meldrum DR, Moore FA et al (1997) Prospective characterization and selective management of the abdominal compartment syndrome. Am J Surg 174:667; discussion 672
Mendez Gallart R, Gomez Tellado M et al (1996) Blunt abdominal trauma. Nonoperative management. Cir Pediatr 9:60
Meng MV, Brandes SB et al (1999) Renal trauma: indications and techniques for surgical exploration. World J Urol 17:71
Meria P, Mazeman E (2000) Immediate and delayed management of renal trauma. Eur Urol 37:121
Merrot T, Portier F et al (2000) Trauma of the renal pedicle in children. Report of 2 cases of late revascularization with endovascular prosthesis. Prog Urol 10:277
Meyer DM, Thal ER et al (1989) The role of abdominal CT in the evaluation of stab wounds to the back. J Trauma 29:1226; discussion 1228
Mhiri MN, Trifa M et al (1997) Kidney contusions and traffic accidents. Apropos of the Tunisian experience. Ann Urol (Paris) 31:243
Michel LA, Lacrosse M et al (1996) Blunt renal traumas: contribution of spiral CT with three dimensional reconstruction to the surgical decision process? Int Surg 81:377
Milas ZL, Dodson TF et al (2004) Pediatric blunt trauma resulting in major arterial injuries. Am Surg 70:443
Miller DC, Forauer A et al (2002) Successful angioembolization of renal artery pseudoaneurysms after blunt abdominal trauma. Urology 59:444
Miller KS, McAninch JW (1995) Radiographic assessment of renal trauma: our 15-year experience. J Urol 154:352
Milzman DP, Boulanger BR et al (1992) Pre-existing disease in trauma patients: a predictor of fate independent of age and injury severity score. J Trauma 32:236; discussion 243
Mirvis SE (1996) Trauma. Radiol Clin North Am 34:1225
Mizobata Y, Yokota J et al (2001) Successful evaluation of pseudoaneurysm formation after blunt renal injury with dual-phase contrast-enhanced helical CT. AJR Am J Roentgenol 177:136
Mizzi A, Shabani A et al (2002) The role of follow-up imaging

in paediatric blunt abdominal trauma. Clin Radiol 57:908
Mohammad Naghi T, Kambiz K et al (2005) Musculoskeletal injuries associated with earthquake. A report of injuries of Iran's December 26, 2003 Bam earthquake casualties managed in tertiary referral centers. Injury 36:27
Moiseienko VO, Krasiuk (IV 2001) Potential of current physical investigative methods in the diagnosis of injuries to organs of the abdominal cavity. Lik Sprava:189
Moller CM, Mommsen S et al (1995) The role of haematuria in the diagnosis of blunt renal trauma. Scand J Urol Nephrol Suppl 172:99
Monserrat Monfort JJ, Oliver Amoros F et al (1996) Renal traumatism: diagnostic protocol and therapeutic indications. Actas Urol Esp 20:534
Monstrey SJ, Beerthuizen GI et al (1989) Renal trauma and hypertension. J Trauma 29:65
Montgomery RC, JD Richardson et al (1998) Posttraumatic renovascular hypertension after occult renal injury. J Trauma 45:106
Montravers P, Villamizar J et al (2001) Superinfection of posttraumatic retroperitoneal hematoma secondary to ascending urinary tract infection. J Trauma 50:931
Moore EE, Shackford SR, Pachter HL et al (1989) Organ injury scaling: spleen, liver, and kidney. J Trauma 29:1664
Morey AF, Bruce JE et al (1996) Efficacy of radiographic imaging in pediatric blunt renal trauma. J Urol 156:2014
Morey AF, McAninch JW et al (1999) Single shot intraoperative excretory urography for the immediate evaluation of renal trauma. J Urol 161:1088
Morey AF, Anema JG et al (2001) Treatment of grade 4 renal stab wounds with absorbable fibrin adhesive bandage in a porcine model. J Urol 165:955
Moriarty KP, Lipkowitz GS e t al (1997) Capsulectomy: a cure for the page kidney. J Pediatr Surg 32:831
Morris CS, Bonnevie GJ et al (2001) Nonsurgical treatment of acute iatrogenic renal artery injuries occurring after renal artery angioplasty and stenting. AJR Am J Roentgenol 177:1353
Morse TS (1975) Renal injuries. Pediatr Clin North Am 22:379
Moudouni SM, Hadj Slimen M et al (2001a) Management of major blunt renal lacerations: is a nonoperative approach indicated? Eur Urol 40:409
Moudouni SM, Patard JJ et al (2001b) A conservative approach to major blunt renal lacerations with urinary extravasation and devitalized renal segments. BJU Int 87:290
Mulligan JM, Cagiannos I et al (1998) Ureteropelvic junction disruption secondary to blunt trauma: excretory phase imaging (delayed films) should help prevent a missed diagnosis. J Urol 159:67
Munk M, Hofmockel G et al (1997) Conservative therapy of blunt kidney injuries. Urologe A 36:531
Munoz D, Gutierrez C et al (1998) Traumatic renal artery thrombosis. Scand J Urol Nephrol 32:296
Murphy JT, Borman KR et al (1996) Renal autotransplantation after horseshoe kidney injury: a case report and literature review. J Trauma 40:840
Mutabagani KH, Coley BD et al (1999) Preliminary experience with focused abdominal sonography for trauma (FAST) in children: is it useful? J Pediatr Surg 34:48; discussion 52
Nadvi SS, Mokoena T et al (1996) Prognosis in posttraumatic acute renal failure is adversely influenced by hypotension and hyperkalaemia. Eur J Surg 162:121
Nagel E, Jahne J et al (1997) Aspects relevant for abdominal surgery of attempted suicide. Langenbecks Arch Chir 382:29
Nagy KK, Brenneman FD et al (1997) Routine preoperative one-shot intravenous pyelography is not indicated in all patients with penetrating abdominal trauma. J Am Coll Surg 185:530
Nance ML, Lutz N et al (2004) Blunt renal injuries in children can be managed nonoperatively: outcome in a consecutive series of patients. J Trauma 57:474; discussion 478
Napal Lecumberri S, Pascual Piedrola I et al (1992) Kidney injuries: a review of 149 cases. A change in the diagnostic and therapeutic approaches. Arch Esp Urol 45:305
Nash PA, Bruce JE et al (1995) Nephrectomy for traumatic renal injuries. J Urol 153:609
Navarrete-Navarro P, Rodriguez A et al (2001) Adult respiratory distress syndrome among blunt and penetrating trauma patients: demographics, mortality, and resource utilization over 8 years. J Crit Care 16:47
Navascues del Rio JA, Arrojo Vila F et al (1997) Results of the conservative treatment of severe renal trauma in childhood. Actas Urol Esp 21:747
Nguyen HT, PR Carroll (1995) Blunt renal trauma: renal preservation through careful staging and selective surgery. Semin Urol 13:83
Nguyen MM, Das S (2002) Pediatric renal trauma. Urology 59:762; discussion 766
Nicol AJ, Theunissen D (2002) Renal salvage in penetrating kidney injuries: a prospective analysis. J Trauma 53:351
Nicolaisen GS, McAninch JW et al (1985) Renal trauma: reevaluation of the indications for radiographic assessment. J Urol 133:183
Nijs E, Callahan MJ et al (2005) Disorders of the pediatric pancreas: imaging features. Pediatr Radiol 35:358
Ninomiya H, Kido M et al (1997) A surgical case of intrapericardial inferior vena cava injury complicating liver injury caused by a blunt trauma. Nippon Kyobu Geka Gakkai Zasshi 45:1616
Nisbeth U, Lindh E et al (1999) Increased fracture rate in diabetes mellitus and females after renal transplantation. Transplantation 67:1218
Nishikura T (1999) The clearance of procalcitonin (PCT) during continuous veno-venous hemodiafiltration (CVVHD) Intensive Care Med 25:1198
Noe HN (1996) Imaging in pediatric blunt renal trauma. J Urol 156:2019
Nomura G (1996) Hypertension following renal trauma. Ryoikibetsu Shokogun Shirizu 12:83
Noor MA, Ather MH (2003) Difference in the outcome of patients managed with isolated renal injury and co-existent abdominal organ injury. J Ayub Med Coll Abbottabad 15:29
Novak I (1996) Kidney injuries in childhood. Rozhl Chir 75:599
Novelline RA, Rhea JT et al (1999) Helical CT of abdominal trauma. Radiol Clin North Am 37:591:vi-vii
Novozhilova AP, Kuleshov VI et al (1999) Structural changes in the parenchymatous organs in animals in venous gas embolism of varying intensity and acute decompression disease. Morfologiia 115:41
Nunez D Jr, Becerra JL et al (1996) Traumatic occlusion of the renal artery: helical CT diagnosis. AJR Am J Roentgenol 167:777
Nunez D Jr, Rivas L et al (1998) Helical CT of traumatic arterial injuries. AJR Am J Roentgenol 170:1621
Nussbaum Blask AR, Nicholson HS et al (1999) Sonographic detection of uterine and ovarian abnormalities in female survivors of Wilms' tumor treated with radiotherapy. AJR Am J Roentgenol 172:759
Nygaard IE, Kreder KJ (1996) Spine update. Urological management in patients with spinal cord injuries. Spine 21:128
Obara W, Ohuchi A et al (2001) A case of congenital hydronephrosis suffering from rupture of the renal pelvis due to trauma. Hinyokika Kiyo 47:425
Oderich GS, Panneton JM et al (2004) Iatrogenic operative injuries of abdominal and pelvic veins: a potentially lethal complication. J Vasc Surg 39:931
Oelschlager BK, Boyle EM Jr et al (1997) Delayed abdominal

closure in the management of ruptured abdominal aortic aneurysms. Am J Surg 173:411
Ohashi H, Oda H et al (1999) Predictors of survival in continuous ambulatory peritoneal dialysis patients: the importance of left ventricular hypertrophy and diabetic nephropathy. Adv Perit Dial 15:87
Okita Y, Ando M et al (1999) Early and long-term results of surgery for aneurysms of the thoracic aorta in septuagenarians and octogenarians. Eur J Cardiothorac Surg 16:317
Oldhafer KJ, Frerker M et al (1999) Complex inferior vena cava and renal vein reconstruction after abdominal gunshot injury. J Trauma 46:721
Olofsen-van Acht MJ, Quint S et al (1999) Three-dimensional treatment planning for postoperative radiotherapy in patients with node-positive cervical cancer. Comparison between a conventional and a conformal technique. Strahlenther Onkol 175:462
O'Neill PJ, Feldman DR et al (1996) Trans-jugular extraction of bullet embolus to the heart. Mil Med 161:360
Onen A, Kaya M et al (2002) Blunt renal trauma in children with previously undiagnosed pre-existing renal lesions and guidelines for effective initial management of kidney injury. BJU Int 89:936
Ortega AE, Tang E et al (1996) Laparoscopic evaluation of penetrating thoracoabdominal traumatic injuries. Surg Endosc 10:19
Otte A, Herrmann R et al (1999) Yttrium 90 DOTATOC: a new somatostatin analog for cancer therapy of neuroendocrine tumors. Schweiz Rundsch Med Prax 88:1263
Ozdemir S, Cekirge S et al (1998) A rare complication of renal biopsy in a child with membranoproliferative glomerulonephritis. Int Urol Nephrol 30:689
Ozturk H, Otcu S et al (2003) Retroperitoneal organ injury caused by anterior penetrating abdominal injury in children. Eur J Emerg Med 10:164
Ozturk H, Dokucu AI et al (2004) Non-operative management of isolated solid organ injuries due to blunt abdominal trauma in children: a fifteen-year experience. Eur J Pediatr Surg 14:29
Ozucelik DN, Karcioglu O (1999) Kidney rupture following extracorporeal shock wave lithotripsy. Acad Emerg Med 6:664
Pagano S, Pachera F et al (1999) Complete pyelo-calyceal avulsion as a result of blunt abdominal trauma. Scand J Urol Nephrol 33:66
Park JK, Yang SO et al (2001) Duodenal obstruction by retroperitoneal hematoma induced by severe blunt renal trauma. J Urol 165:1993
Parker CR, Freemont AJ et al (1999) Cross-sectional analysis of renal transplantation osteoporosis. J Bone Miner Res 14:1943
Partrick DA, Bensard DD et al (1999) Nonoperative management of solid organ injuries in children results in decreased blood utilization. J Pediatr Surg 34:1695
Parvathy U, Saldanha R et al (2003) Blunt abdominal trauma resulting in urinothorax from a missed uretero-pelvic junction avulsion: case report. J Trauma 54:187
Pascual Samaniego M, Fernandez Dominguez L et al (2003) Traumatic intrathoracic herniation of the left kidney. Actas Urol Esp 27:229
Patel HP, Bissler JJ (2001) Hematuria in children. Pediatr Clin North Am 48:1519
Patel R, Caruso RP et al (2003) Use of fibrin glue and gelfoam to repair collecting system injuries in a porcine model: implications for the technique of laparoscopic partial nephrectomy. J Endourol 17:799
Patel VG, Walker ML (1997) The role of one-shot intravenous pyelogram in evaluation of penetrating abdominal trauma. Am Surg 63:350
Paul LC (1999) Chronic allograft nephropathy: An update. Kidney Int 56:783
Peacock PR Jr, Souto HL et al (2001) What is gross hematuria? Correlation of subjective and objective assessment. J Trauma 50:1060
Peclet MH, Newman KD et al (1990) Thoracic trauma in children: an indicator of increased mortality. J Pediatr Surg 25:961; discussion 965
Perdue PW, Watts DD et al (1998) Differences in mortality between elderly and younger adult trauma patients: geriatric status increases risk of delayed death. J Trauma 45:805
Perez-Brayfield MR, Gatti JM et al (2002) Blunt traumatic hematuria in children. Is a simplified algorithm justified? J Urol 167:2543; discussion 2546
Perini S, Gordon RL et al (1998) Transcatheter embolization of biopsy-related vascular injury in the transplant kidney: immediate and long-term outcome. J Vasc Interv Radiol 9:1011
Perouansky M, Oppenheim A et al (1999) Effect of haemofiltration on pathological fibrinolysis due to severe sepsis: a case report. Resuscitation 40:53
Perry MJ, Porte ME et al (1997) Limitations of ultrasound evaluation in acute closed renal trauma. J R Coll Surg Edinb 42:420
Pershad J, Gilmore B (2000) Serial bedside emergency ultrasound in a case of pediatric blunt abdominal trauma with severe abdominal pain. Pediatr Emerg Care 16:375
Peterson NE (1991) Re: attempted nonoperative management of blunt renal lacerations extending through the corticomedullary junction: the short-term and long-term sequelae. J Urol 145:154
Peterson NE, Moore EE (1997) Bilateral renal artery thrombosis secondary to blunt trauma. J Trauma 43:561
Petridis A, Pilavaki M et al (1999) CT of hemodynamically unstable abdominal trauma. Eur Radiol 9:250
Phadke RV, Sawlani V et al (1997) Iatrogenic renal vascular injuries and their radiological management. Clin Radiol 52:119
Philpott JM, Nance ML et al (2003) Ureteral stenting in the management of urinoma after severe blunt renal trauma in children. J Pediatr Surg 38:1096
Pickenpack A, Lang B et al (1999) A 63-year-old patient with worsening general condition, bone demineralization, hypocalcemia and excess parathyroid hormone: late manifestations of pseudohypohyperparathyroidism. Dtsch Med Wochenschr 124:551
Pickhardt PJ, Shimony JS et al (1999) The abdominal compartment syndrome: CT findings. AJR Am J Roentgenol 173:575
Pietrera P, Badachi Y et al (2001) Ultrasound for initial evaluation of post-traumatic renal lesions in children. J Radiol 82:833
Pigolkin Iu I, Denisova OP et al (1997) The forensic medical diagnosis of kidney trauma. Sud Med Ekspert 40:6
Pittrow L, Penk A (1999) Special pharmacokinetics of fluconazole in septic, obese and burn patients. Mycoses 42 [Suppl 2]:87
Pollack HM, Wein AJ (1989) Imaging of renal trauma. Radiology 172:297
Porodenko VA (1999) Specific features of kidney injuries altered by disease. Sud Med Ekspert 42:18
Porter JM, Singh Y (1998) Value of computed tomography in the evaluation of retroperitoneal organ injury in blunt abdominal trauma. Am J Emerg Med 16:225
Powell MA, Nicholas JM et al (1999) Blunt ureteropelvic junction disruption. J Trauma 47:186
Prieto Chaparro L, Silmi Moyano A et al (1992) Renal injury on a pathological kidney. Incidence, management, and results of treatment. Arch Esp Urol 45:407
Pruthi RS, Issa MM et al (1998) Renal masses presenting 25 and 50 years following blunt renal trauma. Urol Int 61:43
Purdie KJ, Pennington J et al (1999) The promoter of a novel

human papillomavirus (HPV77) associated with skin cancer displays UV responsiveness, which is mediated through a consensus p53 binding sequence. EMBO J 18:5359
Qin R, Shao G et al (1996) The diagnosis and treatment of blunt renal trauma. Zhonghua Wai Ke Za Zhi 34:505
Qin R, Wang P et al (2002) Diagnosis and treatment of renal trauma in 298 patients. Chin J Traumatol 5:21
Quinlan DM, Gearhart JP (1990) Blunt renal trauma in childhood. Features indicating severe injury. Br J Urol 66:526
Quinones-Baldrich WJ, Panetta TF et al (1999) Repair of type IV thoracoabdominal aneurysm with a combined endovascular and surgical approach. J Vasc Surg 30:555
Rabii R, Joual A et al (2000) Stab wound to the left solitary kidney: report of a case. Ann Urol (Paris) 34:232
Rabinovici R, Ovadia P et al (1999) Abdominal injuries associated with lumbar spine fractures in blunt trauma. Injury 30:471
Radmayr C, Oswald J et al (2002) Blunt renal trauma in children:26 years clinical experience in an alpine region. Eur Urol 42:297
Radovic M, Ostric V et al (1996) Validity of prediction scores in acute renal failure due to polytrauma. Ren Fail 18:615
Rafique M, MH Arif (2002) Management of iatrogenic ureteric injuries associated with gynecological surgery. Int Urol Nephrol 34:31
Rathaus V, Pomeranz A et al (2004) Isolated severe renal injuries after minimal blunt trauma to the upper abdomen and flank: CT findings. Emerg Radiol 10:190
Rebassa Llull MJ, Munoz Velez D et al (2000) Foreign body as renal pseudotumor in a patient with renal polycystic kidney. Arch Esp Urol 53:831
Regel G, Grotz M et al (1996) Pattern of organ failure following severe trauma. World J Surg 20:422
Reilly KJ, Shapiro MB et al (1996) Angiographic embolization of a penetrating traumatic renal arteriovenous fistula. J Trauma 41:763
Rengo M, Bianchi G et al (1997) Renal injury in childhood. G Chir 18:359
Ricard J, Richard L et al (1994) Lesions of the renal pedicle in blunt abdominal trauma in children. 7 cases. Prog Urol 4:76
Richter ER, Shriver CD (2001) Delayed nephrectomy in grade V renal injury with two interesting anatomic variations. Urology 58:607
Rios Gonzalez E, Ramon de Fata Chillon F et al (2002) Iatrogenic injury of the lumbar ureter and iliac vessels after lumbar discectomy: urologic treatment using kidney autotransplantation. Actas Urol Esp 26:504
Robert M, Drianno N et al (1996) Management of major blunt renal lacerations: surgical or nonoperative approach? Eur Urol 30:335
Robles JE, Rosell D (1996) Experimental applications of shock waves. Rev Med Univ Navarra 40:25
Rodriguez Alonso A, Suarez Pascual G e t al (2004) Iatrogenic rupture of the ureter following extracorporeal shock wave lithotripsy. Actas Urol Esp 28:530
Rogers CG, Knight V et al (2004) High-grade renal injuries in children–is conservative management possible? Urology 64:574
Rogers CJ, Barber DB et al (1996) Spontaneous bladder perforation in paraplegia as a late complication of augmentation enterocystoplasty: case report. Arch Phys Med Rehabil 77:1198
Rommens PM, Lacroix H et al (1996) Three vascular lesions in one patient. Injury 27:509
Rosales A, Arango O et al (1992) The use of ultrasonography as the initial diagnostic exploration in blunt renal trauma. Urol Int 48:134
Rosen MA, McAninch JW (1994) Management of combined renal and pancreatic trauma. J Urol 152:22
Rowland JL, Kuhn M et al (2001) Accuracy of emergency department bedside ultrasonography. Emerg Med (Fremantle) 13:305
Roy C, Tuchmann C et al (2000) Helical CT of urinary tract: clinical applications. J Radiol 81 [9 Suppl]:1071
Roy C, Tuchmann C et al (2001) Post-traumatic rupture in ureteropelvic junction obstruction syndrome: two case reports. J Radiol 82:171
Rubulotta S, Garagozzo G et al (1997) Thrombosis of the renal artery of traumatic origin. Minerva Chir 52:309
Russell RS, Gomelsky A et al (2001) Management of grade IV renal injury in children. J Urol 166:1049
Rutsky EA, Dubovsky EV et al (1991) Long-term follow-up of a human subject with a remnant kidney. Am J Kidney Dis 18: 509
Sacco WJ, Copes WS et al (1993) Effect of preinjury illness on trauma patient survival outcome. J Trauma 35:538; discussion 542
Saengsirisuwan V, Phadungkij S et al (1998) Renal and liver functions and muscle injuries during training and after competition in Thai boxers. Br J Sports Med 32:304
Safir MH, McAninch JW (1999) Diagnosis and management of trauma to the kidney. Curr Opin Urol 9:227
Sagalowsky AI, McConnell JD et al (1983) Renal trauma requiring surgery: an analysis of 185 cases. J Trauma 23:128
Sahin H, Akay AF et al (2004) Retrospective analysis of 135 renal trauma cases. Int J Urol 11:332
Saidi A, Bocqueraz F et al (2003) Early revascularization by stent in renal pedicle trauma. Prog Urol 13:123
Saidi A, Bocqueraz F et al (2004) Blunt kidney trauma: a ten-year experience. Prog Urol 14:1125
Saika T, Manabe D et al (1998) Clinical studies on renal trauma. Hinyokika Kiyo 44:697
Sairanen J, Isotalo T et al (2001) Treatment of a renal artery stab wound with selective embolization. Duodecim 117:959
Sakai Y (1999) A case of idiopathic retroperitoneal fibrosis with renal subcapsular urinoma resolved by steroid therapy. Hinyokika Kiyo 45:249
Salzano A, De Rosa A et al (1999) Gunshot wounds of the abdomen studied by computed tomography. The authors' personal experience in 30 cases. Radiol Med (Torino) 98:168
Sandler CM, Amis ES Jr et al (2000) Diagnostic approach to renal trauma. American College of Radiology. ACR Appropriateness Criteria. Radiology 215 [Suppl]:727
Santiago L, Bellman GC et al (1998) Small bowel and splenic injury during percutaneous renal surgery. J Urol 159:2071; discussion 2072
Santucci RA, Langenburg SE et al (2004) Traumatic hematuria in children can be evaluated as in adults. J Urol 171:822
Santucci RA, McAninch JM (2001) Grade IV renal injuries: evaluation, treatment, and outcome. World J Surg 25:1565
Santucci RA, McAninch JW (2000) Diagnosis and management of renal trauma: past, present, and future. J Am Coll Surg 191:443
Santucci RA, McAninch JW et al (2001) Validation of the American Association for the Surgery of Trauma organ injury severity scale for the kidney. J Trauma 50:195
Santucci RA, Wessells H et al (2004) Evaluation and management of renal injuries: consensus statement of the renal trauma subcommittee. BJU Int 93:937
Sarkisian AE, Khondkarian RA et al (1991) Sonographic screening of mass casualties for abdominal and renal injuries following the 1988 Armenian earthquake. J Trauma 31:247
Sartorelli KH, Frumiento C et al (2000) Nonoperative management of hepatic, splenic, and renal injuries in adults with multiple injuries. J Trauma 49:56; discussion 61
Sato M, Yoshii H (2004) Reevaluation of ultrasonography for solid-organ injury in blunt abdominal trauma. J Ultrasound Med 23:1583

Saunders F, Argall J (2002) Investigating microscopic haematuria in blunt abdominal trauma. Emerg Med J 19:322
Savage C, Reabe S et al (2003) Imaging of bilateral ureteropelvic junction laceration from blunt trauma. Emerg Radiol 10:99
Sawczuk I (1996) Renal cell carcinoma–local recurrence/splenic injury. J Urol 155:37
Sayers RD, Thompson MM et al (1997) Surgical management of 671 abdominal aortic aneurysms: a 13 year review from a single centre. Eur J Vasc Endovasc Surg 13:322
Schmidlin FR, Schmid P et al (1996) Force transmission and stress distribution in a computer-simulated model of the kidney: an analysis of the injury mechanisms in renal trauma. J Trauma 40:791
Schmidlin FR, Rohner S et al (1997) The conservative treatment of major kidney injuries. Ann Urol (Paris) 31:246
Schmidlin F, Farshad M et al (1998a) Biomechanical analysis and clinical treatment of blunt renal trauma. Swiss Surg:237
Schmidlin FR, Iselin CE et al (1998b) The higher injury risk of abnormal kidneys in blunt renal trauma. Scand J Urol Nephrol 32:388
Schmiedl UP, Carter S et al (1999) Sonographic detection of acute parenchymal injury in an experimental porcine model of renal hemorrhage: gray-scale imaging using a sonographic contrast agent. AJR Am J Roentgenol 173:1289
Schnarkowski P, Brecht-Krauss D et al (1992) Abdominal sonography in primary diagnosis of blunt abdominal trauma. Ultraschall Med 13:102
Schreyer HH, Uggowitzer MM et al (2002) Helical CT of the urinary organs. Eur Radiol 12:575
Schroeder PL, Francisco LL (1990) Evaluating hematuria in children. Where to start and how to proceed. Postgrad Med 88:171
Sebastia MC, Rodriguez-Dobao M et al (1999) Renal trauma in occult ureteropelvic junction obstruction: CT findings. Eur Radiol 9:611
Sekiguchi Y, Miyai K et al (1998) Nonoperative management of major blunt renal lacerations with urinary extravasation: report of two cases. Hinyokika Kiyo 44:875
Senado-Lara I, Castro-Mendoza A et al (2004) Experience in management of trauma-related acute abdomen at the General Ignacio Zaragoza Regional Hospital in Mexico City. Cir Cir 72:93
Shalev M, Buchumensky V et al (1997) Protective nephrostomy in the treatment of blunt trauma to a congenital hydronephrotic kidney: experience in three patients. Br J Urol 79:643
Shanmuganathan K, Mirvis SE et al (2004) Penetrating torso trauma: triple-contrast helical CT in peritoneal violation and organ injury–a prospective study in 200 patients. Radiology 231:775
Shapiro MB, Nance ML et al (2001) Nonoperative management of solid abdominal organ injuries from blunt trauma: impact of neurologic impairment. Am Surg 67:793
Sharp DS, Ross JH e t al (2002) Attitudes of pediatric urologists regarding sports participation by children with a solitary kidney. J Urol 168:1811; discussion 1815
Sharples EJ, Sobeh M et al (2002) Renal artery dissection after blunt abdominal trauma: a rare cause of acute cortical necrosis. Am J Kidney Dis 40:e11
Shekarriz B, Stoller ML (2002) The use of fibrin sealant in urology. J Urol 167:1218
Shima H, Nosaka S et al (1997) Diagnostic imaging of renal pedicle injury. Nippon Igaku Hoshasen Gakkai Zasshi 57:5
Shimizu T, Yamazaki Y et al (1998) Giant retroperitoneal hematoma in a patient with von Recklinghausen's disease. Nippon Hinyokika Gakkai Zasshi 89:846
Shin M, Momohara C et al (2003) Traumatic rupture of giant hydronephrosis due to ureteral stone: a case report. Hinyokika Kiyo 49:679
Shinojima T, Nakajima Y et al (2004) Evaluation of 115 consecutive patients with blunt renal trauma by using the classification for renal injury of Japanese Association for the Surgery of Trauma. Nippon Hinyokika Gakkai Zasshi 95:783
Siddins M, Rao MM et al (2001) Late laparoscopic nephrectomy following renal trauma. Aust N Z J Surg 71:618
Siebels M, Andrassy K et al (1998) Spontaneous splenic and renal rupture in polyarteritis nodosa. Aktuelle Radiol 8:236
Silberzweig JE, Tey S et al (1998) Percutaneous renal biopsy complicated by renal capsular artery pseudoaneurysm. Am J Kidney Dis 31:533
Singh TM, Hung R et al (2005) Endovascular repair of traumatic aortic pseudoaneurysm with associated celiacomesenteric trunk. J Endovasc Ther 12:138
Sivit CJ, Taylor GA et al (1991) Blunt trauma in children: significance of peritoneal fluid. Radiology 178:185
Skowvron O, Descotes JL et al (1995) Kidney injuries due to skiing. Prog Urol 5:361
Slaton JW, Kropp KA (1996) Proximal ureteral stent migration: an avoidable complication? J Urol 155:58
Smith DP, Klein FA (1997) Renal injury in a child with airbag deployment. J Trauma 42:341
Smith JK, Kenney PJ (2003) Imaging of renal trauma. Radiol Clin North Am 41:1019
Smith M, Johnston B et al (2003) Trauma cases from Harborview Medical Center. Rupture of a ureteropelvic junction-obstructed kidney in a 15-year-old football player. AJR Am J Roentgenol 180:504
Smith SD, Gardner MJ et al (1993) Renal artery occlusion in pediatric blunt abdominal trauma–decreasing the delay from injury to treatment. J Trauma 35:861
Snedeker JG, Barbezat M et al (2005) Strain energy density as a rupture criterion for the kidney: impact tests on porcine organs, finite element simulation, and a baseline comparison between human and porcine tissues. J Biomech 38:993
Sofer M, Kaver I et al (2001) Conservative management of an uncommon renal foreign body secondary to explosion injury. J Trauma 51:594
Sofocleous CT, C Hinrichs et al (2005) Angiographic findings and embolotherapy in renal arterial trauma. Cardiovasc Intervent Radiol 28:39
Soler Soler JL, Nogueras Ocana M et al (1994) Renal trauma in children: our experience and review of the literature. Arch Esp Urol 47:51
Stalker HP, Kaufman RA et al (1990) The significance of hematuria in children after blunt abdominal trauma. AJR Am J Roentgenol 154:569
Stampfer DS (1997) Free intraperitoneal rupture of hydronephrotic kidney. J Urol 157:2242
Stawicki SP, Hoff WS et al (2005) Human immunodeficiency virus infection in trauma patients: where do we stand? J Trauma 58:88
Steffens MG, Bode PJ et al (1996) Selective embolization of pseudo-aneurysms of the renal artery after blunt abdominal injury in a patient with a single kidney. Injury 27:219
Stein JP, Kaji DM et al (1994) Blunt renal trauma in the pediatric population: indications for radiographic evaluation. Urology 44:406
Steinberg DL, Jeffrey RB et al (1984) The computerized tomography appearance of renal pedicle injury. J Urol 132:1163
Stevenson J, Battistella FD (1994) The 'one-shot' intravenous pyelogram: is it indicated in unstable trauma patients before celiotomy? J Trauma 36:828; discussion 833
Strohmaier WL, Lahme S et al (1999) Reduction of high-energy shock-wave-induced renal tubular injury by selenium. Urol Res 27:382
Sullivan MJ, Stables DP (1972) Renal artery occlusion from trauma. JAMA 221:1282

Surana R, Khan A et al (1995) Scarring following renal trauma in children. Br J Urol 75:663
Suzuki N, Mori I et al (1995) Analysis of 42 patients with renal trauma-radiographic assessment of surgical application. Hinyokika Kiyo 41:965
Swain R, Ross D (1999) Lower extremity compartment syndrome. When to suspect acute or chronic pressure buildup. Postgrad Med 105:159
Swana HS, Cohn SM et al (1996) Renal artery pseudoaneurysm after blunt abdominal trauma: case report and literature review. J Trauma 40:459
Swischuk, LE (1999) I fell today and then there was blood in my urine. Pediatr Emerg Care 15:457
Sy WM, Seo IS et al (1999) A patient with three kidneys: a correlative imaging case report. Clin Nucl Med 24:264
Tahmaz L, Yalcin O et al (2000) Isolated ureteropelvic junction laceration following blunt body trauma. Ulus Travma Derg 6:266
Takeda M, Katayama Y et al (1994) Value of dimercaptosuccinic acid single photon emission computed tomography and magnetic resonance imaging in detecting renal injury in pediatric patients with vesicoureteral reflux. Comparison with dimercaptosuccinic acid planar scintigraphy and intravenous pyelography. Eur Urol 25:320
Tanaka M, Ozono S et al (1994) Clinical studies of renal trauma. Hinyokika Kiyo 40:975
Tang E, Berne TV (1994) Intravenous pyelography in penetrating trauma. Am Surg 60:384
Taviloglu K, Gunay K et al (1998) Abdominal stab wounds: the role of selective management. Eur J Surg 164:17
Tazi K, el Fassi J et al (2000) Major renal trauma: report of 18 cases. Ann Urol (Paris) 34:249
Thall EH, Stone NN et al (1996) Conservative management of penetrating and blunt Type III renal injuries. Br J Urol 77:512
Thomason RB, Julian JS et al (1989) Microscopic hematuria after blunt trauma. Is pyelography necessary? Am Surg 55:145
Thompson-Fawcett M, Kolbe A (1996) Paediatric renal trauma: caution with conservative management of major injuries. Aust N Z J Surg 66:435
Thomsen TW, Brown DF et al (2004) Blunt renal trauma. J Emerg Med 26:331
Thorelius L (2004) Contrast-enhanced ultrasound in trauma. Eur Radiol 14 [Suppl 8]:P43
Tillou A, Romero J et al (2001) Renal vascular injuries. Surg Clin North Am 81:1417
Titton RL, Gervais DA et al (2002) Renal trauma: radiologic evaluation and percutaneous treatment of nonvascular injuries. AJR Am J Roentgenol 178:1507
Tong YC, Chun JS et al (1992) Use of hematoma size on computerized tomography and calculated average bleeding rate as indications for immediate surgical intervention in blunt renal trauma. J Urol 147:984
Touiti D, Paparel P et al (2001) Retroperitoneal foreign body mimicking pararenal tumor. Ann Urol (Paris) 35:151
Toutouzas KG, Karaiskakis M et al (2002) Nonoperative management of blunt renal trauma: a prospective study. Am Surg 68:1097
Trainavicius K, Siaurusevicius B et al (2002) Renal trauma in children. Medicina (Kaunas) 38 [Suppl 1]:18
Traxer O, Lottmann H et al (1999) Extracorporeal lithotripsy in children. Study of its efficacy and evaluation of renal parenchymal damage by DMSA-Tc 99m scintigraphy: a series of 39 children. Arch Pediatr 6:251
Traxer O, Smith TG 3rd et al (2001) Renal parenchymal injury after standard and mini percutaneous nephrostolithotomy. J Urol 165:1693
Trivez Boned MA, Oliva Encina J et al (2001) Thrombosis of the renal artery secondary to closed abdominal trauma. Actas Urol Esp 25:295
Troisi R, Hesse UJ et al (1999) Functional, life-threatening disorders and splenectomy following liver transplantation. Clin Transplant 13:380
Trunkey DD (2000) History and development of trauma care in the United States. Clin Orthop Relat Res (374):36
Tucak A, Lukacevic T et al (1995) Urogenital wounds during the war in Croatia in 1991/1992. J Urol 153:121
Turnock RR, Sprigg A et al (1993) Computed tomography in the management of blunt abdominal trauma in children. Br J Surg 80:982
Udekwu PO, Gurkin B et al (1996) The use of computed tomography in blunt abdominal injuries. Am Surg 62:56
Ugras M, Gunes A et al (2002) Severe renal bleeding caused by a ruptured renal sheath: case report of a rare complication of percutaneous nephrolithotomy. BMC Urol 2:10
Ungania S (2003) Conservative... and non conservative... treatment of renal blunt injuries. Ann Ital Chir 74:445
Uribe CA, Castellanos RI et al (2002) Unusual cause of a mass in the superior pole of the kidney: report of a case. Arch Esp Urol 55:958
Valkema R, Pauwels SA et al (2005) Long-term follow-up of renal function after peptide receptor radiation therapy with (90)Y-DOTA(0),Tyr(3)-octreotide and (177)Lu-DOTA(0), Tyr(3)-octreotate. J Nucl Med 46 [Suppl 1]:83S
Varga A, Salah M et al (2001) Renal tumor-like pyonephrosis with foreign body. J Urol 165:891
Vasile M, Bellin MF et al (2000) Imaging evaluation of renal trauma. Abdom Imaging 25:424
Veenstra DL, Best JH et al (1999) Incidence and long-term cost of steroid-related side effects after renal transplantation. Am J Kidney Dis 33:829
Velazquez OC, Bavaria JE et al (1999) Emergency repair of thoracoabdominal aortic aneurysms with immediate presentation. J Vasc Surg 30:996
Velmahos GC, Degiannis E (1997) The management of urinary tract injuries after gunshot wounds of the anterior and posterior abdomen. Injury 28:535
Velmahos GC, Demetriades D et al (1998) Selective management of renal gunshot wounds. Br J Surg 85:1121
Velmahos GC, Chahwan S et al (2000) Angiographic embolization for intraperitoneal and retroperitoneal injuries. World J Surg 24:539
Velmahos GC, Toutouzas KG et al (2003) Nonoperative treatment of blunt injury to solid abdominal organs: a prospective study. Arch Surg 138:844
Vignali C, Lonzi S et al (2004) Vascular injuries after percutaneous renal procedures: treatment by transcatheter embolization. Eur Radiol 14:723
Villard J (1997) Atheromatous aneurysms of the thoracic aorta. Arch Mal Coeur Vaiss 90 [Suppl]:1741
Villas PA, Cohen G et al (1999) Wallstent placement in a renal artery after blunt abdominal trauma. J Trauma 46:1137
Vogelzang NJ (1999) Re: Radiation induced renal cell cancer: a report of 4 cases and review of the literature. J Urol 162:1388
Voisard R, von Eicken J et al (1999) A human arterial organ culture model of postangioplasty restenosis: results up to 56 days after ballooning. Atherosclerosis 144:123
Vuckovic I, Tucak A et al (1995) Croatian experience in the treatment of 629 urogenital war injuries. J Trauma 39:733
Wah TM, Spencer JA (2001) The role of CT in the management of adult urinary tract trauma. Clin Radiol 56:268
Wahlgren CM, Wahlberg E (2005) Management of thoracoabdominal aneurysm type IV Eur J Vasc Endovasc Surg 29:116
Waldrop J, Ciraulo DL et al (2005) A comparison of continuous renal replacement therapy to intermittent dialysis in the

management of renal insufficiency in the acutely III surgical patient. Am Surg 71:36
Wang KT, Hou CJ et al (1998) Late development of renal arteriovenous fistula following gunshot trauma–a case report. Angiology 49:415
Watterson JD, Mahoney JE et al (1998) Iatrogenic ureteric injuries: approaches to etiology and management. Can J Surg 41:379
Welling RE, Kremchek TE et al (1989) Blunt arterial injuries associated with multiple trauma. Ann Vasc Surg 3:345
Wessells H, McAninch JW (1996) Effect of colon injury on the management of simultaneous renal trauma. J Urol 155:1852Wessells H, McAninch JW et al (1997a) Criteria for nonoperative treatment of significant penetrating renal lacerations. J Urol 157:24
Wessells H, Deirmenjian J et al (1997b) Preservation of renal function after reconstruction for trauma: quantitative assessment with radionuclide scintigraphy. J Urol 157:1583
Wessells H, Suh D et al (2003) Renal injury and operative management in the United States: results of a population-based study. J Trauma 54:423
West OC, Anderson J et al (2002) Patterns of diagnostic error in trauma abdominal CT. Emerg Radiol 9:195
Wicky S, Wintermark M et al (2000) Imaging of blunt chest trauma. Eur Radiol 10:1524
Wilkinson AG, Haddock G et al (1999) Separation of renal fragments by a urinoma after renal trauma: percutaneous drainage accelerates healing. Pediatr Radiol 29:503
Willis LR, Evan AP et al (1999) Relationship between kidney size, renal injury, and renal impairment induced by shock wave lithotripsy. J Am Soc Nephrol 10:1753
Willmann JK, Roos JE et al (2002) Multidetector CT: detection of active hemorrhage in patients with blunt abdominal trauma. AJR Am J Roentgenol 179:437
Wilson RF (1994) Pre-existing peripheral arterial disease in trauma. Crit Care Clin 10:567
Wolfman NT, Bechtold RE et al (1992) Blunt upper abdominal trauma: evaluation by CT. AJR Am J Roentgenol 158:493
Wu CL, Chou MC (1993) Surgical management of blunt renal trauma. Zhonghua Yi Xue Za Zhi (Taipei) 52:184
Xu DM, Xu QM et al (2000) Evaluation of organ function monitoring and supporting during the treatment of multiple trauma. Hunan Yi Ke Da Xue Xue Bao 25:288
Yadin O (1994) Hematuria in children. Pediatr Ann 23:474
Yao DC, Jeffrey RB Jr et al (2002) Using contrast-enhanced helical CT to visualize arterial extravasation after blunt abdominal trauma: incidence and organ distribution. AJR Am J Roentgenol 178:17
Yu NC, Raman SS et al (2004) Fistulas of the genitourinary tract: a radiologic review. Radiographics 24:1331
Zeisberg M, Shah AA et al (2005) Bone morphogenic protein-7 induces mesenchymal to epithelial transition in adult renal fibroblasts and facilitates regeneration of injured kidney. J Biol Chem 280:8094
Zhang P, Zheng SB et al (2003) Selection of the imaging modalities for diagnosis of renal trauma: experience with 74 cases. Di Yi Jun Yi Da Xue Xue Bao 23:872
Zink RA, Muller-Mattheis V et al (1990) Results of the West German multicenter study Urological traumatology. Urologe A 29:243
Zozikov B, Naoumov N et al (2002) Associated trauma with urinary tract injuries. Ann Urol (Paris) 36:290
Zygun DA, Kortbeek JB et al (2005) Non-neurologic organ dysfunction in severe traumatic brain injury. Crit Care Med 33:654

Trauma of the Ureter

15.5

J. Pfitzenmaier, Ch. Gilfrich, A. Haferkamp, M. Hohenfellner

Ureteral trauma is rare, and due to its anatomical location accounts for only 1 % of all urinary tract injuries (Dobrowolski et al. 2002; Lynch et al. 2003). The ureter is protected by the dorsal muscle group and the vertebral column and by the abdominal muscles laterally and anteriorly. Moreover, the ureter is moveable and flexible. Ureteral injuries may be partial or complete and may be caused by blunt or penetrating trauma. However, iatrogenic ureteral injuries are the most common form of trauma to the ureter. A delay in diagnosis is the most important contributory factor in morbidity related to this kind of injury (Armenakas 1999).

15.5.1 Anatomy

The ureter is a thick-walled narrow tube measuring approximately 25 – 30 cm in length and varying in diameter from 1 to 10 mm, in cases of urinary obstruction even larger. It has three different layers (Fig. 15.5.1): The inner mucosal layer which is built of transitional epithelium, the middle layer which consists of circular and longitudinal muscular fibers, and the outer adventitial sheath where the vessels run which are responsible for the blood supply of the ureter. This supply comes from a network of vessels with different origins: the upper part of the ureter receives its blood mainly from the renal arteries, the midportion from the aorta and the iliac vessels, and the lower part from the superior vesical, vaginal, middle hemorrhoidal, and the uterine arteries. Since this vascular source can vary, it is mandatory to perform ureteral dissection cautiously.

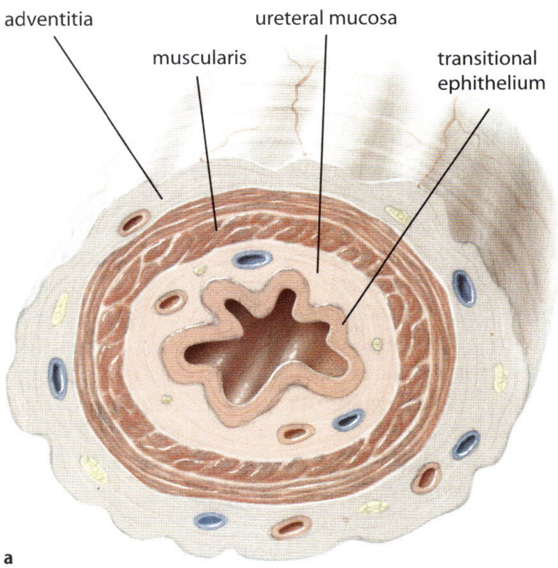

a

Fig. 15.5.1a. Anatomy of the ureter (© Hohenfellnet 2007)

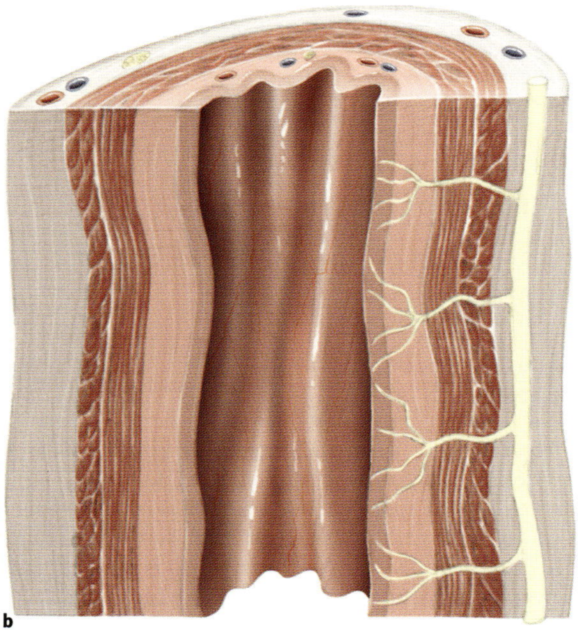

b

Fig. 15.5.1b

15.5.2 Clinical Diagnosis

The most important step toward a successful outcome after ureteral trauma is prompt diagnosis. Therefore, the physician has to have a high index of suspicion based on the injury mechanism and location for this type of trauma to reduce the rate of complications and to perform the appropriate radiographic and intraoperative evaluations in time (Medina et al. 1998). This may be complicated by the presence of multiple organ injuries, and at the same time, the absence of any clinical and laboratory findings associated with the ureteral trauma. For example, hematuria, which is a common diagnostic tool in urological disorders, is absent in approximately 30%–45% of these cases (Lynch et al. 2003; Bright et al. 1977; Campbell et al. 1992; Carlton et al. 1971; Liroff et al. 1977; Pitts and Peterson 1981; Presti et al. 1989; Brandes et al. 2004). Therefore, the diagnosis of ureteral injuries is delayed in 66% (for days or weeks) (Teber et al. 2005), which manifest by fever, flank pain, urinoma, elevated serum creatinine levels, obstruction of the upper urinary tract, fistula formation, vaginal leakage, prolonged ileus, and sepsis (Dobrowolski et al. 2002; Armenakas 1999; Dor airajan et al. 2004; McGinty and Mendez 1977; Palmer et al. 1999). Ureteral trauma should be suspected in all cases of penetrating abdominal injuries, especially gunshot wounds, and also in cases of blunt deceleration trauma, in which the kidney and the renal pelvis can be torn away from the ureter. This type of deceleration injury is more likely to occur in children due to their hyperextensible vertebral column (Lynch et al. 2003; Brandes et al. 2004; Palmer et al. 1999).

15.5.3 Radiographic Diagnosis

In recent years computed tomography (CT scan) has become the most accurate radiographic modality to diagnose ureteral injuries (Lynch et al. 2003; Armenakas 1999; Brandes et al. 2004; Teber et al. 2005). The use of helical CT scan for urinary stone disease is becoming more widespread, and its utility in evaluating the patient with thoracic (Gavant et al. 1995) or abdominal (Janzen et al. 1998) trauma is well documented. Its use in evaluating the upper urinary tract has been documented for staging renal trauma (Carl 1997), vascular trauma (Nunez et al. 1996), and disruption of the ureteropelvic junction (Mulligan et al. 1998). It especially is important to request delayed excretory images to be able to completely judge the renal pelvis, the ureter, and the bladder(Mulligan et al. 1998). Extravasation of contrast confined predominantly to the medial perirenal space is the most consistent finding (Kenney et al. 1987). For example, the absence of contrast material in the distal ureter on delayed films may be diagnostic of a complete ureteral transsection.

The intravenous urogram (IVU) was the standard tool for the evaluation before the widespread use of CT scan. It is still the modality of choice if a CT scan is not available. It can be obtained by using high-dose (2 ml contrast/kg body weight) imaging using a "one-shot" technique if desired. Extravasation also is a certain sign of ureteral injury. Unfortunately, in most cases the findings are more subtle, showing delayed kidney function, mild dilation, or deviation of the ureter (Armenakas 1999).

If the results of IVU and the CT scan are inconclusive, the next step would be an invasive diagnostic procedure with cystoscopy and a retrograde ureterogram (Lynch et al. 2003; Armenakas 1999). As the most accurate procedure to diagnose ureteral injuries, the retrograde ureterogram is very often impractical in the acute trauma setting.

15.5.4 Intraoperative Diagnosis

Usually, penetrating injuries to the ureter are diagnosed intraoperatively when initial laparotomy is performed to manage any complications associated with abdominal injuries. Intraoperative recognition of ureteral injury in penetrating trauma differs depending on the authors, and ranges between 39% and 92% (Liroff

Table 15.5.1. AAST organ injury severity scale for the ureter (Moore et al. 1992)

Grade	Description of injury
I	Hematoma only
II	Laceration 50% of circumference
III	Laceration >50% of circumference
IV	Complete tear 2 cm of devascularization
V	Complete tear >2 cm of devascularization

et al. 1977; Pitts and Peterson 1981; Presti et al. 1989; Brandes et al. 1994; Rober et al. 1990). Most injuries were generally found within the first 24 h after trauma (Liroff et al. 1977; Pitts and Peterson 1981; Presti et al. 1989; Brandes et al. 1994; Rober et al. 1990). In the intraoperative setting, direct visual inspection is the most reliable means of assessing ureteral integrity. To perform appropriate assessment, the bowel needs to be reflected sufficiently to expose the ureter. Besides urinary extravasation, more subtle findings may suggest a ureteral injury, such as contusion, discoloration, lack of bleeding, and decreased peristalsis of the ureter. The severity of the injury is shown in Table 15.5.1. Intraoperative detection of a ureteral injury may be facilitated by the intravenous or intraureteral application of indigo carmine or methylene blue (Lynch et al. 2003; Armenakas 1999).

15.5.5 External Trauma

Blunt and penetrating trauma to the ureter is rare, and occurs in 1% and 4% after external violence, respectively (Campbell et al. 1992). Blunt trauma is usually seen in children during rapid deceleration (Lynch et al. 2003), causing excessive hyperextension of the vertebral column and disruption at the ureteropelvic junction. It may easily be missed because patients often do not exhibit hematuria and the injury is difficult to palpate during intraoperative manual examination (Campbell et al. 1992; Boone et al. 1993).

The incidence of penetrating injuries largely depends on the number of bullet and stab wounds, which are on the increase because of increasing social disorder and the availability of guns (Dobrowolski et al. 2002; Palmer et al. 1999). Best et al. reported that most (97%) trauma to the ureter in a level I trauma center were caused by penetrating injuries, mainly gunshot wounds (55%) (Best et al. 2005). The anatomical location was the left side in 58%, right side in 40%, and bilateral in 2% of patients. The distribution of injuries was proximal in 26%, mid in 37%, and distal in 37% (Best et al. 2005). Only 2%–3% of gunshot wounds to the abdomen result in ureteral injuries (Presti et al. 1989; Azimuddin et al. 1998). These injuries are often associated with multiple organ injuries in up to 98% (Best et al.2005), which include the small bowel (39%–65%), colon (28%–33%), liver, spleen, kidney (10%–28%), bladder (5%), and iliac vessels (Medina et al. 1998; Campbell et al. 1992; Pitts and Peterson 1981; Presti et al. 1989; Robert et al. 1990; Eickenberg and Amin 1976; Holden et al. 1976). The mortality rate in these patients is high: 33% (Campbell et al. 1992). There are two main ways for a bullet to injure the ureter. One is the direct destruction or disruption of the ureter and the other is the disruption of the ureteral blood supply with subsequent necrosis. In an experimental setting, such damage to the vessels was found up to 2 cm below and above of the transection area (Campbell et al. 1992). These experimental studies have shown that the transected ureter back to a bleeding edge must be debrided to remove tissue that may cause invisible damage to the surrounding microvessels.

15.5.6 Iatrogenic/Intraoperative Trauma

Most often ureteral trauma is iatrogenic. It can be caused by open surgery, laparoscopic surgery, and ureterorenoscopy. The most common mechanisms of operative ureteral injury are:

1. Crushing from misapplication of a clamp
2. Ligation with suture
3. Transsection (partial and complete)
4. Angulation of the ureter with secondary obstruction
5. Ischemia from ureteral stripping or electrocoagulation
6. Resection of a ureteral segment
7. Any combination of the above

15.5.6.1 Open Surgery

In a large retrospective study by Dobrowolski et al. (2002) reporting 340 iatrogenic injuries to the ureter, 73% were gynecological, 14% were general surgical (Fig. 15.5.2), and 14% were urological in origin. The source of iatrogenic ureteral injury is urologic surgery in up to 21% of reported cases (Selzman and Spirnak 1996). Injury to the lower third of the ureter is the most common site due to its anatomical location.

The incidence of trauma during gynecological procedures is reported to range from 0.02% to 1.5% (Yeong et al. 1998; Carley et al. 2002; Daly and Higgins 1988; Liapis et al. 2001; St Lezin et al. 1991) to as high as 2.3% (Gambone et al. 1990) and in colorectal surgery from 0.3% to 5.7% (Fig. 15.5.3). Predisposing factors for ureteral injury in gynecologic surgery have

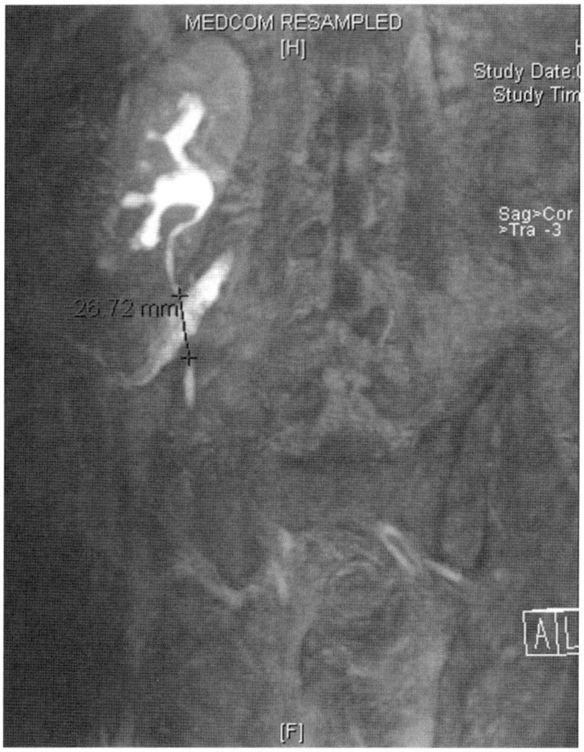

Fig. 15.5.2. Right ureteral injury in a single kidney in the proximal ureter after a Whipple procedure and revision and abscess drainage. The MRI urogram shows the ureteral leakage and urinoma surrounding the right ureter. The left kidney was taken out because of the primary tumor. Because of the abscesses, a nephrostomy tube was placed and the proximal ureter was closed with coils. After recovery from these procedures, the patient will be scheduled for ureteroureterostomy, and if not possible for ureteral replacement with an intestinal segment in approximately 3–6 months

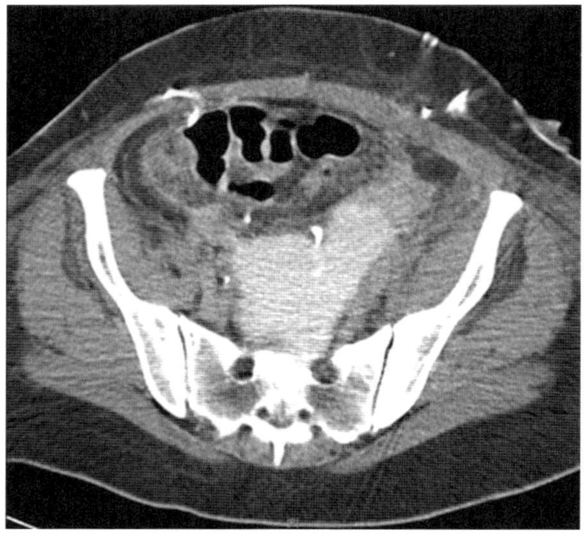

Fig. 15.5.3. Pelvic abscess after colonic surgery and ureteral injury with delayed recognition. This case shows a female patient after laparoscopic resection of the sigmoid colon, who was admitted with injury of the left ureter. An end-to-end anastomosis had already been performed. Afterward, she developed a leakage of the colonic anastomosis. When the second laparotomy was performed to revise the colon and create a colostomy, the left ureter also still showed a huge defect. A second end-to-end-anastomosis of the ureter was performed. Two days later she presented with a large abscess. The abscess was drained and a ureterocutaneostomy was created. Six months later, the colostomy was reversed and ureteral reimplantation using a psoas hitch technique was performed. The result showed good kidney function (Fig. 15.5.5)

been identified. These factors include uterus size larger than 12 weeks' gestation, ovarian cysts 4 cm or larger, radiation therapy, advanced stage of malignancy, and anatomical anomalies of the urinary tract. Nevertheless, there is a slight risk of ureteral injury even without risk factors. Hurd et al. (2001) showed that the ureter runs within 0.5 cm of the cervix in 12% of women.

Vascular surgery in the abdomen can cause hydronephrosis in up to 12%–20%, usually with a benign course, and only 1%–2% will end up with ureteral stenosis in the long run (Campbell et al. 1992; St Lezin et al. 1991; Adams et al. 1992). The risk factors for intraabdominal vascular surgery are:

1. Reoperation
2. Graft placement anterior to the ureter
3. Large dilated arterial aneurysms, which can cause retroperitoneal inflammation involving the ureter.

15.5.6.2 Laparoscopic Surgery

In laparoscopic surgery, especially gynecologic surgery, injuries occur most frequently during electrocoagulation of endometriosis (Grainger et al. 1990). This may be caused because this disease can involve the ureter intrinsically and extrinsically. Injuries mainly occur in the area of the uterosacral ligaments (Grainger et al. 1990). Because of the inflammatory adhesions, visualization of the ureter might be difficult, with a higher risk of injury. After an increase in ureteral injuries in the beginning of laparoscopy, the rate today is equal to that of open surgery: 1% (Harkki-Siren et al. 1999). In laparoscopic surgery, special attention must be paid to ureteral injuries because in contrast to open surgery where approximately one-third of ureteral damage is recognized during the first procedure, the rate is lower in laparoscopy (Grainger et al. 1990).

Overall, intimate knowledge of the ureteral location is mandatory to avoid ureteral injuries. Especially for gynecologic surgery, the relation to the uterine and ovarian vessels, which are often ligated during these procedures, is of special interest (Fig. 15.5.4). In obviously difficult cases, for example large malignancies or

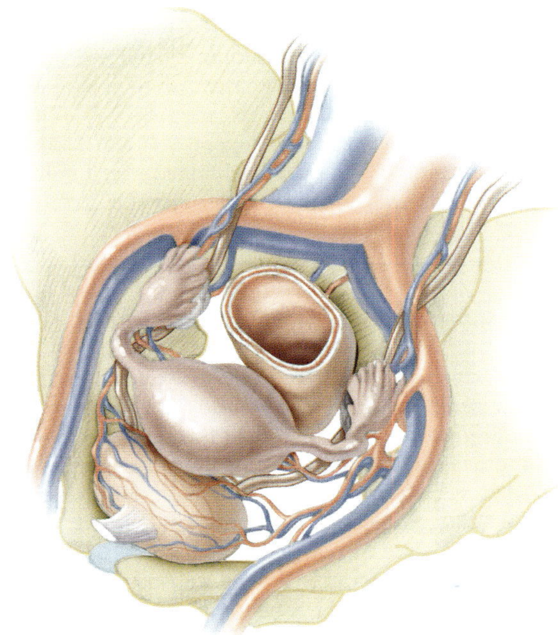

Fig. 15.5.4. Relation of the ureter to nearby structures (© Hohenfelnner 2007)

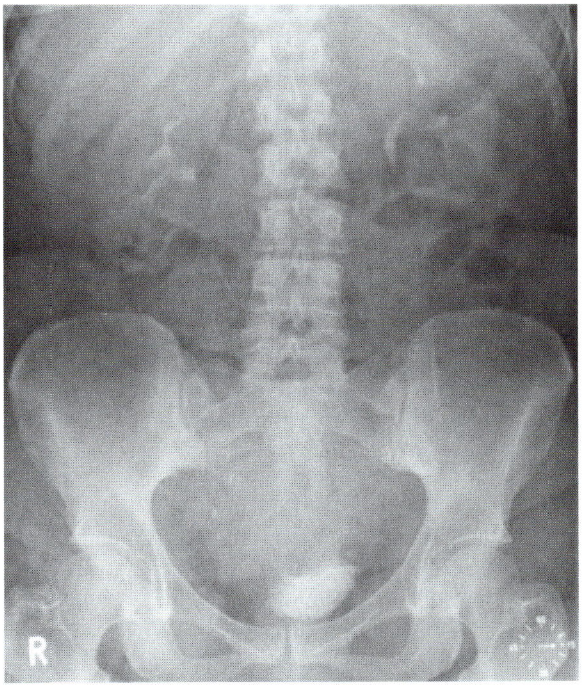

Fig. 15.5.5. IVU shows the same patient as in Fig. 15.5.3, after drainage of the pelvic abscess and left ureteral reimplantation using a Boari technique

reoperation, preoperative insertion of ureteral stents might reduce the risk of ureteral injuries, although published data in the gynecologic population do not confirm this theory (Kuno et al. 1998).

15.5.6.3 Ureterorenoscopy

Ureterorenoscopy is a widespread technique to treat ureteral stones. Since the very beginning, reports of ureteral injury after ureteroscopy have been documented. Nowadays the rate is decreasing because equipment, operative technique, and the surgeon's experience have been improved. Ranging from 0% to 28%, the complication rate has averaged at 7% (McAninch and Santucci 2002). Recommendations to avoid injuries are:

1. Stop stone basket attempts after recognition of ureteral tear.
2. Perform ureterorenoscopy alongside or over a wire.
3. Use smaller or flexible ureterorenoscopes.
4. Avoid ureterorenoscopy in previously irradiated patients (Flam et al. 1988; Huffman 1989).

15.5.7 Techniques of Trauma Repair

Depending on the patient's condition, the site, the extent of the injury, and the time of diagnosis, the appropriate management of the ureteral injury must be selected. Trauma patients with an external trauma mechanism may require prompt operative exploration to manage associated abdominal injuries. At the same time, the ureter should be meticulously inspected for any injury or ischemia. Nevertheless, complex abdominal organ or vascular injuries should not preclude ureteral reconstruction (Spirnak et al. 1989). In these cases, the reconstructive procedure can be performed and an omental or peritoneal flap can be interposed to protect the reconstructed ureter. In unstable patients, it may be necessary to ligate the injured ureter and to put in a nephrostomy tube. Reconstruction can be performed in a later approach after the patient is stable and other sequelae of the trauma have healed. In these complex trauma cases, the approach is in general a midline transperitoneal incision. In patients with delayed repair, the incision can be tailored to the specific procedure that is planned for reconstruction of the ureter. Another reason for ureteral repair in two steps is indicated for cases where an immediate repair is not possible because of massive infection (Fig. 15.5.3) and some kind of transient diversion is performed. Then, in a second step performed after infection has resolved, the patient can undergo definitive treatment (Fig. 15.5.5).

Ureteral injuries with delayed diagnosis or in an unstable patient are initially best managed by percutaneous nephrostomy drainage or endoscopic ureteral stenting by a double-J or a single-J stent. Here the single-J stent is advantageous in that the renal function of the injured ureter and/or kidney can be measured easily. While nephrostomy placement is more easily applied and safer, ureteral stenting should only be used for selected patients with grade I and II injuries or injuries after ureterorenoscopy. In these cases, the stenting procedure may be therapeutic (Armenakas 1999).

15.5.7.1 General Considerations

In general, if ureteral reconstruction is performed, the procedure must include careful debridement and the creation of a watertight, tension-free, spatulated anastomosis. Protection for the reconstructed ureter can be achieved by interposition of an omental or a peritoneal patch. Transient stenting of the ureter and retroperitoneal suction-free drainage are mandatory (Table 15.5.2).

The type of reconstructive procedure chosen by the surgeon depends on the nature and site of the injury. An overview is shown in Fig. 15.5.6. In general, the drain can be removed when drainage is low. Checking the creatinine level of the drain fluid to ensure it is not urine may be prudent before drain removal. The bladder catheter can be removed after 7–10 days, if the bladder had to be opened for the procedure. Voiding cystourethrogram (VCUG) at the time of catheter removal to ensure adequate healing of the bladder is advisable. The stent should be removed 6 weeks postoperatively and a follow-up renogram and IVU should be obtained after 3 months to assess the patency of the repair (Lynch et al. 2003).

Table 15.5.2. Principles of repair for grade III–V injuries (Lynch et al. 2003)

Principle of reconstruction of complete ureteral injuries
Debridement of ureteral ends to fresh and bleeding tissue
Spatulation of the ureteral ends
Internal stenting of the ureter
Watertight, tension-free anastomosis with absorbable suture
External, retroperitoneal, and nonsuction drainage
Protection of the anastomosis by omental or peritoneal flap

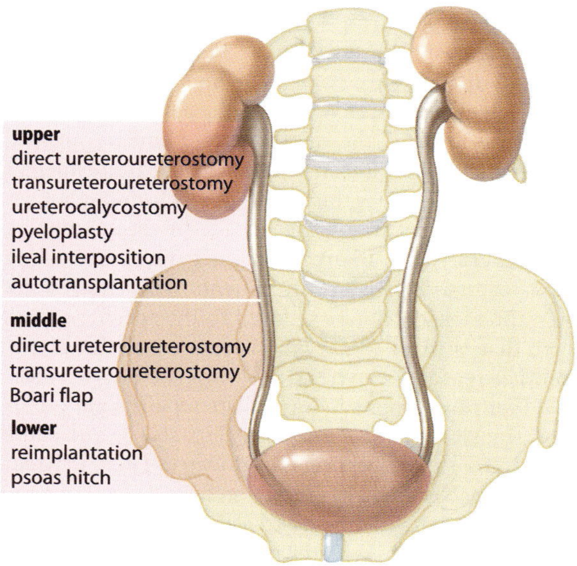

Fig. 15.5.6. Options for ureteral repair of complex injuries, based on its location (© Hohenfellner 2007)

15.5.8 Ureteroureterostomy and Primary Closure

Primary closure is of limited use for external grade II injuries stemming from stab wounds. On the contrary, it should never be used in gunshot wounds because of the microvascular destruction of the surrounding tissue. In these cases a careful debridement is indicated to avoid later complications because of delayed tissue breakdown caused by blast damage.

Ureteroureterostomy, so-called end-to-end anastomosis (Fig. 15.5.7), can be used for the repair of ureteral

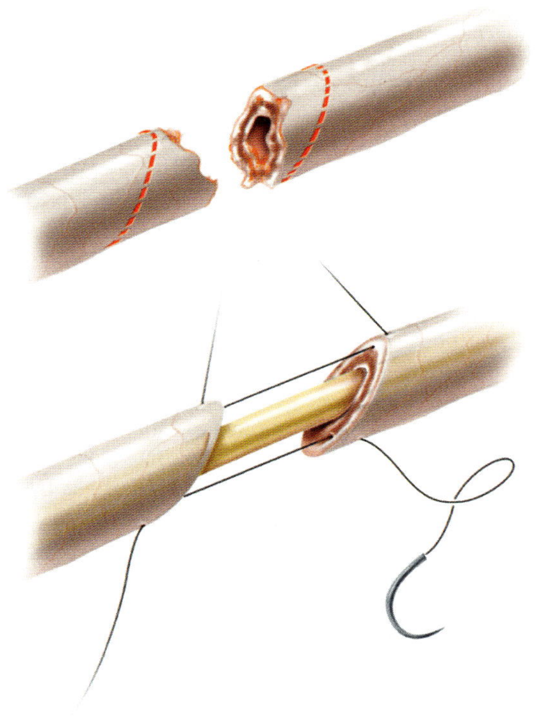

a

b

Fig. 15.5.7. Ureteroureterostomy, end-to-end anastomosis of the ureter. Careful debridement is indicated to avoid later complications caused by delayed tissue breakdown. The well-vascularized ureteral ends are spatulated (**a**), a stent is inserted (**b**) and an anastomosis is performed with a thin (e.g., 5-0 or 6-0) monofilament (e.g., Monocryl or PDS) suture (**c**). The stent should be removed 6 weeks postoperatively and a follow-up renogram and IVU should be obtained after 3 months to assess the patency of the repair

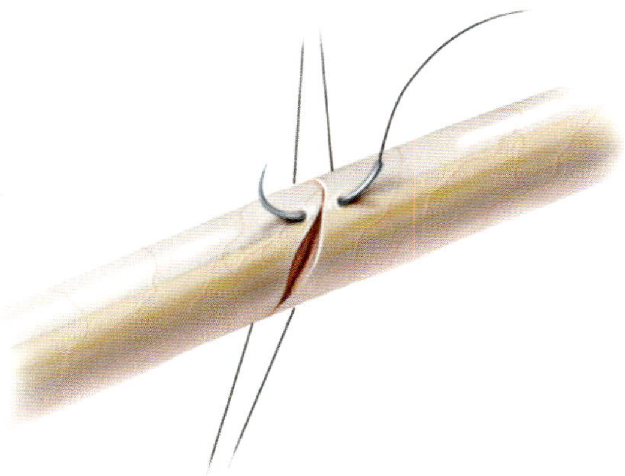

c

Fig. 15.5.7 (Cont.) (© Hohenfellner 2007)

injuries to the upper and middle third of the ureter (Lynch et al. 2003; McAninch and Santucci 2002). The general principles of ureteral trauma surgery as shown in Table 15.5.2 are highly relevant for this procedure. Optical loop magnification may be helpful for optimal suture placement. Maintenance of ureteral vascularity minimizes postoperative fistula and stricture formation (Armenakas 1999). With this procedure, which is very common in ureteral trauma repair (Presti et al. 1989), the success rate is relatively high: up to 90% (Carlton et al. 1969, 1971). Typical complications for this operation are urinary leakage in 10%–24% (Medina et al. 1998; Bright and Peters 1977; Pitts and Peterson 1981; Presti et al. 1989; Velmahos et al. 1996), which can leak into fistula and abscess. A chronic ureteral stenosis is less common (5%–12% incidence (Palmer et al. 1999; Velmahos et al. 1996). Even in patients with prolonged postoperative urine drainage, a watchful waiting strategy should be followed because leakage has a high chance of stopping within several days after repair.

15.5.9 Ureterocalycostomy and Pyeloplasty

For extensive injuries to the ureteropelvic junction and the proximal ureter, either pyeloplasty or, if the renal pelvis is severely injured, ureterocalycostomy can be the treatment of choice. For the latter procedure, the lower pole of the kidney must be amputated to expose the infundibulum of the inferior calyx. The ureter is then spatulated and a direct end-to-end ureterocalyceal anastomosis is performed after stent insertion. Since this operation involves extensive renal dissection and has a high chance of stenosis, it only should be used as a last resort (Lynch et al. 2003; Armenakas 1999). The principle of repair is the same as in ureteroureterostomy with spatulation, stenting, and an anastomosis with a thin monofilament suture.

15.5.10 Transureteroureterostomy and Transureteropyelostomy

Ureteral injuries of the distal half of the ureter and an insufficient bladder capacity or other severe pelvic complications can be managed by transureteroureterostomy or transureteropyelostomy. It is a rarely used procedure. It is mainly performed as a secondary or delayed procedure. For this procedure, the posterior peritoneum is incised to expose both ureters. The injured and debrided ureter is then transposed to the contralateral renal pelvis or ureter, where it is anastomosed via a 1.5 cm longitudinal ureterotomy or incision into the renal pelvis with an end-to-side technique. The course of the ureter should be above the inferior mesenteric artery to avoid ureteral angulation or impingement. These procedures will leave the injured and transposed ureter difficult or impossible to intubate. This is why most authors feel this operation is contraindicated in patients with known urothelial carcinoma or recurrent urolithiasis (Armenakas 1999; McAninch and Santucci 2002). Another problem is the potential to injure the contralateral ureter. Therefore, we prefer ureteral replacement with bowel, and avoid using transureteroureterostomy. The principle of repair is the same as in ureteroureterostomy; with spatulation, stenting, and an anastomosis with a thin monofilament suture (Fig. 15.5.8).

15.5.11 Psoas Hitch

Injuries involving the lower third of the ureter are best managed by a ureteral reimplantation using a psoas-hitch technique. For this procedure, the bladder is mobilized and freed from the peritoneal reflection. When needed, contralateral and in some cases the ipsilateral superior pedicle must be ligated to improve mobilization of the bladder. Stay sutures are placed. A cystostomy is performed perpendicular to the line of the ureter. The bladder is then stretched to the ipsilateral psoas muscle and attached to the psoas tendon with nonabsorbable sutures. Care must be taken to avoid injury to the genitofemoral nerve. The ureter is then reimplanted in a submucosal tunnel and the bladder is closed in two layers (Fig. 15.5.9). This procedure has a high success rate of almost 95% (Middleton 1980). Recent studies show that traumatic disruption of the ureter owing to gynecological procedures can be repaired by a laparoscopic approach using the psoas-hitch technique. None of the patients treated by laparoscopic repair showed an obstruction during the follow-up period, and in five out of six patients reimplantation was nonrefluxing (Modi et al. 2005).

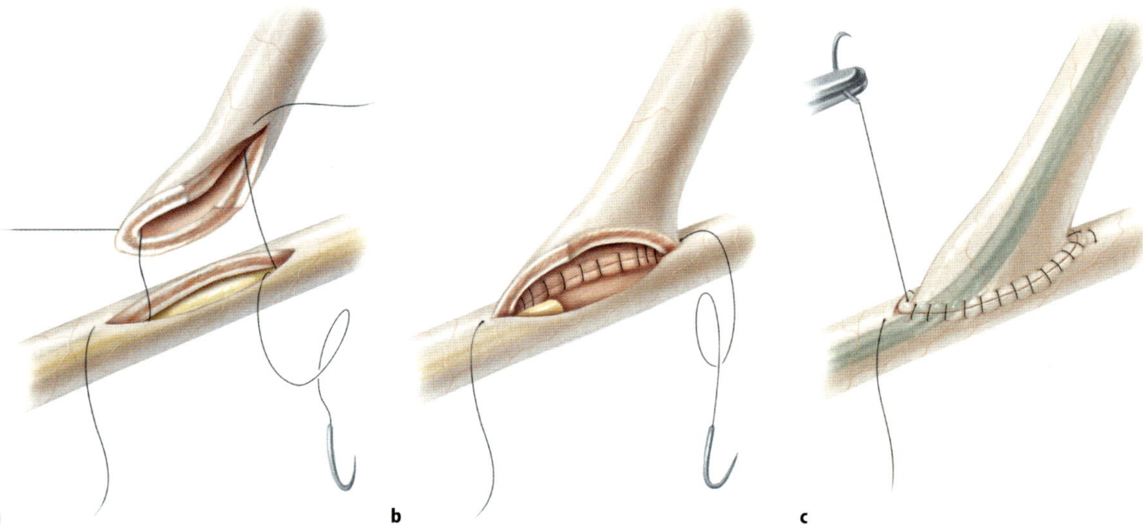

a b c

Fig. 15.5.8. For transureteroureterostomy, the donor ureter is passed retroperitoneally above the inferior mesenteric artery. Then the donor ureter is spatulated and the recipient ureter is incised. Thin monofilament sutures are placed at the cranial and distal end of the incision (**a**). Then the posterior wall of the donor ureter is sewn to the medial wall of the recipient ureter (**b**). A double-J stent is inserted to stent the anastomosis (**c**) and the anastomosis is completed with a 5-0 monofilament running suture. The stent should be removed 6 weeks postoperatively and a follow-up renogram and IVU should be obtained after 3 months to assess the patency of the repair (© Hohenfellner 2007)

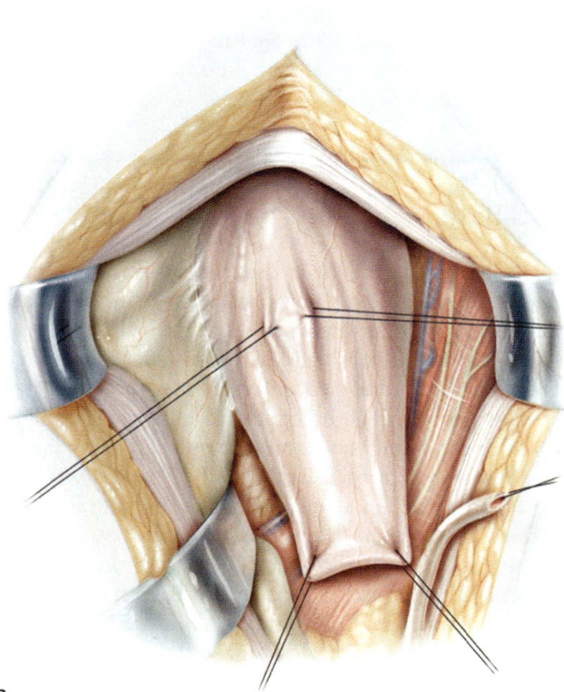

a

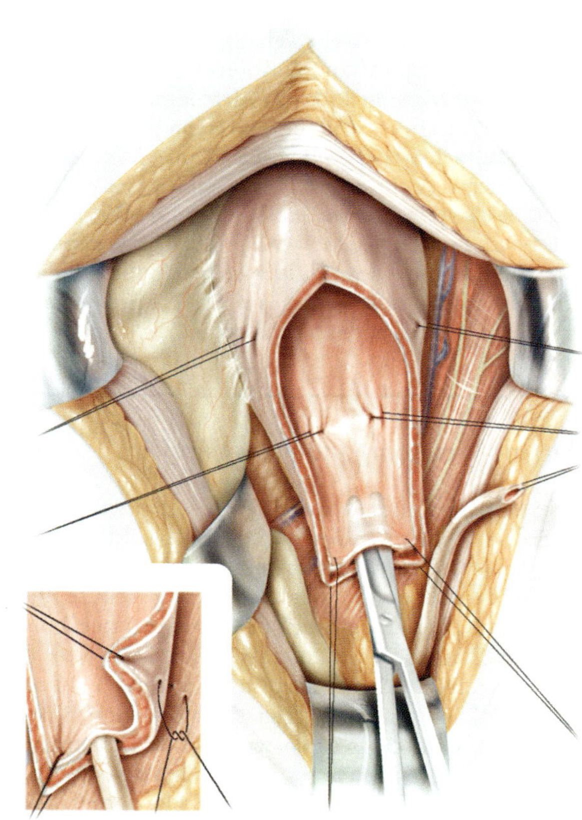

b

Fig. 15.5.9a, b. Longitudinally opened bladder with flap hitched to the fascia of psoas muscle (**a**) forming a submucosal tunnel. Ureteral implantation in a submucosal tunnel with the ureter fixed to the bladder (**b**). Catheter and stent are placed to drain the bladder followed by a two-layer bladder closure. **c** The anastomosis is stented for 14 days. The bladder catheter can be removed after 7–10 days. A follow-up renogram and IVU should be obtained after 3 months to assess the patency of the repair

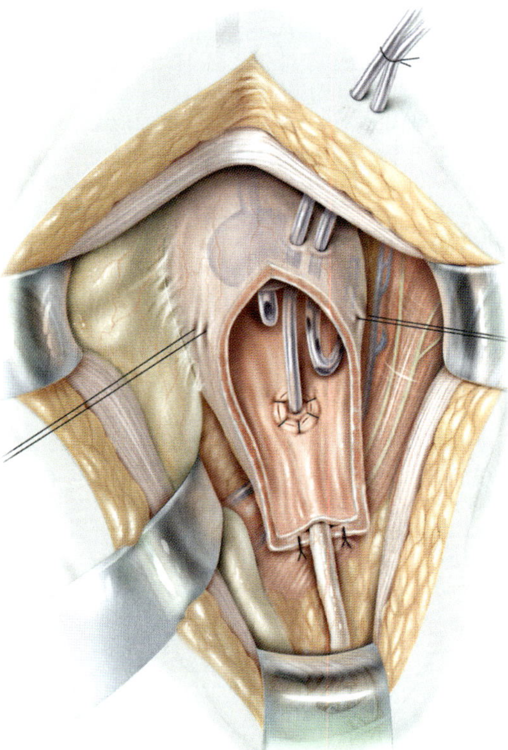

c

Fig. 15.5.9c (© Hohenfellner 2007)

15.5.12 Boari Flap

If the injury encompasses the lower two-thirds of the ureter with a very long defect, which can not be managed using the psoas hitch technique, reimplantation can be successful with the Boari flap technique. As described for the psoas hitch, the bladder is mobilized. Then a full-thickness U-shaped incision is made in its anterior wall. The width of the flap is about four times the diameter of the ureter that has to be reimplanted, with a wider base being maintained to ensure adequate blood supply. The posterior bladder is then hitched to the psoas tendon and the flap is raised to the level of the proximal ureteral stump. The ureter is implanted in a submucosal tunnel and the flap closed in a tubularized fashion. A two-layer bladder closure follows. With this technique, defects of up to 15 cm can be managed. Although it is not commonly performed, the success rate is high (Benson et al. 1990) (Fig. 15.5.10).

15.5.13 Intestinal Replacement of the Ureter

For complete ureteral destruction, small or large bowel can be used as interposition to bridge the space be-

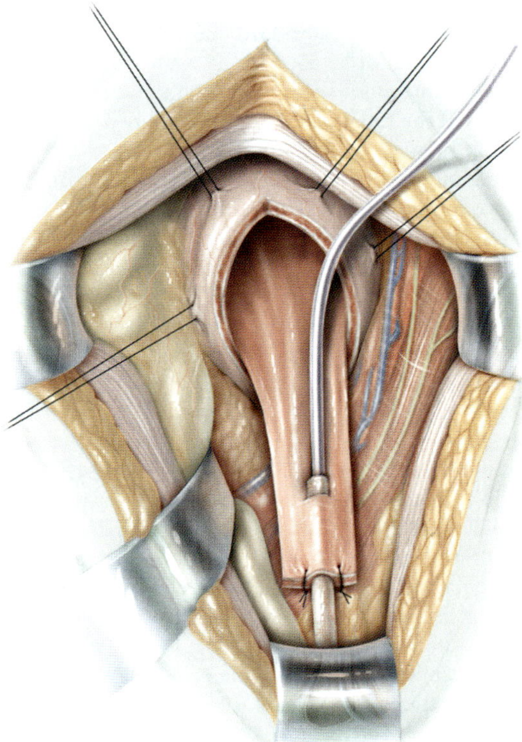

a

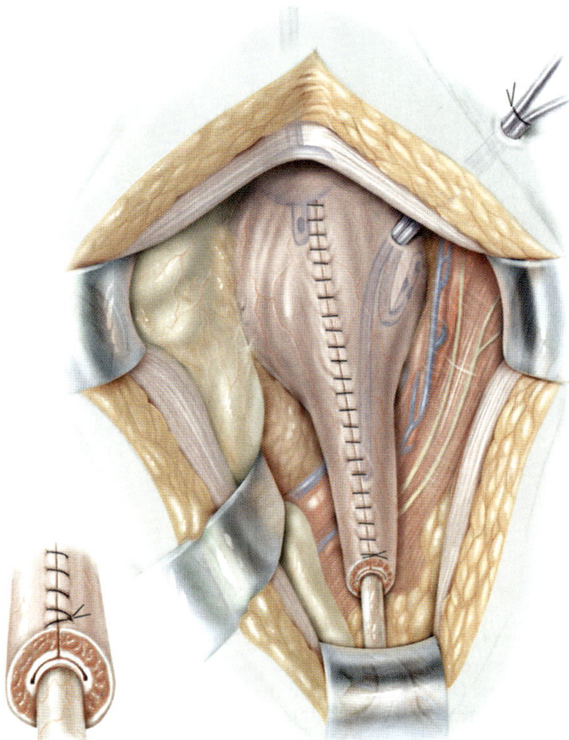

b

Fig. 15.5.10. a Opened bladder with raised Boari flap and submucosal ureteral implantation. b Tubularized bladder after bladder closure (© Hohenfellner 2007) tween the renal pelvis and the bladder. Certainly, this procedure needs standard bowel preparation and therefore cannot be used in the acute trauma setting. It is an operation for secondary repair and should only be chosen if the renal function is relatively normal (creatinine <2.5 mg/dl) (Armenakas 1999).

Usually, a 15- to 25-cm segment of terminal ileum approximately 15–20 cm proximal to the ileocecal valve is used. But especially on the left side, even the sigmoid colon can be used for ureteral replacement. In both cases, the technique is the same as for urinary diversion. After isolation of the segment with vascular integrity, bowel continuity is resumed by either end-to-end or side-to-side anastomosis. The mesenteric window is closed to prevent internal visceral herniation. The "neoureter" is then positioned retroperitoneally in an isoperistaltic fashion. The next step is a pyeloileal-colonic end-to-end anastomosis. A nephrostomy tube as well as a stent is placed for drainage. In a combined intravesical and extravesical or simple extravesical approach, the bowel segment is then anastomosed in a refluxing fashion into the posterior bladder wall. The likelihood of bacteriuria and reflux is very high, but the procedure has not shown deleterious complications on renal function (Bejany et al. 1991; Boxer et al. 1979). Using either small or large bowel, there is a chance of developing metabolic derangements that usually manifest as hyperchloremic metabolic acidosis, but can be corrected with adequate hydration and if necessary, oral alkalization therapy (Pfitzenmaier et al. 2003). In rare cases where the patient presents with a bilateral complete ureteral trauma, the segment can be tailored for both kidneys. Potential long-term complications include obstruction, prolonged mucous formation, stone formation, recurrent urinary tract infection, and (uncommonly) ischemic bowel necrosis (Armenakas 1999). Overall, studies show a success rate of up to 81% (Benson et al. 1990; Boxer et al. 1979; Reznichek et al. 1973; Archbold et al. 1981; Kochakarn et al. 2000) (Fig. 15.5.11).

Tips and Tricks. In rare cases we have used Meckel's diverticulum for ureteral replacement. The advantage is that there is no need for bowel anastomosis and the diverticulum should be ablated anyway. It cannot be used in the 10% of cases where the diverticulum contains gastric mucosa.

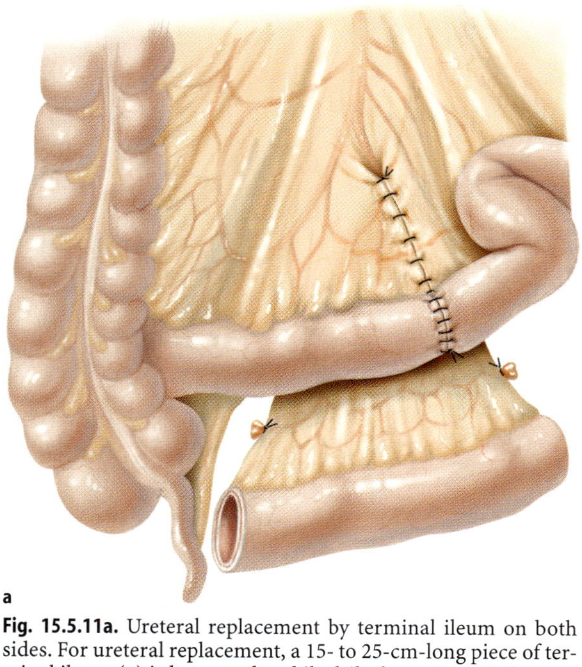

a

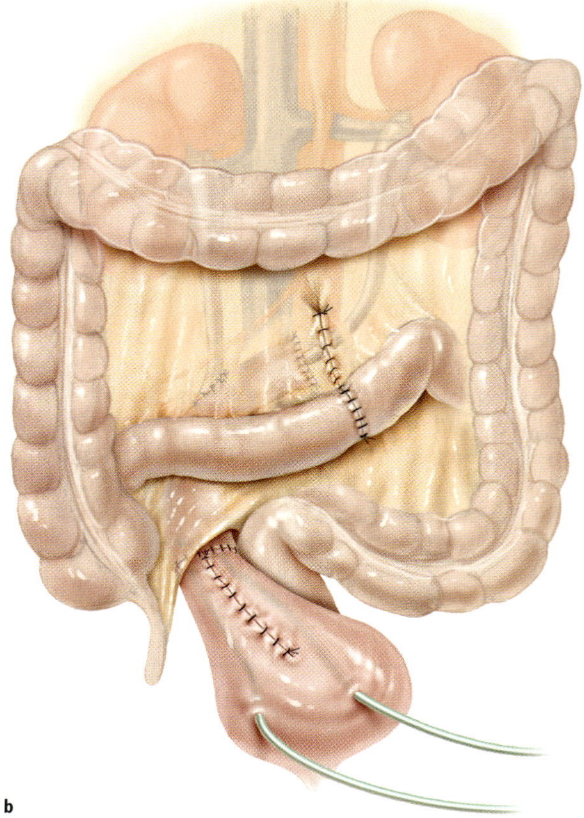

b

Fig. 15.5.11a. Ureteral replacement by terminal ileum on both sides. For ureteral replacement, a 15- to 25-cm-long piece of terminal ileum (**a**) is harvested and ileal-ileal anastomosis is completed. The ileum segment is then connected to the renal pelvis or the proximal ureter (whatever is needed) and anastomosed to the bladder in an isoperistaltic manner (**b**). Both anastomoses are stented. This stent and the bladder catheter can be removed after 3 weeks and an IVU is performed to assess the patency of the repair (© Hohenfellner 2007)

15.5.14 Autotransplantation of the Kidney

In cases with a solitary kidney and a complete ureteral avulsion, renal autotransplantation can be used to manage the trauma. The affected kidney is transplanted into the iliac fossa in a classical fashion with vascular anastomosis and with a pyelovesicostomy. Although this is a procedure with the potential for many minor and major complications, preservation of renal function can be achieved in the long term (Benson et al. 1990; Al Ali and Haddad 1996; Gomella et al. 1997; Bodie et al. 1986). Renal loss can occur in up to 8% (Bodie et al. 1986).

For renal autotransplantation, which can be performed open or laparoscopically (Bulebond-Langner et al. 2004), nephrectomy must be performed retroperitoneally or transperitoneally by identification and transection of the renal vessels. All branch vessels, especially adrenal, lumbar, and gonadal branches that run into the left renal vein, must be clipped or ligated. Then after taking out the kidney, it is perfused with cold University of Wisconsin preservation solution extracorporally through the artery until the venous efflux is clear and the kidney cold. Then the kidney is transplanted using a lower quadrant abdominal incision and preparation of the iliac fossa. The iliac vessels are dissected and transposed. Vessel anastomosis is performed depending on the iliac vessels. First the renal vein is anastomosed to either the common iliac and if too small to the inferior vena cava in an end-to-side technique. All vascular anastomoses are completed with 5-0 running, monofilament, nonabsorbable suture. The renal artery can be anastomosed either to the internal iliac artery in an end-to-end technique or to the external or common iliac artery in an end-to-side technique depending on the status of the iliac vessels. Then reperfusion is accomplished immediately after completion of the vascular anastomosis. Finally, the remnant of the ureter or the renal pelvis is anastomosed to the bladder in a nonrefluxing technique (Fig. 15.5.12).

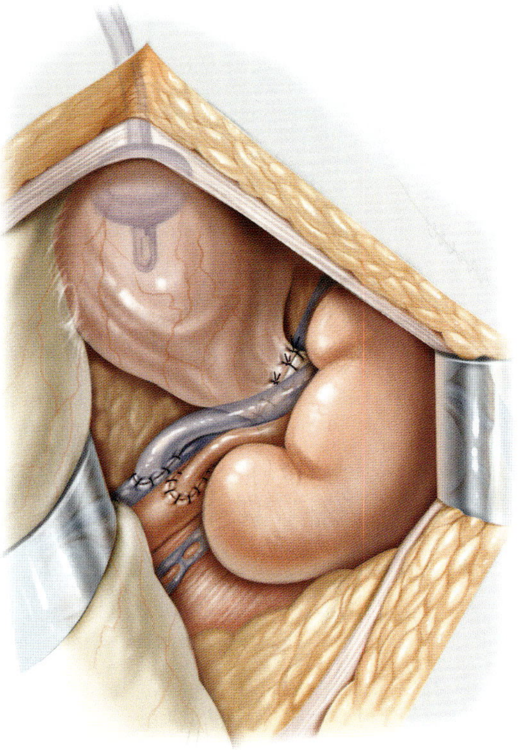

Fig. 15.5.12. Autotransplantation can be indicated in cases with a solitary kidney and a complete ureteral avulsion, or comprised kidney function. The affected kidney is transplanted into the iliac fossa in a classical fashion with vascular anastomosis and with a pyelovesicostomy. The bladder catheter can be removed after 3 weeks. A follow-up renogram and IVU should be obtained after 3 months to assess the patency of the repair (© Hohenfellner 2007)

15.5.15 Nephrectomy

Nephrectomy is rarely required for the treatment of ureteral injuries. It must mainly be performed when the ureteral trauma is associated with massive renal trauma, e.g., in cases of life-threatening bleeding where repair is not possible or severe associated visceral injuries (McGinty and Mendez 1977). Another indication for nephrectomy can be seen for kidneys with poor renal function after delayed diagnosis of ureteral injuries (Campbell et al. 1992). In the acute setting, nephrectomy may also be indicated when the ureteral injury complicates the repair of an abdominal aortic aneurysm or other vascular procedure in which a vascular prosthesis has to be implanted. This is to avoid and lower the chance of urinary leakage, urinoma, sepsis, and graft infection (Lynch et al. 2003). However, most experts suggest the kidney be preserved whenever possible.

15.5.16 Stricture Repair

Ureteral strictures can develop when the blood supply of the ureter is compromised. This can happen after adventitial dissection and disruption of the periureteral blood supply, and may be more common after radiation or gunshot wounds. The ischemic ureter heals with the development of scar tissue. Later the patient will present with complications from ureteral obstruction. Ureteral strictures that are recognized relatively early, that are distal and relatively short (< 2 cm) can be managed endoscopically by dilatation, incision, or stenting. For endoscopic failure, long strictures, or radiated tissue, open surgery should be performed. The size and location of the stricture are the important points to consider when selecting the appropriate surgical procedure.

15.5.17 Future

Prospective studies that investigate ureteral trauma are lacking. In the near future, large trauma centers should consolidate their experience and conduct multi-institutional prospective trials on several issues concerning ureteral injuries (Brandes et al. 2004). These studies must not only include blunt and penetrating trauma, but also iatrogenic injury to the ureter.

References

Adams JR Jr, Mata JA, Culkin DJ et al (1992) Ureteral injury in abdominal vascular reconstructive surgery. Urology 39:77

Al Ali M, Haddad LF (1996) The late treatment of 63 overlooked or complicated ureteral missile injuries: the promise of nephrostomy and role of autotransplantation. J Urol 156:1918

Archbold JA, Barros d'sa AA, Morrison E (1981) Genito-urinary tract injuries of civil hostilities. Br J Surg 68:625

Armenakas NA (1999) Current methods of diagnosis and management of ureteral injuries. World J Urol 17:78

Azimuddin K, Milanesa D, Ivatury R et al (1998) Penetrating ureteric injuries. Injury 29:363

Bejany DE, Lockhart JL, Politano VA (1991) Ileal segment for ureteral substitution or for improvement of ureteral function. J Urol 146:302

Benson MC, Ring KS, Olsson CA (1990) Ureteral reconstruction and bypass: experience with ileal interposition, the Boari flap-psoas hitch and renal autotransplantation. J Urol 143:20

Best CD, Petrone P, Buscarini M et al (2005) Traumatic ureteral injuries: a single institution experience validating the American Association for the Surgery of Trauma-Organ Injury Scale grading scale. J Urol 173:1202

Bluebond-Langner R, Rha KH, Pinto PA et al (2004) Laparoscopic-assisted renal autotransplantation. Urology 63:853

Bodie B, Novick AC, Rose M et al (1986) Long-term results with renal autotransplantation for ureteral replacement. J Urol 136:1187

Boone TB, Gilling PJ, Husmann DA (1993) Ureteropelvic junction disruption following blunt abdominal trauma. J Urol 150:33

Boxer RJ, Fritzsche P, Skinner DG et al (1979) Replacement of the ureter by small intestine: clinical application and results of the ileal ureter in 89 patients. J Urol 121:728

Brandes SB, Chelsky MJ, Buckman RF et al (1994) Ureteral injuries from penetrating trauma. J Trauma 36:766

Brandes S, Coburn M, Armenakas N et al (2004) Diagnosis and management of ureteric injury: an evidence-based analysis. BJU Int 94:277

Bright TC III, Peters PC (1977) Ureteral injuries due to external violence:10 years' experience with 59 cases. J Trauma 17:616

Campbell EW Jr, Filderman PS, Jacobs SC (1992) Ureteral injury due to blunt and penetrating trauma. Urology 40:216

Carl P (1997) Diagnosis and therapy of kidney traumas. Urologe A 36:523

Carley ME, McIntire D, Carley JM et al (2002) Incidence, risk factors and morbidity of unintended bladder or ureter injury during hysterectomy. Int Urogynecol J Pelvic Floor Dysfunct 13:18

Carlton CE Jr, Guthrie AG, Scott R Jr (1969) Surgical correction of ureteral injury. J Trauma 9:457

Carlton CE Jr, Scott R Jr, Guthrie AG (1971) The initial management of ureteral injuries: a report of 78 cases. J Urol 105:335

Daly JW, Higgins KA (1988) Injury to the ureter during gynecologic surgical procedures. Surg Gynecol Obstet 167:19

Dobrowolski Z, Kusionowicz J, Drewniak T et al (2002) Renal and ureteric trauma: diagnosis and management in Poland. BJU Int 89:748

Dorairajan G, Rani PR, Habeebullah S et al (2004) Urological injuries during hysterectomies: a 6-year review. J Obstet Gynaecol Res 30:430

Eickenberg HU, Amin M (1976) Gunshot wounds to the ureter. J Trauma 16:562

Flam TA, Malone MJ, Roth RA (1988) Complications of ureteroscopy. Urol Clin North Am 15:167

Gambone JC, Reiter RC, and Lench JB (1990) Quality assurance indicators and short-term outcome of hysterectomy. Obstet Gynecol 76:841

Gavant ML, Menke PG, Fabian T et al (1995) Blunt traumatic aortic rupture: detection with helical CT of the chest. Radiology 197:125

Gomella LG, Raj GV, Moreno JG (1997) Reverse transcriptase polymerase chain reaction for prostate specific antigen in the management of prostate cancer. J Urol 158:326

Grainger DA, Soderstrom RM, Schiff SF et al (1990) Ureteral injuries at laparoscopy: insights into diagnosis, management, and prevention. Obstet Gynecol 75:839

Harkki-Siren P, Sjoberg J, Kurki T (1999) Major complications of laparoscopy: a follow-up Finnish study. Obstet Gynecol 94:94

Holden S, Hicks CC, O'Brien DP et al (1976) Gunshot wounds of the ureter: a 15-year review of 63 consecutive cases. J Urol 116:562

Huffman JL (1989) Ureteroscopic injuries to the upper urinary tract. Urol Clin North Am 16:249

Hurd WW, Chee SS, Gallagher KL et al (2001) Location of the ureters in relation to the uterine cervix by computed tomography. Am J Obstet Gynecol 184:336

Janzen DL, Zwirewich CV, Breen DJ et al (1998) Diagnostic accuracy of helical CT for detection of blunt bowel and mesenteric injuries. Clin Radiol 53:193

Kenney PJ, Panicek DM, Witanowski LS (1987) Computed tomography of ureteral disruption. J Comput Assist Tomogr 11:480

Kochakarn W, Tirapanich W, Kositchaiwat S (2000) Ileal interposition for the treatment of a long gap ureteral loss. J Med Assoc Thai 83:37

Kuno K, Menzin A, Kauder HH et al (1998) Prophylactic ureteral catheterization in gynecologic surgery. Urology 52:1004

Liapis A, Bakas P, Giannopoulos V et al (2001) Ureteral injuries during gynecological surgery. Int Urogynecol J Pelvic Floor Dysfunct 12:391

Liroff SA, Pontes JE, Pierce JM Jr (1977) Gunshot wounds of the ureter:5 years of experience. J Urol 118:551

Lynch D, Martinez-Pineiro L, Plas E et al (2003) Ureteral trauma. EAU Guidelines on urological trauma, p 25

McAninch JW, Santucci RA (2002) Genitourinary trauma. In: Campbell's urology, 8th edn. Walsh PC, Retik AB, Vaughan AJn et al (eds) Saunders, Philadelphia, p 3707

McGinty DM, Mendez R(1977) Traumatic ureteral injuries with delayed recognition. Urology 10:115
Medina D, Lavery R, Ross SE et al (1998) Ureteral trauma: preoperative studies neither predict injury nor prevent missed injuries. J Am Coll Surg 186:641
Middleton RG (1980) Routine use of the psoas hitch in ureteral reimplantation. J Urol 123:352
Modi P, Goel R, Dodiya S (2005) Laparoscopic ureteroneocystostomy for distal ureteral injuries. Urology 66:751
Moore EE, Cogbill TH, Jurkovich GJ et al (1992) Organ injury scaling. III: Chest wall, abdominal vascular, ureter, bladder, and urethra. J Trauma 33:337
Mulligan JM, Cagiannos I, Collins JP et al (1998) Ureteropelvic junction disruption secondary to blunt trauma: excretory phase imaging (delayed films) should help prevent a missed diagnosis. J Urol 159:67
Nunez D Jr, Becerra JL, Fuentes D et al (1996) Traumatic occlusion of the renal artery: helical CT diagnosis. AJR Am J Roentgenol 167:777
Palmer LS, Rosenbaum RR, Gershbaum MD et al (1999) Penetrating ureteral trauma at an urban trauma center:10-year experience. Urology 54:34
Pfitzenmaier J, Lotz J, Faldum A et al (2003) Metabolic evaluation of 94 patients 5 to 16 years after ileocecal pouch (Mainz pouch 1) continent urinary diversion. J Urol 170:1884
Pitts JC III, Peterson NE (1981) Penetrating injuries of the ureter. J Trauma 21:978
Presti JC Jr, Carroll PR, McAninch JW (1989) Ureteral and renal pelvic injuries from external trauma: diagnosis and management. J Trauma 29:370
Reznichek RC, Brosman SA, Rhodes DB (1973) Ureteral avulsion from blunt trauma. J Urol 109:812
Rober PE, Smith JB, Pierce JM Jr (1990) Gunshot injuries of the ureter. J Trauma 30:83
Selzman AA, Spirnak JP (1996) Iatrogenic ureteral injuries: a 20-year experience in treating 165 injuries. J Urol 155:878
Spirnak JP, Hampel N, Resnick MI (1989) Ureteral injuries complicating vascular surgery: is repair indicated? J Urol 141:13
St Lezin MA, Stoller ML (1991) Surgical ureteral injuries. Urology 38:497
Teber D, Egey A, Gozen AS et al (2005) Ureteral injuries Diagnostic and treatment algorithm.. Urologe A 44:870
Velmahos GC, Degiannis E, Wells M et al (1996) Penetrating ureteral injuries: the impact of associated injuries on management. Am Surg 62:461
Yeong CT, Lim TL, Tan KH (1998) Ureteral injuries in an obstetric and gynaecology teaching hospital. Med J Malaysia 53:51

15.6 Bladder Trauma

N.L. Türkeri

15.6.1 Introduction

Traumatic injury to the bladder is relatively uncommon in adults as well as children. However, the incidence of blunt trauma is rising as a result of modern transportation preferences and increasing reliance on motor vehicles that travel at higher speeds in parallel with advances in engine and mobile parts technology. Therefore, the incidence of intraabdominal and bladder injuries can be expected to rise as well (Espinoza and Rodriguez 1997; Dobrowolski et al. 2002; McGahan et al. 2005). Also, domestic or professional accidents and violence of any sort, including terrorist activities, may contribute to the increasing frequency of intraabdominal and related bladder injury.

Bladder injury seldom represents an immediate threat to life; however, it is often associated with pelvic fractures and other organ injuries, which indicates a major force as the source of injury. Mortality rates over 40% can be expected depending on the severity of accompanying injuries (Rehm et al. 1991). Also, failure of prompt and proper evaluation with subsequent treatment may result in significant and long-term morbidity (Dreitlein et al. 2001).

15.6.2 Etiology and Incidence

Bladder injury may be caused by either external (blunt or penetrating) or iatrogenic trauma, with similar frequencies in general. There is only limited data available in the literature comparing the frequency of external and iatrogenic bladder injuries in the general population. During a 5-year multi-institutional survey from 61 urological departments, Dobrowolski et al. identified 512 cases of bladder injuries, 41% of which resulted from motor vehicle collisions (MVC), 8% from a fall from a height, 2% from crush injury, 0.6% from penetrating injury, and 49% from iatrogenic injury (Dobrowolski et al. 2002).

Similarly, in a retrospective review of hospital charts over a 10-year period, Khan et al. identified 260 patients with bladder injuries, where MVC was responsible in 35% and iatrogenic causes in another 35% of the cases. Falls were responsible in 20% and gunshot wounds in 10% of the injuries (Khan et al. 2004).

15.6.2.1 External Trauma

Blunt Trauma

Approximately 10% of all trauma patients manifest genitourinary involvement (Schneider 1993), and among abdominal injuries that require surgical repair 2% involve the bladder (Carlin and Resnick 1995). Blunt trauma accounts for 67%–86% of traumatic bladder ruptures (McConnell et al. 1982; Carroll and McAninch 1984; Sagalowsky 1998); the rest occur by penetrating or crush injuries. The most common cause (90%) of bladder rupture by blunt trauma is motor vehicle accidents (Flancbaum et al. 1988; Sandler et al. 1998; Morgan et al. 2000). Bladder injury may result from a direct blow to the lower abdomen during the event, usually when the bladder is distended with urine. Transfer of even slight traumatic forces may rupture a urine-filled bladder. When the intravesical pressure is acutely elevated by the traumatic forces, the bladder ruptures at its weakest point, i.e., the dome. A classical example of this type of rupture occurs without associated pelvic ring disruption as a result of seat-belt injury during MVC (Wolk et al. 1985). In contrast, an empty bladder is usually well protected within the bony pelvis and injured by a sharp bony spicule when fractures occur to the bony pelvis (Sandler et al. 1981). However, this classical concept was challenged by Carrol and McAninch, who noted only one-third of bladder injuries occurred on the same side as the pelvic fracture(s) (Carroll and McAninch 1984). This was supported further by Cass and Luxenberg, who proposed that rupture of the empty bladder due to lower abdominal trauma follows a mechanism similar to that involved in intraperitoneal rupture (Cass and Luxenberg 1987). Penetrating or crush injuries may injure the bladder even when it is empty.

Approximately 25% of intraperitoneal bladder ruptures occur in patients without pelvic fracture. These injuries usually occur in patients with a full bladder. The degree of distension of the bladder with urine determines its shape and to some degree the injury it may sustain. An exceedingly light blow may rupture the fully distended bladder, but the empty bladder is seldom injured except by crushing or penetrating wounds (Ben-Menachem et al. 1991). Combined intra- and extraperitoneal rupture may be present in 2%–20% of cases (Sandler et al. 1998; Dreitlein et al. 2001).

Approximately 70%–95% of patients with bladder injuries from blunt trauma have associated pelvic fractures (McConnell et al. 1982; Cass 1989; Aihara et al. 2002). Conversely, up to 30% of patients with pelvic fractures will have some degree of bladder injury due to the major force required to disrupt the integrity of the pelvic ring (Ochsner et al. 1989; Eastridge and Burgess 1997; Dreitlein et al. 2001; Inaba et al. 2004). Pubic symphysis diastasis, sacroiliac diastasis, and sacral, iliac, and pubic rami fractures are significantly associated with bladder rupture, whereas isolated acetabular fractures are not (Morgan et al. 2000; Aihara et al. 2002). The majority of the associated pelvic fractures are of the pubic ramus (Cass 1989), and widening of symphysis pubis is the strongest predictor of bladder injury (Aihara et al. 2002). However, a major bladder injury occurs only in 5%–10% of patients suffering from pelvic fractures (Reed 1976; Bond et al. 1991). Thus, there is a strong association between pelvic fractures and bladder injury, and these fractures are a major cause of death and long-term morbidity in blunt trauma (Coppola and Coppola 2000; Inaba et al. 2004). Motor vehicle accidents remain the leading cause of pelvic fractures, accounting for 44%–64% of these injuries (Gokcen et al. 1994; Ferrera and Hill 1999; Coppola and Coppola 2000). The force required to disrupt the pelvic ring is easily achieved by the massive energy transfer from colliding vehicles, especially in lateral-impact crashes on the occupant's side (Siegel et al. 1993; Loo et al. 1996). This force has also been shown to result in associated damage to the surrounding abdominal organs (Fallon et al. 1984; Failinger and McGanity 1992; Muir et al. 1996). Up to 90% of patients with pelvic fractures may have associated injuries (an average of 2.9) in multiple organ systems (Flancbaum et al. 1988; Poole et al. 1992; Brenneman et al. 1997; Adams et al. 2002), with a mortality rate of 22%–44% (Cass 1989; Rehm et al. 1991; Siegmeth et al. 2000). Analysis of 42,283 trauma admissions from a registry at Los Angeles County and the University of Southern California identified the incidence of pelvic fractures as 9.3% (1,545 patients) among 16,630 blunt trauma cases (Demetriades et al. 2002). Pedestrians involved in an accident comprise the largest group (41.8%), followed by car occupants in MVC (39.1%), falls from a height (12.9%), and motorcycle accidents (3%). In this population, motorcycle injuries were associated with the highest incidence of pelvic fractures (15.5%) followed by pedestrian injuries (13.8%). Only 8.9% (137/1,545) of the pelvic fractures were classified as severe [Abbreviated Injury Impairment Scale (AIS)$\geq$4] and the overall incidence of bladder and urethral injuries was 5.8% (90/1,545), second after liver injuries(6.1%). Although no details were provided on bladder injury alone, the authors identified bladder and urethra as the most commonly injured organs (14.6%) in the presence of severe pelvic fractures (AIS $\geq$4).

Similar pelvic fracture rates (11.9%–12.1%) were observed in trauma patients admitted to American level 1 and 2 centers (Clancy et al. 2001). These figures were also corroborated by trauma registry data (8%–14%) from the UK (Muir et al. 1996; Bircher and Giannoudis 2004).

Penetrating Trauma

Incidence of penetrating trauma due to firearms is rare in the general population (Selikowitz 1977; Tiguert et al. 2000). However, a rising incidence can be expected due to their increasing use in society. A survey in Poland reported the incidence of penetrating injuries as 0.6%; all were due to gunshots (Dobrowolski et al. 2002). In contrast, a series from South Africa (Madiba and Haffejee 1999) reported the incidence of penetrating injuries as 55.8%; 89.5% of them were firearm injuries. Penetrating bladder injuries are also commonly associated with major abdominal and vascular injuries, with a mortality rate of 12%–14% in stable patients and 50% in those presenting with shock (Duncan et al. 1989; Madiba and Haffejee 1999).

15.6.2.2 Pediatric Trauma

It has been proposed that children have lower incidence of lower urinary tract injuries due to the elastic nature of their pelvis. Comparison of data for 23,700 children registered in the National Pediatric Trauma Registry with 10,720 adults recorded over a period of 5 years in a level I trauma center (Ismail et al. 1996) revealed significantly lower pelvic fracture and mortality rates in children (3% vs 5%; $p<0.001$ and 5.7% vs 17.5%; $p<0.001$). Several studies in the pediatric population investigating pelvic fractures and associated injuries similarly reported a lower incidence of urogenital injury ranging from 0.5% to 18.6%, in comparison to adult series (Rehm et al. 1991; Coppola and Coppola 2000). Data from seven different pediatric series identified the average rate of bladder injury as 3.6% (26/711) in patients with pelvic fractures (Reed 1976; Reichard et al. 1980; Torode and Zieg 1985; Musemeche et al. 1987; Bond et al. 1991; Koraitim et al. 1996; Tarman et al. 2002) (Table 15.6.1). The mechanisms of injury in these series were motor vehicles striking pedestrians (59%–90%), MVCs involving occupants (10%–32%), and falls from a height (2%–9%).

15.6.2.3 Iatrogenic Trauma

The bladder is the most frequently injured genitourinary organ during lower abdominal operations (Armenakas et al. 2004). Most of the iatrogenic injuries occur during open abdominal or pelvic surgery (85%), anterior vaginal surgery (9%), and laparoscopy (6%), as reflected by a single-institution series over 12 years. The majority (92%) of the cases were American Association for the Surgery of Trauma (AAST) grade III–IV. Most of the injuries resulted from obstetric and gynecological procedures (61.5%), followed by general surgical (26.2%) and urological (12.3%) interventions (Armenakas et al. 2004). In a multi-institutional study from Poland, the incidence of iatrogenic bladder injuries was 49%, and these were due to gynecologic procedures in 52%, urological in 39%, and general surgical in 9% of the cases (Dobrowolski et al. 2002).

Classic gynecological operations have a reported incidence of bladder injury in 0.3%–5% of cases in different series (Harkki-Siren et al. 1998; Gilmour et al. 1999; Makinen et al. 2001; Mendez 2001). In a prospective multicenter study, where cystoscopy was performed universally at the end of every procedure, Vakili et al. recorded the incidence of urinary tract injuries in 471 patients undergoing abdominal (TAH), vaginal (TVH) or laparoscopic hysterectomy (LH) for benign diseases over 3 years and reported the overall incidence of bladder injuries to be 3.6% (Vakili et al. 2005). Although there was a trend toward a higher incidence of bladder injury with TVH, there was no statistically significant difference in the rate of bladder injury among TAH, TVH, and LH procedures (2.5%, 6.3%, and 2.0%, respectively; $p=0.123$) in this series. However, concurrent anti-incontinence surgery was significantly associated with injury to the bladder (12.5% vs 3.1%; $p=0.049$). The limitations of transvaginal exposure, the variable thickness of the anterior vaginal wall and the proximity of the bladder base to the operative field may explain the potential for bladder injury in transvaginal procedures (Armenakas et al. 2004). Routine cystoscopy is an important adjunct to the major gynecological procedures and its omission may result in underestimation of iatrogenic bladder injury. An extensive review of the literature by Gilmour et al. indicated that in the reports of studies not involving routine cystoscopy, the frequency of bladder injury varied from 0.2 to 19.5 per 1,000, with an overall frequency of 2.6 per 1,000, and consequently only 51.6% of bladder injuries were identified and managed intraoperatively (Gilmour et al. 1999). In the reports of studies involving routine cystoscopy, the frequency of bladder injury varied from 0 to 29.2 per 1,000, with an overall frequency of 10.4 per 1,000; up to 85% of unsuspected bladder injuries were identified with the use of cystoscopy and were managed successfully intraoperatively (Gilmour et al. 1999).

It has also been proposed that the recent increase in laparoscopic procedures might result in an increase in the incidence of iatrogenic bladder injuries. In more than 10,000 cases, Makinen et al. found the highest incidence of bladder injury with laparoscopic hysterectomy (1.3%) compared to TAH (0.5%) and TVH (0.2%), with a relative risk of 2.7 ($p<0.0001$) (Makinen et al. 2001). It was also noted that surgeons' increasing experience had an effect on decreasing the incidence of

Table 15.6.1. Incidence of bladder injury in children with pelvic fractures

Study	Bladder injury rate
Reichard et al.	4.2%
Reed	5.9%
Torode and Zieg	2.8%
Musemeche et al.	1.8%
Bond et al.	3.7%
Koraitim et al.	18.6%
Tarman et al.	0.5%

severe urinary tract injuries. In a thorough review of the literature, Ostrzenski and Ostrzenska found an incidence of laparoscopic bladder injury ranging from 0.02 % to 8.3 %, with the majority occurring during laparoscopic hysterectomy (40 %) and diagnostic laparoscopy (24 %) (Ostrzenski and Ostrzenska 1998). An intraoperative diagnosis of bladder injury was made in 53.2 % of all bladder injury cases and the bladder dome was the most commonly injured structure. Most of the injuries occur by sharp electrosurgical dissection leading to laceration during mobilization of the bladder from the diseased adjacent organ, although it may result from devascularization as well (Ostrzenski and Ostrzenska 1998; Armenakas et al. 2004).

Surgical procedures for the correction of stress urinary incontinence may result in bladder trauma as well. The tension-free vaginal tape (TVT) procedure is a relatively new treatment modality (Ulmsten 2001), and bladder injury is the most common complication of this procedure, with an incidence of 2 %–11.5 % reported in published series (Olsson and Kroon 1999; Meschia et al. 2001; Soulie et al. 2001; Tamussino et al. 2001). This rate can be as high as 19 % in patients with prior failed incontinence surgery (Azam et al. 2001). In a survey of 12,280 TVT procedures in France, Agostini et al. reported a bladder injury rate of 7.4 % (Agostini et al. 2005). This was slightly higher than two previously reported series that reported bladder injuries in 3.8 % (Kuuva and Nilsson 2002) and 2.7 % (Tamussino et al. 2001) of cases in nation-wide analysis in Finland and Austria, respectively.

The transobturator tape (TOT) procedure as described by Delorme minimizes the retropubic needle passage (Delorme 2001) and a decrease in the incidence of bladder injury can be expected. However, early experience with this technique similar rates of injury showed to the TVT procedure. Minaglia et al. reported their incidence of bladder injury with TOT as 4.9 % and recommended routine cystoscopy since it allowed identification of unsuspected bladder injury in two-thirds of patients (Minaglia et al. 2004).

General surgical procedures account for 23 %–26 % of the iatrogenic cases (Dobrowolski et al. 2002; Armenakas et al. 2004). The majority of these operations involve resection of bowel due to malignancy, diverticulitis, or inflammatory diseases.

Urological interventions are responsible for 12 %–39 % of the cases of iatrogenic bladder injury. Vaginal operations and laparoscopy are the type of interventions in most of these instances. Although the incidence of bladder wall perforation varies among different series, it is generally low (1 %) during transurethral resection of bladder tumors; the great majority (88 %) can be managed by catheter drainage (Murshidi 1988; Skolarikos et al. 2005). Transurethral resection of the prostate has even lower rates of injury (Weber et al. 1987).

15.6.3 Classification

Injury to the bladder can be classified based on the anatomical site (extraperitoneal with leakage of urine limited to the perivesical space, intraperitoneal in which the peritoneal surface has been disrupted with concomitant urinary extravasation or combined), etiologic factors such as external trauma (blunt or penetrating injuries), iatrogenic or spontaneous bladder injury. A classification of bladder injury based on cystographic patterns of extravasation has been developed with the following characteristic imaging features (Sandler et al. 1986) (Table 15.6.2). In bladder contusion (type 1), findings are normal. In intraperitoneal rupture (type 2), cystography demonstrates intraperitoneal contrast material around bowel loops, between mesenteric folds, and in the paracolic gutters. Manifestations of interstitial injury (type 3) include intramural hemorrhage and submucosal extravasation of contrast material without transmural extension. In extraperitoneal rupture (type 4), extravasation is confined to the perivesical space in simple extraperitoneal ruptures, whereas in complex extraperitoneal ruptures, contrast material extends beyond the perivesical space and may dissect into a variety of fascial planes and spaces. Combined intra- and extraperitoneal rupture (type 5) usually demonstrates extravasation patterns that are typical for both types of injury. A rather simplistic classification based on the mechanism of injury has also been defined (Dreitlein et al. 2001) (Table 15.6.3). The Committee on Organ Injury Scaling of the American Association for the Surgery of Trauma has developed a bladder injury scaling system that defines the anatomical location as well as the extent of injury (Moore et al. 1992), and it is suggested to be used for greater accuracy in trauma staging (Armenakas et al. 2004). This may make it possible to standardize and compare the acquired data on bladder trauma research. The AAST organ injury severity scale for the bladder appears in Table 15.6.4 (Figs. 15.6.1–6).

Table 15.6.2. Classification of bladder injury

Type 1	Bladder contusion
Type 2	Intraperitoneal rupture
Type 3	Interstitial bladder injury
Type 4	Extraperitoneal rupture
	A. Simple
	B. Complex
Type 5	Combined injury

The pelvic fractures that are seen in the majority of the patients with bladder trauma can be classified either mechanistically using the Young-Burgess system (Young et al. 1986; Young and Resnik 1990) or based on the stability and mechanism, e.g., the Tile and Pennal

Table 15.6.3. Classification of bladder injury based on the type of trauma

Classification of injury		Mechanism of injury	Associated injuries
Blunt trauma	Extraperitoneal	Blunt pelvic trauma with laceration by bone fragment(s)	Pelvic fractures
		Shearing at ligamentous attachment(s)	Other long bone fractures
	Intraperitoneal	High velocity blunt lower abdominal trauma	High rate of associated intraabdominal injuries
		High intravesical pressure with rupture at dome	High mortality
Penetrating trauma		Direct injury to the bladder wall	Associated injury to other organs is common

Table 15.6.4. AAST organ injury severity scale for the bladder and Associated Abbreviated Injury Scale of the American Association for Automotive Medicine, 1990 (AIS-90)

Grade[a]	Injury type	Description of injury	AIS-90
I	Hematoma	Contusion, intramural hematoma	2
I	Laceration	Partial thickness	3
II	Laceration	Extraperitoneal bladder wall laceration <2 cm	4
III	Laceration	Extraperitoneal (>2 cm) or intraperitoneal (<2 cm) bladder wall laceration	4
IV	Laceration	Intraperitoneal bladder wall laceration >2 cm	4
V	Laceration	Intraperitoneal or extraperitoneal bladder wall laceration extending into the bladder neck or ureteral orifice (trigone)	4

[a] Advance one grade for multiple injuries to same organ up to grade III

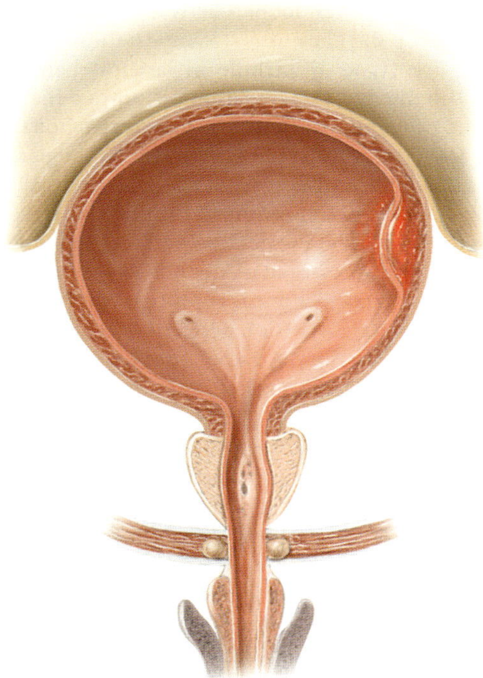

Fig. 15.6.1. AAST classification of bladder injury. Grade 1: contusion, intramural hematoma or partial thickness laceration of the bladder wall (Fig. 15.6.1–6 © Hohenfellner 2007)

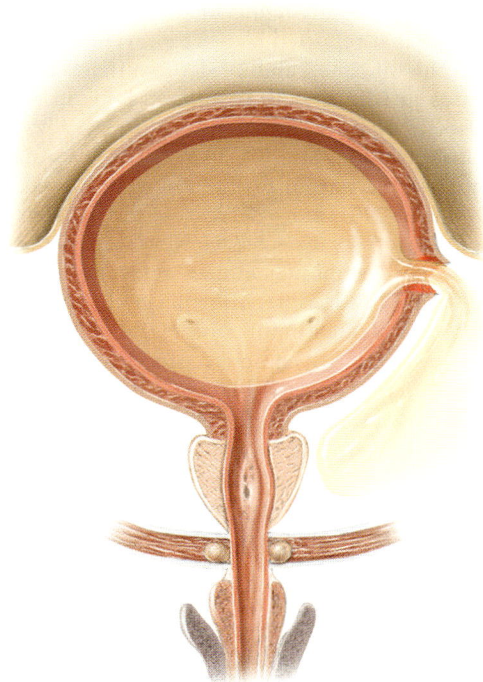

Fig. 15.6.2. AAST classification of bladder injury. Grade 2: extraperitoneal laceration of the bladder wall <2 cm

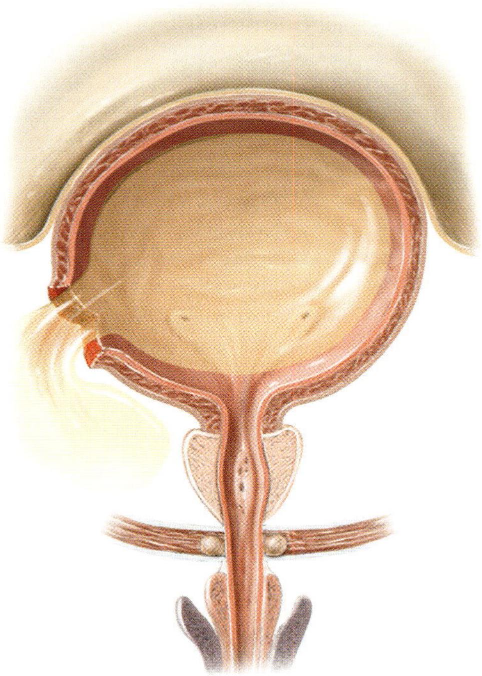

Fig. 15.6.3. AAST classification of bladder injury. Grade 3: extraperitoneal laceration of the bladder wall > 2 cm

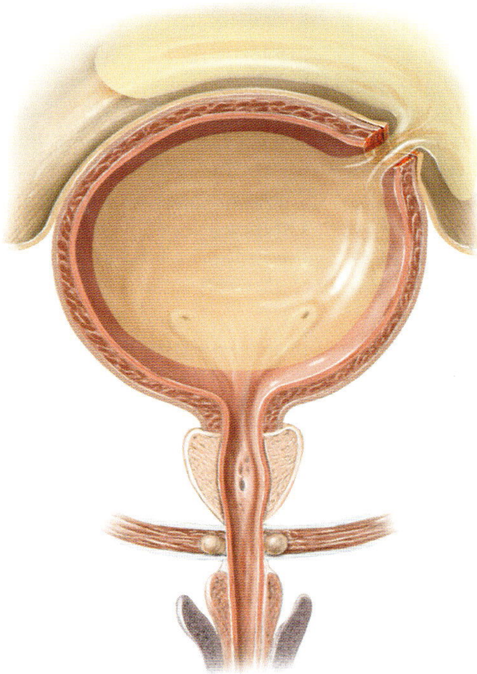

Fig. 15.6.4. AAST classification of bladder injury. Grade 3: intraperitoneal laceration of the bladder wall < 2 cm

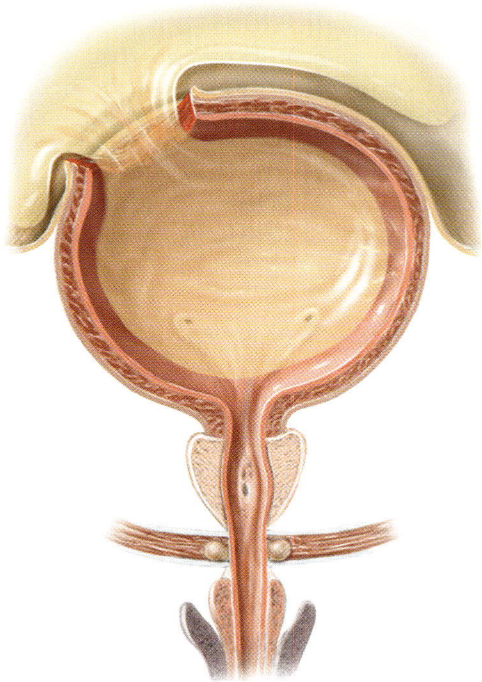

Fig. 15.6.5. AAST classification of bladder injury. Grade 4: intraperitoneal laceration of the bladder wall > 2 cm

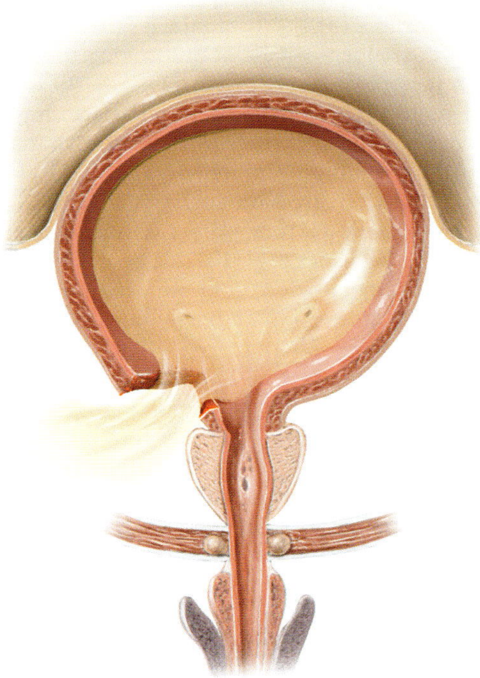

Fig. 15.6.6. AAST classification of bladder injury. Grade 5: intraperitoneal or extraperitoneal laceration of the bladder wall extending in to the bladder neck or trigone

classification, which was adopted, modified, and recommended by the Orthopaedic Trauma Association (OTA) (Tile 1988, 1996; OTA 1996). The OTA classification groups pelvic injuries into three main categories: A-type injuries have a stable pelvic ring, B-type have a partial posterior disruption, and C-type have a complete posterior disruption. Within this classification, the severity of injury increases from type A to type C (Tile 1999), with a higher injury severity score (ISS), incidence of associated injuries, and mortality rate with the latter (Poole et al. 1991; Adams et al. 2002).

15.6.4 Risk Factors

15.6.4.1 Blunt Trauma

Driving under the influence of alcohol predisposes to motor vehicle accidents and to a distended bladder as well. Thus it is a risk factor for bladder injury (Dreitlein et al. 2001).

Lateral-impact MVC are known to be associated with an increased incidence of pelvic fractures (Siegel et al. 1993; Loo et al. 1996; Inaba et al. 2004; Rowe et al. 2004), and therefore may result in bladder injury. Crash impact data in trauma registry for MVC occupants with AIS ≥ 4 pelvic injuries identified the lateral impact as the most common crash variable, accounting for more than 80 % of injuries to drivers and front seat passengers (Inaba et al. 2004). An evaluation of risk factors for severe pelvic injuries (AIS ≥ 4) suggested motorcycle injuries to result in the highest incidence of pelvic fractures, with bladder and urethra as the most commonly injured organs. In this study, stepwise logistic regression analysis identified male gender and pelvic fracture AIS ≥ 4 as independent risk factors (Demetriades et al. 2002). These patients also had significantly more genitourinary injuries, the bladder being the most common (25 %) intraabdominal organ injured.

15.6.4.2 Iatrogenic Trauma

Risk factors for iatrogenic bladder injury include adhesions and pelvic scarring from previous surgery, inflammation, endometriosis, exposure to radiation, presence of malignant disease, pregnancy, pelvic organ prolapse, multiple cesarean sections, congenital abnormalities, hemorrhage, or failure to empty the bladder before the operation (Daly and Higgins 1988; Harris et al. 1997; Davis 1999; Armenakas et al. 2004; Gomez et al. 2004; Yossepowitch et al. 2004). In a multicenter study, concurrent surgery for stress incontinence along with gynecological procedures was found to be the only independent variable for bladder injury in a stepwise logistic regression model, with a relative risk of 4.42 (Vakili et al. 2005). The type of incision during cesarean section is also a risk factor. In a retrospective analysis of data from 3,164 women undergoing cesarean section revealed that the type of incision, the presence of adhesions, and anterior placenta previa were independently associated with increased risk of bladder injury (Makoha et al. 2005). The bladder was injured almost seven times as frequently with the midline subumbilical (MLSU) as with the Pfannenstiel incision ($p < 0.0001$; OR, 6.7). This study has also confirmed the observation that for both types of incision the risk of bladder injury increases with the number of cesarean sections (Makoha et al. 2004) and for a given number the risk is higher with MLSU than Pfannenstiel incision.

15.6.5 Diagnosis

The two most common signs and symptoms of major bladder injuries are gross hematuria (82 %) and abdominal tenderness (62 %) (Carroll and McAninch 1984). Other findings may include inability to void, bruises over the suprapubic region, and abdominal distention (Sagalowsky 1998). Extravasation of urine may result in swelling in the perineum, scrotum, and thighs, as well as along the anterior abdominal wall within the potential space between the transversalis fascia and the parietal peritoneum. Hematuria at the conclusion of an otherwise uneventful procedure, clear fluid in the operative field, gas distention of the urinary drainage bag during laparoscopy, and/or visible bladder laceration should alarm the surgeon to iatrogenic bladder injury (Armenakas et al. 2004; Gomez et al. 2004)

15.6.5.1 Macroscopic (Gross) Hematuria

Gross hematuria indicates urologic trauma. Review of the existing literature reveals that traumatic bladder rupture is strongly correlated with the combination of pelvic fracture and gross hematuria. Morey et al. reported gross hematuria in all of their patients with bladder rupture, and 85 % had pelvic fractures (Morey et al. 2001). Therefore, the classic combination of pelvic fracture and gross hematuria constitutes an absolute indication for immediate cystography in blunt trauma victims (Carroll and McAninch 1984; Rehm et al. 1991; Morey 2005). While grossly clear urine in a trauma patient without a pelvic fracture virtually eliminates the possibility of a bladder rupture, up to 2 % – 10 % of patients with bladder rupture may have only microhematuria or no hematuria at all (Schneider 1993).

Tarman et al. (2002) reviewed 8,021 pediatric trauma patients retrospectively, including 212 consecutive patients with pelvic fractures. Among patients with pelvic fractures, only one patient (0.5%) had an extraperitoneal bladder rupture. Lower urogenital injury occurred in six patients (2.8%). The absence of gross hematuria effectively ruled out serious injury in this cohort. Consequently, these authors concluded that further urological work-up is unnecessary in stable patients with pelvic fractures and isolated microhematuria. Patients with gross hematuria, multiple associated injuries, or significant abnormalities found on their physical examination are recommended to undergo further urological evaluation with appropriate imaging modalities such as retrograde urethrography and cystography.

15.6.5.2 Microscopic Hematuria

In the trauma patient with a pelvic ring fracture, microscopic hematuria should be considered as a possible indicator of bladder laceration, and further investigation is warranted. Existing data do not support lower urinary tract imaging in all patients with either pelvic fracture or microscopic hematuria alone. Also, the threshold of red blood cells in urine that triggers further investigation is a point of controversy. A threshold ranging from 25 to 200 red blood cells per high power field (rbc/phf) has been suggested to indicate significant injury to the bladder (Werkman et al. 1991; Fuhrman et al. 1993; Morgan et al. 2000). These observations seems not to be valid for pediatric trauma patients, as indicated previously in a clinical series (Tarman et al. 2002). In contrast, Abou-Jaoude et al. found that a threshold of 20 rbc/hpf as an indication for radiological evaluation would have missed 25% of cases with bladder injury. In contrast to other reported series, they suggested that lower urogenital tract evaluation in pediatric trauma patients, especially in the presence of pelvic fractures, should be based as much on clinical judgment as on the presence of hematuria (Abou-Jaoude et al. 1996).

15.6.5.3 Cystography

Retrograde cystography in evaluation of bladder trauma is considered the standard diagnostic procedure (Stine et al. 1988; Rehm et al. 1991; Baniel and Schein 1994). Cystography is accepted as the most accurate radiological study for diagnosing bladder rupture (Deck et al. 2000). When adequate bladder filling and post-void images are obtained, they have an accuracy rate of 85%–100%. The diagnosis of bladder rupture is usually made easily on cystography when the injected contrast medium is identified outside the bladder

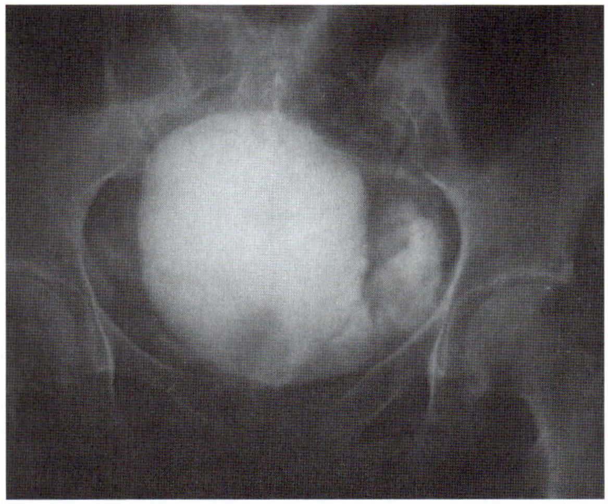

Fig. 15.6.7. Extraperitoneal rupture demonstrated on cystography. Extravasation of contrast material is limited to the perivesical space

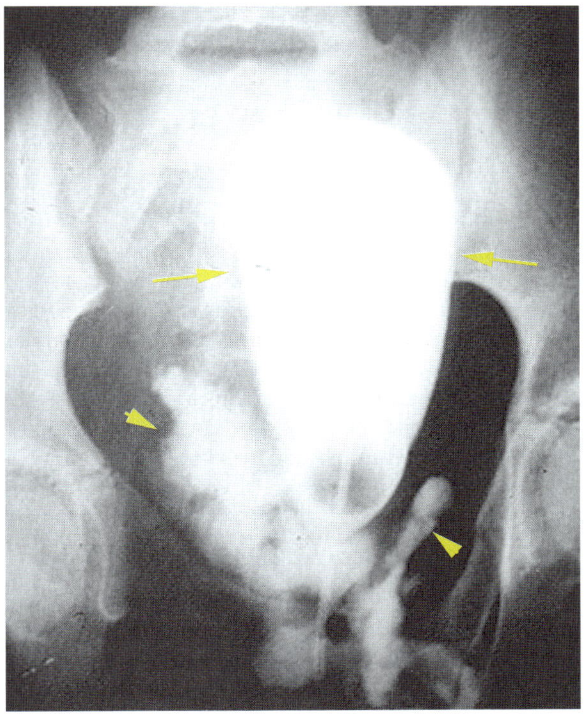

Fig. 15.6.8. Extraperitoneal rupture on cystography

(Figs. 15.6.7–9). Adequate distention of the urinary bladder is crucial to demonstrate perforation, especially in instances of penetrating trauma, since most instances of a false-negative retrograde cystography were found in this situation (Cass 1984; Baniel and Schein 1994). Cystography requires at least plain films, filled films, and postdrainage films. Half-filled film and obliques are optional. For the highest diagnostic accuracy, the bladder must be distended by instillation of at

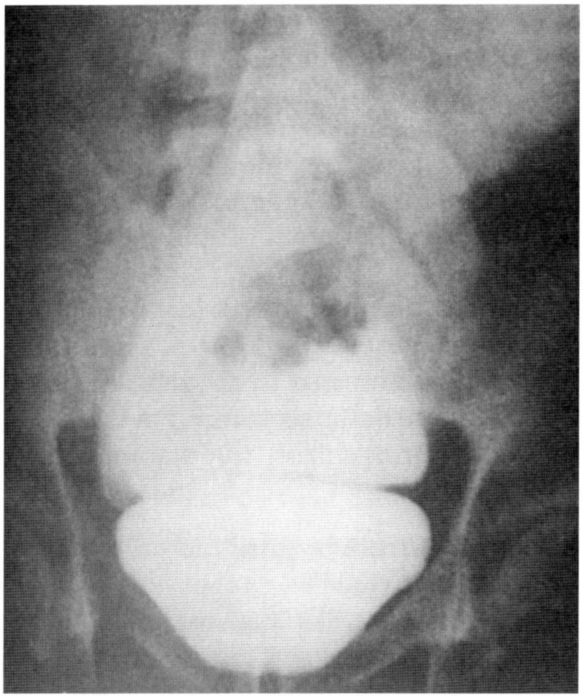

Fig. 15.6.9. Intraperitoneal bladder rupture on cystography. Bowel loops are outlined by the extravasated contrast in the abdominal cavity

least 350 cc of contrast medium with gravity. Bladder injury may be identified only on the postdrainage film in approximately 10 % of the cases. False-negative findings may result from improperly performed studies with instillation of less than 250 ml of contrast medium or omission of a postdrainage film (Morey et al. 1999). Only a properly performed cystography should be used to exclude bladder injury.

15.6.5.4 Excretory Urography (Intravenous Pyelography)

Intravenous pyelography (IVP) is inadequate for evaluation of bladder and urethra after trauma because of dilution of the contrast material within the bladder, and resting intravesical pressure is simply too low to demonstrate a small tear (Ben-Menachem et al. 1991) IVP has a low accuracy, on the order of 15 % – 25 % and various clinical studies indicated that IVP has an unacceptably high false-negative rate of 64 % – 84 %, which precludes its use as a diagnostic tool in bladder injuries (Werkman et al. 1991).

15.6.5.5 Ultrasound

Although the use of US in bladder rupture has been described (Bigongiari et al. 2000), it has not been routinely used for evaluation of bladder injury. The presence of peritoneal fluid in the presence of normal viscera or failure to visualize the bladder after the transurethral introduction of saline is considered highly suggestive of bladder rupture (Bigongiari et al. 2000). In practice, US is not definitive in bladder or urethral trauma and is not routinely used. Focused abdominal sonography for trauma (FAST) has gained popularity in the evaluation of blunt abdominal trauma in adults to detect free intraperitoneal fluid, with a sensitivity of 63 % – 99 % in published series (Fernandez et al. 1998; Yoshii et al. 1998; Nunes et al. 2001; Von Kuenssberg Jehle et al. 2003).

Several reports have indicated that FAST can also reliably detect free intraperitoneal fluid in children, with acceptable sensitivity and specificity rates (Holmes et al. 2001; Soudack et al. 2004). However, a positive FAST in a hemodynamically stable child is of limited use, because in one survey only 26 % (5/19) of pediatric emergency attending physicians considered ultrasound equally available with CT, and none considered it more readily available than CT (Baka et al. 2002). The inability of FAST to distinguish the origin of free fluid in the abdomen such as blood, ascites, or urine remains another disadvantage of this modality (Jones et al. 2003).

Therefore, the exact role of FAST in detection of bladder injury remains to be determined.

15.6.5.6 Computed Tomography

CT is clearly the method of choice for the evaluation of patients with blunt or penetrating abdominal and/or pelvic trauma. However, routine CT is not reliable in the diagnosis of bladder rupture even if an inserted urethral catheter is clamped. CT demonstrates intraperitoneal and extraperitoneal fluid but cannot differentiate urine from ascites. As with IVP, the bladder is usually inadequately distended to cause extravasation through a bladder laceration or perforation during routine abdominal and pelvic studies. Therefore, a negative study cannot be entirely trusted, and routine CT therefore cannot rule out bladder injury (Mee et al. 1987; Cass 1989; Ben-Menachem et al. 1991). Horstman et al. reviewed the cystograms and CT scans of 25 patients who had both studies as the initial evaluation of blunt abdominal trauma (Horstman et al. 1991). Five out of 25 had bladder rupture, three extraperitoneal and two intraperitoneal. All injuries were detected by both studies. The authors felt that delayed imaging or contrast instillation (CT cystography) can provide the adequate bladder distention needed to demonstrate contrast extravasation from the injury site during CT. Similarly, in a series of 316 patients, Deck et al. diagnosed 44 cases with bladder ruptures. In patients who underwent formal surgical repair, 82 % had operative findings that exactly matched the CT cystography interpretation (Deck et al. 2000). Thus, either retrograde cystography or CT cystography are the diagnostic procedures of choice for suspected bladder injury (Schneider 1993). CT cystography may be used in place of a conventional cystography (overall sensitivity 95% and specificity 100%), especially in patients undergoing CT scanning for other associated injuries (Deck et al. 2001). However, this procedure should be performed using retrograde filling of the bladder with a minimum of 350 cc of dilute contrast material (Wah and Spencer 2001).

CT cystographic features may lead to accurate classification of bladder injury (Figs. 15.6.10, 11) and allow prompt, effective treatment with less radiation exposure and without the added cost of conventional cystography (Vaccaro and Brody 2000).

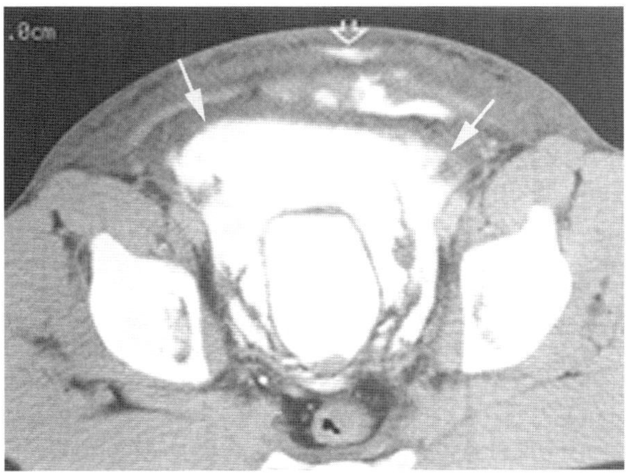

Fig. 15.6.10. CT cystography demonstrating extraperitoneal extravasation of contrast material

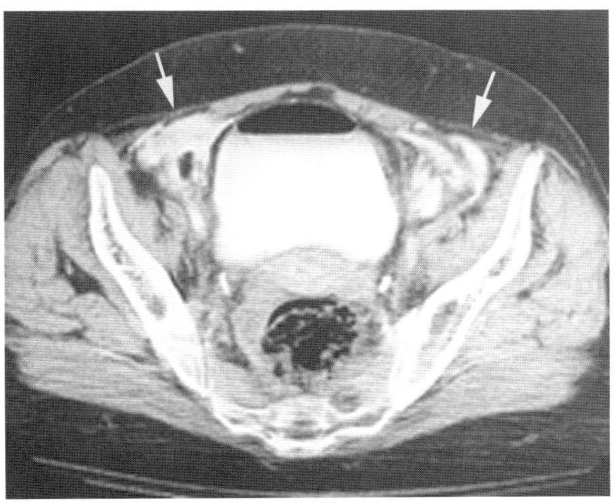

Fig. 15.6.11. Extraperitoneal rupture on CT cystography

15.6.5.7 Angiography

Angiography is rarely if ever indicated. It can be useful in identifying an occult source of bleeding and for therapeutic embolization (Ben-Menachem et al. 1991).

15.6.5.8 Magnetic Resonance Imaging

Since it is extremely difficult to monitor a seriously injured patient in a strong magnetic field, MRI currently has little place in the evaluation of acute bladder (Ben-Menachem et al. 1991).

15.6.5.9 Cystoscopy

Cystoscopy appears an extremely useful tool in the diagnosis of iatrogenic bladder injuries. The results of a multicenter study as well as a comprehensive review of the literature indicated that the majority (49.4%–64.7%) of bladder injuries during gynecological operations would be missed if cystoscopy were not performed at the end of each procedure (Gilmour et al. 1999; Vakili et al. 2005). The detection rate of bladder injury by cystoscopy ranges from 85% to 94.1% in different series (Harris et al. 1997; Vakili et al. 2005).

15.6.6 Treatment

The first priority in the treatment of bladder injuries is stabilization of the patient and treatment of associated life-threatening injuries.

15.6.6.1 Blunt Trauma: Extraperitoneal Rupture

Most patients with extraperitoneal rupture can be managed safely by catheter drainage only, even in the presence of extensive retroperitoneal or scrotal extravasation. Virtually all ruptures are healed in 3 weeks (Morey et al. 1999). However, involvement of the bladder neck (Carroll and McAninch 1984), the presence of bone fragments in the bladder wall, or entrapment of the bladder wall necessitate surgical intervention (Dreitlein et al. 2001). In the absence of bladder neck involvement and/or associated injuries that require surgical intervention such as open pelvic fractures and rectal or vaginal lacerations, extraperitoneal bladder ruptures caused by blunt trauma are managed by catheter drainage only (Cass and Luxenberg 1987). The presence of open pelvic fractures and/or rectal injuries precludes conservative management due to the high risk of serious infectious complications (Cass and Luxenberg 1989). In patients undergoing surgery for other organ injuries, the laceration of the bladder wall should also be repaired transvesically, if the patient is stable at the time of the operation (Gomez et al. 2004).

15.6.6.2
Blunt Trauma: Intraperitoneal Rupture

Intraperitoneal ruptures occurring after blunt trauma should always be managed by surgical exploration. This type of injury involves a high degree of force, and because of the severity of associated injuries carries a high mortality rate of 20 % – 40 % (Cass 1989; Rehm et al. 1991). Lacerations are usually large in these instances with potential risk of peritonitis due to urine leakage, if left untreated (Deck et al. 2000). Abdominal organs should be inspected for possible associated injuries, and urinoma must be drained. The technique of surgical repair depends on the surgeon's preference but a two-layer closure with absorbable sutures achieves a safe repair of the bladder wall. A suprapubic catheter can be used in addition to a urethral catheter to ensure the adequacy of the drainage. However, in a recent study, patients with Foley catheter drainage alone had equally good outcome (Volpe et al. 1999).

15.6.6.3
Penetrating Trauma

All bladder perforations due to a penetrating trauma should undergo emergency exploration and repair (Deck et al. 2000). Penetrating trauma to the pelvis presents a serious challenge because of the complex anatomy of the region. Penetrating trauma patients presenting with shock have a high incidence of vascular injury and subsequent exsanguination, and associated visceral injuries may complicate their management, resulting in a high mortality rate. However, stable patients can be managed without operation, when appropriate diagnostic techniques fail to demonstrate an injury (Duncan et al. 1989). Gunshot wounds to the bladder usually result in intraperitoneal leaks, which require proper drainage and repair of the associated lacerations of the bladder wall as well as adjacent organs. However, in the occasional patient with extraperitoneal rupture, nonoperative management with Foley catheter drainage can be used successfully (Velmahos and Degiannis 1997).

15.6.6.4
Iatrogenic Trauma

In patients with immediate diagnosis, bladder repair accomplished by a transabdominal or transvaginal two-layer closure effectively treats 98 % of cases and the rest are managed by Foley catheter drainage (Armenakas et al. 2004).

15.6.6.5
Complications

In patients with bladder trauma, complications are usually the result of failure to diagnose the injury and repair promptly. This may result in urinoma formation, urinary leakage into the peritoneal cavity, ileus, peritonitis, hematoma, abscess formation, fistula formation (rectal, vaginal, or cutaneous), and urinary tract infection.

Bladder injury with extravasation of urine with or without prostatic injury may complicate the course of recovery by impairing the coagulation mechanism. The prostatic capsule contains abundant activators of plasminogen and urine contains high levels of urokinase, a potent plasminogen activator (Andersson 1980). Both tissue activator and urokinase accelerate the dissolution of clots and may consequently increase and prolong hemorrhage (Hedlund 1969). Epsilon amino caproic acid (EACA) can be effective in controlling hematuria after surgical procedures compared with placebo, and its use was not accompanied by significant complications (Miller et al. 1980). Tranexamic acid (aminomethyl cyclohexane carboxylic acid, AMCA) is a stronger inhibitor of plasminogen activation than EACA and may significantly decrease the amount of blood loss and control the bleeding when administered in a total dose of 3 – 12 g for 4 – 21 days (Hedlund 1975; Dunn and Goa 1999) without any increase in the incidence of thrombosis compared to placebo (Hedlund 1975).

Early angiography and transcatheter embolization in patients with major blood requirements after pelvic trauma may help to avoid the need for and complications of multiple transfusions and large pelvic hematomas. Precise localization of bleeding sites and occlusion of the bleeding artery by either an injection of autologous clot or Gelfoam embolization can be successfully achieved (Matalon et al. 1979; Wong et al. 2000; Ben-Menachem 1988).

15.6.7
Damage Control

Severe multiple traumatic injuries may cause acidosis, hypothermia, and coagulopathy, which have been associated with very high mortality rates (Zacharias et al. 1999). Focusing the initial resuscitative efforts to stabilize the patient with the control of the hemorrhage (temporary packing) and gross contamination along with appropriate bladder drainage with and subsequent intensive care may allow for later definitive repair of the injuries in a patient who will otherwise die.

References

Abou-Jaoude WA et al (1996) Indicators of genitourinary tract injury or anomaly in cases of pediatric blunt trauma. J Pediatr Surg 31:86; discussion 90
Adams JE et al (2002) Analysis of the incidence of pelvic trauma in fatal automobile accidents. Am J Forensic Med Pathol 23:132
Agostini A et al (2006) Immediate complications of tension-free vaginal tape (TVT): results of a French Survey. Eur J Obstet Gynecol Reprod Biol 124:237
Aihara R et al (2002) Fracture locations influence the likelihood of rectal and lower urinary tract injuries in patients sustaining pelvic fractures. J Trauma 52:205; discussion 208
Andersson L (1980) Antifibrinolytic therapy in genitourinary tract surgery. J Clin Pathol Suppl (R Coll Pathol) 14:60
Anonymous (1996) Fracture and dislocation compendium. Orthopaedic Trauma Association Committee for Coding and Classification. J Orthop Trauma 10 [Suppl 1]:v, 1
Armenakas NA et al (2004) Iatrogenic bladder perforations: longterm followup of 65 patients. J Am Coll Surg 198:78
Azam Uet al (2001) The tension-free vaginal tape procedure in women with previous failed stress incontinence surgery. J Urol 166:554
Baka AG et al (2002) Current use and perceived utility of ultrasound for evaluation of pediatric compared with adult trauma patients. Pediatr Emerg Care 18:163
Baniel J, Schein M (1994) The management of penetrating trauma to the urinary tract. J Am Coll Surg 178:417
Ben-Menachem Y (1988) Pelvic fractures: diagnostic and therapeutic angiography. Instr Course Lect 37:139
Ben-Menachem Y et al (1991) Hemorrhage associated with pelvic fractures: causes, diagnosis, and emergent management. AJR Am J Roentgenol 157:1005
Bigongiari LR et al (2000) Trauma to the bladder and urethra. American College of Radiology. ACR Appropriateness Criteria. Radiology 215:733
Bircher M, Giannoudis PV (2004) Pelvic trauma management within the UK: a reflection of a failing trauma service. Injury 35:2
Bond SJ et al (1991) Predictors of abdominal injury in children with pelvic fracture. J Trauma 31:1169
Brenneman FD et al (1997) Long-term outcomes in open pelvic fractures. J Trauma 42:773
Carlin BI, Resnick MI (1995) Indications and techniques for urologic evaluation of the trauma patient with suspected urologic injury. Semin Urol 13:9
Carroll PR, McAninch JW (1984) Major bladder trauma: mechanisms of injury and a unified method of diagnosis and repair. J Urol 132:254
Cass AS (1984) False negative retrograde cystography with bladder rupture owing to external trauma. J Trauma 24:168
Cass AS (1989) Diagnostic studies in bladder rupture. Indications and techniques. Urol Clin North Am 16:267
Cass AS, Luxenberg M (1987) Features of 164 bladder ruptures. J Urol 138:743
Cass AS, Luxenberg M (1989) Management of extraperitoneal ruptures of bladder caused by external trauma. Urology 33:179
Clancy TV et al (2001) A statewide analysis of level I and II trauma centers for patients with major injuries. J Trauma 51:346
Coppola PT, Coppola M (2000) Emergency department evaluation and treatment of pelvic fractures. Emerg Med Clin North Am 18:1
Daly JW, Higgins KA (1988) Injury to the ureter during gynecologic surgical procedures. Surg Gynecol Obstet 167:19
Davis JD (1999) Management of injuries to the urinary and gastrointestinal tract during cesarean section. Obstet Gynecol Clin North Am 26:469
Deck AJ et al (2000) Computerized tomography cystography for the diagnosis of traumatic bladder rupture. J Urol 164:43
Deck AJ et al (2001) Current experience with computed tomographic cystography and blunt trauma. World J Surg 25:1592
Delorme E (2001) Transobturator urethral suspension: mini-invasive procedure in the treatment of stress urinary incontinence in women. Prog Urol 11:1306
Demetriades D et al (2002) Pelvic fractures: epidemiology and predictors of associated abdominal injuries and outcomes. J Am Coll Surg 195:1
Dobrowolski ZF et al (2002) External and iatrogenic trauma of the urinary bladder: a survey in Poland. BJU Int 89:755
Dreitlein DA et al (2001) Genitourinary trauma. Emerg Med Clin North Am 19:569
Duncan AO et al (1989) Management of transpelvic gunshot wounds. J Trauma 29:1335
Dunn CJ, Goa KL (1999) Tranexamic acid: a review of its use in surgery and other indications. Drugs 57:1005
Eastridge BJ, Burgess AR (1997) Pedestrian pelvic fractures:5-year experience of a major urban trauma center. J Trauma 42:695
Espinoza R, Rodriguez A (1997) Traumatic and nontraumatic perforation of hollow viscera. Surg Clin North Am 77:1291
Failinger MS, McGanity PL (1992) Unstable fractures of the pelvic ring. J Bone Joint Surg Am 74:781
Fallon B et al (1984) Urological injury and assessment in patients with fractured pelvis. J Urol 131:712
Fernandez L et al (1998) Ultrasound in blunt abdominal trauma. J Trauma 45:841
Ferrera PC, Hill DA (1999) Good outcomes of open pelvic fractures. Injury 30:187
Flancbaum L et al (1988) Blunt bladder trauma: manifestation of severe injury. Urology 31:220
Fuhrman GM et al (1993) The single indication for cystography in blunt trauma. Am Surg 59:335
Gilmour DT et al (1999) Lower urinary tract injury during gynecologic surgery and its detection by intraoperative cystoscopy. Obstet Gynecol 94:883
Gokcen EC et al (1994) Pelvic fracture mechanism of injury in vehicular trauma patients. J Trauma 36:789; discussion 795
Gomez RG et al (2004) Consensus statement on bladder injuries. BJU Int 94:27
Harkki-Siren P et al (1998) Urinary tract injuries after hysterectomy. Obstet Gynecol 92:113
Harris RL et al (1997) The value of intraoperative cystoscopy in urogynecologic and reconstructive pelvic surgery. Am J Obstet Gynecol 177:1367; discussion 1369
Hedlund PO (1969) Antifibrinolytic therapy with Cyklokapron in connection with prostatectomy. A double blind study. Scand J Urol Nephrol 3:177
Hedlund PO (1975) Postoperative venous thrombosis in benign prostatic disease. A study of 316 patients, using the 125I-fibrinogen uptake test. Scand J Urol Nephrol 27 [Suppl]:1
Holmes JF et al (2001) Emergency department ultrasonography in the evaluation of hypotensive and normotensive children with blunt abdominal trauma. J Pediatr Surg 36:968
Horstman WG et al (1991) Comparison of computed tomography and conventional cystography for detection of traumatic bladder rupture. Urol Radiol 12:188
Inaba K et al (2004) The increasing incidence of severe pelvic injury in motor vehicle collisions. Injury 35:759
Ismail N et al (1996) Death from pelvic fracture: children are different. J Pediatr Surg 31:82
Jones AE et al (2003) Sonographic intraperitoneal fluid in patients with pelvic fracture: two cases of traumatic intraperitoneal bladder rupture. J Emerg Med 25:373

Khan RM et al (2004) A survey of urinary bladder injuries in Abbottabad. J Ayub Med Coll Abbottabad 16:47
Koraitim MM et al (1996) Risk factors and mechanism of urethral injury in pelvic fractures. Br J Urol 77:876
Kuuva N, Nilsson CG (2002) A nationwide analysis of complications associated with the tension-free vaginal tape (TVT) procedure. Acta Obstet Gynecol Scand 81:72
Loo GT et al (1996) Airbag protection versus compartment intrusion effect determines the pattern of injuries in multiple trauma motor vehicle crashes. J Trauma 41:935
Madiba TE, Haffejee AA (1999) Causes and outcome of bladder injuries in Durban. East Afr Med J 76:676
Makinen J et al (2001) Morbidity of 10 110 hysterectomies by type of approach. Hum Reprod 16:1473
Makoha FW et al (2004) Multiple cesarean section morbidity. Int J Gynaecol Obstet 87:227
Makoha FW et al (2005) Choice of abdominal incision and risk of trauma to the urinary bladder and bowel in multiple cesarean sections. Eur J Obstet Gynecol Reprod Biol
Matalon TS, Athanasoulis CA et al (1979) Hemorrhage with pelvic fractures: efficacy of transcatheter embolization. AJR Am J Roentgenol 133:859
McConnell JD et al (1982) Rupture of the bladder. Urol Clin North Am 9:293
McGahan PJ et al (2005) Ultrasound detection of blunt urological trauma: a 6-year study. Injury 36:762
Mee SL et al (1987) Computerized tomography in bladder rupture: diagnostic limitations. J Urol 137:207
Mendez LE (2001) Iatrogenic injuries in gynecologic cancer surgery. Surg Clin North Am 81:897
Meschia M et al (2001) Tension-Free vaginal tape: analysis of outcomes and complications in 404 stress incontinent women. Int Urogynecol J Pelvic Floor Dysfunct 12 [Suppl 2]: S24
Miller RA, May MW et al (1980) The prevention of secondary haemorrhage after prostatectomy: the value of antifibrinolytic therapy. Br J Urol 52:26
Minaglia S et al (2004) Bladder injury during transobturator sling. Urology 64:376
Moore EE et al (1992) Organ injury scaling. III: Chest wall, abdominal vascular, ureter, bladder, and urethra. J Trauma 33:337
Morey AF (2005) Sonographic intraperitoneal fluid in patients with pelvic fracture: two cases of traumatic intraperitoneal bladder rupture. J Urol 174:2264
Morey AF et al (1999) Reconstructive surgery for trauma of the lower urinary tract. Urol Clin North Am 26:49
Morey AF et al (2001) Bladder rupture after blunt trauma: guidelines for diagnostic imaging. J Trauma 51:683
Morgan DE et al (2000) CT cystography: radiographic and clinical predictors of bladder rupture. AJR Am J Roentgenol 174:89
Muir L et al (1996) The epidemiology of pelvic fractures in the Mersey Region. Injury 27:199
Murshidi MS (1988) Intraperitoneal rupture of the urinary bladder during transurethral resection of transitional cell carcinoma. Acta Urol Belg 56:68
Musemeche CA et al (1987) Selective management of pediatric pelvic fractures: a conservative approach. J Pediatr Surg 22:538
Nunes LW et al (2001) Diagnostic performance of trauma US in identifying abdominal or pelvic free fluid and serious abdominal or pelvic injury. Acad Radiol 8:128
Ochsner MG Jr et al (1989) Pelvic fracture as an indicator of increased risk of thoracic aortic rupture. J Trauma 29:1376
Olsson I, Kroon U (1999) A three-year postoperative evaluation of tension-free vaginal tape. Gynecol Obstet Invest 48:267
Ostrzenski A, Ostrzenska KM (1998) Bladder injury during laparoscopic surgery. Obstet Gynecol Surv 53:175
Poole GV et al (1991) Pelvic fracture from major blunt trauma. Outcome is determined by associated injuries. Ann Surg 213:532; discussion 538
Poole GV et al (1992) Complications of pelvic fractures from blunt trauma. Am Surg 58:225
Reed MH (1976) Pelvic fractures in children. J Can Assoc Radiol 27:255
Rehm CG et al (1991) Blunt traumatic bladder rupture: the role of retrograde cystogram. Ann Emerg Med 20:845
Reichard SA et al (1980) Pelvic fractures in children-review of 120 patients with a new look at general management. J Pediatr Surg 15:727
Rowe SA et al (2004) Pelvic ring fractures: implications of vehicle design, crash type, and occupant characteristics. Surgery 136:842
Sagalowsky AI, Peters PC (1998) Genitourinary trauma. In: Walsh PC, Retik AB, Vaughn ED, Wein AJ (eds) Campbell's urology, 7th edn. WB Saunders, Philadelphia, p 3116
Sandler CM et al (1981) Radiology of the bladder and urethra in blunt pelvic trauma. Radiol Clin North Am 19:195
Sandler CM et al (1986) Bladder injury in blunt pelvic trauma. Radiology 158:633
Sandler CM et al (1998) Lower urinary tract trauma. World J Urol 16:69
Schneider RE (1993) Genitourinary trauma. Emerg Med Clin North Am 11:137
Selikowitz SM (1977) Penetrating high-velocity genitourinary injuries. Part II: Ureteral, lower tract, and genital wounds. Urology 9:493
Siegel JH et al (1993) Safety belt restraints and compartment intrusions in frontal and lateral motor vehicle crashes: mechanisms of injuries, complications, and acute care costs. J Trauma 34:736; discussion 758
Siegmeth A et al (2000) Associated injuries in severe pelvic trauma. Unfallchirurg 103:572
Skolarikos A et al (2005) Does the management of bladder perforation during transurethral resection of superficial bladder tumors predispose to extravesical tumor recurrence? J Urol 173:1908
Soudack M et al (2004) Experience with focused abdominal sonography for trauma (FAST) in 313 pediatric patients. J Clin Ultrasound 32:53
Soulie M et al (2001) The tension-free transvaginal tape procedure in the treatment of female urinary stress incontinence: a French prospective multicentre study. Eur Urol 39:709; discussion 715
Stine RJ et al (1988) Diagnostic and therapeutic urologic procedures. Emerg Med Clin North Am 6:547
Tamussino KF et al (2001) Tension-free vaginal tape operation: results of the Austrian registry. Obstet Gynecol 98:732
Tarman GJ et al (2002) Lower genitourinary injury and pelvic fractures in pediatric patients. Urology 59:123; discussion 126
Tiguert R et al (2000) Management of shotgun injuries to the pelvis and lower genitourinary system. Urology 55:193
Tile M (1988) Pelvic ring fractures: should they be fixed? J Bone Joint Surg Br 70:1
Tile M (1996) Acute pelvic fractures: I causation and classification. J Am Acad Orthop Surg 4:143
Tile M (1999) The management of unstable injuries of the pelvic ring. J Bone Joint Surg Br 81:941
Torode I, Zieg D (1985) Pelvic fractures in children. J Pediatr Orthop 5:76
Ulmsten U (2001) An introduction to tension-free vaginal tape (TVT)–a new surgical procedure for treatment of female urinary incontinence. Int Urogynecol J Pelvic Floor Dysfunct 12 [Suppl 2]:S3
Vaccaro JP, Brody JM (2000) CT cystography in the evaluation of major bladder trauma. Radiographics 20:1373

Vakili B et al (2005) The incidence of urinary tract injury during hysterectomy: a prospective analysis based on universal cystoscopy. Am J Obstet Gynecol 192:1599

Velmahos GC, Degiannis E (1997) The management of urinary tract injuries after gunshot wounds of the anterior and posterior abdomen. Injury 28:535

Volpe MA et al (1999) Is there a difference in outcome when treating traumatic intraperitoneal bladder rupture with or without a suprapubic tube? J Urol 161:1103

Von Kuenssberg Jehle D et al (2003) Sensitivity in detecting free intraperitoneal fluid with the pelvic views of the FAST exam. Am J Emerg Med 21:476

Wah TM, Spencer JA (2001) The role of CT in the management of adult urinary tract trauma. Clin Radiol 56:268

Weber S et al (1987) Transurethral prostatectomy complicated by intraperitoneal extravasation of irrigating fluid. Can J Anaesth 34:193

Werkman HA et al (1991) Urinary tract injuries in multiply-injured patients: a rational guideline for the initial assessment. Injury 22:471

Wolk DJ et al (1985) Extraperitoneal bladder rupture without pelvic fracture. J Urol 134:1199

Wong YC, Wang LJ et al (2000) Mortality after successful transcatheter arterial embolization in patients with unstable pelvic fractures: rate of blood transfusion as a predictive factor. J Trauma 49:71

Yoshii H et al (1998) Usefulness and limitations of ultrasonography in the initial evaluation of blunt abdominal trauma. J Trauma 45:45; discussion 50

Yossepowitch O et al (2004) Urological injuries during cesarean section: intraoperative diagnosis and management. J Urol 172:196

Young JW, Resnik CS (1990) Fracture of the pelvis: current concepts of classification. AJR Am J Roentgenol 155:1169

Young JW et al (1986) Lateral compression fractures of the pelvis: the importance of plain radiographs in the diagnosis and surgical management. Skeletal Radiol 15:103

Zacharias SR et al (1999) Damage control surgery. AACN Clin Issues 10:95; quiz 141

15.7 Genital Trauma

E. Plas, I. Berger

15.7.1 Introduction

Traumatic injuries to the genitourinary tract are seen in 2.2%–10.3% of patients admitted to emergency units (Brandes et al. 1995; Marekovic et al. 1997; Salvatierra et al. 1969; Tucak et al. 1995; Archbold et al. 1981). Of these injuries, between one-third and two-thirds are associated with injuries to the external genitalia (Brandes et al. 1995). Due to anatomy and prevalence of accidents, men have a higher incidence of genital trauma than women, since men have an increased exposure to violence, performance of aggressive sports and motor vehicle accidents. In addition, a worldwide increase in domestic violence has led to rising numbers of gunshot and stab wounds over the last few years (Tiguert et al. 2000; Cline et al. 1998; Jolly et al. 1994; Bertini and Corriere 1988), with as many as 35% of all gunshot wounds affecting also the external genitalia (Monga and Hellstrom 1996).

Genitourinary trauma is seen in all age groups, most frequently in males between 15 and 40 years of age. However, 5% of trauma patients are less than 10 years old, again undermining the broad spectrum of traumatic injuries requiring different specialists for management (Monga and Hellstrom 1996).

There are certain popular sports with an increased risk for blunt and/or penetrating genital trauma, such as off-road bicycling, horse-back riding, motorcycle riding, especially on bikes with a dominant gas tank (Leibovitch and Mor 2005). In addition, blunt testicular trauma has been reported in in-line hockey skating and rugby players (Frauscher et al. 2001; de Peretti et al. 1993; Herrmann and Crawford 2002; Lawson et al. 1995; McAninch et al. 1984). Any type of full-contact sport, without the use of necessary protective aids, may be associated with genital trauma.

Besides these risk groups, severe trauma to the external genitalia is seen in female genital mutilation and self-mutilation in psychotic patients and transsexuals (McAninch et al. 1984).

Genitourinary trauma is commonly caused by blunt injuries (80%), whereas 20% result from penetrating lesions. For the above-mentioned reasons, blunt injuries to the external genitalia are more frequently seen in men than in women. Although the incidence of traumatic injuries is higher in males than females, the risk of associated injuries to neighboring organs (bladder, urethra, vagina, and rectum) after blunt genital trauma is higher in females than in males.

In men, blunt genital trauma frequently occurs unilaterally, with only 1% of cases presenting as bilateral scrotal and/or testicular injuries (Monga and Hellstrom 1996). However, penetrating scrotal injuries affect both testes in 30% of cases (Monga and Hellstrom 1996; Cass et al. 1988). Besides locally extended lesions associated with penetrating trauma, there is a 70% risk of additional injuries in both genders.

Table 15.7.1. American Association for the Surgery of Trauma (AAST) organ injury severity scale for the vagina

Grade[a]	Description of injury
I	Contusion or hematoma
II	Laceration, superficial (mucosa only)
III	Laceration, deep into fat or muscle
IV	Laceration, complex, into cervix or peritoneum
V	Injury into adjacent organs (anus, rectum, urethra, bladder)

[a] Advance one grade for multiple injuries up to grade III

Table 15.7.2. AAST organ injury severity scale for the vulva

Grade[a]	Description of injury
I	Contusion or hematoma
II	Laceration, superficial (skin only)
III	Laceration, deep into fat or muscle
IV	Avulsion; skin, fat, or muscle
V	Injury into adjacent organs (anus, rectum, urethra, bladder)

[a] Advance one grade for multiple injuries up to grade III

Table 15.7.3. AAST organ injury severity scale for the testis

Grade[a]	Description of injury
I	Contusion or hematoma
II	Subclinical laceration of tunica albuginea
III	Laceration of tunica albuginea with <50% parenchymal loss
IV	Major laceration of tunica albuginea with ≥50% parenchymal loss
V	Total testicular destruction or avulsion

[a] Advance one grade for bilateral lesions up to grade V

Table 15.7.4. AAST organ injury severity scale for the scrotum

Grade	Description of injury
I	Contusion
II	Laceration <25% of scrotal diameter
III	Laceration ≥25% of scrotal diameter
IV	Avulsion <50%
V	Avulsion ≥50%

Table 15.7.5. AAST organ injury severity scale for the penis

Grade	Description of injury
I	Cutaneous laceration/contusion
II	Buck's fascia (cavernosum) laceration without tissue loss
III	Cutaneous avulsion/laceration through glans/meatus/cavernosal or urethral defect <2 cm
IV	Cavernosal or urethral defect ≥2 cm/partial penectomy
V	Total penectomy

Because of this high incidence of associated lesions, accurate diagnosis and treatment of patients with penetrating injuries are of utmost importance. The classification of male and female genital trauma according to the American Association for the Surgery of Trauma is given in Tables 15.7.1 – 15.7.5.

One aspect that may not be forgotten in treating trauma patients is the associated increased risk of infection of the emergency staff dealing with these patients, especially hepatitis B and C. Recently, a 38% infection rate with hepatitis B and/or C in males with penetrating gunshot or stab wounds to the external genitalia was reported (Cline et al. 1998). This incidence was significantly higher compared with the normal population, thus exposing emergency staff to an increased risk. It is emphasized that standardized preventive procedures must be in place and available for the emergency staff not only to save the patient's life but also to guarantee co-workers' health. Besides the risk of hepatitis infection, which is still higher than for HIV, the possible transmission of HIV by trauma patients must be taken into consideration. In a recent report by Xeroulis et al., a total of 287 consecutive trauma patients in Canada were tested for Hep B/C and HIV infection (Xeroulis et al. 2005). One patient was positive for hepatitis B, eight for hepatitis C, and none for HIV. This revealed a threefold higher seroprevalence for hepatitis C compared with the general population. More than half of the hepatitis C-positive patients were men injured in a motor vehicle crash with a mean Injury Severity Score of 19, determining that hepatitis C poses the highest risk to the trauma team. Although these numbers appear small, there may be demographic differences at different centers, again emphasizing the importance of precautions necessary for physicians and nursing staff.

15.7.2 Pathophysiology of Trauma to External Genitalia

15.7.2.1 Blunt Penile Trauma

Blunt trauma to the flaccid penis may result in subcutaneous hematoma resulting from injury to the subcutaneous veins. Because the penile subcutaneous layers (superficial, Colles fascia; deep, Buck's fascia) meld into lower abdominal fascial layers (superficial Camper's fascia, deep: Scarpa's fascia), hematomas may spread to the lower abdomen or to the penoscrotal base. Descending hematoma of the penile shaft can cause preputial swelling that may cause obstructive voiding, requiring transient catheterization.

Because of the thickness of the tunica albuginea in the flaccid state (approximately 2 mm), blunt trauma to the penis does not usually cause tearing of the tunica albuginea when there is no tumescence and rigidity. During erection, increasing rigidity and tumescence cause a thinning of the tunica, reducing the thickness of the tunica in the fully erect state. In these cases, a direct blow to the erect penis may cause penile fracture, frequently occurring during consensual intercourse, which accounts for approximately 60 % of penile fractures (Haas et al. 1999). This usually occurs if the erect penis slips out of the vagina and strikes against the symphysis pubis or perineum, most frequently if the women sits on top of the man. Penile fracture primarily affects the corporeal tunica by rupturing the tunica but may be associated with lesions of the corpus spongiosum and urethra in 10 % – 22 % (Nicolaisen et al. 1983; Tsang and Demby 1992).

15.7.2.2
Blunt Testicular Trauma

Approximately 85 % of testicular injuries result from blunt trauma (Morey et al. 2004). Blunt trauma to the scrotum can cause testicular dislocation, testicular rupture, and/or subcutaneous scrotal hematoma.

Overall, traumatic dislocation of the testicle occurs rarely, commonly only unilaterally and in victims of car or motorcycle accidents, or in pedestrians run over by a vehicle (Lee et al. 1992; Shefi et al. 1999; Pollen and Funckes 1982; Nagarajan et al. 1983). Bilateral dislocation of the testes has been reported in up to 25 % of cases (Nagarajan et al. 1983). It can result in subcutaneous or internal dislocation of the testis. Subcutaneous dislocation defines a subcutaneous epifascial displacement of the testis, whereas during internal dislocation of the testis it is positioned in the superficial external inguinal ring, inguinal canal, or abdominal cavity.

Depending on the magnitude of blunt power acting on the scrotum, testicular rupture may occur in approximately 50 % of blunt scrotal traumas (Cass and Luxenberg 1991). It can occur under intense, traumatic compression of the testis against the inferior pubic ramus or symphysis, resulting in a rupture of the tunica albuginea of the testis. Wasko and Goldstein estimated that a force of approximately 50 kg is necessary to cause testicular rupture (Wasko and Goldstein 1996).

15.7.2.3
Blunt Vulvar Trauma

Blunt trauma to the vulva is rarely reported and may be caused by obstetric, athletic, or sexual trauma or rarely by car or bicycle accidents. The rich vulvar vascular supply can be damaged by contusive frontal impacts, which crush the vulvar tissues against the osseous planes (Virgili et al. 2000).

In obstetrics, incidence of traumatic vulvar hematomas after vaginal deliveries was reported in only one out of 310 deliveries (Sotto and Collins 1958). The frequency in nonobstetric vulvar hematomas is even lower, with only several cases reported (Propst and Thorp 1998). Although the incidence of vulvar hematoma is generally low, its presence indicates further investigations for associated lesions since vulvar hematoma is closely related to an increased risk of vaginal, pelvic, or abdominal injuries. Goldman et al. reported on the frequency of blunt injuries of female external genitalia associated with pelvic trauma in 30 %, consensual intercourse in 25 %, sexual assault in 20 %, and other blunt trauma in 15 % (Goldman et al. 1998). Besides the presence of perforating associated lesions, blunt perineal trauma may result in female sexual dysfunction classified as orgasmic disorders and/or hyposensitivity (Munnarriz et al. 2002).

15.7.2.4
Penetrating Trauma of the External Genitalia

Penetrating trauma to the external genitalia is frequently associated with complex injuries in other organs. In children, penetrating injuries are most frequently seen after straddle-type falls or laceration of genital skin due to falls on sharp objects (Monga and Hellstrom 1996; Okur et al. 1996). In any penetrating trauma, the tetanus immunization status of the patient has to be clarified. According to a recent review by Rhee et al., tetanus toxoid booster was recommended in the US for patients with the last immunization given more than 10 years before. Since toxoid booster does not protect against the current injury, no urgency for the administration of tetanus toxoid in the acute setting has been suggested. This is divergent to suggestions by the World Health Organization recommending tetanus toxoid booster if tetanus immunization was received more than 5 years before in patients with an open wound (World Health Organization 2000). Tetanus immunoglobulin should be reserved only for previously nonimmunized injured patients (Rhee et al. 2005).

Stab and Gunshot Genital Injuries

Increasing worldwide domestic violence has led to a rising incidence of stab and/or gunshot injuries associated with injuries of the genitourinary tract. The extent of injuries associated with guns is related to the caliber and velocity of the missile (Jolly et al. 1994). Handguns or pistols range from 0.22 to 0.45 caliber, with a velocity of 200 – 300 m/s. In addition, magnum handguns transmit 20 % – 60 % more energy than a standard handgun to the tissue due to the higher velocity of the missile. Injuries by rifles cause even more extensive lesions. Rifles have a caliber ranging from 0.17 to 0.46 with a kinetic energy transmission of up to 1,000 m/s.

Missiles with a velocity of approximately 200–300 m/s are considered as low velocity inducing a permanent cavity by entering the body. The energy along the projectile path transmitted to the tissue is much less than in high-velocity missiles, so that tissue destruction in low-velocity guns is less extensive (Jolly et al. 1994). On the contrary, high-velocity missiles (velocity of 800–1,000 m/s) have an explosive effect with high-energy transmission to the tissue causing a temporary cavity. Due to the high-energy released, gaseous tissue vaporization induces extensive damage, often associated with life-threatening injuries.

In relation to the weapon, caliber and configuration of the missile, gunshot wounds are classified as penetrating, perforating, and avulsive.

a. Penetrating injuries with low-velocity missiles often retain the projectile in the tissue, causing a small, ragged entry wound.
b. Perforating gunshot wounds are frequently seen in low- to high-velocity missiles. In these cases, the missile passes through the tissue with a small entry wound, but larger exit wound.
c. Serious injuries are associated with avulsive gunshot wounds caused by high-velocity missiles, with a small entry wound comparable to the caliber but a large tissue defect at the exit wound.

Genital Injuries Due to Bites

Although animal bites are common, bites involving injury to the external genital are rare. Wounds are usually minor but there is a potential risk of serious wound infection. The nature of local tissues and polymicrobial microbiology of bite wounds make genital bites a potentially morbid event. Animal bites to external genitalia, especially to males, are rare. Of the affected patients, 60%–70% are boys aged under the age of 15 years (Gomes et al. 2000). Time to presentation since trauma, severity of injury, and the type of management have a direct influence on the outcome. A few small series (Gomes et al. 2001) and case reports (Kyriakidis et al. 1979; Cummings and Boullier 2000) of genital bites by different animals and humans have been reported. But the lack of large retrospective or even prospective trials make it difficult for a broad consensus on the management of these injuries (Nabi and Mishriki 2005).

Approximately 30% of animal bite wounds already present signs of infection within 48 h. The most common bacterial infection by a dog bite is *Pasturella multicida*, which accounts for up to 50% of infections (Donovan and Kaplan 1989). Other microorganisms commonly involved are *Escherichia coli*, *Streptococcus viridans*, *Staphylococcus aureus*, *Bacteroides*, and *Fusobacterium* spp. (Donovan and Kaplan 1989; McAninch et al. 1984). The first choice of antibiotics is penicillin followed by cephalosporin or erythromycin. In addition to antibiotics, proper wound management including surgical exploration with debridement and daily wound care are recommended (Kerins et al. 2004).

In animal bites, the possibility of rabies infection must always be considered. In case of domestic presence of rabies infection in animals, vaccination must be given to prevent life-threatening infections (Dreesen and Hanlon 1998). The estimated worldwide number of deaths due to rabies infection amounted to approximately 55,000 in 2004, most commonly in rural areas of Africa and Asia. In addition to vaccination, local wound management is an essential part of postexposure rabies prophylaxis. If rabies infection is suspected, vaccination should be considered in relation to the animal involved, the specific nature of the wound and attack (provoked/unprovoked), and the appearance of the animal (aggressive, foam at the mouth). Presently, vaccination with human rabies immunoglobulin and human diploid cell vaccine is recommended (Dreesen and Hanlon 1998; Anderson 1992).

Human bites to external genitalia include an even broader range of possible infections with an additional risk of sexually transmitted diseases, such as syphilis, hepatitis, HIV, herpes, actinomycosis, or tuberculosis (Franke et al. 1999).

Straddle-Type Genital Injuries

Straddle-type injuries may cause genitourinary trauma, such as vaginal hematoma, vaginal contusion, penile laceration, or urethral injuries. In children, playground equipment-specific injuries are attributed in majority to monkey bars, jungle gyms, swings, and slides (Waltzman et al. 1999).

Genital Mutilation

Female genital mutilation, often referred to as female circumcision, comprises all procedures involving partial or total removal of the external female genitalia (labia majora/minora, clitoris) and/or other injuries to the female genitalia (World Health Organization 2000). It is still commonly performed in some parts of Africa and the Middle East (Collinet et al. 2004). Some case reports even reported genital mutilation performed in Europe (Sheldon 2005; Holmgren et al. 2005; Turone 2004).

According to a recent report from southwestern Nigeria, the majority of genital mutilations were performed by medically untrained personnel (89%) with a complication rate up to 67% (Dare et al. 2004). The procedure is generally performed in young adrenarchal women without anesthesia, with a high rate of hemorrhagic shock, urinary retention, and ulceration of the genital region. Late complications include vulvar introital stenosis, HIV transmission, retention cysts and abscesses, keloid scar formation, urinary incontinence, dyspareunia, and sexual dysfunction, as well as difficulties with childbirth (World Health Organization 2000).

15.7.3 Diagnosis and Management of Genital Trauma

Proper management of genital trauma requires a detailed history, if possible, physical examination, and imaging techniques. Especially in penetrating wounds, information concerning the accident, possibly involved persons, animals, vehicles, and weapons (knife, gun, etc.) are important to estimate the extent of injury, the potential risk of associated lesions, and subsequent infections.

In addition to the history and physical examination, a urine analysis is mandatory. Since an abusive assault may be related to genital injuries, physicians must consider the emotional difficulty for the patient as well as their privacy in such examinations. This requires the investigation of the patient alone without persons related with the patient and may require short term anesthesia for physical examination. In case of suspicion, taking swabs or vaginal smears for detection of spermatozoa is mandatory (Okur et al. 1996). Additionally, other specialists may be requested (pediatrician, gynecologist) for proper management of the patient. In order to follow domestic rules and regulations, it is mandatory to be aware of local guidelines such as the 2002 National Guidelines on the Management of Adult Victims of Sexual Assault (2002).

15.7.4 Blunt Trauma of the Male Genitalia

15.7.4.1 Blunt Penile Trauma

An essential part in the evaluation of blunt penile trauma is the status of penile rigidity at injury. In case of a flaccid penis at trauma, cavernosal and/or spongiosa corporeal injuries are unlikely. Penile ultrasonography with or without Duplex sonography and/or penile MRI are not indicated.

If the patient reports on an erection at injury, diagnosis of penile fracture can be made after a thorough history and examination in most cases. Patients most commonly report a sudden cracking or popping sound of the erect penis associated with moderate local pain but immediate penile detumescence. As a result, local swelling of the penile shaft develops with progressive hematoma that may occur along fascial layers of the penile shaft extending to the lower abdominal wall in case of rupture of Buck's fascia. Depending on the extent of the hematoma, rupture of the tunica may be palpated (Morey et al. 2004).

In case of macro- or microhematuria, retrograde urethrography is mandatory to determine the presence of urethral injury (Morey et al. 2004). Presence of microhematuria without radiographic lesion of the urethra requires no further intervention. In case of radiographic urethral lesion, a transurethral catheter can be placed for bladder drainage.

Besides history and clinical examination, imaging techniques may be performed by cavernosography and magnetic resonance imaging (MRI) (Aboloyosr et al. 2005; Karadeniz et al. 1996; Pretorius et al. 2001). Both techniques may identify laceration of the tunica albuginea. Recent reports support the role of MRI as particularly helpful in investigating the integrity of the tunica albuginea, and presence of intracavernosal or extratunical hematoma (Uder et al. 2002). Associated injuries to adjacent structures (e.g., corpus spongiosum, urethra) may also be found.

It remains uncertain whether the routine use of contrast material-enhanced MRI is justified in these cases (Choi et al. 2000). Presently, cavernosography and/or MRI are the most accurate imaging procedures in cases where penile fracture is suspected but the clinical findings are unclear (Fedel et al. 1996).

15.7.4.2 Blunt Testicular Trauma

Patients report posttraumatic immediate scrotal pain, nausea, vomiting, and sometimes they faint. They often present with a tender, swollen scrotum and a impalpable testis. High-resolution, real-time ultrasonography with a 7.5- to 10-MHz probe should be performed to determine intra- and/or extratesticular bleeding, testicular contusion or rupture (Tsang and Demby 1992; Pavlica and Barozzi 2001; Micallef et al. 2001; Patil and Onuora 1994; Corrales et al. 1993; Mulhall et al. 1995; Martinez-Pineiro et al. 1992; Fournier et al. 1989; Kratzik et al. 1989).

Controversial results have been presented regarding the usefulness of ultrasonography in testicular trauma. Some reported convincing results emphasizing the importance of sonography with accuracy reaching 94% (McAninch et al. 1984; Pavlica and Barozzi 2001; Martinez-Pineiro et al. 1992; Fournier et al. 1989), whereas others presented only low specificity (78%) and sensitivity (28%) in determining testicular rupture (Corrales et al. 1993). Some reported an overall accuracy of scrotal ultrasound for testicular rupture of only 56%, irrespective of the investigator (Corrales et al. 1993). So far, it is the authors' opinion that gray-scale ultrasonography with 7.5- to 10-MHz remains a noninvasive technique with good reliability in experienced hands and should be performed in case of blunt testicular trauma. Information may be increased by color Doppler duplex ultrasonography to evaluate testicular perfusion. In case of inconclusive scrotal sonography, testicular computed tomography (CT) or MRI may be helpful in elucidating scrotal dilemmas (Muglia et al. 2002). However, these techniques did not specifically increase the detection of testicular rupture. The time delay associated with imaging studies has to be weighed against the reliability of information in order to decide whether or not surgical exploration is indicated. If imaging studies cannot exclude testicular rupture, surgical exploration should be initiated.

15.7.4.3 Blunt Female Trauma

In women, colposcopy and vulvovaginoscopy are a valid way of identifying genital injuries and are mandatory if sexual assault is suspected (Mancino et al. 2003). The presence of micro- or macrohematuria should not be misinterpreted as menstrual bleeding. In women with genital injuries and blood at the vaginal introitus, it has been repeatedly emphasized that this may not only result from menstrual bleeding, but further investigation is required to exclude vaginal injuries (Hussman 1998). As already mentioned, blunt genital trauma in women seldom occurs, but if vulvar hematoma develop there is a high chance of associated injuries. The performance of flexible or rigid cystoscopy has been recommended to exclude urethral and bladder injury (Goldman et al. 1998; Hussmann 1998). Complete vaginal inspection with specula is mandatory and, because of pain, should be carried out under sedation or general anesthesia in most cases. In case of suspected assault, vaginal smears must be taken for determination of spermatozoa.

As blunt trauma to the vulva is often associated with pelvic trauma, imaging studies of the pelvis with CT or MRI should be performed to exclude intrapelvic pathologies (Okur et al. 1996; Hussmann 1998).

15.7.4.4 Penetrating Trauma of the External Genitalia

As already mentioned in Sect. 15.7.2, "Pathophysiology of Trauma to External Genitalia," the importance of a thorough history concerning the penetrating injury must again be emphasized. Especially for gunshot wounds, information concerning the type of weapons used, the approximate distance of the missiles entrance, caliber, and size of the bullet is helpful for further treatment.

Penetrating Trauma in Men

Any kind of penetrating trauma of the external genital requires urethrography irrespective of urine analysis to exclude urethral lesion. Additionally, abdominal and a pelvic CT scan, with or without cystography, may be performed in those cases that do not require immediate surgery.

Penetrating Women Trauma

Penetrating lesions of the external genitalia without lesions of adjacent organs are extremely rare, requiring an abdominal and pelvic CT scan in any case. If the CT scan cannot exclude associated bowel injuries or intraabdominal bleeding, exploratory laparoscopy has been suggested in hemodynamically stable patients prior to exploratory laparotomy (Okur et al. 1996). In the hemodynamically unstable patient, exploratory laparotomy is indicated.

15.7.5 Treatment of External Genital Trauma

15.7.5.1 Blunt Trauma

Blunt Penile Trauma

Blunt trauma to the flaccid penis usually develops only subcutaneous hematoma requiring no surgical intervention. The presence of subcutaneous hematoma, without rupture of the cavernosal tunica albuginea and no immediate detumescence of the erect penis, does not require surgical intervention. In these cases, nonsteroidal analgetics and ice packs are recommended.

Preputial swelling and edema may require transient catheterization with the need for percutaneous cystostomy only in a few selected cases with an increased risk of local inflammatory complications (i.e., necrotizing fasciitis). In case of necrotizing fasciitis, rapid extensive surgical debridement is very important in addition to broad-spectrum antibiotic therapy.

In the case of penile fracture, immediate surgical intervention with closure of the tunica albuginea is recommended. Closure of the tunica can be obtained by using either absorbable or nonabsorbable sutures, with good long-term outcome and protection of potency. Postoperative complications were reported in 9%, including superficial wound infection and impotence in 1.3% (Haas et al. 1999; Orvis and McAninch 1989). Conservative management of penile fracture is not recommended because of early and long-term complications, including penile abscess, missed partial urethral disruption, penile curvature, and persistent hematoma requiring delayed surgical intervention (Orvis and McAninch 1989). In addition, fibrosis and penile angulation were reported in 35% after conservative management of penile fracture (Haas et al. 1999; Orvis and McAninch 1989).

Blunt Testicular Trauma

Blunt trauma to the scrotum can cause significant hematocele without testicular rupture. Conservative management with ice packs, nonsteroidal analgetics, and bed rest is recommended in hematoceles smaller than three times the size of the contralateral testis (Tiguert et al. 2000). Several authors reported the risks of conservative management in blunt scrotal trauma requiring delayed interventions (> 3 days) in many cases, with a significantly higher rate of orchiectomy even in the nonruptured testis (Monga and Hellstrom 1996; Cass and Luxenberg 1988, 1991; McAninch et al. 1984; Altarac 1994). The reasons for delayed interventions requiring surgery were local infections and pain. It was repeatedly reported that early surgical intervention, i.e., within 72 h, resulted in more than 90% preservation of the testis, whereas delayed surgery necessitated orchiectomy in 45%–55% (Cass and Luxenberg 1991). If the integrity of testicular tunica albuginea cannot be clearly visualized or duplex ultrasonography shows reduced perfusion in the injured testicles, scrotal exploration is indicated.

Additionally, pain and duration of hospital stay may be markedly reduced by early surgical intervention for large hematoceles. Because of the long convalescence in large hematoceles, surgical exploration is recommended, irrespective of testicle contusion or rupture. By evacuation of the blood clot from the tunica vaginalis, testicular pain is relieved and rehabilitation will be more rapid (Altarac 1994).

In cases of testicular rupture, surgical exploration with excision of necrotic testicular tubules, closure of the tunica albuginea is mandatory and suction drainage should be applied. By early intervention, 80% of injured testicles can be saved (Fowler et al. 1992) and normal testicular endocrine function can be maintained. By applying intravenous antibiotics and nonsteroidal anti-inflammatory drugs within 6 h after injury, a reduction in infectious risk has been seen (Whelan et al. 2005).

Traumatic dislocation of the testis can be repositioned manually followed by delayed surgical orchidopexy. In cases of insufficient positioning of the dislocated testis posttraumatically, primary orchidopexy is indicated.

Blunt Vulvar Trauma

Blunt trauma to the vulva is rare and commonly presents as extended hematomas. Management of vulvar hematomas may range from conservative treatment to surgical decompression. In most cases, vulvar hematomas after blunt trauma do not require surgical intervention, but they may cause significant blood loss requiring transfusion. Reported data are scarce, and recommendations for vulvar wound management are based on empirical experience (Propst and Thorp 1998; Goldman et al. 1998; Okur et al. 1996; Husmann 1998). In hemodynamically stable women, nonsteroidal anti-inflammatories and cold packs relieve pain, requiring no surgical intervention in the majority of cases.

In extended vulvar hematoma or in unstable patients, hospitalization may be indicated for surgical intervention, stabilization, and reduction of infectious risks. The additional use of antibiotics is recommended in major vulvar trauma.

However, blunt trauma to the female external genitalia may be associated with voiding problems and/or lesions to adjacent organs. Therefore, transurethral catheterization for dip stick testing is indicated to exclude hematuria requiring further investigations.

15.7.5.2
Penetrating Trauma

Penetrating trauma to the external genitalia require surgical exploration in most cases, including debridement and reconstruction in order to prevent late complications such as urethral strictures, penile curvature and erectile dysfunction, and testicular atrophy (Morey et al. 2004). In complex wounds with persistent infection, negative-pressure wound therapy (vacuum devices) complements surgical and medical intervention (Whelan et al. 2005).

Penetrating Penile Trauma

Surgical exploration and conservative debridement of necrotic tissue is recommended with primary closure in most cases. Even in extended injuries of the penis or complete dissection, primary repair should be tried with only minor excision of necrotic tissue due to the excellent blood supply of penile corpora. In complete dissection of the penis, vascular and neuronal realignment should be performed by a skilled microsurgeon in addition to corporeal and urethral reconstruction (McAninch et al. 1984; Van der Horst et al. 2004).

In extended loss of penile shaft skin, split-thickness grafts can be utilized after infectious control. McAninch et al. recommended the use of a skin graft thickness of at least 0.001 inch in order to reduce the risk of skin contractions restricting penile enlargement during erection (McAninch et al. 1984). Additionally, during reconstruction grafts should be placed circumferentially to the artificially erected penis to prevent contracture, shortening, or deviation. In case of proper surgical management, potency rates of more than 80% can be achieved (Goldman et al. 1996). Excellent clinical results are also reported on the use of autologous rectus fascia graft for coverage of a tunica or corporeal defect (Pathak et al. 2005).

Besides postsurgical transient urethral stenting, a suprapubic cystostomy may be placed in addition to broad-spectrum antibiotics.

15.7.5.3 Penetrating Testicular Trauma

Penetrating injuries to the scrotum require surgical exploration with conservative debridement of nonviable tissue. Primary realignment can be easily obtained, in most cases. Only in severe infection or necrotizing fasciitis would debridement with subcutaneous femoral displacement of the testicles be required initially. After proper wound granulation, reconstructive surgery either by secondary closure of the scrotal skin and replacement of the testis can be obtained or split thickness grafts may be used for scrotal reconstruction (Rapp et al. 2005). In cases of high-velocity gunshot injuries, the testicle could not be saved in almost 90% of the reported cases (Gomez et al. 1993).

Complete disruption of the spermatic cord occurs and is treated with vascular realignment if possible. Microsurgical reconstruction of the vas deferens either by vasovasostomy or tubulovasostomy should only be performed in the hemodynamically stable patient or secondarily after rehabilitation of the patient (Altarac 1993). If there is extensive destruction of the tunica albuginea, mobilization of a free tunica vaginalis flap can be obtained for testicular closure. If the patient is unstable or reconstruction cannot be achieved, orchiectomy should be performed. If both testicles are severely damaged, prior to surgery or even after orchiectomy, testicular epididymal sperm extraction (TESE) mapping may be considered for future artifical reproduction (Baniel and Sella 2001; Negri et al. 2002).

Extended laceration of scrotal skin requires surgical intervention for skin closure after removal of any foreign material. Due to the elasticity of the scrotum, most defects can be primarily closed, even if the lacerated skin is only minimally attached to the body (McAninch et al. 1984). The recreative capacity of scrotal skin is high, indicating conservative debridement and primary realignment in most cases. However, local wound management with extensive rinsing of the wound is an important fact for scrotal convalescence. Even in cases of complete disruption of scrotal skin, it can be realigned in most cases after debridement and washing. In fact, there is an associated risk of harming the vascular plexus in the stratum reticulare of the skin, causing partial necrosis of full-thickness skin grafts. This in turn may require resection and staged closure with split-thickness grafts or, depending upon the extent of the defect, secondary granulation of the wound. It must be noted that using thick skin flaps, or burying the testicle are not recommended for patients who wish to remain fertile, as the spermatogenesis deteriorates substantially after a period of 2 years (Wang et al. 2003).

Although the rehabilitative capacity of the scrotum is very good, the use of antibiotics is indicated in any case of penetrating trauma.

15.7.5.4 Penetrating Vulvar Trauma

Although penetrating vulvar trauma is rarely seen, it is even more important to emphasize that vulvar hematoma and/or blood at the vaginal introitus are an indication for vaginal exploration in order to identify possible associated vaginal and/or rectal injuries under sedation or general anesthesia (Husmann 1998). In case of vulvar laceration, realignment after conservative debridement is indicated. If there are associated injuries to the vagina, these can be repaired immediately by primary suturing. Additional injuries to the bladder, rectum, or bowel may require laparotomy for closure and, in case of rectal injuries, may necessitate transient colostomy.

References

Aboloyosr A, Moneim AE, Abdelatif AM, Abdalla MA, Imam HM (2005) The management of penile fracture based on clinical and magnetic resonance imaging findings. BJU Int 96:373

Altarac S (1993) A case of testicle replantation. J Urol 150:1507

Altarac S (1994) Management of 53 cases of testicular trauma. Eur Urol 25:119

Anderson CR (1992) Animal bites. Guidelines to current management. Postgrad Med 92:134

Archbold JA, Barros d'sa AA, Morrison E (1981) Genito-urinary tract injuries of civil hostilities. Br J Surg 68:625

Baniel J, Sella A (2001) Sperm extraction at orchiectomy for testis cancer. Fertil Steril 75:260

Bertini JE Jr, Corriere JN Jr (1988) The etiology and management of genital injuries. J Trauma 28:1278

Brandes SB, Buckman RF, Chelsky MJ, Hanno PM (1995) External genitalia gunshot wounds: a ten-year experience with fifty-six cases. J Trauma 39:266

Cass AS, Luxenberg M (1988) Value of early operation in blunt testicular contusion with hematocele. J Urol 139:746

Cass AS, Luxenberg M (1991) Testicular injuries. Urology 37:528

Cass AS, Ferrara L, Wolpert J, Lee J (1988) Bilateral testicular injury from external trauma. J Urol 140:1435

Choi MH, Kim B, Ryu JA, Lee SW, Lee KS (2000) MR imaging of acute penile fracture. Radiographics 20:1397

Cline KJ, Mata JA, Venable DD, Eastham JA (1998) Penetrating trauma to the male external genitalia. J Trauma 44:492

Collinet P, Sabban F, Lucot JP, Boukerrou M, Stien L, Leroy JL (2004) Management of type III female genital mutilation. J Gynecol Obstet Biol Reprod 33:720

Corrales JG, Corbel L, Cipolla B, Staerman F, Darnault P, Guille F, Lobel B (1993) Accuracy of ultrasound diagnosis after blunt testicular trauma. J Urol 150:1834

Cummings JM, Boullier JA (2000) Scrotal dog bites. J Urol 164:57
Dare FO, Oboro VO, Fadiora SO, Orji EO, Sule-Odu AO, Olabode TO (2004) Female genital mutilation: an analysis of 522 cases in South-Western Nigeria. J Obstet Gynaecol. 24:281
De Peretti F, Cambas PM, Veneau B, Argenson C (1993) Fuel tanks of motorcycles. Role in severe trauma of the pelvis. Presse Med 22:61
Donovan JF, Kaplan WE (1989) The therapy of genital trauma by dog bite. J Urol 141:1163
Dreesen DW, Hanlon CA (1998) Current recommendations for the prophylaxis and treatment of rabies. Drugs 56:801
Fedel M, Venz S, Andreessen R, Sudhoff F, Loening SA (1996) The value of magnetic resonance imaging in the diagnosis of suspected penile fracture with atypical clinical findings. J Urol 155:1924
Fournier GR Jr, Laing FC, McAninch JW (1989) Scrotal ultrasonography and the management of testicular trauma. Urol Clin North Am 16:377
Franke M, Lenk S, Petras T (1999) Genitalverletzung durch Hundebisse. Extr Urol 22:15
Frauscher F, Klauser A, Stenzl A, Helweg G, Amort B, zur Nedden D (2001) US findings in the scrotum of extreme mountain bikers. Radiology 219:427
Goldman HB, Dmochowski RR, Cox CE (1996) Penetrating trauma to the penis: functional results. J Urol 155:551
Goldman HB, Idom CB Jr, Dmochowski RR (1998) Traumatic injuries of the female external genitalia and their association with urological injuries. J Urol 159:956
Gomes CM, Ribeiro-Filho L, Giron AM, Mitre AI, Figueira ER, Arap S (2000) Genital trauma due to animal bites. J Urol 165:80
Gomes CM, Ribeiro-Filho L, Giron AM, Mitre AI, Figueira ER, Arap S (2001) Genital trauma due to animal bites. J Urol 165:80
Gomez RG, Castanheira ACC, McAninch JW (1993) Gunshot wounds to the male genitalia. J Urol 150:1147
Haas CA, Brown SL, Spirnak JP (1999) Penile fracture and testicular rupture. World J Urol 17:101
Herrmann B, Crawford J (2002) Genital injuries in prepubertal girls from inline skating accidents. Pediatrics 110:e16
Holmgren H, Almroth L, Berggren V, Bergstrom S (2005) Genital mutilation of children is an offence. Do health services have a sufficient knowledge to see the problem? Lakartidningen 102:1637
Husmann DA (1998) Editorial Comment. J Urol 159:959
Jolly BB, Sharma SK, Vaidyanathan S, Mandal AK (1994) Gunshot wounds of the male external genitalia. Urol Int 53:92
Karadeniz T, Topsakal M, Ariman A, Erton H, Basak D (1996) Penile fracture: differential diagnosis, management and outcome. Br J Urol 77:279
Kerins M, Greene S, O'Connor N (2004) A human bite to the scrotum: a case report and review of the literature. Eur J Emerg Med 11:223
Kratzik C, Hainz A, Kuber W, Donner G, Lunglmayr G, Frick J, Schmoller HJ (1989) Has ultrasound influenced the therapy concept of blunt scrotal trauma? J Urol 142:1243
Kyriakidis A, Karydis G, Yannopoulos P (1979) An unusual trauma of the glans penis. Br J Urol 51:161
Lawson JS, Rotem T, Wilson SF (1995) Catastrophic injuries to the eyes and testicles in footballers. Med J Aust 163:242
Lee JY, Cass AS, Streitz JM (1992) Traumatic dislocation of testes and bladder rupture. Urology 40:506
Leibovitch I, Mor Y (2004) The vicious cycling: bicycling related urogenital disorders. Eur Urol Mar 47:277
Mancino P, Parlavecchio E, Melluso J, Monti M, Russo P (2003) Introducing colposcopy and vulvovaginoscopy as routine examinations for victims of sexual assault. Clin Exp Obstet Gynecol 30:40
Marekovic Z, Derezic D, Krhen I, Kastelan Z (1997) Urogenital war injuries. Mil Med 162:346
Martinez-Pineiro L Jr, Cerezo E, Cozar JM, Avellana JA, Moreno JA, Martinez-Pineiro JA (1992) Value of testicular ultrasound in the evaluation of blunt scrotal trauma without haematocele. Br J Urol 69:286
McAninch JW, Kahn RI, Jeffrey RB, Laing FC, Krieger MJ (1984) Major traumatic and septic genital injuries. J Trauma 24:291
Micallef M, Ahmad I, Ramesh N, Hurley M, McInerney D (2001) Ultrasound features of blunt testicular injury. Injury 32:23
Monga M, Hellstrom WJ (2005) Testicular trauma. Adolesc Med 1996 7:141
Morey AF, Metro MJ, Carney KJ, Miller KS, McAninch JW (2004) Consensus on genitourinary trauma: external genitalia. Br J of Urol Int 94:507
Muglia V, Tucci S Jr, Elias J Jr, Trad CS, Bilbey J, Cooperberg PL (2002) Magnetic resonance imaging of scrotal diseases: when it makes the difference. Urology 59:419
Mulhall JP, Gabram SG, Jacobs LM (1995) Emergency management of blunt testicular trauma. Acad Emerg Med 2:639
Munarriz R, Talakoub L, Somekh NN, Lehrfeld T, Chudnovsky A, Flaherty E, Goldstein I (2002) Characteristics of female patients with sexual dysfunction who also had a history of blunt perineal trauma. J Sex Marital Ther 28 [Suppl 1]:175
Nabi G, Mishriki SF (2005) Bite wounds of genitalia: clinical presentation and management. Hosp Med 66:112
Nagarajan VP, Pranikoff K, Imahori SC, Rabinowitz R (1983) Traumatic dislocation of testis. Urology 22:521
National Guideline Clearinghouse (2002) 2002 National guidelines on the management of adult victims of sexual assault. http://www.guideline.gov/summary/summary.aspx?doc_id=3050. Cited 5 December 2006
Negri L, Albani E, Di Rocco M, Levi-Setti PE (2002) Aspermia and chronic testicular pain after imperforate anus correction. Cryopreservation of sperm cells extracted from whole orchiectomized testis: case report. Hum Reprod 17:2935
Nicolaisen GS, Melamud A, Williams RD, McAninch JW (1983) Rupture of the corpus cavernosum: surgical management. J Urol 130:917
Okur H, Kucikaydin M, Kazez A, Turan C, Bozkurt A (1996) Genitourinary tract injuries in girls. Br J Urol 78:446
Orvis BR, McAninch JW (1989) Penile rupture. Urol Clin North Am 16:369
Pathak AS, Chang JH, Parekh AR, Aboseif SR (2005) Use of rectus fascia graft for corporeal reconstruction during placement of penile implant. Urology 65:1198
Patil MG, Onuora VC (1994) The value of ultrasound in the evaluation of patients with blunt scrotal trauma. Injury 25:177
Pavlica P, Barozzi L (2001) Imaging of the acute scrotum. Eur Radiol 11:220
Pollen JJ, Funckes C (1982) Traumatic dislocation of the testes. J Trauma 22:247
Pretorius ES, Siegelman ES, Ramchandani P, Banner MP (2001) MR imaging of the penis. Radiographics 21:S283; discussion S2989
Propst AM, Thorp JM Jr (1998) Traumatic vulvar hematomas: conservative versus surgical management. South Med J 91:144
Rapp DE, Cohn AB, Gottlieb LJ, Lyon MB, Bales GT (2005) Use of tissue expansion for scrotal sac reconstruction after scrotal skin loss. Urology 65:1216
Rhee P, Nunley MK, Demetriades D, Velmahos G, Doucet JJ (2005) Tetanus and trauma: a review and recommendations. J Trauma 58:1082
Salvatierra O Jr, Rigdon WO, Norris DM, Brady TW (1969)

Vietnam experience with 252 urological war injuries. J Urol 101:615
Shefi S, Mor Y, Dotan ZA, Ramon J (1999) Traumatic testicular dislocation: a case report and review of published reports. Urology 54:744
Sheldon T (2005) Dutch doctors should tackle female genital mutilation. BMJ 330:922
Sotto LSJ, Collins RJ (1958) Perigenital Hematomas. Obstet Gynecol 12:259
Tiguert R, Harb JF, Hurley PM, Gomes De Oliveira J, Castillo-Frontera RJ, Triest JA, Gheiler EL (2000) Management of shotgun injuries to the pelvis and lower genitourinary system. Urology 55:193
Tsang T, Demby AM (1992) Penile fracture with urethral injury. J Urol 147:466
Tucak A, Lukacevic T, Kuvezdic H, Petek Z, Novak R (1995) Urogenital wounds during the war in Croatia in 1991/1992. J Urol 153:121
Turone F (2004) Controversy surrounds proposed Italian alternative to female genital mutilation. BMJ 328:247
Uder M, Gohl D, Takahashi M, Derouet H, Defreyne L, Kramann B, Schneider G (2002) MRI of penile fracture: diagnosis and therapeutic follow-up. Eur Radiol 12:113
Van der Horst C, Martinez Portillo FJ, Seif C, Groth W, Jünemann KP (2004) Male genital injury: diagnosis and treatment. Br J Urol Int 93:927
Virgili A, Bianchi A, Mollica G, Corazza M (2000) Serious hematoma of the vulva from a bicycle accident. A case report. J Reprod Med 45:662
Waltzman ML, Shannon M, Bowen AP, Bailey MC (1999) Monkeybar injuries: complications of play. Pediatrics 103:e58
Wang D, Zheng H, Deng F (2003) Spermatogenesis after scrotal reconstruction. Br J Plast Surg 56:484
Wasko R, Goldstein AG (1966) Traumatic rupture of the testicle. J Urol 95:721
Whelan C, Stewart J, Schwartz BF (2005) Mechanics of wound healing and importance of vaccum assisted closure in urology. J Urol May 173:1463
World Health Organization (2000) Fact sheet No. 241, June 2000
Pan American Health Organization (2000) Epidemiologic surveillance and disease control. In: Natural disasters: protecting the public health. World Health Organization, Pan American Health Organization, Washington, DC, p 43
Xeroulis G, Inaba K, Stewart TC, Lannigan R, Gray D, Malthaner R, Parry NG, Girotti M (2005) Human immunodeficiency virus, hepatitis B, and hepatitis C seroprevalence in a Canadian trauma population. J Trauma 59:105

15.8 Management of Penile Amputation

G.H. Jordan

15.8.1 Introduction

When one reviews the literature surrounding penile amputation, most of what is found is individual case reports or reports of small series. Thus what is considered to be state-of-the-art management is gleaned from literature review, and frankly reliant on expert opinion. An exception to this statement is a series of penile amputation from Thailand published in 1983 (Bhanganada et al. 1983) in the *American Journal of Surgery*. That report described the management of approximately 100 cases of penile amputation, many of which preceded the description of microreplantation techniques and validated much of what literature reviews have proposed.

In Western culture, penile amputation injuries are seen primarily as a result of felonious assault or self-emasculation in the psychotic individual who is responding to command hallucinations. One will also find descriptions of penile amputation as a consequence of circumcision. In most cases, however, in circumcision trauma, what is amputated is the penile skin and/or only a portion of the glans (Neulander et al. 1996; Strimling 1996). True penile amputation is seen in cultures that still perform ritual circumcision, but again the literature reveals only sporadic reports (Ameh et al. 1997; Ozkan and Gurpinar 1997; Hashem et al. 1999; Silfen et al. 2000; Izzidien 1981).

In a review by Greilsheimer and Groves (1979), it was found that patients who amputate or mutilate their genitalia represent a heterogenous group. Eighty-seven percent are believed or shown to be psychotic at the time of the accident, with 51% in a decompensated schizophrenic state. The other group represents individuals with severe character disorders or in some cases gender identity problems. Those individuals are often under the influence of drugs or alcohol at the time of their genital amputation event. While many psychotic individuals have a long history of mental illness, usually the act of self-mutilation occurs during an acute psychotic decompensation. There are some individuals who during their first psychotic break will attempt the amputation of the penis or another body part. In a paper by Hall et al. (1981), it was reported that the psychotic individual often has a history of preexisting conflicts about his role as a male; but with a psychotic break, the individual comes under the effect of hallucinations commanding him to amputate all of his genitalia, or some other form of partial self-mutilation.

Blacker and Wong (1963) show that many of these patients are born to a domineering older mother in the home where there is no male influence. In many cases, the families are impoverished, thus limiting the association of the child with other adults and in particular adult males. It was found that many of these individuals were made to feel guilty or inadequate as males in their childhood. Blacker and Wong have described self-mutilation as a form of focal suicide. Dogma would say that in the case of self-mutilation, replantation is contraindicated, as the patient, when capable, will "just pull the replanted part off again." This has not been the experience of the author, and Stewart and Lowery (1980) in their review state that self-inflicted injury is not an absolute contraindication. The literature in fact attests to a high degree of successful mental rehabilitation in these patients. I believe that the dictum should be replantation first and psychiatry second. Greilsheimer and Groves' (1979) review of over 40 patients of penile amputation show that in that group there was only one postoperative suicide and one repeat attempt at genital self-mutilation. That said, however, when one is confronted in the emergency room with a patient who has undertaken genital self-mutilation, one must be very careful to know the laws of the venue in which one is "operating." In some cases, court order is required, in some states only the agreeing opinion of two practitioners is required, and certainly many other variations of this theme exist from state to state. Often times, getting consent from the patient is possible and where possible should absolutely be done.

At our center, we have also become aware of another interesting phenomenon, probably best described as focal homicide by proxy. We have treated two cases in whom a male child was the victim of penile amputation by his mother. The motivation, however, for the attack on the child was the behavior of the father. In one case, the father was actively physically abusive of the woman; and in another case the father had been discovered to be having an affair. In neither case was replantation possible, as the child's mother took steps to ensure that the amputated part was not available.

With regards to the patient with command hallucinations, the hallucinations not uncommonly involve God or God's representative telling the patient to mutilate himself (Schweitzer 1990; Clark 1981; Waugh 1986; Culliford 1987). Ames (1987) has suggested the eponym of Klingsor syndrome for the phenomenon. In some cases, the delusions involve the notion that there is promise of great things currently denied the individual because of sexual thoughts or sexual indiscretion. Many of these patients find, initially, the hallucinations to be troublesome. Many patients look to the Bible for "confirmation of the will of God." Examples of scripture which seem to support the notions of the hallucinations can be found in Matthew 5:9, Matthew 18:9, and Mark 9:47. The delusional individual obviously misrepresents, to himself, the intent of scripture, thus interpreting the scripture as reaffirmation of the commands. In talking with these patients, once the patient has his affirmation, it is only a matter of time before he proceeds with the act of genital mutilation.

The patient, often times, reports the commands to doctors or other medical personnel, but in vague terms. It is trite to say, however, that the best way to treat a penile amputation is to prevent it. Thus all primary care practitioners, primary healthcare or not, must be alert to the vagueness of these comments; and when they are heard, they must be regarded as very serious and not absurd and trifling, as in many cases they may seem.

15.8.2 History of Penile Replantation

In 1929, the first case of replantation of an amputated penis was reported (Ehrich 1929). The patient had amputated his penis using a radial saw. During the trauma, the patient's penile skin was avulsed; the penis was replanted by macroscopic techniques and buried in the patient's scrotum. Two years later, with liberation of the penis from the scrotum, the patient had a penis that looked quite normal cosmetically and functioned very normally. In 1976, two groups independently reported the first successful microreplantation of an amputated penis (Cohen et al. 1977; Tamai et al. 1977). Neither group was aware of the other's work, and since these landmark reports, other cases using similar techniques have been published with excellent, reproducible results. A review by Carroll and associates in 1985 (Carroll et al. 1985) proposed a logical sequence of care for the patient with penile amputation. In that review, patients were reported to have excellent sensation; ability to achieve intromission was not specifically addressed. Using techniques that vary little from the initial reports of 1977, microreplantation of the penis has been changed from reportable to essentially nonreportable. In 1968, McRoberts reported a case and review of the literature (McRoberts et al. 1968). He then summarized the technique for replantation of the amputated penis using macrotechniques. In that technique, all structures that could be coapted were coapted; this included a repair of the urethra, coaptation of the erectile bodies, and later it was proposed that anastomosis of the dorsal vein was possible under loop magnification with improved results. McRoberts had noted that using these techniques, the skin of the penis if it was avulsed at the time of trauma was frequently sloughed during the postoperative period. He thus recommended debriding the skin of the penis to the coronal margin and burying the penis in the scrotum. The penis could later be liberated, and with the development of microsurgical techniques, nerve repair could later be undertaken. In these cases, often times the glans will develop an eschar; however, uniformly the spongy erectile tissue seems to survive and will re-epithelialize. In the abovementioned series from Thailand, 18 of the 100 cases were managed with microreplantation techniques, many were managed by macroreplantation techniques, and of course in some cases, the end of the penis of some unfortunate patients did not manage to make it to the hospital with the patient.

15.8.3 Anatomy of the Penis

The deep vasculature of the penis is totally dependent on branches of the deep internal pudendal arteries. These are branches of the hypogastric artery. The pudendal artery courses to the perineum via Alcock's canal, and in the perineum gives off the posterior scrotal arteries and the perineal arteries. The vessels then continue as the common penile artery (Fig. 15.8.1) where the artery goes on to multiply bifurcate to provide vasculature to the corpus spongiosum and urethra, as well as the corporal bodies and the glans penis (Kodos 1967). The skin of the penis is dependent on a fasciocutaneous blood supply based on the superficial external pudendal artery (Fig. 15.8.2) (Quartey 1983). The venous drainage of the penis has likewise been nicely de-

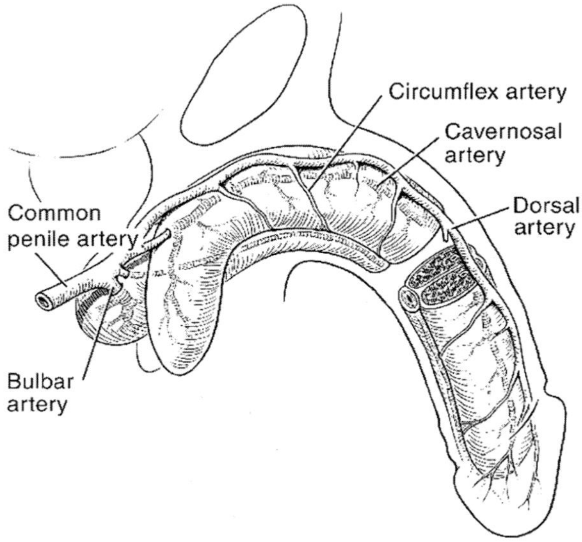

Fig. 15.8.1. Illustration of the common penile arterial system. This is the vasculature to the deep structures of the penis

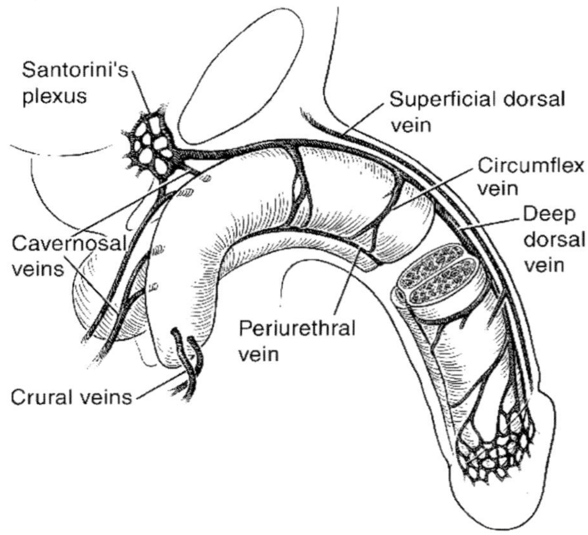

Fig. 15.8.3. Illustration of the venous drainage of the deep structures of the penis (Aboseif 1983)

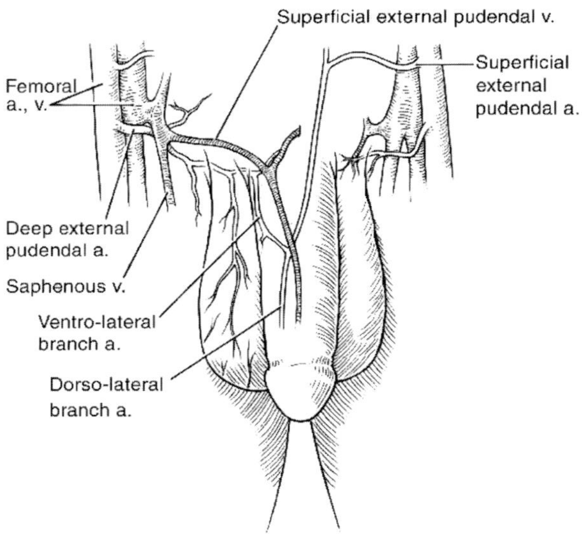

Fig. 15.8.2. Illustration of the superficial external pudendal artery as described by the microinjection studies of Quartey (Quartey 1983)

scribed. The venous system has been divided into three systems: 1) the superficial dorsal system, 2) the deep dorsal venous system, and 3) the crural vessels, which depart from the corporal cavernosa at the crus of the corpora and go on to drain into the periprostatic plexus, and the cavernosal venous system, which likewise departs from the proximal crura and becomes part of the dorsal vein to the penis and the periprostatic plexus (Fig. 15.8.3) (Aboseif et al. 1993).

15.8.4 Penile Replantation

When one is alerted, as a surgeon, that a patient with penile amputation is being brought in, the initial attention must be directed to the preservation of the amputated portion of the penis. Hypothermia prolongs the ischemic survival times of all tissues (Hayhurst et al. 1974). The amputated penis must be regarded as a free flap. Literature that has examined the no-reflow phenomena in a rabbit flap survival model shows that ischemia time clearly affects these phenomena (May et al. 1978). This has been shown in a number of other flap models. In a study examining digital replantation, Hayhurst and his associates demonstrated that hypothermia prolonged the ischemia time or was compatible with eventual survival from 6 to 24 h (Hayhurst et al. 1974). The precise response to hypothermia of the penis has not been studied; however, penile replantation after 16 h, much of which was normal thermic ischemia time, has been reported to be successful (Hashem et al. 1999; Mosahebi et al. 2001; Jezior et al. 2001). At our center, a penis was successfully replanted after 18 h, much of which was hypothermic ischemia time.

Thus I would recommend the following technique: the penis should be placed in saline-soaked gauze and then placed in a sterile plastic bag. The plastic bag can then be placed in slush and the amputated part then transported (Fig. 15.8.4).

The process that we have used in our patients begins with obtaining approval to proceed with surgery. The amputated organ remains in hypothermic preservation. It is essential that the patient be well hydrated, and throughout the procedure, the patient's body tempera-

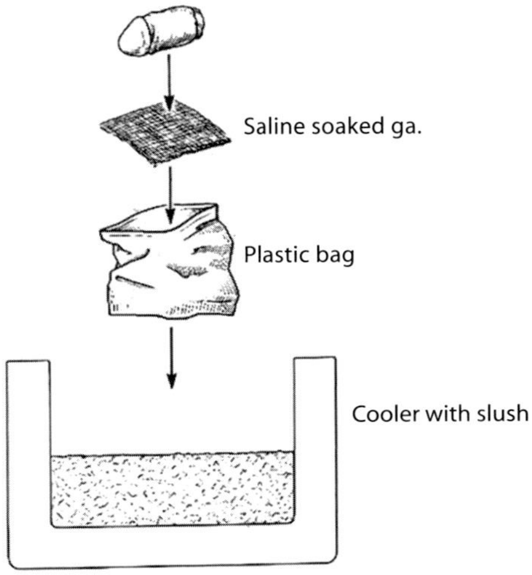

Fig. 15.8.4. Illustration of the technique of "cold ischemic" preservation of organs. In the case of the penis, the amputated part should be placed on a saline-soaked sponge and put into a sterile (if none is available, clean) plastic bag. The bag is then immersed in iced slush

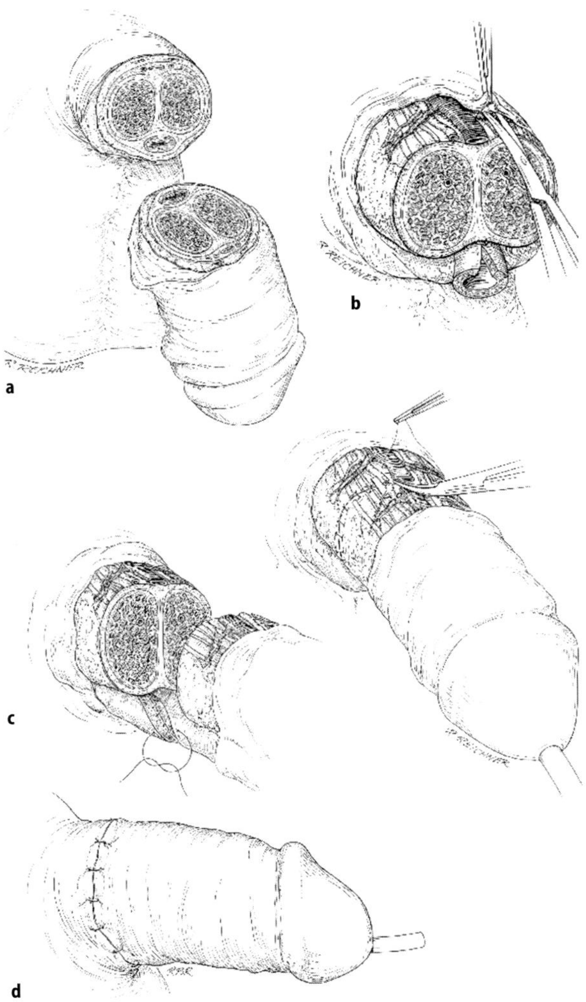

ture should be kept normal. Thus we aggressively use heat lamps and heating devices to keep the patient warm and peripherally vasodilated.

Without question, microsurgical techniques have been demonstrated to be superior and hence are the preferred method of replantation whenever possible. The technique has been well described. The structures that must be anastomosed are the deep dorsal vein, the dorsal arteries, and the dorsal nerves (Fig. 15.8.5). The erectile bodies are coapted, and a two-layer spatulated urethral reanastomosis is performed. Thus, minimal debridement is required to expose these structures (Fig. 15.8.5d). We proceed with the urethral reconstruction first, and a Foley catheter is then placed through the urethra to stabilize the two parts (Fig. 15.8.5d). The urethral epithelium is approximated with small polyglycolic acid (PGA) sutures, and the body of the corpus spongiosum reapproximated with a small suture of poly diaxanone (PDS). While proximally the cavernosal arteries can be identified, it is not recommended to try to do a microanastomosis of these arteries, as the technique is difficult, control of the proximal arteries almost impossible, and nothing has shown improved results with the attempts at coaptation. Next, the corpora cavernosa are reapproximated. This is done with small interrupted sutures of polydiaxanone (PDS).

The dorsal neurovascular structures are then addressed (Fig. 15.8.5d). The vascular integrity of the corpora cavernosa has been reestablished, and because the corpus spongiosum has been reopposed, there will be some venous drainage of the penis. Hence, one can proceed with the anastomosis of the dorsal arteries; 10-0 or 11-0 nylon suture is used for these anastomoses. The dorsal vein is then reanastomosed and a 9-0 or 10-0 nylon suture can be used. After the penis has been revascularized, the surgeon can then direct his attention to the coaptation of the dorsal nerves. Proximally the epineurium can be coapted using 9-0 or 10-0 nylon suture. If the amputation is very distal, then the surgeon may find that, in some areas, fascicular coaptation may be required. The Foley catheter is then removed, a urethral stent of soft silicone silastic is placed in the distal urethra, to serve as a drain. The urine is diverted via a suprapubic cystostomy catheter. We have kept our pa-

◁
Fig. 15.8.5a–d. Collage illustrating the technique of microreplantation of the penis. **a** The amputated part is placed on the operating table. **b** Minimal dissection and debridement of Buck's fascia, the tunica albuginea in some cases, and the urethral edges are required. The urethra is mobilized somewhat both distally and proximally to allow for a spatulated anastomosis. **c** The Foley catheter is placed through the urethra and a two-layer spatulated anastomosis is performed. **d** The corpora cavernosa have been reapproximated using an interrupted long-acting absorbable suture. The microvasculature and nerves are then anastomosed and coapted

tients at bed rest for approximately 1 week and have maintained their urinary diversion for 2–3 weeks, depending on wound healing, i.e., the presence or lack of presence of associated skin loss. We do not do pericatheter urethrograms, but rather at the time of the voiding trial with contrast, the stent is removed, the patient's bladder is filled, and as mentioned a voiding film using contrast is obtained. We do not routinely use anticoagulation in these patients. As mentioned, during the early postoperative period, the patients are kept in a warm room, ostensibly keeping them peripherally dilated and somewhat hyperdynamic. They are kept well hydrated, the hematocrit is kept at a level in the low 30s, in other words, the vast majority of these patients do not require transfusion. The patient is closely monitored using Doppler.

If the patient is transferred to a facility without microreplantation capabilities or if the patient's other physical conditions would preclude the time required for a microreplantation, then the technique described by McRoberts and associates (McRoberts et al. 1968) has also yielded surprisingly good and consistent results. Briefly, as already mentioned, they suggest that the distal penile skin be removed, and the reapproximated penile shaft be buried in the scrotum with the glans protruding. The corpora cavernosa are coapted, and the urethra is reconstructed; if possible the dorsal vein can be coapted, and one must be careful to ensure that the proximal ends and the distal ends of the dorsal arteries are ligated. A urethral stent is placed, a urethral Foley catheter is not used, and a suprapubic cystostomy is placed.

If the patient presents without the amputated end of his penis, hemostasis must be obtained, and the issue then is how to close the penis. In many cases, a great deal of skin has been amputated, but not much of the erectile bodies, and in these cases, primary grafting with a split-thickness skin graft is acceptable. To avoid subsequent meatal stenosis, the neomeatus must be widely spatulated, no matter what technique of skin coverage is employed.

15.8.5 Summary

The development of microsurgery techniques has drastically modified the management of these injuries. The results reported in the literature have been astonishingly good (Stewart and Lowery 1980; Cohen et al. 1977; Tamai et al. 1977; Aboseif et al. 1993; Jezior et al. 2001; Yamano and Tanaka 1983; Wei et al. 1983; Tuerk and Weir 1971; Strauch et al. 1983; Schulman 1973; Jordan and Gilbert 1988; Heymann et al. 1977; Henriksson et al. 1982; Evins et al. 1977; Einarsson et al. 1983; Goldstein 1978; Szasz et al. 1990; Peterson 1992; Zenn et al. 2000; Darewics et al. 2001; Yeniyol et al. 2002). After microreplantation, the patient can be expected to be left with a penis that is cosmetically very normal in appearance and function, with almost undetectable abnormalities, if any.

References

Aboseif S, Gomez R, McAninch JW (1983) Genital self-mutilation. J Urol 150:1143

Ameh EA, Sabo SY, Muhammad I (1997) Amputation of the penis during traditional circumcision. Trop Doct 27:117

Ames D (1987) Autocastration and biblical delusions in schizophrenia (letter) Br J Psychiatry 150:407

Bhanganada K, Chayavatana T, Pongnumkul C et al (1983) Surgical management of an epidemic of penis amputations in Siam. Am J Surg 146:376

Blacker KH, Wong N (1963) Four cases of autocastration. Arch Gen Psychiatry 8:189

Carroll PR, Leu TF, Schmidt RA et al (1985) Penile replantation: current concepts. J Urol 133:281

Clark RA (1981) Self-mutilation accompanying religious delusion: a case report and review. J Clin Psychiatry 42:243

Cohen BE, May JW, Daly JS et al (1977) Successful clinical replantation of an amputated penis by microneurovascular repair. Plast Reconstr Surg 59:276

Culliford L (1987) Autocastration and biblical delusions in schizophrenia (letter) Br J Psychiatry 150:407

Darewicz B, Galek L, Darewicz J, Kudelski J, Malczyk E (2001) Successful microsurgical replantation of an amputated penis. Int Urol Nephrol 33:385

Ehrich WS (1929) Two unusual penile injuries. J Urol 21:239

Einarsson G, Goldstein M, Laungani G (1983) Penile replantation. Urology 22:404

Evins SC, Whittle T, Rous SN (1977) Self-emasculation: review of the literature, report of a case and outline of the objectives of management. J Urol 188:775

Goldstein M (1978) Microsurgical reimplantation of amputated penis. Urol 12:237

Greilsheimer H, Groves JE (1979) Male genital self-mutilation. Arch Gen Psychiatry 36:441

Hall DC, Lawson BX, Wilson LG (1981) Command hallucinations and self-amputation of the penis and hand during a first psychotic break. J Clin Psychiatry 42:322

Hashem FK, Ahmed S, al-Malaq AA, AbuDaia JM (1999) Successful replantation of penile amputation (post-circumcision) complicated by prolonged ischaemia. Br J Plast Surg. 52:308

Hayhurst JW, O'Brien BM, Ishida H et al (1974) Experimental digital replantation after prolonged cooling. Hand 6:143

Henriksson TG, Hahne B, Hakelius S et al (1982) Microsurgical replantation of an amputated penis. Scand J Plast Reconstr Surg Suppl 19:75

Heymann AD, Bell-Thomson J, Rathod DM et al (1977) Successful reimplantation of the penis using microvascular techniques. J Urol 118:879

Izzidien AY (1981) Successful replantation of a traumatically amputated penis in a neonate. J Pediatr Surg 16:202

Jezior JR, Brady JD, Schlossberg SM (2001) Management of penile amputation injuries. World J Surg 25:1602

Jordan GH, Gilbert DA (1988) Male genital trauma. Clin Plast Surg 15:431

Kodos AB (1967) The vascular supply of the penis. Arkh Anat Embriol 43:525

May JW Jr, Chait LA, O'Brien BM et al (1978) The no-reflow phenomenon in experimental free flaps. Plast Reconstr Surg 61:256

McRoberts JW, Chapman WH, Ansell JS (1968) Primary anastomosis of the traumatically amputated penis: cast report and summary of literature. J Urol 100:751

Mosahebi A, Butterworth M, Knight R, Berger L, Kaisary A, Butler PE (2001) Delayed penile replantation after prolonged warm ischemia. Microsurgery 21:52

Neulander E, Walfisch S, Kaneti J (1996) Amputation of distal penile glans during neonatal ritual circumcision – a rare complication. Br J Urol. 77:924

Ozkan S, Gurpinar T (1997) A serious circumcision complication: penile shaft amputation and a new reattachment technique with a successful outcome. J Urol 158:1946

Peterson NE (1992) Repair of a traumatically amputated penis with return of erectile function. J Urol 147:1628

Quartey JKM (1983) One-stage penile/preputial cutaneous island flap urethroplasty for urethral stricture : a preliminary report. J Urol 129:284

Schweitzer I (1990) Genital self-amputation and the Klingsor syndrome. Aust N Z J Psychiatry 24:566

Schulman ML (1973) Reanastomosis of the amputated penis. J Urol 109:432

Silfen R, Hudson DA, McCulley S (2000) Penile lengthening for traumatic penile amputation due to ritual circumcision: a case report. Ann Plast Surg 44:311

Strauch B, Sharzer LA, Petro J et al (1983) Replantation of amputated parts of the penis, nose, ear, and scalp. Clin Plast Surg 10:115

Stewart DE, Lowery MR (1980) Replantation surgery following self-inflicted amputation. Can J Psychiatry 25:143

Strimling BS (1996) Partial amputation of glans penis during Mogen clamp circumcision. Pediatrics 97:906

Szasz G, McLoughlin MG, Warren RJ (1990) Return of sexual functioning following penile replant surgery. Arch Sex Behav. 19343

Tamai S, Nakamura Y, Motomiya Y (1977) Microsurgical replantation of a completely amputated penis and scrotum. Plast Reconstr Surg 60:287

Tuerk M, Weir WH Jr (1971) Successful replantation of a traumatically amputated glans penis. Plast Reconstr Surg 48:499

Waugh AC (1986) Autocastration and biblical delusions in schizophrenia. Br J Psychiatry 149:656

Wei FC, McKee NH, Huerta FJ et al (1983) Microsurgical replantation of a completely amputated penis. Ann Plast Surg 20:317

Yamano Y, Tanaka H (1984) Replantation of a completely amputated penis by the microsurgical technique: A case report. Microsurgery 5:40

Yeniyol CO, Yener H, Kececi Y, Ayder AR (2002) Microvascular replantation of a self-amputated penis. Int Urol Nephrol 33:117

Zenn MR, Carson CC 3rd, Patel MP (2000) Replantation of the penis: a patient report. Ann Plast Surg 44:214

15.9 Urethral Trauma

L. Martínez-Piñeiro

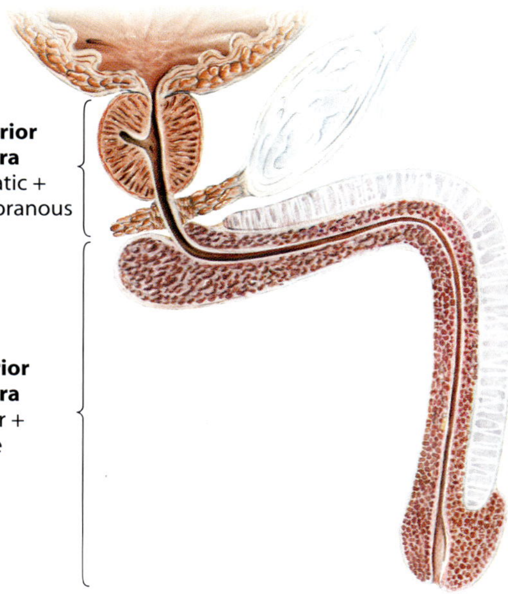

Fig. 15.9.1. Anatomy of the male urethra (© Hohenfellner 2007)

15.9.1 Anatomical and Etiological Considerations

The male urethra is divided into the anterior and posterior sections by the urogenital diaphragm. The posterior urethra consists of the prostatic and the membranous urethra (Fig. 15.9.1). The anterior urethra consists of the bulbar and penile urethra. Only the posterior urethra exists in the female; the anterior urethra corresponds to the labia minora, which results from persistent separation of the urethral folds on the ventral surfaces of the genital tubercle.

15.9.1.1 Posterior Urethral Injuries

Injuries to the posterior urethra occur with pelvic fractures, which are commonly caused by road traffic accidents, crush injuries, or falls from height. Approximately two-thirds (70%) of pelvic fractures occur as a result of motor vehicle accidents, with an incidence of 20% in fatal motor accidents, as a driver or passenger, and nearly 50% in fatal pedestrian accidents. Twenty-five per cent of cases present as a result of a fall from a height (Koraitim et al. 1996; Sevitt 1968) Altogether, blunt trauma accounts for more than 90% of urethral injuries (Dixon 1996). Overall, the male posterior urethra is concomitantly injured in approximately 3.5%–19% and the female urethra in 0%–6% of all pelvic fractures (Carlin and Resnick 1995; Clark and Prudencio 1972; Colapinto 1980; Hemal et al. 2000; Koraitim et al. 1996; Lowe et al. 1988; Palmer et al. 1983; Perry and Husmann 1992; Pokorny et al. 1978; Webster et al. 1983). The female urethra is rarely injured, except by contusion or laceration by bone fragments.

Specifically with a crush or deceleration impact injury, the severe shearing forces necessary to fracture the pelvis are transmitted to the prostatomembranous junction, resulting in disruption of the prostate from its connection to the anterior urethra at the prostatic apex. Retrograde urethrography and magnetic resonance imaging have been correlated with this location of the injury (Colapinto and McCallum 1977; Dixon et al. 1992). Recent cadaveric anatomic studies suggest that in most cases the membranous urethra is torn distally to the urogenital diaphragm (Mouraview and Santucci 2005).

Accurate knowledge of the functional anatomy of the sphincter mechanism is essential to the success of posterior urethral surgery. The feasibility of anastomotic reconstruction of subprostatic pelvic fracture urethral distraction defects depends upon the independent function of the proximal bladder neck and of the distal urethral sphincter mechanism, each of which is competent and independently capable of maintaining continence in the absence of the other (Turner-Warwick 1973).

In order to accurately diagnose and treat pelvic ring disruptions, the surgeon must have a concept of pelvic stability, which should be determined in both the horizontal and vertical planes. A mechanically stable pelvis is defined as one that can withstand normal physiological forces without abnormal deformation (Tile and Pennal 1980). The degree of instability is best indicated by the disruption and posterior displacement at the sacroiliac area and is of extreme importance as a prognostic indicator for the general resuscitation of the patient (Pennal et al. 1980). The anteroposterior and lateral compression types of fracture, while vastly different, may be associated with both stable and unstable subtypes.

The vertical shear fracture is always unstable. The latter described by Malgaigne in 1855 consists of a fracture anteriorly through both rami of the symphysis pubis, in association with massive posterior disruption, either through the sacrum, the sacroiliac joint, or the ilium.

Stable Pelvic Fracture

In a stable pelvic fracture, urethral disruption can occur when the large external force, which has fractured two or all four pelvic rami (straddle fracture), propels the resultant butterfly fragment backward together with the prostate, which is fixed to the back of the pubic bone (Fig. 15.9.2). The shearing force that results disrupts the membranous urethra, as it passes through the perineum and inevitably destroys the distal urethral sphincter mechanism in almost all such cases.

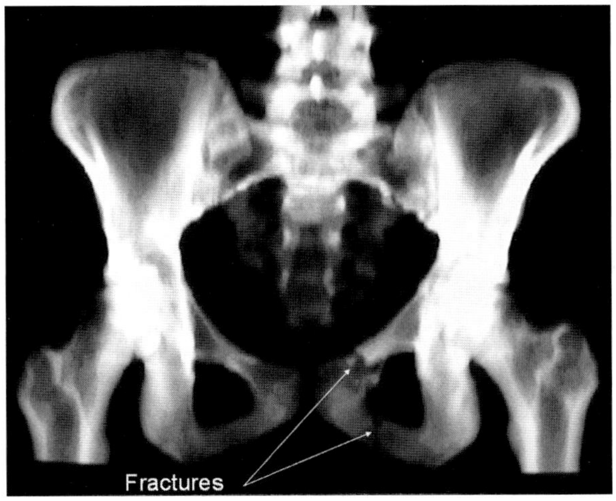

Fig. 15.9.2. Example of stable pelvic fracture. Both pubic rami of the left side are fractured. A mechanically stable pelvis is defined as one that can withstand normal physiological forces without abnormal deformation

Unstable Pelvic Fractures

Unstable fractures that involve the anterior part of the pubic ring and the sacroiliac joint, ileum, or sacrum can also cause injuries to the posterior urethra, either as a result of tears by bony fractures or, more commonly, as a result of disruptions of the urethra caused by distortions of the bony pelvis during major trauma.

This distortion is thought to result in lateral shearing forces, acting on the membranous urethra, as the puboprostatic ligaments and the membranous urethral area are pulled in opposite directions (Pokorny et al. 1978). Unstable diametric pelvic fractures (Conolly and Hedbert 1969; Devine and Devine 1982; Flaherty et al. 1968; Palmer et al. 1983; Pokorny et al. 1978) or bilateral ischiopubic rami fractures have the highest likelihood of injuring the posterior urethra. In particular, the combination of straddle fractures with diastasis of the sacroiliac joint has the highest risk of urethral injury; the odds ratio is about seven times higher than for straddle or Malgaigne fractures (Table 15.9.1) (Fig. 15.9.3) (Koraitim et al. 1996).

Lower urinary tract injury has been reported in about 16% of patients with unilateral rami fractures, but in 41% of patients with bilateral rami fractures (Zorn 1960). Anteroposterior compression injuries from frontal crushes produce more severe pelvic fractures, major retroperitoneal bleeding, and more frequent injury to the lower urinary tract than do lateral crashes (Siegel et al. 1990).

Table 15.9.1. Odds ratio of urethral injury with different types of pelvic fracture

Type of fracture	Odds ratio
Single ramus	0.64
Ipsilateral rami	0.76
Malgaigne's	3.40
Straddle	3.85
Straddle plus sacroiliac	24.02

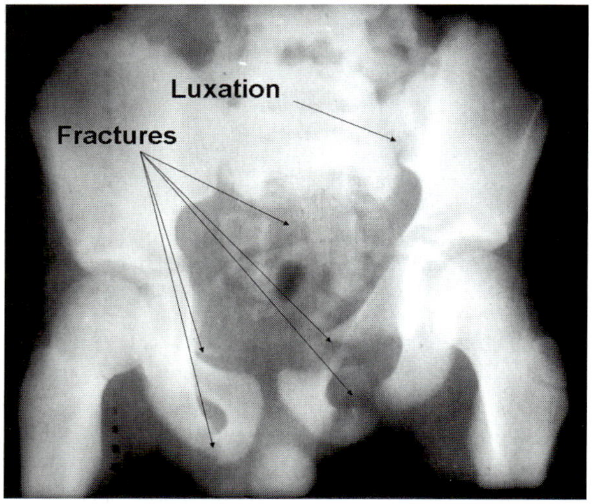

Fig. 15.9.3. Example of unstable pelvic fracture. Unstable fractures involve the anterior part of the pubic ring and the sacroiliac joint, ileum, or sacrum

Prostatomembranous urethral injuries can vary from simple stretching (25%) to partial rupture (25%) or complete disruptions (50%) (Koraitim et al. 1996). The more severe injuries result in prostatourethral displacement, with progressive scar formation encompassing the rupture defect. The incidence of double injuries involving the urethra and the bladder ranges between 10% and 20% of males, and may be intraperitoneal (17%–39%) or extraperitoneal (56%–78%), or both (Carlin and Resnick 1995; Koraitim et al. 1996).

Urethral injuries, by themselves, are never life-threatening, except as a consequence of their close association with pelvic fractures and multiple organ injuries, which occur in about 27% of cases. Initially, the assessment and management of other associated injuries are usually far more important than the assessment and management of the urethral injury (Chapple and Png 1999).

Colapinto and McCallum (1977) classified posterior urethral injuries on the basis of radiographic appearance into three types, depending on the integrity of the membranous urethra and extension of the disruption into the bulbar and membranous urethra. The American Association for Surgery of Trauma (AAST) later proposed the classification given in Table 15.9.2.

Table 15.9.2. Organ injury scaling III classification of urethral injuries

Type	Description	Appearance
I	Contusion	Blood at the urethral meatus; normal urethrogram
II	Stretch injury	Elongation of the urethra without extravasation on urethrography
III	Partial disruption	Extravasation of contrast at injury site with contrast visualized in the bladder
IV	Complete disruption	Extravasation of contrast at injury site without visualization in the bladder; < 2 cm of urethral separation
V	Complete disruption	Complete transection with > 2 cm urethral separation, or extension into the prostate or vagina

From Moore et al. 1992

Table 15.9.3 presents a summary of the different types of blunt trauma of the posterior and anterior urethra, along with their radiographic appearance and different treatment alternatives.

Urethral Injuries in Children

Urethral injuries in children tend to follow the same mechanism of injury as in adults. The only significant difference is that straddle pelvic fractures, Malgaigne's fractures, or the association of straddle plus sacroiliac joint fracture are more common in children than in adults. In addition, posterior urethral injuries can involve the prostatic urethra and the bladder neck, as well as the membranous urethra. The tear is often in the prostatic urethra or at the bladder neck because of the rudimentary nature of the prostate and is more likely to be a complete rupture (69% vs 42%). Urethral stretching is less common than in adults. It has been shown that the more proximal the injury, the greater the risk of incontinence, impotence, and stricture formation in the long term (Chapple and Png 1999; Koraitim 1997, 1999; Koraitim et al. 1996).

Urethral Injuries in Women

These are rare events since the female urethra is short and mobile, without any significant attachments to the pubic bone. They usually occur in children and are accompanied by severe pelvic fractures, where bony fragments of the fractured pelvis provoke lacerations of the urethra, frequently extending into the bladder neck or vagina, and disrupting the normal continence mechanism (Hemal et al. 2000; Perry and Husmann 1992). Injury to the female urethra is usually a partial tear of the anterior wall and is rarely a complete disruption of the proximal or distal urethra (Koraitim 1999).

Table 15.9.3. Different types of blunt trauma of the posterior and anterior urethra, their radiographic appearance and different treatment alternatives

	Description	Management
I	Stretch injury. Elongation of the urethra without extravasation on urethrography	No treatment required
II	Contusion. Blood at the urethral meatus; no extravasation on urethrography	Conservative management with suprapubic cystostomy or urethral catheterization
III	Partial disruption of anterior or posterior urethra. Extravasation of contrast at injury site with contrast visualized in the proximal urethra or bladder	Conservative management with suprapubic cystostomy or urethral catheterization
IV	Complete disruption of anterior urethra. Extravasation of contrast at injury site without visualization of proximal urethra or bladder	Conservative management with suprapubic cystostomy. Open or endoscopic treatment, primary or delayed
V	Complete disruption of posterior urethra. Extravasation of contrast at injury site without visualization of bladder	Conservative management with suprapubic cystostomy. Open or endoscopic treatment, primary or delayed
VI	Complete or partial disruption of posterior urethra with associated tear of the bladder neck or vagina	Primary open repair

Penetrating Injuries to the Perineum

These can occur involving the urethra, as well as being iatrogenic injuries caused by endoscopic instrumentation or during surgery for vaginal repair. In developing countries, urethral and bladder neck damage occur quite often as a result of ischemic injury during obstructed labor.

15.9.1.2 Anterior Urethral Injuries

Anterior urethral injuries result from blunt trauma more frequently than from penetrating trauma (Table 15.9.4).

Blunt Trauma

Most anterior urethral injuries are caused by vehicular accidents, falls, or blows; in contrast to posterior urethral trauma, they are rarely associated with pelvic fractures. They are usually straddle-type injuries caused by blows of blunt objects against the perineum, such as bicycle handlebars or the top of a fence. In this type of accident, the relatively immobile bulbar urethra is trapped and compressed by a direct force on it against the inferior surface of the symphysis pubis. These injuries are more common in children than adults (Koraitim 1997).

Intercourse-Related Trauma

Another less frequent cause of blunt anterior urethral trauma occurs in association with ruptures of the corpora cavernosa, which usually occur with an erect penis, often during intercourse (Fig. 15.9.4). In these injuries, the urethra is involved in 20% of the cases (Nicolaisen et al. 1983). Intraluminal stimulation of the urethra with foreign objects has also been reported to cause anterior urethral trauma. Most are short and incomplete and occur in the distal penile urethra. Surgery is rarely indicated and depends on the degree and extent of injury to the urethra.

Table 15.9.4. Etiology of anterior urethral injuries

Causes
Blunt trauma
Vehicular accidents
Fall astride
Kicks in the perineum
Blows in the perineum from bicycle handlebars, tops of fences, etc.
Sexual intercourse
Penile fractures
Urethral intraluminal stimulation
Constriction bands
Penetrating trauma
Gunshot wounds
Stab wounds
Dog bites
External impalement
Penile amputations
Constriction bands
Paraplegia
Iatrogenic injuries
Endoscopic instrumentations
Urethral catheters, dilators

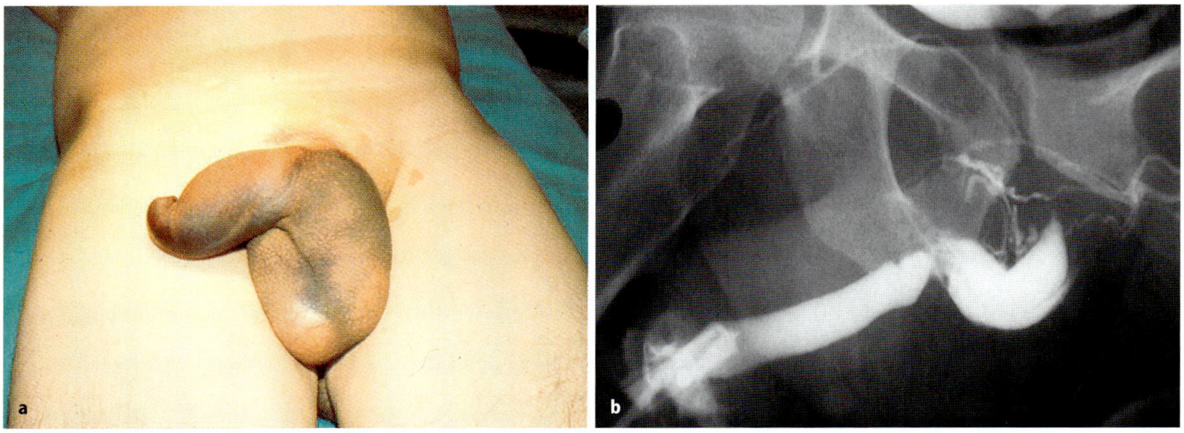

Fig. 15.9.4. **a** Typical aspect of genitalia after rupture of corpora cavernosa during sexual intercourse. **b** In 20% of the cases, the urethra is involved, suffering partial or complete rupture

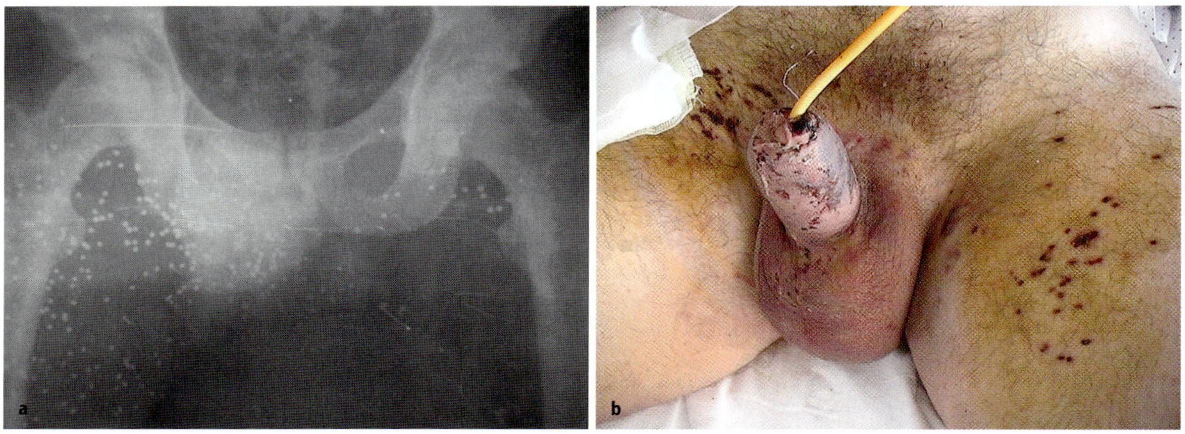

Fig. 15.9.5a, b. Gunshot wound to the genitalia. Penile urethra was involved with only a few pellets and was managed conservatively

Penetrating Trauma

Penetrating injuries to the anterior urethra usually occur from gunshot wounds and involve the pendulous and bulbar urethral segments equally; these injuries are often found with penetrating penile or testicular trauma, depending on the missile tract (Figs. 15.9.5, 15.9.6). These can involve the rectum, which may result in pelvic abscesses and fistulae formation.(Gomez et al. 1993; Pontes and Pierce 1978). Other less frequent causes of external anterior urethral injuries include stab wounds, animal bites (Fig. 15.9.7), penile amputation, and external impalement.

Constriction Band-Related Trauma

Individuals with paraplegia, who use a constriction device for urinary incontinence and forget to release the band due to the lack of sensation, can cause severe ischemic injuries involving the penis and urethra (Fig. 15.9.8).

Iatrogenic Trauma

Iatrogenic urethral injuries caused by instrumentation are by far the most common cause of urethral trauma. Urethral ischemic injuries related to cardiac bypass procedures are not infrequent and can result in long and fibrotic strictures.

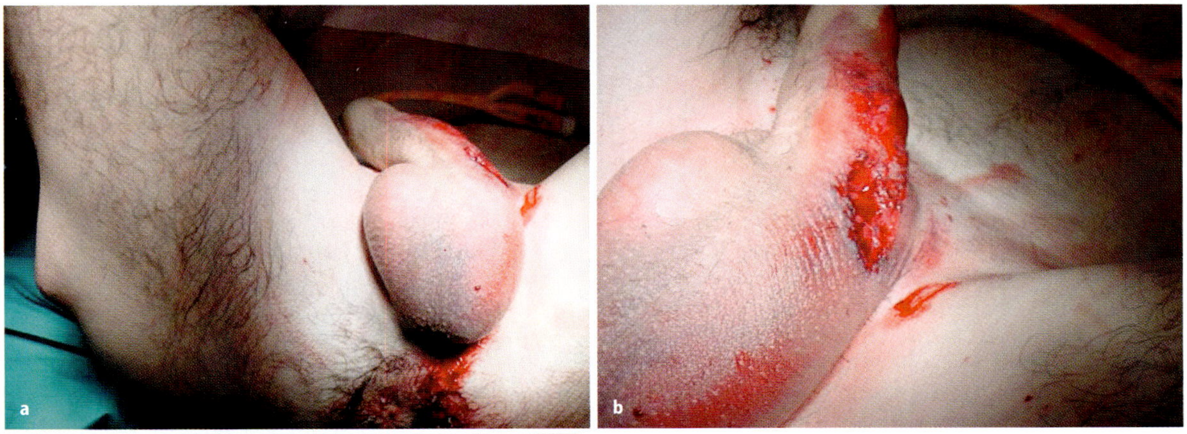

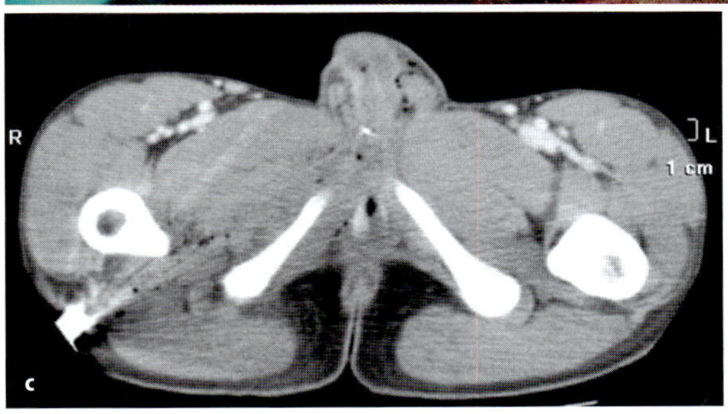

Fig. 15.9.6a–c. Gunshot wound to the penis. The bullet went through the corpora cavernosa, superficially damaged the urethral spongy tissue, and ended in the subcutaneous tissue of the right thigh. Urethroplasty was not required. **a** and **b** Show external aspect at admission. **c** CT scan showing bullet in the posterior aspect of the right thigh. (Courtesy of Dr. J.J. López-Tello)

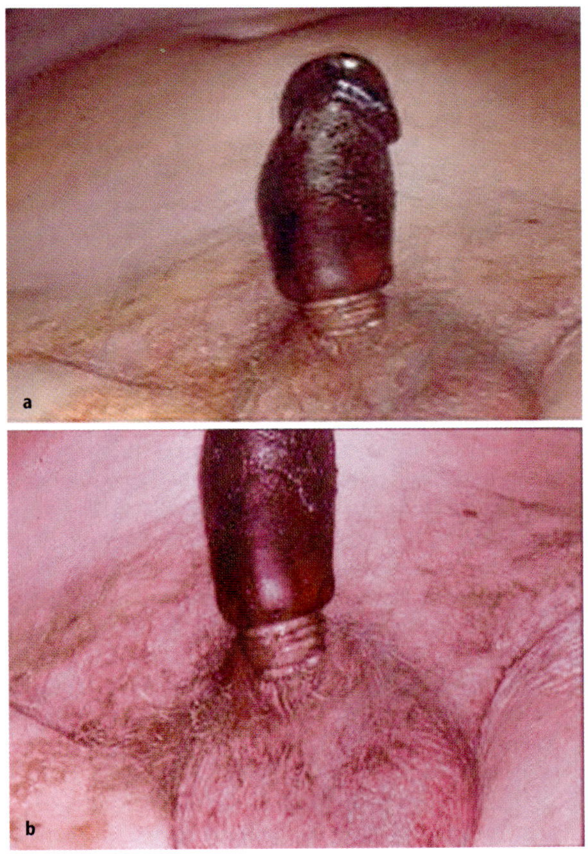

Fig. 15.9.8a, b. Ischemic necrosis of penis due to plastic constriction device (neck of a plastic bottle) used to improve erections (Courtesy of Dr. S. Luengo)

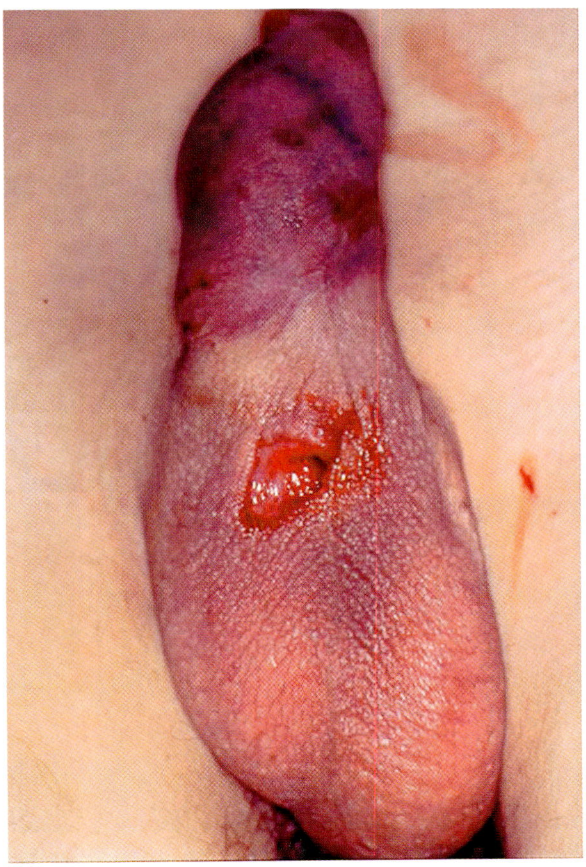

◁

Fig. 15.9.7. Dog bite with urethral laceration at the penoscrotal angle that required immediate open repair.

15.9.2 Diagnosis: Initial Emergency Assessment

15.9.2.1 Clinical Assessment

The initial management of all urethral injuries is resuscitation of the patient as a result of associated possibly life-threatening injuries. In the absence of blood at the meatus or hematoma, a urological injury is very unlikely and will be rapidly excluded by catheterization that promptly occurs in all major trauma victims as part of the process of resuscitation. Airway and respiratory function are maintained, the cervical spine secured in case of polytraumatism, and excessive hemorrhage addressed. This is particularly important in posterior urethral injuries because of their close association with pelvic fractures.

The next step includes taking a complete history and carrying out physical, laboratory, and radiographic evaluations in order to identify all injuries accurately. A diagnosis of acute urethral trauma should be suspected from the history. A pelvic fracture, or any external penile or perineal trauma, can be suggestive of urethral trauma (Armenakas and McAninch 1994, 1996).

For penetrating injuries, the type of weapon used, including the caliber of the bullet with gunshot wounds, is helpful in assessing potential tissue damage. In the conscious patient, a thorough voiding history should be obtained to establish the time of last urination, force of urinary stream, painful urination, and presence of hematuria. The following clinical indicators of acute urethral trauma warrant a complete urethral evaluation:

- Blood at the meatus
  Blood at the meatus is present in 37%–93% of patients with posterior urethral injury and at least 75% of patients with anterior urethral trauma (Lim and Chng 1989; McAninch 1981). Its presence should preclude any attempts at urethral instrumentation, until the entire urethra is adequately imaged. In an unstable patient, an attempt can be made to pass a urethral catheter, but if there is any difficulty a suprapubic catheter is inserted and a retrograde urethrogram performed when appropriate. It is extremely unlikely that gentle passage of a urethral catheter will do any additional damage to that caused by a fracture of the pelvis (Mundy 1996; Venn and Mundy 1998), although it has been suggested that this may convert a partial tear into one that is complete (Corriere and Harris 1981). There are no convincing data indicating a higher rate of infection or urethral stricture after a single attempt at catheterization (Dixon 1996). Indeed, if a urethral injury is suspected, urethrography prior to attempted catheterization is the most prudent approach.
- Blood at the vaginal introitus
  Blood at the vaginal introitus is present in more than 80% of female patients with pelvic fractures and co-existing urethral injuries (Perry and Husmann 1992).
- Hematuria
  Although nonspecific, hematuria on a first voided specimen may indicate urethral injury. The amount of urethral bleeding correlates poorly with the severity of injury, as a mucosal contusion or small partial tear may be accompanied by copious bleeding, while total transection of the urethra may result in little bleeding (Antoci and Schiff 1982).
- Pain on urination or inability to void
  The inability to void suggests urethral disruption.
- Hematoma or swelling
  With anterior urethral trauma, the pattern of the hematoma can be useful in identifying the anatomical boundaries violated by the injury. Extravasation of blood or urine in a sleeve distribution along the penile shaft indicates that the injury is confined by Buck's fascia. Disruption of Buck's fascia results in a pattern of extravasation limited only by Colles fascia, extending therefore up to the coracoclavicular fascia superiorly and the fascia lata inferiorly (Fig. 15.9.9). This results in a characteristic butterfly pattern of bruising in the perineum. In female patients with severe pelvic fractures, the presence

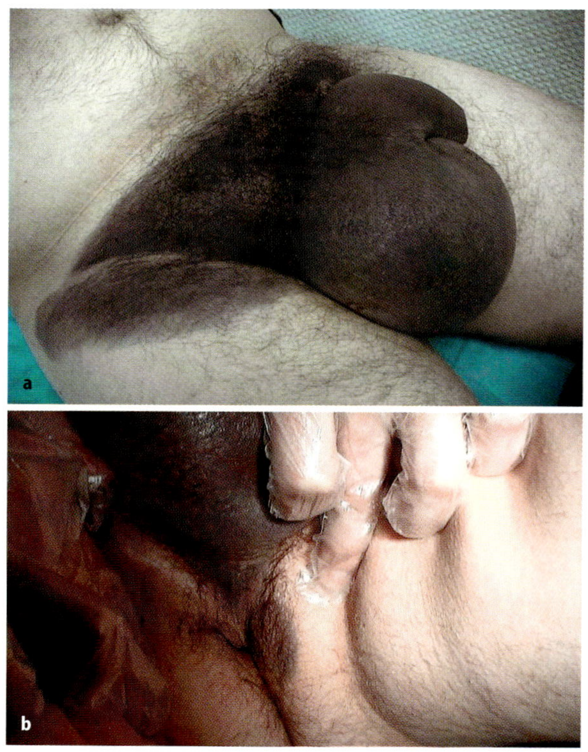

Fig. 15.9.9a, b. Large genital hematoma limited by Colles fascia

of labial swelling may be an indicator of urethral injury. It can be caused by urinary extravasation from a urethral fistula and warrants immediate attention.

- High-riding prostate
  This is a relatively unreliable finding in the acute phase, since the pelvic hematoma associated with pelvic fractures often precludes the adequate palpation of a small prostate, particularly in younger men (Dixon 1996). A boggy mass is usually palpated without recognition of a prostate gland (Fallon et al. 1984). Rectal examination is more important as a tool to screen for rectal injuries, which can be associated with pelvic fractures. Blood on the examination finger is highly suggestive of such an injury. Assessment of concomitant genital injuries is mandatory in every case of external urethral trauma as well.

15.9.2.2 Radiographic Examination

Retrograde urethrography is considered the gold standard for evaluating urethral injury. A scout film should be taken first to assess the radiographic technique and to detect pelvic fractures, as well as the presence of any foreign bodies such as bullets or stones, which may not be delineated once the contrast material has been given. This is taken using a 12- or 14-F Foley catheter in the fossa navicularis, with the balloon inflated using 1 – 2 ml of saline to occlude the urethra. Then, 20 – 30 ml of undiluted contrast material is injected and films taken during the injection in a 30°oblique position. When severe pelvic fractures and associated patient discomfort are present, the oblique position may not always be possible. Radiographic appearance of the urethra permits classification of the injury and facilitates subsequent management.

If posterior urethral injury is suspected, a suprapubic catheter is inserted; a simultaneous cystogram and ascending urethrogram can be carried out at a later date to assess the site, severity, and length of the urethral injury. This is usually done within 1 week of injury, if primary repair is contemplated, or after 3 months if a delayed or late repair is considered (Fig. 15.9.10).

When the proximal urethra is not visualized in a simultaneous cystogram and urethrogram, either magnetic resonance imaging (MRI) of the posterior urethra (McAninch 1996) or endoscopy through the suprapubic tract can be used (Fig. 15.9.11) to define the anatomy of the posterior urethra. Since manipulation in the bladder can cause the bladder neck to open and give the false impression of incompetence; consequently, the endoscopic appearance of the bladder neck should be noted immediately on placing the scope into the bladder (Jordan 1996).

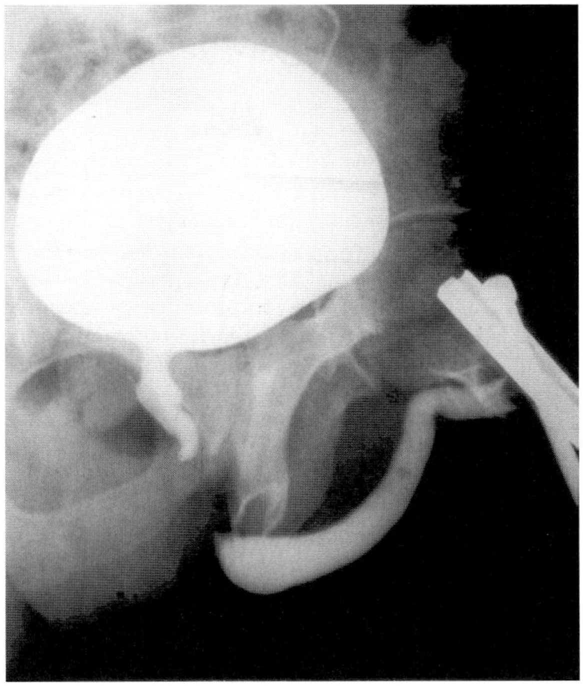

Fig. 15.9.10. Combined micturition and retrograde urethrography to asses the length of the distraction defect after posterior urethral fracture

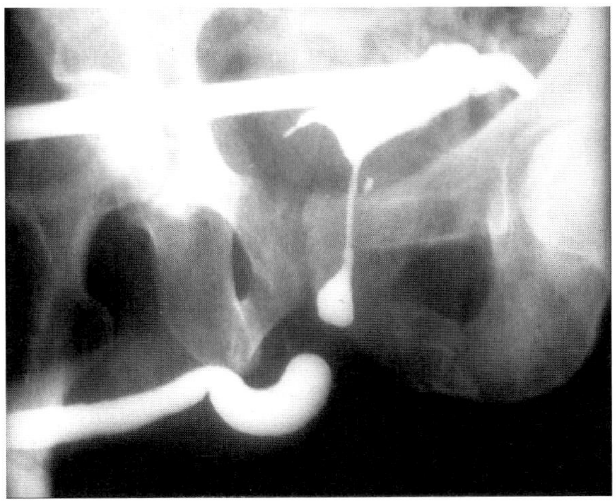

Fig. 15.9.11. After filling the bladder through the suprapubic tube with contrast material, the patient was asked to urinate, but the prostatic urethra was not filled up with contrast. A conventional cystoscope was introduced through the suprapubic tract, the bladder neck inspected and the posterior urethra filled by means of a ureteral catheter introduced into the prostatic urethra. This can be done also with a flexible cystoscope

After assessing the endoscopic appearance of the bladder neck, the flexible endoscope can be advanced through the bladder neck into the posterior urethra to the level of obstruction. If there is a question regarding the length of the distraction, a simultaneous retrograde urethrogram can be performed while the endoscope is in the posterior urethra. The radiographic appearance of the bladder neck is important but not as reliable an indicator of continence as the endoscopic appearance. Furthermore, there are patients who, despite evidence of an open bladder neck or a scar at the bladder neck, will have acceptable continence after reconstruction. For this reason, concomitant bladder neck surgery at the time of urethral reconstruction is debatable (Iselin and Webster 1999; Jordan 1996).

Ultrasonography is not a routine investigation in the initial assessment of urethral injuries but can be very useful in determining the position of the pelvic hematomas and the high-riding bladder when a suprapubic catheter is indicated.

Computed tomography and MRI have no place in the initial assessment of urethral injuries. However, they are useful in defining the distorted pelvic anatomy after severe injury and assessing associated injuries of penile crura, bladder, kidneys, and intraabdominal organs (Dixon et al. 1992; Kane et al. 1989).

15.9.2.3 Endoscopic Examination

Urethroscopy has no role in the initial diagnosis of urethral trauma in males. In females, however, where the short urethra precludes adequate retrograde urethrography, urethroscopy is an important adjunct to the physical examination for the identification and staging of urethral injuries (McAninch 1992).

15.9.3 Management

The management of urethral injuries remains controversial due to the variety of injury patterns, associated injuries, and treatment options available. In addition, urethral injuries are relatively uncommon; hence the limited experience of most urologists worldwide and absence of randomized prospective studies.

15.9.3.1 Anterior Urethral Injuries

Blunt Injuries

Partial tears can be managed with a suprapubic catheter or with urethral catheterization. Suprapubic cystostomy has the advantage of not only diverting the urine away from the site of injury, but also avoiding urethral manipulation (Glassberg et al. 1979). In addition, it allows for a simultaneous study to be carried out at a later date. If the bladder is not easily palpable suprapubically, transabdominal sonography should be used to guide the placement of the catheter. The cystostomy tube is maintained for approximately 4 weeks to allow urethral healing. Voiding cystourethrography is then performed and if normal voiding can be reestablished and no contrast extravasation nor subsequent stricture is present, then the tube can be safely removed.

The potential early complications of acute urethral injuries include strictures and infections. Extravasated blood or urine from the urethral tear produces an inflammatory reaction that can progress to the formation of an abscess. Extension of the infection depends on the fascial planes violated (see Sect. 15.9.2.1 above). Potential sequelae of these infections include urethrocutaneous fistulae, periurethral diverticula, and, rarely, necrotizing fasciitis. Prompt urinary diversion coupled with the appropriate administration of antibiotics decreases the incidence of these complications.

After the patient has adequately recovered from any associated injuries, and the urethral injury has stabilized, the urethra can be thoroughly reevaluated radiographically and, when necessary, the appropriate reconstructive procedure planned. Blunt anterior urethral injuries are associated with important spongiosa contusion, which makes it more difficult to evaluate the limits of urethral debridement in the acute phase. Therefore, acute or early urethroplasty is not indicated and the best management is simply suprapubic diversion. Satisfactory urethral luminal recanalization occurs in approximately 50% of partial anterior urethral disruptions (Cass and Godec 1978; Jackson and Williams 1974). Short and flimsy strictures can be managed with optical urethrotomy or urethral dilation. Denser strictures require formal urethral reconstruction. Anastomotic urethroplasty is indicated in strictures less than 1 cm in length.

Longer strictures of the anterior urethra should not be repaired by an end-to-end anastomosis to avoid chordee. In these cases, flap or graft urethroplasty is indicated. Almost all complete ruptures of the anterior urethra require anastomotic or patch urethroplasty at 3–6 months (Figs. 15.9.12, 15.9.13). The only exception to this is urethral injury associated with penile fracture, which usually results in partial urethral disruption and can be repaired at the time of cavernosal closure.

Open Injuries

Male Urethral Injuries

Stab wounds, gunshot wounds, and dog bites to the urethra often involve the penis and testes, necessitating immediate exploration (Figs. 15.9.5–15.9.7). During this procedure, the urethral injury can be surgically evaluated and repaired as needed, limiting subsequent stricture formation to less than 15% (Husmann et al. 1993).

Primary urethral suturing involves direct visualization of the severed urethral ends, with creation of a wa-

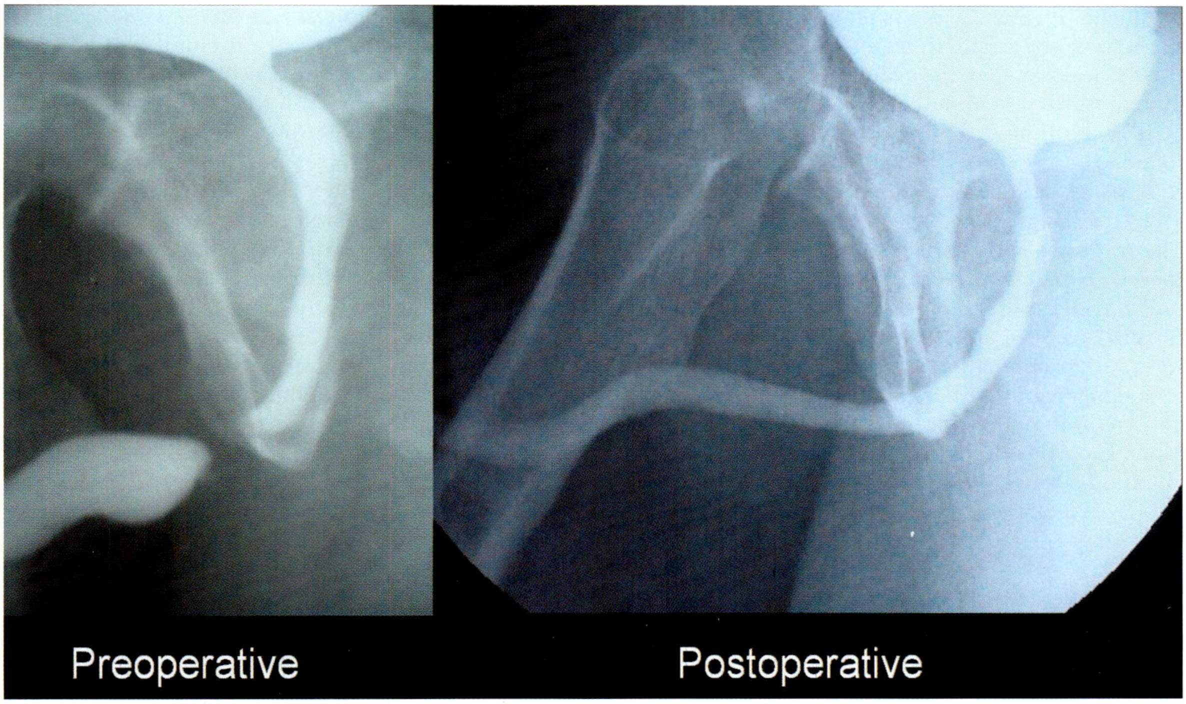

Fig. 15.9.12. Complete bulbar urethral stricture after a straddle injury. Result after delayed end-to-end anastomosis

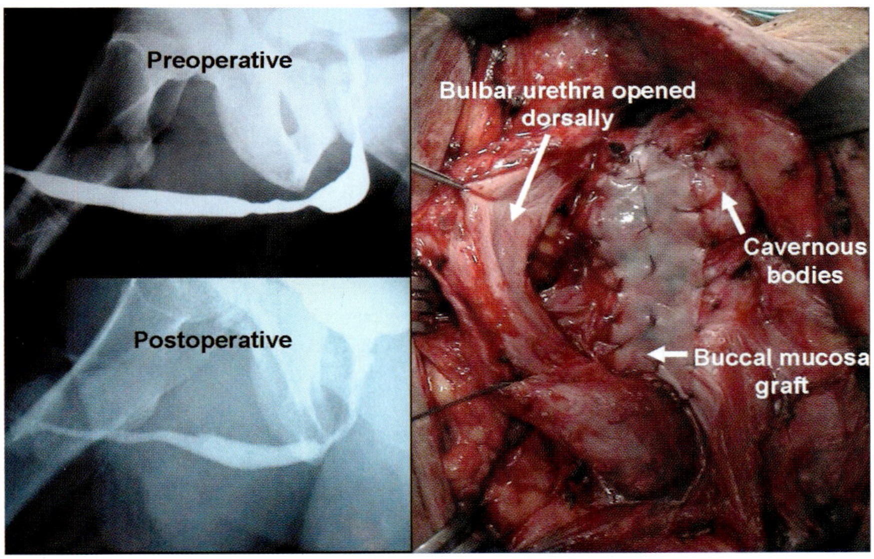

Fig. 15.9.13. Partial traumatic bulbar urethral stricture treated unsuccessfully with internal visual urethrotomy in another center. Dorsal buccal mucosa graft urethroplasty gave good results. The stricture is too long for an end-to-end urethroplasty

ter-tight, tension-free repair. The exposure is obtained using a circumferential subcoronal incision to deglove the penis with the patient in the supine position. In complete disruptions, the corpus spongiosum is mobilized at the level of the injury and the urethral ends dissected distally and proximally. Urethral ends are spatulated and end-to-end anastomosis is fashioned over a 14-F Foley catheter. Small lacerations can be sutured with fine absorbable material. Attention is directed to overclosure of the corpus spongiosum and overlying tissues to minimize subsequent fistulae formation (Chapple and Png 1999). Urethral debridement should be kept to a minimum since the vascular characteristics of the corpus spongiosum will permit excellent healing with a properly performed urethrospongiosal repair.

Perioperative prophylactic antibiotics should be used to avoid infections. At 10 days to 2 weeks, a cystourethrogram should be obtained with the urethral catheter in situ. Provided there is no leakage at the anastomotic site, the urethral catheter can be removed. If there is leakage, then the catheter is left longer and the cystourethrogram should be repeated 1 week later.

If at the time of initial exploration, the urethra is found to be so extensively disrupted that primary anastomosis is not feasible – this occurs with defects over 1–1.5 cm length – the procedure should be aborted. The surgeon should marsupialize the urethra preparatory to a two-stage urethral repair with proximal suprapubic urinary diversion. A delayed elective procedure is usually carried out after a minimum of 3 months after injury. There is no role for urethral substitution, with either a graft or flap, in the initial management of any urethral injury, since contamination or decreased blood supply can compromise such a repair (Armenakas and McAninch 1996).

Female Urethral Injuries

Most female urethral disruptions can be sutured primarily. This is because these injuries occur more frequently in association with bladder ruptures, necessitating prompt exploration. For proximal urethral injuries, urethral exposure is best obtained transvesically, permitting direct visualization of the bladder, bladder neck, and proximal urethra. Distal urethral injuries can be approached via the vaginal route (Koraitim 1999). Early repair of posttraumatic urethral fistulas can be accomplished using a transvaginal approach (Hemal et al. 2000; Perry and Husmann 1992).

15.9.3.2 Posterior Urethral Injuries

It is important to make a distinction between posterior urethral stricture and a subprostatic pelvic fracture urethral distraction defect, as the principles of their surgical management are entirely different. Urethral stricture should be used to indicate a narrowing of the urethral continuity, such as sphincter strictures due to instrumentation or partial urethral tears. In subprostatic complete urethral fractures, a urethral distraction defect exists and there is a gap between the prostatic apex or membranous urethra and the bulbar urethral end. The dismembered end of the urethra retracts and the space between them is filled with fibrous tissue, resulting from organization and healing of the hematoma and urinary extravasation. There is no urethral wall in the scarred space and any lumen represents merely a fistulous tract between the urethral ends. A further difference with inflammatory strictures is that urethral ends, regardless of the length of the distraction defect, present very limited fibrosis and when reanastomosed without tension, usually heal with little potential for restricturing (Fig. 15.9.14) (Martínez-Piñeiro et al. 1997).

Erectile dysfunction occurs in 20%–60% of patients after traumatic posterior urethral rupture.(Corriere 2001; Dhabuwala et al. 1990; Gibson 1970; King 1975; Martínez-Piñeiro et al. 1997). Available data suggest that the severity of the initial injury is the most important determining factor associated with impotence. Only 5% of complete erectile dysfunction follows as a consequence of open surgical repair (Martínez-Piñeiro et al. 1997; Webster 1990). King reported an incidence of 42% in cases of pelvic fracture and urethral injury, but only 5% when the urethra was not injured (King 1975). Barbagli et al. reported an incidence of 60% in patients with posterior urethral injury compared with 14% in patients with bulbar injury (Barbagli et al. 1987).

Factors that correlate with the development of impotence are age, defect length, and the type of fracture; bilateral pubic rami fractures are the most frequent cause of impotence, which is almost always of neurogenic etiology due to bilateral damage of the cavernous nerves at the prostatomembranous urethra behind the symphysis pubis (Mark et al. 1995). Associated vasculogenic erectile failure may occur in up to 80% of cases (Armenakas et al. 1993). Dixon et al. presented evidence that impotence may also be a consequence of avulsion

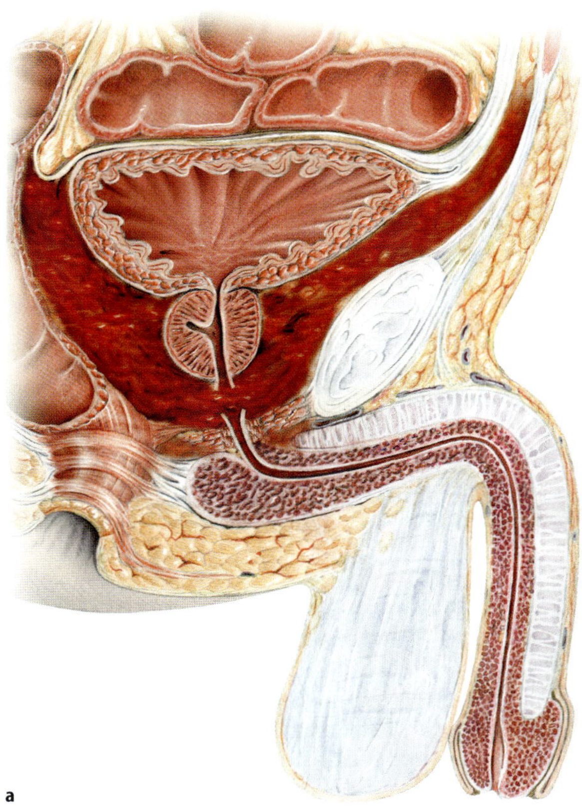

a

Fig. 15.9.14a, b. Difference between urethral distraction defect and urethral stricture. **a** Urethral distraction defect

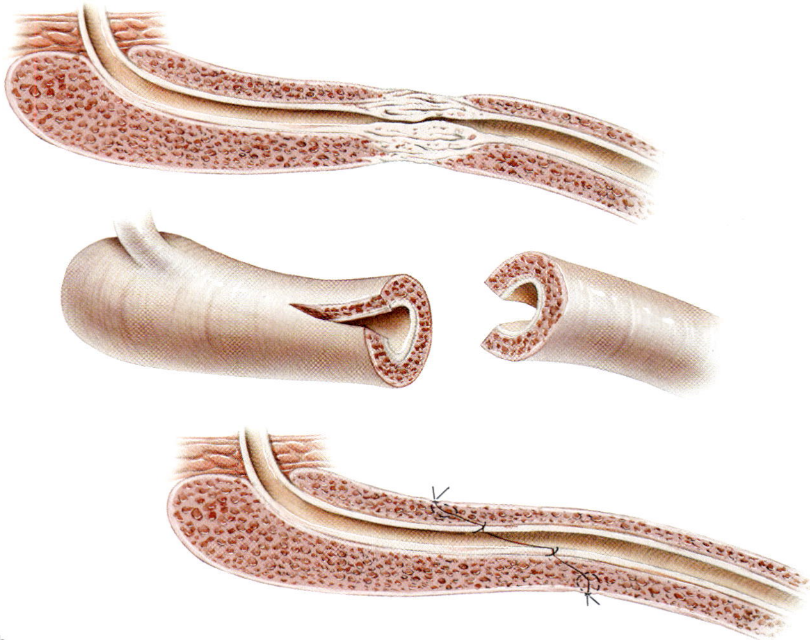

Fig. 15.9.14b. Urethral stricture (© Hohenfellner 2007) **b**

of the corpora cavernosa from the ischium (Dixon et al. 1992). Five of six patients in this series, with avulsion of the corpora cavernosa off the inferior pubic ramus, were impotent. Spontaneous return of potency may occur up to 2 years after injury (McAninch 1996). Gibson reported an incidence of improved sexual function after 18 months in 21 % of patients (Gibson 1970).

Partial Urethral Rupture

Partial tears of the posterior urethra can be managed in most cases with a suprapubic or urethral catheter and repeat retrograde urethrography at 2-week intervals until healing has occurred (Koraitim 1999; Venn and Mundy 1998). They may heal without significant scarring or obstruction if managed by diversion alone (Glassberg et al. 1979; Kielb et al. 2001). Any residual or subsequent stricture can be managed with urethral dilation or optical urethrotomy, if short and flimsy, or by anastomotic urethroplasty if denser (Chapple and Png 1999; Venn and Mundy 1998).

Complete Urethral Rupture

The treatment options available include primary realignment, immediate open urethroplasty, delayed primary urethroplasty, delayed urethroplasty, and delayed endoscopic incision.

Primary Realignment

Urethral realignment can be achieved either transpubically (open realignment) or with endoscopic techniques (endoscopic realignment).

Primary Open Realignment

In posterior urethral injuries associated with concomitant bladder neck or rectal injuries, immediate open exploration, repair and urethral realignment is advisable. Bladder neck injury risks incontinence and infection of the pelvic fractures. Rectal injury carries the obvious risk of sepsis and fistula, and early exploration is indicated to evacuate contaminated hematoma and perform colostomy. Urethral realignment over a stenting catheter is appropriate is such cases (Antoci and Schiff 1982; Berman and Tom 1974; Koraitim 1999; Muhlbauer and Bard 1980; Turner-Warwick 1989).

Primary Endoscopic Realignment

The overall condition of the patient and the extent of associated injuries greatly affect the decision to proceed with primary endoscopic realignment. Most patients with pelvic crush injuries have multiple organ injuries. Associated lower extremity fractures can prevent placement in the lithotomy position, which is often required for primary endoscopic realignment, while head injuries increase the adverse risks of anesthesia. If these conditions are controlled, such that a hemodynamically stable patient can safely undergo a lengthier anesthesia and can be placed in the lithotomy

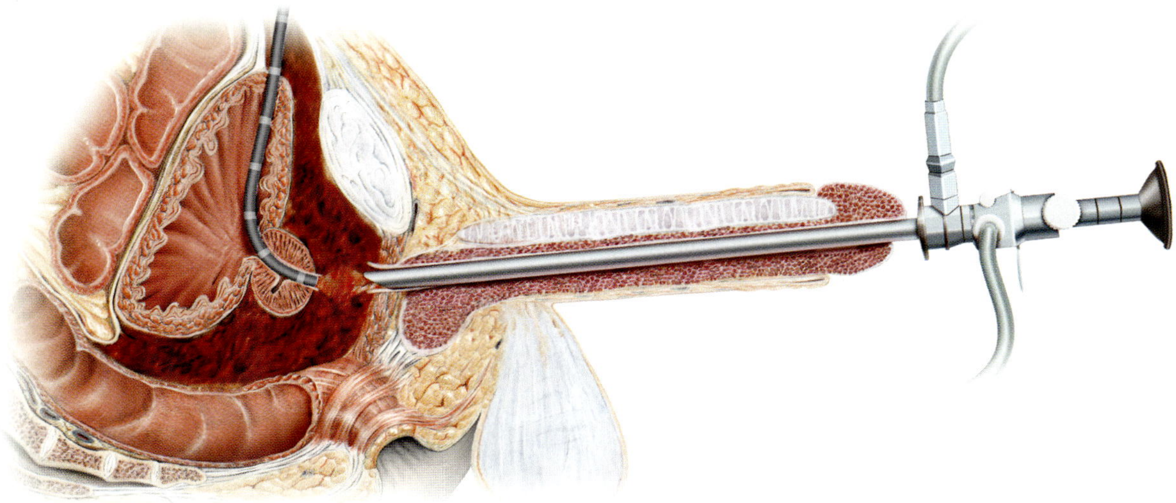

Fig. 15.9.15. Endoscopic realignment in posterior urethral distraction defect by means of a flexible and rigid cystoscope (© Hohenfellner 2007)

position, endoscopic urethral realignment may be considered during the first 2 weeks after trauma (Fig. 15.9.15).

The proposed benefits of primary open or endoscopic alignment follow:

1. There is a lower stricture rate than with suprapubic catheter placement alone (69% vs 10%) (Webster et al. 1983). This avoids a second operation for urethral reconstruction in about one-third of patients (Dixon 1996).
2. If scarring occurs, restoration of urethral continuity is simplified and may be accomplished by endoscopic procedures or dilation.
3. If a urethroplasty is required later, it is technically easier when the prostate and urethra are well aligned.

The disadvantage of open realignment may be a higher incidence of erectile dysfunction and incontinence when compared to delayed reconstruction (Koraitim 1996; Webster et al. 1983). Webster studied 301 patients from 15 series in which primary realignment (open and endourologic) was used, and compared the incontinence, impotence, and stricture rates to those in 236 patients from five series, in which cystostomy and delayed repair was performed (Webster et al. 1983). In this series, primary realignment was performed with different endourologic and open techniques and cannot be used as a valid comparison between open and endoscopic primary realignment. Overall, impotence occurred in 44% of patients treated with primary alignment compared with 11% of patients treated with delayed repair. Incontinence was also higher after primary alignment (20% vs 2%). Stricture rates after cystostomy tube placement approach 100%, whereas after primary realignment, strictures occurred in 64% of patients. In most cases of delayed repair, a stricture-free anastomosis can be achieved with success rates greater than 90% (Coffield and Weems 1977; McAninch 198; Morehouse and Mackinnon 1980; Webster 1989; Webster et al. 1983). In an extensive review of the English literature for the last 50 years, Koraitim came to a similar conclusion. Primary realignment was found to double the incidence of impotence (36% vs 19%) and to have the incidence of stricture compared to suprapubic cystostomy and delayed repair (53% vs 97%) (Koraitim 1999). The implication was that primary realignment led to higher impotence and incontinence rates because of iatrogenic factors and thus should be avoided.

However, the series of primary realignment reviewed by Webster and Koraitim encompassed a number of techniques (open and endourologic), which may explain the poor results of their analysis, compared with those reported by other authors (Elliott and Barret 1997). Recent publications show that the injury itself and not the type of management is probably responsible for the loss of potency and continence after urethral trauma (Asci et al. 1999; Husmann et al. 1990; McAninch 1997; Morey and McAninch 1997). Elliott and Barret (1997) have reported on a series of 57 patients who underwent primary endoscopic urethral realignment, with a mean follow-up of 10.5 years: 21% had some degree of erectile dysfunction, 3.7% had mild stress incontinence, 68% had postalignment strictures. The effects on continence and potency with immediate endourologic realignment following urethral disruption were also reviewed by Kotkin and Koch (1996) in 20 nearly case-matched patients with posterior urethral injuries treated by primary surgical realignment or catheter placement. Continence was preserved in 83% and 80% of patients, respectively, while erectile function returned in 76% and 70%, respectively. A recent series reported by Mouraview et al. (2005) has also shown a lower incidence of impotence and incontinence in patients treated with early realignment than with delayed open reconstruction.

The great variation of techniques used in the past for primary realignment procedures confuses any comparison with delayed repair procedures (Follis et al. 1992; Herschorn et al. 1992; Porter et al. 1997). Primary realignment techniques have included:

- Simple passage of a catheter across the defect (Herschorn et al. 1992)
- Endoscopically assisted catheter realignment using flexible, rigid endoscopes and biplanar fluoroscopy (Gelbard et al. 1989; Guille et al. 1991)
- Use of interlocking sounds ("railroading") or magnetic catheters to place the catheter (Porter et al. 1997)
- Pelvic hematoma evacuation and dissection of the prostatic apex (with or without suture anastomosis) over a catheter
- Catheter traction or perineal traction sutures to pull the prostate back to its normal location (Turner-Warwick 1977)

Realignment, even with traction, may be insufficient to join completely the margins of the severed urethra and 1.5- to 4-cm defects have been observed (Ragde and McInnes 1969). This finding agrees with experimental animal data, which show that when the urethra is transacted and apparently good urethral junction is achieved by catheter traction, there is no evidence of epithelialization of the mucosal gap but rather that the intervening area is filled with fibrous tissue (McRoberts and Radge 1970). Moreover, sustained traction on the balloon catheter has been noted to damage the only remaining sphincter mechanism at the bladder neck from pressure necrosis (Dixon 1996; Turner-Warwick 1989). If series that use true immediate urethral realignment with minimal traction and without suture repair bolsters only are included, the results with immediate realignment are much more favorable (Table 15.9.5).

This type of summary of the literature suggests that immediate realignment is associated with an impotence rate of approximately 35%, an incontinence rate of 5%, and a restricture rate of 60%.

Immediate Open Urethroplasty (< 48 h After Injury)

Immediate open urethroplasty of posterior injuries is not indicated because of poor visualization and the inability to assess accurately the degree of urethral disruption during the acute phase, characterized by extensive swelling and ecchymosis. The difficulty in identifying structures and planes hamper adequate mobilization and subsequent surgical apposition (Chapple and Png 1999). Incontinence and impotence rates are high-

Table 15.9.5. Results of immediate realignment in complete urethral disruption

Series	No. of patients	Follow-up months (range)	Erectile dysfunction *N* (%)	Incontinence *N* (%)	Restricture rate *N* (%)[a]
Gibson 1974	35[b]	NA	12 (34)	1 (3)	26 (74.3)
Crassweller et al. 1977	38	24–240	19/42 (45)	NA	12 (31.6)
Malek et al. 1977[c]	7	168 (96–264)	0	0	1 (14.3)
Gelbard et al. 1989	7	10.2 (2–24)	1/6 (16.7)	0	2 (33)
Cohen et al. 1991	4	28 (17–35)	2 (50)	0	2 (50)
Melekos et al. 1992	4	NA	0	0	4 (100)
Follis et al. 1992	20	42 (1–36)	4 (20)	2 (10)	12 (60)
El-Abd 1995	44	NA	35 (79.5)	0	44 (100)
Gheiler and Frontera 1997	3	6 (5–9)	0	0	1 (33.3)
Londergan et al. 1997	4	20.2 (12–35)	1 (25)	0	3 (75%)
Elliott and Barret 1997	53	126 (1–> 120)	11 (21)	2 (3.8)	36 (68)
Porter et al. 1997	10	10.9 (2–31)	1/7 (14)	0	5 (50)
Rehman et al. 1998	3	(11–26)	1 (16.7)	0	2 (66.7)
Sahin et al. 1998	5	31 (21–53)	1 (20)	1 (20)	4 (80)
Tahan et al. 1999	13	29	3 (23)	0	5 (38.5)
Jepson et al. 1999	8	50.4 (35–85)	3 (37.5)	1 (12.5)	5 (62.5)
Asci et al. 1999	20	39 (19–78)	4 (20)	2 (10)	9 (45)
Ying-Hao et al. 2000	4	56 (39–85)	0	0	1 (25)
Moudouni et al. 2001	23	68 (18–155)	4/29 (14)	0	16 (69.5)
Mouraview et al. 2005	57	< 24 (2–15)	19/57 (34)	10/57 (10)	28/57 (49)
Totals	**362**		**130/368 (35.3)[d]**	**19/362 (5.2)**	**218/362 (60.2)**

[a] Stricture that requires internal urethrotomy or open urethroplasty or more than 1 dilation
[b] Five patients with partial rupture, [c] Children, [d] Some partial ruptures included

er than with the other techniques described in this chapter (impotence 56 %, incontinence 21 %, restricture 49 %) (Cass and Godec 1978; Koraitim 1996, 1999; Mundy 1991; Webster et al. 1983; Weems 1979).

Delayed Primary Urethroplasty (2 – 14 Days After Injury)

The management of complete posterior rupture of the urethra has changed in recent years. There is now more active orthopedic management of pelvic fractures with immediate external and internal fixation, and this has led to an option for early repairs of urethral injuries (Venn and Mundy 1998).

In the absence of indications for immediate exploration, the management of posterior urethral disruption can be in a delayed primary fashion. The delayed primary approach requires placement of a suprapubic tube at the time of initial injury, with repair undertaken when the patient is stable, usually within 10 – 14 days. This is a time when patients are stable and most pelvic bleeding has resolved. The aim of the delayed primary repair is to correct severe distraction injuries rather than to prevent a stricture occurring; however, it will also ensure that if it does occur it is easily treatable (Mundy 1991). Hematomas preventing adequate pelvic descent can be evacuated at this point. Repair at this time can be performed endoscopically, as well as through an abdominal or perineal approach (Cohen et al. 1991; Mundy 1991). Urethral repairs using one-stage perineal anastomotic urethroplasty offer a stricture-free rate of 80 % (Mundy 1996). The progressive perineal technique usually employed in a delayed fashion after 3 or more months of suprapubic drainage is equally useful in the immediate postinjury period for delayed primary repair if the patient is able to tolerate the lithotomy position.

In female urethral disruption, delayed primary urethroplasty is probably the best approach, though no large experience exists. Fewer than 50 cases have been reported so far, with most reports being simple case reports (Hemal et al. 2000). Delayed primary repair tries to preserve as much urethral length as possible and to avoid the urethra being embedded in dense scar, thus trying to avoid subsequent incontinence. Surgical exploration should be attempted via the retropubic route for proximal injuries and the vaginal route for distal injuries (Koraitim 1999).

Delayed Urethroplasty (3 – 6 Months After Trauma)

The most common end result of a subprostatic urethral injury managed by delayed repair is the development of a relatively short prostatobulbar urethral gap. Such a simple short gap defect can generally be resolved by a relatively simple perineal approach anastomotic repair, provided that it is not associated with extensive hematoma and fibrosis and the bladder neck mechanism is occlusive and competent.

After division of the bulbar urethra at the distal point of obliteration, mobilization of a normal bulbar urethra to the base of the penis generally achieves 4 – 5 cm of elastic lengthening. This is usually sufficient to achieve a tension-free, 2 cm spatulated overlap anastomosis with the apical prostatic urethra, after bridging a gap of 2 – 2.5 cm without rerouting (Chapple and Png 1999).

This technique has the advantage that most associated injuries and damaged skin and tissues, in addition to the pelvic hematoma, have resolved by the time it is performed. The only problem with this approach would be the length of the period that the patient must have a suprapubic catheter before definitive treatment.

When the prostatobulbar gap is longer than 2 – 3 cm as a result of a high dislocation of the prostate, or when the available elongation of the mobilized urethra has been foreshortened by damage caused by a previous surgical procedure, the following maneuvers are carried out sequentially to gain sufficient anterior urethral mobility to bridge up to 8 cm of separation (Mark and Webster 1996; Webster and Ramon 1991): midline separation of the proximal corporal bodies, inferior pubectomy and supracorporal urethral rerouting (Fig. 15.9.16).

In addition to its use as initial therapy for posterior urethral distraction injuries, the progressive perineal approach can be applied successfully to salvage procedures following failed repair. There are a number of circumstances that may preclude successful perineal anastomotic repair as either initial or salvage therapy. This group probably represents less than 5 % of cases and includes the following (Mark and Webster 1996; Webster 1987; Webster et al. 1990):

Distraction Defects Longer than 7 – 8 cm. A tubed interposition flap of penile or perineoscrotal skin can be used for reconstruction.

Fistulae. These may require a combined abdominoperineal approach to secure adequate closure.

Synchronous Anterior Urethral Stricture. The presence of associated spongiofibrosis in the anterior urethra may compromise the blood supply to the bulbar urethra following division of the bulbar arteries.

Urinary Incontinence. As the distal urethral sphincter mechanism is usually defunctionalized by urethral distraction, urinary continence must be maintained primarily by the proximal bladder neck sphincter. Concomitant bladder neck injury with the likelihood of incontinence may warrant a combined abdominoperineal procedure to enable simultaneous bladder neck and

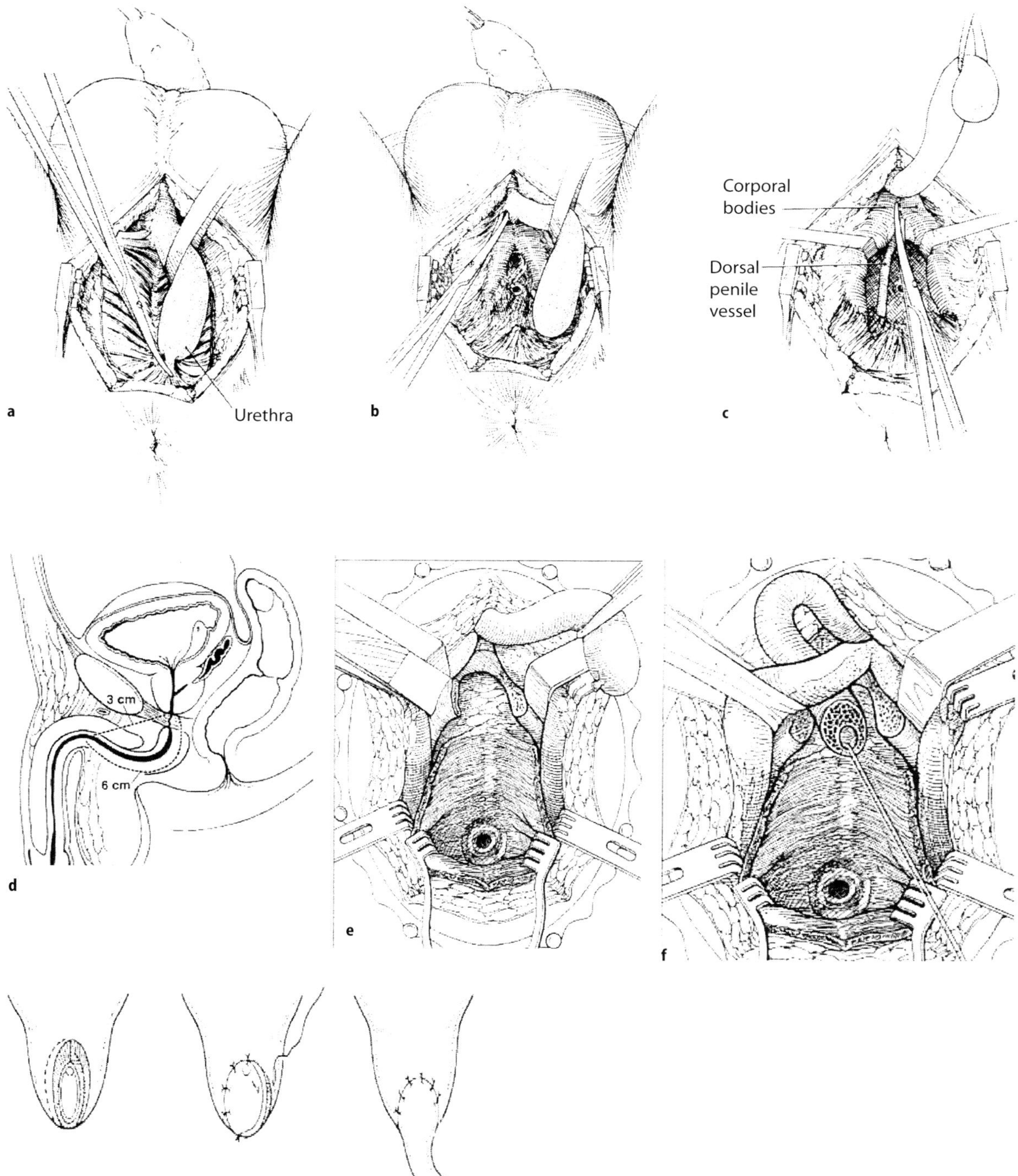

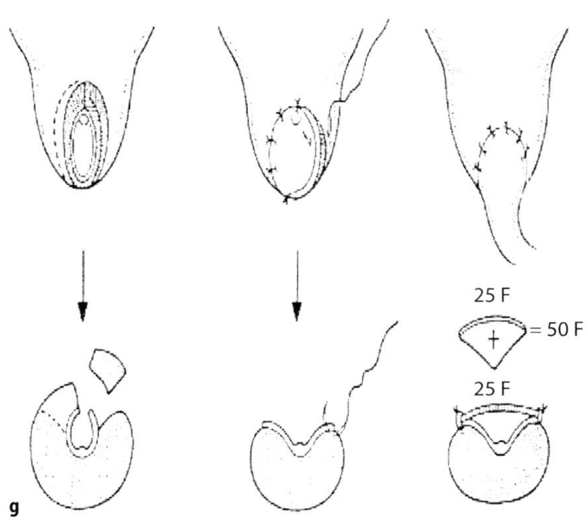

Fig. 15.9.16a–g. Maneuvers carried out sequentially to gain sufficient anterior urethral mobility to bridge up to 8 cm of urethral gap. **a, b** Urethral mobilization, **c** midline separation of the proximal corporal bodies, **d** with the previous maneuvers you can gain more than 3 cm of extra urethral length, **e** inferior pubectomy, **f** supracorporal urethral rerouting, **g** resection of fibrous tissue at the prostatic apex; bulbourethral anastomosis sometimes requires the eversion of the urethral mucosa at the prostatic apex

urethral reconstruction. The most common cause of bladder neck incompetence is the circumferential tethering of an uninjured mechanism by the natural shrinkage or replacement of an extensive pelvic floor hematoma by fibrosis. In such cases, it is usually possible to restore functional competence of the bladder neck by mobilizing it meticulously. This can be accomplished by removal of the dense hematoma/fibrosis anchoring the bladder neck to the pubis, anteriorly and laterally, and prevention of secondary fibrotic reimmobilization by occluding the consequent paraprostatic dead-space cavity with a supple omental pedicle graft, thus preserving the functional mobility of the liberated sphincter mechanism (Iselin and Webster 1999; MacDiarmid et al. 1995).

The results of various techniques are reviewed by Koraitim (1996) in a personal series of 100 patients combined with a review of 771 patients from published reports. Immediate and early realignment ($n=326$) was associated with a 53 % stricture rate, a 5 % incontinence rate, and a 36 % impotence rate. Of the patients successfully managed with immediate realignment, 42 % needed subsequent instrumentation to attempt stricture stabilization. Urethroplasty was ultimately necessary in 33 %. Primary suturing ($n=37$) was associated with a 49 % stricture rate, a 21 % incontinence rate, and a 56 % impotence rate. In comparison, inserting a suprapubic catheter before delayed repair ($n=508$) was associated with a 97 % stricture rate, a 4 % incontinence rate, and a 19 % impotence rate. The restricture rate after delayed anastomotic urethroplasty was less than 10 % (Corriere 2001; Jordan 1996; Koraitim 1997; Martínez-Piñeiro et al. 1997; Mundy 1993, 1996; Santucci et al. 2002; Zinman 1997), and the risk of impotence caused by delayed urethroplasty was approximately 5 % (Corriere 2001; Corriere et al. 1994; Fiala et al. 2001; Koraitim 1995, 1996; Martínez-Piñeiro et al. 1997; Mundy 1996; Webster 1990). On the basis of such results, it is evident that the gold standard remains delayed urethral repair at a minimum of 3 months after trauma, using a one-stage perineal approach.

In children, similar results are obtained as in adults (Podesta et al. 2005); the higher incidence of abdominal surgery simply reflects the greater propensity to damage of the bladder neck in children.

Reconstruction of Failed Repair of Posterior Urethral Rupture

When restenosis occurs after delayed urethral repair, it is identified usually within 6 months. If the anastomosis has a normal caliber at 6 months, then it is extremely unlikely that the patient will develop further stricturing (Mundy 1996).

The principles of a salvage repair are similar to those of the initial procedure. Progressive perineal anastomotic repair alone can be successful in 95 % of salvage urethroplasties. If an anastomotic repair cannot be performed, a one-stage substitution urethroplasty using a pedicle island of penile skin may be possible and may be more desirable than the final alternative, a two-stage scrotourethral inlay procedure or mesh split-thickness skin graft urethroplasty (Mark and Webster 1996; Wadhwa et al. 1998). The presence of fistulous tracts to the bladder base, abdominal wall, or rectum; periurethral epithelialized cavities; and an ability to achieve the lithotomy position are the leading indications for a combined abdominoperineal surgical approach (Webster et al. 1990).

Restenosis to a luminal caliber of 12-F Foley catheter or less is required before a reduction in the urinary flow is perceived as abnormal (Smith 1968). A wide-caliber stricture may be followed expectantly or gently dilated. Optical urethrotomy is an alternative, particularly for a short, narrow stricture.

Delayed Endoscopic Optical Incision

The principles of the procedure were described by Sachse in 1974 (Sachse 1974). A curved metal sound was passed through the suprapubic cystostomy into the blindly ending proximal urethra, the direct vision urethrotome was inserted into the urethra, and cuts were made toward the sound. Blandy subsequently described the suprapubic passage of a cystoscope for transillumination of the thin perineal membrane associated with short urethral defects and transurethral "cutting to the light" with an electrode (Fig. 15.9.17) (Blandy 1980). Today, the cut-to-the-light technique is performed more effectively using c-arm fluoroscopy for stereotactic guidance. The urethral catheter is left in place for between 1 and 3 weeks, and the suprapubic drainage for 2 additional weeks to confirm consistent voiding (Lieberman and Barry 1982).

Results of several small series have been reported and are summarized in Table 15.9.6.

The procedure is only indicated if the urethral defect is short, the bladder neck is competent, and there is minimal displacement of the prostate and proximal bulbous urethra (Barry 1989). Although restoration of urethral continuity is common, and potency is not affected by the procedure, urethral dilation, repeat optical urethrotomy, and transurethral resection of stricture are common and will be required in about 80 % of patients. Most repeat urethrotomies are performed in the 1st year of follow-up. It should be noted that after failure of the initial urethrotomy, alternative treatments should be considered, as repeat urethrotomy achieves only temporary improvement (Pansadoro and Emiliozzi 1996). Urethral false passage and rectal perforation have been reported (De Vries and Anderson 1990; Gupta and Gill 1986; Yasuda et al. 1991). Stents are

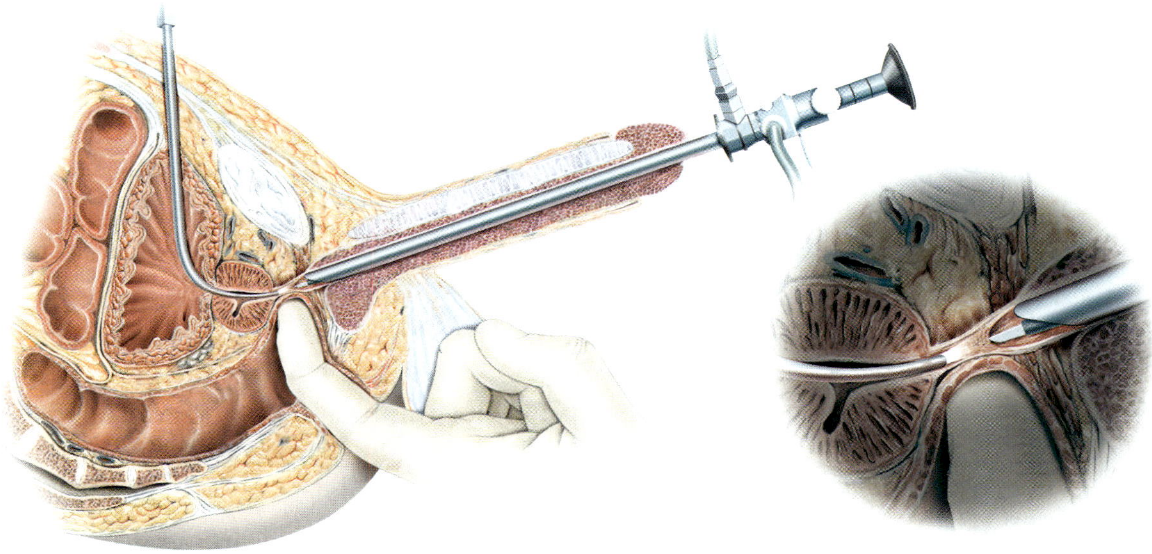

Fig. 15.9.17. Transurethral cutting-to-the-light procedure (© Hohenfellner 2007)

Table 15.9.6. Results of optical urethrotomy for traumatically obliterated pelvic urethra

Series	No. patients	Follow-up months (range)	No. (%) requiring repeat urethrotomy	Erectile dysfunction
Gupta and Gill 1986	10	15.1 (6–24)	10 (100)	0
Chiou et al. 1988	8	43 (12–79)	7 (87.5)	0
Marshall 1989	10	NA	10 (100)	0
Barry 1989	12	22 (1.5–85)	6 (50)	0
DeVries and Anderson 1990	4	<4	1 (25)	0
Leonard et al. 1990	3	31 (13–51)	1 (33.3)	0
Kernohan et al. 1991	7	35 (21–84)	7 (100)	0
Yasuda et al. 1991	17	44 (12–96)	7 (41.2)	0
Quint & Stanisic 1993	10	43 (7–108)	6 (60)	0
El-Abd 1995	284	NA	272 (95.8)	0
Goel et al. 1997	13	17.7 (11–24)	10 (76.9)	NA
Levine and Wessells 2001	6	60	6 (100)	NA
Dogra and Nabi 2002[a]	61	30 (9–44)	11 (18)	NA
Totals	**445**		**354 (79.5)**	

[a] Laser urethrotomy

not currently recommended for patients with strictures following pelvic trauma, as fibrotic tissue tends to grow though into the lumen of the stent (Baert et al. 1993; Jordan 1996; Milroy et al. 1989; Williams 1993).

15.9.4 Recommendations for Treatment: Algorithms

The optimal management of patients with prostatomembranous disruptions should not be thought of as delayed repair vs other types of treatment modalities. Each patient should be assessed and managed according to the initial clinical circumstances. It is impractical to suggest that all patients be managed by one single method, due to the variability of cases and the severity of associated injuries. The intervention should be guided by the clinical circumstances. The following algorithms taken from the European Association of Urology Guidelines (Lynch et al. 2005) are suggested for the treatment of urethral injuries in males and females (Figs. 15.9.18–15.9.20).

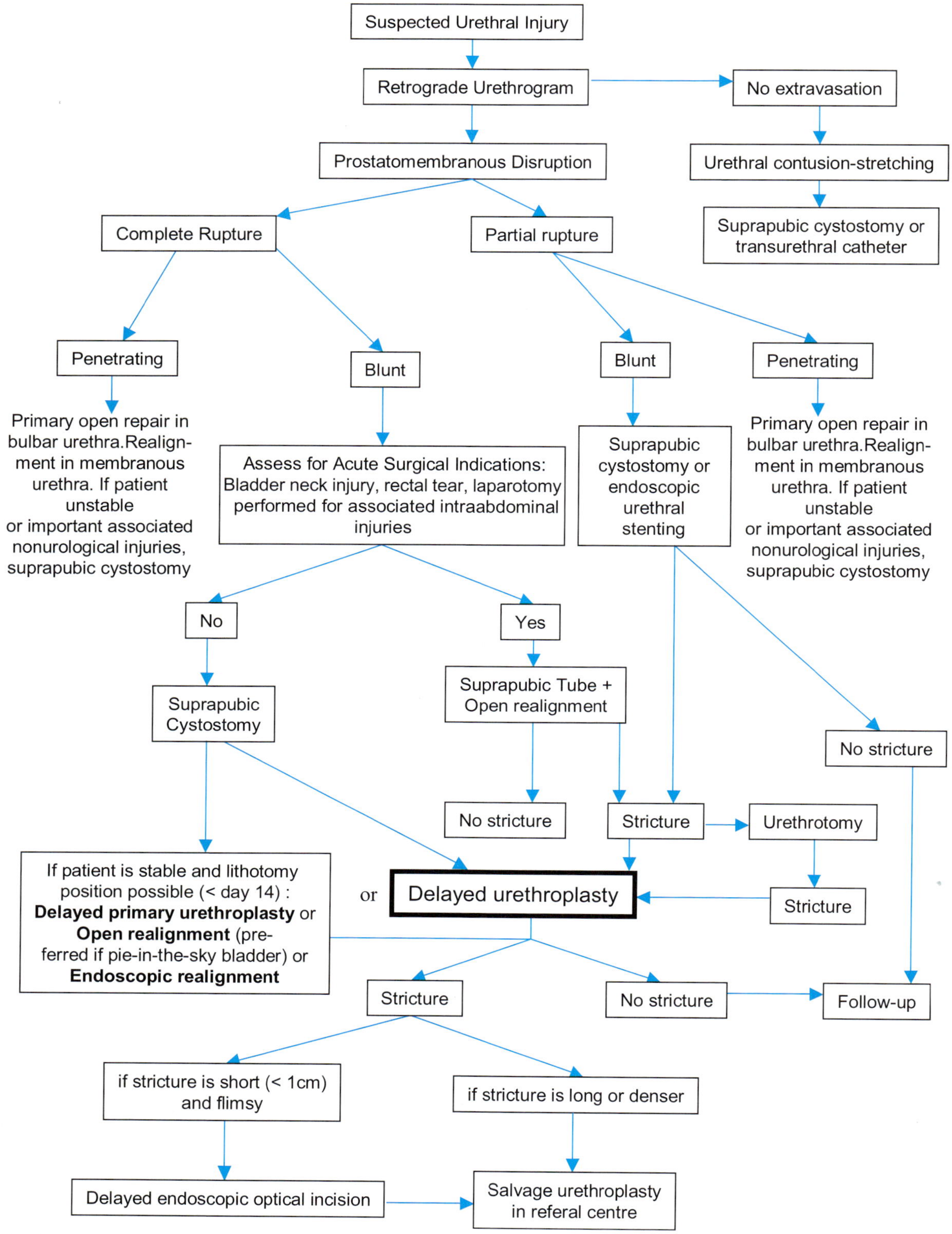

Fig. 15.9.18. Management of posterior urethral injuries in men

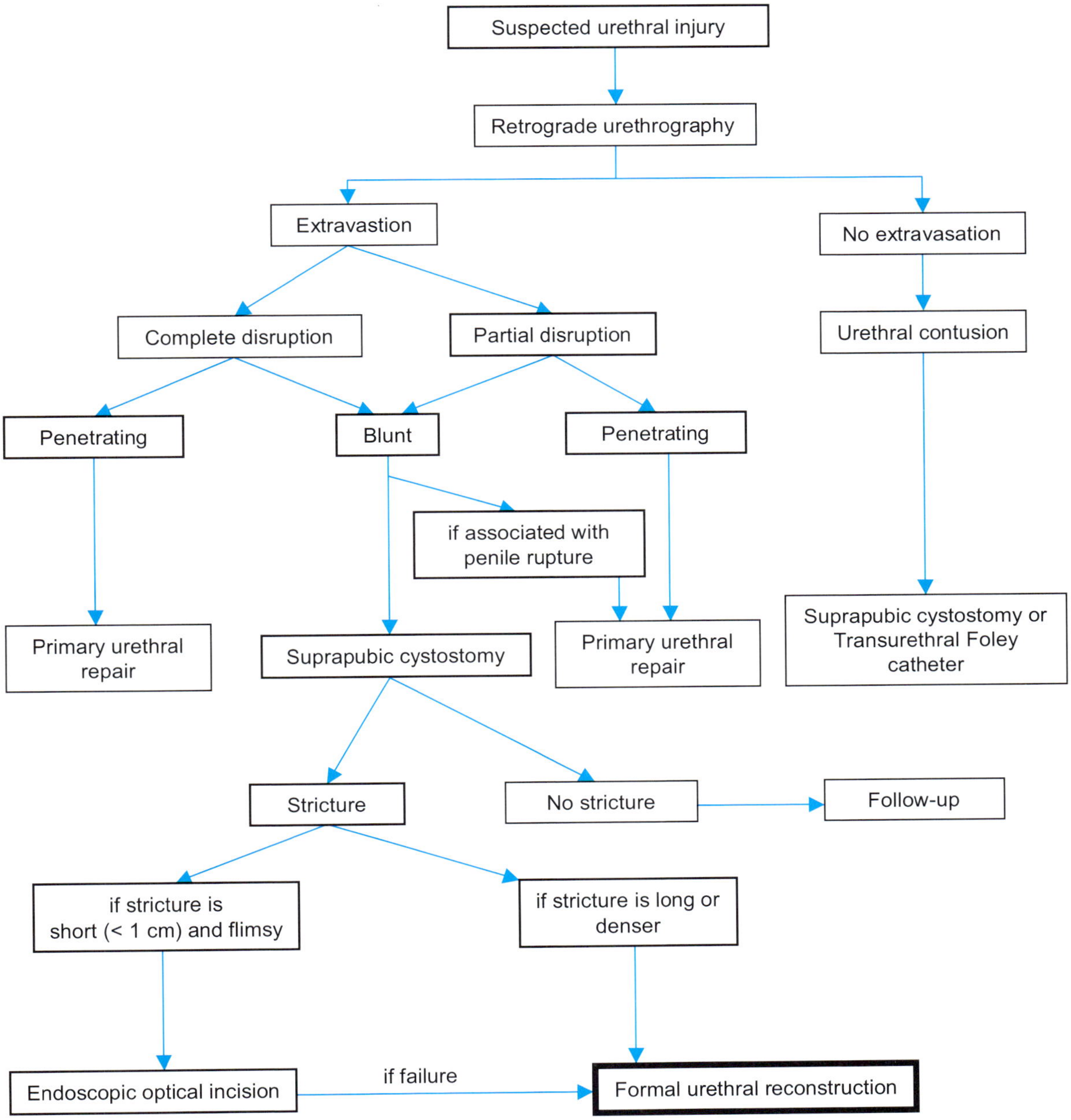

Fig. 15.9.19. Management of anterior urethral injuries in men

References

Antoci JP, Schiff MJ (1982) Bladder and urethral injuries in patients with pelvic fractures. J Urol 128:25

Armenakas NA, McAninch JW (1994) A uniform approach to urethroplasty. Prob Urology 8:254

Armenakas NA, McAninch JW (1996) Acute anterior urethral injuries. In: McAninch JW (ed) Traumatic and reconstructive urology. WB Saunders Philadelphia, p 543

Armenakas NA, McAninch JW, Lue TF, Dixon CM (1993) Posttraumatic impotence: MRI and duplex ultrasound in diagnosis and management. J Urol 149:1272

Asci R, Sarikaya S, Buyukalpelli R, Saylik A, Yilmaz AF, Yildiz S (1999) Voiding and sexual dysfunctions after pelvic fracture urethra injuries treated with either initial cystostomy and delayed urethroplasty or immediate primary urethral realignment. Scand J Urol Nephrol 33:228

Baert L, Verhamme L, Poppel Hv Vandeursen H, Baert J (1993) Long term consequences of urethral stents. J Urol 150:853

Barbagli G, Selli C, Stomaci N, Delle-Rose A, Trippitelli A, Lenzi R (1987) Urethral trauma: radiological aspects and treatment options. J Trauma 27:256

Barry JM (1989) Visual urethrotomy in the management of the obliterated membranous urethra. Urol Clin North Am 16:319

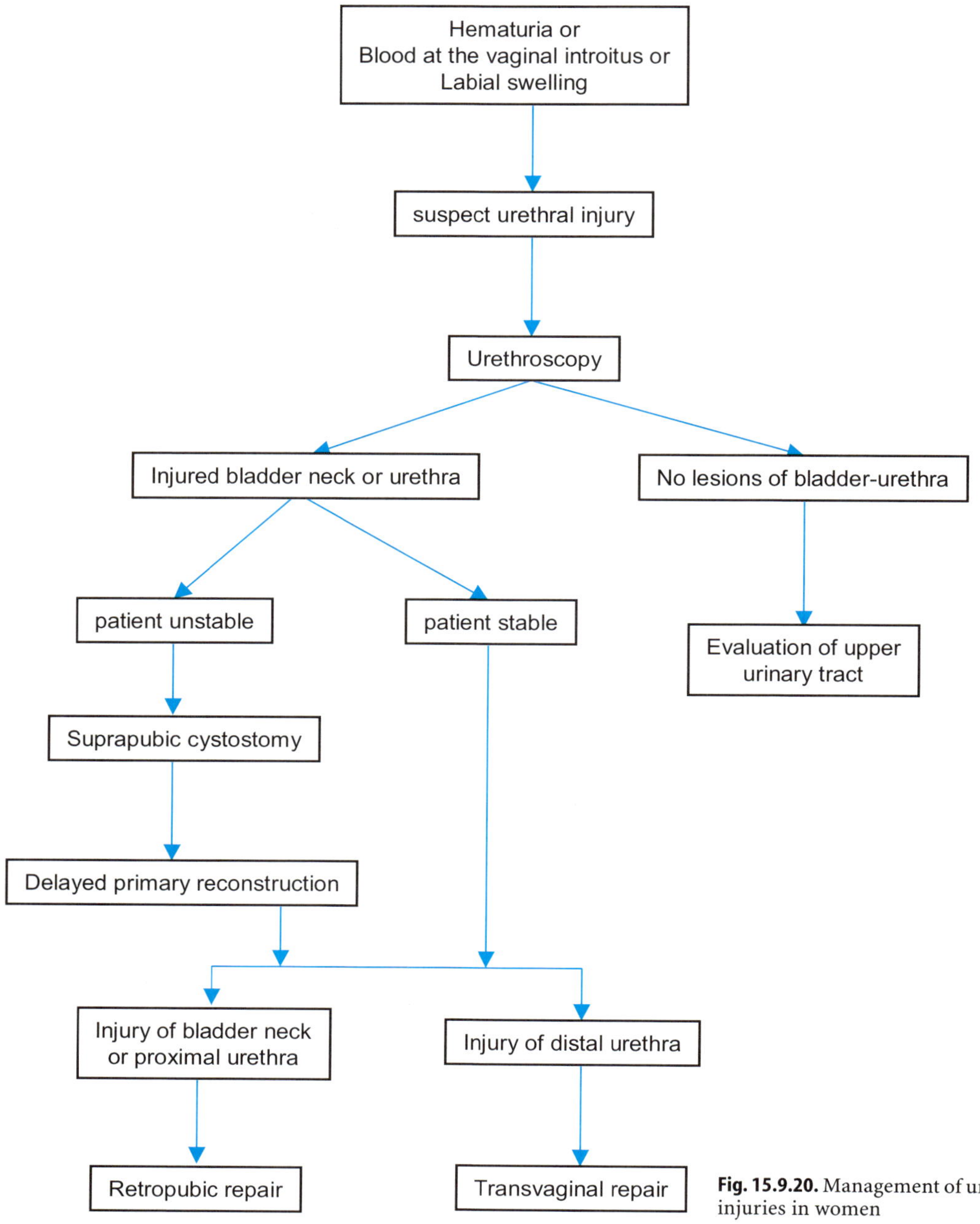

Fig. 15.9.20. Management of urethral injuries in women

Berman AT, Tom L (1974) Traumatic separation of the pubic symphysis with associated fatal rectal tear: A case report and analysis of mechanism of injury. J Trauma 14:1060
Blandy JP (1980) Urethral stricture. Postgrad Med 56:383
Carlin BI, Resnick MI (1995) Indications and techniques for urologic evaluation of the trauma patient with suspected urologic injury. Semin Urol 13:9
Cass AS, Godec CJ (1978) Urethral injury due to external trauma. Urology 11:607
Chapple CR, Png D (1999) Contemporary management of urethral trauma and the post-traumatic stricture. Curr Opin Urol 9:253
Chiou RK, Gonzalez R, Ortlip S, Fraley EE (1988) Endoscopic treatment of posterior urethral obliteration: Long-term follow-up and comparison with transpubic urethroplasty. J Urol 140:508
Clark SS, Prudencio RF (1972) Lower urinary tract injuries associated with pelvic fractures. Surg Clin North Amer 52:183
Coffield KS, Weems WL (1977) Experience with management of posterior urethral injury associated with pelvic fractures. J Urol 117:722
Cohen JK, Berg G, Carl GH, Diamond DD (1991) Primary endoscopic realignment following posterior urethral disruption. J Urol 146:1548

Colapinto V (1980) Trauma to the pelvis: urethral injury. Clin Ortho Rel Res 151:46
Colapinto V, McCallum RW (1977) Injury to the male posterior urethra in fractured pelvis: a new classification. J Urol 118:575
Conolly WB, Hedbert EA (1969) Observations on fractures of the pelvis. J Trauma 9:104
Corriere JN Jr (2001) 1-Stage delayed bulboprostatic anastomotic repair of posterior urethral rupture:60 patients with 1-year followup. J Urol 165:404
Corriere JN Jr, Harris JD (1981) The management of urological injuries in blunt pelvic trauma. Radiol Clin North Am 19:187
Corriere JN Jr, Rudy DC, Benson GS (1994) Voiding and erectile dysfunction after delayed one-stage repair of posterior urethral disruption in 50 men with fractured pelvis. J Trauma 37:587
Crassweller PO, Farrow GA, Robson CJ, Russell JL, Colapinto V (1977) Traumatic rupture of the supramembranous urethra. 118:770
Devine PC, Devine CJ (1982) Posterior urethral injuries associated with pelvic fractures. Urology 20:467
DeVries CR, Anderson RU (1990) Endoscopic urethroplasty: An improved technique. J Urol 143:1225
Dhabuwala CB, Hamid S, Katsikas DM, Pierce J (1990) Impotence following delayed repair of prostate membranous urethral disruption. J Urol 144:677
Dixon CM, Hricak H, McAninch JW (1992) Magnetic resonance imaging of traumatic posterior urethral defects and pelvic crush injuries. J Urol 148:1162
Dixon MD (1996) Diagnosis and acute management of posterior urethral disruptions. In: McAninch JW (ed) Traumatic and reconstructive urology. WB Saunders Philadelphia
Dogra PN, Nabi G (2002) Core-through urethrotomy using the neodynium yag laser for obliterative urethral strictures after traumatic urethral disruption and/or distraction defects: long-term outcome. J Urol 167:543
El-Abd S (1995) Endoscopic treatment of posttraumatic urethral obliteration: experience in 396 patients. J Urol 153:67
Elliott DS, Barret DM (1997) Long-term follow-up and evaluation of primary realignment of posterior urethral disruptions. J Urol 157:814
Fallon B, Wendt JC, Hawtrey CE (1984) Urological injury and assessment in patients with fractured pelvis. J Urol 131:712
Fiala R, Zatura F, Vrtal R (2001) Personal experience with treatment of posttraumatic urethral distraction defects. Acta Chir Orthop Traumatol Cech 68:99
Flaherty JJ, Kelley R, Burnett B, Bucy J, Surian M, Schildkraut D, Clark BG (1968) Relationship of pelvic bone fracture patterns to injuries of urethra and bladder. J Urol 99:297
Follis WH, Koch MO, McDougal WS (1992) Immediate management of prostatomembranous urethral disruptions. J Urol 147:1259
Gelbard MK, Heyman AM, Weintraub P (1989) A technique for immediate realignment and catheterization of the disrupted prostatomembranous urethra. J Urol 142:52
Gheiler EL, Frontera JR (1997) Immediate primary realignment of prostatomembranous urethral disruptions using endourologic techniques. Urology 49:596
Gibson GR (1970) Impotence following fractured pelvis and ruptured urethra. Br J Urol 42:86
Gibson GR (1974) Urological management and complications of fractured pelvis and ruptures urethra. J Urol 111:353
Glassberg KI, Tolete-Velcek F, Ashley R, Waterhouse K (1979) Partial tears of prostatomembranous urethra in children. Urology 13:500
Goel MC, Kumar M, Kapoor R (1997) Endoscopic management of traumatic posterior urethral stricture: early results and follow-up. J Urol 157:95
Goldman SM, Sandler CM, Corriere-Jr, JN, McGuire EJ (1997) Blunt urethral trauma: a unified, anatomical mechanical classification. J Urol 157:85
Gomez RG, Castanheira ACC, McAninch JW (1993) Gunshot wounds to the male external genitalia. J Urol 150:1147
Guille F, Cipolla B, Leveque JM, Guirassy S, Olivo JF, Lobel B (1991) Early endoscopic realignment of complete traumatic rupture of the posterior urethra. Br J Urol 68:178
Gupta NP, Gill IS (1986) Core-through optical internal urethrotomy in management of impassable traumatic posterior urethral strictures. J Urol 136:1018
Hemal AK, Dorairajan LN, Gupta NP (2000) Posttraumatic complete and partial loss of urethra with pelvic fracture in girls: an appraisal of management. J Urol 163:282
Herschorn S, Thijssen A, Radomski SB (1992) The value of immediate or early catheterization of the traumatized posterior urethra. J Urol 148:1428
Husmann DA, Wilson WT, Boone TB, Allen TD (1990) Prostatomembranous urethral disruptions: Management by suprapubic cystostomy and delayed urethroplasty. J Urol 144:76
Husmann DA, Boone TB, Wilson WT (1993) Management of low velocity gunshot wounds to the anterior urethra: the role of primary repair versus urinary diversion alone. J Urol 150:70
Iselin CE, Webster GD (1999) The significance of the open bladder neck associated with pelvic fracture urethral distraction defects. J Urol 162:347
Jackson DH, Williams JL (1974) Urethral injury: a retrospective study. Br J Urol 46:665
Jepson BR, Boullier JA, Moore RG, Parra RO (1999) Traumatic posterior urethral injury and early primary endoscopic realignment: evaluation of long-term follow-up. Urology 53:1205
Jordan GH (1996) Management of membranous urethral distraction injuries via the perineal approach. In: McAninch JW (ed) Traumatic and reconstructive urology. WB Saunders, Philadelphia, p 393
Kane NM, Francis IR, Ellis JH (1989) The value of CT in the detection of bladder and posterior urethral injuries. AJR Am J Roentgenol 153:1243
Kernohan RM, Anwar KK, Johnston SR (1991) Complete urethral stricture of the membranous urethra: A different perspective. Br J Urol 65:51
Kielb SJ, Voeltz ZL, Wolf JS (2001) Evaluation and management of traumatic posterior urethral disruption with flexible cystourethroscopy. J Trauma 50:36
King J (1975) Impotence after fractures of the pelvis. J Bone Joint Surg 57:1107
Koraitim MM (1995) The lessons of 145 posttraumatic posterior urethral strictures treated in 17 years. J Urol 153:63
Koraitim MM (1996) Pelvic fracture urethral injuries: evaluation of various methods of management. J Urol 156:1288
Koraitim MM (1997) Post-traumatic posterior urethral strictures in children: A 20 year experience. J Urol 157:641
Koraitim MM (1999) Pelvic fracture urethral injuries: the unresolved controversy. J Urol 161:1433
Koraitim MM, Marzouk ME, Atta MA, Orabi SS (1996) Risk factors and mechanism of urethral injury in pelvic fractures. Br J Urol 77:876
Kotkin L, Koch MO (1996) Impotence and incontinence after immediate realignment of posterior urethral trauma: results of injury or management? J Urol 155:1600
Leonard MP, Emtaje J, Perez R, Morales A (1990) Endoscopic management of urethral stricture: Cut-to-the-light procedure. Urology 35:117
Levine J, Wessells H (2001) Comparison of open and endoscopic treatment of posttraumatic posterior urethral strictures. World J Surg 25:1597

Lieberman SF, Barry JM (1982) Retreat from transpubic urethroplasty for obliterated membranous urethral strictures. J Urol 128:379
Lim PHC, Chng HC (1989) Initial management of acute urethral injuries. Br J Urol 64:165
Londergan TA, Gundersen LH, Every MJv (1997) Early fluoroscopic realignment for traumatic urethral injuries. Urology 49:101
Lowe MA, Mason JT, Luna GK, Maier RV, Copass MK, Berger RE (1988) Risk factors for urethral injuries in men with traumatic pelvic fractures. J Urol 140:506
Lynch T, Martínez-Piñeiro L, Plas E, Serafetinides E, Türkeri L, Santucci RA, Hohenfellner M (2005) EAU Guidelines on urological trauma. Eur Urol 47:1
MacDiarmid S, Rosario D, Chapple CR (1995) The importance of accurate assessment and conservative management of the open bladder neck in patients with pelvic fracture membranous urethral distraction defects. Br J Urol 75:65
Malek RS, OĎea MJ, Kelalis PP (1977) Management of ruptured posterior urethra in childhood. J Urol 117:105
Mark SD, Webster GD (1996) Reconstruction of the failed repair of posterior urethral rupture. In: McAninch JW (ed) Traumatic and reconstructive urology. WB Saunders, Philadelphia
Mark SD, Keane TE, Vandemark RM, Webster GD (1995) Impotence following pelvic fracture urethral injury: incidence, aetiology and management. Br J Urol 75:62
Marshall FF (1989) Endoscopic reconstruction of traumatic urethral transections. Urol Clin North Am 16:313
Martínez-Piñeiro JA, Carcamo P, García-Matres MJ, Martínez-Piñeiro L, Iglesias JR, Rodriguez-Ledesma JM (1997) Excision and anastomotic repair for urethral stricture disease: experience with 150 cases. Eur Urol 32:433
McAninch JW (1989) Pubectomy in repair of membranous urethral stricture. Urol Clin Norh Am 16:297
McAninch JW (1992) Urethral injuries in female subjects following pelvic fractures (Editorial Comment) J Urol 147:143
McAninch JW (1996) Pubectomy in repair of membranous urethral strictures. In: McAninch JW (ed) Traumatic and reconstructive urology. WB Saunders, Philadelphia
McAninch JW (1997) Editorial: Scars in the urinary system. J Urol 157:817
McAninch JW (1981) Traumatic injuries to the urethra. J Trauma 21:291
McRoberts JW, Radge H (1970) The severed canine posterior urethra: a study of two distinct methods of repair. J Urol 104:724
Melekos MD, Pantazakos A, Daouaher H, Papatsoris G (1992) Primary endourologic re-establishment of urethral continuity after disruption of prostatomembranous urethra. Urology 39:135
Milroy EJG, Chapple CR, Eldrin A, Wallsen N (1989) A new treatment for urethral strictures – A permanently implanted stent. J Urol 141:1120
Moore EE, Cogbill TH, Jurkovich GJ, McAninch JW, Champion HR, Gennarelli TA, Malangoni MA, Shackford SR, Trafton PG (1992) Organ injury scaling III: chest wall, abdominal vascular, ureter, bladder, and urethra. J Trauma 33:337
Morehouse DD, Mackinnon KJ (1980) Management of prostatomembranous urethral disruption: a 13-year experience. J Urol 123:173
Morey AF, McAninch JW (1997) Reconstruction of posterior urethral disruption injuries: outcome analysis in 82 patients. J Urol 157:506
Moudouni SM, Patard JJ, Manuta A, Guiraud P, Lobel B, Guille F (2001) Early endoscopic realignment of post-traumatic posterior urethral disruption. Urology 57:628
Mouraview V, Santucci R (2005) Cadaveric anatomy of pelvic fracture urethral distraction injury: most injuries are distal to the external urinary sphincter. J Urol 173:869
Mouraview V, Coburn M, Santucci R (2005) The treatment of posterior urethral disruption associated with pelvic fractures: comparative experience of early realignment versus delayed urethroplast. J Urol 173:873
Muhlbauer S, Bard R (1980) Early definitive urologic management of patient with crush pelvic trauma and deep perineal laceration. Urology 15:56
Mundy AR (1993) Results and complications of urethroplasty and its future. Br J Urol 71:322
Mundy AR (1991) The role of delayed primary repair in the acute management of pelvic fracture injuries to the urethra. Br J Urol 68:273
Mundy AR (1996) Urethroplasty for posterior urethral strictures. Br J Urol 78:243
Nicolaisen G, Melamud A, Williams RD, McAninch JW (1983) Rupture of the corpus cavernosum: surgical management. J Urol 130:917
Palmer KJ, Benson GS, Corriere JN Jr (1983) Diagnosis and initial management of urological injuries associated with 200 consecutive pelvis fracture. J Urol 130:712
Pansadoro V, Emiliozzi P (1996) Internal urethrotomy in the management of anterior urethral strictures: long-term follow-up. J Urol 156:73
Pennal GF, Tile M, Waddell JP, Garside H (1980) Pelvic disruption: assessment and classification. Clin Orthop 151:12
Perry MO, Husmann DA (1992) Urethral injuries in female subjects following pelvic fractures. J Urol 147:139
Podesta A, Hafez A, El-Assmy A, Sarhan O, El-Hefnawy A, Ghoneim M (2005) Perineal anastomotic urethroplasty for managing post-traumatic urethral strictures in children: the long-term outcome. BJU Int 95:403
Pokorny M, Pontes JE, Pierce JM Jr (1978) Urological injuries associated with pelvic trauma. J Urol 121:455
Pontes JE, Pierce JM Jr (1978) Anterior urethral injuries: four years of experience at the Detroit General Hospital. J Urol 120:563
Porter JR, Takayama TK, Defalco AJ (1997) Traumatic posterior urethral injury and early realigment using magnetic urethral catheters. J Urol 158:425
Quint JH, Stanisic TH (1993) Above and below delayed endoscopic treatment of traumatic posterior urethral disruption. J Urol 149:484
Ragde H, McInnes GF (1969) Transpubic repair of the severed prostatomembranous urethra. J Urol 101:335
Rehman J, Samadi D, Ricciardi R Jr, Kreutzer E (1998) Early endoscopic realignment as primary therapy for complete posterior urethral disruptions. J Endourol 12:283
Sachse H (1974) Zur Behandlung der Harnröhrenstruktur: Die transuretrale Schlitzung unter Sicht mit scharfem Schnitt. Fortschr Med 92:12
Sahin H, Bircan MK, Akay AF, Gocmen M, Bilici A (1998) Endoscopic treatment of complete posterior urethral obliteration. Acta Urol Belg 66:21
Santucci RA, Mario LA, McAninch JW (2002) Anastomotic urethroplasty for bulbar urethral stricture: analysis of 168 patients. J Urol 167:1715
Sevitt S (1968) Fatal road accidents. Injuries, complications, and causes of death in 250 subjects. Br J Surg 55:481
Siegel JH, Dalal SA, Burgess AR (1990) Pattern of organ injuries in pelvic fracture: Impact force implications for survival and death in motor vehicle injuries. Accid Anal Prev 22:457
Smith J (1968) The measurement and significance of the urinary flow rate. Br J Urol 38:701
Tahan H, Randrianantenaina A, Michel F (1999) Treatment of complete rupture of the posterior urethra by endoscopic treatment. Prog Urol 9:489

Tile M, Pennal GF (1980) Pelvic disruptions: Principles of management. Clin Orthop 151:56
Turner-Warwick R (1973) Observations on the treatment of traumatic urethral injuries and the value of the fenestrated urethral catheter. Br J Surg 60:775
Turner-Warwick R (1977) Complex traumatic posterior urethral strictures. J Urol 118:564
Turner-Warwick R (1989) Prevention of complications resulting from pelvic fracture urethral injuries – and from their surgical management. Urol Clin North Am 16:335
Venn SN, Mundy AR (1998) Immediate management of major trauma to the urinary tract. Eur Urol 33:1
Wadhwa SN, Chahal R, Hemal AK, Gupta NP, Dogra PN, Seth A (1998) Management of obliterative posttraumatic posterior urethral strictures after failed initial urethroplasty. J Urol 159:1898
Webster GD (1990) Impotence following delayed repair of prostatomembranous urethral disruption. Editorial comment. J Urol 144:678
Webster GD (1987) The management of complex posterior urethral strictures. Prob Uro 1:226
Webster GD (1989) Perineal repair of membranous urethral stricture. Urol Clin North Am 16:303
Webster GD, Ramon J (1991) Repair of pelvic fracture posterior urethral defects using an elaborated perineal approach. J Urol 145:744
Webster GD, Ramon J, Kreder K (1990) Salvage posterior urethroplasty after failed initial repair of pelvic fracture membranous urethral defects. J Urol 144:1370
Webster GD, Mathes GL, Selli C (1983) Prostatomembranous urethral injuries. A review of the literature and a rational approach to their management. J Urol 130:898
Weems WL (1979) Management of genitourinary injuries in patients with pelvic fractures. Ann Surg 189:717
Williams G (1993) Stents in the lower urinary tract. Am Urol Assoc Update Ser 12:26
Yasuda T, Yamanishi T, Isaka S, Okano T, Masai M, Shimazaki J (1991) Endoscopic re-establishment of membranous urethral disruption. J Urol 145:977
Ying-Hao S, Chuan-Liang X, Xu G, Guo-Qiang L, Jian-Guo H (2000) Urethroscopic realignment of ruptured bulbar urethra. J Urol 164:1543
Zinman LN (1997) The management of traumatic posterior urethral distraction defects. Editorial. J Urol 157:511
Zorn G (1960) Beckenbrüche mit Harnröhrenverletzungen, ihre Behandlung und Ergebnisse. Beitr Klin Chir 1960:147

Priapism

16

W.O. Brant, A.J. Bella, M.M. Gracia, T.F. Lue

16.1 Introduction

Priapism is defined as an erection lasting longer than 4 h that is not associated with sexual stimulation. It is generally classified into two etiologies: ischemic and nonischemic. The former, comprising the vast majority of cases, is considered an emergency due to the associated pain as well as to structural changes in the penis that may lead to penile fibrosis and severe erectile dysfunction. Conservative management is rarely effective except in select circumstances. Interventions may include aspiration of the corpora, injection of vasoconstrictive agents, or surgical procedures. Nonischemic priapism presents fewer emergent risks and may be followed conservatively. If intervention is necessary, angiographic embolization is often the best therapeutic option.

The term "priapism" is derived from Priapus, the Greek god of fertility. Often depicted holding a wooden sickle in his hand, he was also known as the protector of horticulture and viticulture. Priapus was also used in the Roman gardens as a scarecrow, and thieves were often deterred by the enormity of his penis. Priapus's notoriety was secondary to his huge virile member and as such many nicknames were used to refer to his genitals including "column," "12-inch pole," "cypress," "spear," "pyramid," and many others. And just as Zeus shows his thunderbolt, Poseidon his trident, and Hermes his caduceus, so Priapus cannot but proudly exhibit his penis, which best represents him, and without which he is weaponless. This is the reason why his privy parts are always shamelessly displayed in erection (Papadopoulos and Kelami 1988).

Priapism was a condition first described by Tripe in 1845 (Adeyoju et al. 2002). It has been defined as a pathological condition of penile erection that persists beyond or is unrelated to sexual stimulation (Sadeghi-Nejad and Seftel 2002). Priapism is usually painful and fails to subside with orgasm. Pain is often delayed until 6–8 h have elapsed. It has been described in men of all ages including newborns. The peak incidence of priapism is bimodal, with the highest incidence occurring between the ages of 5 and 10, and 20 and 50 years. Generally in the younger age group, priapism is secondary to a neoplasm or sickle cell anemia. Previously, with the common use of intracavernosally injected agents, the incidence of priapism was noted to have increased. With the recent successful introduction of orally acting agents, fewer men are at risk of injection-related prolonged erections. However, even with the success of phosphodiesterase type 5 inhibitors in the older age group, priapism still usually occurs secondary to intracavernous injection or the use of psychotropic drugs (Keoghane et al. 2002).

Priapism must be considered a urological emergency, as it may lead to irreversible penile ischemia, necrosis, and scarring of the intracavernosal erectile tissue, if untreated. A window of opportunity exists when intervention greatly improves the success rate of conservative measures. Delays in treatment greatly compromise success of treatment, and may ultimately lead to significant complications to the patient.

16.2 Classification

Classically, several terms have been used to describe the same condition of priapism. "Low-flow," "venous," and "ischemic" priapism have often been used interchangeably. Correspondingly, "high-flow," "arterial," and "nonischemic" have also been used for the same condition. Doppler ultrasound has become a standard diagnostic tool that may be used to differentiate the various classes of priapism. Important in distinguishing between ischemic and nonischemic priapism, it has also allowed us to clarify the proper terminology that should be adopted when referring to this condition. Whereas historically the term "low-flow" priapism was often used, it is now clear that this is in fact a misnomer as Doppler flow studies demonstrate clearly the complete lack of blood flow in the corpus cavernosum during this condition. Therefore, the more appropriate terms to use are "ischemic" and "nonischemic," as they most accurately describe the pathological condition that exists. Alternatively one could use the terms "no-flow" priapism and "high-flow" priapism.

Ischemic priapism is similar in character to a compartment syndrome. In both conditions there is an occlusion of venous outflow and consequent cessation of arterial inflow that serves to create an acidotic and hypoxic condition in the penis. It is this acidosis and tissue ischemia that leads to a painful prolonged erection. The detumescence mechanism may fail for a number of reasons, including a prolonged relaxation of intracavernosal smooth muscles, malfunction of the intrinsic detumescence mechanism, or anatomical obstruction of the veins draining the penis. Relaxation of the intracavernosal muscles may occur because of an increase in neurotransmitters, exogenous sources causing relaxation of the smooth muscles, or failure to metabolize the neurotransmitters or second messengers. In all cases of ischemic priapism, the end effect is increased penile ischemia and acidosis with resultant pain and inflammation, with subsequent necrosis, fibrosis, and erectile dysfunction if not remedied expeditiously. Various histological studies have been performed to define the pathological pattern during various times of the condition. In the early stages (less then 12 h), interstitial edema and thickening are the most common findings. From 12 to 24 h, thrombocytes start to adhere to the endothelium such that by 48 h necrosis of cavernosal smooth muscle cells and fibroblast proliferation have occurred. The end result is loss of smooth muscle, collapse of sinusoids, and fibrosis of the corpora cavernosa (Spycher and Hauri 1986).

Nonischemic priapism is a different entity than ischemic priapism. Although not technically a urological emergency, it may sometimes be difficult to differentiate from ischemic priapism. Nonischemic priapism is a result of unregulated increased arterial inflow into the penis, which causes penile tumescence. In most cases of nonischemic priapism, a ruptured artery pumps well-oxygenated blood to fill the sinusoids and results in penile erection of various degrees. The injury is most commonly to a branch of the cavernosal artery and usually occurs secondary to perineal or direct penile trauma (McMahon 2002). Significantly less common than ischemic priapism, the condition does not lead to acidosis in the penis and rarely is pain elicited as a major symptom. Because of the relative lack of pain and sometimes only a subtle increase in penile rigidity, these patients tend to seek medical attention much later than those with ischemic priapism.

16.3 Etiology

Although approximately 50 % of all episodes of priapism are thought to be idiopathic, there are a number of known specific causes of this disorder. In adults, intracavernous therapy with papaverine, phentolamine, alprostadil, or combinations of these agents is the most common cause of ischemic priapism (El-Bahnasawy et al. 2002). Zorgniotti and Lefleur (1985) first reported the use of a combination of papaverine (30 mg) and phentolamine (0.5 mg) for self-injection. Prolonged erection occurred in 1.6% during titration and in one patient on home therapy (Zorgniotti and Lefleur 1985). In a review of the published literature, Linet and Neff (1994) found that, in doses of 10–20 μg, alprostadil led to prolonged erection/priapism in 1.3% of patients. The incidence was found to be about five times lower with alprostadil than with papaverine or papaverine/phentolamine (1.3% vs 10% vs 7%), a finding supported by an Australian study (Earle et al. 2003). In the 1996 worldwide clinical trials conducted by the Alprostadil Study group, prolonged erection (4–6 h) was noted in 5%, and priapism (>6 h) was noted in 1% (Linet and Ogrinc 1996). One Argentinean study reported a much higher rate of priapism, reaching 18% and 15% for papaverine plus phentolamine and prostaglandin E1, respectively. These figures are substantially higher than those found in other studies, and this is likely secondary to testing patients with neurologic or psychologic impotence who are often very sensitive to the medication (Bechara et al. 1997).

The introduction of intraurethral alprostadil has emerged as an alternative treatment modality, and the incidence of priapism with its use is less then 0.1% (Ekman et al. 2000). Often it is abuse or inappropriate dosing of these medications that induces a prolonged erection. Dosing of intracavernous agents should be done so that an erection of less than 1 h in duration results. For erections that last longer than 4 h, medical attention should be promptly sought.

Several other medications have been implicated in ischemic priapism. Most notably the psychotropic drugs as a class are over represented. Antipsychotics such as chlorpromazine, phenothiazine, and clozapine are known culprits, as are the antidepressants such as trazodone (Compton and Miller 2001). The antihypertensives hydralazine, prazosin, and guanethidine have also been implicated in ischemic priapism (Avisrror et al. 2000). The high fat content in total parenteral nutrition is also believed to cause priapism (Hebuterne et al. 1992). Various recreational drugs have been associated with ischemic priapism. Drugs of abuse such as alcohol and cocaine have been reported to cause priapism (Kulmala et al. 1995; Altman et al. 1999). Cocaine may be injected intracorporally in intravenous drug abusers, as this is often one of the easier, if not convenient, portals of entry to the venous system. Anticoagulants such as intravenous heparin and oral coumadin have anecdotally been reported to cause priapism (Bschleipfer et al. 2001). In most of these cases, priapism resulted after cessation of the anticoagulant and a resultant rebound hypercoagulable state. Testosterone has also been noted to result in priapism episodes (Zargooshi 2000). Interestingly with the profound increase in use of oral erectogenic agents such as the phosphodiesterase inhibitors, few cases of priapism have been reported from abuse of these agents (Sur and Kane 2000; King et al. 2005; Goldmeier and Lamba 2002).

Hematological diseases, mainly sickle cell disease or trait and leukemia, are well-known causes of ischemic priapism. These hyperviscosity syndromes are considered to be the most common cause of priapism in children. The assumed mechanism is that prolonged nocturnal erections decrease the oxygen tension in the corpora cavernosa, which predisposes the erythrocytes to sickling (Francis and Johnson 1991). The sickled erythrocytes predispose to venous stasis that perpetuates the priapism episode. In one large study, the incidence of priapism in sickle cell diseased patients was 18 % – 27 % (Francis and Johnson 1991). This study also highlighted the lack of knowledge and awareness of this complication by families and patients alike. A unique study by Burnett et al. looked at the magnetic resonance imaging findings of the penis of men with sickle cell anemia and noted a wide range of findings (Burnett et al. 1995). Some of the men had normal corporal anatomy, while others had complete corporal destruction with intense intracorporeal fibrosis and hemosiderin deposition. Anecdotally, other hemoglobinopathies have been associated with priapism, including the rare unstable hemoglobin Hb Olmsted and thrombophilia (Quigley and Fawcett 1999).

Neurological conditions such as cerebrovascular disease and seizure disorders have been implicated as a rare cause of priapism (Baba et al. 1995). Other causes include scuba diving and cord compression (Earle et al. 2003). A variety of malignancies have been associated with priapism. Bladder and prostate cancer (Kvarstein 1996; Schroeder-Printzer et al. 1994) as well as metastases to the corpora cavernosa may present with ischemic priapism. The malignancy is thought to infiltrate and obstruct venous drainage. This type of priapism is usually treated with chemotherapy or radiotherapy.

Nonischemic priapism usually results from an identifiable trauma to the penis, perineum, or pelvis. The trauma tends to cause uncontrolled inflow into the cavernosal sinusoids and bypass the control that the helicine arteries provide and results in priapism. Branches of the cavernosal artery have been identified as the most frequent vessels injured in nonischemic priapism. Because the tissue is well oxygenated, there is the lack of ischemia and necrosis and so patients rarely complain of pain. Several theories have been proposed to explain the common delayed presentation of nonischemic priapism. Witt et al. proposed that after the trauma platelet aggregation and vasospasm may occur, which prevents the immediate development of priapism (Witt et al. 1990). However, subsequent erections may cause enough vascular shearing forces to cause rupture of the arterial wall and priapism. Because the therapy for nonischemic priapism is drastically different than that for ischemic priapism, a systematic approach must be used in evaluating and differentiating all patients who present with priapism.

16.4 Evaluation

Priapism may be a manifestation of a variety of conditions and, therefore, a thorough history and physical examination are necessary in the initial evaluation. Important historical features include duration and quality of erection, presence or absence of pain, and inciting factors of erection. Specific attention should be given to the use of medications as well as recreational drug use. A history of sickle cell anemia as well as other relevant hypercoagulable states should be questioned.

The physical examination is an important component to the evaluation. Specific attention to perineal bruising and lymphadenopathy should be given. Assessment of the erection should be done paying specific attention to the degree of corporal and spongiosal tumescence. The penile examination will typically reveal a rigid and painful erection with a soft glans in cases of ischemic priapism. Patients with nonischemic priapism will have a semi-erect penis that is not painful. A neurological examination should also be included in the routine evaluation of priapism as neurological disease may sometimes initially manifest as priapism.

Diagnosis and classification of the cause of priapism may often be made by history and physical examination alone. Aspiration of penile cavernosal blood may act as both a diagnostic and therapeutic maneuver. In ischemic priapism, corporal blood analysis usually reveals an acidotic and hypoxic blood content (pH <7.25, PO_2 <30, PCO_2 >60). Blood gas values that are similar to arterial levels (pH >7.3, PO_2 >50, PCO_2 <40) suggest nonischemic priapism. It is important to remember that all cases of priapism begin with influx of arterial blood and as such cavernous blood gas measurement, if done early, may be misleading.

A blood sample analysis should also be obtained to include complete blood count, electrolytes, and sickle cell prep for hemoglobin S determination. A complete blood count may also act as a screening tool for patients suspected of having leukemia. Urinalysis and urine toxicology testing may be appropriate in select patients suspected of being illicit drug abusers. To further elucidate the type of priapism, duplex Doppler ultrasound has increasingly been used (Secil et al. 2001). With ultrasound, no cavernosal arterial flow is seen in the ischemic type of priapism, while a ruptured cavernosal artery with unregulated blood flow and blood pooling may be seen in the nonischemic type (Bochinski et al. 2004). Before any form of treatment, informed consent is important, as upwards of 50% of patients will have some form of erectile dysfunction due to underlying tissue changes present at the time of treatment, regardless of treatment approach.

16.5 Management

In general, treatment is aimed at the primary cause of the priapism if it can be identified. The ultimate goal of treatment is to relieve the pain, reverse the erection, and prevent damage to the corporal bodies. A stepwise approach is generally used and the least invasive treatments are used first (Table 16.1).

Table 16.1. Treatment of ischemic priapism

Step	Ischemic priapism, emergency
1	Determine ischemic vs nonischemic
2	Treat priapism, then underlying disorder if present
3	Aspiration and irrigation
4	Injection of sympathomimetic agent, repeat if needed, phenylephrine preferred (dose: 100–500 µg every 3–5 min for up to 1 h)
5	Observe for side effects
6	Consider shunt if injections fail
7	Shunt should be distal (cavernoglanular). Use proximal shunt only if distal fails
8	Oral systemic therapy is not warranted

The first line of treatment is irrigation and evacuation of old blood from the corpora cavernosa using a 19- or 21-gauge butterfly (scalp) needle. To ease the process of evacuating old blood, it may be necessary to milk the blood out of the corporal bodies. If this step is unsuccessful, the next step is injection of a diluted alpha agonist solution into the corporal space. Epinephrine, norepinephrine, norepinephrine with Xylocaine and phenylephrine have all been used with success (Melman and Serels 2002); phenylephrine, a pure alpha-1 adrenergic agonist with minimal cardiac side effects, is recommended. Initially, old blood is aspirated or milked out of the corpora until fresh blood is seen. Then inject 500 µg phenylephrine (250 µg in patients with cardiovascular disease) and observe the penis for 3–5 min. If the penis is still rigid, aspirate 10 ml of blood and inject 500 µg of diluted phenylephrine solution. This procedure is repeated every 3–5 min until detumescence occurs. The phenylephrine solution is made by mixing 1 ml of 10 mg/ml of phenylephrine with 19 ml of normal saline.

The patient should be observed closely during phenylephrine treatment, as complications may ensue if the solution is given in excess or too quickly. Some early complications that are commonly seen include headache, acute hypertension, bradycardia, palpitations, sweating, and arrhythmias. Especially in patients with underlying heart disease, monitoring blood pressure and heart rate during treatment is recommended (Muruve and Hosking 1996).

In an attempt to avoid invasive procedures, a variety of oral agents have been used, such as pseudoephedrine and terbutaline, a beta-2 adrenergic antagonist. However, results have been inconsistent and overall disappointing (Shantha et al. 1989; Ahmed and Shaikh 1997; Lowe and Jarow 1993; Govier et al. 1994). As such, systemic oral agents are not recommended in the treatment of acute ischemic priapism episodes.

The incidence of priapism in the sickle cell population is as high as 35% (Adeyoju et al. 2002). Although there is a high incidence of this problem in the sickle cell population, there continues to be a low level of understanding of the disorder in patients. The treatment of priapism in patients with sickle cell disease should involve a systematic approach. Unfortunately, the literature fails to agree on a standardized therapy protocol and many treatments have been attempted, including hydration, analgesia, oxygen, anesthesia, tranquilizers, estrogen, anticoagulants, blood transfusions, vasodilators, and antifibrinolytics. The American Foundation for Urologic Diseases has assembled a thought panel to discuss and recommend alternatives for the evaluation and treatment of priapism. The treatment options that were considered important in the sickle cell population were analgesia, oxygenation, exchange transfusion, and hydration. It is important to note that, even if a priapism episode is secondary to a general medical condition such as sickle cell, treatment of that condition alone is insufficient. Each individual priapism episode must be treated with intracorporal therapy concurrent with treatment of the underlying disorder. Even with the available treatments, a significant proportion of these patients go on to have stuttering priapism.

16.6 Surgical Treatment of Ischemic Priapism

If conservative measures are unsuccessful, then a surgical approach may be necessary. The goal of surgical treatment is to allow blood to flow in and out of the penis freely to prevent ischemia and fibrosis of the penis. The principles of most of the priapism surgeries involve creation of a fistula between the engorged corpus cavernosum and the glans, corpus spongiosum, and dorsal or saphenous veins. These fistulas are created with the hope that they will spontaneously close after the priapism-inciting factors have abated and the penis is completely detumesced.

16.6.1 Distal Shunts

16.6.1.1 Winter Shunt

This is the least invasive surgical procedure for priapism. With the patient under local anesthesia, a Tru-Cut biopsy needle is inserted through the glans into the corpus cavernosum. A core of tunica albuginea separating the glans and the corpus cavernosum is removed with the needle, thus creating a fistula. Several passes are necessary on each side to create enough communicating channels to achieve a successful outcome (Nelson and Winter 1977).

16.6.1.2 Ebbehoj Procedure

In this procedure, a no. 15 scalpel is used to pierce to the corpus cavernosum through the glans penis (Fig. 16.1). The glans penis may then be closed using a chromic suture (Marx 1981). A variation is to insert a no. 10 blade scalpel vertically through the glans into the corpus cavernosum, turn it 90° laterally, and then pull it out to create a large T-shaped opening in the tunica albuginea (Fig. 16.2). The major advantage is that a single pass on each side creates a large enough shunt for detumescence. The benefits of this procedure are that it can be done with a local anesthetic and has been performed successfully in an emergency department setting.

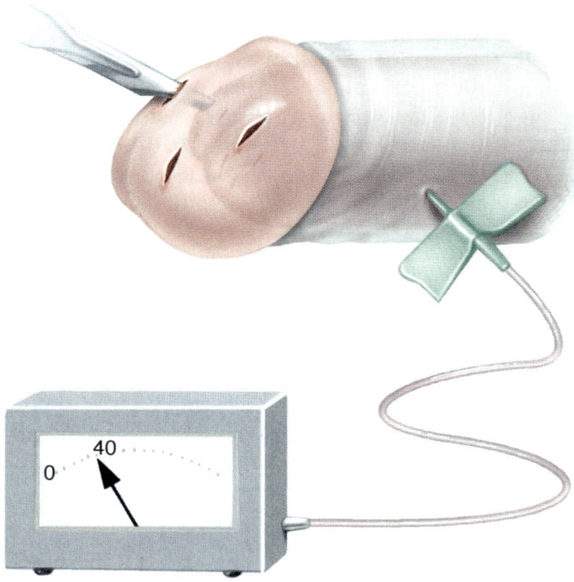

Fig. 16.1. A glans-cavernosal shunt (Ebbehoj) is made with a No. 11 blade. Intracavernosal pressure is monitored via an arterial line set-up. After skin closure, maintenance of pressure at 40 mm Hg or less for 10 min or more is indicative of an adequate shunt (© Hohenfellner 2007)

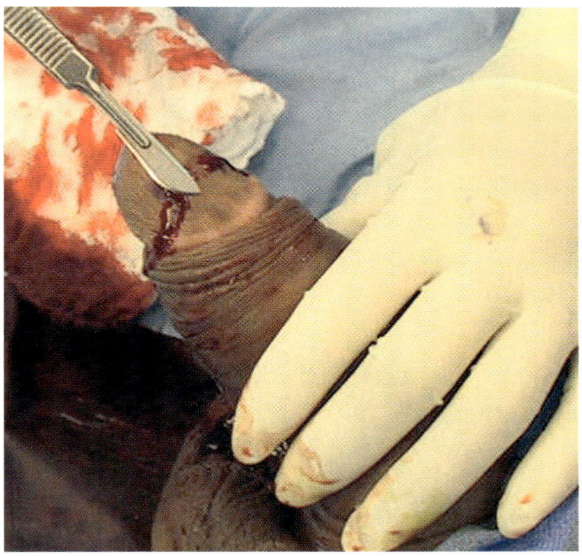

Fig. 16.2. T-shaped glans-cavernosal shunt using a No.10 scalpel. The blade is inserted into each corpus cavernosum from the glans, turned 90 degrees laterally and then pulled out to create a T-shaped shunt

16.6.1.3 Al-Ghorab Shunt

The incision is traditionally made transversely on the dorsal aspect of the glans approximately 1 cm distal to the coronal sulcus. Dissection is carried down to the bulging corporal bodies. A 5-mm elliptical excision is n made at the tips of the corporal bodies and the dark old blood is drained from the corpora cavernosa. When detumescence occurs, the skin is sutured closed with chromic suture. It is important to avoid obliterating the spongy tissue layer of the glans penis with the closure stitches (Benjelloun et al. 1993). Alternatively, two separate vertical incisions can be made, as a transverse incision may cut the sensory nerves to the distal glans.

16.6.2
Proximal Shunts

16.6.2.1
Quackels Cavernoso-Spongiosal Shunt

This shunt is inserted with the patient in the lithotomy position. A longitudinal incision is made in the perineum (Fig. 16.3). The bulb of the corpora spongiosum is dissected free from the bulbospongiosal muscle. This dissection may be aided with the use of a Foley catheter. A 1-cm incision is then made in the corpora cavernosum and corpora spongiosum. This incision should be made close enough to the first so that the two openings can be sutured together (Quackels 1964).

To create a better fistula, some recommend excising an ellipse of tissue from the corpora rather then a simple incision. Once the corpora cavernosa have been opened, the old blood must be milked out until fresh blood is seen. The walls of the fistula may be sutured together using a 5-0 polydioxanone (PDS) suture. A unilateral incision may be sufficient as long as intracavernosal pressures remain below 40 cm H_2O after 10–15 min. If these parameters are not observed a contralateral fistula may be performed.

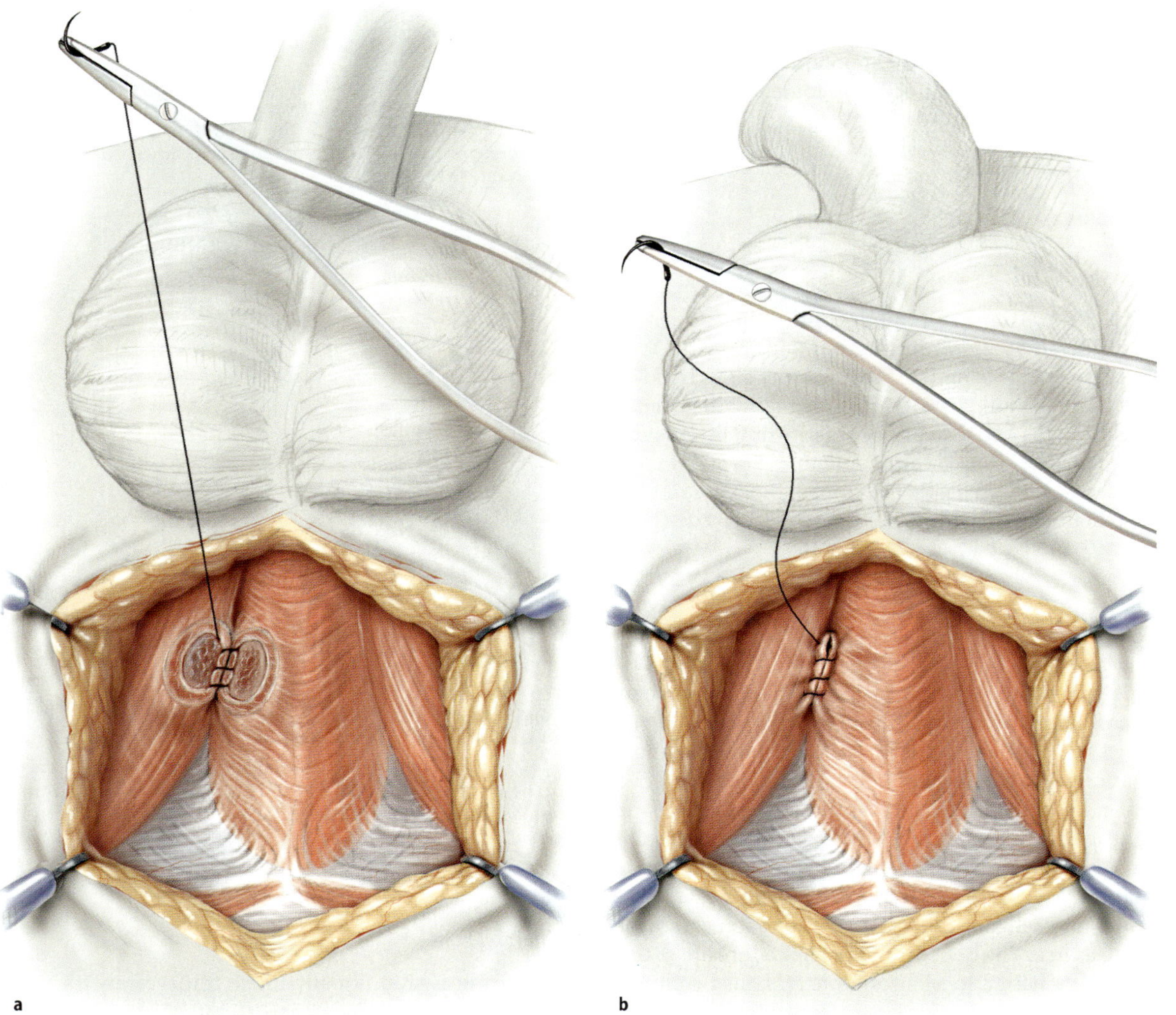

a b

Fig. 16.3. Cavernoso-spongiosal shunt (Quackels). It is important that the shunt is created in the perineum between the urethral bulb and crura. If placed too distal, it will not be effective and will carry a higher risk of urethral injury (© Hohenfellner 2007)

16.6.2.2
Barry Cavernoso-Dorsal Vein Shunt

A 4-cm-long skin incision is made at the base of the penis. The superficial or deep dorsal vein is identified and mobilized to the extent that it can be anastomosed to the tunica albuginea in a tension-free manner (Fig. 16.4). Once again an ellipse of tunica tissue is excised that is proportionate to the size of the dorsal vein. A 5-0 PDS stitch is used for the anastomosis (Barry 1976).

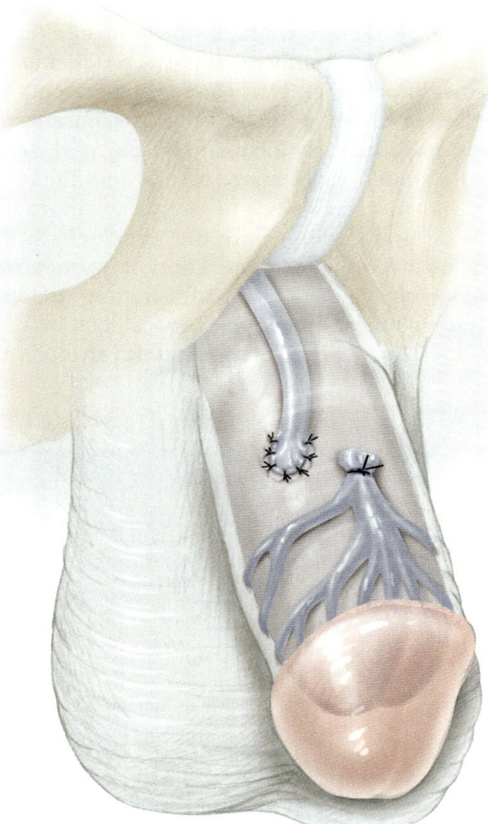

Fig. 16.4. Cavernoso-dorsal vein shunt (Barry). The dorsal vein is sutured to a window in the corpus cavernosum to provide shunting (© Hohenfellner 2007)

16.6.2.3
Grayhack Cavernoso-Saphenous Vein Shunt

For this procedure, the patient is placed in the supine position frog-legged. An incision is made approximately 3–4 cm below the inguinal ligament at the saphenofemoral junction. The saphenous vein is identified and mobilized for approximately 10 cm. After the distal margin of the vein is ligated, a second incision is made on the lateral margin of the shaft at the root of the pe-

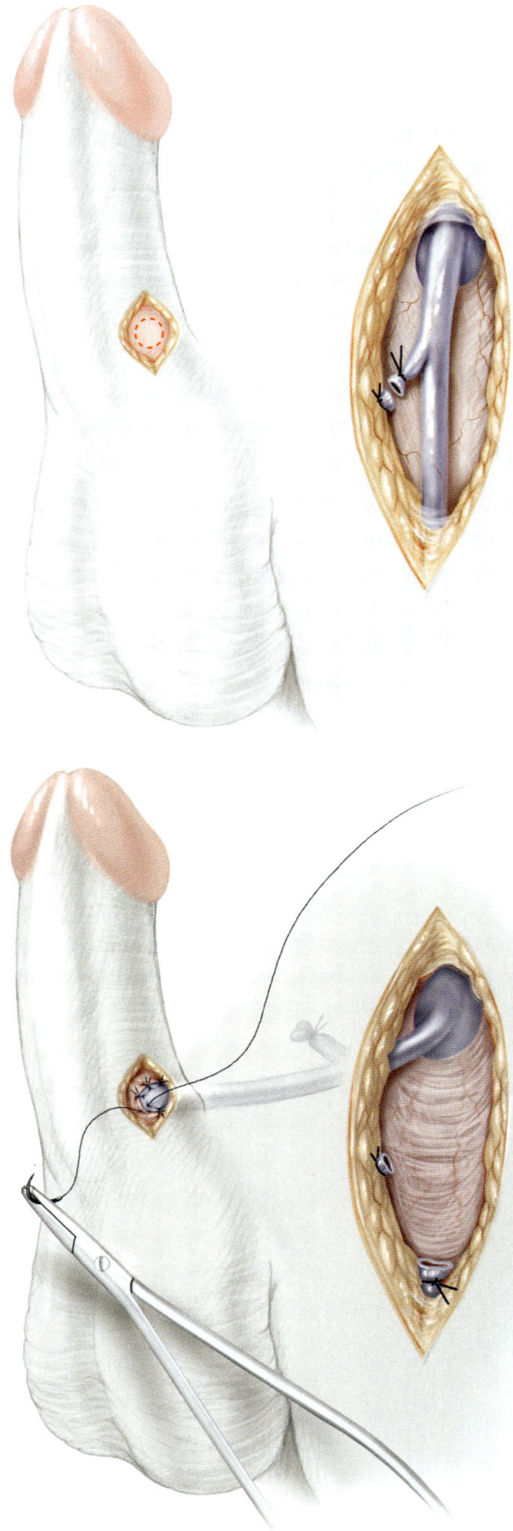

a

b

Fig. 16.5. Cavernoso-saphenous vein shunt (Grayhack). The saphenous vein is mobilized by dividing and ligating the tributaries. It is crucial that the saphenous vein is passed without tension, torsion or angulation (© Hohenfellner 2007) nis. Dissection is continued to the tunica albuginea and the two incisions are connected subcutaneously. The saphenous vein is then passed to the superior incision and a small piece of tunica albuginea is excised (Fig. 16.5). The corporal body is then milked until the old clot is evacuated. The saphenous vein is spatulated and anastomosed to the tunica tissue using a 5-0 PDS stitch (Lehtonen and Tenhunen 1973).

In addition to relieving pain, early treatment of ischemic priapism may preserve erectile function. One study reported that 92 % of men preserve potency with priapism lasting less than 24 h but only 22 % are potent after priapism lasting more than 7 days (Kulmala et al. 1996). In another study, up to 90 % of men had some degree of erectile dysfunction after an episode of priapism as compared to the premorbid state, although this study did not examine the duration of priapism vs subsequent erectile function (Nixon et al. 2003).

16.7 Postoperative Care

If any doubts or concerns arise after the shunt has been created, intracorporal pressure monitoring is an option (Fig. 16.1). Intracorporal pressures less than 40 cm H_2O should be observed consistently; otherwise additional shunts may be required. Initially, the postoperative penis may appear partially erect due to edema and postischemic hyperemia. Penile ultrasound or cavernosal blood gas sampling may be performed if any doubt of perfusion exists. It is important to avoid circular or compressive dressings. Manual milking and squeezing of the penis can be done to ensure that the shunt remains patent and priapism does not recur.

16.8 Treatment of Nonischemic Priapism

With a history of perineal trauma and nonpainful erection with varied rigidity, suspicion should be raised of nonischemic priapism secondary to a ruptured branch of the cavernosal artery. If cavernosal blood gases are measured they will most likely reflect arterial levels. Of interest, patients with nonischemic priapism may have a long delay before consulting a physician (more than 3 years has been reported) (Ilkay and Levine 1995). The priapism is usually painless and if the corporal bodies are aspirated the blood return is bright red and well oxygenated. To confirm the diagnosis, color Doppler ultrasound may identify the high-flow state and the site of arterial rupture. Another diagnostic test that may be performed is arteriography. The most common vessel that is lacerated is a branch of the cavernosal artery, and this may be clearly identified on the arteriogram. Generally around the lacerated area, within the corpora, there is a necrotic space and cavity that allows unrestricted arterial inflow into the cavernous spaces (McMahon 2002). The treatment options for nonischemic priapism range from watchful waiting to autologous clot embolization to open surgical ligation of the ruptured artery. Corporal irrigation with an alpha ago-

Table 16.2. Treatment of nonischemic priapism

Step	Nonischemic priapism, not emergency
1	Aspiration for diagnosis. Do *not* use sympathomimetics
2	Observation
3	Embolization
4	Surgery, aided by intraoperative Doppler ultrasound

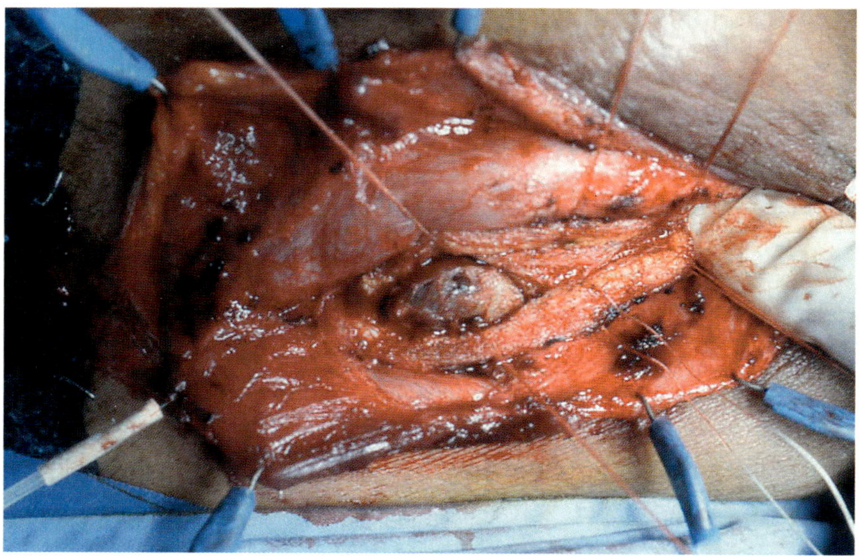

Fig. 16.6. In a case of open repair of traumatic nonischemic priapism, intracavernous pseudocyst filled with clot and a single bleeder was noted

nist is not recommended as a treatment option (Table 16.2).

It is important to note that these patients can be safely followed conservatively for several months, with the hope that the fistula will spontaneously close. In several studies, no permanent erectile dysfunction was noted (Brock et al. 1993; Bastuba et al. 1994).

In the early stages, ice packing or compression may cause sufficient vasospasm and thrombosis of the ruptured artery to effect closure of the fistula. However, in most cases closure does not spontaneously occur and selective angiographic embolization of the ruptured artery is the next step. Localization of the ruptured vessel may be accomplished by ultrasound guidance or an angiographic catheter (Ilkay and Levine 1995). Embolization may be done using one or a combination of Gelfoam, metallic coils, or autologous clot. In the unlikely scenario that the angiographic attempt fails, repeat embolization may be done or open surgical ligation of the ruptured artery may be attempted. Surgical ligation is only indicated in long-standing cases in which a well-formed pseudocapsule can be identified on ultrasound. Open surgery is performed through exploratory corporotomy to identify the pseudocapsule under ultrasound guidance followed by microsurgical closure of the ruptured artery (Hatzichristou et al. 2002; Fernandez et al. 2000).

16.9 Recurrent (Stuttering) Priapism

Stuttering or recurrent priapism is relatively common in patients with sickle cell trait or disease but may occur after an episode of priapism of any etiology (Adeyoju et al 2002; Zisman and Lindner 1993). Recurrent priapism has also been described in patients with nonischemic priapism (de Pablo et al. 1999). The exact mechanism resulting in stuttering priapism is unknown, although some hypothesize that there is an alteration of nerve terminals or receptors or scarring of intracavernous venules.

The goal of the management of recurrent (stuttering) priapism is prevention of future episodes, while management of each episode should follow the specific treatment recommendations for ischemic priapism (Table 16.3). Various therapies have been used to treat stuttering priapism, including oral alpha adrenergic medications (e.g., etilefrine 0.5 mg/kg/day) (Okpala et al. 2002). Other options for treatment include self-intracavernosal injection of an alpha adrenergic agent

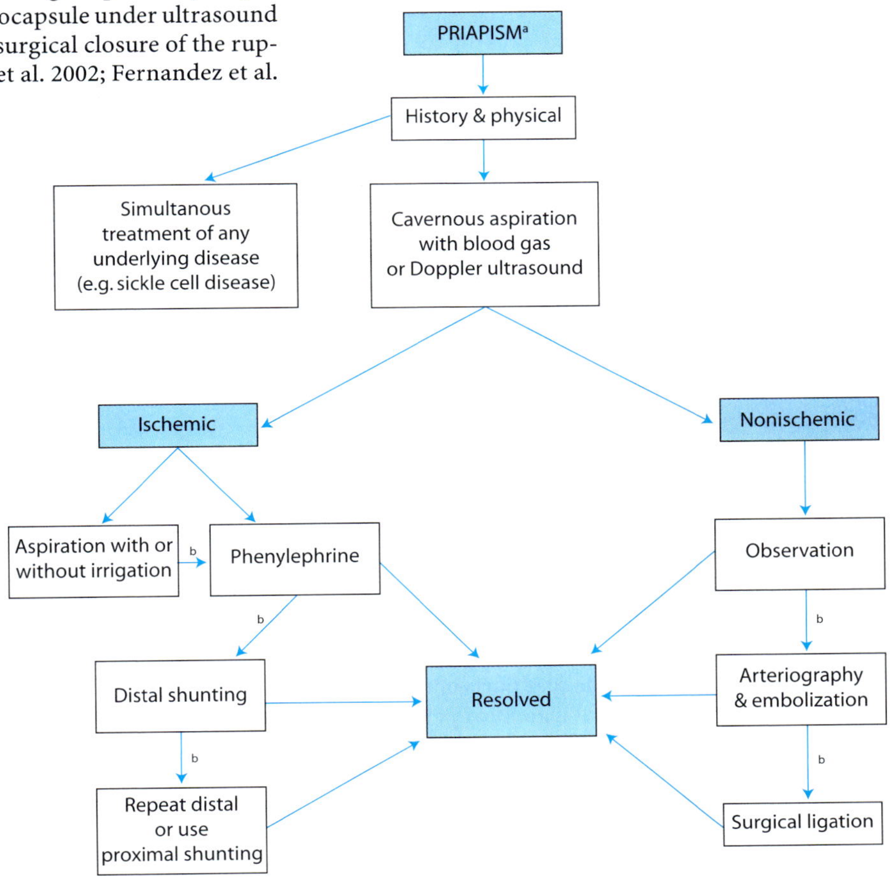

Fig. 16.7. Management algorithm for priapism

[a]Erection greater than 4h duration
[b]Proceed upon treatment failure

Table 16.3. Treatment of stuttering priapism

Step	Stuttering priapism
1	Treat each episode as ischemic priapism
2	Try to prevent future episodes
3	GnRH agonist or antiandrogen (but not in children)
4	Consider intracavernosal self-injection of phenylephrine

such as 500 mg phenylephrine every 5 min until detumescence (Steinberg and Eyre 1995). If the patient has no concerns regarding sexual function and the priapism episodes continue, then an antiandrogen or gonadotropin-releasing hormone agonist may be used (Dahm et al. 2002). These agents suppress nocturnal penile erection and can prevent recurrent episodes of priapism. Oral baclofen, an antispasticity medication, has also recently been shown to treat recurrent priapism (Rourke et al. 2002). It has been shown in patients with sickle cell anemia that red blood cell apheresis does not generally result in detumescence. Anecdotally, sildenafil has been noted to relieve recurrent episodes of priapism in patients with sickle cell disease. It is believed that selective vasodilation of the corporal blood vessels prevents sickling of red cells in the corporal bodies (Bialecki and Bridges 2002).

16.10 Mechanical Priapism

Uncommonly, men present with a variation of priapism resulting from placement of constricting objects over the penis, either excluding or including the scrotum. Patients often place the objects for either sexual enhancement (appearance or performance) or autoerotic stimulation, and use an imaginative variety of objects: rubber bands, metal rings, hammer-heads, barbells (Santucci et al. 2004), plastic bottles (Voegeli and Effert 2005), etc. Although insertion of the penis into the object may be easy, subsequent venous occlusion and lymphedema may prevent egress. Additionally, there have been many case reports and series of children with hair or other thin tourniquets; these may be difficult to identify and these cases may be mistaken for balanitis (Soliman et al. 2003). Morbidity may be considerable, with many reports of urethrocutaneous fistulae, partial or total glans or penile amputation (Soliman et al. 2003). Often, a combination of denial, embarrassment, and fear will cause a delay in presentation that allows aggravation of the edema. The variety of objects used does not lend itself to a straightforward treatment algorithm, and urologists have demonstrated tremendous resourcefulness in applying diverse technologies to these frustrating and challenging scenarios. Although nonmetallic thin objects may be cut off with relative ease, thick and/or hardened materials may be very difficult to cut with standard instruments. In general, four general strategies can be employed when faced with these situations: aspiration (Drachenberg et al. 1999), wrapping (Bucy 1968; Noh et al. 2004; Vahasarja et al. 1993), cutting/drilling (Kimber and Mellon 2004; Santucci et al. 2004), and surgery (Detweiler 2001). Unfortunately, it is difficult to determine the incidence of posttreatment complications in these patients, as they are often lost to follow-up.

16.11 Conclusion

In the evaluation of a pathologically erect penis, the most important initial decision is whether or not it represents a nonischemic or ischemic priapism. This is mainly discerned by history and physical examination, but additional studies such as ultrasonography may clarify or confirm clinical suspicions. If associated conditions are noted, such as hematologic disorders, it is important to address the underlying disorder but also to pursue treatment of the penis acutely. Ischemic priapism usually requires some type of invasive procedure, with treatments proceeding in a step-wise fashion from least to most invasive. Nonischemic priapism may be treated conservatively. When intervention is required, radiologic embolization is usually efficacious, and formal surgery is rarely required. The treatment of recurrent priapism is aimed at both the acute episode as well as prevention of future episodes. Future experience and research will hopefully lead to efficacious oral agents for the treatment of both acute and recurrent episodes of priapism.

Appendix Treatment of Priapism: When and How

Ischemic priapism:
When to treat – as soon as possible
How to treat
a) Evacuation of old blood
b) Injection of diluted phenylephrine 500 µg every 3–5 min
What if medical treatment failed?
a) Distal shunt with pressure monitoring
b) If failed, proximal shunt

Nonischemic priapism
When to treat – not urgent
How to treat – conservative, ice or pressure packing for weeks to months
What if conservative measures failed?

a) Embolization guided by angiography
b) Surgical ligation of ruptured artery

Stuttering priapism
When and how to treat – treat as ischemic priapism with diluted phenylephrine
How to prevent – antiandrogen, gonadotropin releasing hormone agonist, or baclofen

References

Adeyoju AB, Olujohunabe AG, Morris J et al (2002) Priapism in sickle-cell disease; incidence, risk factors and complications – an international multicentre study. BJU Int 90:898
Ahmed I, Shaikh NA (1997) Treatment of intermittent idiopathic priapism with oral terbutaline. Br J Urol 80:341
Altman AL, Seftel AD, Brown SL et al (1999) Cocaine associated priapism. J Urol 161:1817
Avisrror MU, Fernandez IA, Sanchez AS et al (2000) Doxazosin and priapism. J Urol 163:238
Baba H, Maezawa Y, Furusawa N et al (1995) Lumbar spinal stenosis causing intermittent priapism. Paraplegia 33:338
Barry JM (1976) Priapism: treatment with corpus cavernosum to dorsal vein of penis shunts. J Urol 116:754
Bastuba MD, Saenz de Tejada I, Dinlenc CZ et al (1994) Arterial priapism: diagnosis, treatment and long-term followup. J Urol 151:1231
Bechara A, Casabe A, Cheliz G et al (1997) Comparative study of papaverine plus phentolamine versus prostaglandin E1 in erectile dysfunction. J Urol 157:2132Benjelloun S, el Mrini M, Aboutaieb R et al (1993) Priapism. A propos of 10 cases (translation). J Urol (Paris) 99:91
Bialecki ES, Bridges KR (2002) Sildenafil relieves priapism in patients with sickle cell disease. Am J Med 113:252
Bochinski DJ, Dean RC, Lue TF (2004) Erectile dysfunction and priapism. Nat Clin Pract Urol 1:49
Brock G, Breza J, Lue TF et al (1993) High flow priapism: a spectrum of disease. J Urol 150:968
Bschleipfer TH, Hauck EW, Diemer TH et al (2001) Heparin-induced priapism. Int J Impot Res 13:357
Bucy JG (1968) Removal of strangulating objects from the penis. J Urol 99:194
Burnett AL, Allen RP, Tempany CM et al (1995) Evaluation of erectile function in men with sickle cell disease. Urology 45:657
Compton MT, Miller AH (2001) Priapism associated with conventional and atypical antipsychotic medications: a review. J Clin Psychiatry 62:362
Dahm P, Rao DS, Donatucci CF (2002) Antiandrogens in the treatment of priapism. Urology 59:138
De Pablo Cardenas A, Jimenez Calvo JM, Grasa Lanau V et al (1999) High-flow priapism in the pediatric age: review (translation). Arch Esp Urol 52:862
Detweiler MB (2001) Penile incarceration with metal objects–a review of procedure choice based on penile trauma grade. Scand J Urol Nephrol 35:212
Drachenberg D, Nguan C, Norman RW et al. (1999) Penile entrapment injury: a case report. Can J Urol 6:709
Earle CM, Stuckey BG, Ching HL et al (2003) The incidence and management of priapism in Western Australia: a 16 year audit. Int J Impot Res 15:272
Ekman P, Sjogren L, Englund G et al (2000) Optimizing the therapeutic approach of transurethral alprostadil. BJU Int 86:68
El-Bahnasawy MS, Dawood A, Farouk A (2002) Low-flow priapism: risk factors for erectile dysfunction. BJU Int 89:285
Fernandez Arancibia MI, Martinez Portillo FJ, Musial A et al (2000) Diagnosis and therapeutic options for prolonged erection and priapism: up-date review (translation). Arch Esp Urol 53:919
Francis RB Jr, Johnson CS (1991) Vascular occlusion in sickle cell disease: current concepts and unanswered questions. Blood 77:1405
Goldmeier D, Lamba H (2002) Drug points: prolonged erections produced by dihydrocodeine and sildenafil. BMJ 324: 1555
Govier FE, Jonsson E, Kramer-Levien DA (1994) Oral terbutaline for the treatment of priapism. J Urol 151:878
Hatzichristou D, Salpiggidis G, Hatzimouratidis K et al (2002) Management strategy for arterial priapism: therapeutic dilemmas. J Urol 168:2074
Hebuterne X, Frere AM, Bayle J et al (1992) Priapism in a patient treated with total parenteral nutrition. JPEN J Parenter Enteral Nutr 16:171
Ilkay AK, Levine LA (1995) Conservative management of high-flow priapism. Urology 46:419
Keoghane SR, Sullivan ME, Miller MA (2002) The aetiology, pathogenesis and management of priapism. BJU Int 90:149
Kimber RM, Mellon JK (2004) The role of special cutting equipment and corporeal aspiration in the treatment of penile incarceration with a barbell retaining collar. J Urol 172:975
King SH, Hallock M, Strote J et al (2005) Tadalafil-associated priapism. Urol 66:432
Kulmala R, Lehtonen T, Nieminen P et al (1995) Aetiology of priapism in 207 patients. Eur Urol 28:241
Kulmala RV, Lehtonen TA, Tammela TL (1996) Preservation of potency after treatment for priapism. Scan J Urol Nephrol 30:313
Kvarstein B (1996) Bladder cancer complicated with priapism. A case report. Scand J Urol Nephrol Suppl 179:155
Lehtonen T, Tenhunen A (1973) Treatment of idiopathic priapism by Grayhack's caverno-saphenous shunt. Scand J Urol Nephrol 7:233
Linet OI, Neff LL (1994) Intracavernous prostaglandin E1 in erectile dysfunction. Clin Investig 72:139
Linet OI, Ogrinc FG (1996) Efficacy and safety of intracavernosal alprostadil in men with erectile dysfunction. The Alprostadil Study Group. N Engl J Med 334:873
Lowe FC, Jarow JP (1993) Placebo-controlled study of oral terbutaline and pseudoephedrine in management of prostaglandin E1-induced prolonged erections. Urology 42:51
Marx FJ (1981) Therapy of priapism (translation). Urologe A 20:353
McMahon CG (2002) High flow priapism due to an arterial-lacunar fistula complicating initial veno-occlusive priapism. Int J Impot Res 14:195
Melman A, Serels S (2000) Priapism. Int J Impot Res Suppl 12:S133
Muruve N, Hosking DH (1996) Intracorporeal phenylephrine in the treatment of priapism. J Urol 155:141
Nelson JH 3rd, Winter CC (1977) Priapism: evolution of management in 48 patients in a 22-year series. J Urol 117:455
Nixon RG, O'Connor JL, Milam DF (2003) Efficacy of shunt surgery for refractory low flow priapism: a report on the incidence of failed detumescence and erectile dysfunction. J Urol 170:883
Noh J, Kang TW, Heo T et al (2004) Penile strangulation treated with the modified string method. Urology 64:591
Okpala I, Westerdale N, Jegede T et al (2002) Etilefrine for the prevention of priapism in adult sickle cell disease. Br J Haematol 118:918

Papadopoulos I, Kelami A (1988) Priapus and priapism. From mythology to medicine. Urology 32:385
Quigley M, Fawcett DP (1999) Thrombophilia and priapism. BJU Int 83:155
Quackels R (1964) Cure of patient suffering from priapism by cavernospongiosal anastomosis. Acta Urol Belg 32:5
Rourke KF, Fischler AH, Jordan GH (2002) Treatment of recurrent idiopathic priapism with oral baclofen. J Urol 168:2552
Sadeghi-Nejad H, Seftel AD (2002) The etiology, diagnosis, and treatment of priapism: review of the American Foundation for Urologic Disease Consensus Panel report. Curr Urol Rep 3:492
Santucci RA, Deng D, Carney J (2004) Removal of metal penile foreign body with a widely available emergency-medical-services-provided air-driven grinder. Urology 63:1183
Schroeder-Printzen I, Vosshenrich R, Weidner R et al (1994) Malignant priapism in a patient with metastatic prostate adenocarcinoma. Urol Int 52:52
Secil M, Arslan D, Goktay AY et al (2001) The prediction of papaverine induced priapism by color Doppler sonography. J Urol 165:416
Shantha TR, Finnerty DP, Rodriquez AP (1989) Treatment of persistent penile erection and priapism using terbutaline. J Urol 141:1427
Soliman SM, Hafie E, Hassan TA et al (2003) Hair coil induced penile tourniquet injury. Saudi Med J 24:S55
Spycher MA, Hauri D (1986) The ultrastructure of the erectile tissue in priapism. J Urol 135:142
Steinberg J, Eyre RC (1995) Management of recurrent priapism with epinephrine self-injection and gonadotropin-releasing hormone analogue. J Urol 153:152
Sur RL, Kane CJ (2000) Sildenafil citrate-associated priapism. Urology 55:950
Vahasarja VJ, Hellstrom PA, Serlo W et al (1993) Treatment of penile incarceration by the string method: 2 case reports. J Urol 149:372
Voegeli TA, Effert PJ (2005) Pentaethylene-terephthalate (PET) bottles: a new device for autoerotic strangulation of the penis causing serious injury. Arch Sex Behav 34:469
Witt MA, Goldstein I, Saenz de Tejada I et al (1990) Traumatic laceration of intracavernosal arteries: the pathophysiology of non-ischemic, high flow, arterial priapism. J Urol 143:129
Zargooshi J (2000) Priapism as a complication of high dose testosterone therapy in a man with hypogonadism. J Urol 163:907
Zisman A, Lindner A (1993) Recurrent intermittent priapism following priapism (translation). Harefuah 125:85
Zorgniotti AW, Lefleur RS (1985) Auto-injection of the corpus cavernosum with a vasoactive drug combination for vasculogenic impotence. J Urol 133:39

Management of Intraoperative Complications in Open Procedures 17.1

G.H. Yoon, J. Stein, D.G. Skinner

17.1.1 Introduction

Attention to surgical details and a commitment to surgical excellence are two fundamental principles that will help provide the best clinical and functional results following open surgical procedures. Most postoperative complications can be clinically related or traced back to technical errors made in the operating room. Thus, the importance of avoiding or reducing intraoperative surgical complications cannot be overemphasized.

Effective management of intraoperative complications in open surgical procedures begins with the avoidance and prevention of dreaded surgical misadventures. A surgical plan must be devised even before an incision is made. The urologic surgeon must be prepared for any potential changes in plan or alternatives that he may encounter during the course of operating. This preparation often times is derived from personal as well as collective experiences in previous clinical practice where lessons are sometimes best learned from mistakes. In this day and age, when modern urology is shifting toward minimally invasive techniques, there remains a need and requirement for maximally invasive surgery to address specific urologic diseases, especially in urologic oncology and reconstructive surgery. This chapter will describe a philosophical approach and management of specific intraoperative complications that the authors have encountered during open urologic procedures. It is emphasized that the best surgical offense starts with good defense.

Prior to entering the operating room, the urologic surgeon must prepare by mentally reviewing four general principles. Firstly, all necessary imaging studies should be obtained preoperatively to completely delineate the disease process, its extent, and its relation to adjacent organs and structures. This provides a working knowledge of the lay of the land, so to speak, such that few or no surprises are encountered. Radiographic imaging techniques have clearly improved over the past decades and provide the surgeon a road map from an anatomical perspective. Proper imaging preoperatively will reduce the potential for surgical misadventures, identify the anatomy and anomalous structures, as well as help identify the so-called pathology of interest. Preoperative imaging studies may also direct the need for consultations with other surgical specialties as deemed necessary.

Secondly, based on the region of the body involved, total familiarity with and understanding of the basic anatomy and the relations between organs, vessels, bones, and tissue planes are an absolute requirement. This becomes exceedingly important in reoperative surgery and even more so in the irradiated patient where complication rates escalate due to the disruption of normal anatomy. This includes intraabdominal, retroperitoneal, and pelvic anatomy (Touma et al. 2005; Crawford and Skinner 1980).

Thirdly, the most appropriate surgical approach and incisions must be determined in order to provide the necessary operative exposure. In cases of large retroperitoneal masses arising from renal, adrenal, or germ cell tumors, the great vessels and their many branches as well as intestinal segments such as the duodenum may be intimately apposed or involved. Proper exposure is mandatory as normal anatomical relationships may become unrecognizably distorted. Surgeons should utilize a proper incision from a repertoire that is familiar and comfortable. An incision may be extended in situations where poor exposure may limit an appropriate dissection or inhibit the surgeon's ability to operate. Thus, the patient should be properly positioned, prepped, and draped at the start. A general surgical rule is that big cases require big incisions. In addition, the surgical approach and incision provide the operative exposure, which is fundamental in performing the safest surgical procedure.

Lastly, many operative complications can be avoided by simply performing the operation exactly the same way every single time. A routine that is employed each time an operation is performed minimizes the opportunity for mistakes to be made. This approach also increases surgical efficiency as assistants and scrub technicians can anticipate the next operative maneuver.

17.1.2 Vascular Complications

17.1.2.1 General Principles

No other operative mishap is more stressful or feared than a major vascular injury. The surgical management of a number of urologic diseases requires close dissection along major arterial and venous vessels, branches, and networks. In the event of a vascular injury, it is essential that the surgeon remain calm and direct the surgical staff in preparation for control of the injury. Constant communication with the anesthesiology staff should be maintained. A momentary pause may be required of the surgeon as the anesthesiologist prepares for possible rapid and large-volume blood loss. In anticipation of possible rapid volume resuscitation, adequate venous access, with large-bore peripheral venous catheters or central venous catheters, should be obtained by the anesthesiologist prior to surgery. Additional suction tubing and surgical assistants may be necessary to provide a clean working field and additional hands for retraction. Large masses may obstruct vision within the operative field and/or may have large parasitizing vessels themselves that are susceptible to injury. It is prudent and maybe necessary to proceed with first extirpating large tumors while temporarily controlling hemorrhage with manual pressure. After removing the mass and surgical vision is improved, the vascular injury may be more safely and efficiently repaired.

Lymphadenectomy in the treatment of testicular, renal, bladder, and prostatic cancers often requires close dissection along major vessels. It is imperative that subadventitial dissecting planes be avoided, as this weakens the integrity of vessel walls and may lead to rupture. This is especially the case when performing a postchemotherapy retroperitoneal lymph node dissection. A thick and adherent layer of tissue encases the great vessels. In the case of the aorta, the surgeon may inadvertently enter a subadventitial plane and continue dissection before realizing the mistake. This will result in a large surface area of the aortic wall becoming significantly compromised and eventually rupturing. These consequences underscore the important principle of proximal and distal vascular control.

As may be the case in elderly patients with bladder or renal tumors, associated co-morbidities such as peripheral vascular disease and atherosclerosis may result in arteries that are calcified and brittle with intimal plaques. Overhandling these vessels both manually and with instruments may result in plaque embolization or even rupture. Vessels should be palpated for firmness or brittleness prior to placement of vascular clamps. Severe tortuosity of vessels often indicates significant vascular disease.

In anticipation of extensive vascular dissection, the proper instruments, including sutures, forceps, needle holders, and vascular clamps, should be readily available on the sterile field. Nonabsorbable suture such as cardiovascular silk or monofilament polypropylene (Prolene) on a fine vascular needle should be utilized on vessel walls. The choice in suture material is mostly determined by surgeon preference; however, distinct advantages between silk and Prolene exist. Silk is generally easier to handle and tie. Prolene is thought to induce less of an inflammatory response and be less likely to harbor infection. Vascular forceps with fine serrations or interdigitating teeth allow delicate handling of vessel walls. Fine vascular needle holders with diamond jaws allow for precise handling of suture without damaging or distorting the needle.

A variety of different vascular clamps are a vital set of instruments that the urologist must be familiar with. Application of these clamps is best performed in a controlled setting with proximal and distal control of the vessels, a fundamental principle of vascular surgery. Often times dissection of difficult tissue planes or adherent tumors may involve major vessels. Obtaining proximal and distal control of vessels prior to inadvertent injury allows for rapid control of hemorrhage as the operative field is cleared and the injury is addressed. Vascular control may also be obtained using Rummel tourniquets fashioned from red Robinson catheters and moist umbilical tape (Fig. 17.1.1).

Topical hemostatic agents such as oxidized regenerative cellulose (Surgicel), absorbable gelatin sponge (Gelfoam), and microfibrillar collagen (Avitene) are adjunctive agents of hemostasis used in all specialties of surgery, including urology. Newer agents such as NuKnit (Ethicon, Johnson & Johnson, Cincinnati, OH, USA), FloSeal (Baxter, Deerfield, IL, USA), and Tisseel (Baxter) are variations of the original theme with different delivery mechanisms. It should be noted that these agents are supplemental tools of hemostasis and do not substitute for traditional surgical techniques of vessel ligation or suturing to control bleeding. Brisk arterial bleeding must be dealt with in a surgical manner.

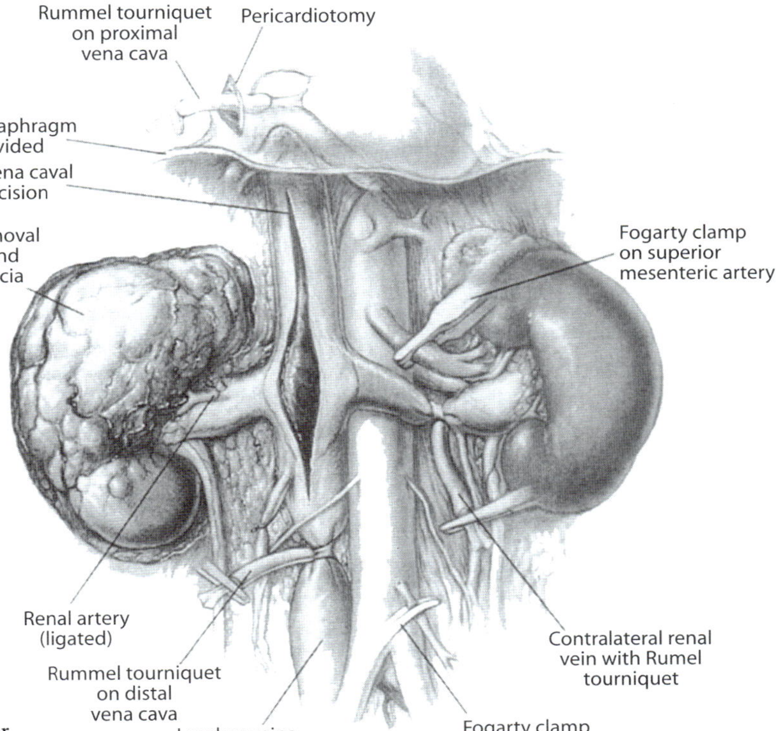

Fig. 17.1.1. Radical nephrectomy with tumor thrombectomy demonstrating proximal and distal vascular control

Topical agents are best used in areas of broad venous oozing or areas that are not easily accessible.

Nu-Knit is a denser-weave version of Surgicel manufactured from regenerated cellulose that is oxidized and woven into gauze-like strips. An advantage of Nu-Knit over Surgicel is its tensile strength, allowing it to be sutured into position or wrapped around structures. It can also cover a broader area of brisk oozing and does not disintegrate immediately during surgery. It is fully absorbed by the body within 14 days. Similar to Surgicel, Nu-Knit has bactericidal effects due to the low pH of its activated form. Both Nu-Knit and Surgicel are most effective when applied to a relatively dry field and held in place with a dry sponge for 5–10 min. Neither will induce a significant foreign body reaction when left in place.

FloSeal is a hemostatic agent in slurry form that must be prepared prior to use. It is a combination of specially engineered collagen-derived particles and topical thrombin. The collagen particles serve as a matrix or lattice in which the thrombin can act to convert fibrinogen into fibrin polymer. This in turn forms a local clot providing hemostasis. FloSeal's advantage over Surgicel or Nu-Knit is its ability to effectively cover an irregular bleeding surface and to fill in defects. Preparation time, advertised as 2 min by the manufacturer, is a disadvantage (Richter et al. 2003).

Tisseel is a versatile agent used for hemostasis and wound healing. It also must be prepared for use and is delivered in liquid form via a double-barreled syringe. It is essentially a fibrin glue formed by the mixture of a highly concentrated fibrinogen aprotinin solution containing factor XIII with a solution of thrombin and calcium chloride. Upon mixing and contact with blood and tissue, a resilient coagulum is formed, providing both rapid hemostasis as well as an adherent tissue bond. Preparation time is longer (10–15 min) and is more labor-intensive, which can delay its availability. Some centers have used Tisseel during repair of collecting system injuries or defects such as in partial nephrectomies with some success (Pruthi et al. 2004).

17.1.2.2 Arterial Injuries

In the event of a major arterial injury there should be no hesitation on the part of the operating urologist to consult a vascular surgeon for assistance if necessary. Injuries can be avoided by keeping in mind the fairly constant branching and orientation of the arterial system and anticipating the take-off of distal arteries. Simpler injuries can often be adequately repaired using standard techniques without intraoperative vascular consultation. Basic principles of vascular repair include maintenance of normal flow and direction with reapproximation and continuity of the intimal layer (Donohue 1989). Through the course of a vascular repair, reduction in luminal surface area must be avoided as well as creation of turbulence from either irregular intimal surfaces or acute changes in direction of blood flow. These technical errors may result in vessel thrombosis. Local heparinized saline flushes in the distal segments of injured vessels may be required if blood flow remains interrupted for an extended period of time while a repair is completed.

Injuries to the abdominal aorta may occur in retroperitoneal surgeries, including retroperitoneal lymph node dissection (RPLND) in the management of testicular germ cell tumors, radical nephrectomy, and resection of primary retroperitoneal tumors. In the event of an aortic wall injury or laceration, the first step in management should focus on proximal and distal vascular control, if possible. In most instances, this should already be established as the operation is set up. Manual pressure or placement of an Allis clamp (for smaller injuries) may be necessary to gain initial control and to assess the extent of injury. A 4-0 or 5-0 nonabsorbable suture should be utilized in repairing the wall injury either in a simple figure-of-8 fashion if possible or a continuous suture. Care must be taken to avoid narrowing the lumen. Occasionally, proper closure of the vessel injury may require the use of Teflon pledgets, which will add additional support to the repair.

In certain cases, the primary tumor may be so intimately attached to the aorta or directly involving the aorta that it is more prudent to resect and replace the damaged or involved segment with a vascular Dacron graft. Ideally, there should be a substantial infrarenal aortic cuff to which a graft may be sewn. An anastomosis can be established using a continuous nonabsorbable suture. Depending on distal involvement, an aortic interposition graft or a bifurcated aortoiliac graft may be utilized. Distal vessel heparinization should be used until revascularization is established. In practice, replacement of a segment of the aorta with a synthetic graft should be performed in conjunction with a vascular surgery consultation.

Injury to the superior mesenteric artery is potentially a devastating and life-threatening complication if unrecognized at surgery. This is especially the case during dissection of the renal arteries and left renal vein while performing a nephrectomy. Anatomical awareness of this vessel and avoidance of injury is paramount. As a point of reference when operating along the great vessels, identification of the left renal vein provides a reliable anatomical landmark to identify other important structures. Knowledge of the location of the left renal vein allows consistent identification of the superior mesenteric artery and both renal arteries and avoidance of injury. The surgeon must also be cognizant, however, of possible variations in renal vein and vena caval anatomy (Hoeltl et al. 1990) (Fig. 17.1.2). Furthermore, preoperative radiographic imaging with specific attention to retroaortic renal veins is also helpful to avoid SMA injury at the time of surgery. When an injury to the superior mesenteric artery is recognized, immediate revascularization should be performed by a vascular surgeon.

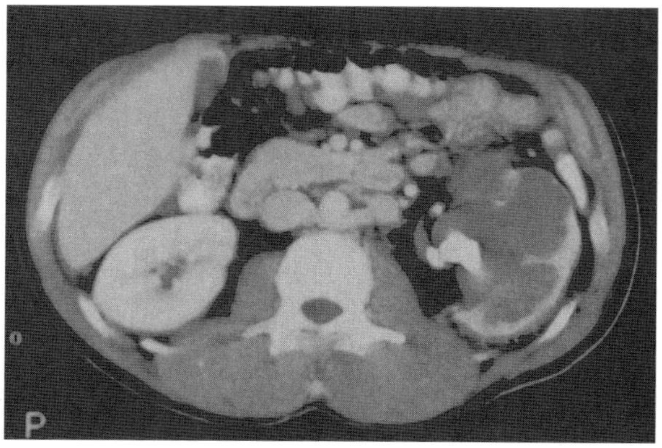

Fig. 17.1.2. Example of retroaortic left renal vein in patient with xanthogranulomatous pyelonephritis

Injury to the inferior mesenteric artery is easily avoidable given its location and ease of identification. It is, however, often involved with lymph node disease or tumor infiltration, necessitating ligation and division. In younger patients, collateral circulation is typically uncompromised and ligation may be performed without untoward effects. In the older patient population, it is prudent to palpate the vascular supply from marginal and rectal vessels when contemplating possible ligation. Careful dissection and preservation of this vessel may prove to be worthwhile in patients with compromised blood supply, preventing ischemic injury to the colonic mucosa.

Injury to the iliac vessels may result from pelvic lymphadenectomy but can be avoided when employing careful and systematic techniques of dissection (Stein and Skinner 2004). An injury to the iliac artery should be primarily repaired in similar fashion to an aortic wall injury incorporating the principals of proximal and distal control. Given the smaller caliber of the iliac vessels, greater attention must be given to avoid reduction of vessel lumen and formation of turbulent flow. If necessary, an autologous vein or Goretex patch may be utilized. Simple ligation should be avoided when possible, especially for injuries of the external iliac branches. The internal iliac (hypogastric) branches may be ligated if repair is not feasible. If possible, preservation of the superior gluteal artery (branch of posterior division of hypogastric artery) should be maintained to prevent development of gluteal claudication (Killion 1989).

Lumbar arteries below the level of the renal pedicle can be systematically ligated during a unilateral template or bilateral RPLND (Yoon et al. 2005). This facilitates the lymph node dissection while also preventing accidental avulsion of the vessels. These branches can be safely ligated below the renal arteries without devascularizing the spinal cord. The feeding arteries to the spinal cord are the longitudinal anterior and posterior spinal arteries, which arise from the vertebral arteries. In the lower thoracic and lumbar regions, the arteria radicularis magna (artery of Adamkiewicz) is the main lower anterior radicular artery and provides collateral blood supply to the anterior spinal artery and allows the lumbar arteries (below the renal arteries) to be ligated without consequence (Smith and Skinner 1976). Preemptive ligation and division of the posterior lumbar vessels can also provide needed mobilization of the great vessels when establishing proximal and distal vascular control. Isolation and pedicalization of the lumbar vessels can be performed using a relatively fine but blunt-tipped right angle clamp. In general, injury to the lumbar arteries can be easily controlled with an Allis clamp and suture ligated without significant detrimental effect.

17.1.2.3 Venous Injuries

In comparison to the arterial system, the venous system follows a less constant pattern of branching, especially in the distal vessels. The venous system is a low-pressure system and is palpably pulseless. In addition, the venous walls are much thinner, lacking the strong muscular fibers seen in arteries. These factors collectively contribute to the higher rate of venous injuries encountered in open surgical procedures. To its advantage, the venous system collateralizes to a greater extent and ligation of injured veins can be safely performed more often to control hemorrhage.

In most situations, the urologist can repair an injury to the vena cava safely and properly. Again, the basic anatomy of venous branches and tributaries along the vena cava must be kept in mind during dissection along its length. In rare cases, preoperative imaging may reveal the presence of a left-sided vena cava, in which case the surgeon should anticipate altered anatomy (Figs. 17.1.3, 17.1.4). Laceration of the caval wall can be addressed in multiple manners. Proximal and distal control can be obtained by manual compression with the operator or assistant's fingers. A gauze sponge on the end of a long-handled clamp may be used for compression. Prior to anticipated vessel injury, proximal and distal control may be obtained by placement of vascular clamps or Rummel tourniquets. In situations where conventional vascular control is unobtainable and there is an injury to a vein or the vena cava with massive hemorrhage, a balloon catheter may be used to temporarily occlude blood flow. The catheter is placed through the open ends of the vessel and inflated, allowing surgical vision and planning. Serrated vascular clamps as opposed to clamps with interdigitating teeth should be used. A C-clamp may also be used to isolate the wall injury or defect without occluding total venous flow. Likewise, an Allis clamp may be utilized on smaller injuries. Once control of bleeding is obtained, a 5-0 or 6-0 monofilament nonabsorbable suture (Prolene) or cardiovascular silk is used to oversew the area of vascular injury.

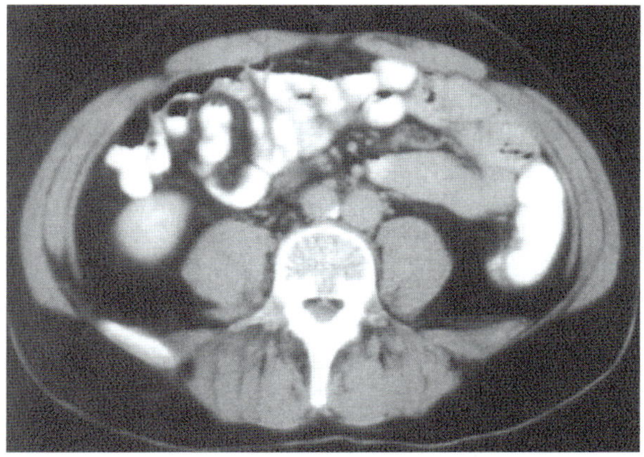

Fig. 17.1.3. Example of left-sided vena cava with abdominal aorta identified by the presence of calcifications

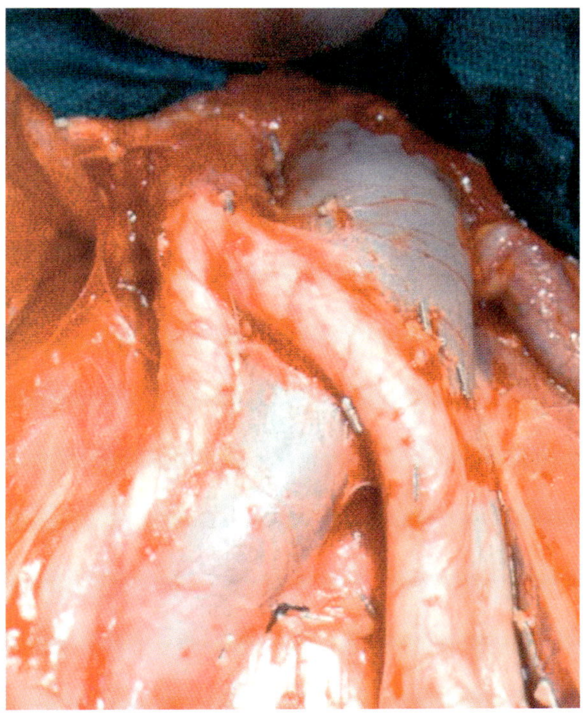

Fig. 17.1.4. Intraoperative photo of the same patient as in Fig. 17.1.3 demonstrating a left-sided vena cava

On occasion, resection of the infrarenal vena cava may be necessary in the setting of a large germ cell tumor in the retroperitoneum, especially following preoperative chemotherapy (Ahlering and Skinner 1989). Proximal and vascular control must first be established and preservation of both common iliac veins is important to avoid postoperative lower-extremity lymphedema. In patients with long-term obstruction of the vena cava, collateral circulation may be well developed; however, in situations where this is not apparent, the vena cava may be best replaced with an interposition polytetrafluoroethylene vascular ring graft. Again, the importance of careful examination of all preoperative imaging studies cannot be over emphasized in order to anticipate such reconstruction needs.

Lumbar veins can be a source of troublesome and significant bleeding if inadvertently avulsed or injured. Complete avulsion may result in retraction of a bleeding vessel into the foramina of the vertebral body. It is nearly impossible to identify and isolate the vessel's edges to control bleeding. An Allis clamp may be used to occlude surrounding tissue so that a vascular suture may be placed. A 2-0 silk or Vicryl suture in a figure-of-8 fashion, which incorporates vertebral periosteum or the aponeurosis of the psoas muscle, should effectively control hemorrhage. Also, sterile bone tacks inserted directly into the periosteum in areas of troublesome bleeding can provide hemostasis. These tacks may be enforced with bone wax as well. To avoid this complication, we routinely ligate and divide the lumbar vessels inferior to the renal vessels when performing a retroperitoneal lymph node dissection. This maneuver allows mobility of the great vessels and facilitates removal of all lymphatic tissue overlying the vertebral column. A right angle clamp with relatively fine tips is useful in pedicalizing the lumbar vessels for ligation. It should be noted that a left-sided posterior ascending lumbar vessel reliably drains into the left renal vein and should be prospectively identified to avoid accidental injury.

The deep dorsal vein complex can be a tenacious source of hemorrhage while performing a radical retropubic prostatectomy or radical cystoprostatectomy. Effective control of the dorsal vein complex can significantly limit blood loss and greatly improve surgical vision in the pelvis. Various techniques to prospectively control the complex are described and detailed elsewhere (Quek et al. 2001). Effective control of the dorsal venous complex begins with proper and adequate exposure of the apex of the prostate. We prospectively identify, ligate, and divide the superficial dorsal vein first. With firm tension on the prostate posteriorly, the puboprostatic ligaments are identified and sharply divided lateral to the dorsal complex just enough to expose the apex of the prostate. The dorsal venous complex can then be controlled either with a right-angle clamp passed around the complex or with an Allis clamp that is used to gather the complex (Figs. 17.1.5, 17.1.6). With the complex controlled, a suture ligature may then be secured.

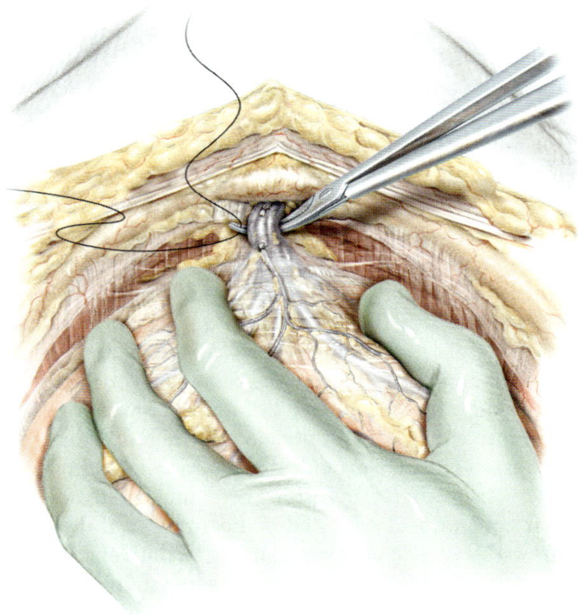

Fig. 17.1.5. Clamp placed between dorsal venous complex and urethra (© Hohenfellner 2007)

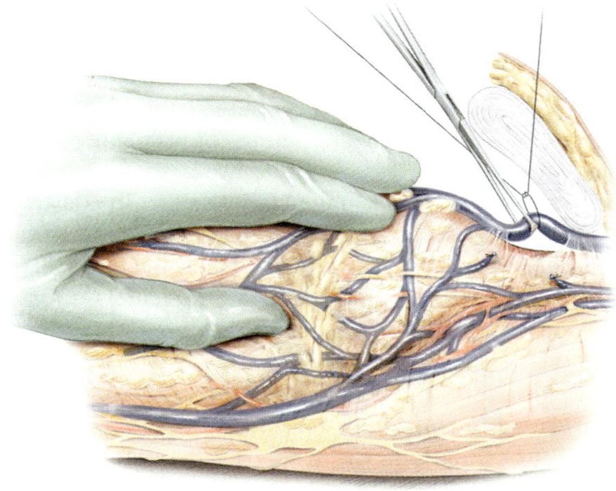

Fig. 17.1.6. Allis clamp used to gather dorsal venous complex (© Hohenfellner 2007)

Occasionally, control of the dorsal venous complex may be lost as a result of dislodgement of a suture. When persistent bleeding occurs from the complex, vascular control may be obtained with suture ligation. This requires proper assistance with constant suction of blood and retraction of pelvic organs posteriorly and cephalad. The leaflets of the complex are usually visible for suture ligation in figure-of-8 fashion. If visualization of the complex is difficult secondary to retraction into the deep pelvis and if patient positioning permits, pressure applied on the perineal body with a spongestick may push the complex into view. When bleeding persists, a large-caliber urinary catheter with a large balloon may be inserted and inflated with 20–30 ml of fluid and placed on temporary traction.

17.1.3 Intestinal Complications

17.1.3.1 Bowel Injury

Reoperative surgery and surgery in irradiated patients can be technically challenging endeavors fraught with potential complications, intestinal injuries being the most common. Extensive intraabdominal and intrapelvic adhesions often require tedious and meticulous lysis of adhesions prior to initiation of the primary operative procedure. This frequently results in a maze of intestinal loops that must be completely sorted out. The surgeon will find that by taking the necessary time initially to release adhesions, the remainder of the operation should proceed with greater ease and less opportunity for injuries. Often times, the surgeon will find that tissue planes will present themselves with a combination of blunt and sharp dissection as the tissue is three-dimensionalized. Again, we emphasize the principle of actively preventing injuries and setting up the operation for success.

Enterotomies may be easily created but often poorly recognized. When bowel injury is noted, immediate repair is most prudent; however, a marking stitch may be placed for later repair. With small rents, a simple inverting or figure-of-8 suture may be sufficient. For more extensive injuries, a short segment of intestine may be discarded with primary anastomosis. The authors prefer a hand-sewn technique using interrupted silk sutures in two layers.

Injury to the second or third portion of the duodenum may occur during a radical nephrectomy, especially on the right. This can be prevented by adequate and careful mobilization of the small bowel mesentery in a cephalad direction starting at the region of the right lower quadrant with careful identification of the retroperitoneal portions of the duodenum. The Kocher maneuver can also be utilized to reflect the duodenum medially and away from the operative field. On the left side, this maneuver will allow careful reflection of the pancreas, thus avoiding injury. Retracting instruments and moist sponges should be utilized to reflect the duodenum and other intestinal loops. Forceful retraction should obviously be avoided to prevent bowel wall injury. In cases of duodenal injury with violation of the bowel wall, careful inspection of the wall edges with sharp debridement of nonviable tissues is necessary prior to repair. A two-layer closure with silk sutures in a transverse fashion should be performed to avoid narrowing of the lumen. An omental patch on the area of duodenal injury provides added security to reduce opportunities for leak. Postoperative gastric decompression with delayed enteral feeding is vital for proper healing. The authors prefer to place a gastrostomy tube when possible for patient comfort, which is detailed elsewhere (Buscarini et al. 2000).

Rectal injuries may occur in the setting of radical prostatectomy or cystoprostatectomy, with increased incidences in those receiving previous definitive radiation (Stephenson et al. 2004). The technique of radical retropubic prostatectomy has been refined over the last two decades based on important anatomical studies detailed by Walsh and Donker (1982). Today, this procedure remains a standard therapeutic option in the treatment of prostatic tumors, affording excellent cancer control with maintenance of sexual function and urinary continence. Rectal injuries are an important potential complication, although they are extremely rare in nonoperated, nonirradiated patients with low-stage disease. An important consideration during a nerve-sparing radical prostatectomy is the entrance into a proper plane of dissection along the lateral prostatic surface. Magnification loupes can aid in the visualization of this plane. Additionally, proper control of the dorsal venous complex and its superficial branch prior to the delicate dissection of the neurovascular bundles will help maintain a relatively bloodless operative field and optimize surgeon vision. Once the lateral pelvic fascia is identified and incised, gentle blunt dissection alternating with sharp dissection will successfully isolate the bundle laterally and allow the posterior surface of the prostate to be freed up (Stein et al. 2001) (Fig. 17.1.7).

The posterior plane between the rectum with the perirectal fat and the posterior surface of the prostate with the leaflets of Denonvilliers fascia can be bluntly dissected when there has been no previous radiation. If this dissection does not occur easily additional force and traction should be avoided, as the correct plane may not be identified and injury to the rectal wall is possible. Following apical dissection of the prostate and transection of the urethra with placement of vesicourethral anastomosis sutures, the rectourethralis fibers and lateral pillars of the prostate are encountered. These attachments should be carefully incised sharply as the apex of the prostate is gently retracted anteriorly and cranially. This maneuver should allow entry into the perirectal fat space previously identified during the lateral dissection.

In patients who have undergone definitive primary radiation therapy for the treatment of prostatic adenocarcinoma or other pelvic malignancies, the normal

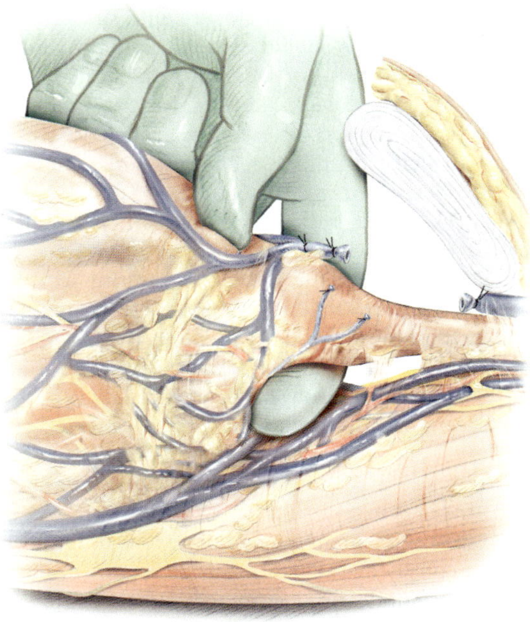

Fig. 17.1.7. Incision of lateral prostatic fascia with blunt dissection along prostatic surface with entry to correct plane posteriorly (Fig. 17.1.7 and 8 © Hohenfellner 2007)

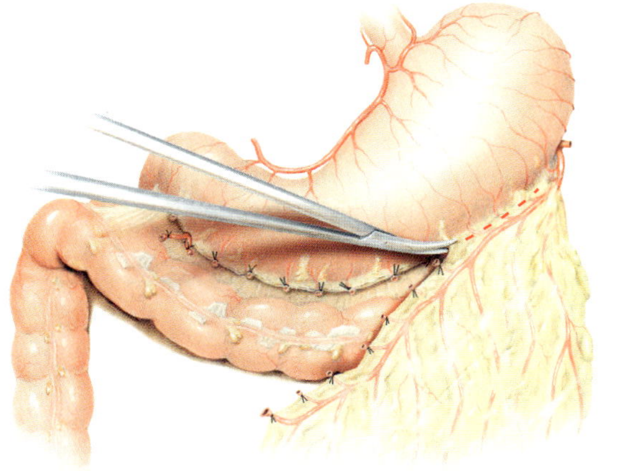

Fig. 17.1.8. Omental pedicle mobilized on left gastroepiploic artery with ligation and division of short gastric arteries

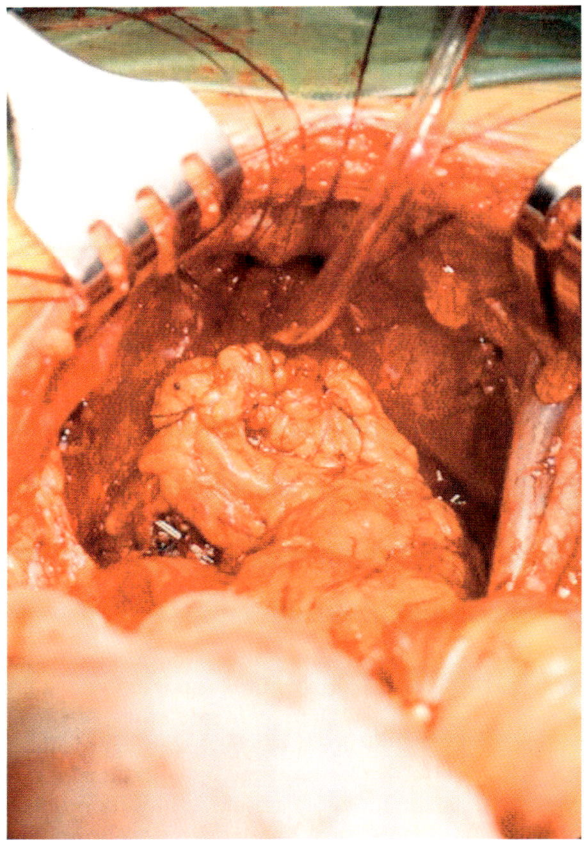

Fig. 17.1.9. Omental pedicle based on left gastroepiploic artery reaches deep pelvis with ease

planes of dissection are often obliterated and indiscernible. A preoperative mechanical bowel prep and enema is prudent in anticipation of possible rectal injury. The technique of radical prostatectomy is not significantly different but greater care must be observed in dissecting the periprostatic planes. Early ligation and division of the dorsal venous complex followed by division of the urethra allows the surgeon to reflect the prostate anteriorly and to visualize the prostate–rectal plane. This plane should be dissected sharply more so than bluntly. In the event of a rectal injury, primary repair and closure (in multiple layers) should be undertaken immediately once the prostate gland is removed. Careful inspection of the rectal wall edges should guide the need for debridement prior to closure. Closure should be performed in a transverse fashion. The closure should be performed in two layers with careful reapproximation of mucosal and seromuscular edges using interrupted 3-0 silk sutures. Alternatively, the closure may be performed in a continuous fashion. If obvious fecal spillage is noted the area should be copiously irrigated and a diverting colostomy should be seriously considered. A diverting colostomy is imperative in patients previously irradiated for prostate cancer resulting from poor healing of tissues. An omental flap interposition may also be necessary in cases of larger injuries or significant fecal contamination. It is our experience that an omental flap based off the left gastroepiploic artery has greater mobility and reach into the deep pelvis (Figs. 17.1.8, 17.1.9).

Suction drains should be considered in cases of fecal spillage with additional postoperative antibiotics to cover Gram-negative and anaerobic organisms. Following completion of the operation, digital dilation of the anal sphincter while the patient remains anesthetized may further serve to protect the repair.

The authors' preferred technique of performing a diverting ileostomy is to use the Turnbull loop method. We utilize this routinely in the creation of ileal conduits, as it provides superior fit for skin appliances and maintains better vascularity to the stoma to help prevent future stomal stenosis. Preoperative preparation for patients undergoing any stoma creation should focus on proper location. The stoma should be located away from bony prominences, skin creases, scars, and areas of chronic skin irritation. It should also be positioned so that an external appliance may be properly seated.

After a suitable segment of bowel is identified and adequately mobilized for creation of the stoma, a circular skin disk is excised by using the butt end of a 20-ml syringe plunger as a template. Underlying subcutaneous fat is incised and retracted using narrow retractors to expose the anterior rectus sheath. Excision of fat from the subcutaneous layer should be routinely avoided, as this may cause retraction of the stoma. The anterior rectus sheath is incised longitudinally over the belly of the rectus abdominus muscle approximately 2–3 cm in length. The muscle is split along the fibers using curved Mayo scissors and the underlying transversalis fascia and peritoneum are incised. A proper opening should accommodate two fingers and avoid injury to the inferior epigastric vessels. The anterior rectus sheath can also be opened transversely for a short distance to create a cruciate. Four 2-0 Vicryl sutures are preplaced in the fascial corners, which will later be placed in the seromuscular layer of the loop.

A narrow Penrose drain is placed through the mesentery at the most mobile location of the ileal loop and the loop is drawn through the opening. The knuckle of bowel should protrude 3–4 cm above the skin level and be secured in place with the preplaced fascial sutures. When properly oriented, the proximal aspect should be cephalad. If necessary, a stoma rod, red Robinson catheter, or Penrose drain may be used to support the loop while the stoma is everted and matured (Fig. 17.1.10). An incision is created along the seromuscular surface on the distal, defunctionalized aspect of the loop at the skin layer approximately four-fifths of the way across. Three 3-0 Vicryl sutures are placed in the subdermal layer on the cephalad aspect of the stoma opening and then passed through the corresponding seromuscular layer and the enterostomy edge of the proximal loop (Fig. 17.1.11). One 3-0 Vicryl suture is placed in the subdermal layer on the caudal aspect and then passed through the enterostomy edge of the distal loop. An Allis clamp is placed into the lumen of the bowel and the mucosa is grasped on the anterior luminal surface. A second clamp is placed on the edge of the enterostomy and the inner clamp is pulled out as the outer clamp is used to evert the bowel edge (Fig. 17.1.12). Once everted, the nipple stoma is matured using a series of inter-

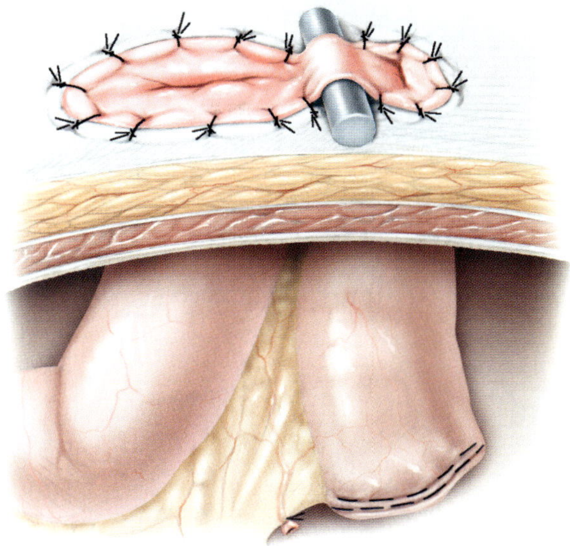

Fig. 17.1.10. Stoma rod used to support loop stoma (Fig. 17.1.10–12 © Hohenfellner 2007)

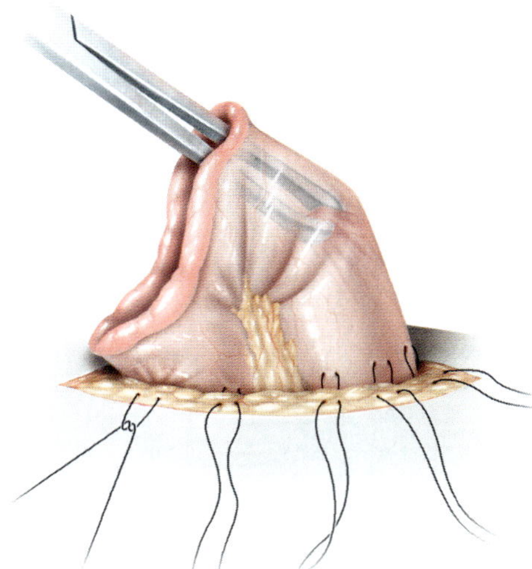

Fig. 17.1.11. Loop ileostomy with Allis clamp grasping inner mucosa

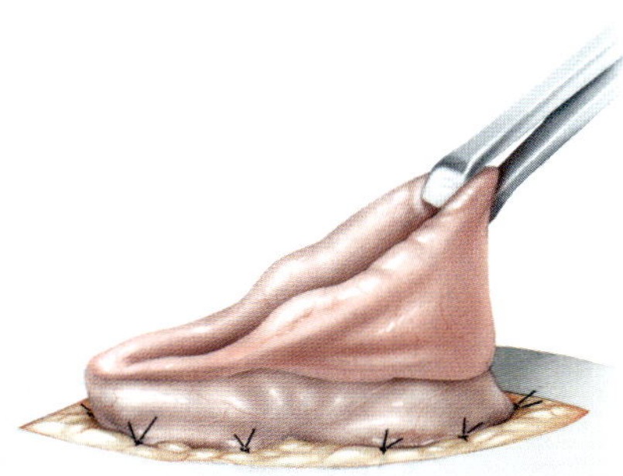

Fig. 17.1.12. Eversion of loop stoma using Allis clamp

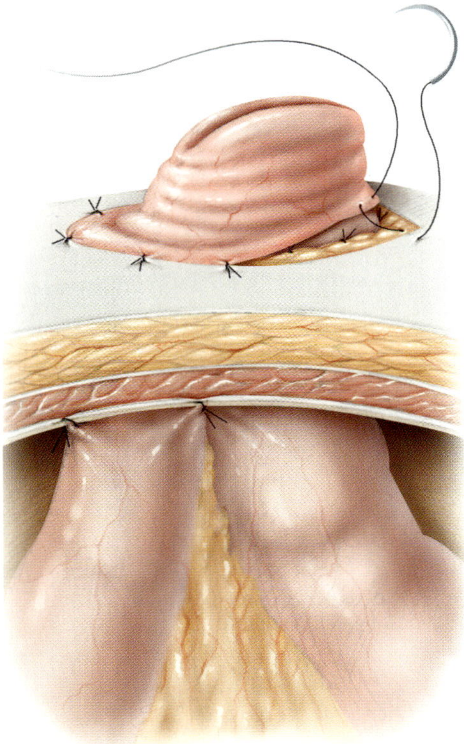

Fig. 17.1.13. Mature Turnbull loop stoma (Fig. 17.1.13 and 14 © Hohenfellner 2007)

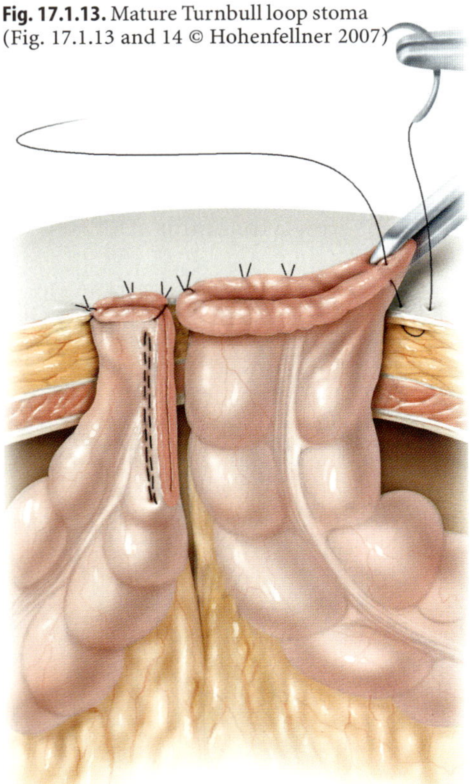

Fig. 17.1.14. Creation of end-loop colostomy

rupted 3-0 Vicryl sutures. Care must be taken to avoid sutures in the mesentery (Fig. 17.1.13).

The ileostomy is closed by excising the stoma and properly mobilizing the proximal and distal loops from the fascial edges. The mesentery of the loop is centrally located and must be avoided to maintain vascularity to the ileal segment. The segment of bowel is excised and the two fresh ends of intestine anastomosed together.

The loop colostomy is constructed in a similar fashion with slight modifications to accommodate the bulkier and occasionally more dilated nature of the colon. Alternatively, an end-loop stoma may be constructed by creating an end stoma flush with the skin using the proximal loop. The distal loop can be brought to the skin as a mucus fistula (Figs. 17.1.14, 17.1.15). This technique still provides the advantages of a loop stoma. Given the more solid nature of output from a colostomy, a nipple stoma is less crucial for appliance fit and surrounding skin care. The closure of a loop or end-loop colostomy is, again, similar to the ileostomy. Resection of the short segment of colon is often unnecessary, as the anterior defect or enterostomy can be closed in two layers.

In the technique of radical cystectomy, the same principle of dissection in proper planes will prevent inadvertent rectal injury. This is particularly important in males, as the bladder, prostate, and seminal vesicles are directly apposed to the rectum. In women, the vagina provides a buffer against any rectal injury. We have previously described our technique of radical cystoprostatectomy and will emphasize key points of the posterior dissection (Fig. 17.1.16). (Stein and Skinner 2004) Following the division of the lateral vascular pedicles (anterior branches of the hypogastric artery), attention is directed toward entry of the pouch of Douglas. The surgeon elevates the bladder anteriorly with a gauze

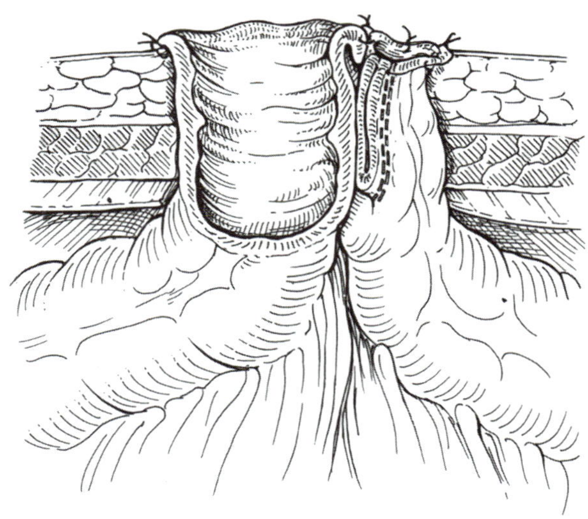

Fig. 17.1.15. End-loop colostomy with mucus fistula

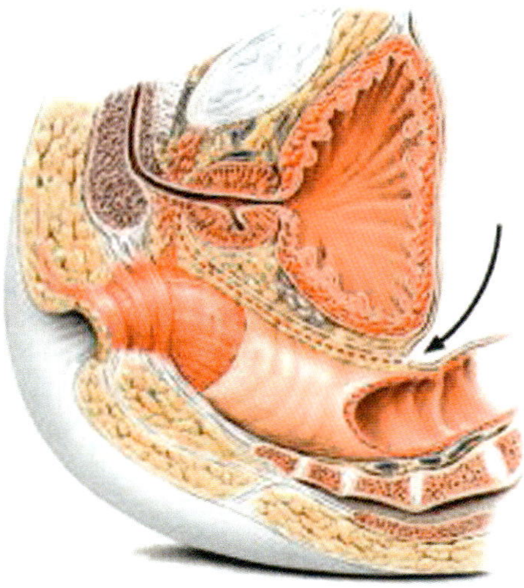

Fig. 17.1.16. Posterior plane of dissection should be carried out between Denonvilliers fascia and the perirectal fat (© Hohenfellner 2007)

sponge in his left hand as the assistant retracts the peritoneum and rectosigmoid colon cephalad. With the peritoneum on tension, it is sharply incised from lateral to medial from both sides. At this point, a clear understanding of fascial planes is critical in the remainder of the dissection. The anterior and posterior peritoneal reflections converge at the pouch of Douglas to form Denonvilliers fascia. Denonvilliers fascia itself is composed of an anterior and posterior sheath with the posterior sheath adjacent to the perirectal fat. This is the correct plane of dissection that must be entered to successfully separate the bladder and prostate specimen from the rectum. The anterior sheath of Denonvilliers fascia is adjacent to the seminal vesicles, vasa, and prostate and does not separate easily. In order to enter the proper plane of dissection, the peritoneum should therefore be incised slightly on the rectal side, rather than on the bladder side. Once the plane between the anterior rectal wall and the posterior sheath of Denonvilliers fascia is entered, a combination of blunt and sharp dissection should reliably carry the dissection down to the apex of the prostate. Again, sharp dissection under direct vision is favored over blind blunt dissection. The assistant's role is critical at this juncture, as the working space is limited and lighting may be less than ideal. Constant retraction on the rectosigmoid colon and suction of blood and fluids will maintain the surgeon's vision. The rectum will more likely be tented up to the prostate in the midline and therefore should be sharply incised in this area. Blunt dissection in a sweeping motion from prostate to rectum is relatively safe on either side of the midline. When the perirectal space has been adequately developed, the posterior pedicles of the bladder will be easily identified for ligation and division.

17.1.4 Solid Organ Injury

17.1.4.1 Spleen

Radical surgery for a left-sided renal cell carcinoma and/or adrenal tumor may sometimes involve injury or removal of the spleen. Not uncommonly, malignant tumors may locally invade or closely abut adjacent organs, including the spleen, pancreas, or duodenum. Injuries can be avoided with judicious use of retracting instruments with blunt edges and soft curves. Assistants should monitor the degree of force placed on retractors, which may frequently become excessive as attention is focused on the operation itself. Mobilization of the spleen may be necessary to expose adrenal and large upper pole renal tumors. This is first accomplished mobilizing the colon and dividing the splenorenal and phrenocolic ligaments. When dividing the attachments of the splenorenal ligament, care must be taken to avoid avulsion or transection of the splenic vessels that run with this ligament. Additionally, mobilization of the spleen can also cause undue mobilization of the tail of the pancreas with subsequent injury.

When a splenic injury does occur, splenorrhaphy should be primarily performed when feasible. Gentle manual compression of the splenic hilum will provide temporary hemostasis for repair. Simple rents in the splenic capsule with concomitant bleeding can usually be controlled with electrocautery followed by suturing of the capsular defect using chromic catgut or silk sutures. Large defects are best repaired with sutures and bolsters of Gelfoam, NuKnit, or Surgicel placed in the defects. Omental patches can also provide substance to both fill and stop bleeding when repairing capsular defects.

With larger injuries not amenable to repair, splenectomy should be and can be safely performed. The postoperative risk of sepsis is rare, especially in nonpediatric patients; however, appropriate prophylactic immunizations should be administered. To safely perform a splenectomy, the entire spleen should be mobilized anteriorly and medially. This is best accomplished by ligating and dividing the short gastric vessels and by rotating the spleen and tail of the pancreas medially to expose the major splenic vessels. The artery and veins should be separately ligated and divided when possible, starting with the artery. This can be performed by utilizing small clamps and free silk or Vicryl sutures. Note that the splenic vessels are best divided close to the hilum of the spleen to prevent injury to the pancreatic tail.

17.1.4.2 Pancreas

As in the case of the duodenum and spleen, specific measures should be taken through the course of an operation to adequately mobilize the pancreatic tail or head to optimize exposure as well as protect the pancreas. This is especially important for large tumors of the kidney and retroperitoneum. Careful mobilization of the tail or head of the pancreas and using padded retractors with gentle force will minimize the opportunity for injury. Gross inspection of the pancreatic surface should alert the surgeon for any signs of contusion, congestion, or laceration. Postoperatively, a prolonged ileus or intense abdominal pain, out of proportion to the site and extent of the incision, should raise suspicion to the possibility of pancreatitis and pancreatic injury.

Occasionally, it may be necessary to resect a portion of the pancreas in the surgical treatment of tumors involving the kidney, adrenal gland, and retroperitoneum (Fig. 17.1.17). For right-sided tumors that involve the head of the pancreas as well as the duodenum, an en bloc resection may be indicated. Preoperative planning and imaging should alert the surgeon for probable consultation with a hepatobiliary surgeon. In cases of left-sided tumors involving the tail of the pancreas, simple resection with repair can be safely performed. In cases of injury to the tail of the pancreas, debridement of the injured portion should be performed followed by visu-

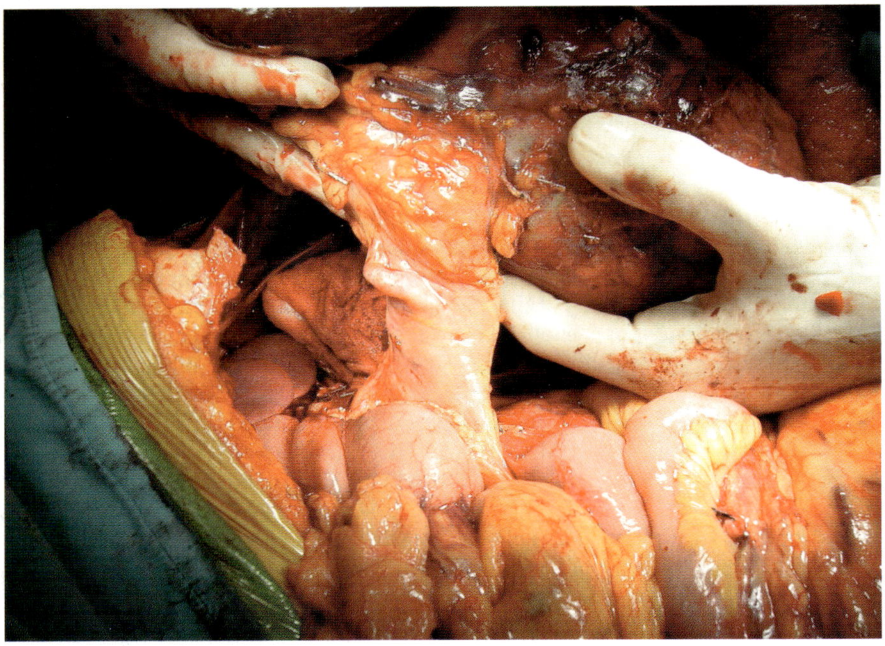

Fig. 17.1.17. Involvement of the pancreatic tail by a large right renal mass

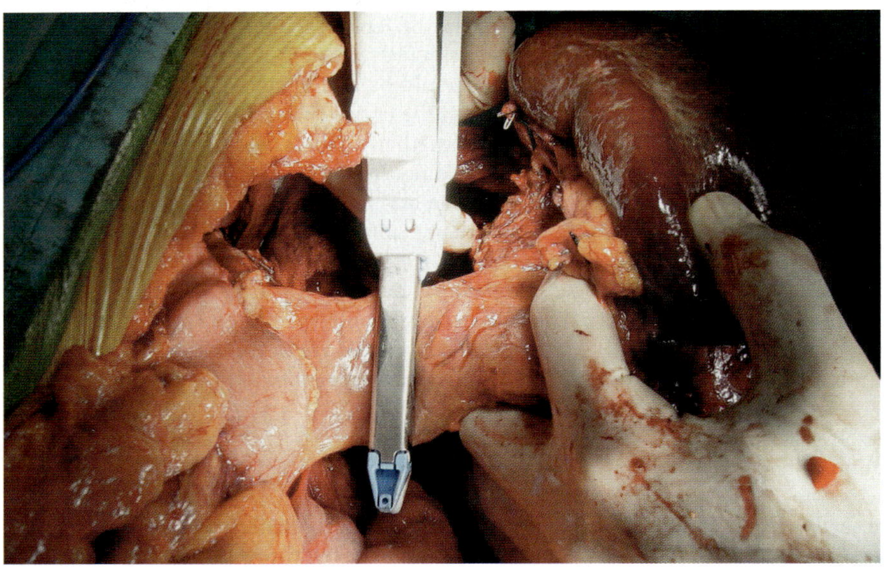

Fig. 17.1.18. Transection of the pancreatic tail using a gastrointestinal stapler

al identification of the pancreatic duct. The duct should be individually ligated or oversewn if visible and the edges of the gland can be reapproximated with interrupted silk sutures. Absorbable sutures should be avoided because of the enzymatic breakdown that may occur prior to complete healing.

When formal resection of the pancreatic tail is necessary, we have found success in using a stapling and cutting device such as a GIA stapler (U.S. Surgical, Norwalk, CT, USA) or Proximate Linear Cutter (Johnson & Johnson, Cincinnati, OH, USA) (Fig. 17.1.18). The transected stump is reinforced with Teflon pledgets securely sewn in place with number-0 silk sutures in a horizontal mattress fashion (Figs. 17.1.19, 17.1.20). The pancreatic duct is effectively ligated and divided with the stapling device. Whenever repair or resection of the pancreas is performed, a closed suction drain should be left in place with close monitoring of outputs postoperatively.

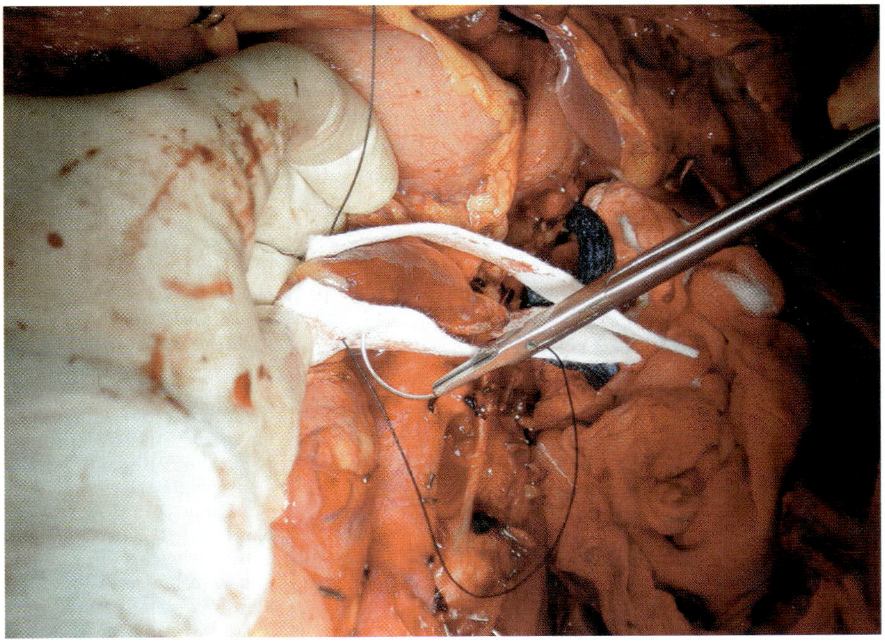

Fig. 17.1.19. Reinforcement of pancreatic tail utilizing Teflon pledgelets

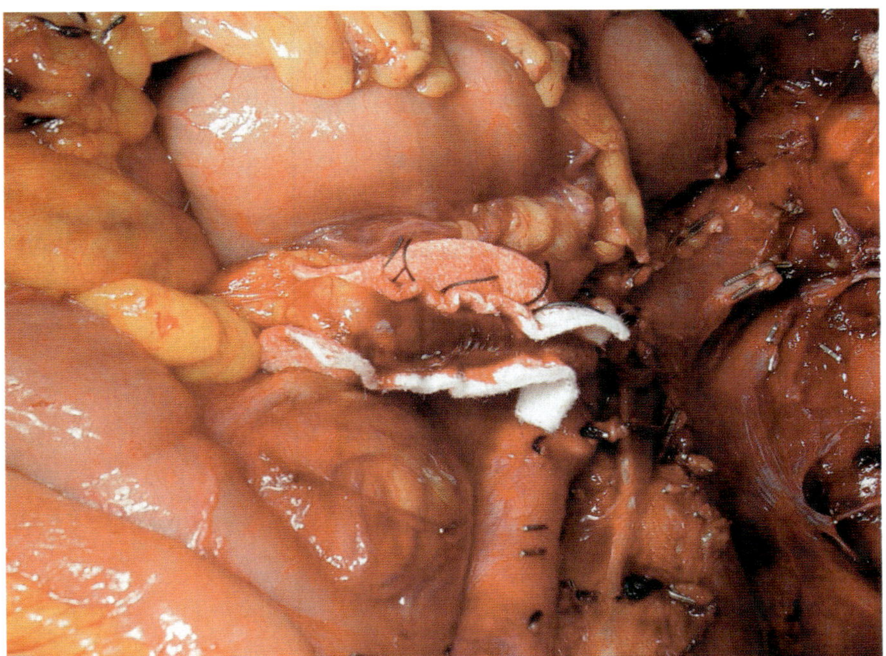

Fig. 17.1.20. Complete repair of pancreatic tail

17.1.4.3 Diaphragm

Resection of large retroperitoneal masses including renal masses may require partial removal of the adjacent diaphragm. Typically, division of the diaphragm is necessary for adequate exposure in the thoracoabdominal incision and can be easily repaired. The diaphragm is reapproximated in two layers with nonabsorbable sutures. Interrupted mattress sutures or an interlocking continuous suture may be used. When a large defect is present because of resection, reconstruction is performed by incorporation of synthetic mesh with nonabsorbable suture to provide stability. We prefer to lay a greater omental apron to cover the mesh on the abdominal side to protect the abdominal organs and facilitate the diaphragm closure. Extended chest tube drainage may be required as intraperitoneal fluid shifts into the ipsilateral thorax during the postoperative period.

17.1.5 Conclusion

Surgical morbidity is significantly minimized with careful surgeon preparation and sound operative techniques. By adhering to basic principles of surgery and patient care, the urologist will avoid many operative misadventures. Thorough preoperative planning with appropriate radiographic imaging will elucidate any potential surprises (vascular or anatomical variances) that may lead to vessel or organ injury. Complete knowledge of anatomical relationships is imperative, especially in situations where normal anatomy is disrupted because of large tumors, previous surgery, infection, or irradiation. The appropriate incision must be employed when patient pathology requires it. Inadequate exposure will not only increase the potential for complications, but will also hamper the efforts to effectively address them. Lastly, when an operation is performed the exact same way each time, the surgeon and assistant will not only operate more efficiently but also prevent many complications.

References

Ahlering TE, Skinner DG (1989) Vena caval resection resection in bulky metastatic germ cell tumors. J Urol 142:1497
Buscarini et al (2000) Tube gastrostomy following radical cystectomy with urinary diversion: surgical technique and experience in 709 patients. Urology 56:150
Crawford ED, Skinner DG (1980) Salvage cystectomy after radiation failure. J Urol 123:32
Donohue JP (1989) Postchemotherapy retroperitoneal lymphadenectomy for bulky tumor including extended suprahilar posterior mediastinal dissection and/or major vessel resection. In: McDougal WS (ed) Difficult problems in urologic surgery. Year Book Medical Publishers
Hoeltl W, Hruby W, Aharinejad S (1990) Renal vein anatomy and its implications for retroperitoneal surgery. J Urol 143:1108
Killion LT (1989) Management of intraoperative hemorrhage from open surgery of bladder and prostate. In: McDougal WS (ed) Difficult problems in urologic surgery. Year Book Medical Publishers
Pruthi RS, Chun, Richman M (2004) The use of a fibrin tissue sealant during laparoscopic partial nephrectomy. BJU Int 93:813
Quek ML, Stein JP, Skinner DG (2001) Surgical approaches to venous tumor thrombus. Sem Uro Onc 19:88
Richter F, Schnorr D, Deger S, Trk I, Roigas J, Wille A, Loening SA (2003) Improvement of hemostasis in open and laparoscopically performed partial nephrectomy using a gelatin matrix-thrombin tissue sealant (FloSeal). Urology 61:73
Skinner DG (1970) Complications of lymph node dissection. In: Smith RB, Skinner DG (eds) Complications of urologic surgery: prevention and management. WB Saunders, Philadelphia, p 422
Stein JP et al (2001) Contemporary surgical techniques for continent urinary diversion continence and potency preservation. Atlas Urol Clin of N Am 9:147
Stein JP, Skinner DG (2004) Surgical atlas radical cystectomy. B J Urol 94:197
Stephenson et al (2004) Morbidity and functional outcomes of salvage radical prostatectomy for locally recurrent prostate cancer after radiation therapy. J Urol 172:2239
Touma NJ, Izawa JI, Chin JL (2005) Current status of loc l salvage therapies following radiation failure for prostate cancer. J Urol 173:373
Walsh PC, Donker PJ (1982) Impotence following radical prostatectomy: Insight into etiology and prevention. J Urol 128:492
Yoon GH, Stein JP, Skinner DG (2005) Retroperitoneal lymph node dissection in the treatment of low-stage nonseminomatous mixed germ cell tumors of the testicle: An update. Urol Oncol 23:168

Complications in Endoscopic Procedures 17.2

F. Wimpissinger, W. Stackl

17.2.1 Complications of Percutaneous Nephrolithotomy

17.2.1.1 Intraoperative and Early Postoperative Complications

The first nephroscope for percutaneous renal access was introduced 1981 by Marberger et al. (1981, 1982). Since that time, percutaneous nephrolithotomy (PCNL) has evolved as a standard procedure in kidney stone therapy. In this chapter, we will focus on the complications of this procedure.

Infection and Sepsis

Infection and sepsis are very rare complications in PCNL, occurring in up to 2.2% (Lewis and Patel 2004). As in all other invasive stone procedures, preexisting urinary tract infection is treated at least 2 days in advance. Cases of obstruction and infection should primarily be managed by percutaneous drainage. PCNL is delayed until the infection has been treated successfully (urinary culture, hematologic signs of recovery from sepsis). During PCNL, we recommend prophylactic antibiotics in all cases. Antibiotic agents are selected according to local bacteria strain spectrum and resistance patterns, which should be monitored on a regular basis. At our institution, we commonly use fourth-generation chinolones, amoxicillin plus clavulanic acid, or an aminoglycoside.

Care must be taken to avoid high-pressure irrigation during the procedure, as this can lead to bacteriemia and subsequent sepsis. To avoid high-pressure irrigation, we use a continuous flow nephroscope. The irrigation container must not be mounted higher than 40 cm above kidney level (Kukreja et al. 2002; Troxel and Low 2002).

Complications with the Percutaneous Nephrostomy Tract

The most severe complication of PCNL is puncturing other organs, especially colon, pleura, liver, gallbladder, or spleen. If the injury is recognized during the procedure, the complication can usually be handled straightforwardly. Unfortunately, most of these complications are diagnosed with a delay of several hours or even days.

Injury of the Colon

Routine preoperative ultrasound shows the anatomical relation of the colon and the kidney and is an important tool to prevent injury. Previous intraabdominal or renal surgery is associated with a higher risk of injury of the colon and may warrant preoperative CT of the abdomen to define anatomic relations.

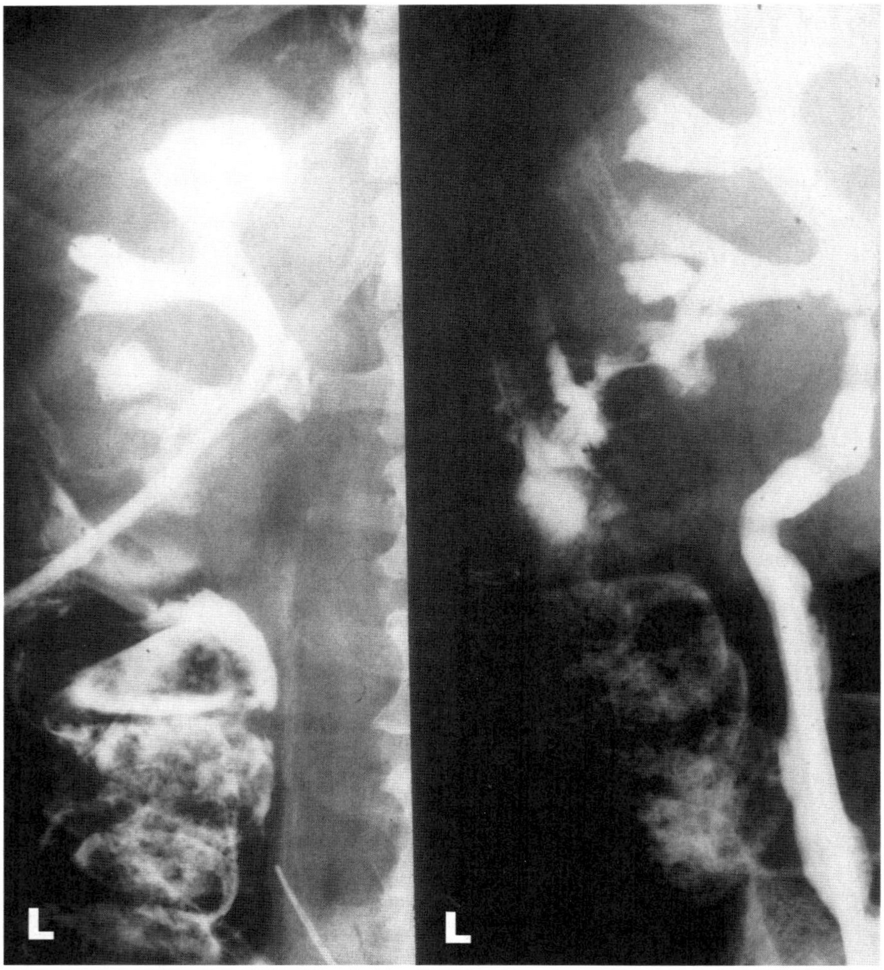

Fig. 17.2.1. Perforation of the left colon during PCNL. Note extravasation of contrast medium from renal collecting system into the descending colon

Needle perforation of the colon is usually not recognized. Colonic perforation with the nephroscope is recognized after contrast filling of bowel at the nephrostogram at the end of the procedure (Fig. 17.2.1). Furthermore, bowel perforation must be suspected in all patients with abdominal pain postoperatively. The anatomic compartment of perforation – retroperitoneal or intraperitoneal – is differentiated by CT scan (distribution of air, fluid; Figs. 17.2.2 – 17.2.4). A water soluble contrast enema study can also be a valuable diagnostic tool.

Needle perforation is usually managed conservatively by observation of the patient. In case of a retroperitoneal perforation of the colon, placement of a nephrostomy tube should be avoided, and the collecting system of the kidney may be drained by a double-J stent. Intraabdominal perforation of the colon requires surgical intervention in almost all cases – usually a transient colostomy (Vallancien et al. 1985).

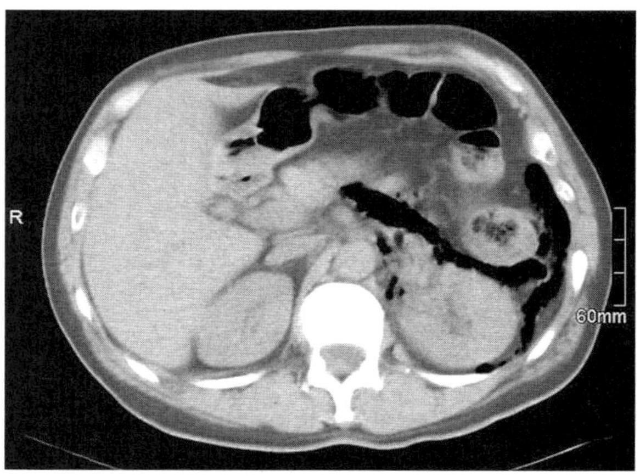

Fig. 17.2.2. Abdominal CT: retroperitoneal air after perforation of the left colon during PCNL

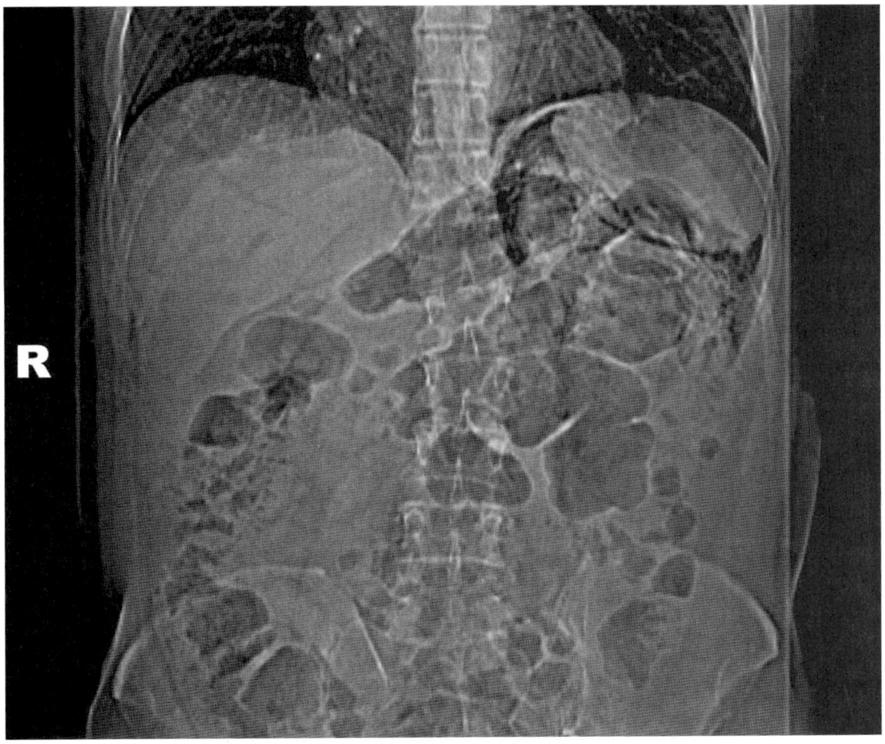

Fig. 17.2.3. Plain abdominal film: retroperitoneal/subphrenic air after perforation of the left colon during PCNL

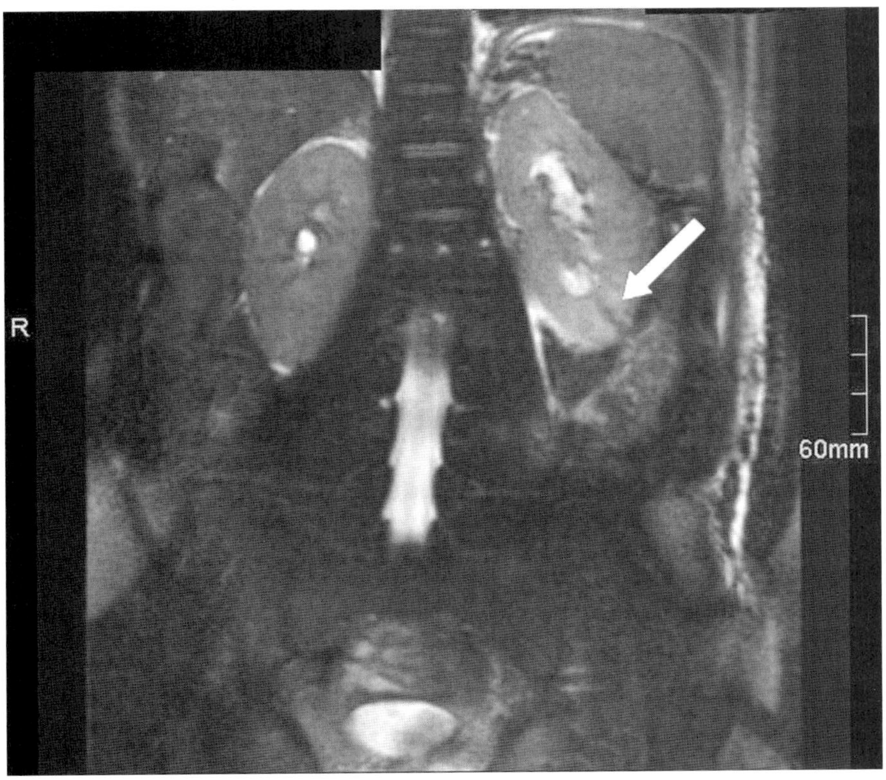

Fig. 17.2.4. MRI of the abdomen (coronal section/reconstruction): Fistula between kidney and left colon and puncture canal in the lower pole of the kidney (*arrow*)

Injury of the Pleura

Injury of the pleura with consecutive pneumo-, fluido-, or hemato-thorax occurs in 0.87% of patients (Lallas et al. 2004). Any dyspnea or thoracic pain must be suspected for puncture of the pleura. Immediate chest x-ray is mandatory in this case. Injury of the pleura can effectively be avoided by puncture below the 12th rib (Munver et al. 2001). Access above the 11th rib significantly increases the risk of pleura injury (Golijanin et al. 1998).

Lesions of the pleura are usually managed conservatively; chest tube drainage can be necessary depending on the extent of pneumo- of hemato-/fluido-thorax.

Injury of the Liver, Gallbladder, or Spleen

Injury of the liver, gallbladder, or spleen are very rare. They are usually not recognized intraoperatively. Bleeding from parenchymatous organ injury can cause hemodynamic problems and abdominal pain. Therapy should follow the same principles as in trauma to these organs. In rare cases of intraoperative recognition of organ injury – usually due to hemodynamic instability – the procedure is terminated and the organ injury managed according to surgical principles.

Bleeding

Bleeding is the most common complication in PCNL, occurring in 0.6%–2.3% (Lewis and Patel 2004; Gremmo et al. 1999). Factors increasing the risk of blood loss have been shown to be diabetes mellitus, multiple-tract procedures, prolonged operative time, and the occurrence of intraoperative complications (Kukreja et al. 2004). Every form of bleeding during or after the procedure requires careful monitoring of hemodynamic and laboratory parameters (red blood count, blood pressure).

The source of bleeding can be renal parenchymal or direct vessel injury. Intraoperative bleeding can make termination and staging of the procedure necessary. Venous bleeding usually stops with plugging the nephrostomy tube leading to tamponade. In contrast to other experts, we recommend insertion of a nephrostomy tube not greater than 14 F. The smaller tube allows for better tissue contraction along the nephrostomy tract. Bleeding from the nephrostomy tract at skin level is managed by a tobacco-pouch suture around the tube. If arterial bleeding causes hemodynamic instability in the patient or a drop in red blood cell count requiring transfusions, angiography and embolization is necessary (Kessaris et al. 1995; Martin et al. 2000). If unsuccessful, open surgery is recommended. However, this situation is exceedingly rare – with a reported rate of 0.1% in one large series (Kessaris et al. 1995).

Perforation of the Renal Pelvis

Perforation of the renal pelvis occurs frequently during PCNL. Intraoperatively, it can lead to increased bleeding and reduced irrigation pressure with impaired visualization. Usually a nephrostomy tube drainage is sufficient to handle this event. In our department, we perform a nephrostogram at the end of the procedure to localize a possible extravasation. An additional nephrostogram is then performed on the second postoperative day to document resolution.

Additional double-J stenting may be necessary to bypass edema of the ureteropelvic junction mucosa or residual stones. Parsons et al. reported infundibular stenosis after PCNL in five of 223 patients treated (2%) as a late sequela of renal pelvis injury in cases with prolonged operating time and large stone burden (Parsons et al. 2002).

Residual Stones

Residual stones after PCNL can be managed by an additional percutaneous procedure or by ESWL.

Absorption of Irrigation Fluid

Problems of irrigation fluid absorption only arise if electrolyte-free solution is used with high pressure and open vessels or renal pelvis perforation. This can lead to water intoxication – also known as TUR syndrome – with hyponatremia and hyposmolarity. It can be prevented by the use of saline and low-pressure irrigation (Schultz et al. 1983). We have never seen problems related to irrigation fluid temperature, even in longer procedures of up to 4 h.

Nephrostomy Tubes

In uneventful cases of PCNL, nephrostomy drainage is not always indicated (Shah et al. 2005). Our indications for a nephrostomy tube drainage are bleeding, extravasation of contrast medium at the end of the procedure, residual stones, obstruction, and infection. Dislocation of a nephrostomy tube must be handled according to symptoms.

17.2.1.2 Late Postoperative Complications

Renal Function Impairment

Renal damage following PCNL usually is insignificant (Chandhoke et al. 1992). An early follow-up study showed no renal function deterioration on split ^{131}I-Hippuran clearance studies 1 year following PCNL in 18 patients (Marberger et al. 1985).

Urinomas

Small – asymptomatic – urinomas are absorbed without late sequelae. Larger and symptomatic urinomas require ultrasound- or CT-guided drainage (Titton et al. 2003). In general, postoperative urinomas are treated in the same way as traumatic urinomas.

17.2.2 Complications of Ureterorenoscopy

Since Pérez-Castro Ellendt and Martínez-Piñeiro introduced the first rigid ureteroscope for endoscopy of the entire ureter including the renal pelvis, ureterorenoscopy has evolved to an indispensable instrument in endourologic surgery. With advanced instruments and experience, safety of the procedure has steadily increased over the last 25 years (Johnson and Pearle 2004).

17.2.2.1 Intraoperative and Early Postoperative Complications

Infection, Sepsis

Postoperative fever higher than 38 °C occurred in 22 % in one large series of 1,575 patients without routine perioperative antibiotic prophylaxis; however, the postoperative infection rate was only 3.7 % (Jeromin and Sosnowski 1998). Sepsis is very rare following URS, with a reported rate of 0.3 % – 2 % (Schuster et al. 2001; Stoller and Wolf 1992). Every effort should be made to avoid retrograde URS in patients with bacteriuria or hematologic signs of infection. In patients with fever and obstruction, a percutaneous nephrostomy drainage or double-J stenting are mandatory.

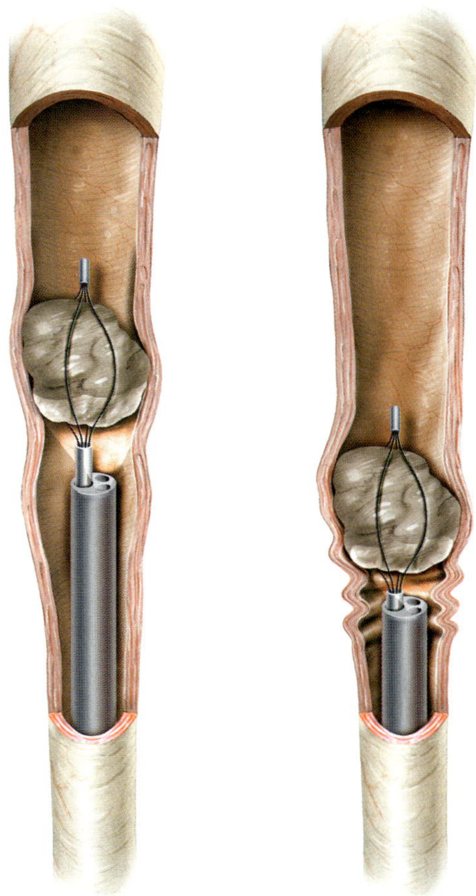

Fig. 17.2.5. Mechanism of avulsion of the ureter with basketed stone during URS (© Hohenfellner 2007)

Avulsion and Intussusception of the Ureter

The most severe complication of ureterorenoscopy is avulsion of the ureter. This usually happens with trapping the ureteral mucosa with a basket (Fig. 17.2.5). Fortunately, avulsion is an extremely rare complication, occurring in 0.0 % – 0.3 % according to three large reviews (Stoller and Wolf 1996; Grasso 2001; Alapont Alacreu et al. 2003). It is usually recognized immediately. Avulsion of the distal ureter is handled by ureteroneocystostomy (psoas hitch, Boari flap). Lesions of the upper ureter require replacement of the ureter by bowel or alternatively autotransplantation (Maier 2002). To prevent ureteral avulsion, baskets should only be used under vision in the lower ureter (Johnson and Pearle 2004). In rare cases of small stones in a dilated ureter, basketing is possible only under direct vision.

Entrapment of a stone in the basket can create a major challenge. In this case, we recommend release of wire and basket and bypassing the wire with the ureteroscope to disintegrate the stone. This should be done with an ultrasound probe or a laser device.

Intussusception of the ureter – the invagination of a mucosal sleeve – is a very rare complication of URS (Bernhard and Reddy 1996). The mechanism is the same as in avulsion (Fig. 17.2.6). It is usually managed by open or laparoscopic reconstruction.

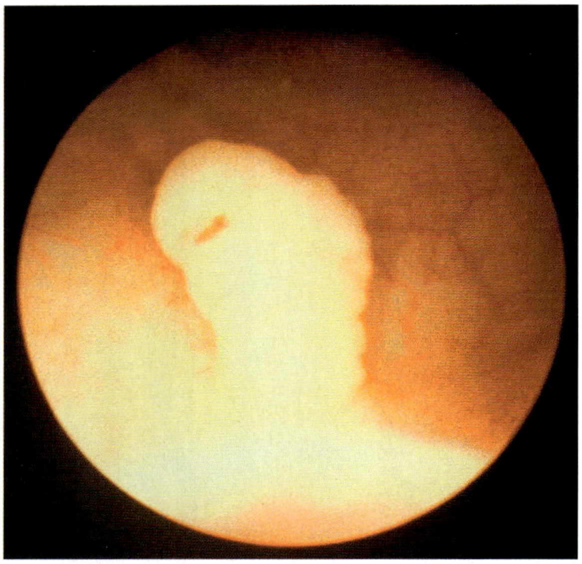

Fig. 17.2.6. Intussesception (and avulsion) of the distal ureter through the ureteral orifice into the bladder

Injury of Neighboring Organs

Injury to other organs is extremely rare. In their series of 4,645 consecutive ureterorenoscopic procedures, Alapont Alacreu and colleagues reported ureteroiliac fistulae in 0.02% (Alapont Alacreu et al. 2003). Management of organ injury has to be individualized based on the same principles as mentioned previously for complications of PCNL.

Ureteric Perforation

Perforation of the ureter during ureterorenoscopy occurs in 1.2%–6.1% according to recent reviews (Fig. 17.2.7) (Alapont Alacreu et al. 2003; Stoller and Wolf 1996). Perforation rate is influenced by instrument diameter and has steadily decreased over time (Johnson and Pearle 2004). Ureteral perforation is usually managed by placement of a double-J stent for 2–3 weeks. If stent placement is not possible, a percutaneous nephrostomy drainage is the therapy of choice. Open surgery is rarely indicated (Jeromin and Sosnowski 1998)

False Passage

False passage – perforation of ureteral mucosa only – occurs in up to 0.9% of ureterorenoscopic procedures (Blute et al. 1988; Grasso 2000). It usually happens during passage of a guidewire and can remain unrecognized. If encountered, it is usually negotiated under direct vision and the ureter is stented at the end of the procedure.

Bleeding

Bleeding during ureterorenoscopy is usually associated with stone disintegration procedures. Its major consequence is impaired vision during the procedure. Major bleeding during ureterorenoscopy is extremely rare. Minor bleeding occurred in 0.3%–2.1% in three large series (Blute et al. 1988; Abdel-Razzak and Bagley 1992; Grasso 2000). Bleeding can require termination of the procedure. It is usually managed by double-J stenting.

Narrowing of the Ureter and Difficult Access

Obstructed segments of ureter can complicate ureterorenoscopy and may require dilation or double-J stenting for at least 48 h. Stenting relaxes and dilates the ureter, facilitating second-stage ureterorenoscopy. The proximal ureter is often more easily accessed via an antegrade percutaneous route (Schmidt 1990).

Difficult ureterorenoscopic access can be expected in patients with previous retroperitoneal or peritoneal surgery with consecutive fixation of the ureter. Flexible ureterorenoscopy can solve this problem.

Residual Stones

Residual stones after ureterorenoscopic stone surgery are rare because of sufficient irrigation and postoperative ureteral stenting in case of small residual fragments. Ureterorenoscopic stone treatment of renal stones constitutes a higher risk for residual ureteric fragments or even steinstrasse (Rudnik et al. 1999). They are usually managed by ESWL or repeat URS depending on size and location. In case of steinstrasse, ESWL of the leading fragment may be sufficient (Kim et al. 1991).

17.2.2.2 Late Postoperative Complications

Ureteric Stricture

Following ureterorenoscopic stone surgery, strictures occur in 0.0%–4.0% (Stackl and Marberger 1986; Beaster 1986). Ureterorenoscopic treatment of upper tract transitional cell carcinoma is associated with a higher stricture rate, ranging from 0% to 16.2% (Elliott et al. 1996, 2001; Martinez-Pinero et al. 1996; Chen and Bagley 2000). Stricture formation should be prevented by minimizing ureteral injury and postoperative stenting in case of perforation of the ureter (Stoller et al. 1992).

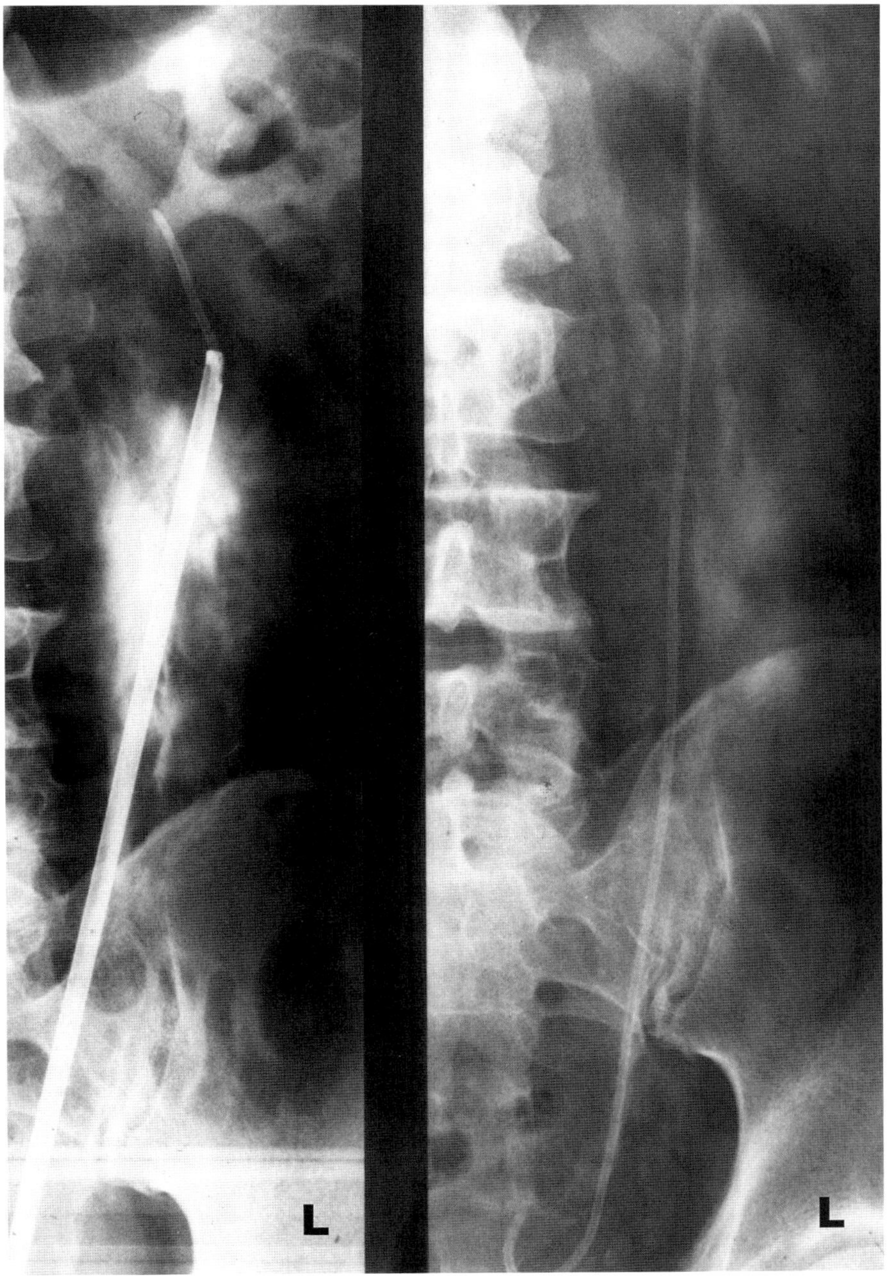

Fig. 17.2.7. Perforation of left ureter with contrast extravasation and management with double-J stent placement

Forgotten Ureteric Stent

A forgotten ureteric stent is a rare but possibly serious complication following urologic procedures. In a series of 31 forgotten indwelling ureteral stents by Monga et al., 68 % were calcified and 14 % were calcified and fragmented (Monga et al. 1995). Half of the patients could be managed by ureteroscopic stent extraction alone; one-third required additional ESWL. The remainder needed either percutaneous nephroscopy, cystoscopic electrohydraulic lithotripsy, open cystolitholapaxy, or simple nephrectomy. To prevent stents from being forgotten, meticulous patient information and close active follow-up are mandatory.

References

Bernhard PH, Reddy PK (1996) Retrograde ureteral intussusception: a rare complication. Endourology 10:349

Blute ML, Segura JW, Patterson DE (1988) Ureteroscopy. J Urol 139:510

Chandhoke PS, Albala DM, Clayman RV (1992) Long-term comparison of renal function in patients with solitary kidneys and/or moderate renal insufficiency undergoing extracorporeal shock wave lithotripsy or percutaneous nephrolithotomy. J Urol 147:1226

Clayman RV, Elbers J, Miller RP, Williamson J, McKeel D, Wassynger W (1987) Percutaneous nephrostomy: assessment of renal damage associated with semi-rigid (24F) and balloon (36F) dilation. J Urol 138:203

Golijanin D, Katz R, Verstandig A, Sasson T, Landau EH, Meretyk S (1998) The supracostal percutaneous nephrostomy for treatment of staghorn and complex kidney stones. J Endourol 12:403

Grasso M (2000) Ureteropyeloscopic treatment of ureteral and intrarenal calculi. Urol Clin North Am 27:623

Grasso M (2001) Complications of ureteropyloscopy. In: Taneja SS, Smith RB, Ehrlich RM (eds) Complications of urologic surgery, 3rd edn. WB Saunders, Philadelphia, p 268

Gremmo E, Ballanger P, Dore B, Aubert J (1999) Hemorrhagic complications during percutaneous nephrolithotomy. Retrospective studies of 772 cases (in French). Prog Urol 9:460

Jeromin L, Sosnowski M (1998) Ureteroscopy in the treatment of ureteral stones: over 10 years' experience. Eur Urol 34:344

Johnson DB, Pearle MS (2004) Complications of ureteroscopy. Urol Clin North Am 31:157

Kessaris DN, Bellman GC, Pardalidis NP, Smith AG (1995) Management of hemorrhage after percutaneous renal surgery. J Urol 153:604

Kim SC, Oh CH, Moon YT, Kim KD (1991) Treatment of steinstrasse with repeat extracorporeal shock wave lithotripsy: experience with piezoelectric lithotriptor. J Urol 145:489

Kukreja RA, Desai MR, Sabnis RB, Patel SH (2002) Fluid absorption during percutaneous nephrolithotomy: does it matter? J Endourol 16:221

Kukreja R, Desai M, Patel S, Bapat S, Desai M (2004) Factors affecting blood loss during percutaneous nephrolithotomy: prospective study. J Endourol 18:715

Lallas CD, Delvecchio FC, Evans BR, Silverstein AD, Preminger GM, Auge BK (2004) Management of nephropleural fistula after supracostal percutaneous nephrolithotomy. Urology 64:241

Lewis S, Patel U (2004) Major complications after percutaneous nephrostomy-lessons from a department audit. Clin Radiol 59:171

Maier U (2002) Autotransplantation der Niere bei Harnleiternekrose nach Ureteroskopie. In: Steffens J, Langen PH (eds) Komplikationen in der Urologie. Steinkopff Verlag, Darmstadt, p 108

Marberger M, Hruby W (1981) Percutaneous litholapaxy of renal calculi with ultrasound. Scientific exhibit at annual meeting of American Urological Association, Boston, MA, May 10–14, 1981.

Marberger M, Stackl W, Hruby W (1982) Percutaneous litholapaxy of renal calculi with ultrasound. Eur Urol 8:236

Marberger M, Stackl W, Hruby W, Kroiss A (1985) Late sequelae of ultrasonic lithotripsy of renal calculi. J Urol 133:170

Martin X, Ndoye A, Konan PG, Feitosa Tajra LC, Gelet A, Dawahra M, Dubernard JM (1998) Hazards of lumbar ureteroscopy: apropos of 4 cases of avulsion of the ureter. Prog Urol 8:358

Martin X, Murat FJ, Feitosa LC, Rouviere O, Lyonnet D, Gelet A, Dubernard J (2000) Severe bleeding after nephrolithotomy: results of hyperselective embolization. Eur Urol 37:136

Monga M, Klein E, Castaneda-Zuniga WR, Thomas R (1995) The forgotten indwelling ureteral stent: a urological dilemma. J Urol 153:1817

Munver R, Delvecchio FC, Newman GE, Preminger GM (2001) Critical analysis of supracostal access for percutaneous renal surgery. J Urol 166:1242

Parsons JK, Jarrett TW, Lancini V, Kavoussi LR (2002) Infundibular stenosis after percutaneous nephrolithotomy. J Urol 167:35

Rudnick DM, Bennett PM, Dretler SP (1999) Retrograde renoscopic fragmentation of moderate-size (1.5–3.0-cm) renal cystine stones. J Endourol 13:483

Schmidt A, Rassweiler J, Gumpinger R, Mayer R, Eisenberger F (1990) Minimally invasive treatment of ureteric calculi using modern techniques. Br J Urol 65:242

Schultz RE, Hanno PM, Wein AJ, Levin RM, Pollack HM, Van Arsdalen KN (1983) Percutaneous ultrasonic lithotripsy: choice of irrigant. J Urol 130:858

Schuster TG, Hollenbeck BK, Faerber GJ, Wolf JS Jr (2001) Complications of ureteroscopy: analysis of predictive factors. J Urol 166:538

Segura JW, Preminger GM, Assimos DG, Dretler SP, Kahn RI, Lingeman JE, Macaluso JN Jr (1997) Ureteral Stones Clinical Guidelines Panel summary report on the management of ureteral calculi. The American Urological Association. J Urol 158:1915

Shah HN, Kausik VB, Hegde SS, Shah JN, Bansal MB (2005) Tubeless percutaneous nephrolithotomy: a prospective feasibility study and review of previous reports. BJU Int 96:879

Stackl W, Marberger M (1986) Late sequelae of the management of ureteral calculi with the ureterorenoscope. J Urol 136:386

Stoller ML, Wolf JS (1996) Endoscopic ureteral injuries. In: McAninch JW (ed) Traumatic and reconstructive urology. WB Saunders, Philadelphia, p 199

Stoller ML, Wolf JS Jr, Hofmann R, Marc B (1992) Ureteroscopy without routine balloon dilation: an outcome assessment. J Urol 147:1238

Titton RL, Gervais DA, Hahn PF, Harisinghani MG, Arellano RS, Mueller PR (2003) Urine leaks and urinomas: diagnosis and imaging-guided intervention. Radiographics 23:1133

Troxel SA, Low RK (2002) Renal intrapelvic pressure during percutaneous nephrolithotomy and its correlation with the development of postoperative fever. J Urol 168:1348.

Vallancien G, Capdeville R, Veillon B, Charton M, Brisset JM (1985) Colonic perforation during percutaneous nephrolithotomy. J Urol 134:1185

Webb DR, Fitzpatrick JM (1985) Percutaneous nephrolithotripsy: a functional and morphological study. J Urol 134:587

TUR-Related Complications

17.3

N. Zantl, R. Hartung

Since the introduction of the transurethral resection of the prostate (TURP) by McCarthy in 1926, instruments, accessories, and surgical technique have changed as a result of improved experience and understanding of pathophysiology, prevention, and treatment of the complications of both TURP and TURB (transurethral resection of bladder tumors). Nevertheless, complications still exist, causing the community of transurethral surgeons to continue to seek innovative techniques and possibilities to secure the instrumental treatment of the lower urinary tract syndrome (LUTS) due to benign prostatic hyperplasia (BPH) and bladder tumors. Borborgoglu et al. recently compared their data on complications following TURP between 1991 and 1998 with earlier published data from the 1980s (Borboroglu et al. 1999; Mebust et al. 1989; Horninger et al. 1996). Their results provide a good overview of the complications to be expected and state that due to recent improvements in how high-frequency current is applied, TURP-related complications significantly decreased in the last decade. The complications are classified in intraoperative and early and late postoperative complications (Tables 17.3.1, 17.3.2).

Table 17.3.1. Intraoperative and early postoperative complications

Complications	Mebust et al. 1989 (%)	Borboroglu et al. 1999 (%)	*P* value
Intraoperative:	272 (6.0)	13 (2.5)	<0.001
Myocardial arrhythmia	(1.1)	7 (1.3)	0.657
TUR syndrome	(2.0)	4 (0.8)	0.055
Transfusion	(2.5)	1 (0.2)	<0.001
Myocardial infarction	2 (0.05)	1 (0.2)	0.392
Death	0 (0)	0 (0)	
Early postoperative:	700 (18.0)	56 (10.8)	<0.001
Failure to void	(6.5)	– (–)	
Discharged home with catheter	93 (2.4)	37 (7.1)	<0.001
Urinary tract infection	(2.3)	11 (2.1)	0.999
Clot retention	(3.3)	7 (1.3)	0.014
Transfusion	(3.9)	1 (0.2)	<0.001
Death	4 (0.1)	0 (0)	0.999
Total mortality	4 (0.1)	0 (0)	0.999
Total transfusions	(6.4)	2 (0.4)	<0.001
Overall	972 (24.9)	69 (13.3)	<0.001

After Borboroglu et al. (1999)

Table 17.3.2. Late postoperative complications after TURP

Complications	Horninger et al. 1996 (%)	Borboroglu et al. 1999 (%)	*P* value
Urinary tract infection	(3.9)	21 (4.0)	0.885
Bladder neck contracture	(1.9)	11 (2.1)	0.842
Urethral stricture	(3.7)	5 (1.0)	0.002
Late postoperative bleeding	(1.7)	7 (1.3)	0.819
Overall:	87 (11.2)	44 (8.5)	0.111

17.3.1 Intraoperative Complications During TURP

After almost 80 years of application, TURP still is referred to as the gold standard in the instrumental treatment of symptomatic BPH. All kinds of operative complications are recognized and current instruments and accessories are specially designed and chosen to prevent these complications. Every surgeon performing transurethral operations should be aware of all the possibilities to make this type of surgery safe and effective.

17.3.1.1 Bleeding

Bleeding is inevitable in TURP. Every cut with the electric current resection loop of the instrument will lead to diffuse tissue bleeding. Other forms of bleeding include bleeding from venous and arterial vessels. Recent technical innovations such as bipolar resection, dry cut, or coagulating intermittent cutting facilitate transurethral resection by means of coagulating most of the diffuse tissue bleeding while cutting. The improvements in electrosurgical units, but also advances and standardization in the resection technique have reduced the actual incidence of major bleeding complications as compared to historical studies (Haupt 2004; Alschibaja et al. 2005; Starkman and Santucci 2005; Berger et al. 2004) (Table 17.3.3). This development should not push transurethral surgeons into feeling safe. Bleeding can lead to severe problems for the surgeon and for the patient, such as:

1. Avoidable blood loss requiring blood transfusions. Especially during the resection of larger glands, continuous bleeding of small amounts may add to a significant blood loss due to the longer resection time.
2. Arterial bleeding can significantly deteriorate the surgeon's view.

These arguments call for meticulous hemostasis already during the resection procedure. Rules that every transurethral surgeon should act upon as a matter of principle include:

1. Observe the operative field with a slow irrigation flow.
2. Siphon or scrape off all blood clots that deteriorate the view.
3. A smooth surface of the resected area always immensely facilitates coagulation.
4. First, coagulate all arterial bleedings before starting to work on the veins. Only coagulate large veins.
5. Close with the observation of the distal and proximal resection margins.

Arterial Bleeding

Under normal conditions, coagulation is not a problem for the transurethral surgeon. However, special techniques are required in certain conditions (Mauermayer 1981):

The Bleeding Spatters into the Instrument

This happens if the artery is cut such that it spatters in the direction of the verumontanum. This problem is managed by:

1. Moving the axis of the instrument out of the spatter
2. Moving the instrument back as far as possible and by carrying out the coagulation with the loop pulled to the front as far as possible (Fig. 17.3.1)

Ricochet Effect Bleeding

If an artery spatters transversely to the opposite side of the resection defect, the bleeding that bounces off can possibly disguise the exit point. The surgeon then recognizes a cloud of blood that may be considered a venous sinus or an unidentifiable bleeding source (Fig. 17.3.2). This problem is managed by:

1. Moving the instrument back into an observation position (approximately around the verumontanum). After emptying the bladder to improve the irrigation flow and irrigating with changing flow intensity, the surgeon must search for the original blood stream (not the ricocheted stream) and follow it back to its origin.

Table 17.3.3. Major bleeding complications in TURP with modern electrosurgical units

Author	Starkman and Santucci 2005	Berger et al. 2004	Haupt et al. 1997	Alschibaja et al. 2005	
Electrosurgical unit	Monopolar	Coagulating intermittent cutting	Microprocessor controlled electrosurgical unit	Coagulating intermittent cutting	
				Multicenter	Munich
No. of patients	18	271	934	778	100
Mean resection weight	18	33	29	33	35
Transfusion rate	0	2.6	2.2	3.2	2.0

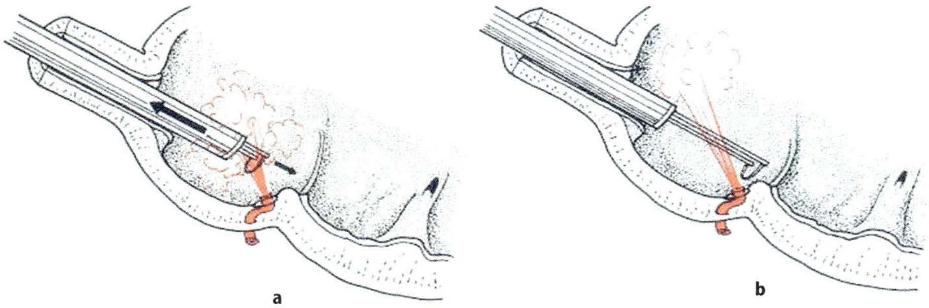

Fig. 17.3.1. a The bleeding spatters into the instrument. **b** By pulling the resectoscope trunk back, the instrument is removed out of the blood spatter, thus providing free visualization onto the bleeding vessel, which can be coagulated with the loop pushed far forward

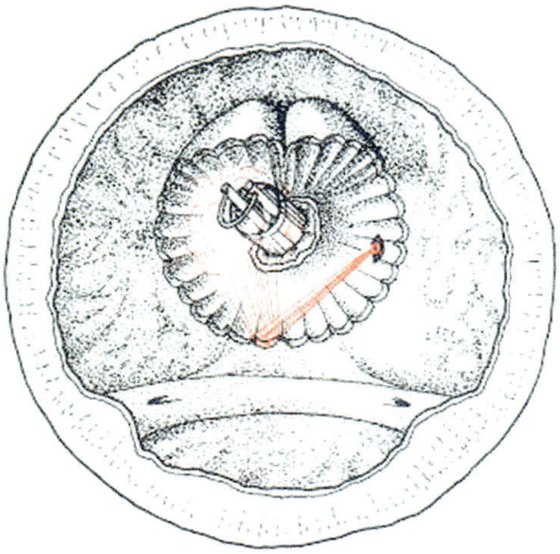

Fig. 17.3.2. Collision bleeding: the blood spatter is bounced off the opposite side of the bleeding vessel

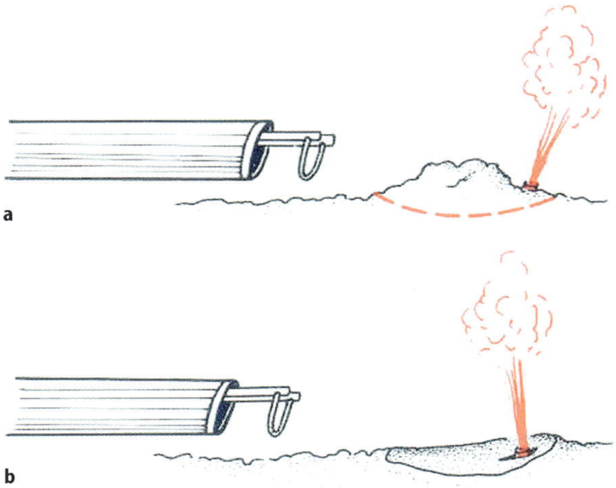

Fig. 17.3.3. a Bleeding behind a tissue rise. **b** The bleeding vessel is visualized after smoothing cuts in the bleeding area

2. Searching the opposite side of the blood cloud. There the resection defect has to be observed in radial segments until the spattering artery is discovered.

Bleeding Behind a Tissue Rise

Sometimes a blood cloud can be seen, but the bleeding vessel is hidden behind a tissue rise. In this case, the problem is managed by:

1. Cutting some smoothing cuts in the region of the bleeding until the vessel is discovered. Subsequently, the vessel is easily coagulated (Fig. 17.3.3).

Bleeding Below Blood Clots

Blood clots may hide the direct signs of arterial bleeding, only coloring the irrigation fluid. This problem is managed by:

1. Removing the blood clots by pushing them away with the resection loop or, if they are already adherent, by resecting them with the loop under current. After that the bleeding sometimes still is not visible; the source must then be visualized by:
2. Smoothing cuts in the respective area, or
3. Observing the area with relevantly reduced irrigation flow.

Pseudohemostasis

Sometimes a blood spatter can clearly be seen, but if the resectoscope is moved to the suspected bleeding source, the bleeding vessel cannot be identified. A possible explanation is that the trunk of the instrument compresses the root of the bleeding vessel. This problem often is not easily managed. It might be helpful to:

1. Move only the loop alone to the bleeding vessel, staying as far as possible away with the trunk of the resectoscope, thus avoiding compression of the root of the vessel.
2. Coagulate without seeing the bleeding, if the lumen of the vessel is visible. Afterwards this must be tested with a different position of the instrument (Fig. 17.3.4).

Bleeding in the Very Distal and Very Proximal Resection Area

This bleeding is frequently difficult to identify, if one does not particularly look for it. When searching over

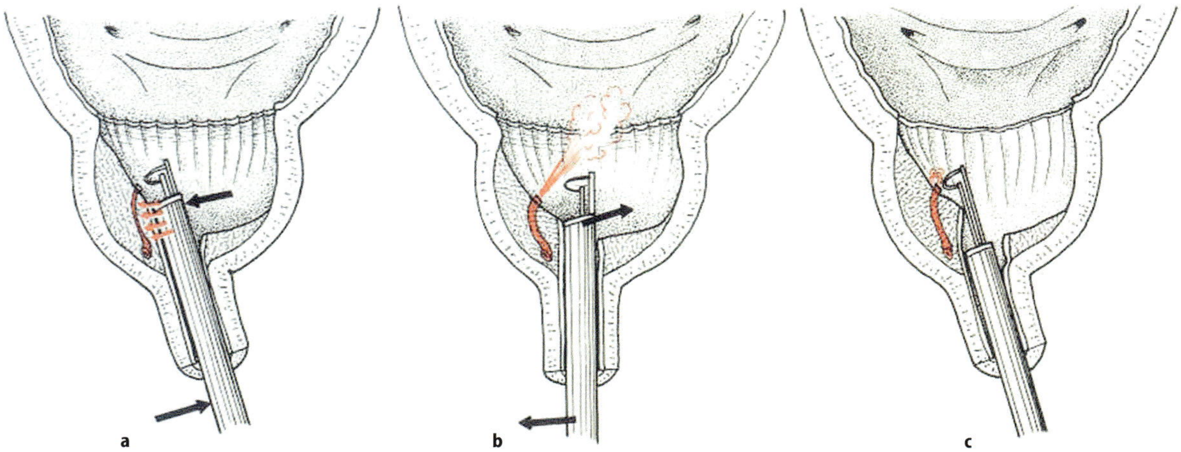

Fig. 17.3.4a–c. Pseudohemostasis. **a** The resectoscope trunk compresses the root of the bleeding vessel on its approach to visualize the vessel. **b** The bleeding continues if the instrument is brought into a different position. **c** After pulling back the instrument, the bleeding vessel can be visualized while bleeding

the resection defect, the instrument often is held a little proximal of the verumontanum. In that case, all vessels further distally cannot be recognized. The same applies to the arteries on the proximal resection edge, since attention is concentrated on the real resection area and not on the periphery. This problem is managed by:

1. Pulling the resectoscope back distal of the verumontanum, or
2. Moving it far to the proximal resection margin in order to particularly look for the distal and proximal resection margins.

Once recognized, the bleeding is easily coagulated.

Venous Bleeding

Venous bleeding often cannot be discovered as long as the irrigation is on high flow, because the hydraulic pressure is higher than the blood pressure in the venous system. Open veins are less in danger of bleeding, but there is greater danger of permitting irrigation fluid to flow directly into the circulating system, possibly leading to hyponatremia and TUR syndrome. Superficial veins normally can be coagulated, but it generally is of no importance. The larger venous sinuses lie in the tissue surrounding the prostatic capsule. They sometimes cannot be coagulated due to their thin wall, but they are easily closed by compression with the catheter balloon.

17.3.1.2 Perforation and Other Injuries

Small perforations of the prostatic capsule and minor levels of extravasation are probably very common but clinically insignificant. Larger perforations of the prostatic capsule with significant extravasation occur in approximately 2 % of patients. Different forms of injuries exist and they must be identified and treated correctly. Every surgeon must therefore be aware of every form of injury and be able to react appropriately.

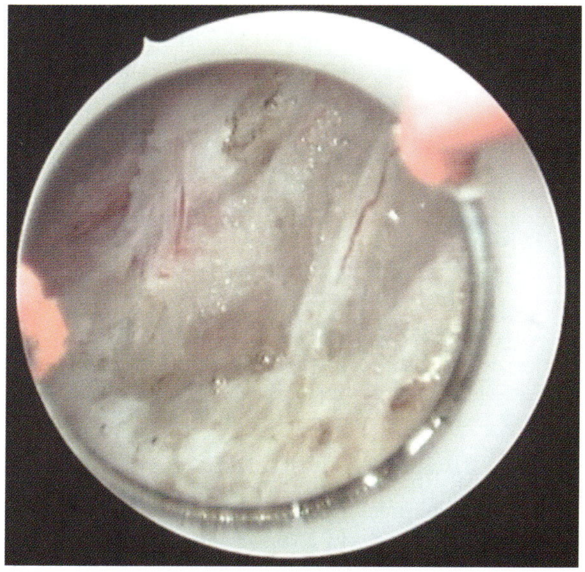

Fig. 17.3.5. Incomplete perforation of the prostatic capsule

Incomplete Perforation of the Prostate Capsule

Most perforations are incomplete perforations with no substantial efflux of irrigating fluid out of the prostate into the surrounding periprostatic and perivesical space. These perforations are characterized by the visualization of fatty tissue in the resection ground. But the fat does not evade backward when hit by the irrigation flush. These injuries arise by tangential cutting into the capsule during resection of the external portions of the prostate (Fig. 17.3.5).

As long as there is no substantial loss of irrigating fluid, there is no special action necessary other than meticulous and careful cessation of the operation, avoiding excessive filling of the bladder, vigorous movement of the resectoscope in the resection defect and performing particularly careful flushing, and removing the resection chips. Normal postoperative care is sufficient with no special change in antibiotic strategy or catheterization time.

Free Perforation (Mostly at the Transition Between Prostate Capsule and Bladder Wall)

The free perforation is an exceptionally rare complication. It is unmistakably seen as a more or less large hole. Irrigating fluid flushes into this hole, but also a flow out of this hole back into the prostatic fossa may be observed. All layers of the capsule are obviously apparent. The periprostatic fat is only seen at the edges of the hole, if at all. This kind of perforation is almost always observed at the transition between the prostatic capsule and the bladder wall but only sporadically at the prostatic capsule itself. Additional signs of a free perforation are a loss of irrigating fluid, suction becoming impossible, abdominal distension, lower abdominal pain, and blood pressure changes. This injury is usually recognized immediately after the cut, assuming the operation is performed under good circumstances including good visual control.

This complication normally means immediately ending the operation, inserting a transurethral catheter into the bladder, and performing CT-guided percutaneous drainage if necessary. In very rare cases, even an open surgical procedure to suture the perforation and insert drainage tubes into the periprostatic and perivesical space can be required. The catheter should be left in the bladder for 1 week and broad-spectrum antibiotic therapy must be given (e.g., a gyrase inhibitor such as a fluoroquinolone or an aminopenicillin with a beta-lactamase inhibitor). The operation must then be completed in a second session after patient recovery (roughly 3 weeks after the injury).

Perforation Under the Trigone

The trigone can be accidentally tunneled at several steps of the surgical procedure:

1. During insertion of the resectoscope, even if this is a rare event.
2. During the resection procedure, if the six o'clock ditch is deeply resected and the remaining thin tissue layer disrupts because of bladder extension due to irrigating fluid or vigorous movement of the resectoscope.
3. During catheter insertion after the resection, it may tunnel under the bladder neck. This is possibly the most dangerous occurrence, because it might be diagnosed only after the influx of a substantial amount of irrigating fluid into the perivesical space.

A lifting of the trigone is often observed in TURP. Endoscopically a separation of capsule fibers is visualized, with fat and loose fibrous tissue appearing between the fibers (Fig. 17.3.6). In this case, the operation can be completed under careful monitoring of the patient, but normally no harmful condition results following this complication. However, the surgical procedure should be immediately interrupted if TUR syndrome (see Sect. 17.3.1.3) is diagnosed or suspected. In that case, a transurethral catheter should be securely inserted into the bladder. In our experience, continuous bladder irrigation to avoid clot retention has never caused additional problems. The catheter can usually also be removed on the second postoperative day, but we presumptively administer broad-spectrum antibiotics for approximately 1 week, although we are not aware of any study that has specifically addressed this question. However, the knowledge that bacteriuria is a finding in approximately 22% of patients after TURP (Wagenlehner et al. 2005) supports our habit of administering this antibiotic prophylaxis. In a subsequent endoscopic follow-up, the bladder neck will be no different from uninjured bladder necks after TURP.

If a tunneling or complete bladder neck perforation is suspected, a cystogram provides an accurate diagnosis.

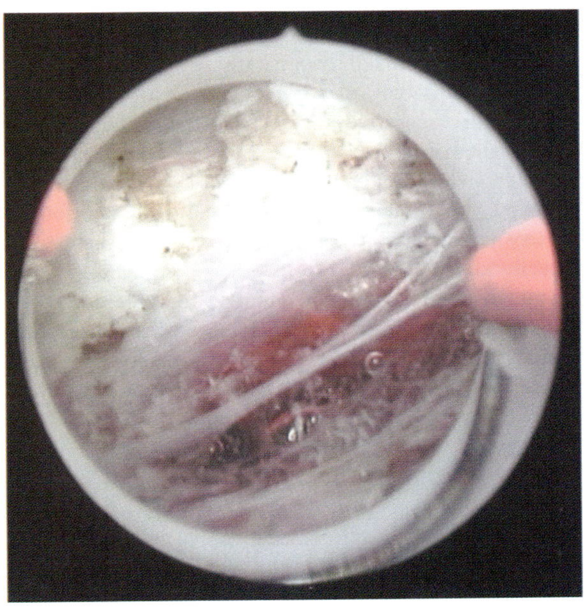

Fig. 17.3.6. Bladder neck perforation

In this case, we recommend a CT scan. If there is free fluid or simply infiltration of the retroperitoneal fatty tissue, we recommend a percutaneous CT-guided drainage, transurethral catheter for 1 week, and a broad-spectrum antibiotic therapy for 1 week. A suture of this injury is not necessary: it always heals spontaneously.

The insertion of the transurethral catheter may be difficult in patients with lifting of the trigone or complete perforation of the bladder neck. Nevertheless, mostly catheterization can be performed using rectal guidance of the catheter with a finger. Only if this procedure is not efficient is insertion of the catheter over a guidewire necessary. If this is abortive, we use an 8-F guiding rod. This is inserted into the bladder through the resectoscope trunk. After removal of the trunk, we carefully push a transurethral catheter with a central opening over the guiding rod. This procedure guides the catheter reliably into the bladder lumen, with an only minimal risk of additional intraperitoneal perforation of the bladder.

Injury of the Ureteral Orifices

An injury of the ureteral orifices is extremely rare. Both stenosis and reflux can occur as well as early or late postoperative complications. If a ureteral orifice is injured, the reduction of the postoperative bladder irrigation to a level as low as possible is recommended in order to avoid reflux and the resulting danger of postoperative pyelonephritis as far as possible. No special antibiotic therapy regimen is necessary.

Prostatorectal Fistulas and Prostate–Symphysis Fistulas

Prostatorectal fistulas are rarely seen urologic complications of TURP. For the most part, they have been managed with colostomy diversion of the fecal stream and suprapubic cystostomy diversion of the urinary stream and in most cases operative closure of the fistula. One recently published case illustrates that a more conservative nonoperative approach utilizing low residue dietary supplements, Foley catheter drainage, and application of broad-spectrum antibiotics can lead to successful closure of such a fistula in selected cases (Evans 1989). Only few cases have been published in literature, making it impossible to give an incidence. However, in cryosurgical ablation of the prostate for prostate cancer prostatorectal fistulas are reported to occur in approximately 0.5 % of patients (Long et al. 2001; Badalament et al. 2000).

A very rare complication observed after TURP is a prostate–symphysis fistula, which may cause an osteitis pubis (Kats et al. 1998).

Complications Due to Suprapubic Trocar Resection

The use of suprapubic drainage of irrigation fluid employing a suprapubic trocar is described to reduce the incidence of the TUR syndrome (Heidler 1999). However, it is of utmost importance that the suprapubic trocar is correctly placed within the bladder and that the trocar tightly seals the puncture hole in the bladder, because otherwise irrigation fluid may leak into the space of Retzius and be absorbed there or after diffusion into the abdominal cavity, thus causing TUR syndrome as a complication in itself. Another possible albeit very rare complication of trocar insertion is the puncture through the abdominal cavity with an injury of a bowel loop.

17.3.1.3
TUR Syndrome

A major complication of TURP is the dilutional hyponatremia resulting from massive absorption of irrigating fluid during the operation. It was first described by Creevy in 1947 and termed TUR syndrome Creevy 1947). Today TUR syndrome occurs in 1 %–7 % of patients undergoing TURP (Mebust et al. 1989; Starkman and Santucci 2005; Collins et al. 2005). The time of risk lasts from 10 min to 24 h after the start of the operation. Mostly simple measures suffice to solve the problem, but sometimes intensive care treatment employing invasive therapy is necessary and the course may even be lethal in 0.2 %–0.8 % of cases (Mebust et al. 1989).

Symptoms and Pathophysiology

The first symptoms of TUR syndrome are usually fatigue and yawning but can include agitation, confusion, and visual changes, if the patient has a spinal anesthesia. In general anesthesia, the first symptoms are a transient hypertension with a reflex bradycardia. The complete picture of the TUR syndrome can comprise symptoms involving the cardiocirculatory system, the lungs, kidney excretion, and the peripheral and central nervous system (Balzarro et al. 2001).

Two mechanisms are suspected to cause the symptoms of TUR syndrome:

1. Hyposmotic hyperhydration as a result of absorption of hyposmotic irrigation fluid. Because the circulating blood is diluted and serum laboratory tests reveal the resulting hyponatremia, this phenomenon is known as dilutional hyponatremia.
2. An increase in ammonia as a result of hyperglycinemia due to absorption of glycine as a component of the irrigation liquid. The absorbed glycine is then metabolized in liver and kidneys to ammonia and glyoxylic acid, which is mainly responsible for

central nervous symptoms such as blurred vision or other vision impairments, which are mainly seen in patients irrigated with glycine.

Interestingly, all symptoms of TUR syndrome are seen in patients irrigated with ether glycine-containing or non-glycine-containing irrigation liquids, proving that the absorption of any irrigant of more than 1.5 l in less than 1 h causes TUR syndrome (Hahn 1997; Ghanem 2003).

Sandfeldt et al. observed after high-dose intravenous infusion of irrigating fluids containing glycine and mannitol in the pig that both glycine 1.5% and mannitol 5% transiently increased cardiac output, the aortic blood flow rate, and arterial pressures, but all of these parameters fell to below baseline after the infusions were ended. The intracranial pressure was significantly lower and the oxygen consumption in the brain significantly decreased during the infusion of mannitol 5%. Glycine 1.5% expanded the intracellular volume significantly more than mannitol did. Signs of myocardial damage were graded glycine 1.5% more than mannitol 5% more than mannitol 3%. Based on these findings, the authors concluded that mannitol 5% seemed to be a more appropriate irrigating fluid to use during endoscopic surgery (Sandfeldt et al. 2001). This glycine-dependent effect was also confirmed in clinical studies, indicating that 5% glucose or mannitol may be superior to 1.5% glycine in respect to TUR syndrome. Therefore, most authors recommend the use of irrigants other than glycine for TURP (Collins et al. 2005; Hahn et al. 1989). Ghanem reported that the fluid type determines the changes of serum solutes and presentation of TUR syndrome: pure water is the most toxic, because it causes hemolysis. The nadir of the hyponatremia is proportional to the severity of TUR syndrome (Ghanem and Ward 1990; Harrison et al. 1956).

The expansion of the intravascular liquid volume due to absorption of the irrigation liquid is responsible for the above-mentioned hypertension with reflex bradycardia. The blood pressure normally rises up to 20–60 mm Hg above the initial value, whereas the heart rate drops down to 10–25 beats per minute below the initial value (Hahn 1990). Retrosternal chest pain may occur concomitantly to hypertension and normally disappears 5–10 min after reduction of hypertension (Hahn 1990).

Rapidly after the hypertensive period, the hyposmolarity leads to a fast transition of the absorbed irrigation fluid into the extravascular, interstitial space. Thus interstitial edema, intravascular hypovolemia, and hyponatremia develop. The first consequence noticed is usually a rapid drop in blood pressure by 50–70 mm Hg with concomitant bradycardia. This condition may even worsen and lead to cardiac arrest (Balzarro et al. 2001).

The resulting interstitial pulmonary edema causes dyspnea, cyanosis, and significant respiratory distress. Even if treated rapidly and correctly, this condition may result in death.

Hypotension may lead to oliguria or anuria. These conditions are difficult to identify, because normally continuous bladder irrigation is necessary after TURP.

The interstitial edema develops especially in the brain, where water but not sodium passes the blood–brain barrier (Gravenstein 1997). Symptoms of the central nervous system include fatigue, yawning, dizziness, nausea, vomiting, confusion, lethargy, unconsciousness, and vision impairment. Itching may appear as a symptom of the peripheral nervous system (Balzarro et al. 2001).

Prevention

Prevention of TUR syndrome involves three mechanisms responsible for the absorption of irrigation fluid:

1. The pressure of the irrigation fluid in the prostatic cavity (depending on the height of the irrigation bag or the adjustment of the irrigation/suction pump)
2. The presence of inflow locations for the irrigation fluid (opened vessels or capsule perforations)
3. The duration of surgery (as over a longer period more liquid may be absorbed by either absorption mechanism).

Therefore it is mandatory to keep the intravesical pressure below 80 cm H_2O. This is achieved by hanging the irrigation fluid bag not higher than 80 cm above the patient's urinary bladder during surgery. Other authors state that the height of the fluid bag over the bladder is of no consequence as long as only a volume corresponding to the almost horizontal first phase of the bladder pressure curve is used (Hubert et al. 1996; Hulten 2002). These authors recommend emptying the bladder as soon as it is only filled to 75% of its capacity to reduce the irrigation absorption in the case of beginning fluid absorption. Other means to control the intravesical pressure are the so called low-pressure TURP. This can be reached using a continuous-flow resectoscope in conjunction with an irrigation/suction pump that controls the irrigation inflow by measuring the intravesical pressure or by the insertion of a suprapubic trocar for continuous drainage of irrigation fluid out of the bladder. Several studies were able to show a reduced fluid absorption in low-pressure TURP; however, none of these studies could clearly prove a significant reduction in TUR syndrome (Bliem et al. 2003; Ekengren and Hahn 1994).

To obtain a secure result in TURP, it is generally important to always perform a fast operation using a rigorous technique. Once the prostatic capsule or large venous blood vessels are opened or if TURP resolves in a large wound field (in the presence of a large prostate), the surgeon should rapidly bring the operation to an end. It should nevertheless be possible to finish the TURP as planned with a complete resection in almost all cases. An additional measure to prevent TUR syndrome in the case of capsule perforations or vessel openings is the prophylactic administration of 20–40 mg furosemide. This measure may also be indicated if the operation time exceeds 45 min. Additionally, it is commonly accepted that the duration of a TURP should not exceed 60–70 min in order to reduce the time of possible fluid absorption. In order to prevent serum sodium levels from decreasing, it is common use to infuse every patient with normal saline (which contains 150 mEq/l NaCl per liter of fluid) during standard TURP and not to use other fluids such as half normal saline. All the prevention measures mentioned so far seem theoretically logical, yet no scientific evidence has proven these hypotheses (Hulten 2002; Norlen and Allgen 1993; Hahn et al. 1990; Weis et al. 1987; Olsson et al. 1995).

It has been shown that changing amounts of irrigation fluid absorption occur in every TURP. Clinical observations suggest that TUR syndrome occurs at a critical absorption of about 2–3 l (Gale and Notley 1985), but symptoms related to glycine may appear even after absorption of as little as 0.5 l (Mebust et al. 1989). A simple and safe method to estimate fluid absorption during TURP is the ethanol breath test. For that purpose, 1%–2% of ethanol should be added into the irrigation fluid; the exhaled ethanol concentration is then measured every 5 min during TURP. It is then easily and reliably possible to calculate the absorbed irrigation fluid from the ethanol concentration in the patients breath (Hahn 1990, 1991a; Hahn et al. 1995; Hulten 2002). Based on the awareness of irrigation absorption, therapy for TUR syndrome can be initiated.

Therapy

Therapy for TUR syndrome must be initiated as early as suspicion of this complication has arisen from laboratory results or clinical symptoms. Some authors recommend stopping the TURP immediately (Borboroglu et al. 1999; Gale and Notley 1985). In our opinion, individual treatment should depend upon time of diagnosis and severity of symptoms. In our experience, it is almost always possible to terminate the operation as planned. But as soon as the symptoms of TUR syndrome aggravate, we immediately finish the operation and proceed with the insertion of the transurethral irrigation catheter.

In general, the treatment of TUR syndrome depends on the symptoms. In severe cases, monitoring and treatment in an intensive care unit become mandatory(Balzarro et al. 2001).

Hypervolemia, hypertension, and dilutional hyponatremia that is not clinically manifest require furosemide in a dose of 20–100 mg. The resulting forced diuresis directly reduces hypervolemia and hypertension; thus furosemide effectively inhibits the passage of fluids into the interstitial space. In severe cases, the additional administration of osmotically active substances such as mannitol may be used to promote diuresis and thus eliminate excess intravascular fluid volume. Dilutional hyponatremia decreases by reduction of the hypervolemic dilution. If the serum sodium level decreases below 125 mEq/l, sodium substitution becomes necessary, even in an asymptomatic state. We then infuse 100 mEq/l sodium added into 1,000 ml of normal saline that includes another 150 mEq/l NaCl, i.e., a total of 250 mEq/l NaCl in 1,000 ml of fluid.

Hypervolemia may lead to pulmonary interstitial edema and thus to an impairment of pulmonary gas exchange. Mechanical impairment of thoracic movement caused by excess free retroperitoneal fluid may add ventilation distress. In such cases, CT-guided drainage of free retroperitoneal fluid may be necessary. Anemia caused by intraoperative bleeding or hemodilution may aggravate hypoxemia. Therefore, blood oxygen saturation must be strictly monitored and blood transfusions are highly recommended. In severe cases, even cannulation and assisted ventilation may become necessary.

Specific correction of the hyponatremia becomes necessary, if clinical symptoms occur such as a decrease in cardiac output volume, a decrease in coronary and organ perfusion, muscle cramps, or central nervous symptoms such as convulsions, impaired consciousness, shock, or coma. Only then can infusions of 250–500 ml of hypertonic saline solution 3%–5% at a rate of up to 100 ml/h be used to normalize sodium plasma levels. In a state of chronic hyponatremia, a serum sodium adjustment faster than 0.5 mEq/h is dangerous, because faster correction exposes the patient to the risk of central pontine myelinolysis, an often fatal complication. However, if hyponatremia occurs as fast as in TUR syndrome (normally within 0.5 h), rapid adjustment may also be done (as described above 250 mEq/l NaCl in 1,000 ml of fluid within 0.5 h, as long as serum sodium levels higher than 125 mmol/l are achieved).

Central nervous system symptoms require appropriate drug treatment. Benzodiazepine, pentobarbital, or phenytoin are appropriate for convulsions. For symptoms related to hyperglycinemia such as temporary blindness, assertion that the problem will resolve spontaneous within 2–4 h is sufficient.

If the TUR syndrome originates from fluid influx due to a misplaced catheter, e.g., retrovesically, a huge amount of fluid may enter the retroperitoneal space. In such a case, sonography or cystography confirms the

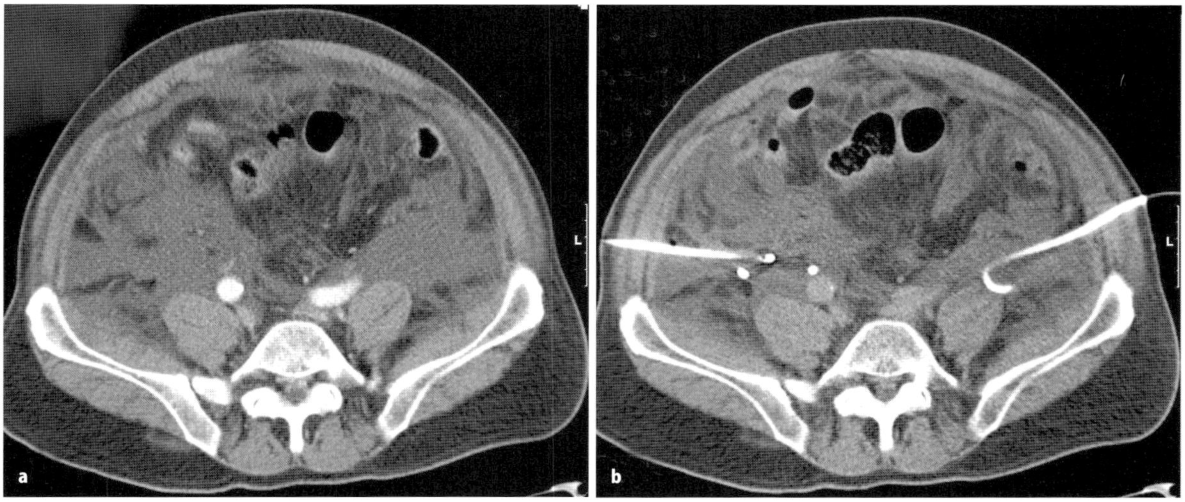

Fig. 17.3.7. a A huge amount of free fluid is diffusely spread within the retroperitoneal space after retrovesical dislocation of the irrigation catheter after TURP. **b** One CT-guided percutaneous drainage is placed on each side within the retroperitoneum

diagnosis and additional CT-guided percutaneous drainage of the retroperitoneum may be a life-saving procedure. It is worth mentioning that the fluid will not constitute a fluid deposit, but it will appear as a diffuse, streaky infiltration of the retroperitoneal fatty tissue. Because of its rare incidence, there are no reports in the literature on percutaneous drainage of free "interstitial" retroperitoneal water. Nevertheless, drainage put into the infiltrated retroperitoneal space at each side might successfully rid the space of the superfluous liquid. In the patient illustrated, 2 l of fluid could be drained after placement of two drainage tubes (Fig. 17.3.7).

The risk of TUR syndrome is theoretically eliminated by using normal saline irrigant with a new bipolar TUR system such as ACMI Vista Controlled Tissue Ablation(ACMI Corporation, Southborough, MA, USA). Gyrus PK Saline TUR (Gyrus Medical, Maple Grove, MN, USA), and Olympus TURis (Olympus America, Melville, NY, USA)

17.3.2 Postoperative Emergencies After TURP

17.3.2.1 Secondary Hemorrhage and Clot Retention

Secondary hemorrhage may be due to arterial or venous bleeding. Arterial bleeding usually attracts attention by constant light red irrigation fluid or by cloudy redness in a more or less clear irrigation fluid. Venous bleeding instead displays a continuous dark red irrigation. Sometimes secondary bleeding may be complicated by retention of blood clots within the bladder, finally causing occlusion of the irrigating catheter. On the other hand, occlusion of the catheter by unextracted resection chips may be the cause of the development of clot retention.

If the bleeding persists after placing the catheter while in the operation room, we recommend an immediate second look with the resectoscope to achieve adequate surgical hemostasis. Nevertheless, light secondary hemorrhage usually can be stopped by conservative measures. The sequence of measures depends upon the primary method of catheter balloon placement. We primarily place the balloon within the prostatic fossa, inflate it there with an amount of water resembling the approximate weight of the resected tissue (i.e., for example about 60 ml of water if 60 g of prostatic tissue are resected) in order to compress residual minor bleeding. In most cases, we take the catheter on gentle traction in order to remain within the prostatic fossa. In this case, we recommend the following order of activities:

1. First of all, blood clots must be extracted from the bladder by suction with a bladder syringe.
2. Then the catheter should be freed of any traction in order to let it slip to the bladder neck and thus enable more compression on the bladder neck.
3. If the bleeding persists, the balloon must be blocked with additional 10 – 20 ml.
4. Then whether renewed traction on the larger balloon can stop the bleeding must be evaluated.
5. If the bleeding persists, the balloon should be emptied, then placed in the bladder and refilled with 100 ml. Then traction pressing the balloon against the bladder neck may control bleeding. The traction is best achieved by fixing an infusion bottle, filled with 500 – 1,000 ml, at the catheter and hanging the bottle over the edge of the patient's bed.

Using this method to apply the traction seems to cause less discomfort to the patient, but it is also possible to simply use tape to achieve the traction. The traction has to be adjusted according to the effect on the bleeding. During this procedure, it is very important not to pull the catheter distally before pushing it into to the bladder, because otherwise it could slip under the inferior bladder neck. Traction can be maintained for about 2–4 h.

6. If the bleeding is controlled with these measures, the above-delineated steps must be reversed in a stepwise fashion, which means removing the catheter tension, decreasing the fluid in the balloon, decreasing continuous bladder irrigation, and removing the catheter.
7. If the bleeding still persists after that, the patient must be returned to the operating room.

Other resectionists place the balloon within the bladder and inflate it with 30–60 ml of water (depending upon the weight of resected tissue) and use gentle traction on the catheter to control bleeding from the bladder neck. Using this method for primary hemostasis after TURP, the steps described should be applied in the following order:

1. First of all, blood clots must be extracted from the bladder by suction with a bladder syringe.
2. The balloon should be filled with 100 ml. Then traction pressing the balloon against the bladder neck may control bleeding. Traction is best achieved by fixing an infusion bottle, filled with 500–1,000 ml, at the catheter and hanging the bottle over the edge of the patient's bed. Using this method to apply the traction seems to cause less discomfort to the patient, but it is also possible to simply use tape to achieve traction. The traction must be adjusted according to the effect on the bleeding.
3. If bleeding is not controlled with these actions, the balloon may be deflated to 15 ml, then pulled into the prostatic fossa and filled with an amount of fluid approximating the resected weight of prostatic tissue.
4. Whether traction on the larger balloon can stop the bleeding should then be evaluated.
5. Then the catheter should be freed of any traction in order to let it slip to the bladder neck and thus enable more compression on the bladder neck.
6. If the bleeding persists, the balloon must be blocked with additional 10–20 ml.
7. If the bleeding is controlled with these measures, the above-delineated steps must be reversed in a stepwise fashion, which means removing the catheter tension, decreasing the fluid in the balloon, decreasing continuous bladder irrigation, and removing the catheter.
8. If the bleeding still persists after that, the patient must be returned to the operating room.

During a second look, transurethral hemostasis inspection always shows adherent blood clots in the prostatic fossa and a partial or complete vesical tamponade. The first step is always to evacuate all blood clots completely with the bladder syringe. Clots adherent in the prostatic fossa often have to be pushed retrograde into the bladder with the resection loop. Normally, minor bleeding remains in the resection area, which should all be coagulated. Most often, a major bleeding event can be found and easily coagulated after all blood clots are removed and after that the irrigation fluid clears immediately from dark red to almost clear, which facilitates the retrospective identification of the coagulated bleeding as the responsible bleeding. However, if the patient's condition permits, the entire prostatic fossa should be thoroughly inspected and subtle coagulation of all identified major and minor bleedings should be performed during a second look transurethral hemostasis!

Usually every bleeding incident caused by TURP should be controllable by a transurethral procedure. However, in desperate situations where conversion to open surgery is necessary, maneuvers used in open prostatectomy such as a suture ligating of the bladder neck at 5 and 7 o'clock to decrease bleeding from prostatic branches of the inferior vesical artery or separation of the bladder from the prostatic fossa using a removable absorbable purse string stitch, as described in 1962 by de la Pena and Alcina (De La Pena and Alcina 1962) and in 1965 by Malament (Malament 1965), can be used to achieve hemostasis. However, open surgery always should remain the last choice after TURP and has in our hands not been necessary over the last 10 years.

17.3.3 Intraoperative and Early Postoperative Complications During TURB

17.3.3.1 Bleeding

Intraoperative and early postoperative bleeding is the most common of all early complications of transurethral resection for superficial bladder tumors. The incidence differs among the published reports in the range from 3.8% to 13% (Collado et al. 2000; Pycha et al. 2003; Dick et al. 1980) (Table 17.3.4). Bleeding accounts for 3.4%–7% of blood transfusions and for most of the repeat interventions (approximately 84%) (Collado et al. 2000; Pycha et al. 2003; Dick et al. 1980). Bleeding mostly occurs in association with large resection areas, but sometimes because the resection area is not thor-

Table 17.3.4. Complications after TURB

Complications	Dick et al. 1980 (%) 373 Patients	Collado et al. 2000 (%) 2,821 Patients	Pycha et al. 2003 (%) 417 Teaching resections
Bladder wall perforation	5	1.3	4
Intraperitoneal	n.d.	0.2	0
Extraperitoneal	n.d.	1.1	4
Hemorrhage requiring transfusion or intervention	13	3.8	8
Overall:	18	5.1	16

oughly coagulated due to the urgent need to stop the operation because of bladder perforation.

The first step in the treatment for postoperative bleeding is blood clot evacuation with a bladder syringe and continuous bladder irrigation. If the bleeding persists, the patient has to be returned to the operating room in order to transurethrally coagulate the bleeding.

17.3.3.2 Bladder Perforation

The incidence of bladder perforation is estimated at 1.3%–5% (Collado et al. 2000; Pycha et al. 2003; Dick et al. 1980). The incidence of bladder perforation is twice as high in women as in men, which, according to Mitchell, results from the female bladder wall being thinner than the male (Collado et al. 2000; Mitchell 1981). From 83% to 88% of bladder perforations are extraperitoneal perforations, and intraperitoneal bladder wall perforations account for about 17% of all bladder perforations or 0.2% of all patients undergoing TURB.

A common cause for lateral bladder perforation is adductor muscle stimulation caused by electrical stimulation of the obturator nerve. If adduction of the lower limb occurs, several measures should be taken to avoid significant perforations of the bladder wall:

1. Avoid overdistension of the bladder.
2. Reduce coagulation energy.
3. Apply coagulation energy in an intermittent manner.
4. Do not extend the resection loop too far.

In the majority of cases, bladder perforations are a visual diagnosis and are usually visualized during resection. Only in a few cases does postoperative pain in the lower abdomen lead to the diagnosis via an extravasation visualized in a cystography (Fig. 17.3.8). If the perforation is seen during resection, resection has to be ended as quickly as possible, but it is usually feasible to finish the operation as planned a priori. However, if the TURB is continued too long after bladder perforation, even TUR syndrome can be the result (Hahn 1995).

Extraperitoneal bladder perforations are usually treated by providing adequate bladder drainage using a transurethral catheter for 2–3 days. A potential perivesical collection only has to be drained in very selected cases with large collections or concomitant bladder infections (Dick et al. 1980). A major concern regarding bladder perforation during TURB for malignant bladder neoplasms is the spillage of tumor cells into the perivesical space with subsequent growth of extravesical tumor and therefore deterioration of the patient's prognosis. Skolarikos published a series of 34 bladder perforations in 3,410 patients undergoing TURB. Thirty patients were treated conservatively, whereas four patients underwent open surgery. All four patients with open surgery presented with extravesical recurrence after a mean follow-up of 7.5 months, whereas none of the 30 patients with conservative treatment showed evidence of extravesical recurrence after a mean follow-up of 60 months (Skolarikos et al. 2005).

Intraperitoneal bladder perforation is a rare but worrisome complication requiring immediate treatment to prevent serious consequences such as peritonitis, uremia, acidosis, hypervolemia due to irrigant fluid reabsorption, and tumor cell spillage into the peritoneal cavity (Pansadoro et al. 2002). Intraperitoneal bladder perforations have traditionally been treated by immediate laparotomy with suture of the bladder breach and peritoneal drainage. However, more recent publications recommend a more conservative treatment employing continuous bladder irrigation and concomitant peritoneal drainage. A very elegant technique to insert the intraperitoneal drainage was published by Pansadoro: the resectoscope is brought forward through the bladder perforation into the peritoneal cavity and up to the ventral abdominal wall. There a limited incision is made above the light of the resectoscope, allowing the resectoscope to pass outside the abdomen. Then a drainage tube (e.g., a Foley catheter) is inserted into the resectoscope sheath, thus bringing the drainage tube easily into the peritoneal cavity by withdrawing the resectoscope. A second catheter was placed within the bladder and antibiotic coverage was administered for 10 days (Pansadoro et al. 2002).

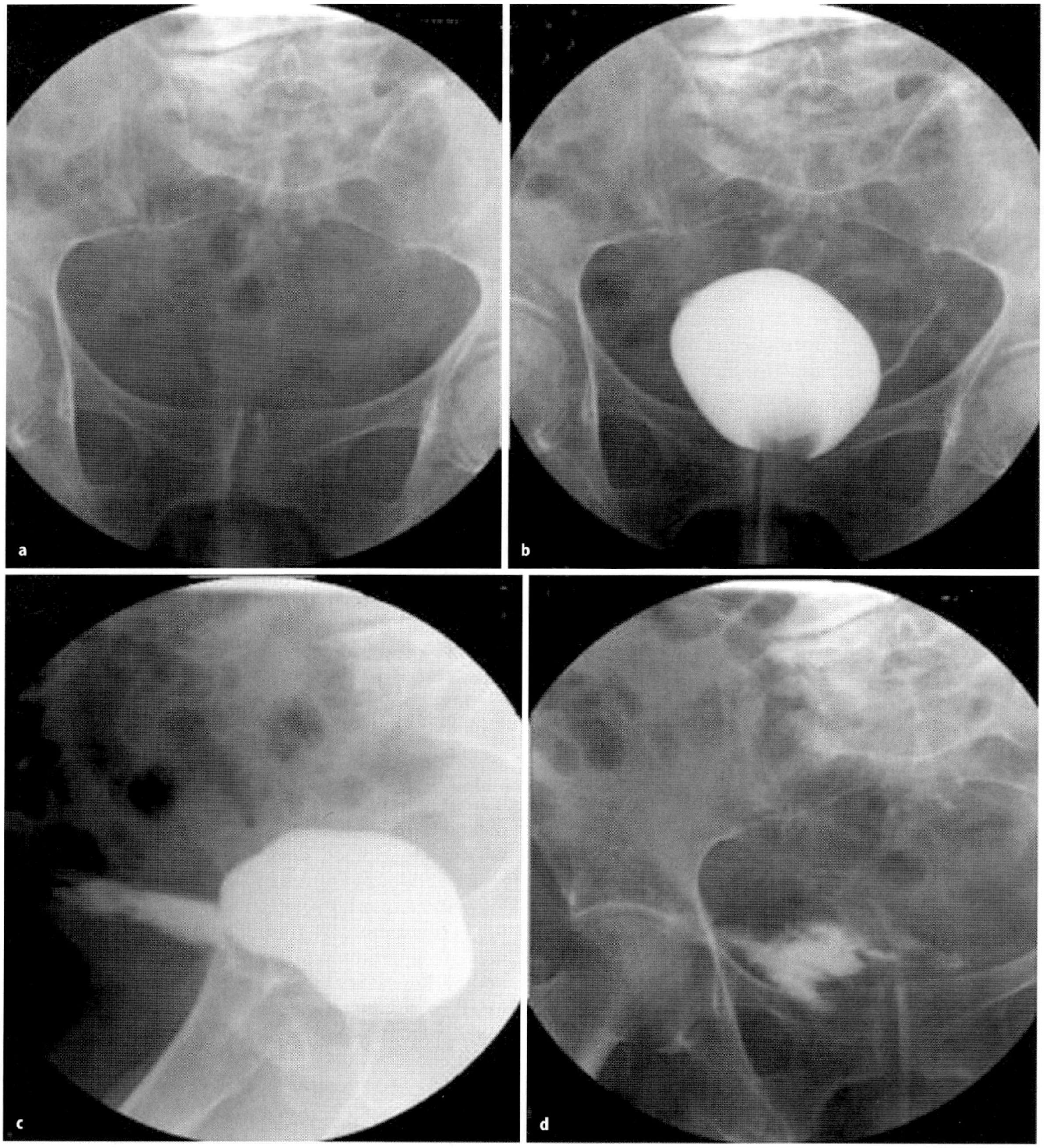

Fig. 17.3.8a–d. Bladder perforation due to TURB. **a** Plain x-ray of the pelvis. **b** Cystogram in anterior-posterior path of rays shows no clear evidence of contrast media extravasation. **c** Lateral path of rays and **d** terminal x-ray of the pelvis after bladder micturition clearly show the ventral bladder perforation with extravasation of contrast media

17.3.3.3 Bladder Explosion

As a consequence of tissue carbonization during contact with the electric loop, a special gas mixture is generated with a potentially hazardous hydrogen and air mixture. Bladder explosion during transurethral electrosurgery is a very rare complication with only two cases fully published in the literature, but can occur as a consequence of sparks igniting this hydrogen and air composition concentrated under the bladder vault (Horger and Babanoury 2004; Di Tonno et al. 2003). These bladder explosions usually result in major laceration of the bladder, therefore requiring careful open surgical exploration, comprehensive reconstruction of the bladder, and thorough drainage of the perivesical space.

To prevent a bladder explosion during transurethral electrosurgery, the following measures are recommended (Di Tonno et al. 2003):

1. Use a current of moderate power during coagulation.
2. Minimize the penetration of air in the bladder by means of a correct and careful liquid irrigation.
3. Carefully evacuate the bladder (either frequently of continuously), especially when operating under the bladder vault.

References

Alschibaja M, May F, Treiber U, Paul R, Hartung R (2005) Transurethral resection for benign prostatic hyperplasia. current developments. Urologe A 44:499

Badalament RA, Bahn DK, Kim H, Kumar A, Bahn JM, Lee F (2000) Patient-reported complications after cryoablation therapy for prostate cancer. Arch Ital Urol Androl 72:305

Balzarro M, Ficarra V, Bartoloni A, Tallarigo C, Malossini G (2001) The pathophysiology, diagnosis and therapy of the transurethral resection of the prostate syndrome. Urol Int 66:121

Berger AP, Wirtenberger W, Bektic J et al (2004) Safer transurethral resection of the prostate: coagulating intermittent cutting reduces hemostatic complications. J Urol 171:289

Bliem F, Lamche M, Janda R, Ilias W, Schramek P (2003) Blood loss and absorption in TURP vs. TUVRP under low pressure and high pressure conditions. Urologe A 42:1477

Borboroglu PG, Kane CJ, Ward JF, Roberts JL, Sands JP (1999) Immediate and postoperative complications of transurethral prostatectomy in the 1990s. J Urol 162:1307

Collado A, Chechile GE, Salvador J, Vicente J (2000) Early complications of endoscopic treatment for superficial bladder tumors. J Urol 164:1529

Collins JW, Macdermott S, Bradbrook RA, Keeley FX Jr, Timoney AG (2005) A comparison of the effect of 1.5% glycine and 5% glucose irrigants on plasma serum physiology and the incidence of transurethral resection syndrome during prostate resection. BJU Int 96:368

Creevy CD (1947) Haemolytic reactions during transurethral resection. J Urol 58:125

De La Pena A, Alcina E (1962) Suprapubic prostatectomy: a new technique to prevent bleeding. J Urol 88:86

Di Tonno F, Fusaro V, Bertoldin R, Lavelli D (2003) Bladder explosion during transurethral resection of the prostate. Urol Int 71:108

Dick A, Barnes R, Hadley H, Bergman RT, Ninan CA (1980) Complications of transurethral resection of bladder tumors: prevention, recognition and treatment. J Urol 124:810

Ekengren J, Hahn RG (1994) Continuous versus intermittent flow irrigation in transurethral resection of the prostate. Urology 43:328

Evins SC (1989) Nonoperative management of iatrogenic prostatorectal fistula. Urology 33:418

Gale DW, Notley RG (1985) TURP without TURP syndrome. Br J Urol 57:708

Ghanem AN (2003) Validation of the ethanol breath test and on-table weighing to measure irrigation absorption during transurethral prostatectomy. BJU Int 92:154

Ghanem AN, Ward JP (1990) Osmotic and metabolic sequelae of volumetric overload in relation to the TUR syndrome. Br J Urol 66:71

Gravenstein D (1997) Transurethral resection of the prostate (TURP) syndrome: a review of the pathophysiology and management. Anesth Analg 84:438

Hahn RG (1990) Prevention of TUR syndrome by detection of trace ethanol in the expired breath. Anaesthesia 45:577

Hahn RG (1991a) Monitoring of TURP with ethanol. Lancet 338:1602

Hahn RG (1991b) The transurethral resection syndrome. Acta Anaesthesiol Scand 35:557

Hahn RG (1995) Transurethral resection syndrome after transurethral resection of bladder tumours. Can J Anaesth 42:69

Hahn RG (1997) Irrigating fluids in endoscopic surgery. Br J Urol 79:669

Hahn RG, Stalberg HP, Gustafsson SA (1989) Intravenous infusion of irrigating fluids containing glycine or mannitol with and without ethanol. J Urol 142:1102

Hahn RG, Algotsson LA, Tornebrandt K (1990) Comparison of ethanol absorption during continuous and intermittent flow irrigation in transurethral resection. Scand J Urol Nephrol 24:27

Hahn RG, Larsson H, Ribbe T (1995) Continuous monitoring of irrigating fluid absorption during transurethral surgery. Anaesthesia 50:327

Harrison RH 3rd, Boren JS, Robison JR (1956) Dilutional hyponatremic shock: another concept of the transurethral prostatic resection reaction. J Urol 75:95

Haupt G (2004) Re: safer transurethral resection of the prostate: coagulating intermittent cutting reduces hemostatic complications. J Urol 172:780

Haupt G, Pannek J, Benkert S, Heinrich C, Schulze H, Senge T (1997) Transurethral resection of the prostate with microprocessor controlled electrosurgical unit. J Urol 158:497

Heidler H (1999) Frequency and causes of fluid absorption: a comparison of three techniques for resection of the prostate under continuous pressure monitoring. BJU Int 83:619

Horger DC, Babanoury A (2004) Intravesical explosion during transurethral resection of bladder tumors. J Urol 172:1813

Horninger W, Unterlechner H, Strasser H, Bartsch G (1996) Transurethral prostatectomy: mortality and morbidity. Prostate 28:195

Hubert J, Cormier L, Gerbaud PF, Guillemin F, Pertek JP, Mangin P (1996) Computer-controlled monitoring of bladder pressure in the prevention of 'TUR syndrome': a randomized study of 53 cases. Br J Urol 78:228

Hulten JO (2002) How to master absorption during transurethral resection of the prostate: basic measures guided by the ethanol method. BJU Int 90:244

Kats E, Venema PL, Kropman RF, Kieft GJ (1998) Diagnosis and treatment of osteitis pubis caused by a prostate-symphysis fistula: a rare complication after transurethral resection of the prostate. Br J Urol 81:927

Long JP, Bahn D, Lee F, Shinohara K, Chinn DO, Macaluso JN Jr (2001) Five-year retrospective, multi-institutional pooled analysis of cancer-related outcomes after cryosurgical ablation of the prostate. Urology 57:518

Malament M (1965) Maximal hemostasis in suprapubic prostatectomy. Surg Gynecol Obstet 120:1307

Mauermayer W (1981) Transurethrale operationen, 1st edn. Springer, Berlin Heidelberg New York

Mebust WK, Holtgrewe HL, Cocked AT, Peters PC (1989) Transurethral prostatectomy: immediate and postoperative complications. A cooperative study of 13 participating institutions evaluating 3,885 patients. J Urol 141:243

Mitchell JP (1981) Transurethral resection for neoplasm of the bladder. In: Mitchell JP (ed) Endoscopic Operative Urology. Wright & Sons, Bristol, p 341

Norlen H, Allgen LG (1993) A comparison between intermittent and continuous transurethral resection of the prostate. Scand J Urol Nephrol 27:21

Olsson J, Nilsson A, Hahn RG (1995) Symptoms of the transurethral resection syndrome using glycine as the irrigant. J Urol 154:123

Pansadoro A, Franco G, Laurenti C, Pansadoro V (2002) Conservative treatment of intraperitoneal bladder perforation during transurethral resection of bladder tumor. Urology 60:682

Pycha A, Lodde M, Lusuardi L et al (2003) Teaching transurethral resection of the bladder: still a challenge? Urology 62:46

Sandfeldt L, Riddez L, Rajs J, Ewaldsson C, Piros D, Hahn RG (2001) High-dose intravenous infusion of irrigating fluids containing glycine and mannitol in the pig. J Surg Res 95:114

Skolarikos A, Chrisofos M, Ferakis N, Papatsoris A, Dellis A, Deliveliotis C (2005) Does the management of bladder perforation during transurethral resection of superficial bladder tumors predispose to extravesical tumor recurrence? J Urol 173:1908

Starkman JS, Santucci RA (2005) Comparison of bipolar transurethral resection of the prostate with standard transurethral prostatectomy: shorter stay, earlier catheter removal and fewer complications. BJU Int 95:69

Wagenlehner FM, Wagenlehner C, Schinzel S, Naber KG (2005) Prospective, randomized, multicentric, open, comparative study on the efficacy of a prophylactic single dose of 500 mg levofloxacin versus 1920 mg trimethoprim/sulfamethoxazole versus a control group in patients undergoing TUR of the prostate. Eur Urol 47:549

Weis N, Jorgensen PE, Bruun E (1987) TUR syndrome after transurethral resection of the prostate using suprapubic drainage. Int Urol Nephrol 19:165

Complications in Laparoscopic Surgery 17.4

M. Muntener, F.R. Romero, L.R. Kavoussi

17.4.1 Introduction

In the last decade, the popularity of laparoscopic surgery has exploded, as evidenced by the dramatic increase in the number of laparoscopically performed urologic procedures. This has been driven by the potential of laparoscopic surgery to achieve the same goals as a standard open approach while offering the patient distinct advantages with regard to perioperative morbidity, length of hospital stay, and convalescence. However, there are also disadvantages to the endoscopic approach. Typically the learning curves for laparoscopic operations are long and there are a number of pitfalls that potentially complicate these procedures. Even for very experienced open surgeons, it is difficult to translate skills and knowledge directly to the endoscopic technique.

Although in laparoscopic surgery the approach is minimally invasive, the complexity of the procedure is generally at least equal to its traditional open counterpart. This is also reflected in the scope of possible complications, which characteristically encompasses all the complications known from open surgery and in addition to that a number of complications that are specific to the endoscopic approach. Knowledge about these complications is essential for their prevention. Additionally, this understanding helps the laparoscopic surgeon to identify possible complications intraoperatively. It is the timely recognition, which in many cases allows the surgeon to manage the complication laparoscopically and thereby preserve the patient some of the benefits of the minimally invasive approach.

This section focuses on the recognition, the management, and the prevention of acute intraoperative and postoperative complications that may be encountered in urologic laparoscopic surgery. Late complications specifically associated with laparoscopic surgery are beyond the scope of this chapter. Since the variety of possible complications is similar for most urologic laparoscopic procedures, this chapter is subdivided by complications rather than procedures.

17.4.2 Intraoperative Complications

17.4.2.1 Complications Related to Access

Establishing a pneumoperitoneum and gaining entry access to the abdomen are prerequisites for laparoscopic surgery. These initial steps of the procedure can be challenging and harbor a unique range of complications. The overall incidence of access-related injuries is relatively small. Large series from general surgery reported incidences below 1% (Champault et al. 1996; Deziel et al. 1993). With increasing experience over the last decade, complications related to the laparoscopic access seem to have become less frequent also in urologic procedures (Gettman 2005). Recent large series showed incidence rates around 0.2% (Fahlenkamp et al. 1999; Soulie et al. 2001). However, the mortality rate reported from these complications is as high as 13% (Chandler et al. 2001).

Recognition

Injury to major blood vessels is probably the most feared complication of gaining laparoscopic access. In those cases, recognition of the complication usually is not a problem. However, in many of the less spectacular complications of trocar placement, the intraoperative recognition of the injury, which is crucial for an optimal management of the situation, is the main difficulty. In their review of 594 laparoscopic entry access injuries, Chandler and colleagues found that nearly 50% of both large- and small-bowel injuries remained unrecognized for at least 24 h. Also, this delayed recognition was found to be an independent, significant predictor of death (Chandler et al. 2001).

If the pneumoperitoneum is established via a Veress needle, correct positioning of the needle should be verified prior to CO_2 insufflation. An irregular finding on aspiration, irrigation, reaspiration, or drop test indicates malpositioning of the needle and may lead to the diagnosis or the suspicion of an injury to an intraabdominal organ. If the intraabdominal pressure reading at the beginning of the insufflation is not below 8–10 mm Hg, incorrect needle position or at least contact of the needle tip with intraabdominal structures must be suspected and the needle should be repositioned. It is particularly important to stay in contact with the anesthesiologist during this phase of initial CO_2 insufflation so that close monitoring can be performed. Any sudden change in the hemodynamics of the patient or end tidal CO_2 reading should lead to cessation of insufflation (Porter 2004). Also, embolization of CO_2 to the right heart, a very rare but potentially catastrophic situation that typically results from inadvertent insufflation of gas into the bloodstream, leads within minutes to a sharp decrease in end tidal CO_2 and oxygen saturation as well as low-output heart failure (Lantz and Smith 1994; Wolf and Stoller 1994). If transesophageal echocardiography is available in the operating room, this may help to visualize the gas embolus in the right heart and make the correct diagnosis.

Once the camera is introduced, a cursory inspection of the peritoneal cavity should be performed in every procedure. In case an access injury is suspected, a very meticulous inspection is mandatory to verify or rule out any intraabdominal lesion.

Not surprisingly, the vast majority of access-related injuries results from the primary entry port. The placement of secondary trocars that are usually placed under direct vision contributed to less than 5% of these injuries (Chandler et al. 2001). It is therefore recommended to routinely inspect the primary trocar as soon as more ports are in place in order to detect a potential problem near that entry site. Because intraabdominal structures can inadvertently become trapped in sutures, this inspection is especially advisable if sutures are used to reduce the loss of CO_2, as is often done after the insertion of a Hasson cannula through a mini-laparotomy (Sadeghi-Nejad et al. 1994).

Management

The optimal management of entry access-related complications obviously varies widely with the severity and acuteness of the problem.

If a complication from the insertion of the Veress needle is suspected, the needle should be withdrawn and the pneumoperitoneum should either be established by introducing the Veress needle at a different site or by open insertion of a Hasson cannula (Hasson 1971). Once the camera is introduced, the suspected intraabdominal needle injury must be verified or ruled out. Injuries caused by the 14-gauge Veress needle can usually be managed laparoscopically even if a major vessel or a parenchymatous organ is involved. If a blood vessel has been punctured by the Veress needle, the bleeding following the withdrawal of the needle is usually not excessive and can be managed by applying pressure for a couple of minutes as well as a oxidized regenerated cellulose and fibrin glue if necessary. Puncture injuries of the liver and the spleen can be managed in the same way or they can be cauterized with the argon beam coagulator. Simple punctures of the bowel or the bladder by the Veress needle do not require any treatment (Bateman et al. 1996; Gill et al. 2002).

If there is any pronounced change in hemodynamics or end tidal CO_2 level at the beginning of the CO_2 insufflation, the gas flow must be stopped and troubleshooting with the anesthesiologist should identify the cause of the problem. If a CO_2 embolization is suspected or diagnosed, the pneumoperitoneum has to be desufflated immediately. The patient should be placed in the Trendelenburg position and a left lateral decubitus position to prevent the gas from entering the pulmonary circulation and to minimize the airlock effect of the embolus within the right ventricle. Additionally, an aspiration of the gas via a central venous catheter can be attempted (See et al. 1993).

Unlike lesions caused by the Veress needle, injuries resulting from initial trocar placement often cannot be managed laparoscopically. Valuable time can be lost if the surgeon attempts to establish full laparoscopic access in order to identify and treat the complication endoscopically. Therefore, it is advisable to convert the case to an open procedure once a trocar lesion of an intraabdominal structure is suspected.

Exceptions to this rule are injuries of small vessels within the abdominal wall. These bleedings typically are inaccessible for electrocautery but they can be stopped by a laparoscopically placed suture ligation or alternatively by a ligation that is placed with the help of a Carter-Thompson fascial closure device (Inlet Medical, Eden Prairie, MN, USA) or similar device, and tied outside the body (Green et al. 1992).

Also, if a trocar-related injury exclusively involves bowel, the lesion can be managed endoscopically by the experienced laparoscopist (see Sect. 17.4.2.3 below).

Prevention

The keys to the prevention of access-related injuries are knowledge of the scope of possible complications as well as the surgeon's skills. Obviously, this comes with experience and Peters reported in a survey of complications in pediatric urological laparoscopy that the surgeon's experience was the best predictor of access-related complications (Peters 1996). However, Cadeddu et al. (2001) showed that intensive laparoscopic training prior to commencing clinical practice decreased the impact of the learning curve. The complication rate (access-related and non-access-related) of surgeons who completed at least 12 months of dedicated training in urological laparoscopy did not differ according to initial vs subsequent surgical experience (Cadeddu et al. 2001).

Proper knowledge of the vascular anatomy of the abdominal wall as well as understanding of the intraabdominal anatomy is necessary to minimize the risk of access-related injuries. Equally important is a thorough preoperative patient evaluation since specific variations of the individual anatomy (e.g., organomegaly, adhesions) can render a patient prone to these complications. Both obese and very slender patients are at higher risk of access-related complications (Chapron et al. 1997; Mendoza et al. 1996). Previous abdominal surgery significantly increases the risk of intraabdominal adhesions and access-related bowel injury (Brill et al. 1995; Lecuru et al. 2001). In these cases, it is advisable to choose the first entry site as far away from the area of previous surgery as possible. Secondary trocars should always be introduced under direct vision.

Careful surgical technique and adequate equipment are prerequisites for a safe laparoscopic access. If a cutting trocar is used, it is important that the cutting edges be very sharp in order to minimize the amount of axial force that has to be applied for trocar insertion. Less force allows for more control during trocar insertion (Kelty et al. 2000). It is not the sharpness of the trocar tip that is most dangerous for intraabdominal structures but inadvertent and uncontrolled movements of the trocar tip that result from excessive axial force. Accordingly, it is important to make sure that the patient's musculature is sufficiently relaxed by the time the first trocar is inserted. This helps to decrease the abdominal wall resistance and thereby reduces the amount of axial force that needs to be applied. Recently developed access systems are also designed to reduce axial forces. Expandable access systems convert axial into radial force (Schulam et al. 1999) and the trocarless rotational access cannula (TRAC) is a threaded, blunt-tip cannula that is radially advanced into the peritoneal cavity (Ternamian 1997).

Other technical advances such as springloaded safety shields that flip over the trocar blade once cutting resistance is no longer detected or visual obturators that permit trocar placement under direct visual control (String et al. 2001) have been brought into use to reduce the number of access-related complications. For the same reason, many laparoscopic surgeons have adopted an open access, where a Hasson cannula is inserted via a mini-laparotomy. The authors of a recent meta-analysis concluded that this open laparoscopy should be the preferred method of peritoneal access (Larobina and Nottle 2005).

However, none of these techniques or instruments is foolproof and none has been able to eliminate access complications in laparoscopic surgery. Also, no particular method of access has convincingly been shown to be superior (Gettman 2005; Moberg and Montgomery 2005). The authors' personal preference is to gain stepwise access under direct laparoscopic vision with the help of a visual obturator with a triggered cutting mechanism.

To decrease the risk of port-site hernias, all fascial defects greater than 10 mm (5 mm in children) need to be closed at the end of the procedure (Colegrove and Ramakumar 2005). If a trocar less than 10 mm in diameter is extensively manipulated during the operation, widening of the respective fascial defect may occur and primary closure should also be considered (Kulacoglu 2000). During closure of the port sites, care must be taken not to entrap bowel or injure other intraabdominal structures. Fascial closure devices such as the Carter-Thompson device allow for easy fascial reapproximation under direct vision. If a port site had to be extended to extract a specimen, fascial closure under direct laparoscopic vision is usually not possible. In these cases, however, the abdomen should be reinsufflated and the suture line inspected laparoscopically after the mini-laparotomy is closed.

17.4.2.2 Vascular Injury

With incidence rates between 1% and 2%, vascular injuries are not common; however, they represent the most frequently encountered and probably the most feared specific complication in urologic laparoscopic surgery. The majority of these injuries are not access-related but occur during dissection (Fahlenkamp et al. 1999; Gill et al. 1995; Meraney et al. 2002; Thiel et al. 1996). Most commonly, this results from inadequate exposure of the vascular structures, leading to either sharp or thermal injury to the vessel (Porter 2004). Additionally, orientation in laparoscopic surgery can be difficult because of a decreased number of reference points as well as a limited field of view, and this may lead to the misidentification of abdominal and retroperitoneal structures. Both transections of the inferior vena cava and the abdominal aorta have been described as rare complications of urologic laparoscopic surgery (McAllister et al. 2004; Sautter et al. 2001). Not surprisingly, the incidence of vascular injuries increases with the complexity of the procedure (Meraney et al. 2002; Nelson et al. 1999; Thiel et al. 1996) and decreases with the surgeon's experience (Guillonneau et al. 2002; Meraney et al. 2002; Peters 1996; Thiel et al. 1996).

Recognition

As in open surgery, early recognition of a vascular complication is the key to its successful management. Whereas the transection of a medium-sized or major artery is usually recognized immediately, the inadvertent ligation or stapler-transection of a vessel can easily go unnoticed during the course of the procedure. In addition, vascular lesions in the retroperitoneum or lacerations of mesenteric arteries often do not bleed briskly into the operative field and only become manifest in the postoperative period. Therefore a high level of suspicion has to be maintained throughout the entire laparoscopic procedure to recognize these injuries intraoperatively. Especially venous lesions can be missed intraoperatively because the pressure created from CO_2 insufflation may compress the injured vein and prevent it from oozing blood. Therefore it is advisable to release the pressure and inspect the operative field prior the completion of any laparoscopic operation.

Since most vascular lesions occur during dissection, the injured vessel typically is not yet fully exposed at the time of laceration. Locating the source of the bleeding can be a very challenging laparoscopic task.

In minor bleeding complications, suction and irrigation may be all that is needed to find the injured vessel, as a trail of blood within the puddle of irrigation fluid will lead directly to the target when the fluid is aspirated. However, if the bleeding is more pronounced, local compression of the respective area (as described below) is advisable. Through an assistant port, pooled blood in the operating field is constantly aspirated, and as soon as the bleeding discontinues one is sure that the compression is applied to the appropriate site. Under constant aspiration, the tamponade is then gradually removed to reveal the exact location of the bleeding source. If exposure is insufficient, the dissection of the field is carefully continued while pressure remains applied to the lesion. When the lacerated vessel cannot be identified and exposed satisfactorily despite these measures, no further time should be lost and conversion to an open procedure should be performed.

Management

Whereas in access-related vascular injuries it is recommended to convert to open surgery in order to control the bleeding, vascular injuries that occur during dissection after all the ports have been placed may be dealt with laparoscopically. The range of appropriate measures goes from simple application of pressure to immediate conversion to open surgery. Obviously, the optimal management of an intraoperative vascular complication depends on the severity of the case and the experience of the surgeon. In the individual case, the surgeon must make this decision based upon the respective situation and must choose the solution that least compromises patient safety and the goals of the actual procedure.

As in open surgery, the first step is the application of pressure to the source of the bleeding. Whereas in open surgery manual compression can be applied very quickly, in a laparoscopic case an effective tamponade requires a small laparotomy pad or at least a sponge gauze to be pressed onto the bleeding site via a laparoscopic instrument (e.g., a grasper). As an alternative, Yurkanin suggested the use of a Foley catheter that is inserted through one of the ports. The inflated catheter balloon can be pressed onto the bleeding site with a catheter guide (Yurkanin et al. 2005). Moreover, the intraabdominal pressure can be increased up to 25 mmHg temporarily to diminish venous bleeding. Blood pooling around the site of the lesion can then be aspirated and a slow retraction of the tamponade should reveal the source of the bleeding.

In a minor vascular injury, application of pressure for a couple of minutes alone may solve the problem. In addition, hemostyptic agents such as oxidized regenerated cellulose and fibrin glue may be applied alone or in combination. If there is adequate exposure of the injured vessel, electrocautery or application of clips can be enough to control the bleeding.

However, in a major vascular lesion these measures are insufficient and are likely to result merely in a loss of time and blood. Here a decision must be made: whether the respective blood vessel has to be repaired or not. If a repair is not necessary, an open or a laparoscopic suture ligation is most likely to stop the bleeding. In case the injured vessel is nicely exposed, the application of a stapling device might also be considered. Clearly, endoscopic management is more likely to be feasible if a repair does not have to be attempted. However, in the patient's best interest, this decision should not be biased by the desire to complete the procedure laparoscopically.

If the vessel needs to be repaired, endoscopic suturing of the laceration may be possible but should only be attempted by the highly experienced laparoscopic surgeon (Kavoussi 2000). The placement of additional ports can be helpful in such a situation, as it creates an opportunity to optimize distance and angle of the instruments toward the site of the lesion. In most cases of major vascular injury, however, it is advisable to convert to an open procedure and consider the consultation of a vascular surgeon.

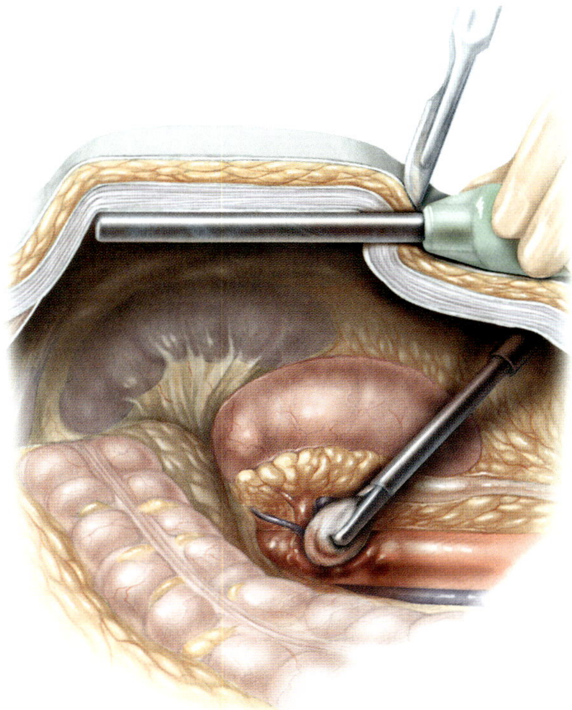

Fig. 17.4.1. Emergency conversion resulting from hemorrhage: The surgeon angles and pulls a midline trocar to the abdominal wall while cutting down on the shaft of this trocar with the other hand to gain open access to the abdomen. At the same time, the bleeding is controlled by compression via a laparoscopic instrument (e.g., grasper holding a small laparotomy pad or a sponge gauze) that has been introduced through another trocar. View from midline toward the left abdominal wall (© Hohenfellner 2007)

How to Perform an Emergency Conversion

In every laparoscopic procedure, however unlikely conversion to an open operation may be, an open laparotomy tray should be available in the room. In case of a vascular injury that necessitates conversion to an open procedure, the first step should be the compression of the bleeding area with a small laparotomy pad or a sponge gauze as outlined in the preceding section. If a major artery has been transected, however, it may be faster and more efficient to clamp the injured vessel with a suitable laparoscopic instrument. To minimize blood loss and to facilitate locating the injury, it is important to leave the instrument and the tamponade in place until the conversion is finished. For the conversion itself, a midline port can be used like a handle to pull the abdominal wall upwards. The incision is then made down to the shaft of this port (Gill et al. 2002) (Fig. 17.4.1). Once the peritoneal cavity is open the respective laparoscopic instrument is followed to the injured vessel.

Prevention

Vascular injuries are potentially catastrophic complications of laparoscopic surgery and they can at least jeopardize the successful outcome of the specific procedure. Therefore, prevention of these injuries is of utmost importance. Key to this prevention is a solid understanding of vascular anatomy in general as well as the vascular anatomy of the specific patient. In this regard, all available radiologic examinations should be carefully studied preoperatively. Especially prior to laparoscopic procedures that involve dissection of major vessels (e.g., renal surgery, retroperitoneal lymph node dissection [RPLND]) a radiologic examination, which shows the vascular anatomy in the region of interest should be obtained. Particularly in laparoscopic surgery with its two-dimensional vision and limited tactile feedback, it is essential to adhere to general surgical principles of a meticulous dissection. Preparation should always lead from the known to the unknown and no structure should be cut unless it is properly dissected and exposed.

17.4.2.3 Bowel Injury

Overall, bowel injury is a rare complication of laparoscopic surgery. In a recent retrospective analysis of 13 laparoscopic series in general surgery, gynecology and urology, 266 bowel complications occurred in a total of 205,969 cases. This corresponds to a combined incidence of 0.13 % (Bishoff et al. 1999). However, gynecologic procedures accounted for more than 50 % and urologic cases for only 0.44 % of the total volume of this review. In the urologic literature, slightly higher incidence rates between 0.2 % and 1.3 % are reported (Fahlenkamp et al. 1999; Guillonneau et al. 2003a; Kavoussi et al. 1993; Parra et al. 1994). This fact is most likely attributable to the higher number of complex surgical cases (e.g., laparoscopic radical prostatectomy, laparoscopic RPLND) included in the urologic series. The most commonly injured part of the intestine is the small bowel followed by the colon and the rarely injured stomach. Injuries of the duodenum are the most serious bowel complications of laparoscopic surgery as they are associated with the highest morbidity and mortality rates (El-Banna et al. 2000).

Recognition

Early recognition is very important for all types of laparoscopic complications, for bowel injuries, however, it is probably most crucial. In this case, a time delay can turn a minor intraoperative problem into a life-threatening condition. Roughly two out of three intestinal lesions that occur during laparoscopy are only diagnosed postoperatively (Bishoff et al. 1999; El-Banna et al. 2000) and up to one out of four patients with delayed presentation of a bowel lesion dies as a result of the complication (Chandler et al. 2001; El-Banna et al. 2000). However, these estimates may be too high since the true incidence of inadvertent and unrecognized bowel injury is not known (Voyles and Tucker 1992).

The bowel can basically be harmed by any kind of sharp or blunt instrument. Given the limited field of view inherent to laparoscopic surgery, such an injury can easily go unnoticed. Manipulation with instruments outside this field (e.g., during instrument changes) is prone to inadvertent violation of bowel and other intraabdominal structures. If a lesion cannot be seen directly, free intestinal contents are proof of a bowel laceration. Additionally, the escape of a fecal smell through an opened port valve must lead to a search for a bowel injury. If such a lesion is strongly suspected, the whole bowel has to be inspected meticulously, since moving small bowel loops and the greater omentum tends to hide an intestinal lesion. Even the spontaneous temporary closure of such defects has been reported (Schafer et al. 2001). Furthermore, the possibility of two or more concomitant injuries has to be taken into consideration.

Electrocautery-induced thermal damage is the single most frequent origin of bowel injury during laparoscopic surgery. In Bishoff's comprehensive review, this form accounted for 50 % of all bowel lesions (Bishoff et al. 1999). Typically, this injury is missed intraoperatively because of the delayed breakdown of the intestinal wall (Philips and Bishoff 2005). So again it is the surgeon's knowledge of possible mechanisms of electrosurgical injury combined with a high index of suspicion throughout the entire procedure that can lead to the detection of as yet invisible bowel lesions. The four mechanisms of electrocautery-induced thermal damage during laparoscopic surgery are inappropriate direct activation of the electrocautery, coupling to another instrument, insulation failure, and capacitive coupling (Gill et al. 2002). The typical situation where capacitive coupling can occur is when an insulated active electrode (e.g., monopolar laparoscopic scissors) is introduced through a metal cannula. Through an electrostatic field that is created between the active electrode and the cannula, the current in the electrode can induce a current in the cannula.

Management

Once an intestinal injury is recognized intraoperatively, it can be safely managed laparoscopically in most cases (Nezhat et al. 1993; Reich 1992). However, if there is any question as to the integrity of the repair or if the patient had prior radiation therapy, open repair and consultation of a general surgeon should be considered (Porter 2004). The laceration should be oversewn in one or two layers if small bowel is involved. Lesions of the colon and the rectum should always be closed in two layers. In simple lesions, it is usually not necessary to resect the injured bowel segment. It is advisable to oversew also small serosal abrasions, since these minor lesions can cause major postoperative complications if they are left unattended during the initial laparoscopic procedure (Bishoff et al. 1999). Immediate repair of a bowel injury does not require intestinal diversion even if the rectum is involved (Guillonneau et al. 2003b; Reich 1992), and it usually does not have a significant impact on the postoperative course and the length of hospital stay.

The management of electrothermal injuries of the bowel differs to some extent from the management of simple lacerations. If a thermal injury is caused by bipolar electrocautery, it may be excised and the bowel wall defect may be simply closed as long as the lesion is small in diameter. If more than half of the circumference of the bowel segment is involved, the respective segment needs to be resected and an end-to-end anastomosis should be performed (Abdel-Meguid and Gomella 1996). In injuries that are caused by monopolar electrocautery, on the other hand, the extension of the tissue damage is typically underestimated. Therefore, any monopolar electrothermal lesion necessitates resection and end-to-end anastomosis of the involved bowel segment. Additionally, a safety margin of several centimeters on either side of the injury should be resected before the completion of the end-to-end anastomosis (Gill et al. 2002).

Again, all these steps may be performed laparoscopically by the highly experienced endoscopic surgeon. Considering the high morbidity of postoperative intestinal complications, a surgeon who does not feel absolutely confident with advanced laparoscopic bowel surgery is strongly advised to convert to an open procedure or consult a general surgeon.

Prevention

Prevention of bowel injuries during urologic laparoscopic surgery seems to be difficult since experienced laparoscopic surgeons are reported to cause an equal rate of intraoperative bowel lesions as inexperienced surgeons (El-Banna et al. 2000). Nevertheless, there are recommendations that may help to avoid these rare but dangerous complications.

Routine use of a nasogastric tube to empty the stomach reduces the risk of injury to the stomach. Also, preoperative bowel preparation may reduce inadvertent intestinal trauma by increasing intraperitoneal free space and by facilitating operative maneuvers (Li et al. 1997). Especially for the inexperienced laparoscopic surgeon and assistant, it is advisable to introduce any new instrument under direct visual control in order to prevent inadvertent bowel injury outside the field of view. Likewise a laparoscopic instrument that is not in use must always be removed from the patient.

To avoid electrothermal trauma, all laparoscopic instruments must be checked for insulation damage prior to their use. Bipolar electrocautery should be used whenever possible and all diathermy must be avoided close to the bowel. Monopolar electrocautery should not be used to take down bowel adhesions. The lowest possible power setting should be used at all times (Saye et al. 1991). The electric energy should only be activated when the entire active part of the instrument is visualized and the tip of the instrument is in contact with the target. To prevent duodenal injury in right-sided renal or adrenal procedures, medial reflection of the duodenum by the Kocher maneuver must be performed using blunt and sharp dissection only. The use of thermal energy must be strictly avoided during this step of the procedure.

Innovative instruments such as Ligasure (Valleylab, Boulder, CO, USA), which uses a high-current low-voltage output, or the Harmonic Scalpel (Johnson & Johnson, Brunswick, NJ, USA), which uses ultrasonic energy for both cutting and coagulation, minimize the spread of thermal energy and thereby may reduce the risk of inadvertent bowel injury.

In patients who are at risk of bowel injury (i.e., patients with a history of abdominal surgery), an adequate means of prevention may be not to offer the patient laparoscopic surgery in the first place. Extensive adhesiolysis must be considered an advanced laparoscopic procedure and it should therefore remain in the hands of the experienced endoscopic surgeon. Alternatively, in patients with prior abdominal surgery and/or radiation therapy, a retroperitoneoscopic approach may be considered. It has recently been shown that retroperitoneoscopic renal and adrenal surgery can be performed in these patients without increasing the perioperative morbidity or the convalescence (Viterbo et al. 2005). However, intraoperative orientation can be very difficult in case a surgeon is unfamiliar with retroperitoneoscopy and bowel complications have also been reported with this approach (Meraney et al. 2002). In a prospective randomized comparison of transperitoneal versus retroperitoneal laparoscopic radical nephrectomy in the general patient population no significant difference in bowel complications was found (Desai et al. 2005).

17.4.2.4 Injuries to Other Intraabdominal Structures

In this subdivision, less common intraoperative complications of laparoscopic surgery are discussed briefly. Lesions of the urinary bladder and the ureter are included for the sake of completeness, although they are not usually an emergency for the urologic surgeon.

Bladder Injury

Bladder injuries during laparoscopic surgery are most commonly associated with gynecological procedures (Hasson and Parker 1998). Incidence rates in the respective literature range from 0.02% to 8.3% (Ostrzenski and Ostrzenska 1998; Vakili et al. 2005). The bladder dome was found to be the most frequent site of bladder injury.

If a bladder lesion is not obvious or not immediately recognized, the finding of gas and/or blood in the urethral catheter bag should cause the laparoscopic surgeon to look for any laceration in the bladder. Irrigation of the bladder via the urethral catheter can help to locate the lesion (Gill et al. 2002). Once detected, any defect in the bladder wall can be closed with an absorbable single-layer running suture, which most endourological surgeons will be able to complete laparoscopically. Depending on the size of the lesion, the Foley catheter should be left to continuously drain the repaired bladder for up to 10 days postoperatively. An easy and effective measure to prevent intraoperative bladder injuries is the routine preoperative placement of a Foley catheter in all patients undergoing laparoscopic procedures.

Ureteral Injury

In a recent review of laparoscopic pelvic surgery, incidences of ureteral injury between 0.03% and 2% were reported (Ostrzenski et al. 2003). The mechanisms of injury include transection, ligation, electrothermal injury, and interruption of the ureteral blood supply (Chow 2005). Unfortunately, the majority of these lesions are not recognized intraoperatively (Ostrzenski et al. 2003; Thomas et al. 1996), which means that a high level of suspicion needs to be maintained throughout a pelvic or retroperitoneal laparoscopic procedure in order to detect a ureteral injury during the initial surgery. If a ureteral injury is suspected, intraoperative diagnosis can be facilitated by the intravenous administration of methylene blue or indigo carmine. Additionally, a retrograde or an antegrade pyelography can help identify the exact location of the lesion. When recognized intraoperatively, laparoscopic repair can be attempted depending on the surgeon's level of expertise. As in open surgery, the optimal management is conditional on the location and the extent of the ureteral lesion. Ureteroureterostomy, ureteroneocystostomy, psoas hitch, or a Boari flap can be performed laparoscopically by the skilled surgeon (Chow 2005). It is important to understand that also nonperforating mechanical (e.g., clamping of the ureter) or thermoelectrical ureteral lesions should be addressed immediately. The respective ureteral segment needs to be excised and the appropriate repair done laparoscopically or in an open procedure. In every case of repair, a ureteral stent should be inserted and left in place for 2–6 weeks.

To prevent ureteral injuries, the laparoscopic surgeon needs a thorough understanding of the intraoperative pelvic and retroperitoneal anatomy. If a surgical procedure involves dissection close to a ureter, this ureter should be identified beforehand. When dissecting a ureter, great care must be taken not to interrupt its blood supply. To avoid electrothermal injury, monopolar current should never be used close to the ureter. Furthermore, routine preoperative ureteral stenting has been advocated in cases where a difficult pelvic dissection is expected (Leff et al. 1982). However, recent reviews have shown that this measure does not affect the rate of ureteral injuries, even though it might help facilitate intraoperative detection of a respective lesion (Bothwell et al. 1994; Kuno et al. 1998).

Injuries of the Liver and the Gallbladder

Non-access-related injury of the liver during urologic laparoscopic surgery is rare. It may complicate right-sided renal or adrenal procedures and it is usually caused by inappropriate retraction of the liver (Ogan and Cadeddu 2005). Alternatively, a tear in the liver surface can result when adhesions to the liver are strained. Usually, liver injuries are easily recognized because of the bleeding, although minor parenchymal bleedings may be concealed by the high intraabdominal pressure due to the pneumoperitoneum. It is therefore advisable to desufflate the abdomen at the end of every laparoscopic procedure and check again for any sources of bleeding.

Injuries of the gallbladder in laparoscopic surgery are very rare and they typically occur during difficult dissection of the right renal upper pole or at the retraction of the liver. In a large single-center experience, these injuries complicated only 0.28% of all laparoscopic procedures performed on the upper urinary tract (Varkarakis et al. 2005).

Minor hepatic injuries may be managed expectantly. If the bleeding is too pronounced or does not stop spontaneously, hemostasis may be achieved with an argon beam coagulator. Additionally, oxidized regenerated cellulose can be sealed onto the laceration using the argon beam coagulator, and fibrin glue can be applied to the lesion. More extensive injuries, which do not respond to these measures, should prompt a general surgical consult and they will typically result in a conversion to an open procedure.

Nonperforating injuries of the gallbladder such as electrothermal lesions can be managed expectantly with placement of a closed suction drain in the gallbladder fossa and observation (Varkarakis et al. 2005). Perforating injuries, on the other hand, should result in cholecystectomy right away with a general surgical consult as needed.

To prevent liver injuries during laparoscopic procedures, all adhesions to the liver must be taken down carefully at the beginning of the dissection. If the liver has to be retracted during the procedure the surgeon has to make sure that this is done in a safe and nontraumatic way. There are a number of different commercially available retractors for this purpose. A sim-

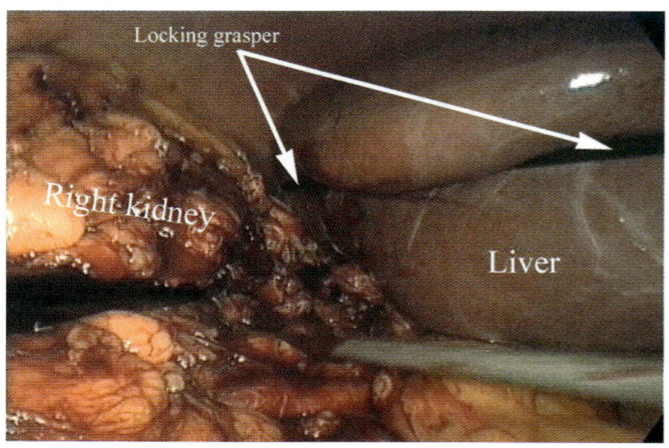

Fig. 17.4.2. To optimize exposure of the right adrenal or upper pole of the right kidney safely, a locking grasper is placed under the edge of the liver from medial to lateral. The liver is then retracted upward and held in place by locking the grasper to the lateral abdominal wall

ple, safe, and very effective way to retract the liver during laparoscopic renal or adrenal surgery is illustrated in Fig. 17.4.2. As long as the respective case and the surgeon's ability allow for it, a retroperitoneal approach can be adopted for another prevention strategy to avoid liver injuries.

Splenic Injury

The mechanisms leading to splenic injuries during laparoscopic surgery are the same as described for laparoscopic liver injuries. Splenic capsular lesions most commonly occur during the exposure of the retroperitoneum in left-sided renal or adrenal procedures. In recent reviews, iatrogenic lesions of the spleen complicated 0.5%–2.5% of laparoscopic and hand-assisted laparoscopic nephrectomies (Hedican 2004; Melcher et al. 2005; Siqueira et al. 2002). In another review that included open nephrectomies, splenic injuries were reported in 4%–13% of the cases, and the authors suspected that iatrogenic splenic injuries are generally underreported in the literature (Cassar and Munro 2002). Intraoperative recognition usually is not a difficulty in splenic lesions but as in other parenchymatous bleedings, reduction of the intraabdominal pressure can help to identify the injury.

The majority of splenic injuries during urologic laparoscopic surgery are minor capsular lesions, which usually can be managed laparoscopically (Hedican 2004). Measures to control these injuries include pressure and the application of oxidized regenerated cellulose, absorbable gelatin sponges, and fibrin glue as well as coagulation with the argon beam coagulator (Canby-Hagino et al. 2000; Hedican 2004; Melcher et al. 2005). More extensive splenic lacerations typically result in open conversion and splenectomy.

The key to preventing intraoperative lesions of the spleen is to avoid traction on the splenic capsule. Therefore any adhesions to the spleen as well as the splenocolic ligaments have to be taken down or incised very carefully during the exposure of the retroperitoneum. Great care must also be taken not to injure the delicate organ with retractors or any pointed laparoscopic instrument, especially when the tip of the respective tool is not in the field of view. If practicable and appropriate, a retroperitoneoscopic approach may reduce the risk of iatrogenic injury to the spleen.

Pancreatic Injury

Due to the close anatomical relationship of the pancreas and the hilum of the spleen, laparoscopic splenectomy is the endoscopic procedure with the highest rate of pancreatic complications. Incidences of up to 15% are reported in the general surgery literature (Chand et al. 2001). Large series of urologic laparoscopic procedures have reported general incidences of pancreatic lesions of 0.2%–0.4% (Fahlenkamp et al. 1999; Gill et al. 1998; Varkarakis et al. 2004). In laparoscopic left radical nephrectomies, however, the incidence of pancreatic complications was found to be 2.1% and in laparoscopic left adrenalectomies this rate was as high as 8.6% (Varkarakis et al. 2004). The pancreatic injury typically occurs during dissection of adjacent structures and it very easily remains unrecognized during the initial operation. Apart from direct observation there is no reliable sign that helps to detect a pancreatic lesion intraoperatively. If a pancreatic injury is recognized intraoperatively, its management depends on the severity of the trauma. Whereas a contusion or a superficial tear without laceration of a pancreatic duct does not need any repair, a more extensive injury has to be oversewn. Alternatively, the lesion can be closed with an endoscopic linear stapler as it is used to close the pancreatic stump in laparoscopic resection of the distal pancreas (Tagaya et al. 2003). Based on the experience gained in a porcine model, the application of a collagen-based sealant has been advocated recently for the treatment pancreatic lesions (Rosen et al. 2004). With every pancreatic injury, a drain must be placed in the peripancreatic region. Postoperatively, this drain should be left in place until the drainage is less than 50 ml/24 h and the amylase levels of the drainage are consistent with serum amylase levels (Varkarakis et al. 2004). Additionally, oral feeding should be withheld until the patient is asymptomatic and has no biochemical evidence of pancreatitis and no evidence of pancreatic fistula. The prevention of pancreatic injury during urologic laparoscopic surgery again demands solid knowledge of the retroperitoneal anatomy and a high level of suspicion during the procedure. Since pancreatic lesions are commonly unrecognized intraoperatively, the placement of a drain into the surgical bed has been proposed if difficulty with the dissection is experienced in an upper tract procedure (Varkarakis et al. 2004). This way the delayed diagnosis of a pancreatic injury can be facilitated and further complications as well as secondary interventions can be prevented.

17.4.2.5 Pleural Injury

Whereas in open nephrectomy inadvertent entry into the pleural space is not uncommon and usually unproblematic, diaphragmatic and pleural injuries are rare but potentially severe complications of urologic laparoscopic surgery. Because of the high intraabdominal pressure associated with laparoscopy, insufflated gas can enter the thorax through a diaphragmatic lesion and lead to ipsilateral pneumothorax and pneumomediastinum. Recently a large multicenter series reported an incidence of pleural injury during laparoscopic renal surgery of 0.6% (Del Pizzo et al. 2003). In this series, two out of ten pleural injuries were access-related and 80% occurred during dissection.

Recognition

Typically a lesion in the diaphragm occurs during the dissection of the renal upper pole. A tear in the diaphragm is not necessarily visible, as electrocautery-induced thermal damage can also injure the pleura. If an injury to the pleura is not directly observed, there are signs of pneumothorax that can be recognized intraoperatively. Voyles and Madden described the floppy diaphragm sign, which refers to the billowing of the diaphragm into the abdomen with every reduction of intraabdominal pressure (Voyles and Madden 1998). This sign reflects a loss of the negative pressure in the pleural space and should prompt a search for a diaphragmatic injury. Additionally, the anesthesiologist may notice a decrease in oxygen saturation, an increase in airway pressures and end-tidal CO_2 as well as reduced breath sounds over the respective hemithorax and hemodynamic instability as a result of the pneumothorax (Potter et al. 2001). Characteristically, these symptoms ameliorate with desufflation of the abdomen and aggravate again when the pneumoperitoneum is reestablished.

Management

Diaphragmatic and pleural injuries that occur during urologic laparoscopic procedures can usually be managed endoscopically and in general an insertion of a thoracostomy tube is not needed. Basically, the diaphragmatic lesion needs to be oversewn and the air or gas needs to be evacuated from the pleural cavity. If the ventilation and the hemodynamic situation of the patient allow it, the procedure may be continued with a lower intraabdominal pressure as needed; the pleural injury may be addressed only at the end of the operation. In doing so (in cases of nephrectomy, upper pole resection, or adrenalectomy), there may be better visualization of the iatrogenic lesion as well as more space to perform the repair than at the time the injury took place. In an extensive injury, a concomitant lesion of the lung may be ruled out or detected by feeding the laparoscope through the diaphragmatic defect.

The diaphragmatic lesion should be sutured with interrupted stitches. This way, the suction device can be passed into the pleural cavity between the sutures and the gas can be evacuated from the thorax before those stitches are tied. Also, the patient can be given a large inspiratory breath before securing the sutures (Del Pizzo 2005). Alternatively, a 6-F central line can be modified by cutting extra side holes and introduced anteriorly through the fifth or sixth intercostal space to evacuate the gas (Del Pizzo et al. 2003).

In case sufficient repair of the diaphragmatic injury cannot be achieved, the placement of a thoracostomy tube must be considered.

Prevention

Diaphragmatic and pleural injuries rarely occur during urologic laparoscopic surgery, but they also happen to the highly experienced laparoscopist. There are no specific preventive measures that can be taken to avoid this type of complication. Probably the best prevention is the awareness of the possibility of this injury, especially during the difficult cases of renal upper pole dissection.

17.4.2.6 Stapler-Related Complications

Successful laparoscopic surgery relies heavily on a variety of sophisticated technical equipment. Laparoscopic endovascular staplers have facilitated the endoscopic control of large vessels and they are widely used in donor nephrectomies as well as in nephrectomies for benign or malignant disease. However, laparoscopic staplers have (as any mechanical device) the potential to malfunction and thereby cause very serious intraoperative complications. In two recent reviews, the incidence of stapler-related complications during laparoscopic nephrectomy was 1.1% and 1.7%, respectively (Chan et al. 2000; Deng et al. 2002). In the majority of the cases, the complication was not caused by a primary mechanical failure of the device but was a result of its inappropriate application and was therefore preventable.

Recognition

The absence of the proximal staple line is likely the scariest failure of a laparoscopic linear cutting stapler. This very rare situation usually leads to the uncontrolled transection of one or more large vessels of the renal hilum, which obviously results in profuse bleeding. Fortunately, most stapler-related problems are less spectacular and less evident. Awareness of situations that lead to device malfunction or inadvertent stapler-induced injury may help to prevent or at least recognize these complications in a timely fashion. The laparoscopic surgeon must be familiar with the proper mechanisms of device closure, activation, and removal in order to recognize any irregularities. If the staple deployment is not smooth, a misfire has to be suspected. No excessive force should be used to activate the device. It has been reported that the safety interlock of the stapler can be overcome and the device can thereby be forced to refire an empty cartridge (Deng et al. 2002), which leads to the drastic complication mentioned above. When the stapler is placed, attention must be paid to the correct closure of the jaws of the instrument. If an abnormal closure is observed, the device must not be fired but must be removed and checked for proper function.

The most common reason for a stapler malfunction, however, is the firing of the staples over a previously placed vascular clip (Chan et al. 2000). If a clip is noticed between the jaws of the instrument after the deployment of the device, misalignment of the staples is likely and an additional ligation of the respective blood vessel should be performed prior to the release of the stapler.

Management

If bleeding is excessive or laparoscopic management is not possible, conversion for open definitive repair should be considered early (Chan 2005). However, most stapler malfunctions can be managed laparoscopically (Chan et al. 2000; Deng et al. 2002). If a stapler malfunction is recognized or suspected, the device should not be opened and the proximal stump of the respective vessel should be additionally controlled by a second stapler, clips, or ligation. If the malfunction is recognized only after the stapler has been removed, direct pressure on the site will stop the bleeding until sufficient overview is reestablished and the source of the bleeding is identified. Definitive control can then be achieved by another stapler, application of vascular clips, or oversewing the lesion.

Prevention

Again prevention of stapler-related complications during urologic laparoscopic surgery starts with the surgeon's complete knowledge regarding the working mechanisms of the stapling device. Intraoperatively, vascular clips should be used sparingly around the renal hilum when the application of an endovascular stapler is considered. Accordingly, when the stapler is brought in, great care must be taken not to place the staple rows over a clip. Before the device is activated, the surgeon must make sure that only the structures that need to be ligated and transected are included between the jaws of the instrument and that these structures are covered by the staple rows to their full extent. Consideration of the issues listed in Sect. 17.4.2.6.1 will also help to prevent stapler malfunction.

To avoid the rare but potentially catastrophic situation of transection of the vessel by the stapler without deployment of the proximal row of staples, a noncutting staple device can be used, allowing the vessel to be cut manually once the appropriate alignment of the staples has been confirmed. Obviously, all stapler-related injuries can be avoided when the transection of the renal hilum or the respective blood vessel is done without the help of a stapling device. For this reason some authors have proposed using vascular clips and ligatures only to control the renal artery and vein (Janetschek et al. 2003).

17.4.3 Postoperative Complications

In laparoscopic surgery with its limited field of view, an intraoperative injury of an abdominal organ is more likely to go unnoticed during the initial procedure than in open surgery. The respective lesions may cause delayed complications and they can lead to an early secondary intervention. Two large series reported reintervention rates after urologic laparoscopic surgery of 0.7 % – 1 % (Soulie et al. 2001; Yaycioglu et al. 2002) and a recent overview of the urologic literature found 1.5 % repeat explorations in a total of more than 4,000 laparoscopic cases (Yaycioglu 2005). This section will not cover the large variety of possible late complications after laparoscopic surgery but only vascular and bowel complications that may need immediate attention.

17.4.3.1 Vascular Complications

Vascular complications contribute to a substantial share of the early postoperative complications after urologic laparoscopic procedures (Yaycioglu 2005). In a recent report, the majority of hemorrhagic complications of laparoscopic partial nephrectomies occurred postoperatively or after the patient's discharge from the hospital (Ramani et al. 2005). Different reasons lead to a delayed manifestation of vascular injuries. An injured vessel can remain undetected during the procedure because of the compression caused by the pneumoperitoneum, due to a vasospasm or a partial ligation. A splenic tear can typically manifest itself only in the postoperative period. A vascular complication that is also prone to delayed recognition is the inadvertent ligation of an artery that will lead to the partial or total infarction and necrosis of the respective organ. A rare but specific vascular complication that can be dangerous and that seems to be more common in laparoscopic surgery than in its open counterpart is the formation of a renal artery pseudoaneurysm following laparoscopic partial nephrectomy (Singh and Gill 2005).

Recognition

As the overall incidence of these complications is low and symptoms may be unspecific. A high index of suspicion is needed in the postoperative period to recognize and treat these potentially dangerous lesions in time. Possible symptoms of late vascular complications include but are not limited to general malaise, abdominal or flank pain, dizziness or syncope, hypotension, tachycardia, decreasing hemoglobin and hematocrit, gross hematuria, bloody drainage from a surgical drain in the operative field, nausea, vomiting, absent pulses, fever, and renal insufficiency.

In patients with clinically significant findings and nondiagnostic routine examinations, a CT scan is the examination of choice (Fig. 17.4.3). A CT can reliably identify the site of postoperative bleeding (Cadeddu et al. 1997). Angiography is a second-line investigation that may provide important additional information if persistent active bleeding is suspected. Angiography also offers the possibility of a concomitant therapeutic intervention (i.e., embolization of a bleeding vessel).

Management

If a postoperative CT scan reveals a hematoma, conservative treatment with transfusion of red blood cells if necessary and observation are often sufficient. With persistent hemodynamic instability, however, active management is needed. If the situation allows it, angiography and possibly embolization of the bleeding vessel is the least invasive intervention. Angiographic embolization is also the treatment of choice for renal artery pseudoaneurysms and arteriovenous malformations (Fig. 17.4.4). If an angiographic procedure is unsuitable or not successful, surgical exploration is necessary. A laparoscopic approach may be attempted, but most cases of significant postoperative bleeding complications ultimately have to be managed by an open approach. With patient safety as the ultimate priority, the surgeon must make sure that no time is wasted with a pointless attempt to treat the complication laparoscopically. In cases of inadvertent ligation of a blood vessel, vascular or general surgery consultation should be obtained as required, and the need for resection of the respective organ or revascularization must be determined based upon the individual situation.

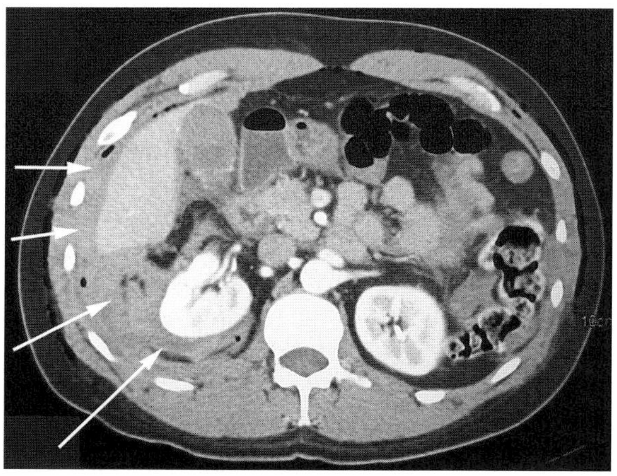

Fig. 17.4.3. Intravenous contrast-enhanced abdominal CT scan of a patient who had a pronounced drop in hematocrit 1 day after right partial nephrectomy. The high-density fluid (*arrows*) that extends from the partial nephrectomy site is compatible with hemorrhage

17.4.3.2 Bowel Complications

In laparoscopic surgery, bowel injuries account for 76% of all complications with a delay in diagnosis of more than 24 h (Chandler et al. 2001). Approximately 50% of all bowel injuries are caused by electrocautery (Bishoff et al. 1999), and thermal injuries typically present later than nonthermal injuries as a result of delayed breakdown of the intestinal wall at the injury site (Philips and Bishoff 2005). Early diagnosis and immediate repair of unrecognized bowel injuries are of utmost importance since longer delays are associated with a significantly higher mortality (Chandler et al. 2001).

Recognition

For unrecognized bowel lesions, the time from surgery to presentation is approximately 5 days on average, and some lesions become clinically apparent more than 4 weeks after the initial procedure depending upon the mechanism of injury as well as the bowel segment involved (Bishoff et al. 1999). Confounding factors such as pain medication and antibiotics can render the postoperative diagnosis of a bowel complication difficult. In addition, delayed bowel complications of laparoscopic surgery have been reported to often present in an atypical way with low-grade temperature, low to normal white blood count, no ileus, and no signs of peritonitis (Philips and Bishoff 2005; Thompson and Wheeless 1973). In a recent review, the initial presenting complaints of all patients with unrecognized bowel injury after laparoscopic surgery was persistent and relatively extreme pain at the trocar site closest to the bowel injury, abdominal distention, diarrhea with persistent bowel sounds, and absence of severe abdominal pain or peritoneal signs. No purulence or erythema was noted at any trocar site (Bishoff et al. 1999).

If an unrecognized bowel injury is clinically suspected, an abdominal CT scan with oral contrast medium should be obtained. This examination reliably identifies bowel perforations as well as other abdominal pathology in the early postoperative period and can help to plan appropriate therapeutic interventions (Cadeddu et al. 1997; Daly et al. 1996).

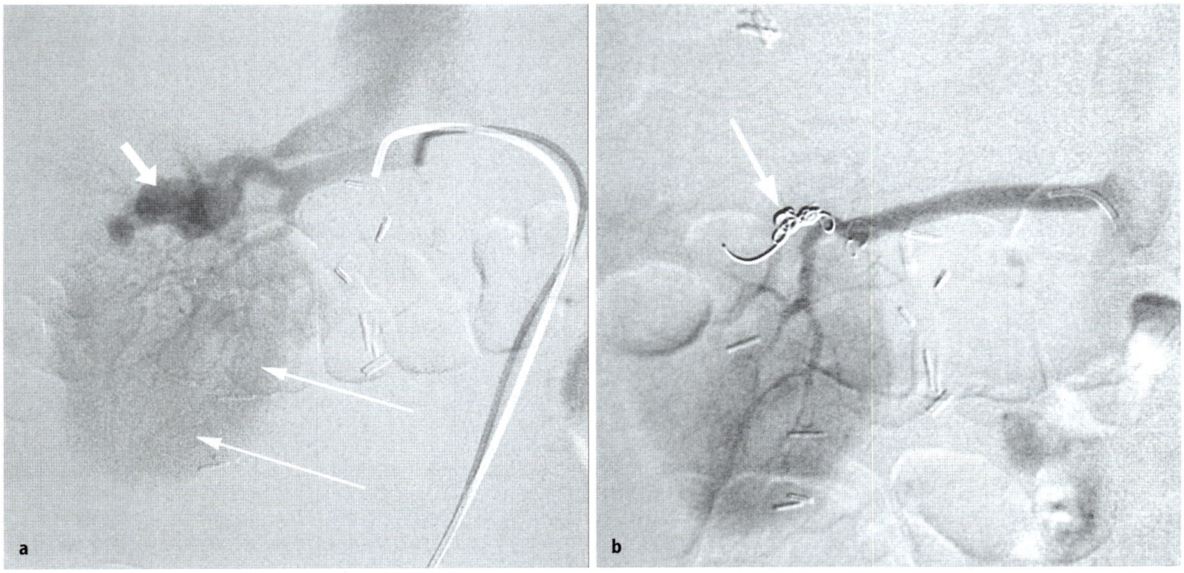

Fig. 17.4.4a, b. Arteriogram of a patient who presented with massive hematuria after right laparoscopic partial nephrectomy. **a** Lower pole (*long arrows*) of the right kidney and arteriovenous malformation (*short arrow*) in the region of the former resection. The contrast media flows immediately into the renal vein. **b** The *arrow* shows the coils in the arteriovenous malformation after successful embolization. No contrast media is seen in the renal vein or the inferior vena cava

Management

Once a previously unrecognized bowel injury is diagnosed, immediate repair is indicated. Whereas in intraoperatively recognized bowel lesions a laparoscopic repair is usually feasible and bowel diversion is generally not necessary, almost all bowel lesions with delayed recognition will need an open repair (Bishoff et al. 1999; van der Voort et al. 2004). Bowel diversion may be necessary depending on the individual case and it may be advisable to obtain a general surgery consultation.

References

Abdel-Meguid TA, Gomella LG (1996) Prevention and management of complications. In: Smith AD, Badlani GH, Bagley DH, Clayman RV, Jordan GH, Kavoussi LR, Lingeman JE, Preminger GM, Segura JW (eds) Smith's textbook of endourology. Quality Medical, St. Louis, p 851

Bateman BG, Kolp LA, Hoeger K (1996) Complications of laparoscopy–operative and diagnostic. Fertil Steril 66:30

Bishoff JT, Allaf ME, Kirkels W, Moore RG, Kavoussi LR, Schroder F (1999) Laparoscopic bowel injury: incidence and clinical presentation. J Urol 161:887

Bothwell WN, Bleicher RJ, Dent TL (1994) Prophylactic ureteral catheterization in colon surgery. A five-year review. Dis Colon Rectum 37:330

Brill AI, Nezhat F, Nezhat CH, Nezhat C (1995) The incidence of adhesions after prior laparotomy: a laparoscopic appraisal. Obstet Gynecol 85:269

Cadeddu JA, Regan F, Kavoussi LR, Moore RG (1997) The role of computerized tomography in the evaluation of complications after laparoscopic urological surgery. J Urol 158:1349

Cadeddu JA, Wolfe JS Jr, Nakada S, Chen R, Shalhav A, Bishoff JT, Hamilton B, Schulam PG, Dunn M, Hoenig D, Fabrizio M, Hedican S, Averch TD (2001) Complications of laparoscopic procedures after concentrated training in urological laparoscopy. J Urol 166:2109

Canby-Hagino ED, Morey AF, Jatoi I, Perahia B, Bishoff JT (2000) Fibrin sealant treatment of splenic injury during open and laparoscopic left radical nephrectomy. J Urol 164:2004

Cassar K, Munro A (2002) Iatrogenic splenic injury. J R Coll Surg Edinb 47:731

Champault G, Cazacu F, Taffinder N (1996) Serious trocar accidents in laparoscopic surgery: a French survey of 103,852 operations. Surg Laparosc Endosc 6:367

Chan D, Bishoff JT, Ratner L, Kavoussi LR, Jarrett TW (2000) Endovascular gastrointestinal stapler device malfunction during laparoscopic nephrectomy: early recognition and management. J Urol 164:319

Chan DY (2005) Stapler malfunction and management. In: Ramakumar S, Jarrett T (eds) Complications of urologic laparoscopic surgery. Taylor & Francis, Boca Raton, p 43

Chand B, Walsh RM, Ponsky J, Brody F (2001) Pancreatic complications following laparoscopic splenectomy. Surg Endosc 15:1273

Chandler JG, Corson SL, Way LW (2001) Three spectra of laparoscopic entry access injuries. J Am Coll Surg 192:478; discussion 490

Chapron CM, Pierre F, Lacroix S, Querleu D, Lansac J, Dubuisson JB (1997) Major vascular injuries during gynecologic laparoscopy. J Am Coll Surg 185:461

Chow GK (2005) Urinary leak complications of laparoscopy. In: S Ramakumar T Jarrett (2005) Complications of Urologic Laparoscopic Surgery. Taylor & Francis Group. Boca Raton

Colegrove P, Ramakumar S, Hernia. In: Ramakumar S, Jarrett T (eds) Complications of urologic laparoscopic surgery. Taylor & Francis, Boca Raton, p 115

Daly B, Sukumar SA, Krebs TL, Wong JJ, Flowers JL (1996) Nonbiliary laparoscopic gastrointestinal surgery: role of CT

in diagnosis and management of complication. AJR Am J Roentgenol 167:455
Del Pizzo JJ (2005) Pleural injury during laparoscopic renal surgery. In: Ramakumar S, Jarrett T (eds) Complications of urologic laparoscopic surgery. Taylor & Francis, Boca Raton, p 83
Del Pizzo JJ, Jacobs SC, Bishoff JT, Kavoussi LR, Jarrett TW (2003) Pleural injury during laparoscopic renal surgery: early recognition and management. J Urol 169:41
Deng DY, Meng MV, Nguyen HT, Bellman GC, Stoller ML (2002) Laparoscopic linear cutting stapler failure. Urology 60:415; discussion 419
Desai MM, Strzempkowski B, Matin SF, Steinberg AP, Ng C, Meraney AM, Kaouk JH, Gill IS (2005) Prospective randomized comparison of transperitoneal versus retroperitoneal laparoscopic radical nephrectomy. J Urol 173:38
Deziel DJ, Millikan KW, Economou SG, Doolas A, Ko ST, Airan MC (1993) Complications of laparoscopic cholecystectomy: a national survey of 4,292 hospitals and an analysis of 77,604 cases. Am J Surg 165:9
El-Banna M, Abdel-Atty M, El-Meteini M, Aly S (2000) Management of laparoscopic-related bowel injuries. Surg Endosc 14:779
Fahlenkamp D, Rassweiler J, Fornara P, Frede T, Loening SA (1999) Complications of laparoscopic procedures in urology: experience with 2,407 procedures at 4 German centers. J Urol 162:765; discussion 770
Gettman MT (2005) Complications of laparoscopic access. In: Ramakumar S, Jarrett T (eds) Complications of urologic laparoscopic surgery. Taylor & Francis, Boca Raton, p 13
Gill IS, Kavoussi LR, Clayman RV, Ehrlich R, Evans R, Fuchs G, Gersham A, Hulbert JC, McDougall EM, Rosenthal T et al (1995) Complications of laparoscopic nephrectomy in 185 patients: a multi-institutional review. J Urol 154:479
Gill IS, Clayman RV, Albala DM, Aso Y, Chiu AW, Das S, Donovan JF, Fuchs GJ, Gaur DD, Go H, Gomella LG, Grune MT, Harewood LM, Janetschek G, Knapp PM, McDougall EM, Nakada SY, Preminger GM, Puppo P, Rassweiler JJ, Royce PL, Thomas R, Urban DA, Winfield HN (1998) Retroperitoneal and pelvic extraperitoneal laparoscopy: an international perspective. Urology 52:566
Gill IS, Kerbl K, Meraney AM, Clayman RV (2002) Basic principles techniques, and equipment of laparoscopic surgery. In: Walsh PC, Retik AB, Vaughan ED, Wein AJ (eds) Campbell's urology. Saunders, Philadelphia, p 3455
Green LS, Loughlin KR, Kavoussi LR (1992) Management of epigastric vessel injury during laparoscopy. J Endourol 2:99
Guillonneau B, Rozet F, Cathelineau X, Lay F, Barret E, Doublet JD, Baumert H, Vallancien G (2002) Perioperative complications of laparoscopic radical prostatectomy: the Montsouris 3-year experience. J Urol 167:51
Guillonneau B, el-Fettouh H, Baumert H, Cathelineau X, Doublet JD, Fromont G, Vallancien G (2003a) Laparoscopic radical prostatectomy: oncological evaluation after 1,000 cases a Montsouris Institute. J Urol 169:1261
Guillonneau B, Gupta R, El Fettouh H, Cathelineau X, Baumert H, Vallancien G (2003b) Laparoscopic [correction of laproscopic] management of rectal injury during laparoscopic [correction of laproscopic] radical prostatectomy. J Urol 169:1694
Hasson HM (1971) A modified instrument and method for laparoscopy. Am J Obstet Gynecol 110:886
Hasson HM, Parker WH (1998) Prevention and management of urinary tract injury in laparoscopic surgery. J Am Assoc Gynecol Laparosc 5:99
Hedican SP (2004) Complications of hand-assisted laparoscopic urologic surgery. J Endourol 18:387
Janetschek G, Bagheri F, Abdelmaksoud A, Biyani CS, Leeb K, Jeschke S (2003) Ligation of the renal vein during laparoscopic nephrectomy: an effective and reliable method to replace vascular staplers. J Urol 170:1295
Kavoussi LR (2000) Complications of laparoscopic surgery. In: Bishoff JT, Kavoussi LR (eds) Atlas of laparoscopic retroperitoneal surgery. Saunders, Philadelphia, p 237
Kavoussi LR, Sosa E, Chandhoke P, Chodak G, Clayman RV, Hadley HR, Loughlin KR, Ruckle HC, Rukstalis D, Schuessler W et al (1993) Complications of laparoscopic pelvic lymph node dissection. J Urol 149:322
Kelty CJ, Super PA, Stoddard CJ (2000) The driving force in trocar insertion: a comparison between disposable and reusable trocars. Surg Endosc 14:1045
Kulacoglu IH (2000) Regarding: small bowel obstruction and incisional hernia after laparoscopic surgery: should 5-mm trocar sites be sutured? J Laparoendosc Adv Surg Tech A 10:227
Kuno K, Menzin A, Kauder HH, Sison C, Gal D (1998) Prophylactic ureteral catheterization in gynecologic surgery. Urology 52:1004
Lantz PE, Smith JD (1994) Fatal carbon dioxide embolism complicating attempted laparoscopic cholecystectomy–case report and literature review. J Forensic Sci 39:1468
Larobina M, Nottle P (2005) Complete evidence regarding major vascular injuries during laparoscopic access. Surg Laparosc Endosc Percutan Tech 15:119
Lecuru F, Leonard F, Philippe Jais J, Rizk E, Robin F, Taurelle R (2001) Laparoscopy in patients with prior surgery: results of the blind approach. JSLS 5:13
Leff EI, Groff W, Rubin RJ, Eisenstat TE, Salvati EP (1982) Use of ureteral catheters in colonic and rectal surgery. Dis Colon Rectum 25:457
Li TC, Saravelos H, Richmond M, Cooke ID (1997) Complications of laparoscopic pelvic surgery: recognition, management and prevention. Hum Reprod Update 3:505
McAllister M, Bhayani SB, Ong A, Jaffe W, Malkowicz SB, VanArsdalen K, Chow GK, Jarrett TW (2004) Vena caval transection during retroperitoneoscopic nephrectomy: report of the complication and review of the literature. J Urol 172:183
Melcher ML, Carter JT, Posselt A, Duh QY, Stoller M, Freise CE, Kang SM (2005) More than 500 consecutive laparoscopic donor nephrectomies without conversion or repeated surgery. Arch Surg 140:835; discussion 839
Mendoza D, Newman RC, Albala D, Cohen MS, Tewari A, Lingeman J, Wong M, Kavoussi L, Adams J, Moore R, Winfield H, Glascock JM, Das S, Munch L, Grasso M, Dickinson M, Clayman R, Nakada S, McDougall EM, Wolf IS, Hulbert J, Leveillee RJ, Houshair A, Carson C (1996) Laparoscopic complications in markedly obese urologic patients (a multi-institutional review) Urology 48:562
Meraney AM, Samee AA, Gill IS (2002) Vascular and bowel complications during retroperitoneal laparoscopic surgery. J Urol 168:1941
Moberg AC, Montgomery A (2005) Primary access-related complications with laparoscopy: comparison of blind and open techniques. Surg Endosc 19:1196
Nelson JB, Chen RN, Bishoff JT, Oh WK, Kantoff PW, Donehower RC, Kavoussi LR (1999) Laparoscopic retroperitoneal lymph node dissection for clinical stage I nonseminomatous germ cell testicular tumors. Urology 54:1064
Nezhat C, Nezhat F, Ambroze W, Pennington E (1993) Laparoscopic repair of small bowel and colon. A report of 26 cases. Surg Endosc 7:88
Ogan K, Cadeddu JA (2005) Liver injury during urologic laparoscopy. In: Ramakumar S, Jarrett T (eds) Complications of urologic laparoscopic surgery. Taylor & Francis, Boca Raton, p 73
Ostrzenski A, Ostrzenska KM (1998) Bladder injury during laparoscopic surgery. Obstet Gynecol Surv 53:175
Ostrzenski A, Radolinski B, Ostrzenska KM (2003) A review of

laparoscopic ureteral injury in pelvic surgery. Obstet Gynecol Surv 58:794
Parra RO, Hagood PG, Boullier JA, Cummings JM, Mehan DJ (1994) Complications of laparoscopic urological surgery: experience at St. Louis University. J Urol 151:681
Peters CA (1996) Complications in pediatric urological laparoscopy: results of a survey. J Urol 155:1070
Philips TM, Bishoff JT (2005) Bowel injury. In: Ramakumar S, Jarrett T (eds) Complications of urologic laparoscopic surgery. Taylor & Francis, Boca Raton, p 49
Porter JR (2004) Management of intra- and postoperative complications. In: Cadeddu JA (ed) Laparoscopic urologic oncology. Humana Press, Totowa, p 329
Potter SR, Kavoussi LR, Jackman SV (2001) Management of diaphragmatic injury during laparoscopic nephrectomy. J Urol 165:1203
Ramani AP, Desai MM, Steinberg AP, Ng CS, Abreu SC, Kaouk JH, Finelli A, Novick AC, Gill IS (2005) Complications of laparoscopic partial nephrectomy in 200 cases. J Urol 173:42
Reich H (1992) Laparoscopic bowel injury. Surg Laparosc Endosc 2:74
Rosen M, Walsh RM, Goldblum JR (2004) Application of a new collagen-based sealant for the treatment of pancreatic injury. Surg Laparosc Endosc Percutan Tech 14:181
Sadeghi-Nejad H, Kavoussi LR, Peters CA (1994) Bowel injury in open technique laparoscopic cannula placement. Urology 43:559
Sautter T, Haueisen H, Stierli P, Kwiatkowski M, Recker F (2001) A severe complication of retroperitoneoscopic nephrectomy. J Urol 165:515
Saye WB, Miller W, Hertzmann P (1991) Electrosurgery thermal injury. Myth or misconception? Surg Laparosc Endosc 1:223
Schafer M, Lauper M, Krahenbuhl L (2001) Trocar and Veress needle injuries during laparoscopy. Surg Endosc 15:275
Schulam PG, Hedican SP, Docimo SG (1999) Radially dilating trocar system for open laparoscopic access. Urology 54:727
See WA, Monk TG, Weldon BC (1993) Complications of laparoscopy: strategies for prevention and treatment. In: Clayman RV, McDougall EM (eds) Laparoscopic Urology. Quality Medical, St. Louis
Singh D, Gill IS (2005) Renal artery pseudoaneurysm following laparoscopic partial nephrectomy. J Urol 174:2256
Siqueira TM Jr, Kuo RL, Gardner TA, Paterson RF, Stevens LH, Lingeman JE, Koch MO, Shalhav AL (2002) Major complications in 213 laparoscopic nephrectomy cases: the Indianapolis experience. J Urol 168:1361
Soulie M, Salomon L, Seguin P, Mervant C, Mouly P, Hoznek A, Antiphon P, Plante P, Abbou CC (2001) Multi-institutional study of complications in 1085 laparoscopic urologic procedures. Urology 58:899
String A, Berber E, Foroutani A, Macho JR, Pearl JM, Siperstein AE (2001) Use of the optical access trocar for safe and rapid entry in various laparoscopic procedures. Surg Endosc 15:570
Tagaya N, Kasama K, Suzuki N, Taketsuka S, Horie K, Furihata M, Kubota K (2003) Laparoscopic resection of the pancreas and review of the literature. Surg Endosc 17:201
Ternamian AM (1997) Laparoscopy without trocars. Surg Endosc 11:815
Thiel R, Adams JB, Schulam PG, Moore RG, Kavoussi LR (1996) Venous dissection injuries during laparoscopic urological surgery. J Urol 155:1874
Thomas R, Steele R, Ahuja S (1996) Complications of urological laparoscopy: a standardized 1 institution experience. J Urol 156:469
Thompson BH, Wheeless CR Jr (1973) Gastrointestinal complications of laparoscopy sterilization. Obstet Gynecol 41: 669
Vakili B, Chesson RR, Kyle BL, Shobeiri SA, Echols KT, Gist R, Zheng YT, Nolan TE (2005) The incidence of urinary tract injury during hysterectomy: a prospective analysis based on universal cystoscopy. Am J Obstet Gynecol 192:1599
Van der Voort M, Heijnsdijk EA, Gouma DJ (2004) Bowel injury as a complication of laparoscopy. Br J Surg 91:1253
Varkarakis IM, Allaf ME, Bhayani SB, Inagaki T, Su LM, Kavoussi LR, Jarrett TW (2004) Pancreatic injuries during laparoscopic urologic surgery. Urology 64:1089
Varkarakis I, Jarrett T, Ramakumar S (2005) Gallbladder, pancreas and splenic injuries. In: Ramakumar S, Jarrett T (eds) Complications of urologic laparoscopic surgery. Taylor & Francis, Boca Raton, p 67
Viterbo R, Greenberg RE, Al-Saleem T, Uzzo RG (2005) Prior abdominal surgery and radiation do not complicate the retroperitoneoscopic approach to the kidney or adrenal gland. J Urol 174:446
Voyles CR, Madden B (1998) The floppy diaphragm sign with laparoscopic-associated pneumothorax. JSLS 2:71
Voyles CR, Tucker RD (1992) Education and engineering solutions for potential problems with laparoscopic monopolar electrosurgery. Am J Surg 164:57
Wolf JS Jr, Stoller ML (1994) The physiology of laparoscopy: basic principles, complications and other considerations. J Urol 152:294
Yaycioglu O (2005) Delayed complications. In: Ramakumar S, Jarrett T (eds) Complications of urologic laparoscopic surgery. Taylor & Francis, Boca Raton, p 149
Yaycioglu O, Ramakumar S, Kavoussi LR, Jarrett TW (2002) Early repeated exploration after laparoscopic urologic surgery: comparison of clinical, radiologic, and surgical findings. Urology 59:190
Yurkanin P, Park E, Ramakumar S (2005) Major vascular injuries of urologic laparoscopic surgery. In: Ramakumar S, Jarrett T (eds) Complications of urologic laparoscopic surgery. Taylor & Francis, Boca Raton, p 33

18.1 Acute Postoperative Complications

M. Seitz, B. Schlenker, Ch. Stief

18.1.1 Postoperative Bleeding

18.1.1.1 Overview

Historically, major bleeding was a significant problem associated with radical retropubic prostatectomy and cystectomy, TUR, and nephrectomy. Nowadays, major life-threatening hemorrhage after urologic open and endoscopic surgery by expert surgeons is a rare event. In some cases, the patient typically becomes hemodynamically unstable soon after arrival in the recovery room. On the other hand, sometimes hemorrhage arises a few hours or days following the initial procedure. The surgeon must make a decision whether to return immediately to the operating room or treat the patient conservatively with blood and volume replacement (Kaufman and Lepor 2005). Reasons for a significant major bleeding later on in the postoperative period may be slipped ligatures or clips (e.g., from the renal pedicle or other major blood vessels) or in case of partial nephrectomy, ruptured kidney. Also, removal of drains days after surgery may induce significant bleeding, if the drains have been put primarily through a major blood vessel (e.g., epigastric). Reasons for early revisions may be insufficient ligatures or hemostasis.

Significant bleeding in a postoperative bleeding setting is defined as patients requiring emergency blood transfusion to maintain blood pressure during the postoperative period (Hedican and Walsh 1994; Kaufman and Lepor 2005).

18.1.1.2 Incidence and Risk Factors

See Table 18.1.1.

18.1.1.3 Detection and Clinical Signs

Clinical findings that can be used to indicate the need for red cell transfusion may be subjective such as fatigue and shortness of breath. Changes in respiratory rate and pulse can be difficult to interpret but can possibly be parameters indicating the need for blood transfusion. Estimated blood loss, blood pressure, as well as the hemoglobin level must be taken into account since the decision to transfuse red cells is a complex one and depends on factors such as the patient's ability to compensate for anemia, the likelihood of further

Table 18.1.1. Incidence[a] of reintervention; incidence[b] of blood transfusion

Surgery	Incidence[a]	Incidence[b]	Author
Laparoscopic radical prostatectomy	0.5%	5%	Rassweiler et al. 2006; Arai et al. 2003
Open radical prostatectomy	0.5%–1.2%	0.4%–2.4%	Hedican and Walsh 1994; Kaufman and Lepor 2005; Koch and Smith 1996
Robotic radical prostatectomy	0%–0.5%	1%–1.3%	Bhandari et al. 2005
Retropubic transvesical prostatectomy	1.1%–3%	8.2%	Adam et al. 2004; Serretta et al. 2002
TURBT	0%–2.2%	2.3%–3.4%	Collado et al. 2000; Nieder et al. 2005
TURP	2.2%–3.5%	2%–8.9%	Gupta et al. 2006; Lim et al. 2004; Montorsi et al. 2004; Muzzonigro et al. 2004
Open nephron-sparing nephrectomy	2.6%–7.6%	5.3%–12%	Becker et al. 2005; Heye et al. 2005; Steffens et al. 2005
Laparoscopic nephron-sparing nephrectomy	0.6%–3.5%	5.2%–17.8%	Albaqami and Janet schek 2005; Desai et al. 2005; Guillonneau et al. 2003
Open radical nephrectomy	0%–2.7%	2.4%–9.8%	Shuford et al. 2004
Laparoscopic radical nephrectomy	1.6%	0.4%	Vallancien et al. 2002; Wille et al. 2004

Table 18.1.2. Classification of hypovolemic shock according to blood loss

	Class I	Class II	Class III	Class IV
Blood loss	<15% (750 ml)	15%–30% (<1500 ml)	30%–40% (<2000 ml)	>40% (>2000 ml)
Blood pressure				
Systolic	Unchanged	Normal	↓	↓↓↓
Diastolic	Unchanged	↑	↓	↓↓↓
Pulse (beats/min)	<100	100–120	120 (thready)	>120 (very thready)
Capillary refill	Normal	Slow (>2 s)	Slow (>2 s)	Undetectable
Respiratory rate	Normal	Normal	>20/min	>20/min
Urinary flow rate	>30 ml/h	20–30 ml/h	10–20 ml/h	0–10 ml/h
Extremities	Normal	Pale	Pale	Pale and cold
Complexion	Normal	Pale	Pale	Ashen

Adapted from Baskett 1990

blood loss, and the severity of the hypovolemic shock (Table 18.1.2). In the early postoperative period, blood loss via the drains may be an important sign as well as an increase in the abdominal girth, unpaired body shape, and blood loss via the surgical incision. Measurement of hemoglobin in the drained fluid may be helpful.

During the very early postoperative period after open urologic surgery, major hemorrhage, although rare, is the most common complication. Patients following nephron-sparing nephrectomy may present with massive hematuria after surgery. Blood loss after partial or radical nephrectomy is associated with acute flank pain or a significant decrease in the hemoglobin level and signs of shock. Hemorrhage in the perirenal space can be found in these patients – recognized either by adequately placed suction drains or by noninvasive imaging techniques such as sonography. Bleeding may be from the kidney or renal pedicle but is occasionally from unrecognized injury to a neighboring structure such as the spleen, the liver, or a mesenteric vessel. Angiography after partial nephrectomy enables not only the exact visualization of extravasation of contrast material, but also the superselective embolization of the feeding arteries within the kidney.

Significant bleeding according to its definition following radical prostatectomy and cystectomy is a rare event, with an incidence between 0.4% and 5% (Arai et al. 2003; Hedican and Walsh 1994; Kaufman and Lepor 2005; Koch and Smith 1996; Rassweiler et al. 2006).

18.1.1.4 Workup

See Table 18.1.3.

18.1.1.5 Management

Acute anemia caused by intra- and postoperative blood loss should be treated by blood and fluid replacement. Clinical experience has shown that losses of up to 30%–40% can be treated by crystalloids alone in young healthy patients. Estimation of actual and likely further blood loss is an important consideration in the decision to administer a red cell transfusion in the treatment of acute blood loss. The benefit of red cell transfusion is usually considered in terms of increasing the oxygen-carrying capacity of the blood, but a more relevant consideration is the avoidance of tissue hypoxia. General complications of blood transfusion are listed in Table 18.1.4. Indications for trans-

Table 18.1.3. Workup with noninvasive and invasive procedures

Hemoglobin level (Hb)	Table 18.1.5	
Classification of hypovolemic shock	Table 18.1.2	
Ultrasound	Coagulum within the bladder	TURP, TURBT
	Fluid in the perirenal spaces, pelvic region	Open and laparoscopic urologic surgery
CT scan	Visualization of extravasation of contrast medium	Open and laparoscopic urologic surgery
Angiography	Exact visualization of extravasation of contrast medium	Open and laparoscopic nephron-sparing nephrectomy

TURP transurethral prostatectomy, *TURBT* transurethral resection of bladder tumors

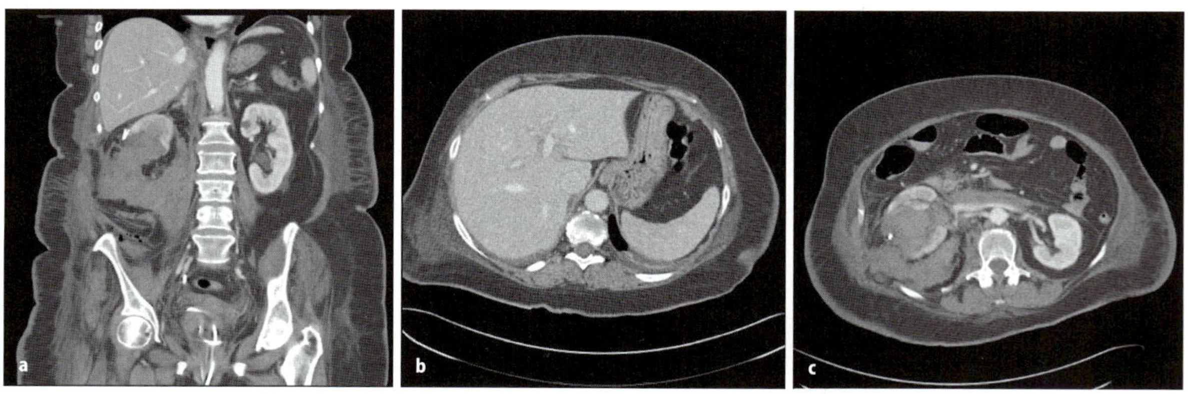

Fig. 18.1.1. CT-scan of a 76 years old female patient 12 days post partial nephrectomy. Postoperatively, no complications were recorded. Due to an elevated creatinine level the patient has not been discharged. On day 12 after the initial surgery she suddenly presented with acute flank pain and a significant decrease in the hemoglobin level. The CT-scan showed a massive retroperitoneal (**a, c**) and subcutaneous (**b**) hematoma. Angio-CT did not show a active bleeding source, the patient remained unstable. Open surgery resulted in a total nephrectomy

Table 18.1.4. Complications of blood transfusion

Complication	Estimated risk per unit	No. of deaths per million units
Hepatitis A	1/1,000,000	0
Hepatitis B	1/50,000 – 1/170,000	0 – 0.14
Hepatitis C	1/200,000	< 0.5
HIV	< 2,000,000	< 0.5
Bacterial contamination	1/500,000	0.1 – 0.25
Acute hemolytic reactions	1/250,000 – 1/1,000,000	0.67
Delayed hemolytic reactions	1/1,000	0.4

Adapted from Murphy et al. 2001

Table 18.1.5. Indications for red cell transfusion and volume replacement in adults

Need based on estimation of blood loss
Estimated blood loss > 40 % (> 2000 ml)
↓
Rapid volume replacement, including RBC transfusion is required, consider emergent control of bleeding source
Estimated blood loss 30 % – 40 % (1,500 – 2,000 ml) and/or presence of symptoms of severe blood loss
↓
Rapid volume replacement with crystalloids or synthetic colloids is required, RBC will probably also be required
Estimated blood loss 15 % – 30 % (800 – 1,500 ml)
↓
Volume replacement with crystalloids or synthetic colloids; need for RBC transfusion is unlikely unless the patient has preexisting anemia, continuing blood loss, or reduced cardiovascular reserve
Estimated blood loss < 15 % (> 750 ml)
↓
Volume replacement or RBC transfusion only in the presence of co-morbid factors
Need based on hemoglobin concentration
Hb < 7 g/dl
↓
RBC transfusion is indicated
In a stable setting the patient should receive 2 U of packed RBC
Hb 7 – 10 g/dl
↓
No clear indication for RBC transfusion
In a stable situation, the patient does not need blood replacement
In the presence of clinical signs of blood loss, consider RBC transfusion
Hb > 10 g/dl
↓
RBC transfusion is not indicated
High-risk patients
↓
Patients > 65 years and/or those with cardiovascular or respiratory disease may tolerate anemia poorly. Such patients may be transfused when Hb < 8 g/dl

Adapted from Murphy et al. 2001

fusion in the acutely bleeding patient are listed in Table 18.1.5.

In some circumstances, it is best to reopen the wound, evacuate the hematoma, and secure the bleeding point. In the event of diffuse bleeding from a clotting disorder, it may be necessary to temporarily pack the wound with gauze, which can then be gradually removed after 24 – 48 h.

After partial nephrectomy, percutaneous superselective embolization (PSE) of the feeding arteries contributing to the bleeding site is preferred to open surgery, which often results in a total nephrectomy (Albani and Novick 2003; Van Poppel et al. 2001). PSE with microcoils as the embolic agent after nephron-sparing renal surgery has a high success rate and a low complication (i.e., major parenchymal infarction) rate (Fisher et al. 1989; Maleux et al. 2003). It is, however, important to avoid occlusion of the proximal great vessels or the adjacent smaller vessels to keep parenchymal loss to a minimum. In case of ruptured kidney, secondary nephrectomy will not be avoidable.

Possible bleeding sources may depend on the surgical approach (transperitoneal or retroperitoneal) and surgical intervention. Partial or radical nephrectomy may develop hemorrhages from neighboring organs such as spleen, adrenal, pancreas, bowel on the right hemiabdomen. On the contralateral side, duodenum, liver, and gallbladder injuries may contribute to postoperative hemorrhage. In general, the bleeding point in a hemodynamic relevant hemorrhage has to be secured (Tables 18.1.6, 18.1.7). Basically, the same applies for retroperitoneal lymphadenectomy (Table 18.1.8). Following radical prostatectomy, two major sites may contribute to a postoperative hemorrhage setting. First is the site of the pelvic lymphadenectomy at which slipped ligatures or clips may be responsible for postoperative bleeding; second is the region of the dorsal vein complex. Patients requiring acute transfusions for hypotension following radical prostatectomy should be explored to evacuate the pelvic hematoma and decrease the likelihood of bladder neck contracture and incontinence (Hedican and Walsh 1994). To secure the bleeding point, bipolar electrocoagulation as well as ligatures or clips can be used (Table 18.1.9). The possible causes of postoperative hemorrhage and its management in simple prostatectomy and radical cystectomy are listed in Tables 18.1.10 and 18.1.11.

In case of bleeding after TURP, venous and arterial bleeding may be controlled conservatively. One can overinflate the balloon of the catheter with 50 – 70 ml,

Table 18.1.6. Right partial and radical nephrectomy with bleeding sources, diagnostic and therapeutic procedures

Surgical procedure	Topographic anatomy and potential bleeding source	Diagnostic procedures	Clinical features
Right transperitoneal nephrectomy	Cutis/subcutis	PE[a]/Lab[b]/US[c]	Hb↓/swelling/hematoma
	Muscle	PE/Lab/US	Hb↓/swelling/hematoma
	Omentum, Peritoneum, Psoas muscle, Gall bladder, Adrenal gland, Duodenum, Bowel, Testicular/ovarian Vessels, branches of lumbalis/iliolumbalis vessels	Lab/US/CT-scan	Check for abnormal coagulation test (see Table 18.1.1.2); Hb↓/intraabdominal fluid/bleeding source/blood pressure↓, pulse↑
		→	Consider relaparotomy in increasing unstable patient
	Renal pedicle, Lumbar veins	→	Unstable patient. Urgent relaparotomy
Right lumbar nephrectomy	Cutis/subcutis	PE/Lap/US	Hb↓/swelling/hematoma
	Muscle	PE/Lab/US	Hb↓/swelling/hematoma
	Intercostal vessels	PE/Lab/US	Hb↓/swelling/hematoma
	Pleural cavity	PE/Lab/US/x-ray	Hb↓/respiratory rate↑/pleural effusion → Consider drainage
	Peritoneum, Psoas muscle, Adrenal gland, Testicular/ovarian vessels, branches of lumbalis/iliolumbalis vessels	Lab/US/CT scan	Hb↓/intraabdominal fluid/bleeding source/blood pressure↓, pulse↑
		→	Consider relaparotomy in increasingly unstable patient
	Renal pedicle, Lumbar veins	→	Unstable patient. Urgent relaparotomy
Partial lumbar/transperitoneal nephrectomy	Same as above	PE/Lab/US/CT scan/CT angiography	Consider PSE
	Additionally:		Consider double-J
	Branches of renal artery		Condsider PSE and/or double-J
	Renal pelvis		
		→	Consider reoperation in increasingly unstable patient
	ruptured kidney	→	Unstable patient. Urgent reoperation

In our institution, although not evidence-based, hemorrhage after partial nephrectomy or nephrectomy is taken very seriously since such conditions may require immediate action. Early CT scan (nephrectomy) or CT angiography (partial nephrectomy) is indicated

[a] Physical examination
[b] Laboratory
[c] Ultrasound

placing it in the bladder, and put traction on it. This compresses the prostate capsule with the remaining prostate tissue, which leads to sufficient hemostasis. A second and technique that is also effective is placing the balloon of the catheter in the resection cavity of the prostate and overinflate the balloon until the bleeding is controlled and the irrigation fluid turns light pink. However, if the irrigation fluid has a continued red color one should reinsert the resectoscope and coagulate the bleeding source.

Practical aspects to approach a postoperative hemorrhage surgically are to keep potential bleeding sources in mind. After reopening the surgical site incision, one should pay attention to the muscle. Carefully, coagula should be removed in order to expose bleeding sources from bruised muscle. Subtile mono- or bipolar coagulation should be performed. The same procedure applies to drainage sites. As one approaches the deeper operation field, hematoma must be evacuated and adherent coagula removed. Washing with 2–3 l of normal saline clears the surgical site and facilitates the search for the bleeding source. Neighboring tissue and organs must be examined carefully. Smaller bleeding sources may be secured by mono- or bipolar electrocoagulation; larger ones need to be clipped or ligated. In case of diffuse bleeding, one can use special devices such as equine-derived, honeycomb-like collagen sponge coated with a layer of coagulation factors: human fibrinogen and human thrombin. When applied to the surface of bleeding tissue, the sponge provides quick, reliable hemostasis. If surgical approaches fail, consider measures as described in Sect. 18.1.6, "Special Conditions."

Table 18.1.7. Left partial and radical nephrectomy with bleeding sources, diagnostic and therapeutic procedures

Surgical procedure	Topographic anatomy and potential bleeding source	Diagnostic procedures	Clinical features
Left transperitoneal nephrectomy	Cutis/subcutis	PE[a]/Lab[b]/US[c]	Hb↓/swelling/hematoma
	Muscle	PE/Lab/US	Hb↓/swelling/hematoma
	Omentum Peritoneum Psoas muscle Spleen Adrenal gland Bowel Pancreas Testicular/ovarian vessels Branches of lumbalis/ iliolumbalis vessels	Lab/US/CT-scan	Check for abnormal coagulation test (see Table 18.1.1.2) Hb↓/intraabdominal fluid/bleeding source/blood pressure↓, pulse↑
		→	Consider relaparotomy in increasingly unstable patient
	Renal pedicle Lumbar veins	→	Unstable patient Urgent relaparotomy
Left lumbar nephrectomy	Cutis/subcutis	PE/Lab/US	Hb↓/swelling/hematoma
	Muscle	PE/Lab/US	Hb↓/swelling/hematoma
	Intercostal vessels	PE/Lab/US	Hb↓/swelling/hematoma
	Pleural cavity	PE/Lab/US/X-ray	Hb↓/respiratory rate↑/pleural effusion → Consider drainage
	Spleen Peritoneum Psoas muscle Adrenal gland Testicular/ovarian vessels Branches of lumbalis/ iliolumbalis vessels	Lab/US/CT scan	Hb↓/intraabdominal fluid/bleeding source/blood pressure↓, pulse↑
		→	Consider relaparotomy in increasingly unstable patient
	Renal pedicle Lumbar veins	→	Unstable patient Urgent relaparotomy
Partial lumbar/ transperitoneal nephrectomy	Same as above additionally: Branches of renal artery Renal pelvis	PE/Lab/US/CT scan/CT angiography	Consider PSE Consider Double-J If PSE or double-J fails condsider PSE and double-J
		→	Consider reoperation in increasing unstable patient
	Ruptured kidney	→	Unstable patient Urgent reoperation

In our institution, although not evidence-based, hemorrhage after partial nephrectomy or nephrectomy is taken very seriously since such conditions may require immediate action. Early CT scan (nephrectomy) or CT angiography (partial nephrectomy) is indicated

[a] Physical examination, [b] Laboratory, [c] Ultrasound

Table 18.1.8. Retroperitoneal lymphadenectomy with bleeding sources, diagnostic and therapeutic procedures

Surgical procedure	Topographic anatomy and potential bleeding source	Diagnostic procedures	Clinical features
Retroperitoneal lymphadenectomy	Cutis/subcutis	PE[a]/Lab[b]/US[c]	Hb↓/swelling/hematoma
	Muscle (due to suture)	PE/Lab/US	Hb↓/swelling/hematoma
	Omentum Bowel Ureter Mesenterium Retroperitoneum Psoas muscle Testicular vessels	Lab/US/CT scan	Check for abnormal coagulation test (see Table 18.1.1.2) Hb↓/extraperitoneal fluid/bleeding source/blood pressure↓, pulse↑
		→	Consider conservative measures: See Table 18.1.5 RBC transfusion
		→	Consider reoperation if conservative measures fail
	Spleen Vessels in the node-bearing areas (caval, aortal, interaortocaval due to slipped ligatures or clips) Renal pedicle Lumbar veins	→	Unstable patient Urgent relaparotomy

[a] Physical examination, [b] Laboratory, [c] Ultrasound

Table 18.1.9. Radical prostatectomy with bleeding sources, diagnostic and therapeutic procedures

Surgical procedure	Topographic anatomy and potential bleeding source	Diagnostic procedures	Clinical features
Radical retropubic prostatectomy (open/extraperitoneoscopic) Plus pelvic lymphadenectomy	Cutis/subcutis	PE[a]/Lab[b]/US[c]	Hb↓/swelling/hematoma
	Muscle (due to suture or drainage)	PE/Lab/US	Hb↓/swelling/hematoma
	Pelvic vessels Dorsal vein complex (due to slipped ligatures or clips) Bladder neck Seminal vesicle vessels Perirectal soft tissue Urethra	Lab/US/CT scan	Check for abnormal coagulation test (see Table 18.1.1.2) Hb↓/extraperitoneal fluid/bleeding source/ blood pressure↓, pulse↑
		→	Consider conservative measures: See Table 18.1.5 RBC transfusion
		→	Consider reoperation in case of pelvic hematoma to prevent bladder neck contracture and incontinence
		→	Unstable patient Urgent reoperation

Although recommended in the literature, we usually do not evacuate pelvic hematoma. In all of the rare cases of pelvic hematoma following radical retropubic prostatectomy that were treated conservatively, we did not find any bladder neck contracture or incontinence. But this a not an evidence-based opinion and prospective randomized trials on this issue are lacking. A condition in patients suspected of acute hemorrhage from pelvic vessels due to slipped ligatures or clips should be taken very seriously since immediate action may be required

[a] Physical examination, [b] Laboratory, [c] Ultrasound

Table 18.1.10. Prostatectomy due to benign prostatic enlargement with bleeding sources, diagnostic and therapeutic procedures

Surgical procedure	Topographic anatomy and potential bleeding source	Diagnostic procedures	Clinical features
Prostatectomy (Mellin/Freyer)	Cutis/subcutis	PE[a]/Lab[b]/US[c]	Hb↓/swelling/hematoma
	Muscle (due to suture or drainage)	PE/Lab/US	Hb↓/swelling/hematoma Check for abnormal coagulation test (see Table 18.1.1.2)
Increase bladder irrigation ↔	Suprapubic cystostomy site and bladder suture	Lab/US/CT scan	Hb↓/extraperitoneal fluid/bleeding source/blood pressure↓, pulse↑
Expand transurethral catheter (50–100 ml) within the bladder and put tension toward bladder neck ↔	Suture of prostate capsule (Mellin)		
Expand transurethral catheter within the prostatic urethra (50–100 ml depending on enucleated prostate volume) ↔	Prostatic urethra (Freyer)	→	Consider conservative measures: See Table 18.1.5 RBC transfusion
		→	Consider reoperation if conservative measures fail
		→	Unstable patient Urgent relaparotomy

[a] Physical examination, [b] Laboratory, [c] Ultrasound

Table 18.1.11. Cystectomy with bleeding sources, diagnostic and therapeutic procedures

Surgical procedure	Topographic anatomy and potential bleeding source	Diagnostic procedures	Clinical features
Cystectomy (Mellin/Freyer)	Cutis/subcutis	PE*/Lab**/US***	Hb↓/swelling/hematoma
Male: pelvic peritoneum ureteral stumps prostate seminal vesicles membranous urethra Female: Uterus Ovaries Fallopian tubes vaginal vault Urethra	Muscle (due to suture or drainage)	PE/Lab/US	Hb↓/swelling/hematoma Check for abnormal coagulation test (see Table 18.1.1.2)
	Vessels in the node-bearing areas (iliac, obturator, caval, aortal, interaortocaval due to slipped ligatures or clips) Dorsal vein complex (due slipped ligatures or clips) Omentum Bowel (anastomosis) Ureter (anastomosis) Mesenterium Perirectal soft tissue Psoas muscle Testicular/ovarian vessels	Lab/US/CT-scan	Hb↓/extraperitoneal fluid/bleeding source/blood pressure↓, pulse↑
		→	Consider conservative measures: See Table 18.1.5 RBC transfusion
		→	Consider reoperation if conservative measures fail
		→	Unstable patient Urgent relaparotomy

The indication for blood transfusion should be posed generously due to the limited prognosis of the underlying disease and Hb↓ is mostly due to diffuse bleeding. Patients generally benefit from RCB transfusion

[a] Physical examination, [b] Laboratory, [c] Ultrasound

18.1.1.6 Special Conditions

Disorders responsible for postoperative hemorrhage are the disseminated intravascular coagulation (DIC) and massive transfusion (MT). MT is commonly defined as the replacement of the entire circulating volume in a period of 24 h. A dynamic definition of MT, such as the transfusion of four or more red cell concentrates within 1 h when ongoing need is foreseeable, or the replacement of 50 % of the total blood volume within 3 h, is more relevant in the acute clinical setting (Crosson 1996; Hardy et al. 2004). A high percentage of massively transfused patients will show evidence of defective hemostasis. The pathophysiology of this phenomena is as complex as the diagnosis is difficult. At present there is no simple, reliable, and rapid diagnostic test. The platelet count is the only indicator of coagulopathy that can be obtained rapidly through the use of automated counters. The prothrombin time (PT) and the activated partial thromboplastin time (aPTT) are expected to become elevated (Turi and Peerschke 1986). Of utmost importance for an intact hemostasis is the fibrinogen concentration. According to the literature, fibrinogen concentration should be at least between 0.5 and 1.0 g/l (Hiippala et al. 1995).

Approaches to treatment initially include crystalloids or colloids, which are infused to maintain normovolemia (Erber 2002). Basic recommendations include the maintenance of normothermia. A low hemoglobin concentration (Hb) should be corrected prior to the administration of hemostatic blood products. The optimal Hb to sustain hemostasis in the context of MT remains unknown but is probably higher than that required for oxygen transport and delivery. The use of fresh frozen plasma (FFP) and/or platelet concentration (PC) should depend on the results of coagulation testing and clinical judgment. A markedly prolonged PT and aPTT as well as decreased levels of fibrinogen will require the administration of FFP. Doses ranging from 5 to 20 ml/kg body weight have been recommended. In an adult, four units FFP (800 – 1,000 ml) should be sufficient, initially (Erber 2002; Hardy et al. 2004; Hiippala 1998). If the fibrinogen concentration remains below 1.0 g/l despite therapy with FFP, the administration of cryoprecipitate, a concentrated source of fibrinogen, factor VIII, factor XIII, and von Willebrand factor may be indicated (10 – 20 U) (Pantanowitz et al. 2003). In Europe, cryoprecipitates are no longer available and when fibrinogen substitution is required, virus-inactivated fibrinogen preparations are administered (e.g., Haemocomplettan 1 – 8 g IV; ZLB Behring, Bern, Switzerland). Platelets should be administered to correct a clinical coagulopathy associated with decreased platelet count and/or platelet function (Tables 18.1.12, 18.1.13).

Pharmacological agents are usually administered relatively late in MT. Protamine sulfate (1,000 – 3,000 IE/day) and desmopressin (Table 18.1.14) have been used, especially in cardiac surgery. Aprotinin (Table 18.1.14)

Table 18.1.12. Abnormal coagulation tests in MT

Fibrinogen concentration	< 1.0 g/l
Prothrombin time (PT)	1.5 – 1.8 times control
Activated partial thromboplastin time (aPTT)	1.5 – 1.8 times control
Platelet count	< 50,000 mm³

Table 18.1.14. Dosage regimes for hemostatic drugs after antiplatelet therapy

Aprotinin	2 million kallikrein inhibitory units (KIU) IV over 20 min, followed by a continuous infusion of 500,000 KIU for the entire duration of the procedure
Tranexamic acid	10 mg/kg IV initially, followed by a continuous infusion of 1 mg/kg for 10 h, alternatively 15 mg/kg, with repeat dosing 4 – 6 h later
Desmopressin	0.3 µg/kg IV, possibly repeated 4 h later (the thrombotic risk must be taken into account)
Platelet transfusion	Transfusion at a dosage of $0.5 – 0.7 \times 10^{11}$, i.e., the standard concentrate per 7 kg of body weight in adults

Table 18.1.13. Proposals for the administration of hemostatic blood products in the massively transfused patient

Presence of clinical bleeding	Yes	No	
Abnormal coagulation test (Table 18.1.12)	Yes	Transfusion of FFP and PC according to the coagulation tests	Possible transfusion of FFP and PC if the hemorrhagic risk related to the surgical procedure is high
	No	Search for a cause other than a hemostatic defect Reevaluate the importance of red cell transfusion and consider FFP and PC if transfusion is massive Repeat coagulation tests	No indication to transfuse
	Unknown	Transfusion guided by clinical probability of a specific hemostatic defect	No indication to transfuse Obtain coagulation tests

FFP fresh frozen plasma; *PC* platelet concentration

has been suggested in the context of MT but its use is not supported by any controlled trial. Recombinant activated factor VII (rFVIIa, Novoseven) is a promising hemostatic agent under investigation. It is a safe and effective tool for the treatment and prevention of hemorrhage in hemophiliacs with circulating inhibitors to replacement factors, and patients with Glanzmann's thrombasthenia refractory to platelet transfusion. By restoring thrombin generation on the surface of tissue-factor-bearing cells, such as activated platelets and monocytes, recombinant activated factor VII has the potential to effect hemostasis in the setting of many coagulopathic states (Hardy et al. 2004; Welsby et al. 2005). Case reports and case series report the successful off-label use of rFVIIa to treat bleeding that could not be controlled by the administration of hemostatic blood components, although only underpowered studies addressing safety concerns have been conducted. Since factor VII must interact with tissue factor to initiate the generation of thrombin, coagulation occurs in the site of injury (Allen et al. 2002) and the risk of thromboembolic effects appears minimal (Hardy et al. 2004; Roberts 1998). In urology, one trial has demonstrated decreasing blood loss and the need for transfusion during retropubic prostatectomy (Friederich et al. 2003). Since there is no established monitoring tool for the effect of rFVIIa, the cessation of bleeding may be the best and only indicator of efficacy (Welsby et al. 2005). Official dosage recommendations for off-label use of rFVII in surgical patients are not available, but doses as low as 20 μg/kg body weight (~60 kIE NovoSeven) have been shown to have some effect, while doses around 40 μg/kg body weight (~120–180 kIE NovoSeven) have been effective in many clinical settings. If ineffective, the dose can be repeated, and larger doses do not necessarily cause more thromboembolic complications (Welsby et al. 2005).

The pathophysiology is complex and coagulopathy associated with MT requires a multidisciplinary approach involving anesthesiologists, blood bankers, hematologists, laboratory specialists, and urologists. Times have changed, blood products have changed, and so has the management of the bleeding patient. Nevertheless, standardized management may not always be possible in massively bleeding patients. Once the initial hemorrhagic phase of coagulopathy is controlled, efforts should be directed toward the prevention of thrombotic complications related to the consumption of coagulation factors associated with DIC.

A very special situation may develop in patients who experience intraoperative myocardial infarction and are in need of immediate therapy with antiplatelet agents. So-called platelet inhibitors are drugs capable of inhibiting platelet function, in particular activation and aggregation. Currently available agents include aspirin, dipyridamole, the thienopyridines (ticlopidine and clopidogrel), and the glycoprotein IIb/IIIa (IIbβ3) receptor antagonists. Recognized indications for antiplatelet therapy (acetylsalicylic acid) are first acute myocardial infarction, which reduces mortality by approximately 20%, and second acute coronary syndrome (minimum recommended initial dose is 160 mg, followed by a maintenance dose of 75–325 mg daily). The perioperative risk of bleeding with antiplatelet agents varies and depends on the surgical procedure (Bertrand et al. 2000). Recommendations with evidence level I can only be given in hip and knee surgery. While in hip surgery low preoperative acetylsalicylic acid doses increase the risk of hemorrhage and exposure to transfusion, this is not seen when acetylsalicylic acid is administered, postoperatively. In urology, only evidence levels II–III are available. Pre- and postoperative ticlopidine/acetylsalicylic acid increases postoperative bleeding and transfusion requirements for TURP and prostate surgery via an abdominal approach. Still, the major issue is how can peri- and postoperative bleeding complications induced by certain antiplatelet agents be avoided. Steroids to reduce or eliminate any possible increase in perioperative blood loss are not recommended Grade E (supported by only Level IV or V studies). Also, prophylactic platelet transfusion should not be given, but platelets must be readily available Grade C (supported by Level II studies). Nonspecific methods to decrease perioperative blood loss are recommended by some physicians such as selecting a surgical approach designed to achieve the most effective hemostatic control. If possible in consultation with the anesthesiologist, a controlled hypotension technique in normothermia should be used. However the surgical procedure hemodilution should be restricted. In addition, hematocrit levels should maintained to ensure normal biological hemostasis, usually at 30%.

In cardiac surgery, established efficacious pharmacological modalities for reducing intra- and postoperative bleeding and transfusion exposure in patients on antiplatelet agents include aprotinin and tranexamic acid (evidence level I) (Castati et al. 2001; Laupacis and Fergusson 1997; Murkin 1994). Aprotinin may be responsible for allergic reaction and even anaphylactic shock (0.3% first exposure and 2.5%–3% after initial contact). Tranexamic acid does not involve this kind of allergic risk and its cost–benefit ratio is more favorable. While aprotinin has been documented with a very low thrombotic risk, desmopressin, a third hemostatic drug, is effective only in patients presenting with major bleeding syndrome (evidence level III), and it is imperative that its thrombotic risk potential be taken into account. Platelet transfusion to reduce or stop postoperative blood loss in patients treated with antiplatelets are effective despite the absence of level I or II evidence (Table 18.1.14).

The lack of data in other types of urological surgery makes it impossible to formulate recommendations.

Whether a patient is in need of antiplatelet therapy perioperatively should always be an on-site decision with an experienced cardiologist, anesthesiologist, and urologist. To stop the surgical procedure after subtile coagulation may be a choice if a cardiovascular intervention is needed. Guidelines concerning this issue do not exist, nor are they wanted since guidelines restrict the margin of individual decisions.

The literature reports two studies on ultrasound-guided transrectal biopsy, and three studies dealing with aspirin-related bleeding complications after transurethral prostatectomy. Although red cell transfusion was never required after prostate biopsy, they were given in 30% of control patients undergoing prostatectomy: two cases of mortality were reported. According to the meta-analysis of Burger et al., aspirin increased this risk of bleeding by a factor of 2.7.

18.1.2 Chest Pain and Dyspnea

18.1.2.1 Overview

Chest pain and dyspnea can be caused by a variety of disorders. After surgery, they are most often due to disorders of the respiratory or cardiovascular system but can also be caused by gastrointestinal disorders (e.g., peptic ulcer disease) or musculoskeletal chest wall pain. The major purpose of diagnosis is to differentiate between cardiac and noncardiac disorders, acute and chronic disorders, and benign and potentially life-threatening disorders (Kurz et al. 2005). Diagnosis must be precise and quick to identify high-risk patients and initiate the appropriate treatment. As symptoms can be misleading, diagnosis should include the following for every patient presenting chest pain and/or dyspnea:

- Evaluation of risk factors for respiratory or cardiovascular disorders (e.g., history of myocardial infarction or thrombosis, diabetes, atherosclerosis, etc.)
- Physical examination
- Vital signs (blood pressure, heart rate, respiratory rate, oxygen saturation)
- 12-Lead electrocardiogram (EKG)
- Complete blood count, electrolytes, creatinine, D-dimer, troponin T
- Chest radiograph (CXR) (optional)
- Chest computed tomography (CT) angiogram (→ pulmonary embolism) (optional)

Table 18.1.15. Cardiovascular system disorders

Acute coronary syndrome/acute ischemia
Systolic dysfunction
Valvular disorders
Pericardial diseases
Anemia
Thoracic aortic rupture
Deconditioning

18.1.2.2 Cardiovascular System Disorders

Table 18.1.15 gives an overview of frequent cardiac disorders. An ECG can reveal acute myocardial ischemia, arrhythmia, signs of left ventricular hypertrophy, bundle branch block, or right ventricular strain.

The presence of ST segment elevation of more than 0.1 mV in at least two corresponding leads or a new complete left bundle branch block indicates a high likelihood of a blockage of a coronary artery with consecutive myocardial infarction (Fig. 18.1.2). Reperfusion therapy by either primary percutaneous coronary intervention (PCI) or thrombolysis can be initiated without any further diagnostic tests, if there are no contraindications due to the history of surgery (Hamm 2004).

It must be remembered that the sensitivity of the 12-lead ECG for detection of myocardial ischemia is only about 50% (Lee et al. 1987; Giannitsis and Katus 2002). Therefore, the measurement of biochemical markers for myocardial necrosis in serum can be considered as standard. Troponin T is widely used as a biochemical marker (Katus et al. 1991; Gerhardt et al. 1992; Bakker et al. 1994b); in addition, troponin I, myoglobin (Ohman et al. 1990; Stone et al. 1977), and creatine kinase MB (CK-MB) (Mair et al. 1991; Van Blerk et al. 1992; Bakker et al. 1994a) are in use.

18.1.2.3 Postoperative Pulmonary Complications

Pulmonary complications are common during the hospital stay and a major cause of morbidity and mortality (Arozullah et al. 2000). The incidence in the perioperative period ranges from 5% to 80% (Fisher et al. 2002; Thompson et al. 2003). Table 18.1.16 gives an overview of frequent postoperative pulmonary complications. In the following sections, management of the most frequent complications is described.

Pulmonary Embolism

Pulmonary embolism (PE) is a complication of deep venous thrombosis (see Chap. 18.1.6, "Deep Venous Thrombosis," for etiology and therapy). Clinical signs include dyspnea, tachypnea, and tachycardia. As a consequence of right heart failure, the jugular veins are dis-

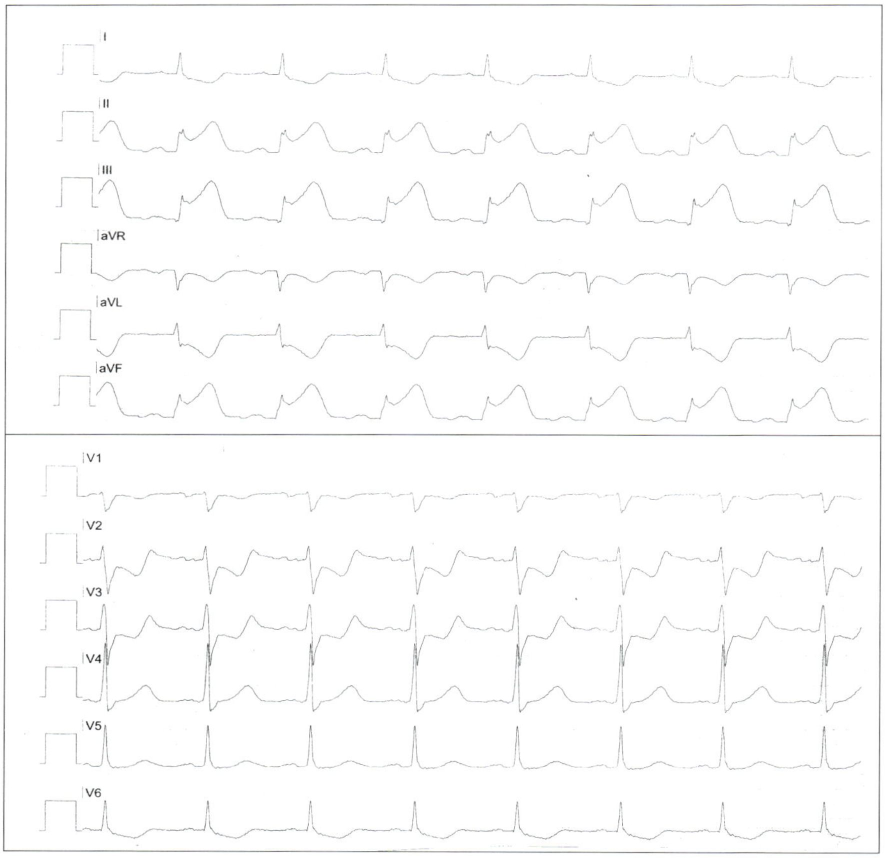

Fig. 18.1.2. ST-Elevation in myocardial infarction

Table 18.1.16. Postoperative pulmonary complications

Pulmonary embolism
Atelectasis
Bronchospasm
Pleural effusions
Hypoxemia
Pneumothorax
Noncardiogenic pulmonary edema
Infection (e.g., pneumonia, bronchitis)
Exacerbation of underlying chronic lung disease
Acute upper airway obstruction
Chemical pneumonitis
Abdominal compartment syndrome (ACS)
Tracheal laceration or rupture

tended, an accentuated pulmonic heart sound and tricuspid regurgitation murmur can be monitored in the physical examination.

Plasma D-dimers have an excellent negative predictive value (Janata 2003); elevated D-dimer levels, however, are frequent after surgery and can be misleading.

The electrocardiogram may show the classic S1Q3T3 pattern (Fig. 18.1.3) as a sign of acute cor pulmonale or a new complete or incomplete right bundle branch block (Chan et al. 2001). However, the majority of patients with PE have normal or unspecific abnormal echocardiograms (Challapalli et al. 2004).

Two-dimensional echocardiography can demonstrate right ventricular hypokinesis with sparing of the right ventricular apex (McConnell's sign [Goldhaber 2002]), tricuspid regurgitation, and lack of collapse of the inferior vena cava during inspiration. Spiral computed tomography is the first-line imaging technique in many hospitals to secure the diagnosis of a PE (Fig. 18.1.4). Patients should be given up to 100% O_2. If the patient is in pain or very distressed, morphine should be administered (10 mg IV). Guidelines suggest a bolus of unfractionated heparin (UFH) 10,000 IU IV over 5 h, followed by a maintenance infusion at 15–25 IU/kg/h as guided by aPTT (for most commercial aPTT reagents, 1.8–3.0 times the control value). Consider streptokinase in the postoperative patient.

The use of inferior vena cava filters reduces the incidence of early pulmonary embolism during the first 12 days, but almost doubles the long-term risk of recurrent DVT (Decousus et al. 1998). Therefore a vena cava filter is only indicated in patients who have a contrain-

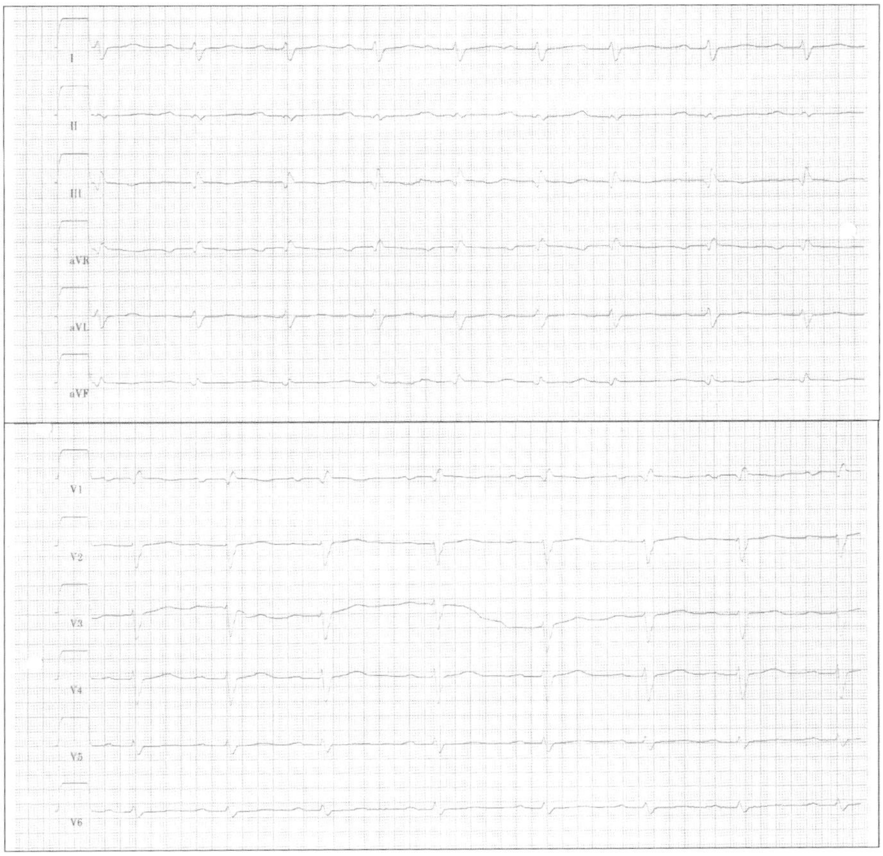

Fig. 18.1.3. S1Q3T3 pattern in pulmonary embolism

dication to anticoagulation or experience pulmonary embolism despite therapeutic anticoagulation (Bates and Ginsberg 2004; Ho et al. 2005).

Pleural Effusions

After abdominal surgery, small pleural effusions can be monitored in up to 50% of patients (Light and George 1976). Most patients have no symptoms: clinical signs due to a restrictive ventilatory defect (Gilmartin et al. 1985) include pleuritic chest pain, dyspnea, and dry nonproductive cough (Yataco and Dweik 2005).

Frontal and lateral chest radiography (Ferrer and Roldan 2000) or sonographic study (McGahan 1985; McLoud and Flower 1991; O'Moore et al. 1987) is usually sufficient to detect a pleural effusion of at least 250 ml of fluid (Yataco and Dweik 2005). In contrast to most other clinical situations, thoracentesis is not mandatory for small effusions after recent surgery but can be indicated if the patient's clinical condition deteriorates. Large and symptomatic effusions causing severe respiratory symptoms should be drained (Yataco and Dweik 2005). A tube thoracostomy can be placed to drain the pleural space continuously. Typical indications for the placement of a tube thoracostomy include pneumothorax, hemothorax, complicated parapneumonic effusion, or empyema (Yataco and Dweik 2005). Additional pharmacological application of antibiotics and diuretics may be indicated.

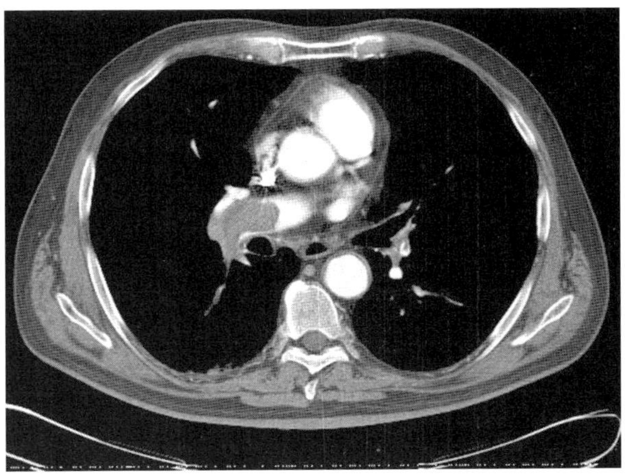

Fig. 18.1.4. Spiral CT scan showing pulmonary embolism

Atelectasis

Atelectasis is one of the most frequent pulmonary complications after abdominal surgery. Most often it is clinically insignificant. The incidence of clinically significant atelectasis is approximately 15% – 20% (Celli et al. 1984; Craven et al. 1974; Platell and Hall 1997). Clinical signs include increased work of breathing and hypoxemia. The development of atelectasis is caused by a variety of processes such as retained airway secretions, the altered compliance of lung tissue, and impaired regional ventilation (Platell and Hall 1997). Standard therapy remains continuous positive airway pressure (CPAP) (Squadrone et al. 2005; Fowler et al. 1978), whereas bronchoscopy may have a role in cases that are unresponsive to CPAP (Wanner et al. 1973; Feldman and Huber 1976; Marini et al. 1979) mucolytic therapy cannot be definitively recommended (Jepsen et al. 1989a, b).

Infection/Pneumonia

See Chap. 18.1.3, "Postoperative Fever."

Tube Thoracostomy

A tube thoracostomy (Fig. 18.1.5) is used to drain air or liquid from the pleural space. Indications to place a tube thoracostomy include large, progressive or symptomatic pneumothorax, tension pneumothorax, hemothorax, chylothorax, and complicated parapneumonic effusion or empyema.

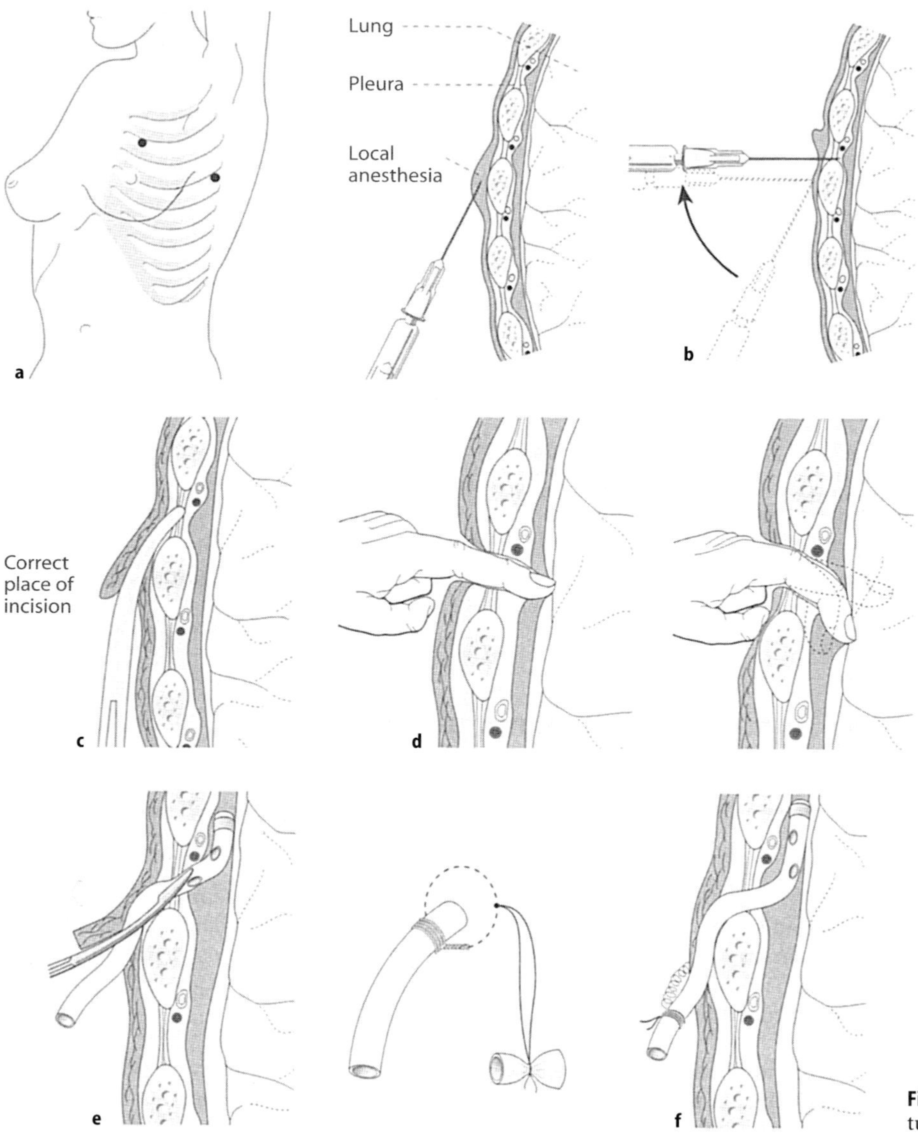

Fig. 18.1.5. Placement of a tube thoracostomy

The silastic tube is most often inserted in the fourth or fifth intercostal space in the anterior axillary or mid-axillary line (Miller and Sahn 1987; Symbas 1989).

For the insertion, the patient's arm is placed behind the head (Fig. 18.1.5a). After disinfection and local anesthesia (combined with general sedation and analgesia if needed), a skin incision is made parallel to the intercostal space. To avoid injuries of nerves or vessels, it is performed immediately above the rib (b). A Kelly clamp is used to penetrate through the intercostal muscle and into the pleural space (c). Using a finger, the correct position is confirmed and adhesions between the lung and the pleural surface are removed (d). After inserting the chest tube (apically for a pneumothorax and inferiorly for a pleural effusion or hemothorax), the distal end is connected to the chest drainage unit (e). The tube is secured by a suture and/or tape (f) (Golden and Hiley 1998). There is no general recommendation on how much suction should be applied, although the most commonly used pressure is 15–20 cm H_2O. Vital signs (blood pressure, pulse, respiration rate, and oxygen saturation) before and after placement of the tube should be monitored and compared. A chest x-ray must be taken to confirm the correct placement of the tube (Schulman et al. 2005).

The drain can be removed when drainage has stopped or an x-ray shows that there is no air or fluid in the intrapleural space. There is controversy over whether the chest tube should be clamped for a few hours before removal. In all events, the patient should have an x-ray immediately after removal to assess for lung reexpansion. The x-ray should be repeated 24 h later.

18.1.3 Acute Abdomen

"Acute abdomen" is a collective term for a variety of disorders, both of intra- and extraabdominal origin. In addition to all the above-mentioned complications after surgery, all non-surgery-related disorders (see Table 18.17) should be kept in mind as differential diagnosis when approaching a patient presenting an acute abdomen.

Signs for an acute abdomen may include (see also the case presentation below):

- Abdominal pain
- Rigid abdomen
- Abdominal distention
- Point tenderness
- Nausea and vomiting
- Signs of shock
- Hypotension
- Anuria
- Inability to pass feces or gas
- Fever
- Free fluid in the abdomen
- Shaking chills

The characteristic expression of the face during an acute abdomen is called facies abdominalis. The patient's face is anxious, furrowed, and pinched with the nose and upper lip drawn up.

Table 18.1.17. Differential diagnosis of acute abdomen

Intraabdominal
Generalized peritonitis: perforated viscus, primary infective peritonitis, rupture of cyst
Localized peritonitis: abscess, appendicitis, cholecystitis, pancreatitis, salpingitis, Meckel diverticulitis
Motility disorders: intestinal obstruction, biliary obstruction, ureteric obstruction, irritable colon, diverticulosis, uterine contraction, urinary retention
Ischemia: acute myocardial infarction (AMI), mesenteric ischemia/infarction/thrombosis, sickle cell crisis, splenic infarction, torsion of ovarian cyst/testicle/omentum, tumor necrosis of hepatoma/fibroid, vasculitides
Infective: urinary tract infection, malaria, tuberculosis, yersinia, cholera, typhoid
Other: peptic ulcer, inflammatory diseases (e.g., ulcerative colitis or Crohn disease), retroperitoneal tumors, ectopic pregnancy
Extraabdominal
Thoracic: lung diseases (e.g., pulmonary embolism, pneumonia), ischemic heart disease, esophageal disease, aortic dissection
Neurological: herpes zoster, spinal arthritis, radiculopathy from tumors, tabes dorsalis, abdominal epilepsy
Metabolic: diabetes mellitus, chronic renal failure, porphyria, acute adrenal insufficiency, thyroid storm, hypercalcemia
Abdominal wall: herniae, rectal sheath hematoma
Retroperitoneal pathologies: hematoma or abscess (with consecutive paralytic ileus)
Nonspecific abdominal pain

Case presentation acute abdomen

A 63-year-old male is developing fever (39.1 °C) and abdominal pain beginning on the 5th day after cystectomy and ileum neobladder construction. The abdomen is becoming increasingly rigid, the blood drains (removed on the 2nd day after surgery) and blood count give no hint of prolonged bleeding. The patients face is pale and covered with cold sweat. He has been complaining about abdominal distention and difficulties passing gas ever since surgery. The vital signs show hypotension (75/45 mm Hg) and an accelerated pulse rate (100/min). The leukocyte count is 18.6 G/l, CRP is 23.2 mg/dl, troponin-T and D-dimer levels are not elevated. The chest x-ray shows no sign for pneumonia; the urine analysis shows a mild infection. The possible reason for acute abdomen: intestinal leakage.

Depending on the preceding type of surgery (open surgery, transurethral surgery, ESWL), postoperative

Table 18.1.18. Postoperative acute abdomen after radical cystectomy

Complications	Incidence
Pyelonephritis (Joniau et al. 2005; Meller et al. 2002; Frazier et al. 1992; Gburek et al. 1998; Madersbacher et al. 2003)	4%–23%
Ileourethral stenosis (Joniau et al. 2005; Knap et al. 2004; Frazier et al. 1992; Gburek et al. 1998; Madersbacher et al. 2003)	3%–14%
Urosepsis (Joniau et al. 2005; Hollenbeck et al. 2005; Rosario et al. 2000)	2%–8%
Ileus (Knap et al. 2004; Hollenbeck et al. 2005; Rosario et al. 2000)[4,5,10]	2%–10%
Intestinal leakage (Eriksen et al. 2005; Matthiessen et al. 2004; Nakada et al. 2004; Piso et al. 2004)	2%–9%

acute abdomen is most often caused by bleeding, abscess, ileus, or intestinal leakage. Extraabdominal disorders induced by physical and mental stress must be considered as well (acute myocardial infarction, pulmonary embolism, peptic ulcer). Most of the surgery-related complications make prompt reintervention necessary.

In urology, a postoperative acute abdomen most often occurs after open surgery, in particular after radical cystectomy. This stems from the long duration of surgery and somewhat high blood loss in combination with bowel surgery. Within the first 30 days after radical cystectomy, complications are reported in 19%–76% (Joniau et al. 2005; Tolhurst et al. 2005; Meller et al. 2002; Knap et al. 2004; Hollenbeck et al. 2005; Stein et al. 2001), most of them may clinically present as acute abdomen (see Table 18.1.18).

After transurethral surgery, an acute abdomen may be attributable to intraperitoneal bladder perforation and bleeding (Nieder et al. 2005; Collado et al. 2000; Kondas and Szentgyorgyi 1992; Pycha et al. 2003). In case of small extraperitoneal perforations, often prolonged catheter drainage is sufficient therapy, whereas larger or intraperitoneal perforations may require abdominal exploration.

Acute abdomen after extracorporeal shockwave lithotripsy (ESWL) is extremely rare, but small bowel perforation, rupture of the kidney, or perforation of the ureter may result in acute abdomen (Klug et al. 2001; Kurtz et al. 1999; Alkibay et al. 1992; Geh et al. 1997; Holmberg et al. 1997).

The main goal after surgery is to monitor the patient to detect early signs for any postoperative complication. According to the above-mentioned probability of postoperative acute abdomen patients with a high risk (e.g., after cystectomy) should be monitored more closely than low-risk patients. The postoperative monitoring should include as a minimal standard:

- Vital signs (blood pressure, heart rate)
- Temperature
- Complete blood count, electrolytes, creatinine
- Fluid balance
- Monitoring of blood drainage

If any of these findings are pathological or the patient presents clinical signs of a postoperative complication (e.g., pain or rigid abdomen), the diagnosis should be extended, which may include:

- Physical examination (auscultation, palpation, percussion)
- Vital signs (blood pressure, heart rate, respiratory rate, oxygen saturation)
- 12-lead electrocardiogram (EKG)
- Complete blood count, electrolytes, creatinine, D-dimer, troponin T, amylase, lipase, glucose, clotting, Ca^{2+}
- Depending on the experience of the surgeon and indication: ultrasound (e.g., bladder, kidneys, abdomen), abdominal x-ray (AXR) or CT scan
- Blood and urine cultures

It must be mentioned that not all examinations are mandatory and some complications such as bleeding may require immediate relaparotomy. Therefore all diagnoses must be tailored to each patient and the individual medical history.

18.1.3.1 Initial Management

As long as the underlying reason for an acute abdomen is unknown, the initial management after surgery should include:

- Nothing by mouth (NBM)
- Intravenous fluids (fluid volume and electrolytes)
- Nasogastric tube
- Stress ulcer prophylaxis
- Antibiotics
- Analgesia

Further therapy depends on the cause of acute abdomen (e.g., reintervention).

18.1.4 Postoperative Fever

18.1.4.1 Overview

Surgical patients are subjected to dramatic alterations in body temperature during the intraoperative and postoperative periods (Sessler 1997). "Postoperative fever" is a recognized term in the literature even though the syndrome has not been clearly characterized. An important question is whether postoperative elevations in body temperature represent true fever or hyperthermia. True fever is an alteration of the thermoregulatory setpoint, which implies a feeling of cold discomfort and active vasoconstriction and shivering until the new setpoint is attained. Hyperthermia occurs when heat gain (usually from an exogenous source) exceeds heat loss, resulting in an elevated Tc that is not regulated.

Elevated core temperature (Tc) in the postoperative period occurs commonly and the mechanism and clinical relevance is poorly understood. It seems that early postoperative elevation in Tc is a normal response after major surgical procedures due to tissue injury and perioperative stress that occurs in proportion to the duration of surgery and is associated with elevated levels of cytokines (Frank et al. 2000). This response satisfies the true definition of fever, i.e., a regulated increase in Tc setpoint. The setpoint for Tc is influenced by endogenous substances, categorized as pyrogens (IL-1, IL-6, tumor necrosis factor, interferon) or cryogens (glucocorticoids, arginine vasopressin), which work by altering the thermoregulatory setpoint in the anterior hypothalamus. The effect of endogenous pyrogens is to increase the Tc setpoint in the anterior hypothalamus.

Although traditional definitions of fever (38.3–38.5 °C) appear to correlate with infection in medical patients (Bates et al. 1990), febrile surgical patients frequently have no identifiable source of infection (Bell et al. 1978; Goodman et al. 1968).

In the past, pulmonary atelectasis has classically been described as the cause of postoperative fever, but more recent studies indicate that the cause of fever in the postoperative period is equally likely to be infectious or noninfectious (Marik 2000; O'Grady et al. 1998a, b). In other words, fever in the postoperative period is neither sensitive nor specific as a clinical sign of infection.

In summary, patients who undergo major surgical procedures experience a regulated increase in Tc setpoint in the early postoperative period, which fits the classic definition of fever. The average Tc setpoint after surgery is elevated by 1.4 °C (2.5°F) above the preoperative baseline. A greater incidence of infection is well recognized when the duration of follow-up is longer. The clinician should therefore use caution when interpreting fever occurring later in the postoperative course when fever may more likely be associated with infection.

Because fever is often the earliest and most easily detected sign of infection in the surgical patient, it is important that in clinical practice there is a clear defined work-up and management.

18.1.4.2 Incidence

Depending on the definition of postoperative fever (see Sect. 18.1.3.1), reviewed literature has estimated its incidence to be between 13 % and 40 %. In general, the procedures with longer surgical incisions and longer duration have the greatest postoperative increase in Tc. Conversely, procedures with shorter incisions and duration have less increase in core temperature (Frank et al. 2000).

18.1.4.3 Definition

See Table 18.1.19.

18.1.4.4 Risk Factors and Prevention

Preoperative identification of risk factors (Table 18.1.3.5) is the best prevention and the most important aspect of therapy.

1. Regarding the pulmonary tract, nosocomial pneumonia is the second most common hospital-acquired infection, after urinary tract infections, and accounts for between 27 % and 47 % of infections within the intensive care unit (ICU) and reported mortality rates between 30 % and 70 % (Kollef 2004). Nosocomial pneumonia is usually defined as hospital-acquired pneumonia that occurs at least 48 h after admission to hospital but excludes any infection that was incubating at the time of admission (Craven and Steger 195). Key risk factors include chronic lung disease, advanced age (> 60 years), smoking, prolonged duration of mechanical ventilation, supine position, and previous antibiotic therapy (Cook and Kollef 1998; Trouillet et al. 1998). Common pathogens responsible for early- (develops after > 2 days but < 4 days of hospitalization) and late-onset nosocomial pneumonia are listed in Table 18.1.20.
2. Catheter-associated urinary tract infection (CAUTI) is the most common nosocomial infection in hospitals worldwide and the incidence has been reported to be approximately 35 %. Although most CAUTIs are asymptomatic (Tambyah and Maki 2000), they often precipitate unnecessary antimicrobial therapy. Numerous studies have documented a high prevalence of resistant pathogens in CAUTI. The association between nosocomial CAUTI and surgical site infections has been made (Krieger et al. 1983).
   The most important risk factors have been prolonged catheterization and being female. Other

Disorder	Definition
Infection	Presence of organisms in a normally sterile site that is usually, but not necessarily, accompanied by an inflammatory host response
Bacteremia	Bacteria present in blood as confirmed by culture may be transient
Septicemia	Same as bacteremia, but implies greater severity Clinical evidence of infection plus evidence of a systemic response to infection. This systemic response is manifested by two or more of the following conditions: Temperature >38 °C or <36 °C Heart rate >90 beats/min Respiratory rate >20 breaths/min or $PaCO_2$ <32 mm Hg (<4.3 kPa) WBC >12,000 cells/mm³ <4,000 cells/mm³ or 10 % immature (band) forms
Sepsis syndrome	Infection plus evidence of altered organ perfusion with at least one of the following: hypoxemia, elevated lactate, oliguria, altered mentation
Hypotension	A systolic blood pressure of <90 mm Hg or a reduction of >40 mm Hg from baseline in the absence of other causes of hypotension
Severe sepsis	Sepsis associated with organ dysfunction, hypoperfusion, or hypotension. Hypoperfusion and perfusion abnormalities may include but are not limited to lactic acidosis, oliguria, or an acute alteration on mental status
Septic shock	Sepsis with hypotension despite adequate fluid resuscitation along with the presence of perfusion abnormalities that may include, but are not limited to, lactic acidosis, oliguria, or an acute alteration in mental status. Patients who are on inotropic or vasopressor agents may not be hypotensive at the time that perfusion abnormalities are measured
Systemic inflammatory response syndrome (SIRS)	Response to a wide variety of clinical insults, which can be infectious, as in sepsis but can be noninfectious in etiology (e.g., burns, pancreatitis)

Table 18.1.19. Clinical diagnostic criteria of sepsis and septic shock

See Chap. 3
Adopted from Naber et al. (2001)

Table 18.1.20. Microbial etiology of nosocomial pneumonia

Pathogen	Onset of pneumonia*	Frequency (%)
Streptococcus pneumoniae	Early	10–20
Haemophilus influenzae	Early	5–15
Anaerobic bacteria	Early	10–30
Staphylococcus aureus	Early/late	20–30
Gram-negative bacilli	Late	30–60
Pseudomonas aeruginosa	Late	17
Klebsiella pneumoniae	Late	7
Acinetobacter spp.	Late	3
Escherichia coli	Late	6
Enterobacter spp.	Late	10
Legionella pneumophila	Late	0–15

Adapted from Craven and Steger (1995)

risk factors identified have included catheterization outside the sterile environment of the operating room, having a urinary tract abnormality, other infections, diabetes, malnutrition, and renal failure. An important factor for preventing infection is the maintenance of a closed sterile drainage system. On the urological ward, it is essential to allow the drainage tube to be above the level of the patient and the collecting tube should be kept from kinking. The collecting bag should be emptied regularly using a separate collecting container. Poorly functioning or obstructed catheters should be irrigated or if necessary, replaced. Meatal care, addition of antimicrobial agents in the drainage device, and vesical irrigation are useless (Leone et al. 2004). Antibiotics are in general protective, but the infections, when they occur, tend to be caused by antibiotic-resistant organisms (Tambyah 2004). The best way of preventing a CAUTI is to remove the catheter or to avoid its use. Suprapubic catheters are associated with a decreased rate of CAUTI (Tambyah 2004).

3. The use of central venous catheters (CVCs) has become an indispensable routine in modern medical practice. It has spread from ICUs and operating rooms to general wards and outpatient clinics. One of the most common and serious complications associated with CVCs is catheter-related infections (CRIs) (Hammarskjold et al. 2006; McGee and Gould 2003). The incidence of CRI varies between 2 and 30 per 1,000 catheter days(Hammarskjold et al. 2006; Fraenkel et al. 2000). Known risk factors for CRI include neutropenia, immunosuppression, ICU admission, shock, parenteral nutrition, long-term hemodialysis, and insertion via the femoral or internal jugular vein (Polerman and Girbes 2002). The mortality rate as a result of CRI is reported to be between 0% and 25% (Polerman and Girbes 2002; Crnich and Maki 2002)). The most common microbiologi-

Table 18.1.21. Risk and protective factors for central venous catheter-related infections

Risk factors	Protective factors
Duration of catheterization	Maximum asepsis
Type of catheter (higher risk with multiple lumen catheter)	Aseptic topical care
Location of insertion (lower risk with subclavian insertion, higher risk with femoral or internal jugular vein	Antiseptic or antibiotic-coated devices
Emergent insertion	
Number of manipulations	
Age	
Disease (benign vs malignant)	
Neutropenia	
Immunosuppression	
ICU admission	
Shock	
Parenteral nutrition	
Long-term hemodialysis	

Table 18.1.22. Microbial etiology of central venous catheter-related infections,

Pathogen	Total
Coagulase-negative staphylococci	~60%
Pseudomonas aeruginosa	~10%
Staphylococcus aureus	5%–6%
Enterobacter	5%
Escherichia coli	2.5%
Enterococcus faecalis	2.5%
Klebsiella pneumoniae	2.5%
Candida albicans	5%

Adapted from Hammarskjold et al. (2006) and Paragioudaki et al. (2004)

cal agents responsible for CRI are *Staphylococcus aureus*, coagulase-negative staphylococci, *Candida* species, and various Gram-negative rods (O'Grady et al. 2002) (refer to Tables 18.1.21 and 18.1.22).

In our institution, the CVC are inserted using maximal sterile precautions (cap, mask, gown, gloves, large drape) with a Seldinger technique by an anesthetic specialist. The insertion site is treated with a solution containing 2% chlorhexidine. The site is dressed with a transparent semipermeable dressing (Tegaderm HP, 3M). Every 3rd day, dressings and stopcocks are changed and the insertion site is treated with the 2% chlorhexidine solution. In a trial performed by Hammarskjöld et al., the median duration of catheterization for the CRI group was 20 days and 15 days for those without infection.

In terms of surgical wound infection, obesity, diabetes, corticosteroids, and stress are the major risk factors. The incidence of surgical site infection (SSI) in the urologic population varies in the literature, with rates ranging from 5.5% to 33% (Takeyama et al. 2005) in patients receiving cystectomy and urinary diversion (Adam et al. 2004; Berger 2005; Hamasuna et al. 2004). Microorganisms originating from the patient and the patient's immediate environment are the primary sources for SSI (*Staphylococcus epidermidis, S. aureus, MRSA*[Methicillin-resistant coagulase-negative *S. aureus*], *Escherichia coli, Proteus mirabilis, Pseudomonas aeroginosa, Enterobacteriaceae*) (Harbarth et al. 1999). The first step in prevention of wound infection starts with the preparation of the operative site. Specifically, avoidance of shaving the skin is emphasized, because the use of a razor increases the risk of skin breakage, which can allow pathogens direct access to the bloodstream. A current review concerning the issue of hair removal policies in clean surgery quotes four randomized, controlled trials, while no eligible meta-analysis was found (Niel-Weise et al. 2005). When hair removal was considered necessary, evidence about the best time for removal was inconclusive. There was some evidence that hair removal by clipper is superior to removal by razor. A Cochrane Database Review in 2006 (Tanner et al. 2006) questioned whether a preoperative hair removal results in a fewer surgical site infections. Only two trials involving 358 patients matched the inclusion criteria of this review. Of people who were shaved, 9.6% developed an SSI compared with 6% who were not shaved. There was no statistically significant difference between shaving and no hair removal; however, the studies were not of high quality and the comparison was underpowered. The same applies to when depilatory cream was compared with no hair removal. When shaving was compared with clipping to reduce SSIs, the difference was statistically significant and shows that people are more likely to develop an SSI when they were shaved than when they were clipped prior to surgery. Unfortunately, no studies were identified which compared clipping with no hair removal.

A different objective is the effect on SSI rates of hair removal immediately before surgery compared with hair removal more than 4 h before surgery. Tanner et al. found no statistically significant difference in his Cochrane Database Review. In conclusion, the review found insufficient evidence for an effect of preoperative hair removal, but if hair removal is considered to be necessary it should be performed with clippers because this results in fewer SSIs.

Preoperative urinary tract infection (UTI) is the major risk factor for SSI in patients undergoing urological surgery. Therefore, urine culture and sensitivities should be available, and UTIs should be treated with appropriate antibiotics preoperatively (Hamasuna et al. 2004).

The etiology of wound complications in obese patients is probably related to the poor vascularity of subcutaneous fat, serous fluid collection, and hematoma formation. Studies have shown that using a subcutaneous suture in all patients with greater than 2-cm subcu-

Table 18.1.23. Risk factors for postoperative fever

Risk factors	Measures taken to reduce risk of infection
Category of surgical procedure	Prophylactic use of antibiotics
Diabetes mellitus	Bowel preparation
Prosthetic heart valve	Bowel preparation
Stress	Bowel preparation
Obesity	Bowel preparation
Corticosteroids	Bowel preparation
	Improvement in general state of patient: Chest physiotherapy Use of bronchodilators

taneous depth significantly reduces the risk of wound disruption. Specifically, closure of excess subcutaneous tissue eliminates dead space, thus reducing the formation of seromas.

Impaired wound healing is frequently seen in patients with diabetes. Cruse and Foord (Cruse and Foord 1973) reviewed infection rates in 23,649 patients and found that diabetics had five times the risk of infection of nondiabetics. Although increased levels of HgA1c do not seem to be positively correlated to surgical site infections in one study, diabetes and postoperative hyperglycemia are independent risk factors for a SSI. It was demonstrated that glucose levels above 200 mg/dl in the immediate postoperative period are associated with an increased SSI rate. Additionally, blood glucose levels above 200 mg/dl at 48 h after surgery are significantly associated with deep wound infection.

No specific recommendations other than avoidance of hyperglycemia (blood glucose <200 mg/dl) and strict regulation of insulin to assist in wound healing can be made (Table 18.1.23).

18.1.4.5 Detection and Work-Up

Concerning etiology of postoperative fever in terms of infection, six different predominant sites are considered.

	Site
1	Pulmonary tract – most common in the immediate postoperative period
2	Urinary tract – common in patients with indwelling catheters
3	Cellulitis in venous access sites
4	Surgical wound infections – generally present 3–7 days postoperatively
5	Intraabdominal sepsis from abscess – generally present after the 5th–7th postoperative day
6	Bacteremia or septicemia

Table 18.1.24. Symptoms and workup in pneumonia

Symptoms and clinical signs	Workup
Systemic upset Fever	Chest x-ray (infiltrate) U&E, FBC (with differential white cell count)
Pleuritic pain, cough, green sputum	Blood cultures
Hemoptysis	Expectorated sputum culture and microscopy (serology)
Confusion (in elderly)	Endotracheal or bronchoscopic aspirate
Crepitation	Quantitatively cultured bronchoscopic bronchoalveolar lavage fluid or brush catheter specimen
Tachypnea	
Sputum purulence	
Degree of oxygenation impairment	

Pulmonary

All patients with suspected pneumonia should have a chest x-ray to assess the severity and complications. Routine blood cultures are also recommended, preferably before initiating antimicrobial treatment. Sputum examination including sputum culture, microscopy, and serology for atypical pneumonia (*Legionella*, *Mycoplasma*, *Chlamydia*, *Coxiella*) should be evaluated (Table 18.1.24).

Urinary Tract

Symptoms are not reliable for the diagnosis of CAUTI. Sometimes it is hard to demonstrate a difference in presence of fever or symptoms related to the urinary tract in catheterized patients with and without CAUTI. The catheter can itself be the source of symptoms. The majority of cases of bloodstream infection associated with CAUTI are in patients where there is significant urinary obstruction. It has also been shown that patients with long-term indwelling catheters rarely have febrile episodes even though they have chronic significant amounts of bacteria in their urine. This changes when obstruction or encrustation occurs in that setting.

Suprapubic aspiration of the bladder represents the gold standard in the diagnosis of urinary tract infection. It is, however, not performed routinely in clinical practice in which urine samples are generally aspirated from the catheter itself or through a port designed specifically for that purpose. Disconnecting the catheter more than absolutely necessary is a violation of the closed drainage principle and is discouraged. The urine sample should be sent immediately to the bacteriology laboratory since bacteria will continue to proliferate in the warm medium, leading to increased bacterial counts. If such immediate referral is not possible, the container should be transported in iced water and then stored in a refrigerator at 40 °C. Cooling stops bacterial growth, but the following day the bacteria can still grow on culture medium. The definition of CAUTI is restricted to the presence of bacteria in the bladder of a patient with an indwelling catheter. Bacteriuria is defined as the detection of more than 10^5 cfu/ml organisms per milliliter of urine with no more than two species of organism (contamination). Because of the prevalence of bacteriuria in patients with urinary catheters, some have advocated daily monitoring of urine in catheterized patients. Routine monitoring of the urine from all catheterized patients is not an effective way to decrease the incidence of symptomatic CAUTI (Garibaldi et al. 1982). Thus, frequent microbiologic monitoring to detect early contamination of the urine in hope of preventing urosepsis cannot be recommended.

From the clinical point of view, a CAUTI can manifest itself as bacteriuria, bacteremia, septicemia, or sepsis syndrome. Sepsis syndrome is diagnosed when clinical evidence of infection is accompanied by signs of inflammation (fever, hypothermia, tachycardia, tachypnea, hypotension, oliguria, leukocyturia, or leukopenia).

Asymptomatic bacteriuria or asymptomatic CAUTI is a microbiologic diagnosis from a patient without symptoms or signs referable to urinary tract infection. The usual quantitative definition is 10^5 cfu/mL or greater in two consecutive urine specimens (Rubin et al. 1992). Acute uncomplicated urinary tract infection is a symptomatic bladder infection characterized by frequency, urgency, dysuria, or suprapubic pain, while acute nonobstructive pyelonephritis is a renal infection characterized by costovertebral angle pain and tenderness, often with fever. In sedated patients, history, complaints, and physical examination are limited. Therefore, urinalysis and culture should be taken; the same applies for blood tests (Tables 18.1.25, 18.1.26). In any case, ultrasound of the bladder as well as the kidneys must be performed. Hydronephrosis, abscesses, and urinary retention needs immediate intervention. If stones are suspected, plain x-ray or native CT scan should be considered. In case of perinephric abscess, abscess of the kidney, or retroperitoneal abscess, a contrast-enhanced CT scan is advised because of the feasibility of a percutaneous intervention and the confirmation of the diagnosis. An algorithm is suggested in Fig. 18.1.3.2.

Table 18.1.25. Symptoms and workup in UTI/CAUTI

Symptoms and clinical signs	Workup
Systemic upset	Urinalysis and culture
Fever	U&E, FBC (with differential white cell count)
Pyuria	Fibrinogen < 1 g/l, platelets < 50,000 mm³, PT and aPTT 1.5–1.8 × control
Suprapubic pain	Blood cultures
Frequency, urgency, dysuria	Sonography of urinary bladder and kidney
Costovertebral angle pain	Consider plain x-ray (abdomen)
Confusion (in elderly)	Consider CT scan (abdomen)
Sepsis signs	Consider MRI

Table 18.1.26. Microbial etiology of UTI/CAUTI (Calandra and Cohen 2005)

Pathogens	Frequency (%)
Escherichia coli	53
Enterococcus	20
Pseudomonas group	8.3
Staphylococcus aureus	6.6
Proteus group	5
Klebsiella	5
Candida	3.3

Central Venous Catheters and Catheter-Related Infections

The diagnosis of CRI is often a diagnosis of exclusion. Clinical findings are nonspecific to establish a diagnosis of catheter-related sepsis. Nevertheless, a diagnostic algorithm is suggested in Fig. 18.1.6. A clinical suspicion of catheter infection in the presence of otherwise unexplained severe sepsis or septic shock, however, should prompt catheter removal and appropriate cultures of the catheter tip, blood cultures, and exit-site or hub cultures depending on the presentation. The clinical probability of CRI increases when a catheter has been in place 7 days. Local signs at the catheter exit site such as erythema, cellulitis along the subcutaneous tract of the catheter, and pus also increase the clinical probability of CRI, although the majority of CRI occurs in the absence of local symptoms.

Surgical (Wound) Site Infection

The diagnosis is SSI is a obvious clinical presentation with calor, dolor, rubor, and tumor (heat, pain, redness, and swelling) as known from textbooks of basic medicine.

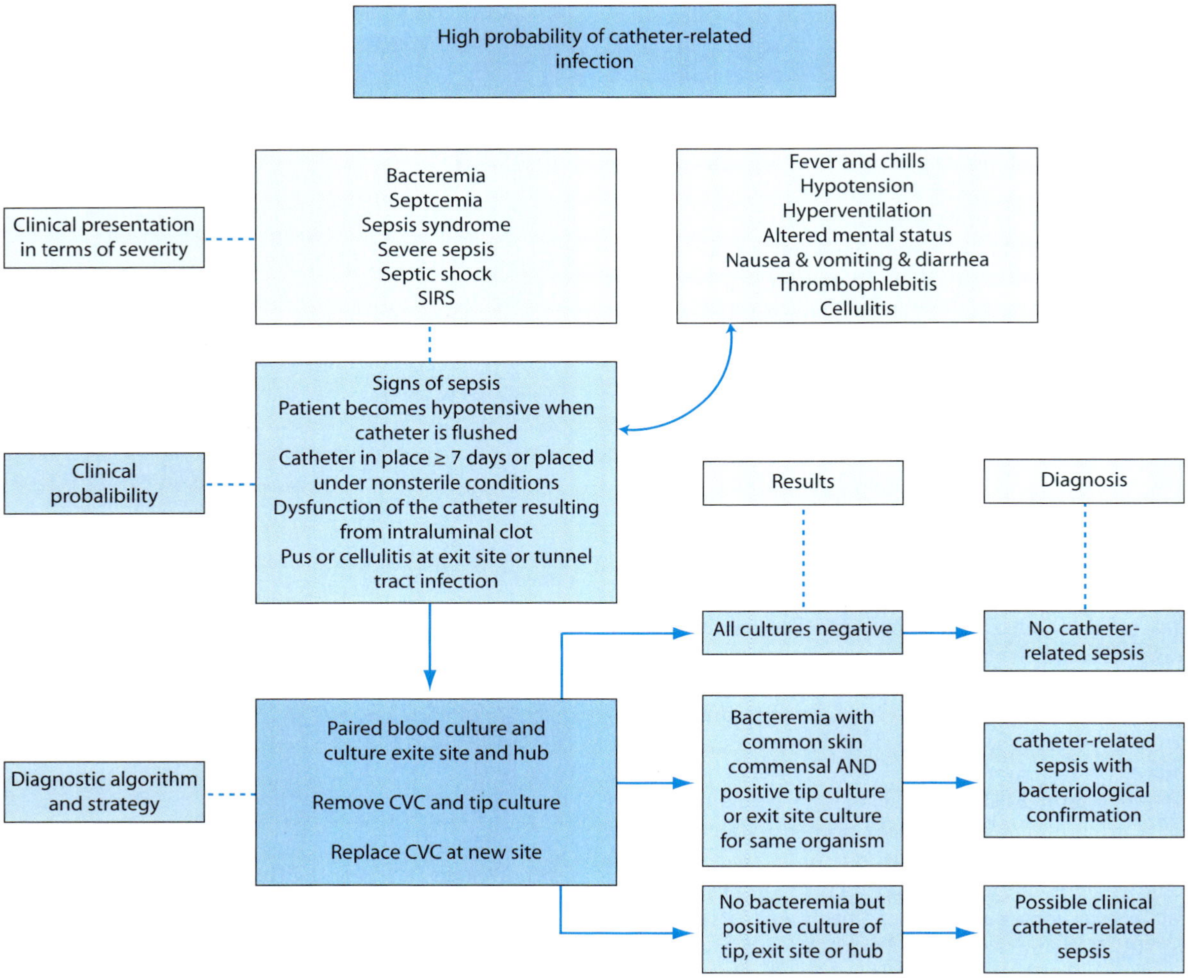

Fig. 18.1.6. Modified diagnostic algorithm in the diagnosis of central venous catheter-related infection (Calandra and Cohen 2005)

Intraabdominal Sepsis from Abscess

Refer to Sect. 18.1.3.7.4.

Bacteremia or Septicemia – Bloodstream Infection

Bloodstream infections (BSIs) account for 30%–40% of all cases of severe sepsis and septic shock (Bochud et al. 2001). However, the incidence of BSI as a cause of severe sepsis is probably underestimated in the hospital setting, since blood cultures are frequently drawn from patients treated with broad-spectrum antibiotics. BSIs can be divided into two categories:

1. Primary BSI comprising BSI of unknown origin in patients without an identifiable focus of infection, and intravascular catheter-related BSI (see Sect. 18.1.3.5.3 above).
2. Secondary BSI defined as a BSI caused by a micro-organism related to an infection at another site.

The patient has a recognized pathogen defined as a microorganism different from a common skin contaminant (i.e., diphtheroids, *Bacillus* species, *Propionibacterium* species, coagulase-negative staphylococci, or micrococci) cultured from one or more blood cultures.

Diagnosis is obtained by blood cultures; for management refer to Sect. 18.1.3.6.3.

18.1.4.6 Management

The treatment of true fever (see Sect. 18.1.3.3) should focus primarily on returning the setpoint toward normal with antipyretics (acetaminophen or cyclooxygenase inhibitors).

Current Treatment of Nosocomial Pneumonia

There are various published guidelines and recommendations for the treatment of nosocomial pneumonia. Generally, nosocomial pneumonia is divided into three levels of severity (Kollef 2004):

- Group (1):
  - Mild/moderate without risk factors, any time of onset (early/late)
  - Severe without risk factors, early onset
- Group (2):
  - Mild/moderate with risk factors, any time of onset (early/late)
- Group (3):
  - Severe pneumonia without risk factors, late onset
  - Severe pneumonia with risk factors, any time of onset (early/late)

Group 1	**Antibiotics**
Enteric Gram-negative bacteria	Third-generation cephalosporins (cefotaxime/ceftriaxone)
Escherichia coli	If *Enterobacter* suspected:
Klebsiella spp.	– β-lactam/β-lactamase inhibitor combination
Proteus spp.	Ampicillin/sulbactam
Serratia marcescens	Ticarcillin/clavulanate
Haemophilus influenzae	Piperacillin/tazobactam
Methicillin-sensitive	If allergic to penicillin:
S. aureus	– Fluoroquinolone
Streptococcus pneumoniae	– Clindamycin plus aztreonam
Group 2	**Antibiotics**
Group 1 organism plus	Group 1 antibiotics plus
Anaerobes	– Clindamycin or β-lactam/β-lactamase inhibitor combination
Staphylococcus aureus	– Vancomycin (until methicillin-resistant *S. aureus* excluded)
Legionella	– Erythromycin
Pseudomonas aeruginosa	– Antipseudomonal penicillin (pieracillin, titarcillin)
Group 3	**Antibiotics**
Group 1 organism plus	Group 1 antibiotics plus
Acinetobacter spp.	– Aminoglycoside or fluoroquinolone plus one of the following:
Pseudomonas aeruginosa	Anti-pseudomonal penicillin (pieracillin, titarcillin)
Methicillin-resistant *S. aureus*	β-lactam/β-lactamase inhibitor combination
	Aztreonam
	– Imipenem/meropenem ± vancomycinllin)

Appropriate empiric antibacterial treatment should be initiated as soon as infection is suspected, since a delay in starting treatment will reduce the effectiveness of therapy and increase the risk of mortality (Iregui et al. 2002; Luna 1997). Following initial therapy, laboratory data on the identification and susceptibility profile of the causative pathogen allow specific therapy. The duration of antibacterial treatment should be limited to the shortest effective course of therapy, to reduce the risk of creating resistance. Seven days of therapy for VAP should be sufficient and could prevent recolonization with resistant pathogens (Kollef 2004), although no prospective randomized controlled trials exist.

Treatment of CAUTI

From expert opinion, asymptomatic bacteriuria does not require treatment (Cravens and Zweig 2000). Indwelling catheters can be changed in this setting, although no evidence is available in the literature. In a randomized comparison of active management including a short course of antibiotic and the replacement of indwelling catheter vs control, no benefit was associated with the active management, and a trend to multiresistant bacterial superinfection was observed in this group (Leone et al. 2004).

There are only a few specific studies of urinary tract infection (UTI) in populations of ICU patients with severe sepsis/septic shock, and although both bacterial CAUTI and candiduria are very common, CAUTI is the most common nosocomial infection. According to the International Conference for the Development of a Consensus on the Management and Prevention of Severe Candidal Infections, colonized patients without evidence of infection do not require treatment. Nevertheless, candiduria can occasionally be the only accessible evidence of deep candidiasis. Candiduria is rare in normal healthy adults, and even in an unselected hospital population only about 2% of urine samples received in the laboratory will show candiduria, although this number rises to 3%–15% in the ICU in catheterized patients (Leone et al. 2003b; Tissot et al. 2001). *Candida albicans* and *Candida glabrata* are found in 46% and 31% of cases, respectively (Leone et al. 2003a). There is considerable uncertainty about the criteria to be used in interpreting the finding of candiduria. The early work of Goldberg et al. (1979) suggesting that *Candida* species counts of 10^4/ml represent clinically significant infection has been supported by others, although there are certainly reports suggesting that lower counts can be associated with symptoms and indeed that lower counts often quickly increase to higher counts if untreated. Hence, in the clinical setting, and in particular on the ICU, clinicians will rarely rely on microbiology alone to decide on the significance of candiduria. They will have to integrate other clinical information. Fluconazole may be the best option for treating candiduria Edwards et al. 1997), but only if the species is *C. albicans*. Voriconazole may be more effective against non-*albicans* species.

In the clinical setting, infected hydronephrosis due to any cause, kidney or perinephric abscesses are

Table 18.1.27. Recommendations for antimicrobial therapy in urology

Diagnosis	Frequent pathogens	Initial, empiric antimicrobial therapy	Therapy duration
UTI with complicating factors	*E. coli*	– Cephalosporin, third-generation (cefotaxime, ceftazidime)	3–5 Days after defervescence or control/elimination of complicating factor
Nosocomial UTI	*Enterococcus*	– Fluoroquinolone (ofloxacin, levofloxacin)	
Pyelonephritis, acute, complicated	*Staphylococcus*	– Anti-*Pseudomonas* active Acylaminopenicllin/ BLI	
Urosepsis	*Klebsiella* *Proteus* *Enterobacter* *Pseudomonas* *Candida* *Serratia*	– Carbapenem – Meropenem ± Aminoglycoside	

Modified according to Naber et al. (2005)
BLI β-lactamase inhibitor

dreaded pathologies because of their potential to turn into severe sepsis. In these cases, it is of utmost importance to come to a rapid diagnosis in order to prelude adequate source control measures. Usually infected hydronephrosis needs to be drained either by a double-J catheter combined with a transurethral catheter or a percutaneous nephrostomy. Early administration of appropriate antimicrobial agents is equally essential. Both kidney and perirenal abscesses need to be drained by inserting a tube (e.g., a pigtail catheter) guided by ultrasound or CT scan. In severe cases, emergency nephrectomy may be indicated in individual cases (refer to Table 18.1.27 and Fig. 18.1.27).

Catheter-Related Infections

The therapy for local CRI such as infection of the insertion site or thrombophlebitis is removing the catheter. Catheter removal is also necessary if *Staphylococcus aureus* is detected in blood cultures. An exchange of the CVC using a guidewire at the infected insertion site may result in bacteremia and septic emboli and therefore should be omitted. In thrombophlebitis and insertion site infection, local and systemic administration of antibiotics is not required unless temperature rises above 38 °C and signs of infection such as purulence are present and cultures are negative. Warm soaks and elevation of the extremity should be sufficient. If any sign of systemic infection is seen, antimicrobial therapy for 7 days or less should be sufficient. If therapy via CVC continues to be necessary and an alternative site for inserting the CVC is unavailable, antimicrobial therapy without removal of the CVC is reasonable in the absence of signs or symptoms of sepsis in the presence of the following pathogens: coagulase-negative staphylococci, *Corynebacterium jeikeium*, *Acinetobacter baumannii*, *Stenotrophomonas maltophilia*, *Pseudomonas aeruginosa*, and *Bacillus* spp. In these cases, it is essential to follow patients up carefully. Attempts to preserve the catheter in patients with CRI due to *S. aureus* have no more than a 20% chance of success (Marr et al. 1997). Catheter preservation is inadvisable in patients with *S. aureus* bacteremia also because of the high risk of secondary complications (endocarditis, osteomyelitis). Catheter removal is likewise necessary in patients with CRI due to *Candida* spp.

Since more than 60% of CRIs are related to staphylococci (coagulase-negative staphylococci), vancomycin (15 mg/kg i.v. every 12 h, if renal function is normal) should be administered as empirical treatment. When cultures grow, a pathogen treatment should be amended accordingly.

The impact of *S. aureus* bacteremia on clinical management has to be stressed specifically. Sufficiently long treatment periods are necessary to adequately address the risk of seeding (e.g., endocarditis, osteomyelitis). Accordingly, 2–4 weeks of treatment with intravenous antibiotics are recommended (Raad and Sabbagh 1992). Therapy with penicillase-resistant penicillin is more effective and therefore preferable to treatment with glycopeptide antibiotics (Siegman-Igra et al. 1997). Glycopeptides are indicated only in patients with penicillin allergy or methicillin-resistant staphylococci. Newer drugs directed against Gram-positive bacteria (linezolid, quinupristin/dalfopristin) should be reserved for patients who are intolerant or infected with organisms resistant to glycopeptide antibiotics. Table 18.1.28 gives an outline of treatment of the most common catheter-related infections.

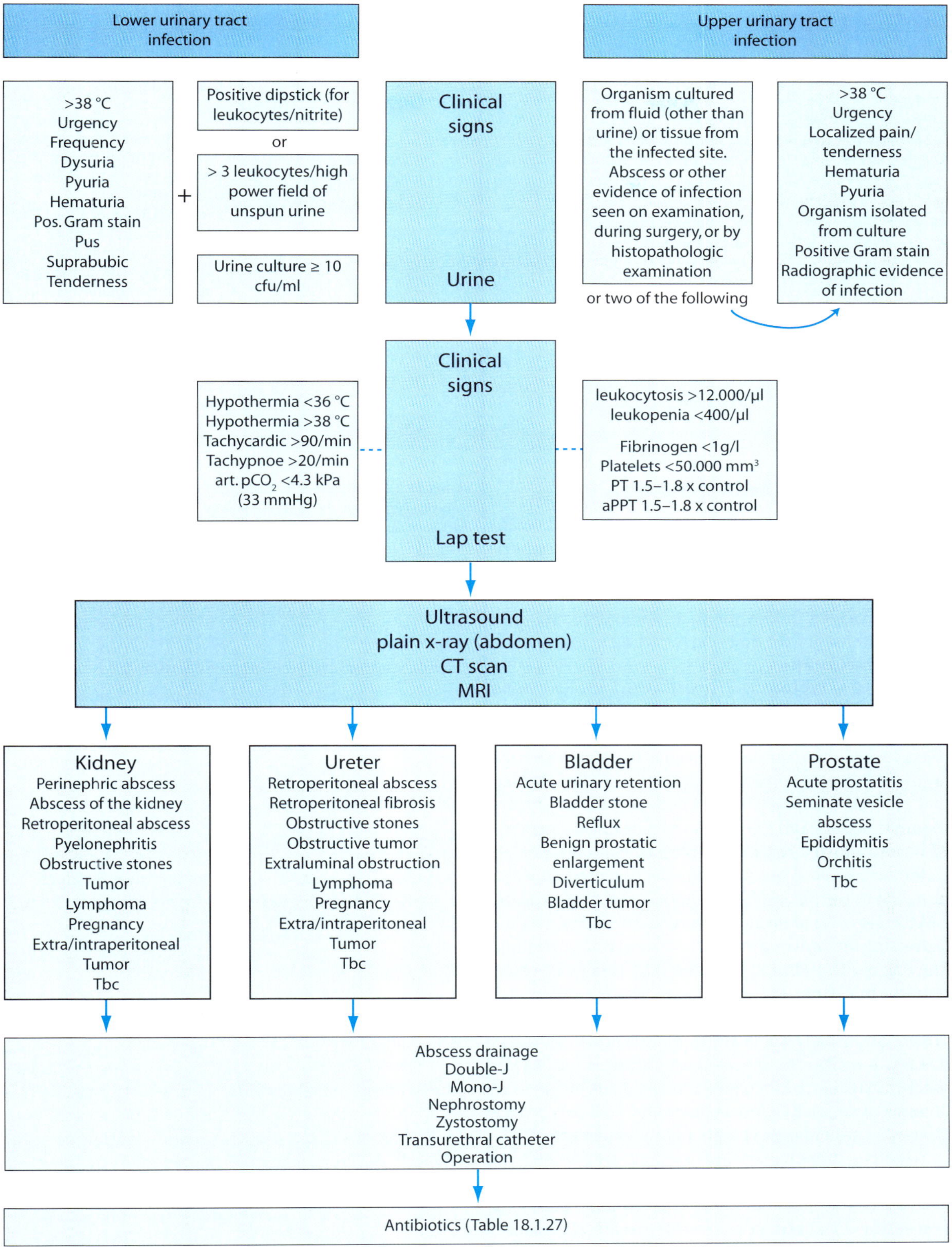

Fig. 18.1.7. Workup and management of urinary tract infection

Pathogen	Therapy	Duration
Staphylococcus aureus (oxacillin-sensitive)	Isoxazolyl penicillin (penicillase-resistant penicillin)[a]	At least 2 weeks i.v. [b]
Staphylococcus aureus (oxacillin-resistant)	Glycopeptide, linezolid, quinupristin + dalfopristin	At least 2 weeks i.v. [b]
Coagulase-negative staphylococci	According to susceptibility pattern; glycopeptide only in oxacillin-resistant cases	For 5–7 days after defervescence
Enterococci	Aminopenicillin plus aminoglycoside	For 5–7 days after defervescence
	Glycopeptide plus aminoglycoside in ampicillin-resistant cases Linezolid or quinupristin/dalfopristin in vancomycin-resistant cases	
Candida albicans	Fluconazole Alternative: amphotericin B or caspofungin	≥ 2 weeks
Non-albicans *Candida* species	Amphotericin B	≥ 2 weeks
	Alternative: caspofungin or Voriconazole or itraconazole	
All other pathogens	According to susceptibility pattern	Not defined

Table 18.1.28. Antimicrobial therapy of venous catheter-related bacteremia depending on identity of pathogen therapy duration

Follow-up blood cultures are always necessary after cessation of antibiotic therapy in order to rule out persistence of infection

From Fatkenheuer et al. (2003)

[a] For oxacillin-sensitive strains (vast majority), treatment with penicillase-resistant penicillin is superior to treatment with a glycopeptide.

[b] High incidence of organ infection if treatment is continued for less than 2 weeks. Catheter removal is required whenever these pathogens are present

Surgical Site Infection: Wound Management

Despite prophylactic measures and good surgical technique, a small percentage of patients will still experience wound complications. SSIs require manual opening of the wounds to allow drainage. An open wound can be managed in two ways: secondary closure, secondary intention with dressings or using negative pressure wound therapy.

Secondary closure can be performed once a wound is free of infection or necrotic tissue and has started to granulate. This procedure is done within 1–4 days after evacuation of hematoma or seroma. The suture may be removed 7 days after reclosure. Several studies showed that patients who were treated with secondary closure required significantly fewer days to heal than patients who were allowed to heal by secondary intention.

Modern wound care dressing selection considers factors such as the phase of healing, the volume of exudate, and the presence of necrotic tissue to determine the type of dressing that will be most supportive of wound healing. The risk of infection can be reduced by using a nontoxic solution to cleanse the wound, e.g., normal saline (Table 18.1.29). Necrotic tissue can be removed by sharp debridement or daily applications of enzymatic debriders that act on necrotic tissue but have no effect on healthy tissue. Drainage can be managed by using highly absorbent dressing material. Calcium alginate and foam are materials used in wound care that are highly absorbent.

Negative pressure wound therapy also known as vacuum-assisted closure uses controlled levels of negative pressure to assist and accelerate wound healing by evacuating localized edema with negative pressure. Bacterial colonization is reduced along with the evacuation of wound drainage. Negative pressure also increases localized blood flow and oxygenation, thereby

Table 18.1.29. Historically used dressing for wound cleansing

Misconceptions about wound healing	
Agent	**Problem**
Povidone iodine	Cytotoxic to white blood cells and other vital wound-healing components
Iodophor gauze	Delays wound healing
Hydrogen peroxide	Delays wound healing
Keeping the wound dry	Moist wounds promote autolytic debridement, support epithelial cell migration

Table 18.1.30. Definition of infective endocarditis

Definite infective endocarditis
Pathologic criteria
– Microorganisms demonstrated by culture or histologic examination of a vegetation, a vegetation that has embolized, or an intracardiac abscess, or
– Pathologic lesions; vegetation or intracardiac abscess confirmed by histologic examination showing active endocarditis
Clinical criteria
– 2 Major criteria or
– 1 Major criterion and 3 minor criteria or
– 5 Minor criterion
Possible infective endocarditis
– 1 Major criterion and 1 minor criterion or
– 3 Minor criteria
Rejected
– Firm alternative diagnosis explaining evidence of infective endocarditis or
– Resolution of infective endocarditis syndrome with antibiotics therapy <4 days or
– No pathologic evidence of infective endocarditis at surgery or autopsy, with antibiotic therapy for <4 days or
– Does not meet criteria for possible infective endocarditis

promoting a nutrient-rich environment that stimulates granulation tissue growth. Such cellular proliferation encourages angioneogenesis, uniform wound size reduction, and reepithelialization.

18.1.4.7 Special Conditions

Fever Due to Infective Endocarditis

Infective endocarditis accounts for about 1% of all cases of severe sepsis and is associated with a mortality rate of 33% (Angus et al. 2001). Diagnostic criteria for infective endocarditis, referred to as the Duke criteria, are based on microbiological data and echocardiographic imaging findings. According to these criteria, patients are classified into three diagnostic categories (definite, possible, and rejected endocarditis; see Tables 18.1.30 and 18.1.31). Recently, modifications of the Duke criteria have been proposed to take into account several identified shortcomings of the original criteria, including the increasing diagnostic role of transesophageal echocardiography and the relative risk of infective endocarditis in bloodstream infections due to *Staphylococcus aureus* (Li et al. 2000).

Clinicians may appropriately and wisely decide to treat or not treat an individual patient, regardless of whether they meet or fail to meet the criteria of "definite" or "possible" infective endocarditis (IE) by the Duke schema. The Duke criteria are meant to be only a clinical guide for diagnosing IE and, certainly, must not

Table 18.1.31. Definition of major and minor criteria of infective endocarditis

Major criteria
Blood culture positive for IE
Typical microorganisms consistent with IE from two separate blood cultures:
Streptococcus viridans, *Streptococcus bovis*, HACEK group, *Staphylococcus aureus* or
Community-acquired enterococci in the absence of a primary focus or
Microorganisms consistent with IE from persistently positive blood cultures, defined as follows:
At least two positive cultures of blood samples drawn >12 h apart or
All of three or a majority of four or more separate cultures of blood (with first and last sample drawn at least 1 h apart)
Single positive blood culture for *Coxiella burnetii* or antiphase I IgG antibody titer >1 : 800
Evidence of endocardial involvement
Echocardiogram positive for IE (TEE recommended in patients with prosthetic valves, rated at least "possible IE" by clinical criteria, or complicated IE (paravalvular abscess); TTE as first test in other patients), defined as follows:
Oscillating intracardiac mass on valve or supporting structures, in the path of regurgitant jets or
On implanted material in the absence of an alternative anatomic explanation or
Abscess or
New partial dehiscence of prosthetic valve
New valvular regurgitation (worsening or changing of preexisting murmur not sufficient)
Minor criteria
Predisposition, predisposing heart condition, or injection drug use
Fever, temperature >37 °C
Vascular phenomena, major arterial emboli, septic pulmonary infarcts, mycotic aneurysm, intracranial hemorrhage, conjunctival hemorrhages, and Janeway lesions
Immunologic phenomena: glomerulonephritis, Osler's nodes, Roth's spots, and rheumatoid factor
Microbiological evidence: positive blood culture but does not meet a major criterion as noted above or serological evidence of active infection with organism consistent with IE
Echocardiographic minor criteria eliminated

IE infective endocarditis, *TEE* transesophageal echocardiography, *TTE* transthoracic echocardiography

Table 18.1.32. Diagnosis of infective endocarditis

History
Prior cardiac lesions
Prior indwelling intravascular catheters
Prior intravenous drug abuse
Physical examination
Auscultation of cardiac murmurs
Neurologic impairment
Petechiae
Splinter hemorrhages
Janeway lesions
Osler's nodes
Roth spots
Clinical evidence of emboli (fundi, conjunctivae, skin, and digits)
Laboratory
Blood cultures – a minimum of three blood cultures should be obtained
Erythrocyte sedimentation rate ↑
CRP ↑
Leukocytes ↑
Rheumatoid factor ↑ (minor criteria in the Duke criteria)
Red blood cell casts in urine plus a low serum complement level (minor criteria in the Duke criteria)
Normochromic normocytic anemia
Organism (see Table 18.1.33)
Electrocardiogram
Heart block
Conduction delay
Baseline electrocardiogram
Chest x-ray
Septic pulmonary emboli with few or multiple focal lung infiltrates
Calcification in a cardiac valve
Echocardiography[a]
Detection of vegetations on valves
Detection of valvular dysfunction
Detection of hemodynamic dysfunction
Detection of associated abnormalities (shunt or abscess)
Histologic examination

[a] Transthoracic echocardiography (TTE) may provide confirmation of the diagnosis of endocarditis. Transesophageal echocardiography (TEE) has a higher spatial resolution than TTE and is much more sensitive for the detection of endocarditis

replace clinical judgment. In the clinical setting the diagnosis is usually obvious when a patient has the characteristic findings of IE:

- Numerous positive blood cultures in the presence of a well-recognized predisposing cardiac lesion
- Absence of infection elsewhere

However, some patients do not have positive blood cultures and 20 % – 30 % of patients have no predisposing cardiac lesion. In this setting, the correct diagnosis may be delayed.

Usually the diagnosis of IE is based upon history and physical examination, blood culture and laboratory results, an electrocardiogram (ECG), a chest x-ray, and an echocardiogram (Table 18.1.32).

Table 18.1.33. Modified therapy of infective endocarditis according to the American Heart Association

Streptococcus viridans and *Streptococcus bovis*	Aqueous crystalline Penicillin G sodium	12 – 18 Million U/24 h IV either continuously or in four or six equally divided doses	4 weeks
History of penicillin allergy Relatively resistant to penicillin	Ceftriaxone sodium plus gentamicin sulfate	2 g/24 h IV/IM in one dose 3 mg/kg per 24 h IV/IM in one dose	4 2
Penicillin-susceptible strains of *S. pneumoniae* and *Streptococcus pyogenes*	Aqueous crystalline Penicillin G sodium	24 Million U/24 h IV either continuously or in four or six equally divided doses	4
Group B, C, G streptococci	Ceftriaxone sodium Aqueous crystalline Penicillin G sodium plus gentamicin sulfate	2 g/24 h IV/IM in one dose 24 Million U/24 h IV either continuously or in four or six equally divided doses 3 mg/kg per 24 h IV/IM in one dose	4 4 2 2
Enterococcus – strains susceptible to penicillin, gentamicin, and vancomycin	Ampicillin sodium or Aqueous crystalline Penicillin G sodium plus gentamycin sulfate	12 g/24 h IV in six equally divided doses 4 – 6 18 – 30 Million U/24 h IV either continuously or in six equally divided doses 3 mg/kg per 24 h IV/IM in three equally divided doses	4 – 12 4 – 6 4 – 6
Staphylococcus – strains susceptible to oxacillin	Nafcillin or oxacillin	12 g/24 h IV in four to six equally divided doses	6
In the absence of prosthetic materials	with optional addition of gentamycin sulfate	3 mg/kg per 24 h IV/IM in two or three equally divided doses	1
History of penicillin allergy	Cefazolin with optional addition of gentamycin sulfate	6 g/24 h IV in three equally divided doses 3 mg/kg per 24 h IV/IM in two or three equally divided doses	6 1
Staphylococcus – strains resistant to oxacillin In the absence of prosthetic materials	Vancomycin	30 mg/kg per 24 h IV in two equally divided doses	6
Staphylococcus – strains susceptible to oxacillin	Nafcillin or oxacillin	12 g/24 h IV in six equally divided doses	6
Therapy for prosthetic valve endocarditis	plus Rifampin	900 mg per 24 h IV/PO in three equally divided doses	6
History of penicillin allergy	plus gentamicin Cefazolin	3 mg/kg per 24 h IV/IM in two or three equally divided doses 6 g/24 h IV in three equally divided doses	2 6
Staphylococcus – strains resistant to oxacillin	Vancomycin	30 mg/kg 24 h in two equally divided doses Adjust vancomycin to achieve 1-h serum concentration of 30 – 45 g/ml and trough concentration of 10 – 15 g/ml	6 6
Staphylococcus – strains resistant to oxacillin	plus Rifampin plus gentamycin	900 mg/24 h IV/PO in 3 equally divided doses 3 mg/kg per 24 h IV/IM in two or three equally divided doses	2
Therapy for both native and prosthetic valve endocarditis caused by HACEK[a] Microorganisms	Ceftriaxone sodium or ampicillin- sulbactam	2 g/24 h IV/IM in one dose 12 g/24 h IV in four equally divided doses	4 4

[a] Haemophilus parainfluenzae, *H. aphrophilus*, *Actinobacillus actinomycetemcomitans*, *Cardiobacterium hominis*, *Eikenella corrodens*, and *Kingella kingae*

From Baddour et al. (2005)

Medical treatment of native valve endocarditis is the domain of antibiotic administration. Basically, the duration of therapy has to be sufficient to eradicate microorganisms. The response to therapy should be assessed by obtaining repeat blood cultures 48–72 h after antibiotics are begun. Thereafter, regular careful serial examinations should be performed to search for signs of heart failure, emboli, or other complications. Most patients with IE generally become afebrile 3–5 days after treatment is begun with an appropriate antibiotic.

Surgical therapy in patients with IE should be individualized, with input from both the cardiologist and the cardiovascular surgeon (Tables 18.1.33, 18.1.34). The incidence of reinfection of newly implanted valves in patients with active IE is 2%–3% (Mills et al. 1974) and is far less than the mortality rate for IE and congestive heart failure (CHF) without surgical therapy, which can be as high as 51% (Sexton and Spelman 2003).

Complications of IE are CHF, which occurs more frequently in aortic valve infections (29%) than with mitral (20%) or tricuspid disease (8%). Systemic embolization occurs in 22%–50% of cases of IE. Emboli often involve the lungs, coronary arteries, spleen, bowel, and extremities. Up to 65% of embolic events involve the central nervous system. Most emboli occur within the first 2–4 weeks of antimicrobial therapy. Splenic abscess is a rare complication of IE. Mycotic aneurysms (MAs) are uncommon complications of IE that result from septic embolization of vegetations to the arterial vasa vasorum or the intraluminal space, with subsequent spread of infection through the intima and outward through the vessel wall. MAs occur most frequently in the intracranial arteries, followed by the visceral arteries and the arteries of the upper and lower extremities. Neurological complications develop in 20%–40% of patients with IE. Intracranial MAs represent an extremely dangerous subset of these complications. The overall mortality rate among IE patients with intracranial MAs is 60%. h antimicrobial therapy. Extracranial MAs (intrathoracic or intraabdominal) are often asymptomatic until leakage or rupture occurs. Presumably, most extracranial MAs (ECMAs) will rupture if not excised. Hematemesis, hematobilia, and jaundice suggest rupture of a hepatic artery MA, arterial hypertension and hematuria suggest rupture of a renal MA, and massive bloody diarrhea suggests the rupture of an ECMA into the small or large bowel (Baddour et al. 2005).

Table 18.1.34. Echocardiographic features that suggest potential need for surgical intervention according to (Baddour et al. 2005)

Vegetation
Persistent vegetation after systemic embolization
Anterior mitral leaflet vegetation, particularly with >10 mm (surgery may be required because of risk of embolization)
≥ Embolic events during first 2 weeks of antimicrobial therapy (surgery may be required because of risk of embolization)
Increase in vegetation size despite appropriate antimicrobial therapy (surgery may be required because of risk of embolization, heart failure, or failure of medical therapy)

Valvular dsyfunction
Acute aortic or mitral insufficiency with signs of ventricular failure
Heart failure unresponsive to medical therapy
Valve perforation or rupture

Perivalvular extension
Valvular dehiscence, rupture, or fistula
New heart block
Large abscess or extension of abscess despite appropriate antimicrobial therapy

Fever Due to Postoperative Appendicitis

The role of incidental appendectomy during elective and nonelective surgery remains controversial. Proponents of this practice argue with the technical ease, the low morbidity of the procedure, and the elimination of future risk and confusion over conflicting diagnosis and therefore for the prophylactic merits (Salom et al. 2003; Silvert and Meares 1976). Epidemiological studies estimate a lifetime risk of acute appendicitis as 8.6% in men and 6.7% in women (Gupta et al. 2002; Hayes 1977). Addis et al. (1990) estimated that for a 60-year-old male, it would require 166 incidental appendectomies to prevent a single lifetime case of appendicitis. Since the cumulative lifetime risk for appendicitis decreases with advancing age (see Table 18.1.35) and patients undergoing radical cystectomy and urinary diversion have a mean age of 64 years (Frazier et al. 1992), the lifetime risk of a postoperative appendicitis is very low (Gupta et al. 2002). The rationale for removing the appendix during urologic surgery is to prevent the future development of appendicitis since anatomical al-

Table 18.1.35. Cumulative lifetime risk for acute appendicitis

Age group (y)	Men (%)	Women (%)
0– 5	9.4	8.4
5– 9	9.2	8.3
10–14	8.6	7.8
15–19	7.2	6.7
20–24	5.9	5.4
25–29	4.9	4.5
30–34	4.1	3.8
35–39	3.4	3.1
40–44	2.8	2.5
45–49	2.3	2.0
50–54	1.9	1.7
55–59	1.6	1.2
60–64	1.2	0.9
65–69	0.8	0.6
70–74	0.4	0.3

From Wang and Sax (2001)

teration of viscera following urinary tract reconstruction makes differential diagnosis of recurrent abdominal pain in the right lower abdominal region difficult. But with the availability of the latest investigative modalities (CT scan) over 95% of painful abdominal conditions can be detected. The value of computed tomography in the diagnosis of appendicitis has been well established in the past few years. This has been advocated as the imaging modality of choice because of its high sensitivity, accuracy, and negative predictive value in diagnosing appendicitis. In a study of patients with suspected appendicitis, computed tomography has shown its superiority in evaluating the extent of inflammation and in differentiating other intraabdominal pathologic findings by demonstrating a normal appendix (Balthazar et al. 1994; Levine et al. 1997). In a study performed by Gupta et al. (2002) on 160 consecutive radical cystectomy patients with urinary diversion in whom appendectomy was not done, patients presenting with acute abdominal pain were easily diagnosed and managed. Moreover, none of the patients who were followed over a period of 10 years developed a appendicitis postoperatively (Table 18.36).

Therefore, routine appendectomy should be abandoned in urologic surgery, due to the evolving role of the appendix in various urinary tract reconstructions and the very low risk of subsequent appendicitis (Gupta et al. 2002; Neulander et al. 2000; Santoshi et al. 2002). The incidence of incidental carcinoid tumors of the appendix between 0.4% and 2% should not change this way of proceeding (Silvert and Meares 1976). Another important point that has not been well documented to date is that, despite performing appendectomy, the dilemma of acute abdominal pain may persist, as reported by varying studies on "stump appendicitis." This is an entity in which inflammation occurs in the remnant tissue of the appendix after appendectomy. The incidence of stump appendicitis is underestimated, and it can occur any time from a few months to 20 years after appendectomy (Feigin et al. 1993; Liang et al. 2006; Watkins et al. 2004).

Table 18.1.36. Causes of acute abdominal pain on follow-up following radical cystectomy

Cause	Incidence (%)
Intestinal obstruction	11
Urinary retention	1.8
Neobladder perforation	0.6
Recurrent colic	1.3
Pyelonephritis	13
Stomal stenosis	1.3
Parastomal hernia	0.6
Postoperative appendicitis	0

Fever Due to Forgotten Foreign Body (Corpus Alienum: Rubber Drain, Gauze Sponge, Forceps, etc.)

"Gossypiboma" refers to retained surgical sponge or swab and is derived from *gossypium* ("cotton" in Latin) and *boma* ("place of concealment" in Swahili) (O'Connor et al. 2003). Because of legal implications, this condition is often underreported and the incidence has been estimated as 1 in 100–5,000 surgeries (Lauwers and Van Hee 2000). The most commonly retained foreign body is the laparotomy sponge. It is often forgotten during operations in the lesser pelvis. Circumstances reported to explain operative loss of sponges are emergencies, hemorrhagic procedures, time-consuming operations, sponge counting while closing, change in operating room personnel, and operations in anatomic regions that are difficult to reach. Fifty percent of gossypibomas are discovered 5 years or more after surgery, and 40% are detected within the 1st year (Lauwers and Van Hee 2000; Rappaport and Haynes 1990).

Migration of gauze sponge has been reported to occur in ileum, duodenum, stomach, urinary bladder, and even by transdiaphragmatic migration into the lung causing lung abscess (Lone et al. 2005). The expulsion of sponge has been seen to occur through laparotomy wound and rectum. A sponge left in usually manifests within weeks to years and the longest duration of concealment has been 24 years (Kokubo et al. 1987). Retained sponge may produce various complications such as obstruction, fistula, peritonitis, abscess, transmural migration, or spontaneous extrusion. Two variants of reaction have been studied. In one there is aseptic fibrinous response, which follows a silent, delayed course, and the second variant is an acute, exudative type leading to abscess formation including bacterial infection with anaerobes.

Usual symptoms include unexplained abdominal distension and pain as well as palpable mass, nausea, vomiting, chronic anemia, rectal tenesmus and bleeding, diarrhea, discharge through a persistent sinus, intestinal obstruction, and pseudotumoral syndrome (Tacyildiz and Aldemir 2004; Ben Meir et al. 2003). These symptoms are often accompanied with general symptoms such as fever and weight loss. Coughing and dyspnea as well as UTI may be the result of exogenous compression on the respiratory or urinary tract. Postoperative septic shock has been described (Lauwers and Van Hee 2000). Plain radiographs fail to delineate the sponge in the absence of a radiopaque marker. Abdominal ultrasonography can demonstrate the gossypiboma by an intense and sharply delineated acoustic shadow that can be present even in the absence of air and calcification. The diagnostic procedure of choice is the CT scan, which shows lesions with densely enhancing wall and a central, low-density, whirl-like zone due to gas trapped in the fiber meshwork of the gossypiboma.

Differential diagnosis includes tumor or tumor recurrence, postoperative adhesions, invagination, intraabdominal abscesses, volvulus, and hematoma.

Treatment consists of thorough surgical exploration of the abdomen, removal of the gossypiboma, drainage of purulent fluid, and treatment of the accompanying lesions such as fistulizations. Complication of a gossypiboma is the development of an angiosarcoma, late abscess formation, chronic fistulas, and erosion into blood vessels. Gossypiboma-associated mortality is as high as 11 % – 35 % (Chorvat et al. 1976). When the foreign body is diagnosed and removed during the immediate postoperative period, morbidity and mortality are low (Le Neel et al. 1994). A gossypiboma is potentially life-threatening. Therefore, extreme care in the handling of gauzes during surgical procedures is highly advisable. Repeated sponge counts before and after each part of the operative procedure and systematic use of large sponges, one by one is recommended. Although the presence of radiopaque markers in all gauzes might give a false feeling of safety, their use is helpful in case of an incomplete sponge count at the end of an operative procedure (Lauwers and Van Hee 2000).

Fever Due to Intraabdominal Infections

Intraabdominal infection continues to be one of the major challenges in surgery and urology. While the term "peritonitis" means an inflammation of the peritoneum regardless of its etiology, intraabdominal infections encompass all forms of bacterial peritonitis, intraabdominal abscesses, and infections of intraabdominal organs. Several classification systems have been suggested for peritonitis and intraabdominal infections, respectively. However, neither phenomenological classifications nor classification systems with respect to the origin of bacterial contamination have a proven relevance for the clinical course of this disease. Moreover, most of the studies dealing with secondary peritonitis or intraabdominal infections are difficult to compare because of wide variations in inclusion criteria. Thus the true incidence of secondary bacterial peritonitis is difficult to assess. With respect to its etiology, perforation of hollow viscus is the leading cause followed by postoperative peritonitis, ischemic damage of bowel wall, infection of intraabdominal organs, and translocation in nonbacterial peritonitis. The anatomic origin of bacterial contamination and microbiological findings are not major predictors of outcome. However, the preoperative physiological derangement, the surgical clearance of the infectious focus and the response to treatment are established prognostic factors. The pathogenesis of intraabdominal infections is determined by bacterial factors that influence the transition from contamination to infection. Intraabdominal adjuvants and the local host response are also important. Bacterial stimuli lead to an almost uniform activation response, which is triggered by reaction of mesothelial cells and interspersed peritoneal macrophages and which also involves plasmatic systems, endothelial cells, and extra- and intravascular leukocytes. The local consequences of this activation are the transmigration of granulocytes from peritoneal capillaries to the mesothelial surface and a dilatation of peritoneal blood vessels resulting in enhanced permeability, peritoneal edema, and lastly the formation of protein-rich peritoneal exudate.

Clinically, peritonitis is often classified either as local or as diffuse. Local peritonitis refers to loculi of infection, usually walled-off or contained by adjacent organs, whereas diffuse is synonymous with generalized peritonitis, i.e., spread to the entire cavity.

The pathogens (Table 18.1.37) normally detected in peritonitis are Gram-negative, e.g., *E. coli*, and anaerobes, e.g., *Bacteroides fragilis*. When peritonitis persists, however, other pathogens may be isolated, e.g., *Pseudomonas aeruginosa*, *Enterobacter*, *Enterococcus* spp. Antimicrobial resistance of operative flora may correlate with postoperative infection. The response to intraabdominal infection depends on five key factors:

1. Inoculum size
2. Virulence of the contaminating organisms
3. Presence of adjuvants within the peritoneal cavity
4. Adequacy of local, regional, and systemic host defenses
5. Adequacy of initial treatment

The immune response mounted against the invading pathogens is the decisive element for outcome. When the inflammatory response gets out of control, multiorgan failure (MOF) will ensue and surgery can no longer limit the immune response, emphasizing the need for

Table 18.1.37. The microbial flora of secondary peritonitis

Type	Organism	Percent
Aerobic bacteria	*E. coli*	60
Gram-negative	*Enterobacter/Klebsiella*	26
	Proteus	22
	Pseudomonas	8
Gram-positive	*Streptococci*	28
	Enterococci	17
	Staphylococci	7
Anaerobic bacteria	*Bacteroides*	72
	Eubacteria	24
	Clostridia	17
	Peptostreptococcus	14
	Peptococcus	11
Fungi	*Candida*	2

From Hau et al. (1979)

timely operation in suspected peritonitis, the mainstay of treatment. Factors affecting prognosis are age, fecal peritonitis, metabolic acidosis, blood pressure, preoperative organ failure, serum albumin, malnutrition, malignoma, cause of infection, site of origin of peritonitis, and the number of organs involved in multiorgan-failure (MOF).

The diagnosis of intraabdominal infection is generally made on physical examination and is supported by clinical signs, e.g., abdominal pain and tenderness, nausea, vomiting, diminished intestine sounds, fever, and shock. Prior performed surgery should raise the suspicion of a complication directly related to the procedure itself (for example, a leak from an intestinal anastomosis or the inadvertent incorporation of a loop of bowel into the abdominal wall closure). A history of hypotension may be suspicious of intestinal ischemia or infarction, especially in patients with co-existing peripheral vascular disease and general atherosclerosis. After major surgery, perforation of a duodenal ulcer is a not uncommon complication, particularly in the patient with known peptic ulcer disease. Occasionally, peritonitis may be due to devices within the peritoneal cavity such as dialysis cannulae or due to postoperative pancreatitis. The physiologic response to the trauma of surgery causes increased levels of antidiuretic hormone (ADH) and aldosterone, leading to fluid retention. In the absence of complications, this process usually resolves by the 3rd day. Should a positive fluid balance persist after this time, the possibility of unrecognized complications should be suspected. Fluid retention is often manifested clinically by signs of organ dysfunction, such as tachypnea and hypoxemia, confusion, or the onset of a new supraventricular dysrhythmia (Marshall 2004). These clinical signs of surgical complications typically become evident on the 3rd postoperative day, but peritonitis usually presents not until 7 – 10 days after the surgical procedure.

Radiographic procedures are the cornerstone of diagnosis and include plain x-ray (intraperitoneal free air, although air may normally be present for up to 7 days following a laparotomy; thumb-printing, which suggests ischemia; evidence of intestinal obstruction; contrast studies, which may demonstrate leaks or delineate the location of an obstruction), ultrasound, and CT scan. Computed tomography combined with oral and intravenous contrast medium is the most reliable imaging modality for evaluating the abdomen (intra- or retroperitoneal fluid collections, abscess formation, intestinal ischemia, clots within larger vessels, etc.) (Velmahos et al. 1999). MRI should also be considered with the possible exception of the evaluation of retroperitoneal pancreatic pathology.

Leukocytes and C reactive protein may be altered but are not direct signs of peritonitis.

Management principles (Marshall 2004) of the patient with intraabdominal infection include three principles:

- Timely hemodynamic resuscitation and support of vital organ function
- Early administration of antimicrobial agents appropriate for the infectious problem
- Rapid anatomic diagnosis and the institution of adequate source control measures

The cornerstone of timely hemodynamic resuscitation is the administration of adequate amounts of fluids to restore adequate intravascular volume and thus optimize oxygen delivery to the tissues. There is no compelling evidence of the superiority of one type of fluid over another. Resuscitation should be guided by frequent assessment of heart rate and blood pressure. Urinary output is a simle and sensitive measure of intravascular volume filling and organ function; an hourly output of 30 – 50 ml/kg should be the minimal objective of therapy. Patients who have significant co-morbidities, who present with more profound hemodynamic instability, or who fail to respond rapidly to fluid replacement should be managed in an ICU setting. The amount of fluid required to achieve hemodynamic stability is variable, and frequently substantial, because of unappreciated third-space losses into the focus of infection and into the GI tract as a consequence of ileus (Madl and Druml 2003; Marshall 2004). Another mainstay is the early administration of systemic antibiotics (Table 18.1.38) without waiting for radiographic or microbiologic confirmation. The spectrum should include Gram-negative aerobic organisms and anaerobes. The optimal duration of antibiotic therapy is unknown, and

Table 18.1.38. Recommended antimicrobial regimens for patients with intraabdominal infections

Single agents
Infection
Ampicillin/sulbactam
Cefotetan
Cefoxitin
Ertapenem
Imipenem/cilastatin
Meropenem
Piperacillin/tazobactam
Ticarcillin/clavulanic acid
Combination regimens
Aminoglycoside plus an antianaerobe agent (clindamycin or metronidazole)
Aztreonam plus clindamycin
Cefuroxime plus metronidazole
Ciprofloxacin plus metronidazole
Third- or fourth-generation cephalosporin (cefepime, cefotaxime, ceftazidime, ceftizoxime, or ceftriaxone) plus an antianaerobe anaerobe (clindamycin or metronidazole)

from Malangoni (2005); Mazuski et al. (2002)

when antibiotics are used in association with adequate source control, the duration of therapy can be short (Wittmann and Schein 1996), and certainly no longer than 5–7 days (Wittmann and Schein 1996).

The term “source control” can be defined as those physical measures undertaken to eradicate a focus of infection, eliminate ongoing microbial contamination, and render the local environment inhospitable to microbial growth and tissue invasion (Jimenez and Marshall 2001). This involves one or more of the following strategies:

- Drainage of abscesses or infected fluid collections
- Debridement of necrotic infected tissue
- Definitive measures to control a source of ongoing microbial contamination and to restore anatomy and function

Drainage converts an abscess to a controlled sinus or fistula. This can be done by percutaneous techniques guided by radiographic imaging.

In general, although no randomized control trial is available, percutaneous drainage seems to be as effective as operative drainage and when percutaneous drainage is feasible it is the preferred initial approach because it is the least invasive procedure (Bufalari et al. 1996). Contraindications for percutaneous drainage include diffuse peritonitis due to the lack of localization of the infectious process, multiple abscesses, and anatomic inaccessibility. Debridement is the physical removal of infected or necrotic tissue and can be accomplished by surgical excision and irrigation. Early aggressive debridement is associated with an improved clinical outcome. Debridement encompasses the excision of necrotic intestine, the removal of feces or fibrin from the peritoneal cavity, and the excision of necrotic and infected fat. Clear demarcation between viable and nonviable tissues is a prerequisite to successful debridement (Marshall et al. 2004). Removal of extensive fibrin deposition on the peritoneal surface of loops of bowel shows no improvement in the clinical outcome. Intraoperative peritoneal lavage, although well entrenched in modern surgical practice, has not yet demonstrated that it decreases clinical mortality. No absolute proof exists that the addition of antibiotics to intraoperative lavage increases the survival rate (Hudspeth 1975). Definitive measures to correct the anatomic derangement are an integral part of source control management. Whether definitive measures should be undertaken during the initial management of the septic episode or preferentially delayed and performed electively when the patient has recovered depends on the stability of the patient and the nature of the intervention that is needed: in general, the simplest intervention that accomplishes the source control objective is the best option. There is a trend in the literature to make a stoma in cases of anastomotic dehiscence and peritoneal infection. While there is general agreement that on-table bowel preparation and primary anastomosis is safe in the presence of localized peritonitis, its use in the presence of generalized peritonitis is controversial and most surgeons opt for a Hartmann’s procedure in this situation. Intestinal reanastomosis is in most instances not performed in peritonitis. The approach employed to treat the immediate problem must take into consideration the consequences of that decision for later reconstruction. Open abdomen approaches, for example, commit the patient to a series of reconstructive procedures to repair abdominal wall hernias or to close enterocutaneous fistulae. The creation of a stoma requires a subsequent procedure if the stoma is to be closed, and the morbidity associated with such procedures can be substantial (Hackam and Rotstein 1995a, b). If a stoma is created, a loop enterostomy or colostomy is easier to close than an end stoma, for it can be accomplished locally without the need for a full laparotomy.

There is increasing evidence that laparoscopy may play a definite role in patients with peritonitis. In patients with generalized peritonitis resulting from perforated diverticular disease, treatment by laparoscopy and peritoneal lavage was successful. However, laparoscopic management of generalized peritonitis needs further assessment.

The most common cause of peritonitis in the hospitalized patient is intraperitoneal infection as a consequence of prior abdominal surgery (Table 18.1.39). If the GI tract has been entered as in radical cystectomy and urinary diversion, then the possibility of an anastomotic leak should be considered. Risk factors for this complication include excessive tension on the suture line, hematoma at the suture line, ischemia related to

Table 18.1.39. Causes of peritonitis in the hospitalized patient

Type	Cause
Postoperative peritonitis	Anastomotic leak (Fig. 18.1.3.4)
Procedural complications	Inadvertent or missed intestinal injury Infected hematoma Intestinal injury secondary to laparoscopic trocar
Spontaneous GI perforation	Perforation of gastric or duodenal ulcer
Intestinal ischemia	Delayed ischemia secondary to low-flow mesenteric venous thrombosis Acalculous cholecystitis
Device-related infection	CAPD peritonitis Infected ventriculoperitoneal shunt
Hematoma	Insufficient coagulation Slipped clips or ligatures Coagulopathy

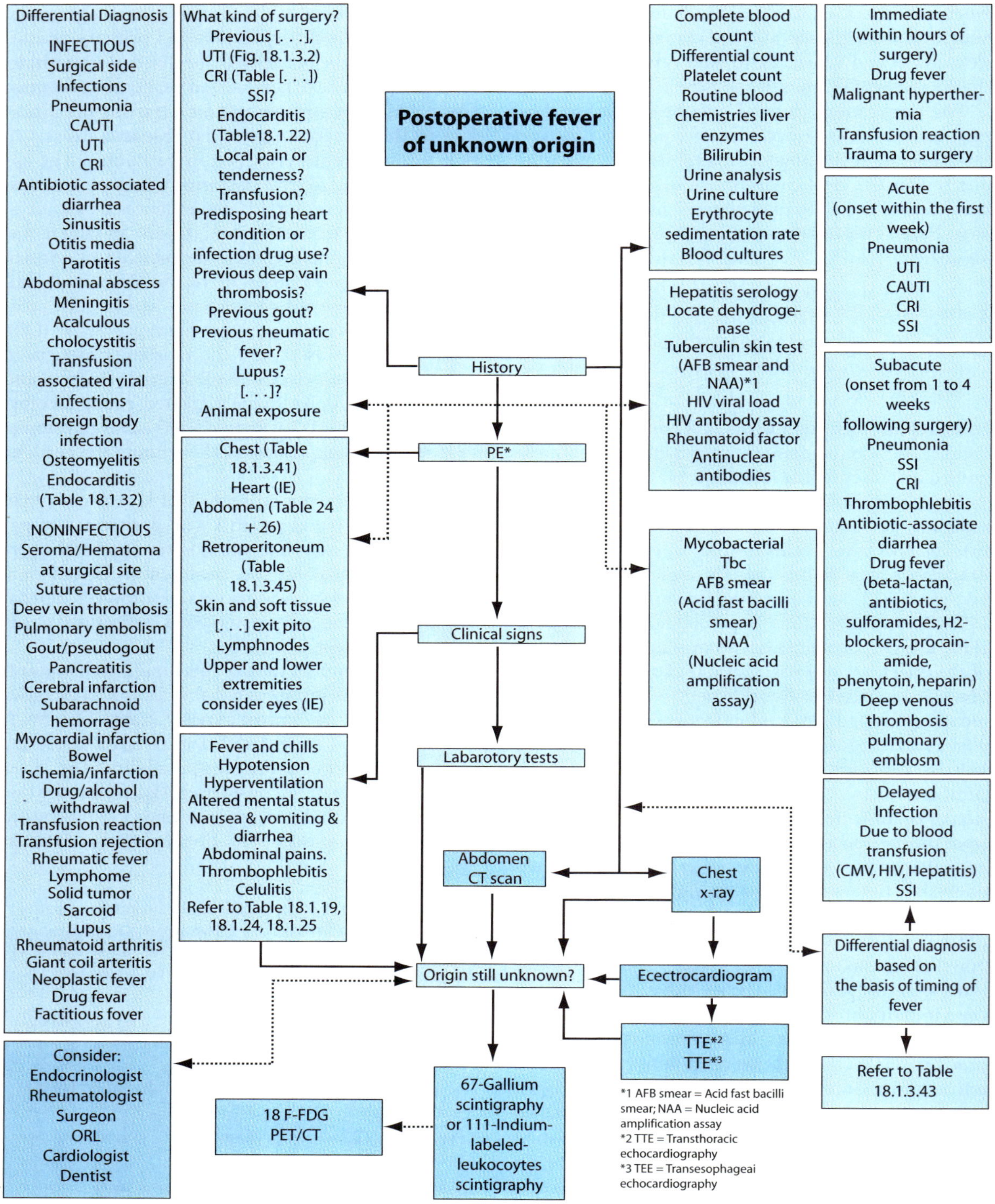

Fig. 18.1.8. Algorithm for postoperative fever of unknown origin

underlying vascular disease, obesity, excessive devascularization of the intestine at the site of the anastomosis, or intestinal distension at the suture line, and technical errors in the creation of the anastomosis. Collections of blood within the peritoneal cavity support the proliferation of bacteria shed at the time of surgery, and is one of the most common predisposing factors to postoperative abscesses (Fig. 18.1.8). Their anatomic location reflects the preceding operative procedure: following nephrectomy, for example, postoperative abscesses are typically found in the subhepatic or subsplenic spaces or along the psoas muscle, whereas an abscess developing following radical prostatectomy or cystectomy most commonly occurs in the pelvis. The same applies to lymphatic fluid and collection from which infected lymphoceles and infected chylogenous ascites can develop (refer to Chaps. 18.1.5, 18.1.7). Unrecognized intraoperative tear of a segment of bowel or the inadvertent incorporation of a loop of bowel into the abdominal wall closure may be another cause of a postoperative peritonitis. Such complications are more frequent in reoperative surgery, since scarring and adhesions distort the intraabdominal anatomy and necessitate a more extensive dissection. Less common complications should also be considered: trocar injury following laparoscopic surgery, inadvertent passage of a drain through a loop of intestine, etc. The morbidity and mortality of postoperative peritonitis is substantial, with mortality rates of up to 60 % for patients having diffuse peritonitis (Bohnen et al. 1983; Marshall 2004; Marshall et al. 2004).

Fever Due to Skin and Soft-Tissue Infections

Infections of the skin and soft tissue are common and encompass a spectrum of illness severity, from focal cellulitis producing only mild symptoms to life-threatening necrotizing infections resulting in extensive tissue loss and substantial acute morbidity and mortality.

Local signs of inflammation are the hallmark of a soft tissue infection. Features of severe sepsis rarely accompany a superficial skin and soft tissue infection and suggest concomitant tissue necrosis, a deep skin and soft tissue infection, or a particularly virulent infecting organism. Fluctuance suggests a subcutaneous abscess. Necrotizing infection is suggested by the presence of pain (usually severe and constant in the case of necrotizing fasciitis), discoloration of the overlying skin, bullous lesions, or soft tissue crepitus; these findings, however, are neither sensitive nor specific for the recognition of tissue necrosis, and extensive necrotizing infection of the subcutaneous tissues may be present with only minimal findings in the overlying skin. The diagnosis of infection of the skin and soft tissues is most commonly accomplished by direct examination, obtaining cultures to identify the infecting organisms and to aid in the selection of an optimal antimicrobial agent. A microbiological diagnosis of cellulitis can sometimes be made by aspiration of the involved area. Biopsy can be used to determine whether tissue necrosis is present and to facilitate quantitative culture, a technique that is useful in the diagnosis of burn wound infection. Radiologic examination – particularly computed tomography – is of value to define the extent of the process and to identify deep sites of infection. The classification of skin and soft-tissue infections can be subdivided into surgical and nonsurgical infections. Surgical site infection is an infection that arises within 30 days of an operative procedure and at the site of surgical intervention. Nonsurgical skin and soft-tissue infections comprise erysipelas, impetigo, folliculitis, cellulitis, pyodermas, abscess, necrotizing cellulitis or fasciitis or myositis, and myositis/pyomyositis/myonecrosis.

Cellulitis is defined as an acute spreading infection of the skin and underlying soft tissue suggested by the presence of a rapidly expanding erythema, local tenderness, pain, swelling, lymphangitis, and lymphadenopathy, which is frequently accompanied by systemic signs and symptoms including malaise, fever (temperature 38.0 °C), and chills.

Necrotizing cellulitis and fasciitis are defined as acute, rapidly progressing, and life-threatening destructive (i.e., necrotizing) infections of the subcutaneous tissues dissecting along tissue planes. Although these two clinical entities exhibit some distinctive clinical and microbial characteristics, they share common features. The symptoms and signs suggestive of necrotizing cellulitis or fasciitis are intense local pain (a cardinal feature), exquisite tenderness, erythema (initially discrete but evolving to red-purple and then blue-gray cutaneous lesions often with hemorrhagic bullae), swelling, edema, crepitations (in the case of necrotizing cellulitis), and extensive tissue necrosis, which are associated with prominent systemic toxicity (toxic shock syndrome, severe sepsis, or septic shock).

Microbiologically confirmed skin and soft tissue infection is defined by the isolation by culture or Gram stain of a microorganism from a skin aspirate or biopsy of the subcutaneous tissues of an erythematous skin lesion or wound. Probable skin and soft tissue infection is defined as compelling clinical and laboratory evidence (such as spreading cutaneous erythema and blanching, or drainage of purulent material on opening a surgical wound, with or without lymphangitis, in association with fever 38.0 °C, or leukocytosis) of the presence of a skin and soft tissue infection based on radiographic, clinical, and surgical findings but without microbiological confirmation. Possible skin and soft tissue infection is defined as clinical (such as mild cutaneous erythema associated with fever of 38.0 °C), laboratory (such as leukocytosis), or radiographic findings suggestive of the presence of a skin and soft tissue infection but with insufficient evidence to confirm diagnosis. Infections are further classified as superficial or deep, based on whether the deep fascia or muscle layers are involved. In mild to moderate cases, antibiotic therapy should be sufficient, while in severe cases radical surgical debridement is required.

Fever Due to Impaired Drainage of Upper Urinary Tract After Urologic Surgery

Urinary tract infection due to urinary diversion with and without cystectomy due to benign and nonbenign diseases is a common problem in this setting. The ileal conduit is colonized postsurgically through the cutaneous opening. During the initial 10-day period after operation, both ureters are stented and antibiotic therapy is discontinued after removal of the ureteral stents in our institution. When fever stemming from impaired drainage of the upper urinary tract occurs in these first 10 days, ultrasound of the kidney may reveal hydronephrosis and urinalysis and culture should be obtained. Correct replacement of the ureteral stent or percutaneous nephrostomy should be performed. When cultures grow, a pathogen treatment should be amended accordingly.

A mixed population of yeast and Gram-positive cocci (*Streptococcus* species, *Staphylococcus epidermis*, and *enterococci*) subsequently develops in the conduit. As antibiotic protection is withdrawn, Gram-negative organisms (*E. coli* and *Proteus*, *Pseudomonas*, and *Klebsiella* species) become part of the mixed microbial flora. Electron microscopic examination showed no bacteria adhering to columnar cells of the conduit, but mucus was heavily colonized with microcolonies of Gram-positive and Gram-negative bacteria (Bruce et al. 1984; Chan et al. 1984), whereas cultures from colonic conduits most often grow a single bacterial species. Because conduit urine is bacteriuric in most cases, clinicians have to decide when to provide antibiotic coverage and when to drain the upper urinary tract. Treatment should be instituted if symptoms suggest upper urinary tract infection such as fever, costovertebral pain or tenderness, pathologic blood test, and coagulopathy (see Fig. 18.1.3.2). Antibiotics should be administered as mentioned above (Table 18.1.3.9), and in case of infected hydronephrosis and/or impaired renal function, ureteral stents or percutaneous nephrostomy must be implemented. Prophylactic antibiotic treatment is justified in patients with the history of recurrent pyelonephritis. The incidence of UTI after noncontinent urinary diversion varies according to the literature and is estimated by Madersbacher et al. to be roughly 23% with a median follow-up of 98% (Madersbacher et al. 2003); causes associated with UTI are anastomotic stricture, stomal stenosis, and urolithiasis.

Basically, as for ileal or colonic conduit, the same applies for orthotopic urinary diversion in terms of clinical signs, diagnostic procedure, and management. A standard 3- to 5-day course of antibiotics (see Table 18.1.27), after removal of the urinary catheter placed intraoperatively after formation of a neobladder, usually sterilizes urine. However, in the following period there is an increased risk for UTIs in this patients because bacteria are more easily able to colonize the neobladder formation in comparison to the normal urinary bladder. Additionally, incomplete emptying of the neobladder may promote infection, even with nonadherent microorganisms. Finally, excessive mucus production by the bowel epithelium accompanying an established infection prevents effective clearance of microorganisms. Microbial flora includes *E. coli* strains (60%), *Klebsiella* species, *Proteus mirabilis*, *Enterococcus* species, *Pseudomonas* species, and *Citrobacter* species. In neobladders, bacterial colonization correlates with residual urine, thus optimal evacuation decreases the bacterial burden as residual volumes reaches 20 ml or less. Controversy exists regarding the appropriate treatment of asymptomatic bacteriuria in patients with ileal neobladder. Wood et al. (2003) stated that although small bowel intestine appears to promote asymptomatic bacterial colonization (39%), urosepsis occurs in 12% of the patients with UTI. The estimated 5-year probability of UTI and urosepsis according to Wood et al. (2003) is around 58% and 18%, respectively. Urine culture with greater than 10^5 cfu bacteria and female gender are the only factors predictive of UTI. Recurrent UTI in this trial is the only predictor for urosepsis. Intermittent catheterization or hydronephrosis are not related to urinary tract infection or urosepsis. Therefore, prophylactic antibiotics are recommended only for patients with recurring UTIs (Wood et al. 2003; Falagas and Vergidis 2005).

In patients with continent nonorthotopic urinary diversion (pouch) pouchitis is a rare complication caused by infection of the urine reservoir. It is manifested by sudden explosive loss of urine through the continence mechanism, associated with pain in the region of the pouch. The explosive urine discharge results from pouch hypercontractility. Mucus production is increased in these infections. Although this is an expected protective response of the intestinal segment to inflammation, the resultant excessive mucus produced potentially contributes to the persistence of the microorganisms (Falagas and Vergidis 2005; N'Dow et al. 2004). The infection must be treated with appropriate antimicrobial treatment for at least 10 days. Benson and Ollson (Benson and Ollson 2002; Falagas and Vergidis 2005) reported that short courses of antibiotics usually are not successful in pouch infections (Falagas and Vergidis 2005).

Postoperative fever due to impaired drainage of the upper urinary tract system may also occur after radical prostatectomy, prostatectomy due to benign prostatic enlargement, TURP, and TURBT. After open surgery (radical prostatectomy, prostatectomy due to benign prostatic enlargement), a surgical failure such as sutures may contribute to obstruction of distal/prevesical ureter. Ultrasound and urinalysis as well as creatinine levels will guide the diagnosis. Management include

Table 18.1.40. Microorganisms isolated and recommended treatment in different types of urinary diversion

Type of Diversion	Microorganisms isolated	Treatment
Noncontinent urinary diversion	Gram-positive mixed skin flora (*Streptococcus* species, *Staphylococcus epidermidis*) Gram-negative Enterobacteriaceae (*E coli*, *Proteus* species, *Pseudomonas* species) *Enterococcus faecalis*	No treatment for asymptomatic bacteriuria, unless history of recurrent pyelonephritis
Continent nonorthotopic urinary diversion	Chronic bacteriuria as patient performs intermittent self-catheterization	No treatment for asymptomatic bacteriuria
Orthotopic urinary diversion	*E. coli* and other Gram-negative Enterobacteriaceae	No treatment for asymptomatic bacteriuria (controversy) Treat for urea-splitting organisms, such as *Proteus* species, even if asymptomatic (potential for stone formation)

From Falagas and Vergidis (2005)

transurethral ureteral stents and percutaneous nephrostomy. Violation of the ureteral orifice at TURP or TURBT may also lead to infected hydronephrosis and when infected has to be drained as described above (Fig. 18.1.17; Table 18.1.40).

Fever Due to Epididymitis After TUR, Brachytherapy, Prostate Biopsy, and Open Surgery

Although epididymitis after TURP and TURBT is an event with an incidence of less than 1% (Uchida et al. 1993, 1999), such testicle pathologies may contribute to postoperative fever. Even in patients receiving brachytherapy of the prostate due to prostate cancer develop postimplantation epididymitis, for example in only 1% of a large patient cohort with 517 patients, and when administered preoperative antibiotics, epididymitis drops to 0.5% (Hoffelt et al. 2004). In TRUS-guided biopsy of the prostate, Donzella et al. (2004) estimated the incidence of approximately 1% and an onset of weeks to months after the procedure, particularly in older patients or those with a greater number of prostate biopsies taken.

After open surgery such as transvesical prostatectomy, the incidence of epididymitis as an early complication has been reported to be around 1.8%–11.5% (Diallo et al. 2001; Tan et al. 1991). For the diagnosis of epididymitis and orchitis, a scrotal ultrasound must be carried out. On physical examination, epididymal swelling and pain and erythema of the scrotal skin may be present. Clinical features also include dysuria, fever, and chills. Laboratory tests will assess leukocytosis and elevated CRP levels and a positive urine bacterial culture. In epididymitis, B-mode ultrasonography shows an enlarged, echo-poor epididymis; color-flow Doppler ultrasonography shows hypervascularity. Bacteriuria-associated causes of acute epididymitis include the following organisms: *E. coli*, *Proteus* species, *Klebsiella pneumoniae, Pseudomonas aeruginosa*, *H. influenzae* type b, *Staphylococcus* spp., and *Streptococcus* spp.

In the management of acute epididymitis, one should consider bed rest, scrotal elevation, and cooling. Also recommended are analgesics and NSAIDs. In men with epididymitis caused by probable urinary pathogens, the use of quinolone antibiotics such as ciprofloxacin 500 mg twice daily for 10–14 days or doxycycline 100 mg twice daily for 10–14 days is recommended. In severe infections with systemic disturbance or features suggesting bacteremia, initial intravenous therapy may be indicated.

Postoperative Fever of Unknown Origin

Physical examination usually starts with the respiratory system. The respiratory examination is normally performed according to Osler's classic sequence of inspection, palpation, percussion, and auscultation. All lobes of the lung should be systematically examined. Findings should be compared left with right, upper with lower, and anterior with posterior. Percussion of the thorax attempts to assess the state of the pulmonary parenchyma. Auscultation assesses the state of the airways and provides additional information about the state of the lung parenchyma. Pulmonary disorders are listed in Table 18.1.41, whereas consolidation and pneumonia secondary to atelectasis and pleural effusion may be the major causes of postoperative fever.

Congenital abnormalities of the heart, previous endocarditis, and valvular disease are typically associated with increased risk of IE. The presence of a new, changing or altered murmur has been reported in as few as 40% of IE patients (Stamboulian and Carbone 1997), but still the auscultation of the heart is essential when dealing with a patient with postoperative fever. When IE is suspected, examination of the nails, which may show splinter hemorrhages, should be performed; the eyes may show retinal hemorrhages and petechiae in the conjunctiva on examination may be present. Janeway lesions are seen in people with acute bacterial endocarditis. They appear as flat, painless, red to bluish-red spots on the palms and soles.

Table 18.1.41. Major diagnostic complexes in the evaluation of pulmonary disorders

	Percussion	Transmission	Quality/intensity	Adventitious sounds
Consolidation	Dull	↑↑↑	Bronchial ↓	Rales
Atelectasis	Dull	±	↓	Rales
Pleural fluid	Dull	Egophony ↓	Vesicular ↓	Rub
Pneumothorax	Tympanitic	↓	Vesicular ↓	–

Lymph nodes should be examined in a systematic fashion. Lymph nodes that are smooth and relatively soft, but slightly enlarged, may be normal or may show hyperplasia. Enlarged lymph nodes that have an irregular shape and a rubbery, hard consistency may be infiltrated by malignant cells. Tender nodes are suggestive of an inflammatory process. Matted nodes or nodes fixed to underlying structures should raise the question of malignancy or infection; freely movable nodes are more likely to occur in benign conditions. Lymphadenitis may occur if the glands are overwhelmed by bacteria, virus, fungi, or other organisms and infection develops within the glands. The location of the affected lymph nodes is usually associated with the site of the underlying lesion. The skin over a node may be reddened and hot. Lymphangitis secondary to lymphadenopathy involves the lymph vessels, with resultant pain and systemic and localized symptoms. It commonly results from an acute streptococcal or staphylococcal infection of the skin (cellulitis), or from an abscess in the skin or soft tissues. Lymphangitis presents with red streaks from infected area to the armpit or groin and throbbing pain along the affected area.

Beginning with the lymph nodes of the neck, cervical lymph node chains should be evaluated including the preauricular, posterior auricular, occipital, superior cervical, posterior cervical, submaxillary, submental, inferior deep cervical, and supraclavicular. Enlargement of specific cervical lymph node groups can be helpful diagnostically. For example, oropharyngeal and dental infections can cause cervical adenopathy. Right-sided supraclavicular nodes drain parts of the lung and mediastinum and are signals of intrathoracic lesions (lung and esophagus). Left-sided supraclavicular nodes (Virchow's nodes) are close to the thoracic duct and often signal intraabdominal lesions, particularly from the stomach, ovaries, testes, or kidneys. The patient should then be examined for axillary adenopathy. Axillary adenopathy may be part of a generalized process or may be localized and secondary to infection in the upper extremity. Next, the patient should be evaluated for lymph nodes that can be found in the vicinity of the umbilicus. These nodes have the eponym "the node of Sister Mary Joseph" and are a signal of significant intraabdominal lymphadenopathy, usually associated with malignant processes or massive abdominal infection. Finally, the inguinal region should be carefully evaluated for significant lymphadenopathy. It is not uncommon for adults to have firm, unfixed lymph nodes that are less than 1 cm in diameter from recurrent infections and insults to the feet and legs. Unilateral enlarged and tender nodes in this region suggest an infection of an ipsilateral lower extremity. Inguinal adenopathy can also be part of systemic processes such as lymphoma or leukemia.

Table 18.1.42. Causes of splenomegaly

Vascular congestion
Cirrhosis
Splenic vein thrombosis
Portal vein thrombosis
Reticuloendothelial hyperplasia
Acute infections (e.g., bacterial endocarditis)
Subacute or chronic infections
Collagen vascular diseases and abnormal immune responses (e.g., systemic lupus erythematosus)
Work hypertrophy
Hemolytic anemias
Infiltrative or replacement processes
Nonmalignant hematologic disorders (e.g., polycythemia vera, myelofibrosis)
Leukemias
Lymphomas
Metastatic solid tumors
Abscess

Table 18.1.43. Time of onset of pain and fever in abdominal disorders

Sudden onset	Perforation of the gastrointestinal tract (duodenal ulcer, a colonic diverticulum, or a foreign body)
	Mesenteric infraction
	Ruptured aortic aneurysm
Rapid onset	Cholecystitis
	Pancreatitis
	Intestinal obstruction
	Diverticulitis
	Appendicitis
	Ureteral stone
	Penetrating gastric or duodenal ulcer
Gradual onset	Neoplasms
	Chronic inflammatory processes
	Large bowel obstruction

The spleen (Table 18.1.42) is part of the lymphatic system and should be carefully evaluated in any patient in whom other lymphadenopathy is present.

The workup in postoperative fever and pain concerning the abdomen includes six features: onset, progression, migration, character, intensity, and location (Table 18.1.43).

Table 18.1.44. Common abnormalities of abdominal examination

Anatomical structure	Abnormality	Common condition
Umbilicus	Mass, pain, or protrusion	Hernia Abdominal wound dehiscence Surgical site infection Sister Mary Joseph's node
	Prominent veins	Portal hypertension
Stomach	Mass or pain in left upper quadrant	Gastric carcinoma Gastric outlet obstruction Ulcer perforation
Pancreas	Mass or pain in right upper quadrant	Pancreatic carcinoma Pancreatitis
Gallbladder	Mass or pain in right upper quadrant	Cholecystolithiasis Hydrops of gallbladder Carcinoma of gallbladder Acute cholecystitis
Small intestine	Mass or pain, decreased bowel sounds	Ileus, anastomosis leakage
	Mass or pain, increased bowel sounds	Obstruction
Liver	Increased size	Hepatitis Metastatic carcinoma Cirrhosis Abscess
	Decreased size	Budd-Chiari
	Nodularity	Cirrhosis Metastatic carcinoma Cirrhosis
Spleen	Increased size	See Table 18.1.3.24
Peritoneal space	Presence of ascites	Portal hypotension Metastatic disease Congestive heart failure Lymphocele (infected) Chylogenous ascites
Anus and rectum	Anal or rectal mass or pain	Anal carcinoma Rectal perforation Douglas abscess Prostatitis Fissure Fistula

Table 18.1.45. Cause of flank pain and postoperative fever

Acute ureteral obstruction	Chronic ureteral obstruction
Stone Blood clot Papillary necrosis	Congenital anomaly Tumor Stricture of ureter Previous surgery Radiation therapy Retroperitoneal fibrosis Stone
Renal inflammation Acute pyelonephritis Perinephric abscess Renal tumor Renal cell carcinoma Transitional cell carcinoma Wilms tumor Kidney trauma Renal infarction Vesicoureteral reflux	 Gallbladder disease Appendicitis Diverticulitis Other gastrointestinal disease Chest disease Salpingitis

For examination of the gastrointestinal system and abdomen, a sequence of steps should be followed (auscultation, palpation, percussion, check for ascites, rectal examination, inguinal examination). Common abnormalities of the abdomen are described in Table 18.1.44.

The characteristic of flank pain is very helpful in determining the cause. Important characteristics include local or referred pain, acute or chronic or recurrent pain, degree of severity, and duration. Associated symptoms such as fever, nausea and vomiting, and atrial fibrillation often help in making the correct diagnosis (Table 18.1.45).

For the evaluation of the suprapubic region, there may be tenderness referring to injury to the bladder or urine leakage mostly in combination with hematuria (bladder augmentation, psoas bladder hitch, Boari plastic, etc.). Other causes may stem from lymphoceles after radical cystectomy, prostatectomy, and retroperitoneal lymphadenectomy.

Evaluation of the external genitalia in males includes examination of the penis, scrotum, and scrotal contents. Postoperatively, most common are epididymitis, orchitis, and paraphimosis.

For a diagnostic algorithm refer to Fig. 18.1.9.

The imaging diagnostic approach in postoperative fever of unknown origin (FUO) includes not only conventional radiographic studies such as plain x-rays, CT scans, or MRI. It has been reported that gallium-67 and 111-indium-labeled leukocyte scanning have an overall higher yield than CT for detecting sites of FUO (Knockaert et al. 1994; Syrjala et al. 1987). At the moment gallium-67 scanning is a commonly used radiotracer for the evaluation of postoperative FUO because it has the advantage of detecting changes at the molecular level in the early stages before any visible structural changes have occurred, and it can also differentiate between necrotic and viable tissues. Therefore, it has higher sensitivity than anatomical imaging techniques (CT, MRI). When performing a ^{67}Ga scintigraphy or a single photon emission computerized tomography (SPECT), some facts should be remembered. Gallium is normally distributed in bone marrow and gut excretion. Also, a faint salivary gland and renal activity is normal. This normal contribution of gallium as well as the poor resolution and the high dosimetry of this imaging modality was the impetus to develop ^{111}In-oxide-labeled leukocyte scintigraphy. A significant disadvantage of the ^{111}In-oxide-labeled leukocytes scintigraphy is the need for in vitro isolation of blood cells, which exposes the patient to an infection hazard (Peters 1998). Positron emission tomography (PET and PET/CT) has the potential to replace other nuclear medicine imaging techniques in the evaluation of patients with FUO. The tracer 18-fluoro-deoxy-glucose (18F-FDG) is

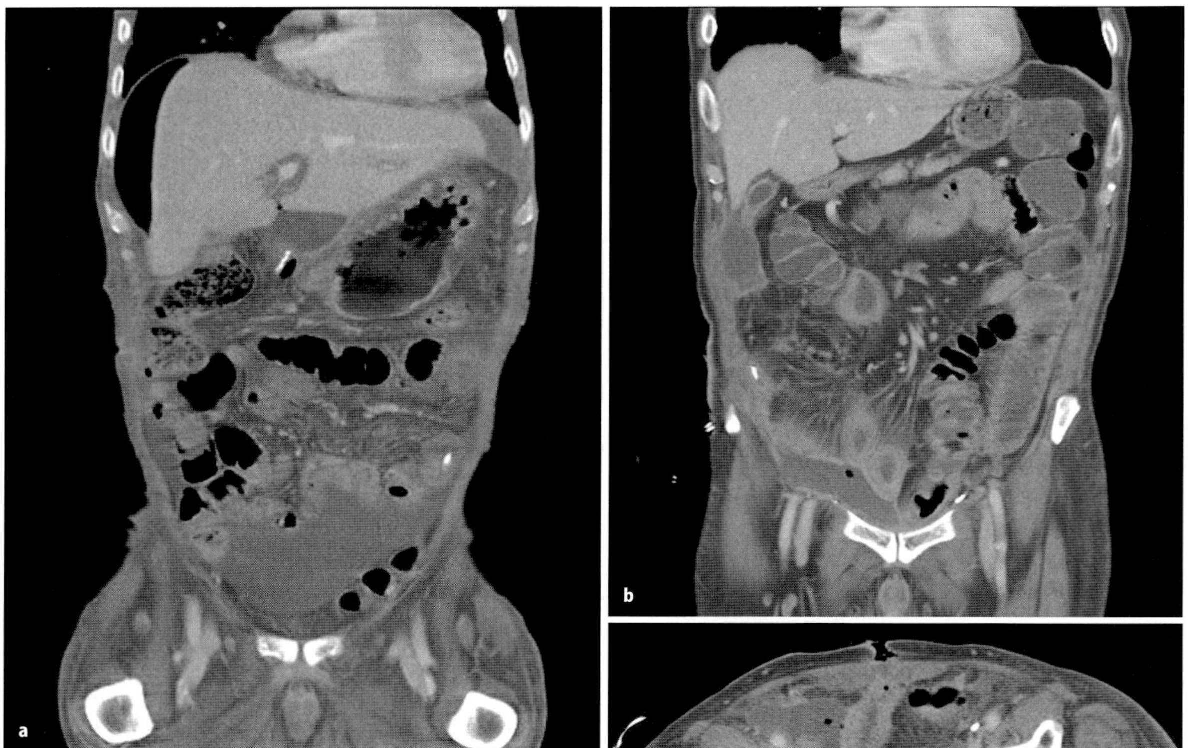

Fig. 18.1.9a–c. CT scan in patients with postoperative fever due to abdominal infection. **a** Patient on day 10 following radical cystectomy with urinary diversion (ileal conduit) with an anastomotic leakage. Note free fluid in the pelvis and upper abdomen. **b, c** Patient following radical cystectomy with urinary diversion (ileal neobladder); a relaparotomy was required because of an acute abdomen and peritonitis due to necrotic neobldder. After conversion to ileal conduit, the patient presented 9 days postoperatively with fever due to abscess formation in the subhepatic (**b**) and lesser pelvic (**c**) spaces

a nonspecific tracer of increased glucose metabolism and does not accumulate only in sites of infection and inflammation. Indeed, its high sensitivity for the detection of malignant cells has led to its successful and extensive use in oncology. Therefore, 18F-FDG-PET is advantageous over gallium-67 and 111-In-oxide labeled leukocyte scintigraphy because it can image the whole body in a short time, has high spatial resolution and provides high-quality images, and delivers a relatively low radiation dose to the patient (Sugawara et al. 1998). Several authors reported sensitivity rates of 81%–98%, specificity of 75%–100%, and accuracy of 91% for FDG-PET(-CT), while scintigraphy revealed sensitivity rates of 67%, specificity of 78%, and accuracy of 84%–86% in patients with suspected infections (El-Haddad et al. 2004; Meller et al. 2000; Stumpe et al. 2000).

In spite of its high spatial resolution, the anatomic information available with stand-alone PET remains limited. Integrated PET/CT systems provide "hardware" coregistered metabolic and structural data. Such a correlated acquisition of metabolic and anatomic data may benefit the precise detection of infected sites. In a feasibility trial with 18F-FDG-labeled leukocyte PET/CT depending on the standardized uptake value (SUV), Dumarey et al. showed a sensitivity of 86%, a specificity of 86%, a PPV of 92%, a NPV of 85%, and an accuracy of 86% in imaging infection (Dumarey et al. 2006). In another current publication comparing PET with FDG-labeled leukocytes vs ^{111}In-oxine-labeled leukocyte scintigraphy, the authors found a sensitivity of 87% vs 73%, a specificity of 82% vs 86%, a PPV of 72% vs 73%, a NPV of 92% vs 86%, and an accuracy of 84% vs 81%. Further investigations and larger trials are necessary to evaluate the superiority of FDG-labeled leukocyte PET/CT over ^{111}In-oxine-labeled leukocyte scintigraphy (Rini et al. 2006).

Appendix

How to Perform Blood Cultures

No microbiologic test is more important for the clinician than the blood culture. Although only 5%–15% of blood cultures drawn in febrile patients are positive, the finding of pathogenic microorganisms in the bloodstream often provides critical clinical information that in turn leads to specific, often life-saving therapy.

Blood cultures should be drawn prior to beginning antibiotics whenever possible. If an empiric treatment is an emergency, blood cultures should be drawn as soon as possible after beginning antibiotics. There are no data to suggest that the timing of culture in relation to appearance of fever or chills will maximize the yield.

After the vessel site is selected, a 5-cm area of skin should be disinfected by swabbing concentrically with 70% alcohol, from the venipuncture site outward. The site should be cleansed once again, this time with 10% povidone-iodine again in a circular motion. Iodine should be dried completely before puncture, which takes between 1 and 2 min. In the meantime, the rubber stopper of the blood culture bottle should be decontaminated with 70% alcohol. One should withdraw 20 ml of blood from the puncture site. Changing the needles between venipuncture and inoculation of the bottles, or between bottles, should be omitted because there might be a chance of needlestick injury without lessening the chance of contamination (Little et al. 1999).

If at all possible, blood for cultures should not be drawn through an intravenous or intraarterial catheter. If blood cultures are drawn from an intravenous line, a second culture should be drawn from a peripheral venipuncture. Single sets of blood cultures should not be used to evaluate any patient with suspected bacteremia or candidemia. The optimal yield is obtained with two – including at least one set of central and peripheral blood cultures taken simultaneously – (in suspected intraabdominal sepsis or pneumonia) or three (in suspected infective endocarditis) sets of blood cultures but no more than three blood cultures within a 24-h period. There is a direct relationship between the volume of blood obtained and the yield of a blood culture set. A total of 20 ml of blood should be obtained per blood culture bottle (Mermel and Maki 1993).

18.1.5 Abdominal Wound Dehiscence

18.1.5.1 Synonyms

Synonyms for abdominal wound dehiscence include burst abdomen, open abdomen, and ruptured abdomen.

18.1.5.2 Overview and Incidence

The open abdomen, although uncommon, is associated with significant morbidity and mortality (Barker et al. 2000). Long-term sequelae include enterocutaneous fistula formation, ventral hernia development, and esthetic problems. Deep abdominal dehiscence involving fascia, otherwise known as a burst abdomen, may occur following a laparotomy. The incidence ranges between 0.4% and 3%, and the mortality rate is 15%–20% (Knight and Griffen 1983; Pool 1985; Swan and Banwell 2005). In some instances, the abdomen is left open after laparotomy when surgical reexploration (second look) is foreseeable, for example if repeated drainage of infectious material is indicated, or in cases of abdominal compartment syndrome where immediate closure is contraindicated.

18.1.5.3 Risk Factors

Postoperative nausea and vomiting (PONV) continues to be a common complication of surgery and one of the leading causes of postoperative abdominal wound dehiscence. Other risk factors are listed in Table 18.1.46. Prevention means reducing risk factors. Local factors such as infection and surgical technique can be influenced easily by the physician in attendance. Systemic factors can be assessed but usually cannot be treated before the surgical procedures. Therefore, attention should be directed to prevent PONV (see also Chap. 3, "New Developments in Anesthesia") and postoperative coughing.

An important goal in prevention is to identify patients at high risk for PONV (Table 18.1.47). The consensus guidelines for managing PONV of the International Anesthesia Research Society differentiates between patient-specific, anesthetic, and surgical risk factors (Gan et al. 2003). A reduction of baseline risk factors can significantly reduce the incidence of PONV. Approaches for this context are the use of regional anesthesia, the use of propofol, supplemental oxygen, and hydration. Nitrous oxide and volatile anesthetics should be avoided. Minimization of intraoperative and postoperative opioids as well as neostigmine is recommended.

Antiemetic therapy for PONV prophylaxis (doses and timing) is shown in Table 18.1.48.

Since coughing represents a way for airway clearance and secretion mobilization there should not be an attempt to inhibit this reflex by drugs because coughing decreases the incidence of pneumonia by reducing the probability of developing postoperative atelectasis. Some authors even propagandize the two-stage cough in the postoperative setting. The first cough raises the secretions, the second cough facilitates expectoration. One may use splinting techniques for coughing, splinting the surgical incision with the use of a pillow or hands.

Table 18.1.46. Risk factors for abdominal wound dehiscence

Local factors	
Infection	
Surgical technique	Type of incision
	Closure technique
	Suture type
	Surgeon's experience
Mechanical	Abdominal distension
	Pulmonary complication
Systemic factors	
Obesity	
Malnutrition	
Medication	Steroids
	Immunosuppression
Smoking	
Anemia	
Hyperbilirubinemia	
Postoperative factors	
Coughing	
Vomiting	

18.1.5.4 Clinical Signs and Complications

From clinical experience, open abdominal wounds can be classified by the wound type and its clinical importance. Superficial skin defects, also known as surgical site infection (SSI), involves only skin and subcutaneous tissue of incision and occurs within 30 days after the operation and at least one of the following features are present:

- Purulent drainage (culture documentation is not required)
- Organisms are isolated from tissue or fluid of the superficial incision
- At least one sign of inflammation (pain or tenderness, induration, erythema, local warmth of the wound

Table 18.1.47. Risk factors for PONV

Patient-specific risk factors
Female sex
Nonsmoking status
History of PONV/motion sickness
Anesthetic risk factors
Use of volatile anesthetics within 0–2 h
Nitrous oxide
Use of intraoperative and postoperative opioids
Surgical risk factors
Duration of surgery (every 30-min increase in duration increases PONV risk by 60%
Type of surgery (laparoscopy, laparotomy)

From Gan et al. (2003)

Table 18.1.48. Antiemetic doses and timing for administration in adults

Drug	Dose	Evidence level	Timing
Ondansetron	4–8 mg i.v.	IA	At end of surgery
Dolasetron	12.5–50 mg i.v.	IA	At end of surgery
Granisetron	0.35–1 mg i.v.	IA	At end of surgery
Tropisetron	2 mg i.v.	IA	At end of surgery
Dexamethasone	5–10 mg i.v.	IIA	Before induction
Droperidol	0.625–1.25 mg i.v.	IA	At end of surgery

Table 18.1.49. Pathogens associated with wound infections

Pathogen	Frequency (%)
Staphylococcus aureus	20
Coagulase-negative staphylococci	14
Enterococci	12
Escherichia coli	8
Pseudomonas aeruginosa	8
Enterobacter species	7
Proteus mirabilis	3
Klebsiella pneumoniae	3
Other streptococci	3
Candida albicans	3
Group D streptococci	2
Other Gram-positive aerobes	2
Bacteroides fragilis	2

Deep incisional SSI also occurs within 30 days of the operation or within 1 year if an implant is present. It involves deep soft tissue such as fascia and/or muscle and at least one of the following features apply:

- Purulent drainage is present from the deep incision but without organ or space involvement
- Fascial dehiscence
- A deep abscess identified by direct examination or by radiologic examination

Open abdomen with fascial dehiscence may show exposed bowel or omentum, and in a rather complex form the patient presents with intraabdominal sepsis or enteric fistulae. Pathogens commonly associated with wound infections and their frequency of occurrence is listed in Table 18.1.49.

Usually, the abdominal wound dehiscence is an on-site diagnosis. Organisms should be isolated by aseptic culturing technique. Any sign of infection should lead the surgeon to open the incision site deliberately. Manually, palpation is performed to ensure the continuity of the closure of the fascia. Any discontinuity in terms of fascial dehiscence (exposed bowel or omentum, any sign of intraabdominal abscess or sepsis) is a dangerous complication that requires emergency operative intervention. Most patients are in poor condition since the cause is mostly an intraabdominal infection. Coagulopathy can manifest as diffuse microvascular bleeding, with abnormal clotting studies and thrombocytopenia (Ferrara et al. 1990; Valeri et al. 1987). Necrotizing fasciitis is a dreaded condition. This rapidly progressive, infective process affecting the deep fascia, with secondary involvement of the subcutaneous tissues, is associated with high morbidity and mortality. Early, aggressive surgical debridement is necessary. Early and late complications are listed in Table 18.1.50.

Table 18.1.50. Complications of the open abdomen

Early	Late
Evisceration	Ventral hernia
Peritoneal contamination	Enterocutaneous fistulae
Third-space fluid loss	Intraabdominal abscesses
Necrotizing fasciitis	Suture sinus/incision pain
Intestinal ileus	
Death	

18.1.5.5 Prevention

Despite of advances in surgical technique and materials, abdominal fascial closure has remained a procedure that often reflects a surgeon's personal preference with a reliance on tradition and anecdotal experience. The best abdominal closure technique should be fast, easy, and cost-effective, while preventing both early and late complications. A meta-analysis by Rucinski delineates the optimal closure technique of the abdominal midline fascia incision. The continuous all-layer closure with absorbable monofilament suture material looped or double-looped (Nasir and Baker 2001) (Polydioxanone [PDS], Ethicon, Inc., Somerville, NJ; Polyglyconate, Maxon, US Surgical, and Davis & Geck, Inc., Danbury, CT) with #1 or #2 suture with a suture-length-to-wound-length ratio of 4:1 (placing the sutures approximately 2 cm away from fascial edge and approximately 2 cm from one another) is the optimal technique for fascial closure after laparotomy and therefore the best prevention of a ruptured abdomen (Rucinski et al. 2001).

18.1.5.6 Management

In the management of open abdomen, primary closure, as long as it is performed without tension and does not lead to abdominal compartment syndrome (ACS), is the preferable form of definitive closure. Although difficult to quantify, the risks of infection, enterocutaneous fistula, and recurrent wound problems appear to be lower if primary closure is possible (Rutherford et al. 2004). As the patient's overall status improves and edema lessens, primary closure can often be performed days to weeks after the original laparotomy.

Primary closure of the abdomen without tension is a main goal, preferable as soon as possible after diagnosis. In most circumstances, the rectus sheath as well as the ventral fascia of the rectus muscle are identifiable. If tension-free closure can be performed one should use the same technique as mentioned above (prevention) after aggressive surgical debridement thoroughly removing necrotic tissue (skin, subcutaneous tissues, fascia, muscle) and cleaning the wound with normal saline or antiseptic fluids (Lavasept). Sometimes it may be necessary to recreate a neofascia by mobilization of skin and subcutaneous tissue. If tension-free closure is not achievable, component separation, described by Ramirez et al. in 1990, reconstructs the midline defect with an innervated advancement of muscle and fascia. The external oblique is transected approximately 2 cm lateral to its insertion into the rectus sheath and separated from the internal oblique (Fig. 18.10). This separation extends 5–7 cm cephalad to the costal margin, and as far laterally as possible. The rectus muscles are advanced medially and sutured to close the defect. Additional mobility in each location can be gained by separating the rectus muscle from the posterior rectus sheath. Bilateral advancement yields enough mobility to close defects of 10 cm in the epigastrium, 20 cm at the umbilicus, and 6 cm at the suprapubic level. Sometimes it may be necessary to place a Vicryl band between fascia closure and subcutaneous tissue in order to strengthen the abdominal wall. The skin is closed

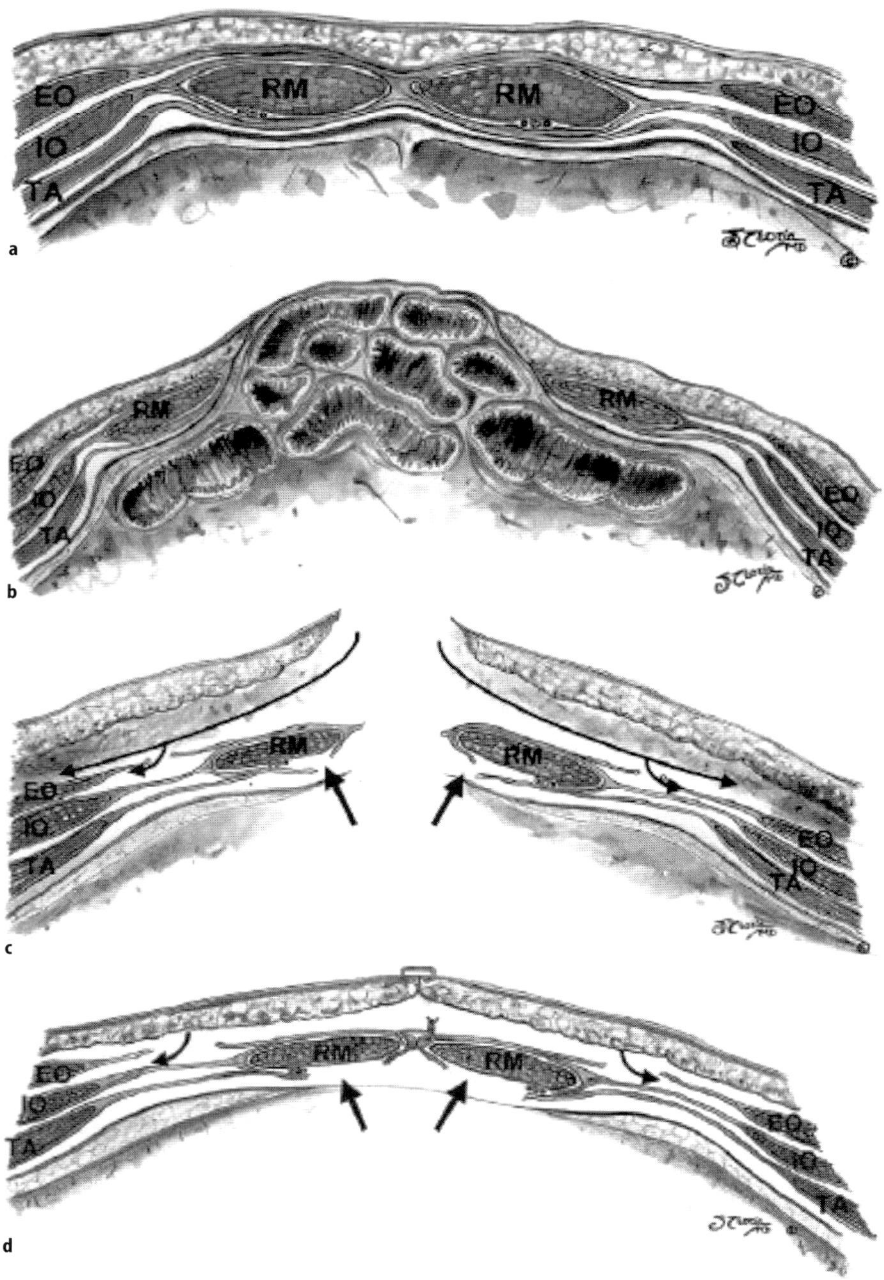

Fig. 18.1.10. **a** Cross-sectional view of the normal anatomy of the abdominal wall. *RM* rectus abdominis muscle, *EO* external oblique muscle, *IO* internal oblique muscle, *TA* transversus abdominis muscle. **b** Open abdomen with ventral hernia. **c** *Arrows* demonstrate the line of dissection between the external oblique muscle and the overlying subcutaneous tissue. Incision in the external oblique muscle lateral to the rectus sheath. Another incision into the posterior sheath. **d** Completed procedure of the components separation

over closed-suction drains, which remain in place 1–2 weeks. Necrosis of the overlying skin can be a common complication because of the extensive mobilization of skin that is required. Component separation can be used in the acute setting, or in a delayed fashion. In times of evidence-based medicine, steel sutures, although recommended by some authors, should no longer be used as reinforcement sutures and are abandoned in our institution.

If primary closure is not possible, the options include closure with a permanent prosthesis (polypropylene, polytetrafluoroethylene [PTFE], composite materials – a sandwich of polypropylene and ePTFE, antiseptic-impregnated materials using chlorhexidine hydrochloride and silver carbonate preservative agents, biologic materials – porcine small intestinal submucosa, human acellular dermis), vacuum-assisted closure, or plastic surgical techniques (tissue expanders, flaps, component separation [Ramirez et al. 1990]), anticipating a hernia (Fig. 18.1.11).

Total parenteral nutrition (TPN) and enteral nutrition are available routes of nutritional support in the recovery of critically ill patients. In patients who have enterocutaneous fistulas, lack of intestinal continuity, dysmotility disorders, or mechanical bowel obstruction, TPN remains the first choice (Rutherford et al. 2004) (Table 18.1.51), although typical complications such as intravenous catheter sepsis, hepatic failure,

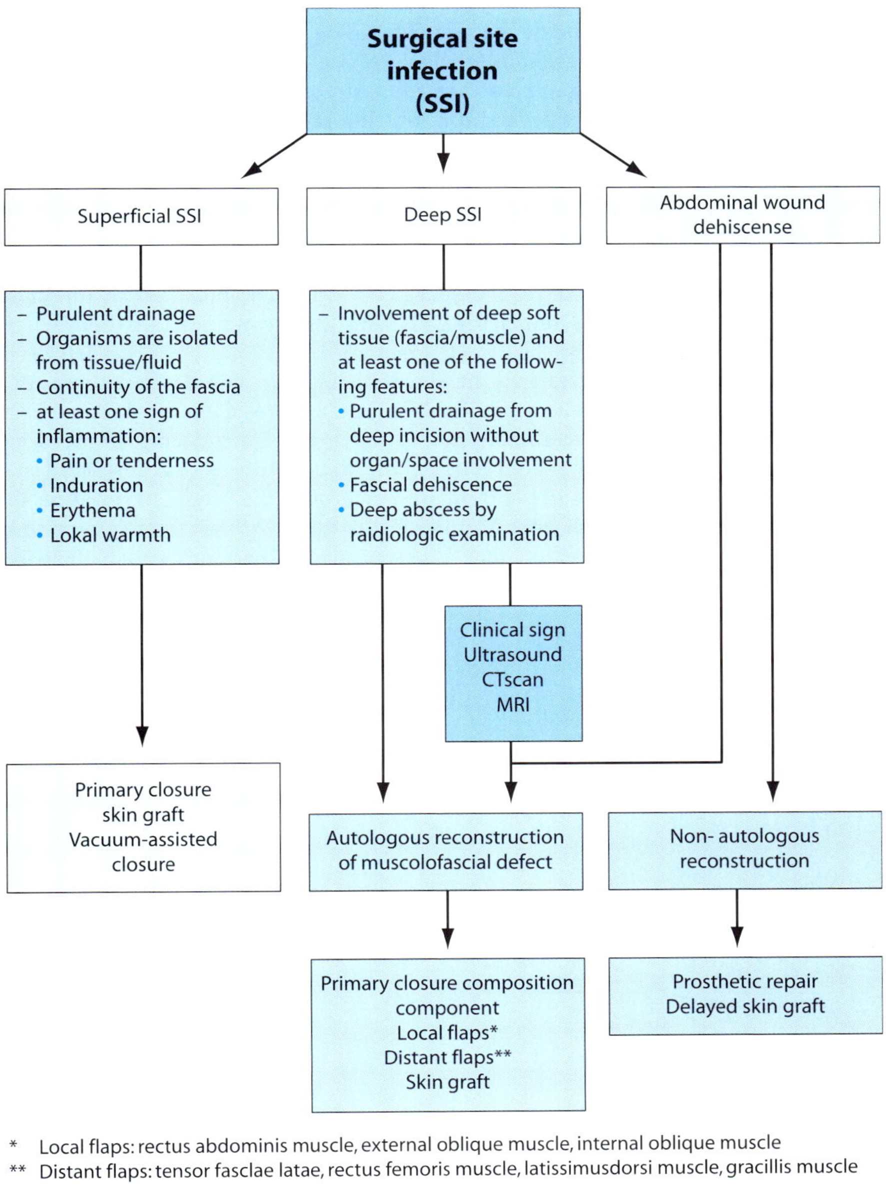

Fig. 18.1.11. Algorithm for surgical repair of abdominal wall defects

Table 18.1.51. Indications for TPN

Severe short bowel syndrome, i.e., less than 100 cm of small bowel
Severe radiation enteritis, including nonoperative strictures
Gastrointestinal fistulas
Persistent postoperative ileus, mechanical bowel obstruction, dysmotility disorders
Lack of intestinal continuity

and metabolic bone disease should be kept in mind. Tight control of blood sugars in the range of 80–110 mg/dl should be maintained (Rutherford et al. 2004).

Findings from a review of the available data published by Jeejeebhoy (2004) show the benefits of enteral nutrition (EN). Enteral diets are usually less expensive, are nutritionally complete, and have a more physiological administration than intravenous feeding. EN is associated with a higher frequency of gastrointestinal adverse effects than parenteral nutrition, but the effects are usually mild (Bozzetti et al. 2001). Patients on EN have significantly fewer complications and a shorter postoperative stay than patients on TPN. Furthermore, EN seems to be favored in terms of duration of complications, time required to recover bowel function, and mortality. A cumulative incidence curve of postoperative complications comparing TPN with EN was published by Bozzetti (Fig. 18.1.12) (Bozzetti et al. 2001). Reasons in this context may be the so-called bacterial translocation, which means that the migration of bacteria from the intestinal lumen to the systemic circulation is limited, thus reducing the incidence of sepsis. Therefore, prevention of bacterial translocation with the use of enteral nutrition is the premise of why enteral nutrition may be associated with fewer infectious complications than TPN (Scolapio 2004).

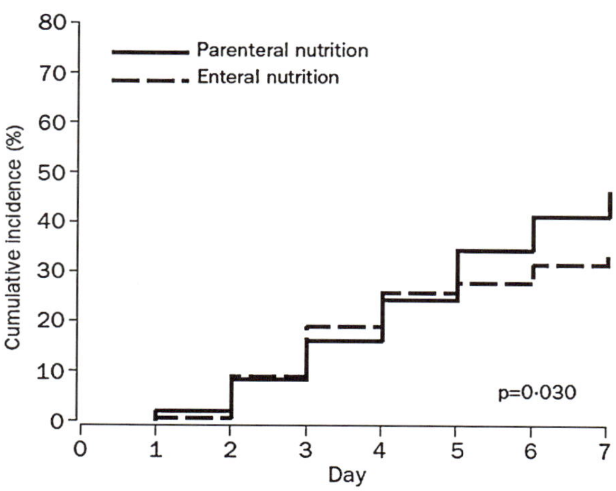

Fig. 18.1.12. Cumulative incidence of postoperative complications (TPN vs EN)

Braunschweig et al. (2001) published a meta-analysis of prospective, randomized, controlled trials to determine both infectious and noninfectious complications associated with EN and TPN in clinical practice. Aggregated results showed a significantly lower rate of infection with tube feeding (0.66; 95% confidence interval [CI], 0.56–0.79) compared with TPN. This lower risk of infection with enteral feeding is independent of whether catheter sepsis is included in the analysis. Noncatheter infections include pneumonia, abdominal abscess, and empyema. The higher risk of infection in TPN patients may be partially explained by a higher incidence of hyperglycemia since increased serum glucose concentrations are a known risk factor for systemic infection of hospitalized patients. In terms of noninfectious complications, a significantly higher risk of nutrition-support complications (parenteral and enteral nutrition technical problems, diarrhea, vomiting, aspiration) was found with tube feeding compared with TPN (relative risk [RR], 1.36; 95% CI, 0.96–1.83). Although many of the complications associated with EN such as diarrhea and abdominal bloating occur, they are considered less severe than catheter sepsis.

If catheter sepsis is included as a nutrition support complication in this meta-analysis, the difference in complications between EN and TPN are eliminated (RR, 1.05; 95% CI, 0.79–1.4).

Others share these observations (Scolapio 2004) and results published in this meta-analysis and speak about downplaying tube feeding complications. Aspiration of tube feeds, misplaced nasal gastric feeding tubes into the lungs, perforation and local infection associated with percutaneous endoscopic gastrostomy (PEG) tube insertion, and inadequate nutrition delivery secondary to tube feeding interruption are just a few examples. Therefore, one can say that EN has advantages over TPN in terms of infections complications, but nevertheless EN has some limitations with respect to its adverse effects and contraindications.

Irrespective of the mode of nutrition support, critically ill patients are also at risk for the development of stress-related mucosal disease that can lead to significant upper gastrointestinal bleeding (Fennerty 2002). Stress gastritis prophylaxis for these patients is strongly recommended with histamine-2-receptor antagonists (H2RA) or even more sufficient with proton pump inhibitors [PPIs]) (Rutheford et al. 2004). Some ICUs still use sucralfate.

Messori et al. (2000) showed in a meta-analysis of placebo-controlled trials of ranitidine or sucralfate a picture of poor effectiveness. Only a few prospective randomized placebo-controlled studies on sucralfate exist, showing rather disappointing results in prophylactic treatment (Ruiz-Santana et al. 1991). The meta-analysis of the trials on ranitidine also showed no difference compared with placebo. Another meta-analysis has been published by Cook et al. (1996). In their assessment of effectiveness of H2RA in terms of stress ulcer prophylaxis, Cook included five trials that used cimetidine and three trials with negative results that used ranitidine. Cimetidine is probably effective at statistical levels, as out of the trials that used cimetidine three had positive results, one had significant results in patients at low risk, and one had negative results.

The results of three meta-analyses that evaluated pneumonia were contradictory in some respects (ranitidine vs placebo and sucralfate vs placebo had the same incidence of pneumonia; for ranitidine vs sucral-

Table 18.1.52. Recommended antibiotics in an abdominal wound dehiscence setting

Cephalosporin first-generation	
Drug name	Cefazolin
Description	First-generation semisynthetic cephalosporin that arrests bacterial cell wall synthesis, inhibiting bacterial growth. Primarily active against skin flora, including *Staphylococcus aureus*. Typically used alone for skin and skin-structure coverage. IV and IM dosing regimens are similar
Adult dose	250 mg to 2 g IV/IM, 6–12 h depending on severity of infection; not to exceed 12 g/day
Pediatric dose	25–100 mg/kg/d IV/IM divided 6–8 h depending on severity of infection; not to exceed 6 g/day
Contraindications	Documented hypersensitivity
Interactions	Probenecid prolongs effect; coadministration with aminoglycosides may increase renal toxicity; may yield false-positive urine dip test for glucose
Pregnancy	Usually safe but benefits must outweigh risks
Precautions	Adjust dose in renal impairment; superinfections and promotion of nonsusceptible organisms may occur with prolonged use or repeated therapy
Cephalosporin second-generation	
Drug name	Cefoxitin (Mefoxin)
Description	Second-generation cephalosporin indicated for Gram-positive cocci and Gram-negative rod infections. Infections caused by cephalosporin- or penicillin-resistant Gram-negative bacteria may respond to cefoxitin
Adult dose	1–2 g IV 6–8 h
Pediatric dose	Infants and children: 80–160 mg/kg/d IV divided every 4–6 h; higher doses for severe or serious infections; not to exceed 12 g/day
Contraindications	Documented hypersensitivity
Interactions	Probenecid may increase effects of cefoxitin; coadministration with aminoglycosides or furosemide may increase nephrotoxicity (closely monitor renal function)
Pregnancy	Usually safe but benefits must outweigh the risks
Precautions	Bacterial or fungal overgrowth of nonsusceptible organisms may occur with prolonged use or repeated treatment; caution in patients with previously diagnosed colitis
Drug name	Cefotetan (Cefotan)
Description	Second-generation cephalosporin indicated for infections caused by susceptible Gram-positive cocci and Gram-negative rods Dose and route of administration depend on condition of patient, severity of infection, and susceptibility of causative organism
Adult dose	1–2 g IV/IM 12 h for 5–10 days
Pediatric dose	20–40 mg/kg/dose IV/IM 12 h for 5–10 days
Contraindications	Documented hypersensitivity
Interactions	Consumption of alcohol within 72 h of cefotetan may produce disulfiram-like reactions; cefotetan may increase hypoprothrombinemic effects of anticoagulants; coadministration with potent diuretics (e.g., loop diuretics) or aminoglycosides may increase
Pregnancy	Usually safe but benefits must outweigh the risks
Precautions	Reduce dose by one-half if CrCl < 10–30 ml/min and by one-fourth if CrCl < 10 ml/min; bacterial or fungal overgrowth of nonsusceptible organisms may occur with prolonged or repeated therapy

fate, there was a significantly higher incidence of pneumonia with ranitidine, $p = 0.012$) (Messori et al. (2000). The large trial by Cook et al. showed a trend toward an increased incidence of pneumonia with ranitidine vs sucralfate.

PPIs are the most potent and reliable acid suppressants available, are well tolerated, and offer the versatility of i.v. administration. Thus, their use in the perioperative setting should be considered when managing patients at high risk for acid-related complications (Pisegna and Martindale 2005). When comparing H2RA with PPI therapy in critical care, nosocomial pneumonia developed in 14% and 3% of patients treated with ranitidine and omeprazole, respectively (Levy et al. 1997). An evaluation of nosocomial pneumonia after trauma demonstrated no difference in patients receiving famotidine i.v. or omeprazole suspension, despite more frequent risk factors for pneumonia in the omeprazole group (Mallow et al. 2004). Adequate prevention of venous thromboembolic disease in this setting must be an important goal, since autopsy series showed an incidence of deep venous thrombosis (DVT) as high as 65% and a 3.8%- to 20%-incidence of pulmonary embolism (Rogers 2001). Still, route and dose of prophylaxis are debatable, but LMWH (low-molecular-weight heparin) should be initiated early in the patient's course of treatment when the risk of bleeding is deemed acceptable (Rutherford et al. 2004). Infection remains a feared complication in these high-risk patients, since they harbor risk factors that increase their septic morbidity, such as hemorrhagic shock, intestinal injuries, and age. With massive volume resuscitation, the potential for antibiotic washout exists and redosing should be considered. In patients with open abdomen without intestinal injury, a first-generation cephalosporin or equivalent is recommended. In patients suffering from open abdomen in combination with intestinal injury a second-generation cephalosporin or equivalent is recommended (Table 18.1.52). Unfortunately, studies are lacking in this population of patients that address antibiotic type, dosage, and duration of therapy. Physicians caring for these patients must be vigilant in the search for infection, but should exercise judgment and common sense in antibiotic usage, since excessive antibiotic use may lead to toxicity and resistance (Fabian 2002; Rutherford et al. 2004).

18.1.6 Chylous Ascites

18.1.6.1 Overview

Chylous ascites (CA), an uncommon disease with an incidence of 1 in 20,000 hospital admissions (Aalami et al. 2000) (Table 18.1.53) usually caused by obstruction or rupture of the peritoneal or retroperitoneal lymphatic glands, is defined as the accumulation of chyle in the peritoneal cavity (Browse et al. 1992). It is a difficult disorder because of the serious mechanical, nutritional, and immunological consequences of the constant loss of protein and lymphocytes (Leibovitch 2002).

Most investigators believe that the incidence of CA is increasing because of more aggressive thoracic and retroperitoneal surgery and with the prolonged survival of patients with cancer (Huang et al. 2004). Some new techniques, such as laparoscopic surgery and transplantation, also have led to increased postoperative CA (Huang et al. 2004; Shafizadeh et al. 2002).

The response to conservative treatment is low, and resolution of the fistula cannot be guaranteed; invasive treatments, including reoperation of the patient, involve additional trauma and may not be successful, and protein malnutrition and immune dysfunction develop from persistent lymph wasting (Giovannini et al. 2005).

Table 18.1.53. Incidence of CA after RPLND and LLDN in the literature

Surgery	CA rate in %
RPLND (primary and secondary)	2–15[a]
LLDN (laparoscopic life donor nephrectomy)	7 reported cases in literature

[a] Baniel and Sella (1999); Sexton et al. (2003)

18.1.6.2 Risk Factors and Pathogenesis

Although CA is a rare condition in urology, reviewing the literature there are some reports on CA, predominantly as casuistics in patients following radical prostatectomy, retroperitoneal lymphadenectomy for testis (Heidenreich et al. 2005), and renal carcinomas (Leibovitch et al. 2002), as well as laparoscopy nephrectomy, including donor and hand-assisted donor nephrectomy (Caumartin et al. 2005; Wu et al. 2004). Figure 18.1.13 illustrates schematically the lymphatic drainage in relation to a human torso. Figure 18.1.14 demonstrates the cisterna chyli, which is the origin of the thoracic duct, lies in the retrocrural space. It arises from several confluent lumbar (right and left lumbar truncal, syn. truncus lumbaris dextra et sinistra), intes-

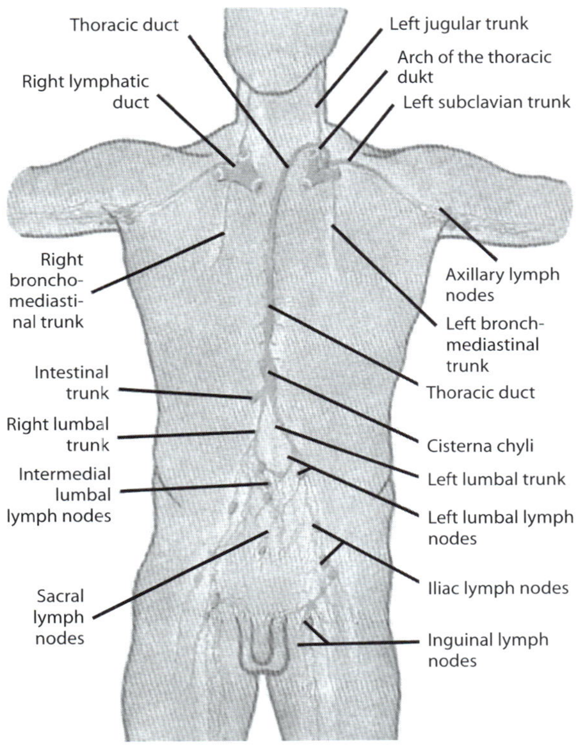

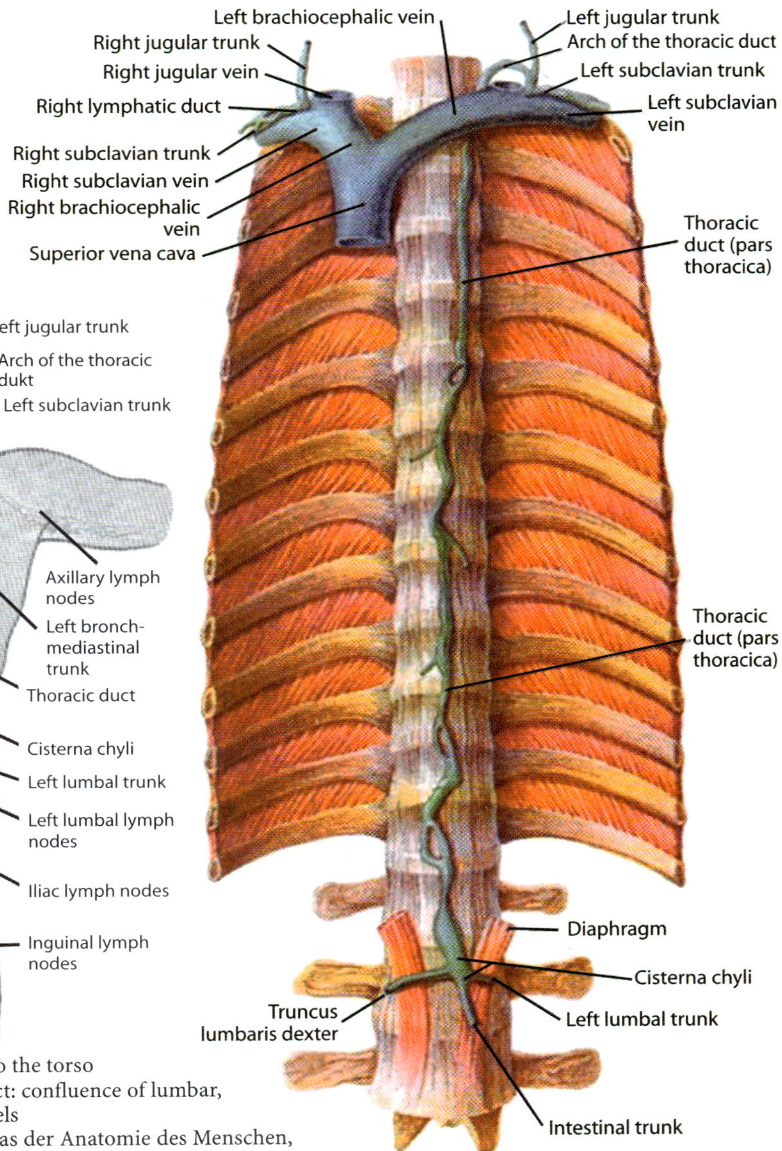

Fig. 18.1.13. Lymphatic vessels in relation to the torso
Fig. 18.1.14. Cisterna chyli and thoracic duct: confluence of lumbar, intestinal, and intercostal lymphatic channels
(Fig. 18.1.13 and 18.1.14 from: Sobotta, Atlas der Anatomie des Menschen, 19. Auflage © 1988 Elsevier GmbH, Urban & Fischer Verlag München)

tinal (intestinal truncal, syn. truncus intestinalis), and intercostal lymphatic channels, and can be seen during lymphangiography and at surgery. It is located to the right of the aorta and anterior to the first and second lumbar vertebrae. Surgical dissections have revealed a range of 5–7 cm in length. Figure 18.1.15 illustrates the anatomy of the retroperitoneal vessels and in combination with the intestinal lymph vessels, it is easy to understand that any surgical intervention to the abdominal cavity and retroperitoneal space can cause crucial damage to this rather little known anatomical structure.

The peritoneal cavity normally contains a small volume of free-circulating fluid. The peritoneal fluid is derived from the transudation of plasma and proteins through capillary membranes into the peritoneal cavity. A delicate balance between the production and reabsorption regulates the volume of peritoneal fluid. The fluid is removed exclusively by way of the lymphatic capillaries lining the diaphragmatic peritoneum. Under normal conditions, the peritoneal fluid and particles are brought to the right hemidiaphragm by a clockwise current. Respiratory movements and elevation of the diaphragm create this current such that a relative vacuum is created in the upper quadrants. From the diaphragm, 80 % of the lymphatic fluid drains by way of anterior mediastinal retrosternal channels to the right thoracic trunk, which ultimately empties into the right

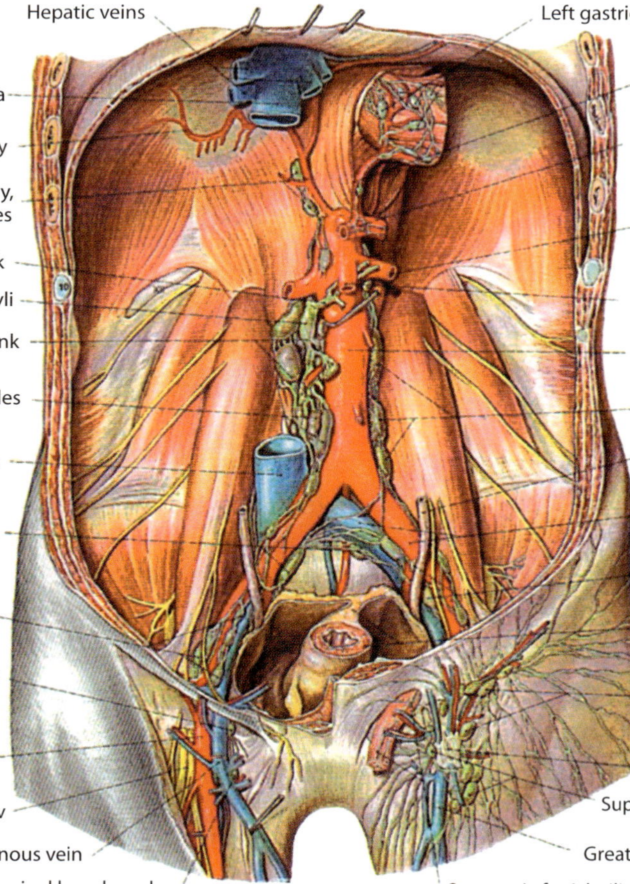

Fig. 18.1.15. Retroperitoneal lymphatic system and cisterna chyli. Anatomic relation of lymphatic system to blood supply and retroperitoneal muscle (From: Sobotta, Atlas der Anatomie des Menschen, 19. Auflage © 1988 Elsevier GmbH, Urban & Fischer Verlag München)

subclavian vein. The principal mechanisms of ascites formation are lymphoperitoneal fistula or leakage from the small bowel and mesenteric lymphatics or through the walls of the retroperitoneal megalymphatics (Amin 2002).

18.1.6.3 Prevention

To prevent the formation of chylogenous ascites, some urologists recommend monopolar and/or bipolar electrocautery dissection with placement of multiple lymphatic ligatures to decrease postoperative lymphorrhea. No prospective comparative studies of the efficacy of these measures have been reported (Olszewski 1991) (see Chap. 18.1.7). If one looks at the histology of lymphatic vessels at the light microscopy level, the lymphatic capillaries (initial lymphatics) have diameters between 10 and 80 μm, whereas the precollectors have a caliber between 100–200 μm. Both lack a basement membrane and muscle layers, but reticular fibers are present. One can imagine that these small lymphatic vessels can be managed by monopolar or bipolar coagulation. Collecting lymphatics, with a diameter of more than 0.2 mm, consist of a tunica intima (endothelium with basement membrane), tunica media (muscular layer), and tunica adventitia (fibrous fibers). Following the management of blood vessels, collecting lymphatics should be clipped or tied by the surgeon with increasing diameter. The intraoperative application of fibrin glue does not reduce the rate of lymphoceles or chylogenous ascites (Pepper et al. 2005; Scholz et al. 2002). Drains routinely placed after surgery to evacuate blood should be used carefully after intraabdominal node dissection, as the absorptive surface of the peritoneum usually serves to mobilize and clear lymphorrhea without stasis or infection. However, some authors recommend their use routinely to minimize lymphocele formation. In our institution, drains are usually removed on the 2nd to 3rd postoperative day independent of the amount of removed fluid. Suction drains with negative pressure are contraindicated in these conditions.

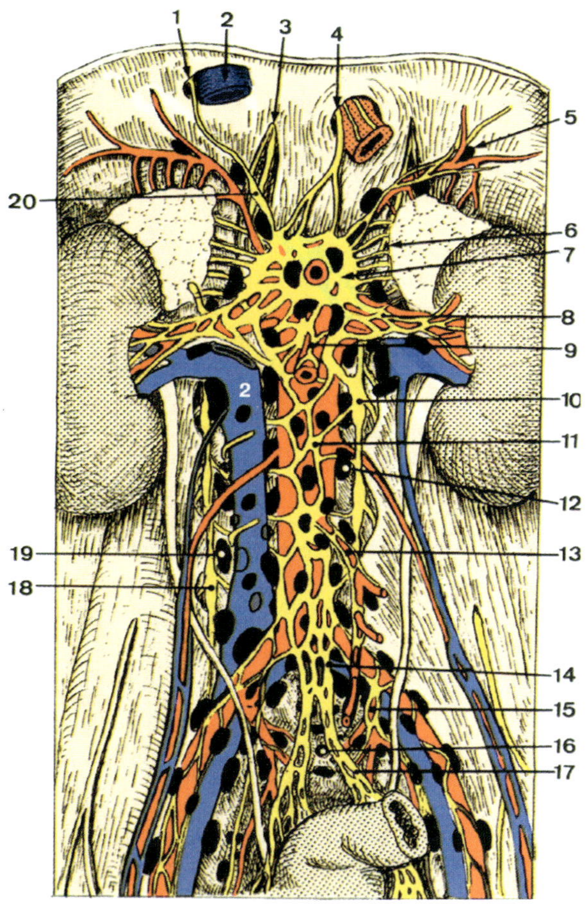

1 Phrenic nerve, **2** Inferior vena cava, **3** Minor and major splanchnic nerves, **4** Vagus nerve, **5** Inferior phrenical artery and inferior diaphragmatic lymph nodes, **6** Suprarenal plexus, **7** Coeliac ganglion and plexus with coeliac lymph nodes, **8** Renal plexus, **9** Superior mesenteric plexus with central mesenteric lymph nodes, **10** Sympathetic trunc, **11** Aortic plexus, **12** Left lumbal lymph nodes, **13** Inferior mesenteric plexus with inferior mesenteric lymph nodes, **14** Superior hypogastric plexus, **15** Internal iliac plexus, **16** Promontory lymph nodes, **17** Left inferior hypogastric plexus, **18** Sympathetic trunc, **19** Right lumbal lymph nodes, **20** Phrenic ganglion

Fig. 18.1.16. Relationship between lumbar and iliac lymph nodes and vegetative nervous system, ganglia, and sympathetic trunk (*black*, lymph nodes) (From: Földi/Földi/Kubik: Lehrbuch der Lymphologie, 6. Auflage © 2005 Elsevier GmbH, Urban & Fischer Verlag München)

18.1.6.4 Detection and Workup

Clinical findings vary from nausea, lack of appetite, and shortness of breath to distended abdomen. These findings, in combination with ultrasound and CT scan results, usually indicate the diagnosis. Other symptoms and clinical signs as well as diagnostic procedures are listed in Table 18.1.54. The diagnosis is usually con-

Table 18.1.54. Clinical findings and workup of CA

Symptoms and clinical findings	Workup
Nausea	Ultrasound
Lack of appetite	Bipedal lymphangiography
Weight gain/weight loss	Lymphoscintigraphy
Shortness of breath/dyspnea	CT scan
Increase in abdominal girth	
Distended abdomen	Total serum protein ↓ (normal, 61–80 g/l)
Dullness to percussion	Albumin ↓ (normal, 30–48 g/l)
Leg swelling (plus upward involving scrotum)	
Diagnostic paracentesis	Milky in color CA culture/microscopy/cytology CA cytochemical: Total protein level 2.5–7.0 g/dl Triglyceride level > 200 mg/dl Specific gravity > serum

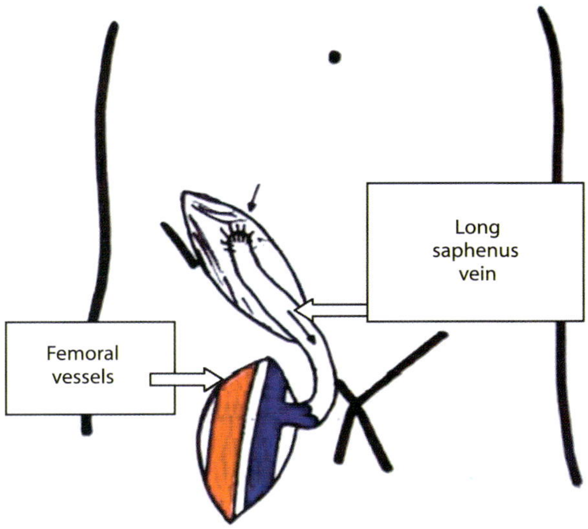

Fig. 18.1.17. Scheme of saphenoperitoneal shunt

firmed by the diagnostic paracentesis, which shows milky fluid with a specific gravity higher of that in serum as well as total protein levels between 2.5–7.0 g/dl and triglyceride levels above 200 mg/dl.

18.1.6.5 Management

Conservative treatment of chylous ascites involves paracentesis and a medium chain triglyceride (MCT) -based diet. Patients should be supplemented with MCT oil, 15 ml orally three times a day. Total parenteral nutrition (TPN) is recommended after dietary manipulation has failed (nonprotein calories, 25 kcal/kg/day; nitrogen, 0.2–0.25 g/kg/day; glucose:fat ratio, 6:4 via central vein) and somatostatin therapy (continuous intravenous infusion at a dose of 6 mg/24 h) is attempted only if chylous ascites has been refractory to all conservative measures. It will take several weeks to 2 months to close the lymphatic fistula adequately with routine conservative regimens (Aalami et al. 2000). Others prefer TPN with somatostatin as first-line therapy, which should be started as soon as possible. Fasting, together with TPN, can decrease the lymph flow in thoracic duct dramatically from 220 ml/kg/h to 1 ml/kg/h. Furthermore, TPN restores nutritional deficits and balances metabolic impairments (Huang et al. 2004). The resolution rate of chyloperitoneum by conservative management is approximately 50%–60% (Caumartin et al. 2005).

Surgery should usually be considered after failure of conservative treatment (Leibovitch 2002). Recently, the laparoscopic approach has been used successfully to resolve postoperative CA (Caumartin et al. 2005) and is thought to be less invasive than the conventional surgical technique. The timing for surgical repair remains controversial. Surgical management of patients with CA should be addressed after 4 weeks of conservative management. This delay will permit small fistula to heal (Baniel et al. 1993; Busch et al. 2000).

Surgical options include placement of a peritoneovenous shunt (Schumpelick and Riesener 1993; Utikal et al. 2004) (Fig. 18.1.14) or repair of the cisterna chyli. Peritoneovenous shunts are considered for patients in whom a definitive leak cannot be identified. A permanent peritoneal cavity drainage with return of ascitic fluid into the circulation based on positive pressure gradient between peritoneal cavity with ascites and central venous pressure is the principle. The long saphenous vein is used as a drainage system. One-way ascites flow is ensured by a natural valve in the saphenous orifice. A suitable long saphenous vein with sufficient orificial valve is required. The procedure is performed under general anesthesia. The long saphenous vein is exposed through vertical incision, its branches are ligated and it is divided at 20 cm. In a simple mechanical manner, (catheterization with saline solution flush) the central patency of the saphenus vein and the sufficiency of its orificial valve (no backflow from the femoral vein) should be checked. The inguinal canal is exposed through an oblique incision and the parietal peritoneum is disclosed after division of the internal oblique muscle fibers laterally from the spermatic cord (funiculus) in the internal ring. This is the place for incision in the peritoneum. The proximal cut end of the long saphenous vein is turned upward and pulled through the subcutis above the inguinal ligament. A slight curve is formed in the venous orifice to prevent a sharp bend. The peritoneum is cut and a watertight anastomosis is performed with an obliquely cut saphenous end using a continuous Prolene 6-0 suture. The wounds are closed in layers with no drainage.

Table 18.1.55. Surgical management and prevention of CA

Technique	
	Clips
	Sutures, direct ligation
	Coagulation
	Biological glue[a]
	Placement of peritoneovenous shunt

[a] Pepper et al. (2005); Scholz et al. (2002)

Surgical exploration to repair the cisterna chyli is most successful when a discrete leak can be found by lymphangiogram. Outcome data are limited to retrospective case studies, but all patients that were treated surgically with direct ligation or placement of a peritoneovenous shunt were reported to be successful (Aalami et al. 2000; Almakdisi et al. 2005; Dewdney et al. 2005) (Table 18.1.55).

18.1.7 Deep Venous Thrombosis

18.1.7.1 Overview and Incidence

Venous thromboembolism (VTE) is common risk for hospitalized patients, especially in general and urological surgery. The annual incidence of VTE is approximately 0.1%–0.2%, most often presented as deep venous thrombosis (DVT) or pulmonary embolism (PE) (Oger 2000). The annual incidence of VTE among young adults is about 0.01%, increasing to about 1% among people who are 60 years and older (Nordstrom et al. 1992; Silverstein et al. 1998).

18.1.7.2 Risk Factors

Several factors – inherited and acquired – influence the risk for developing a VTE (Table 18.1.56). These risk factors accumulate and increase the individual risk for a VTE.

The most effective way to reduce the morbidity of VTE is to identify patients who present the above-mentioned risk factors and to institute an appropriate individual primary prophylaxis (Heyers et al. 2001; Hirsh and Hoak1996).

In urology and general surgery, no consensus on the ideal prophylaxis exists. While in Europe pharmacological thromboprophylaxis in patients undergoing major pelvic surgery can be considered as standard, in the United States intermittent pneumatic compression and early ambulation often is favored (Galvin et al. 2004; Koya et al. 2005). Pharmacological thromboprophylaxis by low-dose unfractionated heparin (LDUH) or low-molecular-weight heparin (LMWH) seems to be the most effective (Kakkar et al. 1993, 1997; Nurmohamed et al. 1995).

Table 18.1.56. Risk factors for venous thromboembolism

Inherited conditions
Protein C, protein S, antithrombin III deficiency
Factor V Leiden mutation
G20210A prothrombin-gene mutation (heterozygous)
Dysfibrinogenemia
Acquired conditions
Major surgery or major trauma
Previous venous thromboembolism
Antiphospholipid antibodies
Cancer (chemotherapy)
Major medical illness
Age
Obesity
Leg paralysis
Estrogen therapy
Pregnancy or puerperium
Major medical illness
Hereditary, environmental or idiopathic conditions
High plasma homocysteine
High plasma coagulation factors VIII, IX, XI

18.1.7.3 Detection and Clinical Findings

Classic signs of a DVT are pain, tenderness, and swelling of the leg. However, these symptoms can be misleading and can be caused by nonthrombotic disorders (Hull et al. 1984; Nicolaides et al. 1971). Therefor, it is essential to confirm the diagnosis of venous thrombosis by reliable objective tests. These objective tests include venography (Lensing et al. 1992), impedance plethysmography (IPG) (Buller et al. 1991; Hull et al. 1990a), and venous ultrasonography. Today, compression ultrasonography can be considered as the diagnostic test of choice in clinical practice, because it is noninvasive, reliable, and widely available (Hirsh and Hoak 1996; Kearon et al. 1998). In patients with clinical symptoms and negative results on ultrasonography, ascending contrast venography may be additionally performed. Another way is to perform a D-dimer assay, but since after surgery the D-dimer test is often false positive, its value is limited in the diagnosis of DVT for surgical patients.

18.1.7.4 Management

The initial therapy of DVT should be a combination of unfractionated (UFH) or low-molecular-weight heparin (LMWH) followed by oral anticoagulants (Hirsh and Hoak 1996; Brandjes et al. 1992). Thrombolytic treatment and surgical thrombectomy is usually only indicated for patients with massive iliofemoral thrombosis or pulmonary embolism (Hyers et al. 2001; Heymans et al. 1998; Verhaeghe et al. 1997). LMWH has become the standard for the initial treatment of DVT because it has been shown to be as effective and safe as

Table 18.1.57. Contraindications for anticoagulation

Absolute contraindications
Active bleeding
Relative contraindications
Recent bleeding, gastrointestinal bleeding (within 2 weeks), intracranial bleeding (within 3 months)
Bleeding diathesis
Coagulation defect
Severe thrombocytopenia
Platelet function defect
Recent major trauma
Uncontrolled hypertension
Endocarditis

continuous intravenous UFH. It can be administered subcutaneously without laboratory monitoring in most patients and is more convenient to use (Ho et al. 2005).

There are contraindications for anticoagulation (Table 18.1.57), but most of them are relative.

Unfractionated Heparin

After an initial loading dose, UFH is given intravenously by continuous infusion. Laboratory monitoring of the activated partial thromboplastin time (aPTT) is necessary, because the anticoagulant response varies due to variable binding of UFH to plasma proteins (Hirsh et al. 2001). There exist many different application schemes for UFH. The therapeutic range is for most commercial aPTT reagents 1.8 – 3.0 times the control value (Monreal et al. 1989) although for less sensitive reagents it is 1.5 – 2.0 (Hirsh and Hoak 1996; Basu et al. 1972; Bjornsson and Nash 1986). To maintain anticoagulation within this therapeutic range, weight-based heparin nomograms can be used (Raschke et al. 1996). Other guidelines suggest a bolus of 5,000 IU i.v. when a DVT is suspected, followed by a rebolus with UFH 80 IU/kg i.v. and a maintenance infusion at 18 IU/kg as soon as a DVT is confirmed[7]. Monitoring of the aPTT after 4 h is mandatory. The duration of heparin therapy should be 4 – 5 days for patients with DVT (Gallus et al. 1986; Hull et al. 1990b). It should be only extended to a 7- to 10-day course in case of large iliofemoral vein thrombi or major pulmonary embolism(Hirsh and Hoak 1996).

Low-Molecular-Weight Heparin

Administration of LMWH in a fixed dose by subcutaneous injection once or twice daily in weight-adjusted doses provides some important advantages compared to UFH. LMWHs have proven to be at least as effective and safe as UHF (Monreal et al. 1994; Hull et al. 1992; Siragusa et al. 1996; Gould et al. 1999). In addition, they seem to cause less heparin-induced thrombocytopenia

(Hirsh et al. 2001; Warkentin et al. 1995) and a lower incidence of osteoporosis than heparin (Monreal et al. 1994; Pettila et al. 2002). As they need no monitoring, LMWHs are more convenient to administer and make an effective outpatient therapy possible (Koopman et al. 1996; Levine et al. 1996). As there are numerous LMWH agents on the market, no general advice on the dosage can be given.

Long-Term Therapy

Initial therapy of venous thromboembolism by either LMWH or UFH should be followed by oral anticoagulation for secondary prophylaxis and to reduce risk of recurrence (Hyers et al. 2001; Prins et al. 1999). Heparin therapy is overlapped with initiation of warfarin or another coumarin until the therapeutic range, indicated by an international normalized ratio (INR) of 2.0–3.0, is reached for 2 consecutive days. In case of massive thrombosis, an extended course of heparin for 7–14 days should be considered (Bates and Ginsberg 2004; Schulman 2003). Because of an increased bleeding risk, it can be essential to delay coumarin therapy after surgery.

The duration of oral anticoagulation treatment should be adapted to the individual patient. In general, a course of 3–6 months is recommended (Hyers et al. 2001). Extending therapy beyond 6 months may be advisable for patients with multiple recurrent episodes of idiopathic VTE or with active malignant disease-associated VTE or antithrombin deficiency (Levine et al. 1988; Hirsh 1995).

18.1.8 Lymphoceles

18.1.8.1 Anatomy and Physiology

The lymphatic system is an anatomical structure composed of channels, where the principal function is to maintain the blood volume by returning fluid and protein molecules that leak from blood capillaries to the interstitial space to the general circulation. In addition, there are circulating lymphocytes and lymphoid organs that play an important role in the process of defense against infection and tumor growth (Olszewski 1991).

The lymph draining system of the body is composed of thin-walled channels that are classified according to the histotopographical position. The smaller channels, commonly called lymphatic capillaries (initial lymphatics), form the roots of this vascular system. Within the organs, the initial lymphatics communicate to precollector ducts. Outside of parenchymatous organs, the lymph is drained by collecting vessels that carry the lymph to the regional nodes. These vessels are referred to as prenodal collecting vessels. After intranodal passage of one node or a set of successive nodes, the lymph is drained by postnodal collecting lymphatics, which converge to larger lymphatic trunks that finally drain into the lymphatic ducts. The largest of them, the thoracic duct, joins the angle between the left subclavian vein and the internal jugular vein (Földi et al. 2005; Olszewski 1991). Figures 18.1.19 and 18.1.20 illustrate the decisive lymphatic vessels and nodes physicians encounter in urology.

At the light microscopy level, initial lymphatic vessels show highly variable diameters, between 10 and 80 µm,

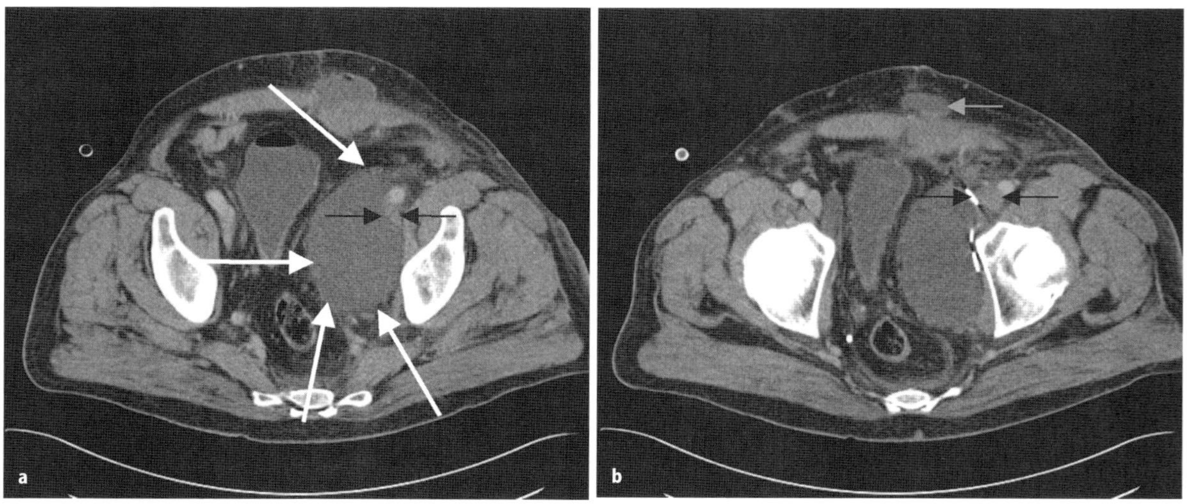

Fig. 18.1.18a–d. CT scan of a patient on day 6 following open radical retropubic prostatectomy with a large (>5 cm) lymphocele in the left pelvic region presenting with pain in the left lower abdomen. *White arrows* show the extension of the lymphocele. *Black arrows* show a partial compression of the common iliac vein (**a**). On the CT scan (**b**), the *black arrows* indicate the stasis of the common iliac vein with no signs of thrombosis. The *grey arrow* is placed to show a small epifascial hematoma

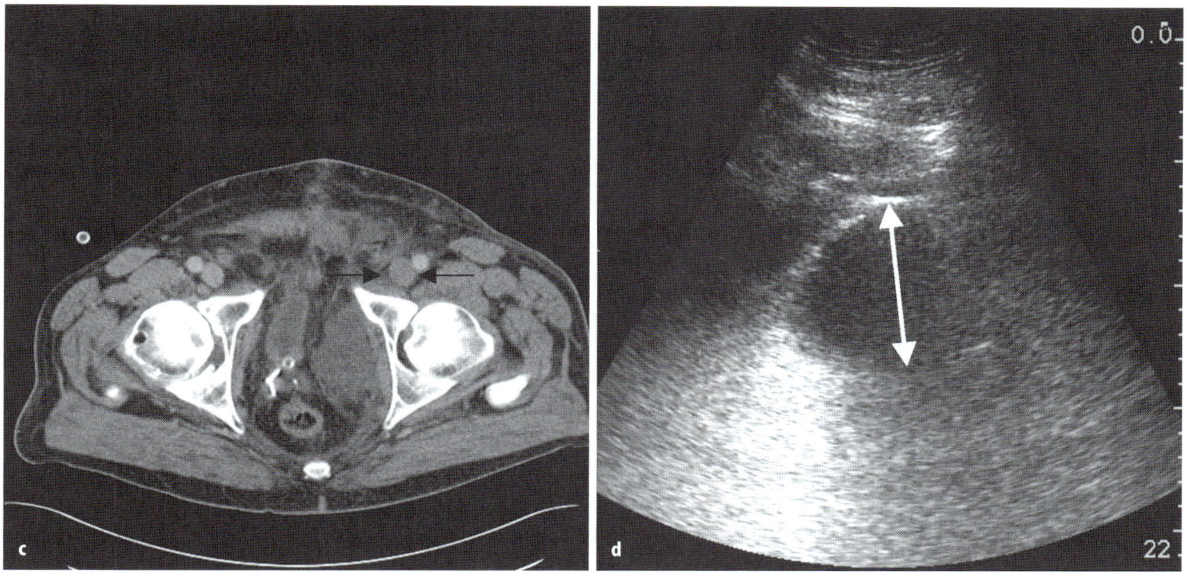

Fig. 18.1.18. c A dilated common iliac vein without thrombosis. **d** Ultrasound of the same patient showing the lymphocele with a diameter of more than 5 cm

which clearly exceed that of blood capillaries, that lack a basement membrane, but reticular fibers are present. The precollectors have a larger caliber (100–200 μm) than the initial lymphatics but the fundamental morphology is similar in both types of vessels. Lymphatic channels have numerous valves and are often slightly distended at these sites. Collecting lymphatics with a diameter of more than 0.2 mm usually have three layers: tunica intima (endothelium with basement membrane),
tunica media (muscular layer with no clear division into circular or longitudinal coats), and tunica adventitia (fibrous fibers). A longitudinal muscular layer is present in the right lymphatic and thoracic ducts. The lymphatic system is an organized network composed of functionally interrelated lymphoid tissue, and transportation pathways of tissue fluid, or lymph, and lymphoid cels. Its main components are

1. Migrating dendritic cells, macrophages and lymphocytes, organized lymphoid tissue such as lymph nodes, thymus, spleen,

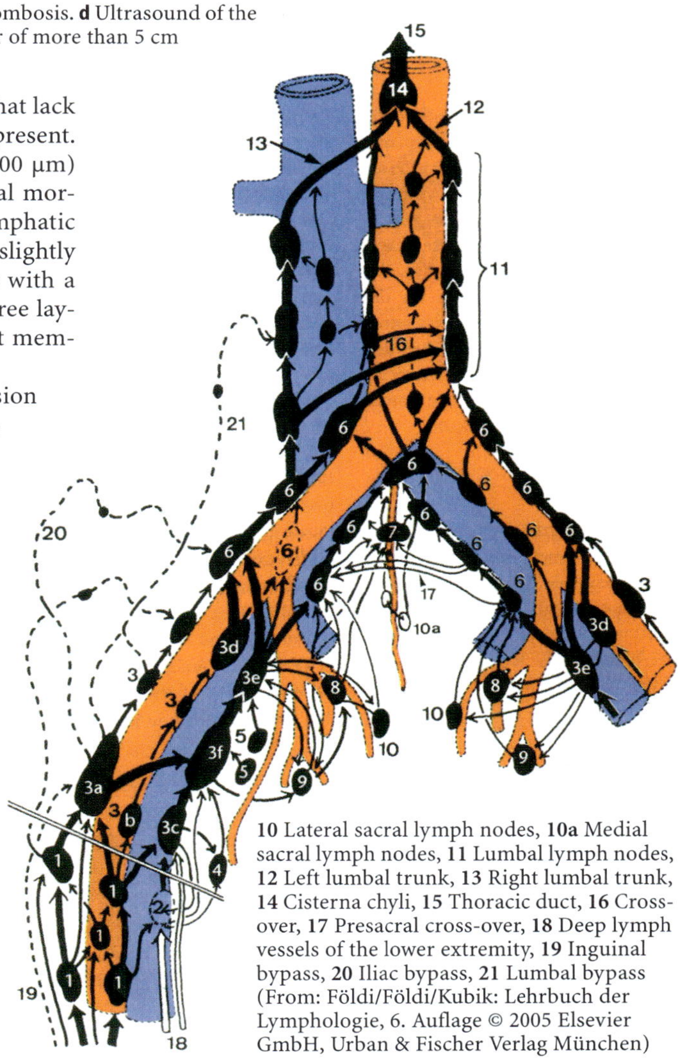

Fig. 18.1.19. Lymphatic drainage of the pelvic region **1** Superficial inguinal lymph nodes, **2** Profund inguinal lymph nodes, **3** External iliac lymph nodes, **3a** Lateral lacunar lymph node, **3b** Intermedial lacunar lymph node, **3c** Medial lacunar lymph node, **3d** Lateral interiliac lymph node, **3e** Medial interiliac lymph node, **3f** Principal lymph node, **4** Obturator canal lymph node, **5** Obturator fossa lymph nodes, **6** Common iliac lymph nodes, **7** Promontory lymph nodes, **8** Superior gluteal lymph nodes, **9** Inferior gluteal lymph nodes, **10** Lateral sacral lymph nodes, **10a** Medial sacral lymph nodes, **11** Lumbal lymph nodes, **12** Left lumbal trunk, **13** Right lumbal trunk, **14** Cisterna chyli, **15** Thoracic duct, **16** Cross-over, **17** Presacral cross-over, **18** Deep lymph vessels of the lower extremity, **19** Inguinal bypass, **20** Iliac bypass, **21** Lumbal bypass (From: Földi/Földi/Kubik: Lehrbuch der Lymphologie, 6. Auflage © 2005 Elsevier GmbH, Urban & Fischer Verlag München)

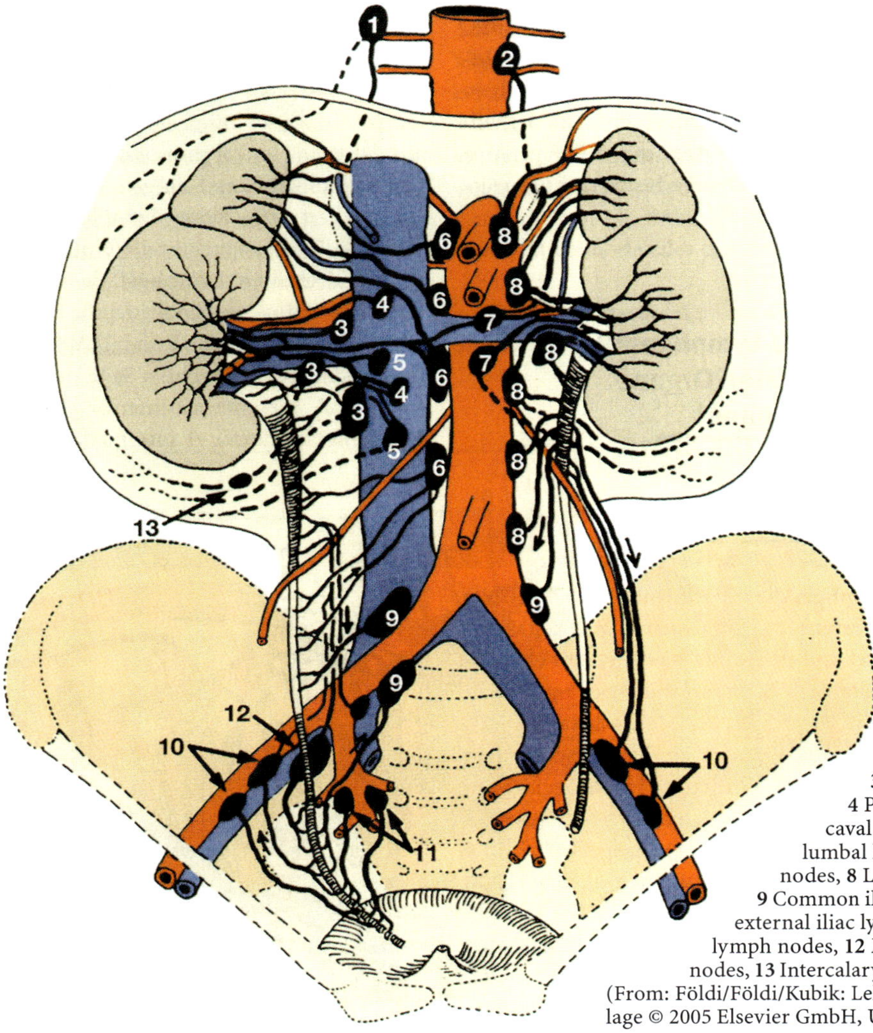

Fig. 18.1.20. Lymphatic drainage of the extraperitoneal region
1 Intercostal lymph node, **2** Juxtavertebral lymph node, **3** Laterocaval lymph nodes, **4** Precaval lymph nodes, **5** Retrocaval lymph nodes, **6** Intermedial lumbal lymph nodes, **7** Preaortic lymph nodes, **8** Lateroaortic lymph nodes, **9** Common iliac lymph nodes, **10** Intermedial external iliac lymph nodes, **11** Internal iliac lymph nodes, **12** Medial external iliac lymph nodes, **13** Intercalary lymph node
(From: Földi/Földi/Kubik: Lehrbuch der Lymphologie, 6. Auflage © 2005 Elsevier GmbH, Urban & Fischer Verlag München

bone marrow, and lymphoid tissue in gut and lungs, liver lymphoid cells, and the dendritic cell network of nonlymphoid organs
2. Vessels (intercellular space, lymphatics, and perivascular spaces)
3. Fluids (tissue fluid and lymph).

The lymphatic system can be divided into the following compartments: peripheral (from the interstitial space to and within the nearest lymph node) and central (efferent lymphatics, cisterna chyli, and the thoracic duct, all lymphoid organs). Organs and tissues with the most active afferent arm of the lymphatic system are skin, gut, and lungs. These are the body structures exposed to the external environment (Földi et al. 2005; Olszewski 1991).

The daily production of lymph goes beyond 2 l/24 h under normal conditions. The chemical composition of lymph is to a large degree different from that of plasma. In addition, it is enriched in products of cell metabolism. Thus the exact composition of lymph is dictated by capillary filtration rate, permeability of the capillary wall, the metabolic state of parenchymal cells, and tissue fluid, and lymph transport away via lymphatics. All these factors change depending on the actual functional state of the tissue or organ from which the lymph is drained. The average amount of proteins is approximately 20 g/l but shows dependence on the topographical areas (Table 18.1.58).

The tissue fluid and lymph constitute a 12-l water and electrolyte compartment containing immune cells and free cellular components, apoptotic bodies, cell lysates, exosomes, bacteria, viruses or virus-like antigens, intracellular pathogens, and proteins (soluble, particulate, or complexed with immunoglobulins, heat shock proteins, complement factors, coagulation factors, cytokines and chemokines, and their receptors and inhibitors, free DNA from the host's destroyed

Table 18.1.58. Proteins in lymph of humans

Source of lymph	Protein	Value g/l	L:S
Thoracic duct	Total protein	35.0	
		31.0–48.9	0.5–0.69
	Albumin	21.1–34.2	0.56–0.82
Hepatic	Total protein	29.0	0.52
		34.0–87.0	0.57–1.0
	Albumin	29.4–42.0	0.93
Intestinal	Total protein	30.0–41.0	0.46–0.65
	Albumin	12.4–25.5	0.4–0.68

L:S lymph to serum ratio

cells, lipoproteins, auto- and foreign antigens encoded by RNA or DNA, and ectoenzymes) (Olszewski 2005).

Mechanisms regulating extravascular coagulation in slow-moving extravascular fluids (interstitial fluids and lymph) are poorly understood since data dealing with this aspect are rare in the literature. Whereas considerable data are available on coagulation factor levels in thoracic duct lymph, which is not surprising, since lymph from the liver, the site of synthesis of most hemostatic factors, very few data are available on the levels of hemostatic factors in peripheral lymph. A recent study on hemostatic factors in peripheral rabbit lymph by Le et al. (1998) showed a mean lymph fibrinogen level of almost 30 % of the mean plasma level. Since fibrin degradation products were not detectable, the authors concluded that fibrin does not form under normal physiological conditions, despite a substantial concentration of fibrinogen in this slow-moving fluid. Additionally, the data are compatible with a basal factor VIIa tissue factor-catalyzed extravascular activation of factor X, which is prevented from progressing to generation of fibrin in limb interstitial fluid and lymph by low levels of factor VIII and factor V and by the inhibitory activity of antithrombin and tissue factor pathway inhibitor (TFPI).

A different study conducted by Olszewski (Olszewski 2005) investigated 17 healthy men and their lymph: plasma ratios. Activated factor VII (FVIIa) and TFPI-Xa complex concentrations were higher in lymph than plasma. Fibrin degradation products were higher in lymph than plasma, up to five times as high. This high level may indicate proteolysis of fibrinogen and may indirectly show hemostatic activity, which may explain the ability of the lymphatic system of spontaneous coagulation following injury or surgery.

18.1.8.2 Overview

Lymphoceles are a collection of lymphatic fluid without an epithelial lining occurring as a consequence of surgical dissection and inadequate closure of afferent lymphatic vessels and subsequent leakage of lymph.

Table 18.1.59. Incidence of symptomatic lymphoceles depending on surgical intervention

Surgery	Incidence (symptomatic)[a] 11–16, 10, 17
Renal transplantation	0.6 %–18 %
RPLND	25 %
Open pelvic lymph node dissection	4.7 %–14.8 %
Laparoscopic pelvic lymph node dissection	1 %–3 %
Inguinal lymphadenectomy	7.5 %–30 %

RPLND retroperitoneal lymph node dissection
[a] Sogani et al. (1981); Bailey et al. (2003); Corvin et al. (2004); Jacobelis (2003); Janetschek et al. (1999); McCullough et al. (1991); Nelson et al. (2004); Solberg et al. (2003)

In renal transplantation, lymphatics can be disrupted in the hilum of the graft either during procurement or graft preparation. Lymphoceles develop in up to 61 % of patients undergoing renal transplantation or pelvic surgery. However, only a small portion of these lymphoceles are clinically significant (Table 18.1.59), causing venous obstruction with subsequent edema and thromboembolic complications (Yablon et al. 2004).

Most lymphoceles are asymptomatic and resolve spontaneously (Pepper et al. 2005; Sogani et al. 1981). Drainage or ablation may be necessary if lymphoceles are large (~5 cm), become infected, are associated with pain, or cause compression of adjacent structures (e.g., ureter, urinary bladder, iliac veins) (Pepper et al. 2005; Sogani et al. 1981). The development of lymphoceles depends on:

1. The number of injured lymphatics and insufficient closure of lymph vessels
2. The speed of development of new lymphatic connections
3. The coexistence of deep thrombophlebitis with venous blood stasis and subsequent lymph overproduction
4. The preexistence of idiopathic lymph stasis
5. Postischemic capillary permeability with high infiltration rate and augmented lymph production.

18.1.8.3 Risk Factors and Prevention

The incidence of lymphoceles can be minimized by meticulous surgical technique and attention to sealing the lymph vessels during lymph node dissection (Pepper et al. 2005; Sogani et al. 1981). The most common nodal operation performed in urology are groin, pelvic, and retroperitoneal node dissection. Lymph node dissections are performed similarly by most surgeons. The margins of dissection are exposed, cleaned of fat and interlying lymphatic structures are removed en bloc.

Table 18.1.60. Risk factors for lymphoceles in surgical urology

Repeat transplantation
Acute graft rejection
Cadaveric donor kidney
Sirolimus immunosuppression
Adult polycystic kidney disease
Previous chemotherapy
Low-molecular-weight heparin
Surgical techniques
Extension of pelvic lymph node dissection

The skin incision is placed along the lines of skin tension and crossing the major flexion of the groin at right angles is avoided. The margins of dissection are dissected sharply and blood vessels are tied or clipped. Some surgeons recommend both monopolar and bipolar electrocautery dissection with placement of multiple lymphatic ligatures to decrease postoperative lymphorrhea. No prospective comparative studies of the efficacy of these measures have been reported (Olszewski 1991). Suction drains are routinely placed in the groin area after dissection to evacuate blood and lymph from divided vessels and to coapt the skin to the exposed structures beneath. The drains used are sterile, closed systems that produce a constant negative pressure of 20–50 mmHg. They are removed when the tissue adheres well and the fluid removed is minimal (<30 ml/day) and without obvious infection. Drains are not always placed after intraabdominal node dissection, as the absorptive surface of the peritoneum usually serves to mobilize and clear lymphorrhea without stasis or infection. However, some authors recommend their use routinely to minimize lymphocele formation. In our institution, suction drains are used as described above for lymphadenectomy of the groin. For extraperitoneal and intraabdominal procedures, the management is identical. Drains (without suction) are removed at day 2 or 3 after surgery independent of the amount of fluid removed. Lymphadenectomy is performed by using clips and/or bipolar electrocoagulation.

Risk factors are listed in Table 18.1.60 (Koch and Jr 1997; Lundin et al. 2002).

18.1.8.4 Clinical Signs

The symptoms of a lymphocele depend on the site, size, and the presence of infection. A visible or palpable pelvic mass may be present, resulting in abdominal or pelvic pain. Symptoms or signs may stem from venous or ureteric compression resulting in unilateral leg edema and leg pain, hydronephrosis with deterioration in renal function, and deep vein thrombosis. Fever and chills should raise the suspicion of an infected collection. Differential diagnosis includes urinoma, hematoma, and abscess formation (Table 18.1.61).

Table 18.1.61. Clinical findings and workup

Clinical findings
Distension or abdominal pain
Secondary infection
Edema of the lower extremity or genitalia
Compressive effect on ureter
Deep vein thrombosis
Graft dysfunction
Diagnostic procedure
Ultrasound/duplex sonography (Fig. 18.1.21)
CT scan (Fig. 18.1.18–18.1.20)
Lymphocele aspirate (microbiology/culture)

18.1.8.5 Diagnosis and Workup

Ultrasound is simple and effective in confirming the position and size of the fluid collection. Occasionally CT scans are used to diagnose lymphoceles (Fig. 18.1.18). Cytological and biochemical analysis of the aspirate can be used to aid in their diagnosis. Fluid chemistry is particularly helpful in differentiating lymphoceles from urinoma since lymphocytes usually can be detected. While electrolytes and creatinine are serum isotone in lymphoceles, in urinoma high creatinine levels are the rule. If there is a discontinuation of the lymphatics in the upper retroperitoneum (celiac axis area), chylous fluid collects. In case of chills and fever, the aspirate should be cultured.

18.1.8.6 Management

Pelvic lymphoceles after radical or transplant surgery can be treated by single or recurrent percutaneous drainage (Pepper et al. 2005; Zanetta et al. 1993), with or without sclerotherapy (Table 18.1.62), percutaneous catheter drainage (Pepper et al. 2005; Kim et al; 1999), laparoscopic surgery (Pepper et al. 2005; Fallick and Long 1996; Thurlow et al. 1996) or open surgical drainage (Pepper et al. 2005; Gruessner et al. 1995).

Table 18.1.62. Suggested agents for sclerotherapy of lymphoceles

Sclerosant
Tetracycline
Doxycycline (e.g., 500 mg doxycycline hyclate powder reconstituted in 100 ml 0.9% NaCl combined with 5 ml 1% lidocaine for 60 min)
Bleomycin (e.g., 60,000 units of bleomycin in 50 ml 0.9% NaCl for 2–3 h)
Ethanol (e.g., 10–100 ml absolute alcohol for 30 min)
Povidone iodine (e.g., 20 ml 5% povidone iodine for 20 min)
Talcum (e.g., 1 g asbestos-free, sterilized talc in 50–100 ml 0.9% NaCl for 60 min)
Fibrin glue (e.g., 5 ml fibrin sealant (Tissucol, Tisseel, Vivostat)

Simple percutaneous aspiration is simple and safe but has recurrence rates ranging from 50%–80% (Teruel et al. 1983). Closed percutaneous drainage systems can be used for a defined period of time, but they introduce the possibility of infection and also carry a recurrence rate of 40%–50%. Additionally, in case of infection antibiotics should be administered. There may be a role for sclerotherapy in treating lymphoceles, especially in recurrent lymphoceles, before surgery is contemplated.

Techniques such as laparoscopic or open fenestration (Pepper et al. 2005; Gill et al. 1995) and marsupialization with or without omentopexy (Pepper et al. 2005; Perrin et al. 1995; Sibert et al. 1994) may be more effective. Success rates for fenestration have been reported to range between 50% and 70%. After peritoneal marsupialization, success rates reach more than 90% (Pepper et al. 2005; Bailey et al. 2003; Meyers et al. 1977).

The intraoperative application of fibrin glue does not reduce the rate of lymphoceles after lymphadenectomy in patients with pelvic surgery or renal transplantation (Pepper et al. 2005; Scholz et al. 2002). The technique of omentoplasty and omentopexy after pelvic lymphadenectomy (Pepper et al. 2005; Fujiwara et al. 2003) results in a lower incidence of lymphoceles.

References

Aalami OO, Allen DB, Organ CH Jr (2000) Chylous ascites: a collective review. Surgery 128:761

Adam C, Hofstetter A, Deubner J, Zaak D, Weitkunat R, Seitz M, Schneede P (2004) Retropubic transvesical prostatectomy for significant prostatic enlargement must remain a standard part of urology training. Scand J Urol Nephrol 38:472

Adam C, Hofstetter A, Deubner J, Zaak D, Weitkunat R, Seitz M, Schneede P (2004) Retropubic transvesical prostatectomy for significant prostatic enlargement must remain a standard part of urology training. Scand J Urol Nephrol 38:472

Addiss DG, Shaffer N, Fowler BS, Tauxe RV (1990) The epidemiology of appendicitis and appendectomy in the United States. Am J Epidemiol 132:910

Albani JM, Novick AC (2003) Renal artery pseudoaneurysm after partial nephrectomy: three case reports and a literature review. Urology 62:227

Albqami N, Janetschek G (2005) Laparoscopic partial nephrectomy. Curr Opin Urol 15:306

Alkibay T, Karaoglan U, Gundogdu S, Bozkirli I (1992) An unusual complication of extracorporeal shock wave lithotripsy: urinoma due to rupture of the renal pelvis. Int Urol Nephrol 24:11

Allen GA, Hoffman M, Roberts HR, Monroe DM 3rd (2002) Recombinant activated factor VII its mechanism of action and role in the control of hemorrhage. Can J Anaesth 49:S7

Almakdisi T, Massoud S, Makdisi G (2005) Lymphomas and chylous ascites: review of the literature. Oncologist 10:632

Altman PL, Dittmer DS (eds.) (1974) Biology Data Book, vol 3 (2nd ed.) Federation of American Societies for Experimental Biology, Bethesda, M.D.

Amin R (2002) Chylous ascites from prostatic adenocarcinoma. Urology 59:773

Angus DC, Linde-Zwirble WT, Lidicker J, Clermont G, Carcillo J, Pinsky MR (2001) Epidemiology of severe sepsis in the United States: analysis of incidence, outcome, and associated costs of care. Crit Care Med 29:1303

Arai Y, Egawa S, Terachi T, Suzuki K, Gotoh M, Kawakita M, Tanaka M, Terada N, Baba S, Okumura K, Hayami S, Ono Y, Matsuda T, Naito S (2003) Morbidity of laparoscopic radical prostatectomy: summary of early multi-institutional experience in Japan. Int J Urol 10:430

Arozullah AM, Daley J, Henderson WG, Khuri SF (2000) Multifactorial risk index for predicting postoperative respiratory failure in men after major noncardiac surgery. The National Veterans Administration Surgical Quality Improvement Program. Ann Surg 232:242

Baddour LM, Wilson WR, Bayer AS, Fowler VG Jr, Bolger AF, Levison ME, Ferrieri P, Gerber MA, Tani LY, Gewitz MH, Tong DC, Steckelberg JM, Baltimore RS, Shulman ST, Burns JC, Falace DA, Newburger JW, Pallasch TJ, Takahashi M, Taubert KA (2005) Infective endocarditis: diagnosis, antimicrobial therapy, and management of complications: a statement for healthcare professionals from the Committee on Rheumatic Fever Endocarditis, and Kawasaki Disease Council on Cardiovascular Disease in the Young, and the Councils on Clinical Cardiology Stroke, and Cardiovascular Surgery and Anesthesia American Heart Association: endorsed by the Infectious Diseases Society of America. Circulation 111:e394

Bailey SH, Mone MC, Holman JM, Nelson EW (2003) Laparoscopic treatment of post renal transplant lymphoceles. Surg Endosc 17:1896

Bakker AJ, Gorgels JP, van Vlies B, Koelemay MJ, Smits R, Tijssen JG, Haagen FD (1994) Contribution of creatine kinase MB mass concentration at admission to early diagnosis of acute myocardial infarction. Br Heart J 72:112

Bakker AJ, Koelemay MJ, Gorgels JP, van Vlies B, Smits R, Tijssen JG, Haagen FD (1994) Troponin T and myoglobin at admission: value of early diagnosis of acute myocardial infarction. Eur Heart J 15:45

Balthazar EJ, Birnbaum BA, Yee J, Megibow AJ, Roshkow J, Gray C (1994) Acute appendicitis: CT, US correlation in 100 patients. Radiology 190:31

Baniel J, Foster RS, Rowland RG, Bihrle R, Donohue JP (1993) Management of chylous ascites after retroperitoneal lymph node dissection for testicular cancer. J Urol 150:1422

Baniel J, Sella A (1999) Complications of retroperitoneal lymph node dissection in testicular cancer: primary and post-chemotherapy. Semin Surg Oncol 17:263

Barker DE, Kaufman HJ, Smith LA, Ciraulo DL, Richart CL, Burns RP (2000) Vacuum pack technique of temporary abdominal closure: a 7-year experience with 112 patients. J Trauma 48:201; discussion 206

Baskett PJ (1990) ABC of major trauma. Management of hypovolaemic shock. BMJ 300:1453

Basu D, Gallus A, Hirsh J, Cade J (1972) A prospective study of the value of monitoring heparin treatment with the activated partial thromboplastin time. N Engl J Med 287:324

Bates DW, Cook EF, Goldman L, Lee TH (1990) Predicting bacteremia in hospitalized patients. A prospectively validated model. Ann Intern Med 113:495

Bates SM, Ginsberg JS (2004) Clinical practice. Treatment of deep-vein thrombosis. N Engl J Med 351:268

Bates SM, Ginsberg JS (2004) Clinical practice. Treatment of deep-vein thrombosis. N Engl J Med 351:268

Becker F, Siemer S, Humke U, Hack M, Ziegler M, Stockle M (2005) Elective Nephron Sparing Surgery Should Become Standard Treatment for Small Unilateral Renal Cell Carcinoma: Long-term Survival Data of 216 Patients. Eur Urol 49:308

Bell DM, Goldmann DA, Hopkins CC, Karchmer AW, Moellering RC Jr (1978) Unreliability of fever and leukocytosis in the diagnosis of infection after cardiac valve surgery. J Thorac Cardiovasc Surg 75:87

Ben Meir D, Lask D, Koren R (2003) Livne PM Intrarenal foreign body presenting as a solid tumor. Urology 61:1035

Benson MC, Ollson CA (2002) Cutaneous continent urinary diversion. In: Walsh PC et al (eds) Campbell's urology. Elsevier, Philadelphia, pp 3806

Berger RE (2005) Bacteria of preoperative urinary tract infections contaminate the surgical fields and develop surgical site infections in urological operations. J Urol 174:2244

Bertrand ME, Rupprecht HJ, Urban P, Gershlick AH; CLASSICS Investigators (2000) Double-blind study of safety of clopidogrel with and without a loading dose in combination with aspirin compared with ticlopidine in combination with aspirin after coronary stenting: the clopidogrel aspirin stent international cooperative study (CLASSICS). Circulation 102:624

Bhandari A, McIntire L, Kaul SA, Hemal AK, Peabody JO, Menon M (2005) Perioperative complications of robotic radical prostatectomy after the learning curve. J Urol 174:915

Bjornsson TD, Nash PV (1986) Variability in heparin sensitivity of APTT reagents. Am J Clin Pathol 86:199

Bochud PY, Glauser MP, Calandra T (2001) Antibiotics in sepsis. Intensive Care Med 27 [Suppl 1]:S33

Bohnen J, Boulanger M, Meakins JL, McLean AP (1983) Prognosis in generalized peritonitis. Relation to cause and risk factors. Arch Surg 118:285

Bozzetti F, Braga M, Gianotti L, Gavazzi, C Mariani L (2001) Postoperative enteral versus parenteral nutrition in malnourished patients with gastrointestinal cancer: a randomised multicentre trial. Lancet 358:1487

Brandjes DP, Heijboer H, Buller HR, de Rijk M, Jagt H, ten Cate JW (1992) Acenocoumarol and heparin compared with acenocoumarol alone in the initial treatment of proximal-vein thrombosis. N Engl J Med 327:1485

Braunschweig CL, Levy P, Sheean PM, Wang X (2001) Enteral compared with parenteral nutrition: a meta-analysis. Am J Clin Nutr 74:534

Browse NL, Wilson NM, Russo F, al-Hassan H, Allen DR (1992) Aetiology and treatment of chylous ascites. Br J Surg 79:1145

Bruce AW, Reid G, Chan RC Costerton JW (1984) Bacterial adherence in the human ileal conduit: a morphological and bacteriological study. J Urol 132:184

Bufalari A, Giustozzi G, Moggi L (1996) Postoperative intraabdominal abscesses: percutaneous versus surgical treatment. Acta Chir Belg 96:197

Buller HR, Lensing AW, Hirsh J, ten Cate JW (1991) Deep vein thrombosis: new non-invasive diagnostic tests. Thromb Haemost 66:133

Busch T, Lotfi S, Sirbu H, Aleksic I, Dalichau H (2000) Chyloperitoneum. A rare complication after abdominal aortic aneurysm repair. J Cardiovasc Surg 41:617

Calandra T, Cohen J (1984) The international sepsis forum consensus conference on definitions of infection in the intensive care unit. Crit Care Med 33 1538

Casati V, Bellotti F, Gerli C, Franco A, Oppizzi M, Calori G, Alfieri O, Torr G (2001) Tranexamic acid administration after cardiac surgery: a prospective, randomized, double-blind, placebo-controlled study. Anesthesiology 94:8

Caumartin Y, Pouliot F, Sabbagh R, Dujardin T (2005) Chylous ascites as a complication of laparoscopic donor nephrectomy. Transpl Int 18:1378

Celli BR, Rodriguez KS, Snider GL (1984) A controlled trial of intermittent positive pressure breathing, incentive spirometry, and deep breathing exercises in preventing pulmonary complications after abdominal surgery. Am Rev Respir Dis 130:12

Challapalli H, Goldhaber SZ, Brown DF, Nadel ES (2004) Shortness of breath in the postoperative patient. J Emerg Med 27:171

Chan RC, Reid G, Bruce AW, Costerton JW (2005) Microbial colonization of human ileal conduits. Appl Environ Microbiol 48:1159

Chan TC, Vilke GM, Pollack M, Brady WJ (2001) Electrocardiographic manifestations: pulmonary embolism. J Emerg Med 21:263

Chorvat G, Kahn J, Camelot G, Henriet P, Gillet JY, Gillet M (1976) The fate of swabs forgotten in the abdomen (author's transl). Ann Chir 30:643

Collado A, Chechile GE, Salvador J, Vicente J (2000) Early complications of endoscopic treatment for superficial bladder tumors. J Urol 164:1529

Collado A, Chechile GE, Salvador J, Vicente J (2000) Early complications of endoscopic treatment for superficial bladder tumors. J Urol 164:1529

Cook DJ, Kollef MH (1998) Risk factors for ICU-acquired pneumonia. JAMA 279:1605

Cook DJ, Reeve BK, Guyatt GH, Heyland DK, Griffith LE, Buckingham L, Tryba M (1996) Stress ulcer prophylaxis in critically ill patients. Resolving discordant meta-analyses. JAMA 275:308

Corvin S, Kuczyk M, Anastasiadis A, Stenzl A (2004) Laparoscopic retroperitoneal lymph node dissection for nonseminomatous testicular carcinoma. World J Urol 22:33

Craven DE, Steger KA (1995) Epidemiology of nosocomial pneumonia. New perspectives on an old disease. Chest 108:1S–16S

Craven JL, Evans GA, Davenport PJ, Williams RH (1974) The evaluation of the incentive spirometer in the management of postoperative pulmonary complications. Br J Surg 61:793

Cravens DD, Zweig S (2000) Urinary catheter management. Am Fam Physician 61:369

Crnich CJ, Maki DG (2002) The promise of novel technology for the prevention of intravascular device-related bloodstream infection. II Long-term devices. Clin Infect Dis 34: 1362

Crosson JT (1996) Massive transfusion. Clin Lab Med 16:873

Cruse PJ, Foord R (1973) A five-year prospective study of 23,649 surgical wounds. Arch Surg 107:206

Decousus H, Leizorovicz A, Parent F, Page Y, Tardy B, Girard P, Laporte S, Faivre R, Charbonnier B, Barral FG et al (1998) A clinical trial of vena caval filters in the prevention of pulmonary embolism in patients with proximal deep-vein thrombosis. Prevention du Risque d'EMBOlie Pulmonaire par Interruption Cave Study Group. N Engl J Med 338:409

Desai MM, Aron M, Gill IS (2005) Laparoscopic partial nephrectomy versus laparoscopic cryoablation for the small renal tumor. Urology 66:23

Dewdney S, Sokoloff M, Yamada SD (2005) Conservative management of chylous ascites after removal of a symptomatic growing retroperitoneal teratoma. Gynecol Oncol 100:608

Diallo MB, Diallo AT, Sow KB, Guirassy S, Balde S, Balde A(2001) Early complications of transvesical prostatectomy for prostatic adenoma at the Conakry urologic department: report of 96 cases. Ann Urol 35:120

Donzella JG, Merrick GS, Lindert DJ, Andreini HJ, Jr Curtis RL, Luna IH, Allen Z, Butler WM (2004) Epididymitis after transrectal ultrasound-guided needle biopsy of prostate gland. Urology 63:306

Dumarey N, Egrise D, Blocklet D, Stallenberg B, Remmelink M, del Marmol V, Van Simaeys G, Jacobs F, Goldman S (2006) Imaging infection with 18F-FDG-labeled leukocyte PET/CT initial experience in 21 patients. J Nucl Med 47:625

Edwards JE Jr, Bodey GP, Bowden RA, Buchner T, de Pauw BE, Filler SG, Ghannoum MA, Glauser M, Herbrecht R, Kauffman CA, Kohno S, Martino P, Meunier F, Mori T, Pfaller MA, Rex JH, Rogers TR, Rubin RH, Solomkin J, Viscoli C, Walsh TJ, White M (1997) International Conference for the Development of a Consensus on the Management and Prevention of Severe Candidal Infections. Clin Infect Dis 25:43

El-Haddad G, Zhuang H, Gupta N, Alavi A (2004) Evolving role of positron emission tomography in the management of patients with inflammatory and other benign disorders. Semin Nucl Med 34:313

Erber WN (2002) Massive blood transfusion in the elective surgical setting. Transfus Apher Sci 27:83

Eriksen MT, Wibe A, Norstein J, Haffner J, Wiig JN (2005) Anastomotic leakage following routine mesorectal excision for rectal cancer in a national cohort of patients. Colorectal Dis 7:51

Fabian TC (2002) Infection in penetrating abdominal trauma: risk factors and preventive antibiotics. Am Surg 68:29

Falagas ME, Vergidis PI (2005) Urinary tract infections in patients with urinary diversion. Am J Kidney Dis 46:1030

Fallick ML, Long JP (1996) Laparoscopic marsupialization of lymphocele after laparoscopic lymph node dissection. J Endourol 10:533

Fatkenheuer G, Buchheidt D, Cornely OA, Fuhr HG, Karthaus M, Kisro J, Leithauser M, Salwender H, Sudhoff T, Szelenyi H, Weissinger F (2003) Central venous catheter (CVC)-related infections in neutropenic patients–guidelines of the Infectious Diseases Working Party (AGIHO) of the German Society of Hematology and Oncology (DGHO) Ann Hematol 82 [Suppl 2]:S149

Feigin E, Carmon M, Szold A, Seror D (1993) Acute stump appendicitis. Lancet 341:757

Feldman NT, Huber GL (1976) Fiberoptic bronchoscopy in the intensive care unit. Int Anesthesiol Clin 14:31

Fennerty MB (2002) Pathophysiology of the upper gastrointestinal tract in the critically ill patient: rationale for the therapeutic benefits of acid suppression. Crit Care Med 30:S351

Ferrara A, MacArthur JD, Wright HK, Modlin IM, McMillen MA (1990) Hypothermia and acidosis worsen coagulopathy in the patient requiring massive transfusion. Am J Surg 160:515

Ferrer J, Roldan J (2000) Clinical management of the patient with pleural effusion. Eur J Radiol 34:76

Fisher BW, Majumdar SR, McAlister FA (2002) Predicting pulmonary complications after nonthoracic surgery: a systematic review of blinded studies. Am J Med 112:219

Fisher RG, Ben-Menachem Y, Whigham C (1989) Stab wounds of the renal artery branches: angiographic diagnosis and treatment by embolization. AJR Am J Roentgenol 152:1231

Földi M, Földi E, Kubik S (2005) Lehrbuch der Lymphologie. Anatomie des Lymphgefäßsystems. Urban Fischer Elsevier, München

Fowler AA 3rd, Scoggins WG, O'Donohue WJ Jr (1978) Positive end-expiratory pressure in the management of lobar atelectasis. Chest 74:497

Fraenkel DJ, Rickard C, Lipman J (2000) Can we achieve consensus on central venous catheter-related infections? Anaesth Intensive Care 28:475

Frank SM, Kluger MJ, Kunkel SL (2000) Elevated thermostatic setpoint in postoperative patients. Anesthesiology 93:1426

Frazier HA, Robertson JE, Paulson DF (1992) Complications of radical cystectomy and urinary diversion: a retrospective review of 675 cases in 2 decades. J Urol 148:1401

Frazier HA, Robertson JE, Paulson DF (1992) Complications of radical cystectomy and urinary diversion: a retrospective review of 675 cases in 2 decades. J Urol 148:1401

Friederich PW, Henny CP, Messelink EJ, Geerdink MG, Keller T, Kurth KH, Buller HR, Levi M (2003) Effect of recombinant activated factor VII on perioperative blood loss in patients undergoing retropubic prostatectomy: a double-blind placebo-controlled randomised trial. Lancet 361:201

Fujiwara K, Kigawa J, Hasegawa K, Nishimura R, Umezaki N, Ando M, Itamochi H, Yamaguchi S, Oda T, Terakawa N, Kohshima I, Kohno I (2003) Effect of simple omentoplasty and omentopexy in the prevention of complications after pelvic lymphadenectomy. Int J Gynecol Cancer 13:61

Gallus A, Jackaman J, Tillett J, Mills W, Wycherley A (1986) Safety and efficacy of warfarin started early after submassive venous thrombosis or pulmonary embolism. Lancet 2:1293

Galvin DJ, Mulvin D, Quinlan DM (2004) Thromboprophylaxis for radical prostatectomy: a comparative analysis of present practice between the USA, the UK, and Ireland. Prostate 60:338

Gan TJ, Meyer T, Apfel CC, Chung F, Davis PJ, Eubanks S, Kovac A, Philip BK, Sessler DI, Temo J, Tramer MR, Watcha M (2003) Consensus guidelines for managing postoperative nausea and vomiting. Anesth Analg 97:62

Garibaldi RA, Mooney BR, Epstein BJ, Britt MR (1982) An evaluation of daily bacteriologic monitoring to identify preventable episodes of catheter-associated urinary tract infection. Infect Control 3:466

Gburek BM, Lieber MM, Blute ML (1998) Comparison of studer ileal neobladder and ileal conduit urinary diversion with respect to perioperative outcome and late complications. J Urol 160:721

Geh JL, Curley P, Mayfield MP, Price JJ (1997) Small bowel perforation after extracorporeal shock wave lithotripsy. Br J Urol 79:648

Gerhardt W, Katus HA, Ravkilde J, Hamm CW (1992) S-troponin-T as a marker of ischemic myocardial injury. Clin Chem 38:1194

Giannitsis E, Katus HA (2002) Acute posterior myocardial infarct. A typical diagnostic error. Internist (Berl) 43:618

Gill IS, Hodge EE, Munch LC, Goldfarb DA, Novick AC, Lucas BA (1995) Transperitoneal marsupialization of lymphoceles: a comparison of laparoscopic and open techniques. J Urol 153:706

Gilmartin JJ, Wright AJ, Gibson GJ (1985) Effects of pneumothorax or pleural effusion on pulmonary function. Thorax 40:60

Giovannini I, Giuliante F, Chiarla C, Ardito F, Vellone M, Nuzzo G (2005) Non-surgical management of a lymphatic fistula, after laparoscopic colorectal surgery, with total parenteral nutrition, octreotide, and somatostatin. Nutrition 21:1065

Godden J, Hiley C (1998) Managing the patient with a chest drain: a review. Nurs Stand 12:35

Goldberg PK, Kozinn PJ, Wise GJ, Nouri N (1979) Brooks RB Incidence and significance of candiduria. JAMA 241:582

Goldhaber SZ (2002) Echocardiography in the management of pulmonary embolism. Ann Intern Med 136:691

Goodman JS, Schaffner W, Collins HA, Battersby EJ, Koenig MG (1968) Infection after cardiovascular surgery. Clinical study including examination of antimicrobial prophylaxis. N Engl J Med 278:117

Gould MK, Dembitzer AD, Doyle RL, Hastie TJ, Garber AM (1999) Low-molecular-weight heparins compared with unfractionated heparin for treatment of acute deep venous thrombosis. A meta-analysis of randomized, controlled trials. Ann Intern Med 130:800

Gruessner RW, Fasola C, Benedetti E, Foshager MC, Gruessner AC, Matas AJ, Najarian JS, Goodale RL (1995) Laparoscopic drainage of lymphoceles after kidney transplantation: indications and limitations. Surgery 117:288

Guillonneau B, Bermudez H, Gholami S, El Fettouh H, Gupta R, Adorno Rosa J, Baumert H, Cathelineau X, Fromont G, Vallancien G (2003) Laparoscopic partial nephrectomy for renal tumor: single center experience comparing clamping and no clamping techniques of the renal vasculature. J Urol 169:483

Gupta N, Kumar R, Dogra PN, Seth A (2006) Comparison of standard transurethral resection, transurethral vapour resection and holmium laser enucleation of the prostate for managing benign prostatic hyperplasia of >40 g. BJU Int 97:85
Gupta NP, Nabi G, Hemal AK, Dogra PN, Seth A, Aron M (2002) Is incidental appendectomy necessary during radical cystectomy? Urol Int 69:181
Hackam DJ, Rotstein OD (1995a) Stoma closure and wound infection: an evaluation of risk factors. Can J Surg 38:144
Hackam DJ, Rotstein OD (1995b) Wound infection during stoma closure. Can J Surg 38:191
Hamasuna R, Betsunoh H, Sueyoshi T, Yakushiji K, Tsukino H, Nagano M, Takehara T, Osada Y (2004) Bacteria of preoperative urinary tract infections contaminate the surgical fields and develop surgical site infections in urological operations. Int J Urol 11:941
Hamm CW (2004) Guidelines: Acute coronary syndrome (ACS) II Acute coronary syndrome with ST-elevation. Z Kardiol 93:324
Hammarskjold F, Wallen G, Malmvall BE (2006) Central venous catheter infections at a county hospital in Sweden: a prospective analysis of colonization, incidence of infection and risk factors. Acta Anaesthesiol Scand 50:451
Harbarth S, Ruef C, Francioli P, Widmer A, Pittet D (1999) Nosocomial infections in Swiss university hospitals: a multicentre survey and review of the published experience. Swiss-Noso Network. Schweiz Med Wochenschr 129:1521
Hardy JF, De Moerloose P, Samama M (2004) Massive transfusion and coagulopathy: pathophysiology and implications for clinical management. Can J Anaesth 51:293
Hau T, Ahrenholz DH, Simmons RL (1979) Secondary bacterial peritonitis: the biologic basis of treatment. Curr Probl Surg 16:1
Hayes RJ (1977) Incidental appendectomies. Current teaching. JAMA 238:31
Hedican SP, Walsh PC (1994) Postoperative bleeding following radical retropubic prostatectomy. J Urol 152:1181
Heidenreich A, Ohlmann C, Hegele A, Beyer J (2005) Repeat retroperitoneal lymphadenectomy in advanced testicular cancer. Eur Urol 47:64
Heye S, Maleux G, Van Poppel H, Oyen R, Wilms G (2005) Hemorrhagic complications after nephron-sparing surgery: angiographic diagnosis and management by transcatheter embolization. AJR Am J Roentgenol 184:1661
Heymans S, Verhaeghe R, Stockx L, Collen D (1998) Feasibility study of catheter-directed thrombolysis with recombinant staphylokinase in deep venous thrombosis. Thromb Haemost 79:517
Hiippala S (1998) Replacement of massive blood loss. Vox Sang 74 [Suppl 2]:399
Hiippala ST, Myllyla GJ, Vahtera EM (1995) Hemostatic factors and replacement of major blood loss with plasma-poor red cell concentrates. Anesth Analg 81:360
Hirsh J (1995) The optimal duration of anticoagulant therapy for venous thrombosis. N Engl J Med 332:1710
Hirsh J, Hoak J (1996) Management of deep vein thrombosis and pulmonary embolism. A statement for healthcare professionals. Council on Thrombosis (in consultation with the Council on Cardiovascular Radiology) American Heart Association. Circulation 93:2212
Hirsh J, Warkentin TE, Shaughnessy SG, Anand SS, Halperin JL, Raschke R, Granger C, Ohman EM, Dalen JE (2001) Heparin and low-molecular-weight heparin: mechanisms of action, pharmacokinetics, dosing, monitoring, efficacy, and safety. Chest 119:S64
Ho WK, Hankey GJ, Lee CH, Eikelboom JW (2005) Venous thromboembolism: diagnosis and management of deep venous thrombosis. Med J Aust 182:476
Ho WK, Hankey GJ, Lee CH, Eikelboom JW (2005) Venous thromboembolism: diagnosis and management of deep venous thrombosis. Med J Aust 182:476
Hoffelt SC, Wallner K, Merrick G (2004) Epididymitis after prostate brachytherapy. Urology 63:293
Hollenbeck BK, Miller DC, Taub D, Dunn RL, Khuri SF, Henderson WG, Montie JE, Underwood W 3rd, Wei JT (2005) Identifying risk factors for potentially avoidable complications following radical cystectomy. J Urol 174:1231; discussion 1237
Holmberg G, Spinnell S, Sjodin JG (1997) Perforation of the bowel during SWL in prone position. J Endourol 11:313
Huang Q, Jiang ZW, Jiang J, Li N, Li JS (2004) Chylous ascites: treated with total parenteral nutrition and somatostatin. World J Gastroenterol 10:2588
Hudspeth AS (1975) Radical surgical debridement in the treatment of advanced generalized bacterial peritonitis. Arch Surg 110:1233
Hull RD, Raskob GE, Carter CJ (1990a) Serial impedance plethysmography in pregnant patients with clinically suspected deep-vein thrombosis. Clinical validity of negative findings. Ann Intern Med 112:663
Hull RD, Raskob GE, LeClerc JR, Jay RM, Hirsh J (1984) The diagnosis of clinically suspected venous thrombosis. Clin Chest Med 5:439
Hull RD, Raskob GE, Pineo GF, Green D, Trowbridge AA, Elliott CG, Lerner RG, Hall J, Sparling T, Brettell HR et al (1992) Subcutaneous low-molecular-weight heparin compared with continuous intravenous heparin in the treatment of proximal-vein thrombosis. N Engl J Med 326:975
Hull RD, Raskob GE, Rosenbloom D, Panju AA, Brill-Edwards P, Ginsberg JS, Hirsh J, Martin GJ, Green D (1990b) Heparin for 5 days as compared with 10 days in the initial treatment of proximal venous thrombosis. N Engl J Med 322:1260
Hyers TM, Agnelli G, Hull RD, Morris TA, Samama M, Tapson V, Weg JG (2001) Antithrombotic therapy for venous thromboembolic disease. Chest 119:176S–193S
Iregui M, Ward S, Sherman G, Fraser VJ, Kollef MH (2002) Clinical importance of delays in the initiation of appropriate antibiotic treatment for ventilator-associated pneumonia. Chest 122:262
Jacobellis U (2003) Modified radical inguinal lymphadenectomy for carcinoma of the penis: technique and results. J Urol 169:1349
Janata K (2003) Managing pulmonary embolism. BMJ 326:1341
Janetschek G, Hobisch A, Hittmair A, Holtl L, Peschel R, Bartsch G (1999) Laparoscopic retroperitoneal lymphadenectomy after chemotherapy for stage IIB nonseminomatous testicular carcinoma. J Urol 161:477
Jeejeebhoy KN (2004) Enteral feeding. Curr Opin Gastroenterol 20:110
Jepsen S, Klaerke A, Nielsen PH, Nielsen ST, Simonsen O (1989) Systemic administration of N-acetylcysteine has no effect on postoperative lung function following elective upper laparotomy in lung healthy patients. Acta Anaesthesiol Scand 33:219
Jepsen S, Nielsen PH, Klaerke A, Nielsen ST, Simonsen O (1989) Peroral N-acetylcysteine as prophylaxis against bronchopulmonary complications of pulmonary surgery. Scand J Thorac Cardiovasc Surg 23:185
Jimenez MF, Marshall JC (2001) Source control in the management of sepsis. Intensive Care Med 27 [Suppl 1]:S49
Jonathan P, Wyatt RI, Clancy M, Munro PT, Robertson C (2005) Oxford handbook of accident and emergency medicine. Oxford University Press, Oxford
Joniau S, Benijts J, Van Kampen M, De Waele M, Ooms J, Van Cleynenbreugel B, Van Poppel H (2005) Clinical experience with the N-shaped ileal neobladder: assessment of compli-

cations, voiding patterns, and quality of life in our series of 58 patients. Eur Urol 47:666; discussion 672

Kaartinen M, Imir T, Klockars M, Sandholm M, Makela O (1978) IgA in blood and thoracic duct lymph: concentration and degree of polymerization. Scand J Immunol 7:229

Kakkar VV, Boeckl O, Boneu B, Bordenave L, Brehm OA, Brukke P, Coccheri S, Cohen AT, Galland F, Haas S et al (1997) Efficacy and safety of a low-molecular-weight heparin and standard unfractionated heparin for prophylaxis of postoperative venous thromboembolism: European multicenter trial. World J Surg 21:2; discussion 8

Kakkar VV, Cohen AT, Edmonson RA, Phillips MJ, Cooper DJ, Das SK, Maher KT, Sanderson RM, Ward VP, Kakkar S (1993) Low molecular weight versus standard heparin for prevention of venous thromboembolism after major abdominal surgery. The Thromboprophylaxis Collaborative Group. Lancet 341:259

Katus HA, Remppis A, Neumann FJ, Scheffold T, Diederich KW, Vinar G, Noe A, Matern G, Kuebler W (1991) Diagnostic efficiency of troponin T measurements in acute myocardial infarction. Circulation 83:902

Kaufman JD, Lepor H (2005) Reoperation versus observation in men with major bleeding after radical retropubic prostatectomy. Urology 66:561

Kearon C (2001) Epidemiology of venous thromboembolism. Semin Vasc Med 1:7

Kearon C, Julian JA, Newman TE, Ginsberg JS (1998) Noninvasive diagnosis of deep venous thrombosis. McMaster Diagnostic Imaging Practice Guidelines Initiative. Ann Intern Med 128:663

Kim JK, Jeong YY, Kim YH, Kim YC, Kang HK, Choi HS (1999) Postoperative pelvic lymphocele: treatment with simple percutaneous catheter drainage. Radiology 212:390

Klug R, Kurz F, Dunzinger M, Aufschnaiter M (2001) Small bowel perforation after extracorporeal shockwave lithotripsy of an ureter stone. Dig Surg 18:241

Knap MM, Lundbeck F, Overgaard J (2004) Early and late treatment-related morbidity following radical cystectomy. Scand J Urol Nephrol 38:153

Knight CD, Griffen FD (1983) Abdominal wound closure with a continuous monofilament polypropylene suture. Experience with 1,000 consecutive cases. Arch Surg 118:1305

Knockaert DC, Mortelmans LA, De Roo, MC Bobbaers HJ (1994) Clinical value of gallium-67 scintigraphy in evaluation of fever of unknown origin. Clin Infect Dis 18:601

Koch MO, Jr JS (1997) Low molecular weight heparin and radical prostatectomy: a prospective analysis of safety and side effects. Prostate Cancer Prostatic Dis 1:101

Koch MO, Smith JA Jr (1996) Blood loss during radical retropubic prostatectomy: is preoperative autologous blood donation indicated? J Urol 156:1077; discussion 1079

Kokubo T, Itai Y, Ohtomo K, Yoshikawa K, Iio M, Atomi Y (1987) Retained surgical sponges: CT, US appearance. Radiology 165:415

Kollef MH (2004) Appropriate empiric antimicrobial therapy of nosocomial pneumonia: the role of the carbapenems. Respir Care 49:1530

Kondas J, Szentgyorgyi E (1992) Transurethral resection of 1250 bladder tumours. Int Urol Nephrol 24:35

Koopman MM, Prandoni P, Piovella F, Ockelford PA, Brandjes DP, van der Meer J, Gallus AS, Simonneau G, Chesterman CH, Prins MH (1996) Treatment of venous thrombosis with intravenous unfractionated heparin administered in the hospital as compared with subcutaneous low-molecular-weight heparin administered at home. The Tasman Study Group. N Engl J Med 334:682

Koya MP, Manoharan M, Kim SS, Soloway MS (2005) Venous thromboembolism in radical prostatectomy: is heparinoid prophylaxis warranted? BJU Int 96:1019

Krieger JN, Kaiser DL Wenzel RP (1983) Nosocomial urinary tract infections cause wound infections postoperatively in surgical patients. Surg Gynecol Obstet 156:313

Kurtz V, Muller-Sorg M, Federmann G (1999) Perforation of the small intestine after nephro-uretero-lithotripsy by ESWL–a rare complication. Chirurg 70:306

Kurz K, Katus HA, Giannitsis E (2005) Acute chest pain.. Internist (Berl) 46:957

Laupacis A, Fergusson D (1997) Drugs to minimize perioperative blood loss in cardiac surgery: meta-analysis using perioperative blood transfusion as the outcome. The International Study of Peri-operative Transfusion (ISPOT) Investigators. Anesth Analg 85:1258

Lauwers PR, Van Hee RH (2000) Intraperitoneal gossypibomas: the need to count sponges. World J Surg 24:521

Le DT, Borgs P, Toneff TW, Witte MH (1998) Rapaport SI hemostatic factors in rabbit limb lymph: relationship to mechanisms regulating extravascular coagulation. Am J Physiol 274:H769

Le Neel JC, De Cussac JB, Dupas B, Letessier E, Borde L, Eloufir M, Armstrong O (1994) Textiloma. Apropos of 25 cases and review of the literature. Chirurgie 120:272; discussion 276

Lee TH, Rouan GW, Weisberg MC, Brand DA, Cook EF, Acampora D, Goldman L (1987) Sensitivity of routine clinical criteria for diagnosing myocardial infarction within 24 hours of hospitalization. Ann Intern Med 106:181

Leibovitch I (2002) Postoperative chylous ascites–the urologist's view. Drugs Today (Barc) 38:687

Leibovitch I, Mor Y, Golomb J, Ramon J (2002)Chylous ascites after radical nephrectomy and inferior vena cava thrombectomy. Successful conservative management with somatostatin analogue. Eur Urol 41:220

Lensing AW, Buller HR, Prandoni P, Batchelor D, Molenaar AH, Cogo A, Vigo M, Huisman PM, ten Cate JW (1992) Contrast venography, the gold standard for the diagnosis of deep-vein thrombosis: improvement in observer agreement. Thromb Haemost 67:8

Leone M, Albanese J, Antonini F, Michel-Nguyen A, Blanc-Bimar MC, Martin C (2003a) Long-term epidemiological survey of Candida species: comparison of isolates found in an intensive care unit and in conventional wards. J Hosp Infect 55:169

Leone M, Albanese J, Garnier F, Sapin C, Barrau K, Bimar MC, Martin C (2003b) Risk factors of nosocomial catheter-associated urinary tract infection in a polyvalent intensive care unit. Intensive Care Med 29:929

Leone M, Garnier F, Avidan M, Martin C (2004) Catheter-associated urinary tract infections in intensive care units. Microbes Infect 6:1026

Levine CD, Gonzales RN, Wachsberg RH, Ghanekar D (1997) CT findings of bowel and mesenteric injury. J Comput Assist Tomogr 21:974

Levine M, Gent M, Hirsh J, Leclerc J, Anderson D, Weitz J, Ginsberg J, Turpie AG, Demers C, Kovacs M (1996) A comparison of low-molecular-weight heparin administered primarily at home with unfractionated heparin administered in the hospital for proximal deep-vein thrombosis. N Engl J Med 334:677

Levine MN, Gent M, Hirsh J, Arnold A, Goodyear MD, Hryniuk W, De Pauw S (1988) The thrombogenic effect of anticancer drug therapy in women with stage II breast cancer. N Engl J Med 318:404

Levy MJ, Seelig CB, Robinson NJ, Ranney JE (1997) Comparison of omeprazole and ranitidine for stress ulcer prophylaxis. Dig Dis Sci 42:1255

Li JS, Sexton DJ, Mick N, Nettles R, Fowler VG Jr, Ryan T, Bashore T, Corey GR (2000) Proposed modifications to the Duke criteria for the diagnosis of infective endocarditis. Clin Infect Dis 30:633

Liang MK, Lo HG, Marks JL (2006) Stump appendicitis: a comprehensive review of literature. Am Surg 72:162
Light RW, George RB (1976) Incidence and significance of pleural effusion after abdominal surgery. Chest 69:621
Lim KB, Wong MY, Foo KT (2004) Transurethral resection of prostate (TURP) through the decades–a comparison of results over the last thirty years in a single institution in Asia. Ann Acad Med Singapore 33:775
Little JR, Murray PR, Traynor PS, Spitznagel E (1999) A randomized trial of povidone-iodine compared with iodine tincture for venipuncture site disinfection: effects on rates of blood culture contamination. Am J Med 107:119
Lone GN, Bhat AH, Tak MY, Garcoo SA (2005) Transdiaphragmatic migration of forgotten gauze sponge: an unreported entity of lung abscess. Eur J Cardiothorac Surg 28:355
Luna CM, Vujacich P, Niederman MS, Vay C, Gherardi C, Matera J, Jolly EC (1997) Impact of BAL data on the therapy and outcome of ventilator-associated pneumonia. Chest 111:676
Lundin C, Bersztel A, Wahlberg J, Wadstrom J (2002) Low molecular weight heparin prophylaxis increases the incidence of lymphocele after kidney transplantation. Ups J Med Sci 107:9
Madersbacher S, Schmidt J, Eberle JM, Thoeny HC, Burkhard F, Hochreiter W, Studer UE (2003) Long-term outcome of ileal conduit diversion. J Urol 169:985
Madersbacher S, Schmidt J, Eberle JM, Thoeny HC, Burkhard F, Hochreiter W, Studer UE (2003) Long-term outcome of ileal conduit diversion. J Urol 169:985
Madl C, Druml W (2003) Gastrointestinal disorders of the critically ill. Systemic consequences of ileus. Best Pract Res Clin Gastroenterol 17:445
Mair J, Artner-Dworzak E, Dienstl A, Lechleitner P, Morass B, Smidt J, Wagner I, Wettach C, Puschendorf B (1991) Early detection of acute myocardial infarction by measurement of mass concentration of creatine kinase-MB. Am J Cardiol 68:1545
Malangoni MA (2005) Contributions to the management of intraabdominal infections. Am J Surg 190:255
Maleux G, Messiaen T, Stockx L, Vanrenterghem Y, Wilms G (2003) Transcatheter embolization of biopsy-related vascular injuries in renal allografts. Long-term technical, clinical and biochemical results. Acta Radiol 44:13
Mallow S, Rebuck JA, Osler T, Ahern J, Healey MA, Rogers FB (2004) Do proton pump inhibitors increase the incidence of nosocomial pneumonia and related infectious complications when compared with histamine-2 receptor antagonists in critically ill trauma patients? Curr Surg 61:452
Marik PE (2000) Fever in the ICU. Chest 117:855
Marini JJ, Pierson DJ, Hudson LD (1979) Acute lobar atelectasis: a prospective comparison of fiberoptic bronchoscopy and respiratory therapy. Am Rev Respir Dis 119:971
Marr KA, Sexton DJ, Conlon PJ, Corey GR, Schwab SJ, Kirkland KB (1997) Catheter-related bacteremia and outcome of attempted catheter salvage in patients undergoing hemodialysis. Ann Intern Med 127:275
Marshall JC (2004) Intra-abdominal infections. Microbes Infect 6:1015
Marshall JC, Maier RV, Jimenez M, Dellinger EP (2004) Source control in the management of severe sepsis and septic shock: an evidence-based review. Crit Care Med 32:S513
Matthiessen P, Hallbook O, Andersson M, Rutegard J, Sjodahl R (2004) Risk factors for anastomotic leakage after anterior resection of the rectum. Colorectal Dis 6:462
Mazuski JE, Sawyer RG, Nathens AB, DiPiro JT, Schein M, Kudsk KA, Yowler C (2002) The Surgical Infection Society guidelines on antimicrobial therapy for intra-abdominal infections: evidence for the recommendations. Surg Infect (Larchmt) 3:175
McCullough CS, Soper NJ, Clayman RV, So SS, Jendrisak MD, Hanto DW (1991) Laparoscopic drainage of a posttransplant lymphocele. Transplantation 51:725
McGahan JP (1985) Aspiration and drainage procedures in the intensive care unit: percutaneous sonographic guidance. Radiology 154:531
McGee DC, Gould MK (2003) Preventing complications of central venous catheterization. N Engl J Med 348:1123
McLoud TC, Flower CD (1991) Imaging the pleura: sonography CT, and MR imaging. AJR Am J Roentgenol 156:1145
Meller AE, Nesrallah LJ, Dall'Oglio MF, Srougi M (2002) Complications in radical cystectomy performed at a teaching hospital. Int Braz J Urol 28:522
Meller J, Altenvoerde G, Munzel U, Jauho A, Behe M, Gratz S, Luig H, Becker W (2000) Fever of unknown origin: prospective comparison of 18FFDG imaging with a double-head coincidence camera and gallium-67 citrate SPET. Eur J Nucl Med 27:1617
Mermel LA, Maki DG (1993) Detection of bacteremia in adults: consequences of culturing an inadequate volume of blood. Ann Intern Med 119:270
Messori A, Trippoli S, Vaiani M, Gorini M, Corrado A (2000) Bleeding and pneumonia in intensive care patients given ranitidine and sucralfate for prevention of stress ulcer: meta-analysis of randomised controlled trials. BMJ 321:1103
Meyers AM, Levine E, Myburgh JA, Goudie E (1977) Diagnosis and management of lymphoceles after renal transplantation. Urology 10:497
Miller KS, Sahn SA (1987) Chest tubes. Indications, technique, management and complications. Chest 91:258
Mills J, Utley J, Abbott J (1974) Heart failure in infective endocarditis: predisposing factors, course, and treatment. Chest 66:151
Monreal M, Lafoz E, Olive A, del Rio L, Vedia C (1994) Comparison of subcutaneous unfractionated heparin with a low molecular weight heparin (Fragmin) in patients with venous thromboembolism and contraindications to coumarin. Thromb Haemost 71:7
Monreal M, Montserrat E, Salvador R, Bechini J, Donoso L, MaCallejas J, Foz M (1989) Real-time ultrasound for diagnosis of symptomatic venous thrombosis and for screening of patients at risk: correlation with ascending conventional venography. Angiology 40:527
Montorsi F, Naspro R, Salonia A, Suardi N, Briganti A, Zanoni M, Valenti S, Vavassori I, Rigatti P (2004) Holmium laser enucleation versus transurethral resection of the prostate: results from a 2-center, prospective, randomized trial in patients with obstructive benign prostatic hyperplasia. J Urol 172:1926
Mossner J (2005) Acute abdomen. Internist (Berl) 46:974
Murkin JM (1994) Con: tranexamic acid is not better than aprotinin in decreasing bleeding after cardiac surgery. J Cardiothorac Vasc Anesth 8:474
Murphy MF, Wallington TB, Kelsey P, Boulton F, Bruce M, Cohen H, Duguid J, Knowles SM, Poole G, Williamson LM (2001) Guidelines for the clinical use of red cell transfusions. Br J Haematol 113:24
Muzzonigro G, Milanese G, Minardi D, Yehia M, Galosi AB, Dellabella M (2004) Safety and efficacy of transurethral resection of prostate glands up to 150 ml: a prospective comparative study with 1 year of followup. J Urol 172:611
Naber KG, Bergman B, Bishop MC, Bjerklund-Johansen TE, Botto H, Lobel B, Jinenez Cruz F, Selvaggi FP (2001) EAU guidelines for the management of urinary and male genital tract infections. Urinary Tract Infection (UTI) Working Group of the Health Care Office (HCO) of the European Association of Urology (EAU) Eur Urol 40:576
Nakada I, Kawasaki S, Sonoda Y, Watanabe Y, Tabuchi T (2004)

Abdominal stapled side-to-end anastomosis (Baker type) in low and high anterior resection: experiences and results in 69 consecutive patients at a regional general hospital in Japan. Colorectal Dis 6:165
Nasir GA, Baker KK (2001) Continuous double loop closure for midline laparotomy wounds. Saudi Med J 22:351
N'Dow J, Pearson, J Neal D (2004) Mucus production after transposition of intestinal segments into the urinary tract. World J Urol 22 178
Nelson BA, Cookson MS, Smith JA Jr, Chang SS (2004) Complications of inguinal and pelvic lymphadenectomy for squamous cell carcinoma of the penis: a contemporary series. J Urol 172:494
Neulander EZ, Hawke CK, Soloway MS (2000) Incidental appendectomy during radical cystectomy: an interdepartmental survey and review of the literature. Urology 56:241
Nicolaides AN, Kakkar VV, Field ES, Renney JT (1971) The origin of deep vein thrombosis: a venographic study. Br J Radiol 44:653
Nieder AM, Meinbach DS, Kim SS, Soloway MS (2005) Transurethral bladder tumor resection: intraoperative and postoperative complications in a residency setting. J Urol 174:2307
Nieder AM, Meinbach DS, Kim SS, Soloway MS (2005) Transurethral bladder tumor resection: intraoperative and postoperative complications in a residency setting. J Urol 174:2307
Niel-Weise BS, Wille JC, van den Broek PJ (2005) Hair removal policies in clean surgery: systematic review of randomized, controlled trials. Infect Control Hosp Epidemiol 26:923
Nordstrom M, Lindblad B, Bergqvist D, Kjellstrom T (1992) A prospective study of the incidence of deep-vein thrombosis within a defined urban population. J Intern Med 232:155
Nurmohamed MT, Verhaeghe R, Haas S, Iriarte JA, Vogel G, van Rij AM, Prentice CR, ten Cate JW (1995) A comparative trial of a low molecular weight heparin (enoxaparin) versus standard heparin for the prophylaxis of postoperative deep vein thrombosis in general surgery. Am J Surg 169:567
O'Connor AR, Coakley FV, Meng MV, Eberhardt SC (2003) Imaging of retained surgical sponges in the abdomen and pelvis. AJR Am J Roentgenol 180:481
Oger E (2000) Incidence of venous thromboembolism: a community-based study in Western France. EPI-GETBP Study Group. Groupe d'Etude de la Thrombose de Bretagne Occidentale. Thromb Haemost 83:657
O'Grady NP, Alexander M, Dellinger EP, Gerberding JL, Heard SO, Maki DG, Masur H, McCormick RD, Mermel LA, Pearson ML, Raad II, Randolph A, Weinstein RA (2002) Guidelines for the prevention of intravascular catheter-related infections. Am J Infect Control 30:476
O'Grady NP, Barie PS, Bartlett J, Bleck T, Garvey G, Jacobi J, Linden P, Maki DG, Nam M, Pasculle W, Pasquale MD, Tribett DL, Masur H (1998a) Practice parameters for evaluating new fever in critically ill adult patients. Task Force of the American College of Critical Care Medicine of the Society of Critical Care Medicine in collaboration with the Infectious Disease Society of America. Crit Care Med 26:392
O'Grady NP, Barie PS, Bartlett JG, Bleck T, Garvey G, Jacobi J, Linden P, Maki DG, Nam M, Pasculle W, Pasquale MD, Tribett DL, Masur H (1998b) Practice guidelines for evaluating new fever in critically ill adult patients. Task Force of the Society of Critical Care Medicine and the Infectious Diseases Society of America. Clin Infect Dis 26:1042
Ohman EM, Casey C, Bengtson JR, Pryor D, Tormey W, Horgan JH (1990) Early detection of acute myocardial infarction: additional diagnostic information from serum concentrations of myoglobin in patients without ST elevation. Br Heart J 63:335
Olszewski WL (1991) Lymph stasis: pathophysiology diagnosis and treatment. In: Olszewski WL (ed) Lymphology and the lymphatic system. CRC Press, Boca Raton, p 1
Olszewski WL (1991) Lymph stasis: pathophysiology diagnosis and treatment. In: Olszewski WL (ed) Lymphology and the lymphatic system. CRC Press, Boca Raton, p 3
Olszewski WL (2005) The innate reaction of the human skin lymphatic system to foreign and self-antigens. Lymphat Res Biol 3:50
Olszewski WL, Loe K, Engeset A (1978) Immune proteins and other biochemical constituents of peripheral lymph in patients with malignancy and postirradiation lymphedema. Lymphology 11:174
O'Moore PV, Mueller PR, Simeone JF, Saini S, Butch RJ, Hahn PF, Steiner E, Stark DD, Ferrucci JT Jr (1987) Sonographic guidance in diagnostic and therapeutic interventions in the pleural space. AJR Am J Roentgenol 149:1
Pantanowitz L, Kruskall MS, Uhl L (2003) Cryoprecipitate. Patterns of use. Am J Clin Pathol 119:874
Paragioudaki M, Stamouli V, Kolonitsiou F, Anastassiou ED, Dimitracopoulos G, Spiliopoulou I (2004) Intravenous catheter infections associated with bacteraemia: a 2-year study in a university hospital. Clin Microbiol Infect 10:431
Pepper RJ, Pati J, Kaisary AV (2005) The incidence and treatment of lymphoceles after radical retropubic prostatectomy. BJU Int 95:772
Pepper RJ, Pati J, Kaisary AV (2005) The incidence and treatment of lymphoceles after radical retropubic prostatectomy. BJU Int 95:772
Perrin LC, Goh J, Crandon AJ (1995) The treatment of recurrent pelvic lymphocysts with marsupialization and functioning omental flap. Aust N Z J Obstet Gynaecol 35:195
Peters AM (1998) The use of nuclear medicine in infections. Br J Radiol 71:252
Pettila V, Leinonen P, Markkola A, Hiilesmaa V, Kaaja R (2002) Postpartum bone mineral density in women treated for thromboprophylaxis with unfractionated heparin or LMW heparin. Thromb Haemost 87:182
Pisegna JR, Martindale RG (2005) Acid suppression in the perioperative period. J Clin Gastroenterol 39:10
Piso P, Dahlke MH, Mirena P, Schmidt U, Aselmann H, Schlitt HJ, Raab R, Klempnauer J (2004) Total mesorectal excision for middle and lower rectal cancer: a single institution experience with 337 consecutive patients. J Surg Oncol 86:115
Platell C, Hall JC (1997) Atelectasis after abdominal surgery. J Am Coll Surg 185:584
Polderman KH, Girbes AR (2002) Central venous catheter use. Part 2: infectious complications. Intensive Care Med 28:18
Poole GV Jr (1985) Mechanical factors in abdominal wound closure: the prevention of fascial dehiscence. Surgery 97:631
Prins MH, Hutten BA, Koopman MM, Buller HR (1999) Long-term treatment of venous thromboembolic disease. Thromb Haemost 82:892
Pycha A, Lodde M, Lusuardi L, Palermo S, Signorello D, Galantini A, Mian C, Hohenfellner R (2003)Teaching transurethral resection of the bladder: still a challenge? Urology 62:46
Raad II, Sabbagh MF (1992) Optimal duration of therapy for catheter-related Staphylococcus aureus bacteremia: a study of 55 cases and review. Clin Infect Dis 14:75
Ramirez OM, Ruas E, Dellon AL (1990) "Components separation" method for closure of abdominal-wall defects: an anatomic and clinical study. Plast Reconstr Surg 86:519
Rappaport W, Haynes K (1990) The retained surgical sponge following intra-abdominal surgery. A continuing problem. Arch Surg 125:405
Raschke RA, Gollihare B, Peirce JC (1996) The effectiveness of implementing the weight-based heparin nomogram as a practice guideline. Arch Intern Med 156:1645

Rassweiler J, Stolzenburg J, Sulser T, Deger S, Zumbe J, Hofmockel G, John H, Janetschek G, Fehr JL, Hatzinger M, Probst M, Rothenberger KH, Poulakis V, Truss M, Popken G, Westphal J, Alles U, Fornara P (2006) Laparoscopic radical prostatectomy – the experience of the german laparoscopic working group. Eur Urol 49:113

Rini JN, Bhargava KK, Tronco GG, Singer C, Caprioli R, Marwin SE, Richardson HL, Nichols KJ, Pugliese PV, Palestro CJ (2006) PET with FDG-labeled leukocytes versus scintigraphy with 111In-oxine-labeled leukocytes for detection of infection. Radiology 238:978

Roberts HR (1998) Clinical experience with activated factor VII focus on safety aspects. Blood Coagul Fibrinolysis 9 [Suppl 1]:S115

Rogers FB (2001) Venous thromboembolism in trauma patients: a review. Surgery 130:1

Rosario DJ, Becker M, Anderson JB (2000) The changing pattern of mortality and morbidity from radical cystectomy. BJU Int 85:427

Rosendaal FR (1999) Venous thrombosis: a multicausal disease. Lancet 353:1167

Rubin RH, Shapiro ED, Andriole VT, Davis RJ, Stamm WE (1992) Evaluation of new anti-infective drugs for the treatment of urinary tract infection. Infectious Diseases Society of America and the Food and Drug Administration. Clin Infect Dis 15 [Suppl 1]:S216

Rucinski J, Margolis M, Panagopoulos G, Wise L (2001) Closure of the abdominal midline fascia: meta-analysis delineates the optimal technique. Am Surg 67:421

Ruiz-Santana S, Ortiz E, Gonzalez B, Bolanos J, Ruiz-Santana AJ, Manzano JL (1991) Stress-induced gastroduodenal lesions and total parenteral nutrition in critically ill patients: frequency, complications, and the value of prophylactic treatment. A prospective, randomized study. Crit Care Med 19:887

Rutherford EJ, Skeete DA, Brasel KJ (2004) Management of the patient with an open abdomen: techniques in temporary and definitive closure. Curr Probl Surg 41 8:5

Salom EM, Schey D, Penalver M, Gomez-Marin O, Lambrou N, Almeida Z, Mendez L (2003) The safety of incidental appendectomy at the time of abdominal hysterectomy. Am J Obstet Gynecol 189:1563; discussion 1567

Santoshi N, Gaitonde K, Patil N, Goyal A, Srinivas V (2002) Incidental appendectomy during radical cystectomy–is it necessary? Urology 59:678

Scholz HS, Petru E, Benedicic C, Haas J, Tamussino K (2002) Winter R Fibrin application for preventing lymphocysts after retroperitoneal lymphadenectomy in patients with gynecologic malignancies. Gynecol Oncol 84:43

Scholz HS, Petru E, Benedicic C, Haas J, Tamussino K, Winter R (2002) Fibrin application for preventing lymphocysts after retroperitoneal lymphadenectomy in patients with gynecologic malignancies. Gynecol Oncol 84:43

Schulman CI, Cohn SM, Blackbourne L, Soffer D, Hoskins N, Bowers N, Habib F, Crookes B, Benjamin B, Pizano LR (2005) How long should you wait for a chest radiograph after placing a chest tube on water seal? A prospective study. J Trauma 59:92

Schulman S (2003) Clinical practice. Care of patients receiving long-term anticoagulant therapy. N Engl J Med 349:675

Schumpelick V, Riesener KP (1993) Peritoneovenous shunt–indications, limits, results. Chirurg 64:11

Scolapio JS (2004) A review of the trends in the use of enteral and parenteral nutrition support. J Clin Gastroenterol 38:403

Serretta V, Morgia G, Fondacaro L, Curto G, Lo Bianco A, Pirritano D, Melloni D, Orestano F, Motta M, Pavone-Macaluso M (2002) Open prostatectomy for benign prostatic enlargement in southern Europe in the late 1990s: a contemporary series of 1800 interventions. Urology 60:623

Sessler DI (1997) Mild perioperative hypothermia. N Engl J Med 336:1730

Sexton DJ, Spelman D (2003) Current best practices and guidelines. Assessment and management of complications in infective endocarditis. Cardiol Clin 21:273, vii-viii

Sexton WJ, Wood CG, Kim R, Pisters LL (2003) Repeat retroperitoneal lymph node dissection for metastatic testis cancer. J Urol 169:1353

Shafizadeh SF, Daily PP, Baliga P, Rogers J, Baillie GM, Rajagopolan PR, Chavin KD (2002) Chylous ascites secondary to laparoscopic donor nephrectomy. Urology 60:345

Shuford MD, McDougall EM, Chang SS, LaFleur BJ, Smith JA Jr, Cookson MS (2004) Complications of contemporary radical nephrectomy: comparison of open vs. laparoscopic approach. Urol Oncol 22:121

Sibert L, Descargues G, Scotte M, Planet M, Thoumas D, Annoot M, Boillot B, Grise P (1994) Laparoscopic drainage of a lymphocele after radical prostatectomy. Ann Urol (Paris) 28:202

Siegman-Igra Y, Anglim AM, Shapiro DE, Adal KA, Strain BA, Farr BM (1997) Diagnosis of vascular catheter-related bloodstream infection: a meta-analysis. J Clin Microbiol 35:928

Silverstein MD, Heit JA, Mohr DN, Petterson TM, O'Fallon WM, Melton LJ 3rd (1998) Trends in the incidence of deep vein thrombosis and pulmonary embolism: a 25-year population-based study. Arch Intern Med 158:585

Silvert MA, Meares EM Jr (1976) Rationale of incidental appendectomy. Urology 7:129

Siragusa S, Cosmi B, Piovella F, Hirsh J, Ginsberg JS (1996) Low-molecular-weight heparins and unfractionated heparin in the treatment of patients with acute venous thromboembolism: results of a meta-analysis. Am J Med 100:269

Sogani PC, Watson RC, Whitmore WF Jr (1981) Lymphocele after pelvic lymphadenectomy for urologic cancer. Urology 17:39

Solberg A, Angelsen A, Bergan U, Haugen OA, Viset T, Klepp O (2003) Frequency of lymphoceles after open and laparoscopic pelvic lymph node dissection in patients with prostate cancer. Scand J Urol Nephrol 37:218

Squadrone V, Coha M, Cerutti E, Schellino MM, Biolino P, Occella P, Belloni G, Vilianis G, Fiore G, Cavallo F et al (2005) Continuous positive airway pressure for treatment of postoperative hypoxemia: a randomized controlled trial. JAMA 293:589

Stamboulian D, Carbone E (1997) Recognition, management and prophylaxis of endocarditis. Drugs 54:730

Steffens J, Humke U, Ziegler M, Siemer S (2005) Partial nephrectomy with perfusion cooling for imperative indications: a 24-year experience. BJU Int 96:608

Stein JP, Lieskovsky G, Cote R, Groshen S, Feng AC, Boyd S, Skinner E, Bochner B, Thangathurai D, Mikhail M et al (2001) Radical cystectomy in the treatment of invasive bladder cancer: long-term results in 1,054 patients. J Clin Oncol 19:666

Stone MJ, Waterman MR, Harimoto D, Murray G, Willson N, Platt MR, Blomqvist G, Willerson JT (1977) Serum myoglobin level as diagnostic test in patients with acute myocardial infarction. Br Heart J 39:375

Stumpe KD, Dazzi H, Schaffner A, von Schulthess GK (2000) Infection imaging using whole-body FDG-PET. Eur J Nucl Med 27:822

Sugawara Y, Braun DK, Kison PV, Russo JE, Zasadny KR, Wahl RL (1998) Rapid detection of human infections with fluorine-18 fluorodeoxyglucose and positron emission tomography: preliminary results. Eur J Nucl Med 25:1238

Swan MC, Banwell PE (2005) The open abdomen: aetiology,

classification and current management strategies. J Wound Care 14:7
Symbas PN (1989) Chest drainage tubes. Surg Clin North Am 69:41
Syrjala MT, Valtonen V, Liewendahl K, Myllyla G (1987) Diagnostic significance of indium-111 granulocyte scintigraphy in febrile patients. J Nucl Med 28:155
Tacyildiz I, Aldemir M (2004) The mistakes of surgeons: "gossypiboma". Acta Chir Belg 104:71
Takeyama K, Matsukawa M, Kunishima Y, Takahashi S, Hotta H, Nishiyama N, Tsukamoto T (2005) Incidence of and risk factors for surgical site infection in patients with radical cystectomy with urinary diversion. J Infect Chemother 11:177
Tambyah PA (2004) Catheter-associated urinary tract infections: diagnosis and prophylaxis. Int J Antimicrob Agents 24 [Suppl 1]:S44
Tambyah PA, Maki DG (2000) Catheter-associated urinary tract infection is rarely symptomatic: a prospective study of 1,497 catheterized patients. Arch Intern Med 160:678
Tan LB, Chiang CP, Huang CH, Chou YH, Wang CJ (1991) Transvesical prostatectomy for benign prostatic hyperplasia–a 364 cases analysis. Gaoxiong Yi Xue Ke Xue Za Zhi 7:599
Tanner J, Woodings D, Moncaster K (2006) Preoperative hair removal to reduce surgical site infection. Cochrane Database Syst Rev CD004122
Teruel JL, Escobar EM, Quereda C, Mayayo T, Ortuno J (1983) A simple and safe method for management of lymphocele after renal transplantation. J Urol 130:1058
Thompson JS, Baxter BT, Allison JG, Johnson FE, Lee KK, Park WY (2003) Temporal patterns of postoperative complications. Arch Surg 138:596; discussion 602
Thurlow JP, Gelpi J, Schwaitzberg SD, Rohrer RJ (1996) Laparoscopic peritoneal fenestration and internal drainage of lymphoceles after renal transplantation. Surg Laparosc Endosc 6:290
Tissot E, Woronoff-Lemsi MC, Cornette C, Plesiat P, Jacquet M, Capellier G (2001) Cost-effectiveness of urinary dipsticks to screen asymptomatic catheter-associated urinary infections in an intensive care unit. Intensive Care Med 27:1842
Tolhurst SR, Rapp DE, O'Connor RC, Lyon MB, Orvieto MA, Steinberg GD (2005) Complications after cystectomy and urinary diversion in patients previously treated for localized prostate cancer. Urology 66:824
Trouillet JL, Chastre J, Vuagnat A, Joly-Guillou ML, Combaux D, Dombret MC, Gibert C (1998) Ventilator-associated pneumonia caused by potentially drug-resistant bacteria. Am J Respir Crit Care Med 157:531
Turi DC, Peerschke EI (1986) Sensitivity of three activated partial thromboplastin time reagents to coagulation factor deficiencies. Am J Clin Pathol 85:43
Uchida T, Adachi K, Ao T, Fujino A, Omata T, Yoshizawa K, Kurokawa J, Kadowaki K, Shoji K, Yokoyama E et al (1993) Preoperative, operative and postoperative complications in 2266 cases of transurethral resection of the prostate. Nippon Hinyokika Gakkai Zasshi 84:897
Uchida T, Ohori M, Soh S, Sato T, Iwamura M, Ao T, Koshiba K (1999) Factors influencing morbidity in patients undergoing transurethral resection of the prostate. Urology 53:98
Utikal P, Drac P, Bachleda P, Klein J, Kral V, Hrabalova M (2004) Peritoneovenous shunt – modification with the use of long saphenous vein. Biomed Pap Med Fac Univ Palacky Olomouc Czech Repub 148:89
Valeri CR, Feingold H, Cassidy G, Ragno G, Khuri S, Altschule MD (1987) Hypothermia-induced reversible platelet dysfunction. Ann Surg 205:175
Vallancien G, Cathelineau X, Baumert H, Doublet JD, Guillonneau B (2002) Complications of transperitoneal laparoscopic surgery in urology: review of 1,311 procedures at a single center. J Urol 168:23
Van Blerk M, Maes V, Huyghens L, Derde MP, Meert R, Gorus FK (1992) Analytical and clinical evaluation of creatine kinase MB mass assay by IMx: comparison with MB isoenzyme activity and serum myoglobin for early diagnosis of myocardial infarction. Clin Chem 38:2380
Van Poppel H, Dilen K, Baert L (2001) Incidental renal cell carcinoma and nephron sparing surgery. Curr Opin Urol 11:281
Velmahos GC, Kamel E, Berne TV, Yassa N, Ramicone E, Song Z, Demetriades D (1999) Abdominal computed tomography for the diagnosis of intra-abdominal sepsis in critically injured patients: fishing in murky waters. Arch Surg 134:831; discussion 836
Verhaeghe R, Stockx L, Lacroix H, Vermylen J, Baert AL (1997) Catheter-directed lysis of iliofemoral vein thrombosis with use of rt-PA. Eur Radiol 7:996
Wang HT, Sax HC (2001) Incidental appendectomy in the era of managed care and laparoscopy. J Am Coll Surg 192:182
Wanner A, Landa JF, Nieman RE Jr, Vevaina J, Delgado I (1973) Bedside bronchofiberscopy for atelectasis and lung abscess. JAMA 224:1281
Warkentin TE, Levine MN, Hirsh J, Horsewood P, Roberts RS, Gent M, Kelton JG (1995) Heparin-induced thrombocytopenia in patients treated with low-molecular-weight heparin or unfractionated heparin. N Engl J Med 332:1330
Watkins BP, Kothari SN, Landercasper J (2004) Stump appendicitis: case report and review. Surg Laparosc Endosc Percutan Tech 14:167
Welsby IJ, Monroe DM, Lawson JH, Hoffmann M (2005) Recombinant activated factor VII and the anaesthetist. Anaesthesia 60:1203
Wille AH, Roigas J, Deger S, Tullmann M, Turk I, Loening SA (2004) Laparoscopic radical nephrectomy: techniques, results and oncological outcome in 125 consecutive cases. Eur Urol 45:483; discussion 488
Wittmann DH, Schein M (1996) Let us shorten antibiotic prophylaxis and therapy in surgery. Am J Surg 172:S26–S32
Wood DP Jr, Bianco FJ Jr, Pontes JE, Heath MA, DaJusta D (2003) Incidence and significance of positive urine cultures in patients with an orthotopic neobladder. J Urol 169:2196
Wu CT, Chiang YJ, Liu KL, Chu SH (2004) Laparoscopic donor nephrectomy: new combination of hand-assisted and standard approaches. Transplant Proc 36:1909
Yablon CM, Banner MP, Ramchandani P, Rovner ES (2004) Complications of prostate cancer treatment: spectrum of imaging findings. Radiographics 24 [Suppl 1]:S181
Yataco JC, Dweik RA (2005) Pleural effusions: evaluation and management. Cleve Clin J Med 72:854, 858, 862 passim
Zanetta G, Trio D, Lissoni A, Dalla Valle C, Rangoni G, Pittelli M, Marzola M, Pellegrino A (1993) Early and short-term complications after US-guided puncture of gynecologic lesions: evaluation after 1,000 consecutive cases. Radiology 189:161

18.2 Preventing and Managing Infectious Emergencies of Urologic Surgery

T.J. Walsh, M.A. Dall'Era, J.N. Krieger

18.2.1 Introduction

This chapter reviews our approach to preventing and managing infectious emergencies complicating urological surgery from our perspective as practicing urologists. We focus on the surgical site and urinary tract infections that are of most interest to practicing urologists. Because of limited space, we omitted important postoperative problems that are less relevant to urological practice, such as respiratory infections and antibiotic-associated bowel problems. When appropriate, we highlight studies of special interest and outline our own clinical approach to management of urological patients with postoperative infectious complications.

18.2.2 Surgical Site Infections

In the late 1800s, Sir Joseph Lister hypothesized that microbes from the air caused most of his patients to die from wound sepsis shortly after surgery (Townsend 2004). After learning that carbolic acid was being used successfully to treat raw sewage, Lister began to practice antiseptic surgery. He used carbolic acid-soaked dressings and soaked the surgical instruments and surgeons' hands in carbolic acid. He also sprayed carbolic acid around the operating room and into his patients' wounds. The result was a dramatic decrease in postoperative wound infection rates.

Even in today's era of aseptic surgery, surgical site infections (SSIs) still cause significant morbidity and mortality. After pneumonia, SSIs are the second most common nosocomial infections with approximately 500,000 documented infections per year in the US (National Nosocomial Infections Surveillance System 2004). Large series show that SSIs complicate 1%–2% of clean, extraabdominal procedures and up to 12% of abdominal procedures (National Nosocomial Infections Surveillance System 2004). In addition to increasing patient morbidity and mortality, SSIs significantly increase hospital stays and health care costs (Kirkland et al. 1999).

18.2.2.1 Definition and Classification of SSIs

The Centers for Disease Control and Prevention (CDC) defines an SSI as any infection occurring between 0 and 30 days after a surgical procedure or up to 1 year after insertion of prosthetic materials (www.cdc.gov). Superficial wound infections are diagnosed by the classical signs and symptoms of infection, such as erythema, pain, or localized swelling. Diagnosis of a wound infection can also be based on a positive, aseptically obtained bacterial wound culture. SSIs are further classified as incisional (superficial and deep) and organ or surgical space-related, such as abdominal or retroperitoneal.

18.2.2.2
Risk Factors for SSI

Traditionally, SSI risk was estimated based solely on the wound category. Rates ranged from 1%–4% for clean wounds to 12%–40% for dirty wounds (Table 18.2.1) (Culver et al. 1991). Evidence now suggests that a combination of patient factors, surgical factors, and microbiological factors must be assessed to accurately estimate SSI risk (Gaynes et al. 2001).

Patient Factors

Data show that certain intraoperative factors are associated with reduced SSI risk, including high inhaled oxygen tension (80%), tight control of perioperative blood glucose, and maintenance of normothermia (Kurz et al. 1996; Belda et al. 2005; Grey and Perdrizet 2004). Presence of co-morbid conditions, medications, or drug usage must also be considered (Table 18.2.2) (Heinzelmann et al. 2002). Chemotherapy and steroids, for example, significantly increase SSI risk due to their immunosuppressive effects (Heinzelmann et al. 2002; Fuenfer et al. 1975). Some data show that heparin and coumadin prophylaxis for venous thrombosis may also be associated with higher rates of prosthetic joint infections after joint replacement (Asensio et al. 2005). Based on these findings, similar risk factors may also increase prosthetic infection rates after urological surgery.

Table 18.2.1. Surgical wound category definitions and surgical site infection (SSI) risk

Wound category	Definition	SSI risk
Clean	GI/GU/respiratory tract not entered	1%–4%
Clean-contaminated	GI/GU/respiratory tract entered without gross contamination	3%–8%
Contaminated	Open accidental wounds, gross GI contamination, inflammation	8%–15%
Dirty	Old traumatic wounds, perforated viscous, existing infection	12%–40%

After Culver et al. (1990)

Surgical Factors

Surgical factors that affect SSI risk include the presence of foreign bodies, seroma/hematoma prevention, methods of preoperative hair removal, and wound drainage (Heinzelmann et al. 2002; Alexander et al. 1983; Raves et al. 1984). Appropriate wound irrigation is important to decrease bacterial counts after surgical procedures, especially those involving the genitourinary or gastrointestinal tracts. Prevention of hematomas or seromas with appropriate drains is also critical for reducing SSI risk (Heinzelmann et al. 2002). Hematoma formation may account for some of the increased risk found in patients given subcutaneous heparin prophylaxis or coumadin after prosthetic joint surgery. Clipping hair immediately before surgery has clearly been shown to result in fewer SSIs than shaving, which is no longer recommended (Alexander et al. 1983). In general, closed suction drains are associated with lower SSI rates than more passive drainage systems (Raves et al. 1984).

Microbiological Factors

The degree of wound contamination, or overall bacterial load, at the surgical site clearly influences SSI risk. Other important microbiological factors include virulence-associated traits of the particular organisms involved. Microorganisms have developed a variety of survival methods to flourish in specific environments. Perhaps the most commonly encountered bacteriolog-

Table 18.2.2. Traditional risk factors for surgical site infection

Patient-related	Procedure-related	Microorganism-related
Hypothermia Hyperglycemia Advanced age (>70 years) Diabetes mellitus Malnutrition Immunosuppression Obesity Chronic alcohol use Malignancy	Seroma/hematoma Hair removal method Closed suction drains Foreign bodies Wound irrigation	Wound contamination Extent of contamination Antibiotic resistance

Documented univariate risk factors for surgical site infection risk (Kurz et al. 1996; Belda et al. 2005; Grey and Perdrizet 2004; Heinzelmann et al. 2002; Fuenfer et al. 1975; Alexander et al. 1983; Raves et al. 1984; Furuno et al. 2005). Estimating an individual patient's risk is based on the interaction among several risk factors.

ic survival mechanism in the health-care environment is the evolution and transmission of antibiotic resistance. With increased numbers of compromised patients and the widespread use of antibiotics, multiple drug-resistant organisms, including methicillin-resistant *Staphylococcus aureus* and vancomycin-resistant *Enterococcus* species, are encountered with increasing frequency in many practice situations (Furuno et al. 2005).

Coagulase-negative *Staphylococcus* species and *Enterococcus* remain the most common causative agents in SSI followed by *S. aureus* and *Candida albicans*; all ubiquitous components of the normal human flora (Weiss et al. 1999). *Bacteroides fragilis*, *Pseudomonas aeruginosa*, and enterics such as *Escherichia coli* are also commonly causes of SSI. Many other bacteria may be encountered depending on wound type. It is exceedingly important to consider local antimicrobial sensitivity patterns and trends in individual practice settings to select optimal antimicrobial therapy because bacterial resistance patterns differ substantially in various practice settings.

Need for a Comprehensive Approach

Accurate SSI risk assessment requires a comprehensive evaluation of several factors simultaneously. A large multivariate analysis identified several independent risk factors for SSI: wound type, length of procedure, American Society of Anesthesiology (ASA) score, hypothermia, hypoxia, presence of remote site infection, and preoperative shaving (Christou et al. 1987). Integrating multiple variables to estimate SSI risk proved complex. Therefore, a more practical and objective measure for individual risk assessment was needed.

The National Nosocomial Infection Surveillance System (NNIS) Score was devised to more accurately reflect the interaction among multiple factors and to more easily classify an individual patient's risk (Culver et al. 1991). The NNIS score integrates three primary risk factors: wound category, ASA score, and length of procedure (>75th percentile is considered high-risk). The total NNIS score predicts an individual's SSI risk (Table 18.2.3). Contaminated or dirty wounds are scored as one point, ASA score of III, IV, or V is scored as one point, and above the 75th percentile for procedure length is scored as one point.

Table 18.2.3. National Nosocomial Infection Surveillance System (NNIS) score predicts surgical site infection risk

NNIS score[a]	SSI risk[b]
0	1.5%
1	2.9%
2	6.8%
3	13.0%

[a] To calculate an individual patient's NNIS score, contaminated and dirty wounds are given 1 point, an ASA score of III or greater is given 1 point, and length of procedure over the 75th percentile is given 1 point

[b] Since it is difficult to estimate an individual patient's SSI risk based on the traditional risk factors outlined in Table 18.2.2, the NNIS score was developed to consider the interactions among multiple risk factors and provide individualized SSI risk assessments. Estimates are based on over 84,000 procedures with 2,376 documented SSIs (Culver et al. 1991)

18.2.2.3 Diagnosing SSIs

One should entertain the diagnosis of SSI when a patient is not recovering as expected after a surgical procedure. Redness, swelling, and pain over the incision, with purulent drainage or foul odor represent the classical physical signs of infection. These findings occur most frequently with superficial SSIs. Deeper wound infections often present initially with more systemic symptoms, including fever, chills, and rigors. Laboratory findings of leukocytosis, C-reactive protein elevation, hyperglycemia, acidosis, and procalcitonin elevation all support the diagnosis of infection (Folcoz et al. 2005; Tegnell et al. 2002).

When needed to document and localize an SSI, useful imaging procedures include ultrasound, computerized tomography (CT), and magnetic resonance imaging (MRI) (Noone et al. 1998, 2004; Bydder and Kreel 1980). All three modalities have equal sensitivity for detecting large, drainable abdominal and subcutaneous fluid collections (Noone et al. 2004). Ultrasound imaging is very operator-dependent and is less accessible than computerized tomography in many practice settings. We prefer CT and MRI because these methods have proven more sensitive for detecting small, deeper abscesses. Both imaging modalities provide excellent anatomic detail for diagnosis and safe, percutaneous drain placement near vital structures (Bydder and Kreel 1980; Noone et al. 2004). Since MRI is significantly more expensive than CT, we reserve MRI for patients with absolute contraindications to iodinated intravenous contrast agents.

18.2.2.4 Managing SSIs

Initial SSI management depends on the depth and location of infection along the surgical tract. Cellulitis and other superficial infections respond well to antimicrobial therapy and local wound care alone. Superficial abscesses are drained easily by opening the surgical wound. Deeper fluid collections or abscesses usually require more aggressive drainage maneuvers for diagnosis and management. In these situations, our preference is percutaneous radiologically guided drainage, reserving open surgical procedures for cases with contraindications to percutaneous drainage or when more conservative measures have failed. With this paradigm, up to 85% of intra-abdominal abscesses can be managed by percutaneous drainage and appropriate antimicrobial therapy (Khurrum Baig et al. 2002). Purulent material should be carefully collected and evaluated with Gram stain, culture, and antimicrobial sensitivity testing.

Empirical antimicrobial therapy should be chosen using the Gram stain results and the suspected pathogens based upon the wound type and local sensitivity patterns. Such therapy may be modified, if needed, depending on subsequent culture and sensitivity results. Most patients respond rapidly to appropriate therapy. Therefore, lack of the expected clinical improvement or subsequent clinical deterioration should prompt re-evaluation of the diagnosis and therapy. Such re-evaluation includes careful physical examination in conjunction with other diagnostic maneuvers such as repeated imaging, culturing, or a change in antimicrobial coverage. Fungal or mycobacterial infections and undrained abscess must also be considered when patients do not respond to therapy as expected.

18.2.2.5 Preventing SSIs

Any procedure with an estimated SSI risk greater than 1% warrants preoperative prophylactic antimicrobial therapy (Bratzler and Houck 2005). Therefore, prophylactic antimicrobial therapy should be strongly considered for:

1. Any clean procedure in a patient with an NNIS score > 1
2. Any clean-contaminated procedure
3. Any procedure in an immunocompromised patient
4. When any prosthetic material is inserted
5. When the operative area contains high bacterial counts, such as the axilla or scrotum

Timing of preoperative antibiotic administration is crucial for SSI prevention. Stone et al. (1979) reported the lowest SSI risk when therapy was initiated within 1 h of the start of surgery (Stone et al. 1979). Patients who received antibiotics after the incision had nearly the same SSI risk as patients who did not receive prophylaxis. Other data corroborate the conclusion that timely preoperative antimicrobial administration can reduce SSI rates (Classen et al. 1992). These data demonstrate the importance of obtaining therapeutic serum antimicrobial levels before bacterial exposure occurs during the operation. NNIS guidelines also suggest that prophylactic antimicrobials should be redosed appropriately for lengthy procedures to maintain therapeutic drug levels and that therapy should stop within 24 h of surgery when used for prophylaxis (Bratzler and Houck 2005).

NNIS guidelines also support prophylactic antimicrobial therapy for transscrotal surgery based on high bacterial counts on the scrotum and perineum. In a retrospective review of 131 outpatient scrotal procedures, Kiddoo et al. (2004) found a 9.3% overall SSI rate among patients who did not receive prophylactic therapy. In a separate study using prophylactic antibiotics, Swartz et al. found a 4% SSI rate in over 100 transscrotal procedures with a mean follow-up of 36 months (Swartz, personal communication). Although, the benefit of prophylactic antimicrobials in transscrotal surgery can not be proven by such retrospective surgical series, these data do suggest that scrotal wounds merit consideration as clean-contaminated wounds that may warrant prophylaxis.

Appropriate antimicrobial agents should be selected based on the most likely organisms encountered during the particular surgical procedure. Beta-lactam antibiotics, such as the cephalosporins, are the most common agents used for general prophylaxis against normal skin flora. Recommendations include cefazolin for clean abdominal procedures or cefotetan for clean-contaminated abdominal procedures involving the GI tract (Bratzler and Houck 2005). Clindamycin or vancomycin may be used for Gram-positive coverage in patients with documented beta-lactam allergies (Bratzler and Houck 2005). Other possible regimens include combinations of either metronidazole or clindamycin with gentamicin or a fluoroquinolone. Even in hospitals with perceived high rates of bacterial resistance, there is no evidence supporting the routine use of vancomycin rather than other agents. Recommendations for specific urologic procedures are presented below.

Surgical patients with prosthetic joints who are at risk for joint infections or patients with certain cardiac anomalies who are at risk for life-threatening endocarditis warrant special consideration. The American Urological Association (AUA), the American Academy of Orthopedic Surgeons, and the American Heart Association (AHA) have published guidelines for prophylaxis in these patient populations (Dajani et al. 1997a; American Urological SocietyAmerican Academy of Orthopaedic Surgeons 2003).

Transient bacteremia often occurs after urological procedures, especially if patients are instrumented during active UTI. Identification and treatment of active infections is strongly recommended prior to any elective procedure. Bacteremia is commonly associated with urological procedures, with rates of 31% for patients undergoing TURP, 24% for patients undergoing urethral dilations, 44% for patients having prostate biopsies, and 7% for patients having office urodynamics (Onur et al. 2004; Sullivan et al. 1973; Lindert et al. 2000).

Following total joint replacements, an expert panel from the AUA and the American Academy of Orthopedic Surgeons recommended that patients at highest risk for joint infection included those who had had joint implant surgery within 2 years, immunocompromised patients, patients with previous joint infections, or medical conditions such as diabetes or malignancy. This panel recommended either a single oral quinolone dose taken 1 – 2 h before biopsy or 2 g of parenteral ampicillin (or 1 g intravenous vancomycin for patients allergic to penicillin) plus 80 mg of gentamicin at least 30 min before the procedure (American Urological Society/American Academy of Orthopaedic Surgeons 2003).

The AHA recommends endocarditis prophylaxis for patients undergoing prostatic surgery, urethral dilation, cystoscopy, or ureteroscopy (Dajani et al. 1997a). Prophylaxis is not necessary for urethral catheterization or circumcision in the absence of clinical infections (Dajani et al. 1997a). Perioperative ampicillin (or vancomycin for allergic patients) plus gentamicin is recommended for high-risk patients. Moderate-risk patients can be treated with single agent ampicillin or vancomycin (Dajani et al. 1997a). High-risk patients are defined by having prosthetic heart valves, previous histories of endocarditis, or complex congenital anomalies. Currently, the AUA recommends assessing patients' overall risk for artificial joint infection based on a combination of patient-related and procedure-related factors (as outlined above) (American Urological Society/American Academy of Orthopaedic Surgeons 2003).

18.2.2.6 Examples of Our Approach to Urological SSIs

Infected Artificial Urinary Sphincter

Prevention and Clinical Presentation

Because prevention of artificial urinary sphincter (AUS) infections is always preferable to treatment of an infected AUA, appropriate perioperative antimicrobial administration is imperative. We favor broad-spectrum coverage with particular attention to coverage of *Staphylococcus epidermidis* using either a cephalosporin or beta-lactam agent. Again, it is imperative that therapy be administered within 1 h of surgery. The literature does not support prolonged postoperative antimicrobial administration. As outlined above, control of intraoperative risk factors to limit SSI risk is also important.

Infections complicate between 4% and 21% of AUS insertions and there is no difference in infection rates between men and women (Venn et al. 2000; Hajivassiliou 1999; Petero and Kiokno 2006; Martins and Boyd 1995). AUS infections represent some of the most difficult and frustrating complications to deal with in urology. *S. aureus* and coagulase-negative *Staphylococcus* species cause the vast majority of AUS infections (Martins and Boyd 1995; Bryan et al. 2002). Patient risk factors for infection include previous sphincter insertion, previous radiotherapy, and previous procedures for bladder neck incisions (Martins and Boyd 1995). Recent series with modern focused radiotherapy for cancer report no increased risk for AUS infections compared to other patient populations (Martins and Boyd 1995; Gomha and Boone 2002). Other important risk factors for AUS infections include improper urethral catheterization or endoscopy in patients with artificial sphincters. Prior to any urethral instrumentation, it is critical that the sphincter be deflated and inactivated to reduce the risk of intraurethral cuff erosion.

Multiple authors debated the risks and benefits of simultaneous bladder augmentation and AUS insertion for patients with neurogenic bladders. Depending on the bowel segment used, reported infection rates after such combined procedures range from 5% to 50% (Miller et al. 1998; Holmes et al. 2001; Catto et al. 2005). Miller et al. (1998) described an overall infection rate of 6.9% in 29 patients undergoing simultaneous AUS insertion and bladder augmentation. Nineteen (66%) of the 29 patients in this series underwent gastrocystoplasty with no reported AUS infections. In contrast, two (20%) of ten patients had sphincter infections following ileal or colonic augmentations (Miller et al. 1998). Other studies report similar findings, suggesting that the relatively sterile stomach environment allows simultaneous procedures to be performed with no increased risk of sphincter infection (Holmes et al. 2001; Ganesan et al. 1993).

Most patients with infected sphincters present with persistent pain over the prosthetic parts, however, other symptoms, including dysuria, hematuria, or pump fixation against the scrotal wall, may represent the first indication of an infection (Bryan et al. 2002). Others present with more obvious signs of infection, such as purulent drainage from the scrotum or exposed prosthetic parts. Same patients present with few systemic symptoms and only a mild leukocytosis or low-grade fever.

In summary, AUS infections have highly variable presentations. Urologists must have a high index of suspicion for infection when any patient with an AUS presents with local signs and symptoms, vague symptoms, or symptoms of systemic infection or inflammation with no clear source.

Clinical Management

Initial management of an infected AUS depends on the clinical presentation and extent of infection. Patients with suspected infections who are otherwise stable may undergo a trial of oral or parenteral antimicrobial therapy. However, resolution of true prosthetic infections with medical management alone is extremely rare.

Persistent symptoms or progressive clinical deterioration necessitates prompt surgical exploration and removal of the infected prosthesis. More than half of patients have infections involving all three device components, supporting complete device removal (Venn et al. 2000; Hajivassiliou 1999). Standard management includes removal of all parts with thorough washout and debridement of any devitalized tissue. Several months later, after the infection has completely resolved and all wounds have healed, select patients may undergo AUS reinsertion.

Successful salvage protocols for removal and immediate replacement of an infected AUA have been described by several investigators similar to that outlined below for infected penile prostheses (Bryan et al. 2002). Bryan et al. (2002) reported the outcomes of eight patients with infected AUSs who underwent a salvage protocol with complete device removal, followed by extensive washout of the wound with multiple solutions, then immediate replacement. Most series describe men with postradical prostatectomy incontinence and all patients were given an oral fluoroquinolone for 1 month after reinsertion. With a mean follow up of 33 months, seven (88%) of eight patients had no evidence of recurrent infection.

The advantages offered by immediate removal and replacement of an infected AUS are not as pronounced as those seen for an infected penile prosthesis. Reinsertion once the infection has completely resolved is often not much more technically difficult than primary AUS insertion. Further, overall outcomes with regard to comfort and continence appear similar with primary and secondary insertions (Raj et al. 2005). With immediate reinsertion of a new AUS, patients enjoy immediate return of continence and observations suggest that a salvage protocol for AUS infections might be feasible for highly selected patients. Further data on long-term follow-up and patient selection are needed to determine if the risk-to-benefit ratio with immediate reinsertion warrants general adoption of such salvage protocols for infected AUSs.

Infected Penile Prosthesis

Prevention and Clinical Presentation

As with urinary sphincters, we believe that the urologist's first goal should be to prevent infections. Perioperative antimicrobial administration is paramount in preventing penile prosthesis infections. In 1978, Small et al. reported a significantly decreased infection rate in men undergoing placement of penile prostheses with the administration of prophylactic antimicrobial therapy (Small 1978). In this series, five (25%) of 20 patients without antimicrobial prophylaxis developed prosthetic infections compared to one (<1%) of 140 patients given prophylaxis.

It is imperative to ensure the absence of any urinary tract, cutaneous, or systemic infection prior to penile prosthesis insertion. The patient should be carefully shaved just before surgery. Schwartz et al. (1996) investigated the merits of different prophylactic antibimicrobial regimens and found no difference between oral and IV therapy for penile prosthesis insertion in 20 men. This study showed a clear overall cost reduction with oral therapy, as these men did not require hospital admission.

Current AUA guidelines recommend preoperative broad spectrum Gram-positive and Gram-negative prophylactic antimicrobial coverage using a combination of an aminoglycoside plus a cephalosporin or vancomycin administered 1 h prior to surgery (Montague et al. 2005). Broad-spectrum coverage should be continued for 24–48 h postoperatively, which often requires an overnight hospital stay for intravenous administration. There is no evidence that prolonged prophylaxis results in lower infection rates.

Industry has produced antimicrobial-impregnated and hydrophilic coatings for penile prostheses in hopes of further reducing the infection risk (Carson 2004). Hopefully, long-term data will show clear clinical advantages for these modifications. It has long been recognized that revision surgery of for noninfectious problems with penile prostheses is associated with a significantly higher risk for infection than primary insertions. Multiple factors are likely responsible for this finding; however, extensive washout procedures similar to the salvage protocol can significantly reduce reinfection rates from 12% to 3% (Henry et al. 2005). In 140 penile prostheses removed for mechanical failure followed by extensive wound irrigation and immediate replacement, Henry et al. (2005) reported infections in only four (3%) compared with five (12%) infections in 43 men who were not irrigated prior to reinsertion (Henry et al. 2005).

Finding subclinical bacterial colonization within protective biofilms covering prosthetic devices corroborates these observations and supports extensive washout during any revision surgery, even for clinically noninfected prostheses (Nickel et al. 1986). Multiple organisms are known to produce biofilms that protect them from host defenses and antibiotics (Nickel et al. 1986; Silverstein and Donatucci 2003). Within biofilms, bacteria exist in colonies where individual organisms often have a low metabolic rate, substantially increasing antimicrobial resistance. Microbial biofilms facilitate subclinical bacterial persistence on the prosthesis for extended periods. Studies of clinically uninfected prostheses removed for mechanical failure report a 70% colonization rate, most commonly with *S. epidermidis* (Henry et al. 2004).

A number of series report postoperative infections complicating 1% – 8% of primary penile prosthesis insertions and up to 18% of reinsertions performed for mechanical failure (Darouiche 2004; Mulcahy 2000; Merrill 1988; Kabalin and Kessler 1988; Montague 1987; Minervini et al. 2006). Most infections presumably result from device contamination during initial implantation (Henry et al. 1994). Less commonly, late hematogenous bacterial seeding of the prosthesis has been described (Carson and Robertson 1988). *S. epidermidis* is the most common isolate from prosthetic infections (Henry et al. 1994; Mulcahy 2000; Montague 1987). Infections with *E. coli*, *Pseudomonas* species, *Proteus* species, and *Enterobacter* species have also been documented (Henry et al. 1994; Jarow 1996).

The most common signs and symptoms of prosthesis infections include fever, erythema, swelling, and pain over the affected parts (Jarow 1996). Other patients present with more indolent symptoms, as described previously for AUS.

Clinical Management

As with infected sphincters, staged procedures were used traditionally to manage penile prosthesis infections with complete device removal, wound debridement, and antimicrobial administration (Kaufman et al. 1982). Patients are typically candidates for reinsertion several months later, once the infection has resolved completely.

In contrast to AUS infections, reinsertion of penile prostheses several months after removal is technically challenging, with significantly higher morbidity. Corporal scar formation typically results in penile shortening with a substantially higher chance for perforation during corporal dilation and generally poorer outcomes (Wilson and Delk 1995). After failure of penile prostheses, men typically have few options for management of their erectile dysfunction, which may substantially reduce their quality of life.

The ability to perform simultaneous removal of an infected prosthesis with immediate successful insertion of a new device holds obvious appeal. Difficult dissections are avoided and penile length is often maintained. Unfortunately, early attempts at salvage procedures with penile prostheses were largely unsuccessful (Wilson and Delk 1995). However, the orthopedic literature described successful direct exchange salvage protocols for infected hip arthroses (Buchholz et al. 1981; Miley et al. 1982). In many ways, orthopedic prosthetic joint infections parallel urological prosthetic infections. In both situations, *S. epidermidis* is the most common pathogen and traditional management involved complete removal, wound washout, and delayed replacement (Ure et al. 1998). Realizing the advantages of direct exchange protocols, orthopedic surgeons began performing successful salvage procedures in the 1970s by removing the infected joint followed by extensive wound washout prior to insertion of a new prosthetic (Buchholz et al. 1981). Carefully selected patients greatly benefit from immediate joint replacement (Minervini et al. 2006). Re-infection rates after direct exchange arthroplasty are now on the order of 1% – 2%, especially with the widespread use of antimicrobial-impregnated cements (Ure et al. 1998). With modern techniques, the lower infection rates occur in patients undergoing direct removal and replacement of infected joints than for patients undergoing debridement with joint retention or joint removal with delayed reinsertion, although surgical case selection likely accounts for part of this difference (Berbari et al. 2006).

In 1991, Mulcahy et al. published a salvage protocol for managing infected penile prostheses; since then, many groups have adopted this strategy (Mulcahy et al. 1995; Kaufman et al. 1998). The original Mulcahy protocol includes extensive irrigation with sequential use of seven solutions, followed by immediate insertion of a new device (Table 18.2.4). With a mean follow-up of 35 months, they described an 82% successful salvage rate for 65 men undergoing the salvage protocol. They identified several risk factors for failure, including early infection after initial placement of the prosthetic, extensive cellulitis upon presentation, and the isolation of particularly virulent organisms, such as methacillin-resistant *S. aureus* or vancomycin-resistant *Enterococcus* (Mulcahy 2000). Severe necrotizing infections, sepsis, or patient immunosuppression are absolute contraindications to performing this salvage protocol.

Table 18.2.4. Sequence of irrigation solutions used prior to immediate reinsertion following removal of infected penile prostheses

1. Antimicrobial irrigation (bacitracin 50,000 units/l and kanamycin 500 mg/l)
2. Half-strength hydrogen peroxide
3. Half-strength povidone-iodine
4. Pressure irrigation with 1 g vancomycin and 80 mg gentamicin per liter of solution
5. Half-strength povidone-iodine
6. Half-strength hydrogen peroxide
7. Antimicrobial irrigation

Solutions are used in sequence after removal of an infected prostheses (after Mulcahy et al. 1995; Dajani et al. 1997)

18.2.3 Urinary Tract Infections Complicating Urological Procedures

The risk of UTI associated with urological procedures is controversial. Some of this controversy reflects the difficulties inherent in classifying and defining UTI. Further, there are difficulties in distinguishing among the various types urological procedures. We begin by defining and categorizing UTI and urological endoscopic procedures. We then provide an overview of the pertinent literature and offer a systematic approach for diagnosing and managing postoperative UTIs.

18.2.3.1 Post-procedural UTIs – A Clinical Approach

UTI is defined as the inflammatory response of the urothelium to microbial invasion. Typically, UTI is associated with bacteriuria and with pyuria. Although a seemingly straightforward definition, further categorization of UTI is necessary to facilitate clinical decision making.

We prefer to classify UTI into three simple categories: asymptomatic bacteriuria, uncomplicated UTI, and complicated UTI, which includes urinary sepsis syndrome. This classification facilitates determination of the appropriate clinical approach.

Asymptomatic Bacteriuria

Asymptomatic bacteriuria is defined as bacteria present in the urine of a patient who has no symptoms or signs. This definition presumes that such bacteria are not contaminants from the skin, vagina, or prepuce. This presumes that the specimen has been "handled properly" and that it has been transported promptly to the laboratory for processing. Asymptomatic bacteriuria represents one of the most commonly measured and reported urological infections.

There is considerable debate in the literature regarding the concentration of bacteria in urine that is considered "significant." Traditionally, the threshold has been more than 100,000 colony forming units (cfu)/ml of a single species. This definition was based on older population surveys where patients were required to have repeated samples showing more than 10^5 cfu/ml (Kunin 2003). Contemporary literature suggests that greater than 10^2 cfu/ml may represent significant bacteriuria in a patient with urinary tract symptoms. Importantly, the criterion for definition of "significant" bacteriuria in an asymptomatic patient remains debatable (Stamm 2003).

Complicated Versus Uncomplicated Urinary Tract Infection

Historically, UTIs were classified based upon organ of origin (pyelonephritis, cystitis, epididymitis, etc). However, this subjective classification contributes little to clinical management. Localization studies have shown that it is exceedingly difficult to distinguish bladder infection from renal infection in many populations based upon clinical signs and symptoms (Kunin 2003). Additionally, such distinction may be arbitrary because patients with upper and lower UTIs may do equally well on similar antibiotic regimens if the infections are uncomplicated.

We classify patients with clinical signs or symptoms of UTI into two distinct groups; uncomplicated UTIs or complicated UTIs. Uncomplicated UTIs occur in patients with structurally and functionally normal urinary tracts. Such UTIs include most isolated or recurrent bacterial cystitis as well as acute, uncomplicated pyelonephritis in women.

In contrast, complicated UTIs occur in patients with structural or functional impairment of the urinary tract. Such impairments include urinary tract obstruction from edema, stone, or foreign body, presence of renal disease, or the loss of normal voiding, as is the case with neurological impairment or bladder outlet obstruction. Such a clinical approach to UTI is preferable, because it reflects the efficacy of antimicrobial therapies: complicated infections often do not respond to antimicrobial therapy alone and require relief of structural or functional obstruction, abscess drainage, or other urological measures (Krieger 2002).

Urosepsis

Urosepsis is a syndrome that results from a complicated UTI and includes one or more of the following clinical signs: tachypnea, tachycardia, hyper- or hypothermia, or evidence of inadequate end-organ perfusion. The clinical hallmarks of inadequate tissue perfusion are oliguria and hypoxemia, which may be accompanied by elevated plasma lactate. Septic shock refers to sepsis syndrome in a hypotensive patient. Fortunately, septic shock following urological procedures is rare (often termed "urosepsis"). Urosepsis has a more favorable prognosis than septic shock.

18.2.3.2 UTI Risk Associated with Urological Procedures

The procedures performed by urologists are widely varied and are associated with varied risks for infection. Below, we consider the risks with common urological procedures.

Urethral Catheterization

The placement of urinary catheters represents an essential part of medical care. Urinary catheters are widely employed to relieve structural or functional obstructions of the urinary tract. When used inappropriately or left in place too long, urethral catheters pose a significant risk for development of UTI. Catheter-associated UTIs account for approximately 40 % of nosocomial infections and increase the duration, morbidity, and costs of hospitalization. The use of antimicrobial therapy with concomitant placement of indwelling urethral catheters often leads to selection of antibiotic-resistant microorganisms and nosocomial infection caused by multidrug resistant strains (Kunin 2001).

The bottom line is that catheters should be placed for a sound clinical reason and left in place for the minimal amount of time. Efforts to decrease catheter-associated UTI rates by improving meatal care, instillations into the catheter drainage bags, use of antimicrobial coatings, valves in the drainage bags, and other measures have generally proven disappointing in carefully conducted clinical trials.

Cystoscopy

Historically, cystoscopy was considered a clean procedure that did not merit routine prophylactic antimicrobial therapy. Symptomatic infections likely occur following fewer than 5 % of procedures, if the urine is sterile preoperatively (Grabe 2001). Asymptomatic bacteriuria has been reported after as many as 35 % of cystoscopic procedures; however, most series are in the 10 % range (Kraklau and Wolf 1999; Rane et al. 2001).

Rane and colleagues compared preoperative, intramuscular gentamicin to no antimicrobial therapy. In a randomized controlled trial of 162 patients undergoing office cystoscopy. Only 4.9 % of the gentamicin group developed postcystoscopy bacteriuria, compared to a 21.3 % bacteriuria among untreated controls ($p = 0.004$) (Rane et al. 2001). There was no adverse reaction to gentamicin. However, this study did not evaluate patients' symptoms and results were based solely on a single urine specimen from each patient.

In a study of 104 patients having office cystoscopy without prophylaxis, Kortmann et al. (1999) determined the symptomatic UTI rate. Outcomes included both urine culture and a follow-up symptom questionnaire. The authors found a 3 % symptomatic UTI rate and a 9 % asymptomatic bacteriuria rate (Kortmann et al. 1999). In contrast, Manson and colleagues found a 2.2 % asymptomatic bacteriuria rate among 138 patients who had cystoscopy without antimicrobials (Manson 1988). These low symptomatic UTI rates following cystoscopy led Kraklau and colleagues to conclude that low-risk patients undergoing cystoscopy are not likely to benefit from prophylactic antimicrobials (Kraklau and Wolf 1999).

These and other data have led us to conclude that patients with a history of UTI, voiding dysfunction, presence of a foreign body, or immunosuppression should be considered at high risk for symptomatic UTI. Such high-risk patients merit either a single dose or short course of antimicrobial prophylaxis. We agree that low-risk patients do not require prophylactic antibiotics.

Ureteroscopy

Ureteroscopy is a first-line approach for treating renal and ureteral calculi, as well as for diagnosis and treatment of upper tract urothelial tumors. As such, ureteroscopy is now one of the most common outpatient urological procedures. In contrast to cystoscopy and other transurethral procedures, there are few data on the infectious complications of ureteroscopy. Reported UTI rates following ureteroscopy range from 3.9 % to 25 %, despite almost ubiquitous use of routine prophylactic antimicrobials.

In a case series of 378 patients undergoing ureteroscopy, Puppo and colleagues reported postoperative fever after 3.9 % of procedures for ureterolithiasis (Puppo et al. 1999). Because the focus of this report was not on infectious complications, routine postoperative urine cultures were not obtained and antimicrobial use was not described. In 1991, Rao et al. (1991) described 117 patients undergoing endoscopic treatment of renal and ureteral stones (Rao et al. 1991). Bacteremia occurred in nearly one-quarter of patients; however, the authors included many more invasive procedures such as percutaneous nephrolithotomy in this series. Thus, the information is of limited utility. Hendrikx and colleagues collected infection data in a randomized trial comparing extracorporeal shock wave lithotripsy to ureteroscopy for treatment of mid-to-distal ureteral stones. Among 156 patients undergoing ureteroscopy, 3.5 % had signs of pyelonephritis with septicemia, including fever greater than 38.5 °C and symptomatic UTI (Hendrikx et al. 1999). As infection rates were not the focus of their study, details of prophylactic antimicrobial regimens were not provided. In 2003, Knopf randomized 113 patients undergoing ureteroscopy for stone treatment, without clinical evidence of UTI to a single oral dose of levofloxacin vs no prophylaxis (Knopf et al. 2003). Although no patient in either group developed a symptomatic UTI, there was a significant reduction in postoperative bacteriuria from 12.5 % to 1.8 % in the antimicrobial therapy group.

These data are limited; however they support the standard practice of prophylactic antimicrobial therapy for patients undergoing ureteroscopy and suggest that treatment is associated with lower rates of infectious complications.

Nephroscopy

Percutaneous entry to the renal collecting system is necessary for the treatment of large renal calculi, for patients who fail shock-wave lithotripsy, or for stones in kidneys with anatomic abnormalities. As with ureteroscopy, very limited data are available on the infectious risks of nephroscopy. With the need to traverse the renal parenchyma, there is elevated concern for causing bacteremia and sepsis syndrome.

Rao and colleagues described a series of 27 patients undergoing percutaneous nephrolithotomy (Rao et al. 1991). Nearly 40% of patients developed sepsis syndrome despite routine use of prophylactic antibiotics. The clinical importance of this observation was underscored by O'Keefe's series of 700 patients undergoing percutaneous procedures for upper tract stones. In this series, sepsis syndrome occurred in 1.3% of patients, with a 66% associated mortality rate (O'Keeffe et al. 1993). Mariappan and colleagues described 54 patients undergoing percutaneous nephrolithotomy. Patients were monitored closely for sepsis syndrome using very strictly defined criteria. Despite routine perioperative intravenous gentamicin therapy, nearly 6% developed sepsis syndrome (Mariappan et al. 2005).

These observations support the routine use of antimicrobial prophylaxis for patients undergoing nephroscopy. Infectious complications are common, and it may be difficult to identify patients with risk factors such as positive renal pelvis urine or culture-positive stones preoperatively.

Transurethral Prostatic Resection

Benign prostatic hypertrophy (BPH) is a common urologic problem affecting older men. With the development of selective alpha-antagonists and 5-alpha reductase inhibitors, the need for surgical intervention has decreased dramatically. However, TURP remains the gold standard therapy for medically refractory prostatic obstruction.

Traditionally, TURP was considered a "clean-contaminated" procedure that did not require routine perioperative antimicrobial therapy (Childs 1986). However, postoperative bacteriuria rates up to 60% have been reported following TURP (Berry and Barratt 2002; Colau et al. 2001). The pathophysiology of infection after TURP is unknown, but likely results from urethral abrasion and disruption of the prostatic bed (Berry and Barratt 2002). The sources of bacteria leading to infection include bladder colonization, prostatic adenoma, urethral flora, or perioperative contamination (Qiang et al. 2005).

Asymptomatic bacteriuria following TURP is of debatable clinical significance. In contrast, reported urosepsis rates post-TURP bacteriuria range from 1% to 4%, with an associated mortality rate of 13%. In cases of post-TURP sepsis, mortality rates increase to more that 20% in men over 65 years old. Further postoperative hospital stays may be prolonged by 0.6–5 days as a result of bacteriuria (Raz et al. 1994).

In 2002, Berry et al. reported a meta-analysis of 32 randomized controlled trials evaluating antimicrobial prophylaxis for TURP in patients with negative urine cultures (Berry and Barratt 2002). The meta-analysis included 4,260 patients, with 1,914 randomized to receive no antimicrobials, and 2,346 randomized to receive various perioperative antimicrobial regimens. The primary endpoints for the study were the development of bacteriuria, symptomatic infection, or urosepsis. Patients receiving prophylaxis had reduced rates of bacteriuria (9.1% vs 26%; $p<0.01$), and postoperative sepsis syndrome (0.7% vs 4.4%; $p<0.01$), corresponding to relative risk reductions of 65% and 77%, respectively. The effectiveness of particular agents was also analyzed, with aminoglycosides, co-trimoxazole, and cephalosporins all decreasing relative risks by 55% to 67%. Fluoroquinolones were evaluated in fewer studies; however, their administration was associated with a relative risk reduction of 92%. The duration of prophylactic antimicrobial therapy appeared important, with short course (<72 h) therapy proving more effective than a single preoperative dose. Extension of antibiotic therapy beyond 72 h was of little benefit. Of the 2,346 patients who received prophylactic antimicrobials, 19 (0.8%) had treatment-related adverse events, with only two (0.09%) considered moderate or severe.

More recently, Qiang confirmed Berry's findings in a systematic review of 28 randomized clinical trials of antimicrobial prophylaxis for TURP (Qiang et al. 2005). Additionally, they noted a reduced rate of postoperative fever in patients receiving prophylaxis (13.5% vs 2.6%). To identify potential risk factors for postoperative bacteriuria, Colau and colleagues collected prospective data on 101 men undergoing TURP. All patients had negative preoperative urine cultures and received a single preoperative cephalosporin dose (Colau et al. 2001). Nearly one-quarter of patients developed bacteriuria; however, all were easily treated, with no patient developing urosepsis. On multivariate analysis, the authors found that risks for bacteriuria included long operative times, increased duration of postoperative catheterization, and disruption of closed urethral catheter drainage.

In summary, these studies support the following conclusions on antimicrobial prophylaxis for patients undergoing TURP:

1. Assure that the patient has a negative urine culture preoperatively, if possible.
2. A single dose of perioperative antimicrobial therapy may decrease rates of postoperative bacteriuria and perhaps postoperative symptomatic UTIs.

3. Maintaining closed urinary drainage and minimizing the duration of postoperative catheterization substantially reduce postoperative infection rates.

Transurethral Resection of Bladder Tumor

Compared with TURP, little has been published on the infectious complications of TURBT. In 1990, Badenoch and colleagues prospectively analyzed TURBT complications in 51 patients. Interestingly, infected tumors were identified in 75 % of females and 18 % of males. In most cases, tumor infections correlated with preoperative urine culture results (Badenoch et al. 1990).

Extrapolating from the data on TURP, we recommend the following:

1. Avoid TURBT in patients with positive urine cultures, if possible.
2. Despite few data suggesting that routine antimicrobial prophylaxis results in improved results, such therapy should be recommended for high-risk patients.
3. Maintain sterile closed urinary drainage.
4. Minimize the duration of postoperative catheterization.

Prostate Needle Biopsy

Over the past 15 years, advances in screening and diagnosis of prostate cancer have changed the practice of urology. In 1989, Hodge and colleagues introduced the concept of sextant biopsies for detecting prostate cancer. This represented a marked improvement from the earlier practice of directed biopsies of palpable lesions or abnormalities visualized by transrectal ultrasound (Hodge et al. 1989).

Data supporting prophylactic antimicrobials for prostate biopsy are conflicting. Aron and colleagues randomized 231 men into three groups: placebo for 3 days, single dose oral antimicrobial therapy, or oral prophylaxis for 3 days. Significantly more patients in the placebo group developed infectious complications. They found no benefit from increasing duration of prophylaxis from single dose to 3 days (Aron et al. 2000). Additional studies have noted similar results and support the routine use of single-dose therapy (Griffith et al. 2002; Kapoor et al. 1998; Enlund and Varenhorst 1997).

For patients with valvular heart disease, the American Heart Association recommends 2 g of intravenous ampicillin plus 80 mg of gentamicin, administered 30 min before the procedure to prevent bacterial endocarditis (Dajani et al. 1997b).

Following total joint replacements, patients at highest risk for joint infection (see above) should receive either a single oral quinolone dose taken 1–2 h before biopsy or 2 g of parenteral ampicillin (or 1 g intravenous vancomycin for patients allergic to penicillin) plus 80 mg of gentamicin at least 30 min before the procedure (American Urological Society/American Academy of Orthopaedic Surgeons 2003).

Historically, an enema was routine prior to prostate biopsy. This practice has been examined by multiple investigators. Recently, Carey and Korman analyzed 410 patients who received 3 days of oral ciprofloxacin. Two hundred twenty-five patients received enemas prior to biopsy while 185 did not. The authors concluded that a prebiopsy enema provided no significant clinical advantage (Carey and Korman 2001). Lindbert et al. (2000) randomized 50 patients to receive either a prebiopsy enema or no enema. In this study, both arms received postbiopsy oral antibiotics, and patients were evaluated with post-biopsy urine and blood cultures prior to antibiotic administration. Although the authors found no difference in postbiopsy bacteriuria rates, patients who had received enemas were less likely to develop bacteremia (16 %) than those who had not received enemas (87 %, $p = 0.003$).

In summary, prophylactic antimicrobial therapy (e.g., an oral quinolone) is recommended prior to prostate biopsy. There is no consensus on the value of enemas to decrease infectious complications.

18.2.3.3 Presentation and Clinical Approach

The clinical presentation of UTI varies widely depending on the organs involved, bacterial virulence, the patient's urological anatomy and immune function, and the patient's sensory and communication capabilities. Further, irritative urinary symptoms and hematuria are present routinely following urological procedures, further complicating diagnosis of UTI.

In cases where there is concern for postoperative infection, clinicians should take a history focusing on details of the operative procedure and the patient's anatomy. In addition to the usual symptoms of UTI, attention to systemic symptoms and signs aids in determining if the patient has developed bacteremia or is progressing to sepsis syndrome. For some patients, it may prove difficult to determine whether symptoms result from the procedure itself or whether symptoms result from UTI. Other patients may experience no symptoms at all in the setting of UTI.

Physical examination should focus on the genitourinary tract. A more general exam may often be indicated as UTI can ascend from the lower to the upper urinary tract and local infections can cause systemic symptoms and signs. A patient's vital signs and urine production must be monitored closely for evidence of bacteremia or impending sepsis. Typically, such a systemic infection is typically heralded by fever, tachycardia, or low urinary output. When accompanied by hypotension, these findings indicate that septic shock is present.

Urine cultures are crucial to making a diagnosis. However, urinalysis may be of limited value. The urinalysis routinely shows erythrocytes, pyuria, and proteinuria following instrumentation of the genitourinary tract. When possible, a mid-stream, clean-catch urine sample is the optimal specimen.

Depending upon the specific procedure or the patient's presentation, additional studies may be indicated. For example, in the setting of suspected pyelonephritis following ureteroscopy or nephroscopy, radiographic studies should be performed to determine if the collecting system is obstructed or if there are signs of an abscess. Potential imaging modalities include antegrade nephrostogram, renal-bladder ultrasonography, computerized tomography, or abdominal plain film to assess the position of a previously placed stent or tube. The optimal imaging study depends on the clinical setting.

In the setting of fever and presumed bacteremia, we recommend obtaining a complete blood count and serum chemistries, as well as two peripheral blood cultures.

We have several general recommendations:

1. In all cases of presumed postprocedure UTI, quantitative urine cultures should be speciated, and antimicrobial sensitivities obtained. Ideally, these urine specimens should be obtained prior to initiating therapy.
2. Always ensure the patency of urethral catheters, nephrostomy, stents, or other urological tubing.
3. If started prior to availability of culture results, antimicrobial therapy must be modified based on sensitivity data and the patient's clinical response.
4. Additional imaging may indicate other factors that require attention, such as relief of obstruction or drainage of an abscess.

References

Alexander JW, Fischer JE, Boyajian M, Palmquist J, Morris MJ (1983) The influence of hair-removal methods on wound infections. Arch Surg 118:347

American Urological Association; American Academy of Orthopaedic Surgeons (2003) Antibiotic prophylaxis for urological patients with total joint replacements. J Urol 169:1796

Anonymous (2004) National Nosocomial Infections Surveillance (NNIS) System Report, data summary from January 1992 through June 2004, issued October 2. Am J Infect Control 32:470

Aron M, Rajeev TP, Gupta NP (2000) Antibiotic prophylaxis for transrectal needle biopsy of the prostate: a randomized controlled study. BJU Int 85:682

Asensio A, Ramos A, Munez E, Vilanova JL, Torrijos P, Garcia FJ (2005) Preoperative low molecular weight heparin as venous thromboembolism prophylaxis in patients at risk for prosthetic infection after knee arthroplasty. Infect Control Hosp Epidemiol 26:903

Badenoch DF, Murdoch DA, Tiptaft RC (1990)Microbiological study of bladder tumors, their histology and infective complications. Urology 35:5

Belda FJ, Aguilera L, Garcia de la Asuncion J et al (2005) Supplemental perioperative oxygen and the risk of surgical wound infection: a randomized controlled trial. JAMA 294:2035

Berbari EF, Osmon DR, Duffy MC et al (2006) Outcome of prosthetic joint infection in patients with rheumatoid arthritis: the impact of medical and surgical therapy in 200 episodes. Clin Infect Dis 42:216

Berry A, Barratt A (2002) Prophylatic antibiotic use in transurethral prostatic resection: a meta-analysis. J Urol 167:571

Bratzler DW, Houck PM (2005) Antimicrobial prophylaxis for surgery: an advisory statement from the National Surgical Infection Prevention Project. Am J Surg 189:395

Bryan DE, Mulcahy JJ, Simmons GR (2002) Salvage procedure for infected noneroded artificial urinary sphincters. J Urol 168:2464

Buchholz HW, Elson RA, Engelbrecht E, Lodenkamper H, Rottger J, Siegel A (1981) Management of deep infection of total hip replacement. J Bone Joint Surg Br 63-B:342

Bydder GM, Kreel L (1980) Computed tomography in the diagnosis of abdominal abscess. J Comput Tomogr 4:132

Carey JM, Korman HJ (2001) Transrectal ultrasound guided biopsy of the prostate. Do enemas decrease clinically significant complications? J Urol 166:82

Carson CC 3rd (2004) Efficacy of antibiotic impregnation of inflatable penile prostheses in decreasing infection in original implants. J Urol 171:1611

Carson CC, Robertson CN (1988) Late hematogenous infection of penile prostheses. J Urol 139:50

Catto JW, Natarajan V, Tophill PR (2005) Simultaneous augmentation cystoplasty is associated with earlier rather than increased artificial urinary sphincter infection. J Urol 173:1237

Childs SJ (1986) Appropriate surgical prophylaxis in transurethral genitourinary surgery and potential reduction in nosocomial infections. Urology 27:415

Christou NV, Nohr CW, Meakins JL (1987) Assessing operative site infection in surgical patients. Arch Surg 122:165

Classen DC, Evans RS, Pestotnik SL, Horn SD, Menlove RL, Burke JP (1992) The timing of prophylactic administration of antibiotics and the risk of surgical-wound infection. N Engl J Med 326:281

Colau A, Lucet JC, Rufat P, Botto H, Benoit G, Jardin A (2001) Incidence and risk factors of bacteriuria after transurethral resection of the prostate. Eur Urol 39:272

Culver DH, Horan TC, Gaynes RP et al (1991) Surgical wound infection rates by wound class, operative procedure, and patient risk index. National Nosocomial Infections Surveillance System. Am J Med 91:152S

Dajani AS, Taubert KA, Wilson W et al (1997a) Prevention of bacterial endocarditis: recommendations by the American Heart Association. Clin Infect Dis 25:1448

Dajani AS, Taubert KA, Wilson W et al (1997b) Prevention of bacterial endocarditis. Recommendations by the American Heart Association. JAMA 277:1794

Darouiche RO (2004) Treatment of infections associated with surgical implants. N Engl J Med 350:1422

Enlund AL, Varenhorst E (1997) Morbidity of ultrasound-guided transrectal core biopsy of the prostate without prophylactic antibiotic therapy. A prospective study in 415 cases. Br J Urol 79:777

Falcoz PE, Laluc F, Toubin MM et al (2005) Usefulness of procalcitonin in the early detection of infection after thoracic surgery. Eur J Cardiothorac Surg 27:1074

Fuenfer MM, Olson GE, Polk HC Jr (1975) Effect of various cor-

ticosteroids upon the phagocytic bactericidal activity of neutrophils. Surgery 78:27
Furuno JP, Perencevich EN, Johnson JA et al (2005) Methicillin-resistant Staphylococcus aureus and vancomycin-resistant Enterococci co-colonization. Emerg Infect Dis 11:1539
Ganesan GS, Nguyen DH, Adams MC et al (1993) Lower urinary tract reconstruction using stomach and the artificial sphincter. J Urol 149:1107
Gaynes RP, Culver DH, Horan TC, Edwards JR, Richards C, Tolson JS (2001) Surgical site infection (SSI) rates in the United States, 1992: the National Nosocomial Infections Surveillance System basic SSI risk index. Clin Infect Dis 33 [Suppl 2]:S69
Gomha MA, Boone TB (2002) Artificial urinary sphincter for post-prostatectomy incontinence in men who had prior radiotherapy: a risk and outcome analysis. J Urol 167:591
Grabe M (2001) Perioperative antibiotic prophylaxis in urology. Curr Opin Urol 11:81
Grey NJ, Perdrizet GA (2004) Reduction of nosocomial infections in the surgical intensive-care unit by strict glycemic control. Endocr Pract 10 [Suppl 2]:46
Griffith BC, Morey AF, Ali-Khan MM, Canby-Hagino E, Foley JP, Rozanski TA (2002) Single dose levofloxacin prophylaxis for prostate biopsy in patients at low risk. J Urol 168:1021
Hajivassiliou CA (1999) A review of the complications and results of implantation of the AMS artificial urinary sphincter. Eur Urol 35:36
Heinzelmann M, Scott M, Lam T (2002) Factors predisposing to bacterial invasion and infection. Am J Surg 183:179
Hendrikx AJ, Strijbos WE, de Knijff DW, Kums JJ, Doesburg WH, Lemmens WA (1999) Treatment for extended-mid and distal ureteral stones: SWL or ureteroscopy? Results of a multicenter study. J Endourol 13:727
Henry GD, Wilson SK, Delk JR 2nd et al (2004) Penile prosthesis cultures during revision surgery: a multicenter study. J Urol 172:153
Henry GD, Wilson SK, Delk JR 2nd et al (2005) Revision washout decreases penile prosthesis infection in revision surgery: a multicenter study. J Urol 173:89
Hodge KK, McNeal JE, Terris MK, Stamey TA (1989) Random systematic versus directed ultrasound guided transrectal core biopsies of the prostate. J Urol 142:71
Holmes NM, Kogan BA, Baskin LS (2001) Placement of artificial urinary sphincter in children and simultaneous gastrocystoplasty. J Urol 165:2366
Jarow JP (1996) Risk factors for penile prosthetic infection. J Urol 156:402
Kabalin JN, Kessler R (1988) Infectious complications of penile prosthesis surgery. J Urol 139:953
Kapoor DA, Klimberg IW, Malek GH et al (1998) Single-dose oral ciprofloxacin versus placebo for prophylaxis during transrectal prostate biopsy. Urology 52:552
Kaufman JJ, Lindner A, Raz S (1982) Complications of penile prosthesis surgery for impotence. J Urol 128:1192
Kaufman JM, Kaufman JL, Borges FD (1998) Immediate salvage procedure for infected penile prosthesis. J Urol 159:816
Khurrum Baig M, Hua Zhao R, Batista O et al (2002) Percutaneous postoperative intra-abdominal abscess drainage after elective colorectal surgery. Tech Coloproctol 6:159
Kiddoo DA, Wollin TA, Mador DR (2004) A population based assessment of complications following outpatient hydrocelectomy and spermatocelectomy. J Urol 171:746
Kirkland KB, Briggs JP, Trivette SL, Wilkinson WE, Sexton DJ (1999) The impact of surgical-site infections in the 1990 s: attributable mortality, excess length of hospitalization, and extra costs. Infect Control Hosp Epidemiol 20:725
Knopf HJ, Graff HJ, Schulze H (2003) Perioperative antibiotic prophylaxis in ureteroscopic stone removal. Eur Urol 44:115
Kortmann BB, Sonke GS, D'Ancona F C, Floratos DL, Debruyne FM, De La Rosette JJ (1999) The tolerability of urodynamic studies and flexible cysto-urethroscopy used in the assessment of men with lower urinary tract symptoms. BJU Int 84:449
Kraklau DM, Wolf JS Jr (1999) Review of antibiotic prophylaxis recommendations for office-based urologic procedures. Tech Urol 5:123
Krieger JN (2002) Urinary tract infections: what's new? J Urol 168:2351
Kunin CM (1994) Guidelines for urinary tract infections. Rationale for a separate strata for patients with "low-count" bacteriuria. Infection 22 Suppl 1:S38
Kunin CM (2001) Nosocomial urinary tract infections and the indwelling catheter: what is new and what is true? Chest 120:10
Kunin CM (2003) Definition of acute pyelonephritis vs the urosepsis syndrome. Arch Intern Med 163:2393
Kurz A, Sessler DI, Lenhardt R (1996) Perioperative normothermia to reduce the incidence of surgical-wound infection and shorten hospitalization. Study of Wound Infection and Temperature Group. N Engl J Med 334:1209
Lindert KA, Kabalin JN, Terris MK (2000) Bacteremia and bacteriuria after transrectal ultrasound guided prostate biopsy. J Urol 164:76
Manson AL (1988) Is antibiotic administration indicated after outpatient cystoscopy. J Urol 140:316
Mariappan P, Smith G, Bariol SV, Moussa SA, Tolley DA (2005) Stone and pelvic urine culture and sensitivity are better than bladder urine as predictors of urosepsis following percutaneous nephrolithotomy: a prospective clinical study. J Urol 173:1610
Martins FE, Boyd SD (1995) Post-operative risk factors associated with artificial urinary sphincter infection-erosion. Br J Urol 75:354
Merrill DC (1988) Clinical experience with the Mentor inflatable penile prosthesis in 301 patients. J Urol 140:1424
Miley GB, Scheller AD, Jr Turner RH (1982) Medical and surgical treatment of the septic hip with one-stage revision arthroplasty. Clin Orthop Relat Res (170):76
Miller EA, Mayo M, Kwan D, Mitchell M (1998) Simultaneous augmentation cystoplasty and artificial urinary sphincter placement: infection rates and voiding mechanisms. J Urol 160:750
Minervini A, Ralph DJ, Pryor JP (2006) Outcome of penile prosthesis implantation for treating erectile dysfunction: experience with 504 procedures. BJU Int 97:129
Montague DK (1987) Periprosthetic infections. J Urol 138:68
Montague DK, Jarow JP, Broderick GA et al (2005) Chapter 1: The management of erectile dysfunction: an AUA update. J Urol 174:230
Mulcahy JJ (2000) Long-term experience with salvage of infected penile implants. J Urol 163:481
Mulcahy JJ, Brant MD, Ludlow JK (1995) Management of infected penile implants. Tech Urol 1:115
Nickel JC, Heaton J, Morales A, Costerton JW (1986) Bacterial biofilm in persistent penile prosthesis-associated infection. J Urol 135:586
Noone TC, Semelka RC, Worawattanakul S, Marcos HB (1998) Intraperitoneal abscesses: diagnostic accuracy of and appearances at MR imaging. Radiology 208:525
Noone TC, Semelka RC, Chaney DM, Reinhold C (2004) Abdominal imaging studies: comparison of diagnostic accuracies resulting from ultrasound, computed tomography, and magnetic resonance imaging in the same individual. Magn Reson Imaging 22:19
O'Keeffe NK, Mortimer AJ, Sambrook PA, Rao PN (1993) Severe sepsis following percutaneous or endoscopic procedures for urinary tract stones. Br J Urol 72:277

Onur R, Ozden M, Orhan I, Kalkan A, Semercioz A (2004) Incidence of bacteraemia after urodynamic study. J Hosp Infect 57:241
Petero VG, Jr Diokno AC (2006) Comparison of the long-term outcomes between incontinent men and women treated with artificial urinary sphincter. J Urol 175:605
Puppo P, Ricciotti G, Bozzo W, Introini C (1999) Primary endoscopic treatment of ureteric calculi. A review of 378 cases. Eur Urol 36:48
Qiang W, Jianchen W, MacDonald R, Monga M, Wilt TJ (2005) Antibiotic prophylaxis for transurethral prostatic resection in men with preoperative urine containing less than 100,000 bacteria per ml: a systematic review. J Urol 173:1175
Raj GV, Peterson AC, Toh KL, Webster GD (2005) Outcomes following revisions and secondary implantation of the artificial urinary sphincter. J Urol 173:1242
Rane A, Cahill D, Saleemi A, Montgomery B, Palfrey E (2001) The issue of prophylactic antibiotics prior to flexible cystoscopy. Eur Urol 39:212
Rao PN, Dube DA, Weightman NC, Oppenheim BA, Morris J (1991) Prediction of septicemia following endourological manipulation for stones in the upper urinary tract. J Urol 146:955
Raves JJ, Slifkin M, Diamond DLA (1984) bacteriologic study comparing closed suction and simple conduit drainage. Am J Surg 148:618
Raz R, Almog D, Elhanan G, Shental J (1994) The use of ceftriaxone in the prevention of urinary tract infection in patients undergoing transurethral resection of the prostate (TUR-P). Infection 22:347
Schwartz BF, Swanzy S, Thrasher JB (1996) A randomized prospective comparison of antibiotic tissue levels in the corpora cavernosa of patients undergoing penile prosthesis implantation using gentamicin plus cefazolin versus an oral fluoroquinolone for prophylaxis. J Urol 156:991
Silverstein A, Donatucci CF (2003) Bacterial biofilms and implantable prosthetic devices. Int J Impot Res 15 [Suppl 5]:S150
Small MP (1978) Small-Carrion penile prosthesis: a report on 160 cases and review of the literature. J Urol 119:365
Stamm WE (2003) Urinary tract infections. Infect Dis Clin North Am 17:xiii-xiv
Stone HH, Haney BB, Kolb LD, Geheber CE, Hooper CA (1979) Prophylactic and preventive antibiotic therapy: timing, duration and economics. Ann Surg 189:691
Sullivan NM, Sutter VL, Mims MM, Marsh VH, Finegold SM (1973) Clinical aspects of bacteremia after manipulation of the genitourinary tract. J Infect Dis 127:49
Tegnell A, Aren C, Ohman L (2002) Wound infections after cardiac surgery–a wound scoring system may improve early detection. Scand Cardiovasc J 36:60
Townsend CM Jr (ed) (2004) Sabiston textbook of surgery, 17th edn. Saunders Elsevier, Philadelphia
Ure KJ, Amstutz HC, Nasser S, Schmalzried TP (1998) Direct-exchange arthroplasty for the treatment of infection after total hip replacement. An average ten-year follow-up. J Bone Joint Surg Am 80:961
Venn SN, Greenwell TJ, Mundy AR (2000) The long-term outcome of artificial urinary sphincters. J Urol 164:702
Weiss CA 3rd Statz CL, Dahms RA, Remucal MJ, Dunn DL, Beilman GJ (1999) Six years of surgical wound infection surveillance at a tertiary care center: review of the microbiologic and epidemiological aspects of 20,007 wounds. Arch Surg 134:1041
Wilson SK, Delk JR 2nd (1995) Inflatable penile implant infection: predisposing factors and treatment suggestions. J Urol 153:659

18.3 Emergencies in Continent Bladder Replacement

M.C. Schumacher, F.C. Burkhard, U.E. Studer

18.3.1 Introduction

Following continent bladder substitution, acute life-threatening situations are rare, but there are complications that require immediate attention. In this chapter we focus on emergencies that are specific for continent bladder replacement. Emergencies specific to surgery, such as blood loss, lymphoceles, thrombosis, abscess, and anastomotic insufficiency are not discussed.

18.3.2 Continent Urinary Diversion

Continent urinary diversion has become a widely accepted surgical procedure in patients after cystectomy. Although continent urinary diversion is certainly appropriate in selected patients, these procedures are technically more demanding and are associated with specific postoperative and long-term complications compared to noncontinent urinary diversion procedures. Continent, nonorthotopic urinary diversion can be divided into two major categories: ureterosigmoidostomy and its variations, such as ileocecal sigmoidostomy, rectal bladder, and sigmoid Hemi-Kock operation with colonic intussusception, allowing the excretion of urine by bowel evacuation; and continent cutaneous diversions requiring clean intermittent catheterization of the reservoir at regular intervals.

18.3.3 Diversion-Related Emergencies

18.3.3.1 Acute Metabolic Disturbances Requiring Immediate Attention

Metabolic disturbances are a frequent early complication after bladder substitution with an intestinal segment, which can present with severe symptoms and require immediate attention. Overall metabolic complications occur in approximately 6 % following ileal bladder substitution (Hautmann et al. 1999; Studer et al. 2006; Stein et al. 2004). In large series incorporating colon segments, metabolic complications appear to be lower, around 2 % (Table 18.3.1) (Elmajian et al. 1996).

The pathophysiological mechanism behind metabolic disturbances is the ileum's normal function, namely to produce iso-osmotic contents by rapidly absorbing or secreting sodium and chloride ions in response to the osmolarity of its contents (Mills and Studer 1999). This can result in a counteraction to the renal regulation of body sodium and acid base balance, and particularly patients with renal impairment are at great risk of metabolic complications. If long or proximal ileal segments are used, salt loss can also occur, especially in the early postoperative phase when the patient is encouraged to drink a lot of liquid and therefore produces hypotonic urine. The ileal bladder substitute then shifts sodium and chloride from the blood stream to the urine to restore urinary iso-osmolality. Thus, unless the patient takes sufficient extra salt, a salt-losing hypovolemic state can occur. Potassium absorption from the reservoir, in exchange for sodium, saturates the renal exchange mechanism and reduces hydrogen ion excretion and thus a hyperkalemic, hypochloremic acidosis ensues. Hyperchloremic, hypokalemic acidosis, as seen

Table 18.3.1. Severe metabolic complications requiring hospitalization as an early (<30 days) and late (>30 days) postoperative emergency in patients after continent urinary diversion

Authors	Type of continent urinary diversion	Metabolic acidosis and salt loss syndrome Early N (%)	Late N (%)
Studer et al. 2006 ($n=482$)	Ileal orthotopic	9 (1.9)	21 (4.4)
Hautmann et al. 1999 ($n=363$)	Ileal orthotopic	0[a]	4 (1.1)[a]
Stein et al. 2004 ($n=209$)	Ileal orthotopic (T-pouch)	10 (4.8)	0
D'Elia et al. 2004 ($n=123$)	Mainz pouch II	0	0
Elmajin et al. 1996 ($n=295$)	Kock pouch	6 (2.0)[a]	1 (0.3)[a]
Abol-Enein et al. 2004 ($n=109$)	Cutaneous ileal pouch	0	0
Leissner et al. 1999 ($n=103$)	Mainz pouch I	–[b]	–[b]

[a] Early <3 months, late >3 months
[b] no information

with an ureterosigmoidostomy, may also occur. This arises from sodium and chloride reabsorption, with potassium secretion. Absorbed ammonium ions are the principal source of acidosis and responsible for acute acidosis and ensuing vomiting. The resulting chronic acidosis may produce osteoporosis or osteomalacia.

In contrast, the main absorptive function of the colon is water recovery through active sodium and chloride reabsorption. This may lead to serum hyperosmolarity with an increased antidiuretic hormone release, resulting in highly concentrated urine from which the colon will absorb more sodium and chloride. At the same time, ammonium is absorbed, which is thought to be the main mechanism leading to metabolic acidosis, the result being hyperchloremic metabolic acidosis.

Diagnosis and Management

Patients generally feel lethargic, tired, and nauseous and have no appetite. In severe cases vomiting, dehydration, weight loss, and a grayish skin coloring can be noted. A venous blood gas analysis will show metabolic acidosis with a negative base excess.

Table 18.3.2. Clinical signs of acute metabolic acidosis in patients with ileal orthotopic bladder substitution

Early signs	Late signs
Fatigue	Vomiting
Loss of appetite	Dehydration
Nausea	Weight loss
Lethargic state	Grayish skin color

The immediate therapy is drainage of the bladder with a transurethral catheter, to minimize the contact time of the urine with the reservoir. An intravenous fluid substitution with ringer lactate combined with per oral sodium bicarbonate substitution with 2–3 g/day should be initiated. Any negative base excess combined with symptoms should be treated. An infection of the urinary tract should be excluded, as urease splitting bacteria produce ammonium, which interacts with the sodium and proton transport through the cell membrane and can accentuate an already existing acidosis. Any bacteriuria should be treated with antibiotics (Table 18.3.2).

18.3.3.2 Urinary Tract Infection with Fever

In continent urinary diversion, data concerning upper urinary tract infection is sparse. In two large series, postoperative pyelonephritis was reported by Hautmann and Studer et al. in 4%–6% of their patients (Hautmann et al. 1999; Studer et al. 2006) (Table 18.3.3). Urinary sepsis was reported as a rare complication. In a series from Leissner et al. (1999), acute obstructive pyelonephritis as a consequence of uretero-intestinal stenosis occurred in 1% of their 103 patients with a Mainz pouch bladder substitute, as an early complication requiring emergency treatment with

Table 18.3.3. Urinary tract infection as an early (<30 days) and late (>30 days) postoperative emergency in patients after continent urinary diversion

Authors	Type of continent urinary diversion	Pyelonephritis Early N (%)	Late N (%)	Sepsis Early N (%)	Late N (%)
Studer et al. 2006 ($n=482$)	Ileal orthotopic	28 (5.8)	19 (3.9)	7 (1.5)	10 (2.1)
Hautmann et al. 1999 ($n=363$)	Ileal orthotopic	22 (6.1)[a]	23 (6.3)[a]	–	–
Stein et al. 2004 ($n=209$)	Ileal orthotopic (T-pouch)	–	–	4 (1.9)	0
D'Elia et al. 2004 ($n=123$)	Mainz Pouch II	–	–	–	–
Elmajin et al. 1996 ($n=295$)	Kock pouch	–	–	5 (1.7)[a]	0
Abol-Enein et al. 2004 ($n=109$)	Cutaneous ileal pouch	–	–	–	–
Leissner et al. 1999 ($n=103$)	Mainz pouch I	1 (1.0)	0	–	–

[a] early <3 months, late >3 months, – no information

placement of a percutaneous nephrostomy tube. If drainage is neglected a life-threatening sepsis can be the consequence. The cause of urinary tract infection and ascending pyelonephritis is most often reservoir outlet obstruction with increased residual urine and the cause of obstruction must be treated appropriately (see below). The diagnosis and treatment of infection should always be based on urinary cultures, and if these are positive patients must be treated. Most patients with urinary diversion using bowel segments have leukocyte esterase on dipstick examination and dipstick examination is only reliable if negative.

18.3.3.3 Urinary Retention (Acute or Chronic)

Orthotopic Bladder Substitutes

In orthotopic bladder substitutes, retention or incomplete emptying is observed overall in 6%–25% (Stein et al. 2004; Leissner et al. 1999; Abol-Enein and Ghoneim 2001). This rate is higher in women: approximately 8%–40%. The number of patients performing intermittent self-catheterization is 3%–20% (Hautmann et al. 1999; Studer et al. 2006; Stein et al. 2004; Abol-Enein and Ghoneim 2001) in men and up to 40% (Stein et al. 2004) in women. The reasons for development of retention are outlet obstruction because of infection due to increased mucous production, urethral strictures, ileo-urethral stenosis, recurrent prostatic adenoma, and protrusion of reservoir mucosa into the outlet. In women, voiding dysfunction is most likely the combined effect of anatomical mechanical and neurological components (Table 18.3.4) (Studer et al. 2006; Stein et al. 2004; Abol-Enein and Ghoneim 2001). Denervation of the proximal urethra in females leads to a flaccid hypotonic urethra with a tendency to kink, causing outlet obstruction. This may be avoided by resection of the proximal urethra, however, possibly at the cost of continence (Mills and Studer 2000).

Diagnosis and Management

Increased mucous production is often the first clinical sign of bacterial colonization and infection of the reservoir. Whenever bacteriuria and/or residual urine is found, endoscopy should be performed to determine the cause of outlet obstruction, which needs to be treated before complications from reservoir overdistension occur.

Bacterial infection should be treated in all cases by antibiotics until the urine is sterile. Most cases of mechanical outlet obstruction can be treated endoscopically. Mucosal protrusion into the bladder outlet requires transurethral resection of the protruding mucosa. In women, resection of the hypertrophic bladder neck, in our hands, has improved emptying in most cases.

18.3.3.4 Continent Catheterizable Reservoirs

In these patients, the main reason for acute retention is difficult catheterization and nipple stenosis, which occurs in 3%–25% (Holmes et al. 2002; Rowland 1995; Webster et al. 2003; Barqawi et al. 2004; De Ganck et al. 2002). Umbilical stomas have a higher tendency to nipple stenosis than abdominal stomas, whereas the material used for stoma construction does not appear to be of importance (Barqawi et al. 2004; De Ganck et al. 2002). A difference between the various continence mechanisms has been described, with 18% stenosis after a tunneled appendix, 9% after an intussuscepted valve, and 3% after stapled plicated valves (Table 18.3.5). Necrosis of both ileum and appendix stomas can occur, leading to the inability to catheterize (De Ganck et al. 2002). Attention to surgical detail may help

Table 18.3.4. Urinary retention in continuous urinary diversion

Authors	Type of continent urinary diversion	Number of patients (%)							
		Men/women	Retention/incomplete voiding	Urethral stricture	Ileo-urethral stenosis	Mucous retention	Mucosal prolapse	Recurrent prostate adenoma	Hypercontinence in women
Studer et al. 2006 ($n=482$)	Ileal orthotopic	442/40	22 (4.5%)[b]	18 (3.7)	12/447 (2.7)[c]	28 (5.8)	34 (7)	8 (1.7)	12/40 (30)
Hautmann et al. 1999 ($n=363$)	Ileal orthotopic	363/0	6 (1.7%)	11 (3.0)	17 (5.2)	17 (5.2)	–	–	–
Stein et al. 2004 ($n=209$)	Ileal orthotopic (T- Pouch)	169/40	49 (25%)	2 (1)	9 (4.3)	–	–	–	0
Abol-Enein et al. 2001 ($n=450$)	Ileal orthotopic	264/80 (344[a])	–	4/264 (1.5)	7 (2.7)	2 (0.6)	–	–	9/80 (11.2)
Elmajin et al. 1996 ($n=295$)	Kock pouch	295/0	8 (5.3%)	2 (0.7)	1 (0.3)	1 (0.3)	–	–	0

[a] Evaluable patients, [b] Three of these 22 patients required ISC, [c] Only patients without antireflex anastomosis

Table 18.3.5. Postoperative complications with ileal pouches after cystectomy

Authors	Type of continent urinary diversion	Number of patients with appendix/ileal nipple	Nipple stenosis appendix (%)	Nipple stenosis ileum (%)
Gerharz et al. 1997	Ileocecal pouch	96/106	18	2
Webster et al. 2003	Indiana pouch	0/74	–	4
Holmes et al. 2002	Indiana pouch	0/125	–	15
Abol-Enein et al. 2004	Ileal pouch	40/69	2	1.5
Lampel et al. 1996	Mainz pouch I	440[a]	15	12

[a] Total number of patients included

with fixation and stabilization of the continence mechanism to avoid angulations or kinking. Creation of a tension-free mucocutaneous anastomosis is important, as well as maintaining an adequate blood supply by avoiding compression of the mesoappendix or mesoileum. Chronic overdistension may be the result of patients not adhering to strict intervals of self-catheterization, resulting in an increased reservoir volume and as a consequence infection and increased mucous production, which in turn makes efficient emptying more difficult and supports infection.

Diagnosis and Management

In the acute situation, ultrasound shows a distended reservoir and placement of a guidewire, in some cases cystoscopically, before catheterization can be attempted. If this is not possible, ultrasound-guided placement of a drainage catheter parallel to the continence mechanism may be necessary. Some patients will present with difficulty catheterizing, which can clearly be located to the skin level. About half of these cases can be treated by placing three or four radiating incisions in an outpatient setting(De Ganck et al. 2002). Alternatively, open repair by a Y-V plasty or reimplantation of the nipple may be required. In the case of necrosis, complete reconstruction is necessary. Intermediately, some form of continuous drainage needs to be achieved.

18.3.3.5 Pouch Rupture or Perforation

Spontaneous rupture of augmentation cystoplasties are more frequently reported (4%–13%) than in bladder replacement. In a series from Scandinavia, 1,720 patients were followed by questionnaires sent to the urological departments performing continent urinary reservoirs (Mansson et al. 1997). Overall, 20 episodes of perforation occurred in 18 patients (1.5%), 17 of 1,070 patients with continent urinary diversion and only 1 of 650 with an orthotopic bladder substitute, where the urethra and the external sphincter may act as an overflow valve. Nippgen et al. reported on four spontaneous ruptures in 93 patients (4.3%) who underwent an ileal bladder substitution at their institute (Nippgen et al. 2001). In a relatively recent report on a patient with a ruptured sigmoid colon bladder substitute, Gupta stated that 13 cases of spontaneous rupture of ileal or ileocolonic bladder substitutes had been reported (Gupta et al. 2002). In most other large series, the authors report at most one case (Hautmann et al. 1999; Stein et al. 2004; Abol-Enein and Ghoneim 2001).

The cause of perforation or rupture is most likely acute retention of the reservoirs. In the case of an orthotopic bladder substitute, the urethra serves as an overflow valve. Once the pressure in the reservoir exceeds the urethral closing pressure, leakage occurs, causing overflow incontinence. In certain cases, this mechanism may fail and one report of a rupture of an ileal bladder was secondary to urinary retention caused by a mucosal plug in the bladder neck (Haupt et al. 1990). In contrast, in continent catheterizable reservoirs complete continence is achieved, which may explain the higher rate of spontaneous ruptures if the patient fails to catheterize. Some authors also consider chronic retention and overdistension to be a risk factor for rupture. Mechanically, a reservoir will rupture when the maximum wall tension is exceeded. According to Laplace's law, tension = 1/2 pressure × radius. Therefore at large volumes, the wall tension is higher at a given reservoir pressure. In reservoirs constructed from intestinal segments there may be areas of weakness (suture lines) as well as areas with suboptimal vascularization, possibly as a result of increased pressure. Another proposed cause for decreased wall strength in bowel segments is chronic bacterial colonization and inflammation as a result of continuous exposure to urine. This theory is controversial since in continent reservoirs chronic infection can be avoided, and the inflammatory infiltrate has been shown to be limited to the lamina propria and submucosa with the smooth muscle remaining unaffected.

The etiology of acute urinary retention in the sigma-rectum pouch is similar to other forms of continent urinary diversion. However, in our experience mucous from the large bowel tends to be of thicker consistency compared to mucous from the small bowel. This can be explained by the physiological function of the large bowel, namely to reabsorb sodium and fluid (Noble et al. 1990; Laguna et al. 2005).

Diagnosis and Management

Patients generally present with abdominal pain and distension. However, symptoms can range from mild, localized tenderness to severe generalized peritonitis and fever. These symptoms together with urinary retention should be treated as perforation until proven otherwise. In the case of incapacitated patients (unconscious) unable to empty their reservoirs, rupture of the reservoir should also be suspected.

For diagnosis, a cystogram should be performed; however, it can fail to show the perforation. The reservoir must be filled adequately, and multiple views should be taken in different positions. After emptying, no contrast should remain in the abdomen. Ultrasonography or CT imaging my reveal free intraperitoneal fluid. In case of acute overdistension of the pouch, postrenal azotemia occurs with increased urea and serum creatinine values. In case of pouch perforation, serum creatinine values are often normal, whereas urea is increased.

Surgical exploration (Mansson et al. 1997) is generally considered necessary for the management of rupture or perforation of intestinal reservoirs; however, conservative management has been described (Gupta et al. 2002; Parsons and Schoenberg 2001). Conservative management may be applicable in hemodynamically stable patients with localized abdominal symptoms under vigilant clinical monitoring and continuous drainage of the reservoir for 2–3 weeks combined with broad-spectrum antibiotics. Abdominal exploration is mandatory if there is progressive peritonitis, hemodynamic instability, or when sepsis develops.

18.3.4 Emergencies Not Related to Diversion

18.3.4.1 Bowel Obstruction

Early postoperative bowel obstruction is defined as an obstruction occurring within 30 days after surgery and is often difficult to differentiate from postoperative paralytic ileus (D'Elia et al. 2004). Adhesions are most often the cause for obstruction of the small bowel in the early postoperative period, but one must consider other possible etiologies requiring surgical intervention, such as pouch rupture (see Sect. 18.3.3.5 above), urinary extravasation, and abscess formation (Leissner et al. 1999).

In a series from Studer et al. (2006), ileus as an early complication (<30 days) after cystectomy and orthotopic bladder substitution occurred in 16 of 482 patients (3.3%). Conservative management was successful in 13 of these 16 patients (2.7%), whereas three patients (0.6%) were reoperated because of adhesions with consecutive mechanical bowel obstruction. Stein et al. (2004) reported on small bowel obstruction after cystectomy and construction of a T-pouch ileal neobladder in 13 of 209 patients (6.2%). Dividing the onset of complications not related to diversion into early (<30 days) and late (>30 days), they found that one of the most common late complications was small bowel obstruction. Seven of 209 patients (3.4%) had small-bowel obstruction and four patients (1.9%) required surgical intervention. In Studer et al.'s series, ileus occurred as a late complication in 34 of their 482 patients (7%) (Studer et al. 2006). Of these patients, two-thirds were managed conservatively, whereas 13 of 482 patients (2.7%) needed surgical intervention. Pickleman et al. (1989) reported on five of 109 patients (4.6%) with intestinal obstruction after cystectomy and continent cutaneous ileal pouch; of these five patients, one required surgical intervention (Table 18.3.6).

Urinary diversion not using small-bowel segments seems to be associated with less risk of postoperative small-bowel obstruction, as reported in a series from D'Elia et al. (2004) on 123 patients with Mainz pouch II ureterosigmoidostomy, with only two of 123 patients (1.6%) developing an acute abdomen. One patient presented with a mechanical ileus due to adhesions and required surgical reintervention with a thereafter uneventful course (Stein et al. 2004). Another patient developed acute peritonitis by dehiscence of a single-layer running suture of the anterior pouch wall and required

Table 18.3.6. Ileus as an early (<30 days) and late (>30 days) postoperative emergency in patients after continent urinary diversion

Authors	Type of continent urinary diversion	Conservative treatment Early N (%)	Conservative treatment Late N (%)	Surgical treatment Early N (%)	Surgical treatment Late N (%)
Studer et al. 2006 (n=482)	Ileal orthotopic	13 (2.7)	21 (4.3)	3 (0.6)	13 (2.7)
Hautmann et al. 1999 (n=363)	Ileal orthotopic	4 (1.1)[a]	–	7 (1.9)[a]	6 (1.6)[a]
Stein et al. 2004 (n=209)	Ileal orthotopic (T-pouch)	5 (2.4)	3 (1.4)	1 (0.5)	4 (1.9)
D'Elia et al. 2004 (n=123)	Mainz pouch II	–	–	1 (0.8)	–
Elmajin et al. 1996 (n=295)	Kock pouch	7 (2.4)[a]	1 (0.3)[a]	–	–
Abol-Enein et al. 2004 (n=109)	Cutaneous ileal pouch	4 (3.7)	–	1 (0.9)	–
Leissner et al. 1999 (n=103)	Mainz pouch I	–	–	–	1 (0.9)

[a] Early <3 months, late >3 months, – no information

emergency laparotomy and colostomy. Five months later, the anterior wall was revised and the colostomy closed (Table 18.3.6).

Intra- and postoperative management after urinary diversion is of great importance to minimize the risk of bowel obstruction. Minimal trauma during surgery, restricted use of electrocautery and covering the pelvic walls with peritoneal flaps are essential to achieve low complication rates. Another key issue regarding bowel function is to keep fluid input reasonably low. Crystalloids and plasma expanders used during surgery move into the third space, resulting in tissue edema hindering healing of the bowel anastomosis. Bowel edema may further prolong the paralytic state of the bowel after surgery. Therefore, a strict fluid balance with daily weight measurement is necessary to avoid these complications. The administration of intravenous glucose 5% and Furosemide at 10–20 mg per day will lower the serum osmolarity and help mobilization and excretion of retained fluids from the third space (Varol and Studer 2004).

Placement of an epidural catheter the day of surgery is recommended for two reasons: 1) to avoid the systemic use of analgesics (morphine derivates), which would increase the risk of ileus, and 2) because application of local anesthetics by an epidural catheter indirectly causes, via blockade of the sympathetic nervous system, a stimulation of the bowel movements and reduces the risk of paralytic ileus. Subcutaneous injections of Neostigmine methylsulphate 0.5 mg three times daily from the third postoperative day actively stimulates bowel movement and reduces gaseous distension (Kahi and Rex 2003; Saunders and Kimmey 2005). The most common side effects of Neostigmine methylsulphate are abdominal cramping due to bowel movements, excessive salivation, and bradycardia. In patients who smoke, a similar benefit can be obtained with nicotine patches, which directly stimulates bowel movements.

Intraoperative placement of a gastrostomy tube instead of a nasogastric tube not only has the advantage of increasing patient comfort, facilitating breathing, and allowing patients to drink the first postoperative day, but also stimulates the gastrocolic reflex and bowel peristalsis. After cystectomy a prolonged bowel paralysis often occurs, mainly due to the resection of peritoneum and to a lesser extent the small bowel anastomosis. Transferring the ureter in the retroperitoneal space from the left to the right side, while constructing an orthotopic ileal bladder or catheterizable pouch, as well as the incision of the mesoileum for isolation of the intestinal segment, increases the likelihood of prolonged paralysis of the intestine. The risk of possible complications by intraoperative placement of a gastrostomy tube after suturing the anterior gastric wall to the abdominal wall, which prevents any leakage of gastric fluid into the abdominal cavity, seems to be very low, at least in our experience.

Diagnosis and Management

Mechanical bowel obstruction is a surgical emergency and its diagnosis is often delayed or confused with that of postoperative paralytic ileus. The clinical features of early obstruction may be less apparent and analgesics may mask the clinical picture. A nasogastric tube, if not already in situ, should be placed to decompress the stomach and to prevent vomiting and aspiration pneumonia. Electrolyte imbalances, which promote ileus, should be excluded or corrected. Opiates are the most common promoters of ileus; therefore their use should be restricted. The first radiological study performed is plain abdominal radiography with the patient erect and supine. The presence of distended small bowel loops with fluid levels and paucity of colonic gas suggests small bowel ileus. The presence of free air indicates bowel perforation. Subsequent abdominal computerized tomography with oral Gastrografin (triple-contrast study) has the advantage of being able to identify possible intraabdominal causes of ileus, such as intestinal strangulation by adhesion, abscess, perianastomotic phlegmon, or leakage of bowel anastomosis. In case of persistent ileus with no clinical and radiological evidence of strangulating intestinal obstruction, conservative management with stimulation of the bowel activity should be attempted initially in every patient.

To avoid the occurrence of postoperative mechanical ileus, a thorough surgical operating technique with gentle dissection and handling of tissues, careful hemostasis to avoid hematoma formation, not denuding the peritoneum unnecessarily and avoiding potential orifices for internal hernias are essential.

18.3.5 Conclusions

Emergencies following continent urinary diversion are rare and often can be managed conservatively. The most common complications requiring immediate attention are pyelonephritis, metabolic acidosis, and retention, especially in continent catheterizable reservoirs. The risk that these problems occur can be lowered by meticulous patient follow-up, allowing recognition and treatment of increased postvoid residuals and urinary tract infection as well as providing an adequate sodium bicarbonate substitution. Pouch rupture is a rare emergency, which generally will require surgical treatment.

References

Abol-Enein H, Ghoneim MA (2001) Functional results of orthotopic ileal neobladder with serous-lined extramural ureteral reimplantation: experience with 450 patients. J Urol 165:1427

Abol-Enein H, Salem M, Mesbah A, Abdel-Latif M, Kamal M, Shabaan A et al (2004) Continent cutaneous ileal pouch using the serous lined extramural valves. The Mansoura experience in more than 100 patients. J Urol 172:588

Barqawi A, de Valdenebro M, Furness PD 3rd, Koyle MA (2004) Lessons learned from stomal complications in children with cutaneous catheterizable continent stomas. BJU Int 94:1344

De Ganck J, Everaert K, Van Laecke E, Oosterlinck W, Hoebeke P (2002) A high easy-to-treat complication rate is the price for a continent stoma. BJU Int 90:240

D'Elia G, Pahernik S, Fisch M, Hohenfellner R, Thuroff JW (2004) Mainz Pouch II technique:10 years' experience. BJU Int 93:1037

Elmajian DA, Stein JP, Esrig D, Freeman JA, Skinner EC, Boyd SD et al (1996) The Kock ileal neobladder: updated experience in 295 male patients. J Urol 156:920

Gerharz EW, Kohl U, Weingartner K, Melekos MD, Bonfig R, Riedmiller H (1997) Complications related to different continence mechanisms in ileocecal reservoirs. J Urol 158:1709

Gupta NP, Nabi G, Ansari MS (2002) Conservative management of spontaneous rupture of a sigmoid colon neobladder. Urol Int 69:325

Haupt G, Pannek J, Knopf HJ, Schulze H, Senge T (1990) Rupture of ileal neobladder due to urethral obstruction by mucous plug. J Urol 144:740

Hautmann RE, de Petriconi R, Gottfried HW, Kleinschmidt K, Mattes R, Paiss T (1999) The ileal neobladder: complications and functional results in 363 patients after 11 years of followup. J Urol 161:422

Holmes DG, Thrasher JB, Park GY, Kueker DC, Weigel JW (2002) Long-term complications related to the modified Indiana pouch. Urology 60:603

Kahi CJ, Rex DK (2003) Bowel obstruction and pseudo-obstruction. Gastroenterol Clin North Am 32:1229

Laguna MP, Brenninkmeier M, Belon JA, Marrero R, Wijkstra H, de la Rosette J et al (2005) Long-term functional and urodynamic results of 50 patients receiving a modified sigmoid neobladder created with a short distal segment. J Urol 174:963

Lampel A, Fisch M, Stein R, Schultz-Lampel D, Hohenfellner M, Eggersmann C et al (1996) Continent diversion with the Mainz pouch. World J Urol 14:85

Leissner J, Stein R, Hohenfellner R, Kohl U, Riedmiller H, Schroder A et al (1999) Radical cystoprostatectomy combined with Mainz pouch bladder substitution to the urethra: long-term results. BJU Int 83:964

Mansson W, Bakke A, Bergman B, Brekkan E, Jonsson O, Kihl B et al (1997) Perforation of continent urinary reservoirs. Scandinavian experience. Scand J Urol Nephrol 31:529

Mills RD, Studer UE (1999) Metabolic consequences of continent urinary diversion. J Urol 161:1057

Mills RD, Studer UE (2000) Female orthotopic bladder substitution: a good operation in the right circumstances. J Urol 163:1501

Nippgen JB, Hakenberg OW, Manseck A, Wirth MP (2001) Spontaneous late rupture of orthotopic detubularized ileal neobladders: report of five cases. Urology 58:43

Noble JR, Mata JA, Humble RL, Culkin DJ (1990) Maxi-pouch: a new technique for ileal conduit conversion to continent urinary reservoir. J Urol 143:116

Parsons JK, Schoenberg MP (2001) Successful conservative management of perforated ileal neobladder. J Urol 165:1214

Pickleman J, Lee RM (1989) The management of patients with suspected early postoperative small bowel obstruction. Ann Surg 210:216

Rowland R (1995) Complications of continent cutaneous reservoirs and neobladders-series using contemporary techniques. AUA Update Ser 14:202

Saunders MD, Kimmey MB (2005) Systematic review: acute colonic pseudo-obstruction. Aliment Pharmacol Ther 22:917

Stein JP, Dunn MD, Quek ML, Miranda G, Skinner DG (2004) The orthotopic T pouch ileal neobladder: experience with 209 patients. J Urol 172:584

Studer U, Burkhard F, Schumacher M, Kessler T, Thoeny H, Fleischmann A et al (2006) Twenty years experience with an ileal orthotopic low pressure bladder substitute – Lessons to be learned. J Urol 176:161

Varol C, Studer UE (2004) Managing patients after an ileal orthotopic bladder substitution. BJU Int 93:266

Webster C, Bukkapatnam R, Seigne JD, Pow-Sang J, Hoffman M, Helal M et al (2003) Continent colonic urinary reservoir (Florida pouch): long-term surgical complications (greater than 11 years). J Urol 169:174

Emergencies Following Renal Transplantation 18.4

M.A. Ghoneim, A.A. Shokeir

18.4.1 Introduction

Despite the remarkable improvement in the results of renal transplantation during the last decade, surgical and medical complications continue to contribute significantly to the morbidity and mortality of allograft recipients. Moreover, in live-donor renal transplantation the risks to living donors are small, but real. The objective of the present chapter is to review the complications that may affect the safety of both the donors and recipients as well as the efficacy of the graft. A special emphasis on the surgical complications in both the donors and recipients will be done. Other medical problems that may interfere with the proper diagnosis and prompt management of surgical emergencies will be discussed shortly.

18.4.2 The Living Donor: Surgical Emergencies

18.4.2.1 Mortality

Five deaths among 19,368 open nephrectomies were documented in US between January 1980 and January 1991; an incidence of 0.03 % (Najarian et al. 1992). Pulmonary emboli were the major cause of death, but none of the donors died intra- or postoperatively due to technical problems. In the Mansoura Urology and Nephrology Center, no mortality among 1,800 open nephrectomies was reported.

Matas et al. (2003) surveyed mortality and morbidity after living kidney donation in the US between 1 January 1999 and 1 July 2001. The survey included 171 US transplantation centers, which carried out 10,828 living-donor nephrectomies: 53 % open, 20.7 % hand-assisted, and 27 % non-hand assisted laparoscopic nephrectomy. Two donors died from surgical complications and one was in a persistent vegetative state; all after laparoscopic nephrectomy. Therefore, according to Matas et al., the mortality rate after laparoscopic nephrectomy is 0.1 %; triple the incidence of mortality after the conventional open technique. Vastag (2003) reported five donor deaths, all after laparoscopic nephrectomy in the US. Two kidney donors died from embolism, another from acute hemorrhage, and a fourth from respiratory failure. The cause of death of the fifth donor is uncertain. In addition, one donor death after laparoscopic nephrectomy resulting from cerebral gas embolism has been recently reported in a specialized transplantation center (Boghossian et al. 2005).

18.4.2.2 Morbidity: Intraoperative

Some recent series reported major intraoperative complications particular to laparoscopic nephrectomy. In a large single-center series including 738 laparoscopic nephrectomies, major intraoperative complications occurred in 6.8 % (Jacobs et al. 2004). The authors defined major complications as those representing significant risk to the donor's life. One graft was lost due to extensive vascular injury and in two donors nephrectomy was aborted due to colonic injury in one and mesenteric vein injury in the other. Recognized intraoperative injuries to the future allograft included seven injuries of arterial branches, four parenchymal lacerations, two large perinephric hematoma, and four renal vein injuries requiring intracorporeal suturing. The endovascular stapler also created 37 extra arteries for implantation. Graft malfunction due to technical issues occurred in 81 donors (11%). The authors concluded that the risks of laparoscopic nephrectomy to the donor must not be minimized.

On the other hand, there was a trend toward higher estimated blood loss in the open procedures than in laparoscopic procedures, although the difference was not always found to be statistically significant. Whether the laparoscopic procedure was hand-assisted did not seem to make a difference in these comparisons (Huynh and Hollander 2005).

18.4.2.3 Morbidity: Postoperative

Major postoperative complications such as pneumothorax, pneumonia, hemorrhage, deep vein thrombosis, pulmonary embolism, and wound problems were reported at rates of 1.4%–2.5% after live-donor nephrectomy (Blohme et al. 1992). Pulmonary and thrombotic complications occur more often with open nephrectomy. On the other hand, gastrointestinal complications such as bowel injury, bowel obstruction, internal hernia, and pancreatitis are more common with laparoscopic nephrectomy (Matas et al. 2003).

18.4.3 Recipients: Surgical and Nonsurgical Emergencies

Emergencies in the renal allograft recipient are defined as complications representing a significant risk to the survival of the patient and/or the graft. These emergencies could be classified as hemorrhagic complications, disorders causing early graft dysfunction, pathologies leading to late graft dysfunction, and surgical complications secondary to certain immunosuppressive medications. Table 18.4.1 provides a summary of these four broad categories.

Table 18.4.1. Emergencies of renal allograft recipient

Hemorrhagic emergencies
Primary hemorrhage
Secondary hemorrhage
Rupture of renal allograft
Rupture of mycotic aneurysm of renal allograft artery
Hematuria
Early graft dysfunction
Volume contraction
Acute tubular necrosis
Hyperacute, accelerated, and acute rejection
Renal artery thrombosis
Renal vein thrombosis
Urinary leakage
Ureteric obstruction
Drug toxicity
Early recurrence of the original kidney disease
Late graft dysfunction
Renal artery stenosis
Lymphocele
Ureteric obstruction
Chronic rejection
Surgical complications related to immunosuppressive drugs
Sirolimus: wound complications
Mycophenolate mofetil: intestinal bleeding or perforation
Cyclophosphamide: hemorrhagic cystitis.

18.4.3.1 Hemorrhagic Emergencies

Hemorrhagic complications may include primary hemorrhage occurring in the first 24–48 h after transplantation or secondary hemorrhage that may occur within a few weeks after transplantation due to rupture of the renal allograft or rupture of mycotic aneurysm of the renal allograft artery. Moreover, hematuria is not an uncommon complication occurring either early after transplantation or late as a complication of graft biopsy.

Primary Hemorrhage

As with all surgeries, postoperative bleeding may complicate renal transplant outcomes. Primary hemorrhagic complications have been little reported in the literature. In a recent study, we have reported a primary hemorrhage incidence of 23 out of 1,200 (1.9%) after live-donor renal transplantation (Osman et al. 2003). We observed a statistically significant association of such complications and grafts with multiple renal arteries.

Primary bleeding generally occurs during the first 24–48 h after the transplantation and is diagnosed by tachycardia, hypotension, a falling hematocrit level, swelling over the graft with a bulging incision, or significant bleeding coming through the incision or from the tube drain. Most often, this bleeding occurs in patients taking anticoagulation agents. If the hematoma is not clinically evident, a US or CT scan can define the size and help determine whether or not surgical evacuation is appropriate. Treatment includes immediate surgery and blood transfusion as necessary. The beeding site is identified and secured. Common sites of bleeding are the suture line of the vascular anastomosis, particularly with interrupted sutures, the exit site of the tube drain, and slipped ligature of the inferior epigastric artery. Additional stitches are usually sufficient to control the bleeding.

18.4.3.1.2 Secondary Hemorrhage

Spontaneous Renal Allograft Rupture

Spontaneous renal allograft rupture is one of the most dangerous complications following kidney transplantation and can result in graft loss. Its prevalence varies from 0.3% to 3% (Shahrokh et al. 2005). Rupture usually occurs in the first few weeks after transplantation. Predisposing factors for graft rupture include acute rejection, acute tubular necrosis, and renal vein thrombosis (Sanchez de la Nietra et al. 2004; Veroux et al. 2003). The condition usually manifests as sudden acute pain and swelling over the graft. Gray-scale US and noncontrast CT confirm presence of a large hematoma surrounding the graft. Rupture of the graft needs immediate surgical intervention with the evacuation of the hematoma and identification of the bleeding sites. The renal allograft vein and artery should be inspected and palpated to ensure their patency. Intraoperative power Doppler US is an excellent tool of assessment of renal perfusion. If the kidney is well perfused, a release incision of the renal allograft capsule (capsulotomy) will decrease the intrarenal tension of the excessive associated edema of the graft. A biopsy should be taken, bleeding sites are secured, and the wound is drained. On the other hand, a graft nephrectomy is carried out if it is proved to be nonvascularized.

Rupture of Mycotic Aneurysm of Renal Allograft Artery

Arterial mycotic aneurysm may develop as a result of sepsis within a few days to several weeks after transplantation at the site of the arterial anastomosis of the renal allograft. Mycotic aneurysms of the renal allograft artery are rarely detected before their rupture. The diagnosis currently relies on arteriography, but a high degree of suspicion is required to make the correct diagnosis. Rupture of the mycotic aneurysm is a life-threatening condition that needs immediate surgical exploration and graft nephrectomy. This dangerous event can be avoided by preventing infective complications of the wound (Laouad et al. 2005; Kyriakides et al. 1976).

Hematuria

Gross hematuria is not an uncommon observation immediately after transplantation, particularly with the use of anticoagulants. It is usually related to the method of ureteroneocystostomy. It is more common with the transvesical technique of Politano-Leadbetter than the extravesical method of Lich-Gregoir. Minor hematuria without clots is common in the first 2 days after transplantation and does not require treatment since it resolves spontaneously. Occasionally, hematuria is severe enough to cause clot retention, which is considered an emergency and is best managed by gentle intermittent manual irrigation and suction. It is better to avoid continuous bladder irrigation and cystoscopy for fear of leakage from the bladder suture line. It is advisable to withdraw anticoagulants during hematuria.

Transplant biopsy, which is frequently required in the posttransplantation period, may be complicated by hematuria, which can be severe enough to cause clot retention. Moreover, clots descending from the kidney and passing through the ureter may cause obstructive anuria (Rao 1986). In such situations, the cause of hematuria is accidental traumatic injury of a small blood vessel, which may lead to the development of arteriovenous fistula (Fig. 18.4.1). Normally, the bleeding resolves spontaneously, but occasionally it may be necessary to pass an irrigating catheter into the bladder to evacuate blood clots. In cases complicated with anuria, a graft percutaneous nephrectomy (PCN) is placed for a few days until spontaneous resolution of the intrarenal hematoma (Fig. 18.4.2).

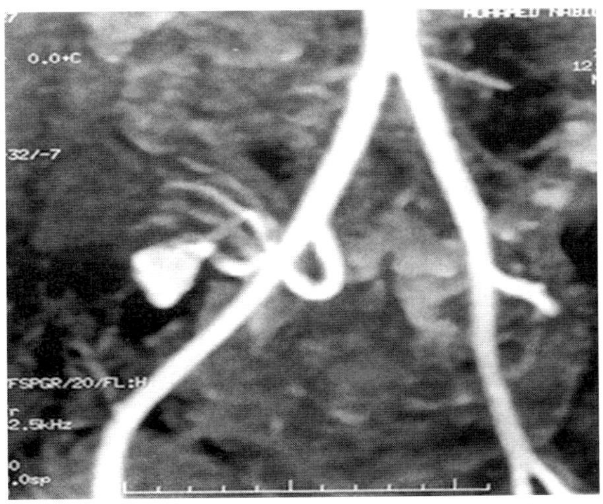

Fig. 18.4.1. Magnetic resonance angiography (MRA) showing arteriovenous communication in the lower pole of the graft following biopsy

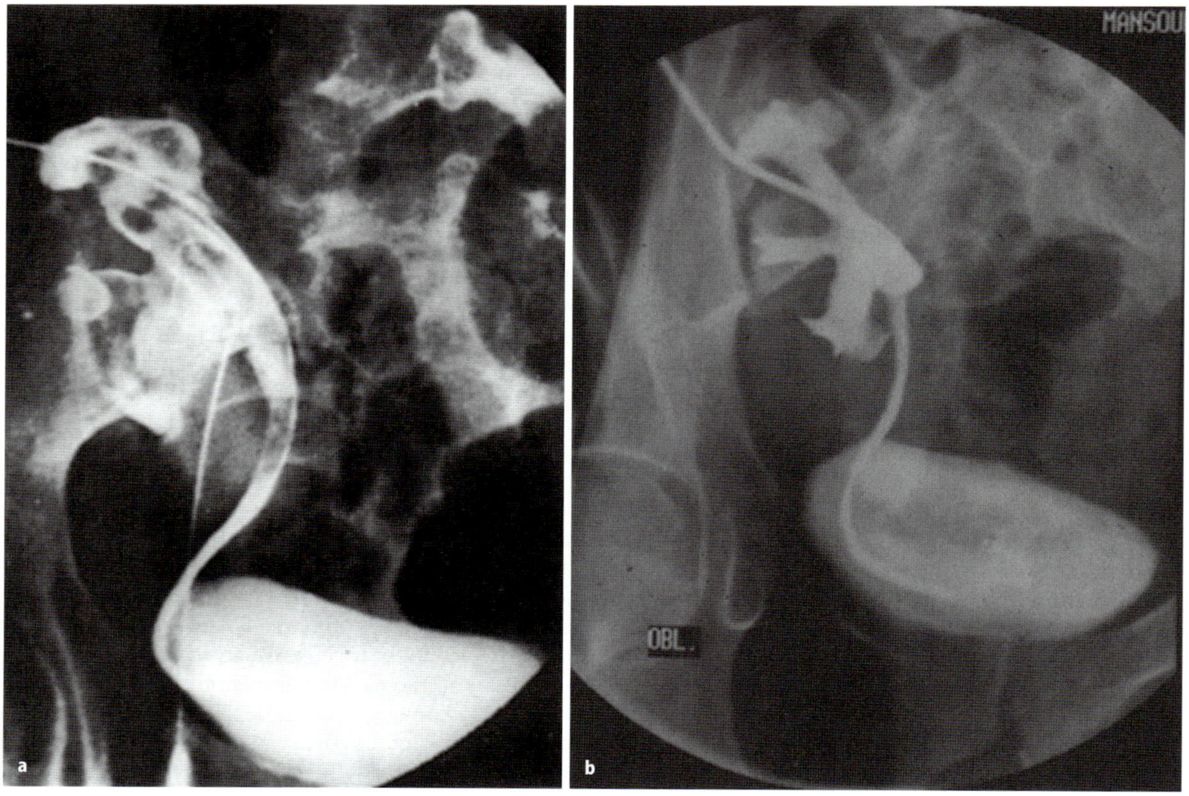

Fig. 18.4.2a, b. Clot anuria following graft biopsy. **a** Antegrade study showing blood clots obstructing the ureter of the transplanted kidney. **b** Antegrade study of the same patient a few days after drainage of the graft by percutaneous nephrostomy (PCN) showing the patent ureter

18.4.3.2
Early Graft Dysfunction

Early graft dysfunction is usually manifested by falling or absent urine output in the first few days after transplantation with elevation of serum creatinine. Early anuria or oliguria could be caused by a variety of conditions, including volume contraction (prerenal azotemia), acute tubular necrosis (ATN), rejection (hyperacute, accelerated, or acute), renal artery or renal vein thrombosis, urine leak, ureteral obstruction, drug toxicity, and early recurrence of the original kidney disease.

Identification of the cause of early graft dysfunction is paramount for proper treatment. Improper diagnosis will result in mismanagement that may aggravate the condition. Therefore, the key of success is to start the proper treatment at the optimal time depending upon precise identification of the cause of dysfunction. A simple algorithm to reach the diagnosis of early graft dysfunction is depicted in Fig. 18.4.3. The first step is to confirm patency of the Foley catheter by gentle irrigation and suction. Then the patient's volume status and fluid balance must be assessed by measuring the pulse, blood pressure, hematocrit, central venous pressure,

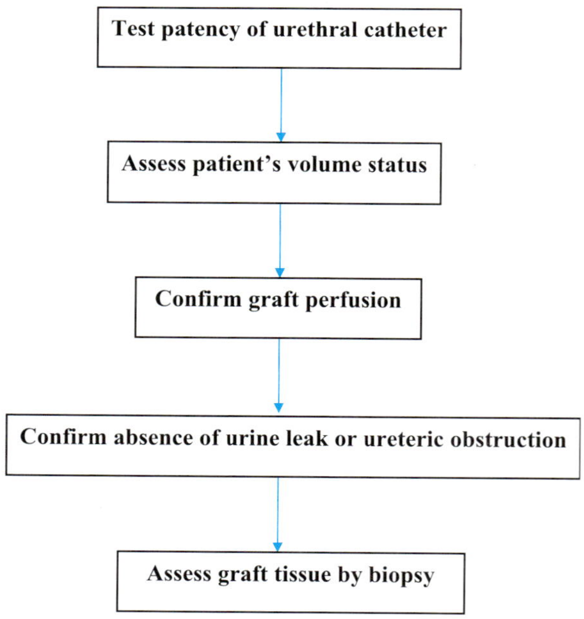

Fig. 18.4.3. Algorithmic approach to posttransplantation anuria or oliguria

and by reviewing the fluid balance charts of intake and output. US is a very helpful tool in the differential diagnosis of early oliguria or anuria. Gray-scale US excludes urological complications, while Doppler US is used for assessment of graft perfusion to exclude vascular thrombosis. If there are no urological or vascular problems, the next step is to assess the graft tissue by biopsy, which will differentiate between a variety of conditions such as ATN, rejection, drug toxicity, and early recurrence of the original kidney disease. The onset of a rejection episode on top of another complication such as ATN, urological complication, drug toxicity, or recurrence of the original kidney disease is confusing and renders the diagnosis more difficult. Nevertheless, repeated graft biopsy is very helpful in this situation.

Volume Contraction

Prerenal azotemia or volume contraction often may lead to allograft deterioration during the immediate postoperative period. Excessive diuretics and uncontrolled blood glucose are two of the commonest causes of the development of prerenal azotemia from volume contraction. Because most of these patients are already receiving calcineurin inhibitors, which decrease renal blood flow, the concomitant insult of volume contraction may lead to an elevated level of blood urea nitrogen and serum creatinine, which may be difficult to distinguish from an episode of acute rejection. Careful attention to central venous pressure, daily weight, intake and output, and assessment of orthostatic blood pressure changes can reliably diagnose volume contraction as a contributing factor for renal allograft dysfunction. Volume repletion with intravenous or oral fluid is indicated.

Acute Tubular Necrosis

Acute tubular necrosis (ATN) is the most frequent posttransplantation complication. Other than hyperacute rejection, ATN is the earliest posttransplantation complication. The incidence of ATN is significantly higher in cadaveric vs living donor transplants. An incidence of 25 % for cadaver donors vs 5 % for living donors has been reported (Shoskes and Cecka 1997). An increase in the incidence of ATN has also been noted with advancing donor age. Prolonged cold ischemia time, up to 30 h, does not appear to have a significant impact on the incidence of ATN unless there is an episode of rejection.

The diagnosis of ATN usually is apparent during the first 24 h after transplantation. Although some kidneys may produce urine initially, a fall off in urine output that is unresponsive to fluid challenge is the commonest clinical scenario indicating ATN. The major differential diagnostic consideration in a patient with a falling or absent urine output is an acute vascular or urological complication. The differential diagnosis can be determined easily with urgent US and radionuclide renal scanning. Gray-scale US shows a large swollen graft, compressed pelvicalyceal system and an empty bladder. Moreover, Doppler US reveals perfect graft perfusion. A radioisotope scan may also help in diagnosis; typically, a transplantation with ATN shows good renal perfusion, good parenchymal uptake of $^{99\text{-m}}$ Tc MAG_3 with poor or no renal excretion (Fig. 18.4.4). In case of doubt, a biopsy is taken. Once the diagnosis of ATN is established, careful attention to fluid status is paramount to decrease the frequency and necessity for dialysis. The usual course of ATN is 10 – 14 days, and patients may require supportive dialysis for management of fluid and electrolyte disturbances. Moreover, the immunosuppressive drugs and antibiotics need to be modified.

The major concern for transplant recipients with ATN is the potential onset of a concomitant acute rejection. The diagnosis of rejection in patients with ATN may be hindered because the primary clinical monitoring tool is a fall in serum creatinine. For this reason, some centers use antilymphocyte therapy to prevent early acute rejection in patients with ATN. Alternatively, frequent biopsies of patients with ATN have been proposed as a means for detection of acute rejection episodes. An early acute rejection episode after ATN

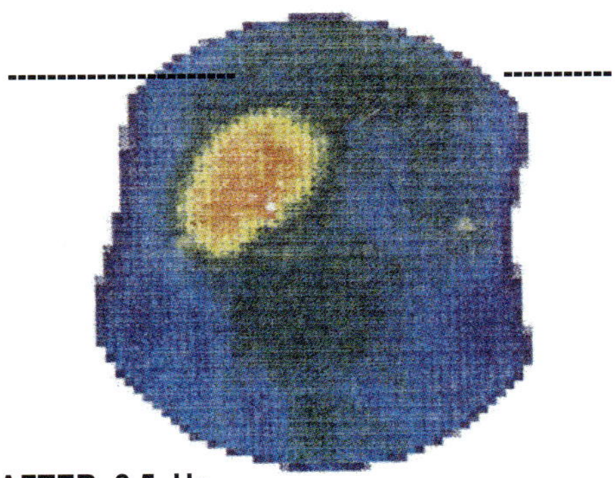

AFTER 2.5 Hr

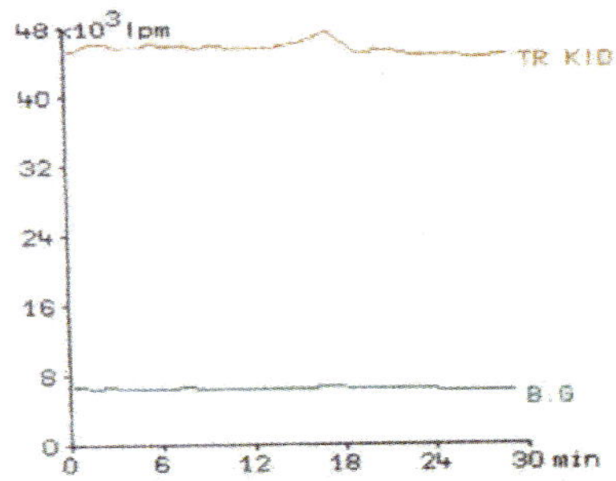

RENOGRAM AFTER 2.5 Hr

Fig. 18.4.4. Radioisotope renal scan ($^{99m}Tc\text{-}MAG_3$) in a patient with acute tubular necrosis (ATN) showing good perfusion, good uptake, and no excretion significantly lowers short- and long-term survival (Land 1998).

Rejection

Rejection that occurs early after transplantation includes hyperacute, accelerated, and acute rejection. Hyperacute rejection occurs if renal transplantation is performed in the setting of an ABO mismatch or a positive lymphocytotoxic crossmatch. Hyperacute rejection is manifested intraoperatively as soft blue kidney immediately after release of the vascular clamps. A hyperacutely rejected kidney has no perfusion on Doppler US or renal scan because of the microvascular thrombosis. There is no effective treatment and the graft needs to be removed.

Despite a negative T cell crossmatch test preoperatively, some patients may develop an early aggressive form of rejection, termed accelerated vascular rejection. This rejection is seen most often in patients with a previous transplant or in those with high panel-reactive antibody. Accelerated rejection typically occurs within 2–5 days of the transplant. Histologically, renal transplant biopsy shows fibrin deposition and endotheliitis. Accelerated rejection is poorly responsive to steroids and may be resistant to all forms of antirejection therapy. Because of the likely contribution of the humoral immune response, a combination of plasmapheresis and anti-CD_{20} monoclonal antibody (rituximab) have been recently used as a rescue therapy of accelerated rejection. The rationale of this combined therapy is that plasmapheresis gets rid of the existing antibodies, while rituximab prevents further formation of new antibodies through inhibition of B lymphocytes (Pescovitz, 2004; Garrett et al. 2002).

Acute cellular rejection is the most common form of rejection in the early posttransplantation period. It is mediated predominantly by host lymphocytes responding to the allogenic donor kidney. Acute rejection typically occurs 5–7 days after transplantation, but can occur at virtually any time thereafter. The highest incidence of acute rejection is within the first 3 months and overall rates of rejection vary from 10 % to 50 % within the first 6 months depending on HLA matching and the immunosuppressive protocol. The clinical manifestation of acute rejection includes a rising serum creatinine, weight gain, fever, and graft tenderness. Since the introduction of cyclosporine and tacrolimus, the latter two signs are seldom present. The diagnostic gold standard is kidney biopsy that shows cellular infiltration. The first line of treatment is bolus steroid therapy. Approximately 85 %–90 % of acute cellular rejection episodes are steroid responsive. If the patient's serum creatinine does not start decreasing by day 4 of therapy, alternative treatments should be considered, such as ALG or OKT_3. Rejection that does not respond to treatment with steroids, ALG, or OKT_3 occurs in less than 5 % of patients. This is observed more frequently in sensitized patients or retransplantations.

Vascular Thrombosis

Renal allograft vascular thrombosis is a serious complication of kidney transplantation that ultimately leads to graft loss. The reported incidence of thrombotic complications varies from 0.8 % to 6 % (Bakir et al. 1996; Groggel 1991). In our series, an incidence of 0.5 % was observed (Osman et al. 2003). Many factors have been associated with thrombotic sequelae, such as pediatric recipients, preoperative hypercoagulable states, pretransplantation peritoneal dialysis, the type of fluid used for perfusion, and the pro-coagulant effect of OKT_3 or cyclosporine (van Lieburg et al. 1995; Murphy et al. 1994; Benoit et al. 1994). Thrombotic complications usually occur very early after transplantation and manifest by sudden anuria. The diagnosis is confirmed by Doppler US (Fig. 18.4.5a), MRA (Fig 18.4.5b), and/or radioisotope scan, which demonstrate absence of renal perfusion. Exploration must be performed immediately and rarely can the graft be salvaged by thrombectomy, but most cases will end in a graft loss.

In a series of 1,200 consecutive live-donor renal transplantations, we recorded renal artery thrombosis in five patients (0.5 %) and renal vein thrombosis in one (0.1 %) (Osman et al. 2003). Patients with renal artery thrombosis were treated by graft nephrectomy in four and renal artery thrombectomy in one in whom the graft could be persevered. The patient with renal vein thrombosis was managed by graft nephrectomy (Osman et al. 2003).

Routine prophylactic heparinization has been greatly debated over the years. Ubhi et al. (1989) recommended routine subcutaneous heparin to decrease postoperative thromboembolic complications in renal transplantation patients based in a prospective randomized study. Broyer et al. (1991) observed the effectiveness of low-molecular-weight heparin for decreasing the incidence of graft thrombosis in pediatric kidney transplantation. On the other hand, in a more recent study the role of intraoperative heparin was questioned. Moreover, it was associated with a significant increase in postoperative hemorrhagic complications and the need for blood transfusion (Mohan et al. 1999). In our opinion, the use of posttransplantation anticoagulants must be reserved for patients at high risk of developing vascular thrombosis such as pediatric recipients, diabetics, patients with hypercoagulable state, or those with multiple vessels.

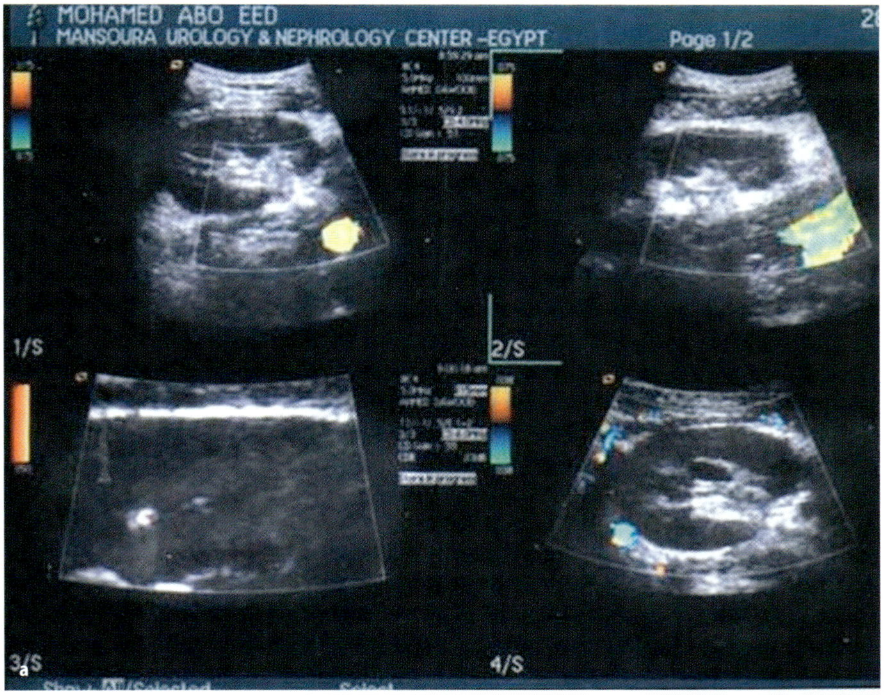

Fig. 18.4.5a, b. Renal artery thrombosis. **a** Power Doppler US showing nonperfused transplanted kidney. **b** Magnetic resonance angiography (MRA) showing nonvascularized right iliac renal allograft

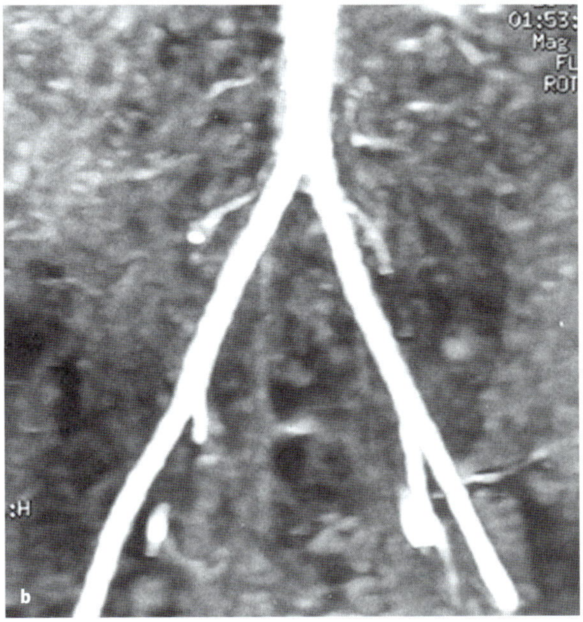

Urinary Leakage

The reported incidence of urinary leakage varies between 1.2% (Ghasemian et al. 1996; Makisalo et al. 1997) and 8.9% (Loughlin et al. 1984). In our series, an incidence of 3% was observed (El-Mekresh et al. 2001). Urinary leakage is generally evident early after transplantation and commonly caused by vascular insufficiency secondary to inadvertent damage to the vessels that supply the ureter during organ harvesting. It may also occur as a result of technical problems during ureteroneocystostomy, particularly with transvesical procedures. The rate is slightly higher in patients who received kidneys from living donors than in those who received organs from cadavers (Loughlin et al. 1984; Cimic et al. 1997). This is presumably a result of more extensive hilar dissection required during harvesting from the living donor, with the attendant risks of injury to the blood supply of the ureter. With the early learning curve of laparoscopic live-donor nephrectomy, the incidence of ureteral complications was significantly higher in comparison to open liver-donor nephrectomy (Rawlins et al. 2002; Ratner et al. 1999). The higher incidence of ureteral complications with laparoscopic nephrectomy was attributed to extensive dissections close to the wall of the ureter. With the current knowledge of the necessity for a meticulous preparation of the ureter and its surrounding fatty tissue, the proportion of ureteral complications no longer differs between laparoscopic and open live-donor nephrectomy. Some authors even describe fewer ureteral complications with the laparoscopic approach (Ratner et al. 1999).

Symptoms of ureteric leak generally include sudden oliguria or anuria, an increasing serum creatinine level, and perigraft swelling. The urine may collect around the graft or leak from the wound or through the tube drain. Gray-scale US is important to diagnose a perigraft collection; if found, the collection should be drained. Determining the nature of the fluid collecting around the graft or leaking from the wound is para-

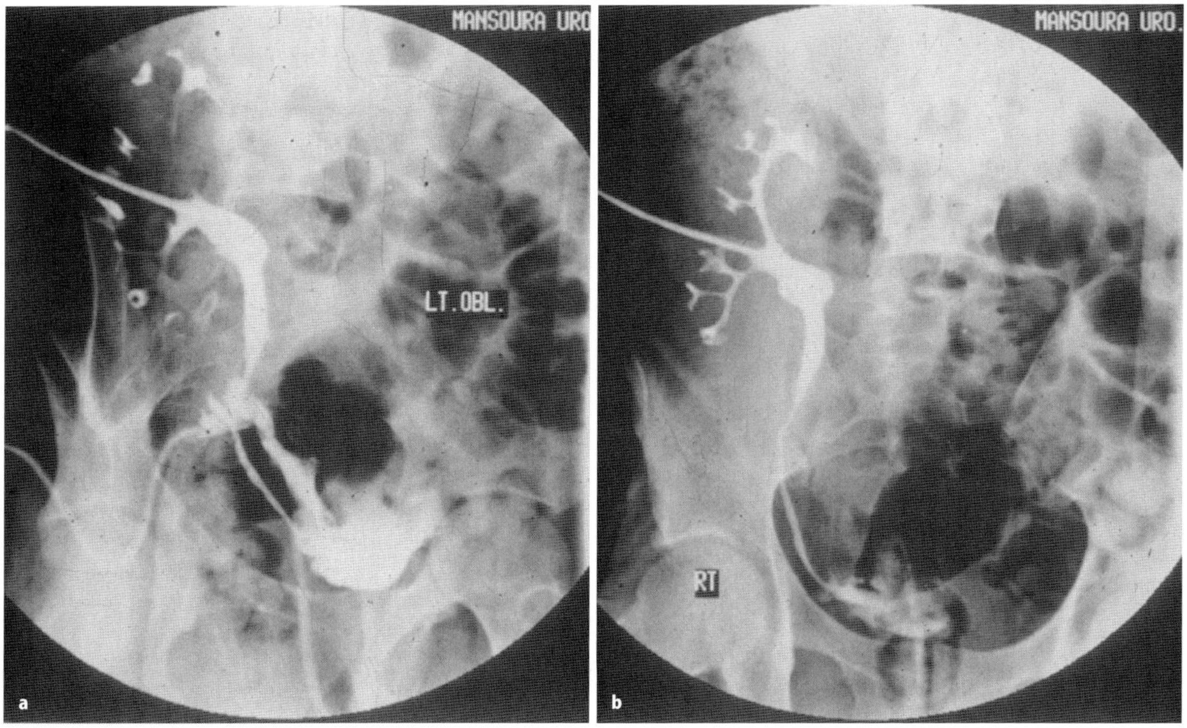

Fig. 18.4.6a, b. Urinary leakage. **a** Antegrade study showing leakage from the middle part of the ureter of the transplanted kidney. **b** Antegrade study of the same patient a few days after drainage of the graft by PCN showing intact patent ureter with absence of extravasations

mount. A quantitative estimation of the creatinine content of this fluid differentiates between urine and lymph. If urine leakage is diagnosed, its possible sources could be either the site of the ureterovesical anastomosis or a ureteric fistula. A few days of watchful waiting with proper drainage of the wound and the bladder usually result in cessation of the urine leak if its source is the bladder. However, if urine continues to leak, then a ureteric fistula is suspected. The diagnosis is usually confirmed by fixation of a graft PCN and antegrade study (Fig. 18.4.6).

Leakage from the urinary bladder is usually easily treated by prolonged catheter drainage. Almost half of ureteric leaks are managed by percutaneous techniques, which are currently used as the initial management in all cases. Open surgical revision can be used subsequently if this fails. The choice of the reconstructive procedure depends on the operative findings. Distal pathologies can be corrected by ureterovesical reimplantation. For more proximal lesions, a Boari tube or ureteroureteral reanastomosis can be used. Early diagnosis and prompt treatment usually result in salvage of the graft with no harmful effect on either the graft or on the patient's survival (Shokeir et al. 1993c).

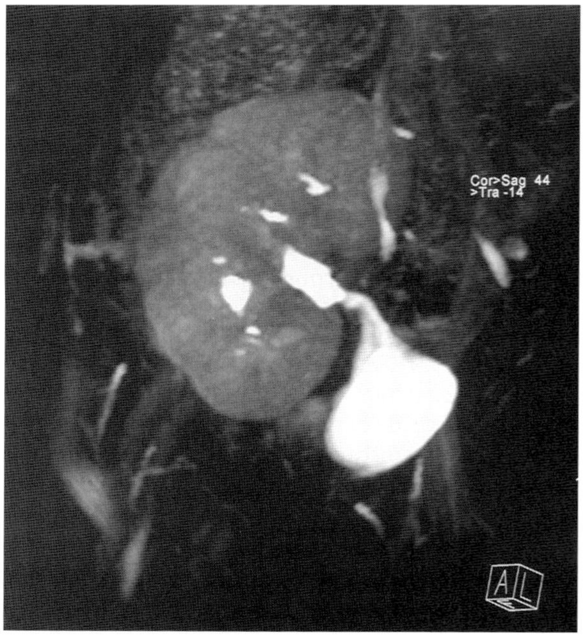

Fig. 18.4.7. MRU following a Boari flap from the bladder to the pelvis of the graft for treatment of extensive fibrosis of the ureter

In a recent study, we reported 37 cases of urinary leakage among 1,200 live-donor renal transplantations. The conservative management of vesical leaks by prolonged catheter drainage was successful in six patients. Three patients (with ureters reimplanted using the Politano-Leadbetter technique) required open repair and closure in two layers. Several methods were used to manage ureteric leaks. For minor leaks at the vesicoureteric junction, definitive treatment by PCN drainage was attempted in 14 patients. Two patients required subsequent reconstructive procedures. Open surgical revision was required in 16 patients. For distal pathologies, a ureterovesical reimplantation was possible. Leaks resulting from more ischemic damage of the ureter required either a ureteroureteric anastomosis (five), a Boari flap ureteroneocytostomy (two) (Fig. 18.4.7) or an anastomosis between the renal pelvis of the donor's kidney and the ureter of the recipient (one patient). In one patient with total necrosis of the ureter, interposition of a segment of ileum between the renal pelvis and the bladder was necessary (El-Mekresh et al. 2001).

Drug Toxicity

Both of the calcineurin inhibitors, cyclosporine and tacrolimus, are effective in preventing acute rejection episodes but clearly can lead to nephrotoxicity, primarily by decreasing renal blood flow in the afferent arteriole, leading to tubular injury (Pirsch and Friedman 1994). Because of variability in intestinal absorption in the early transplant period, underdosing may result in rejection episodes and overdosing can lead to nephrotoxicity. Although there are many clinical parameters that have been advocated to differentiate calcineurin inhibitor nephrotoxicity from rejection, most clinical parameters are not of sufficient sensitively to predict the cause of the transplant dysfunction confidently. In patients with ATN, it is be more difficult to diagnose acute rejection or calcineurin nephrotoxicity reliably. Monitoring cyclosporine and tacrolimus levels is of value in preventing significant increases in blood levels, which may lead to nephrotoxicity. Controversy remains regarding the time of sample collection for monitoring of cyclosporine level using either a trough level sample (12 h after the previous dose) or a C_2 level sample (2 h after the previous dose). The most reliable way of differentiating calcineurin nephrotoxicity from rejection is percutaneous renal allograft biopsy. Early functional nephrotoxicity is manifested most often by evidence of tubular injury characterized by vacuolation (Fig. 18.4.8). In patients with established calcineurin nephrotoxicity, lowering the dose or temporary discontinuation of cyclosporine or tacrolimus can lead to reversal of the renal injury.

Recurrence of the Original Kidney Disease

Most causes of renal failure do not recur in the transplant kidney, when they do, it is usually later in the posttransplant course. Two diseases may occur in the immediate posttransplant period and lead to significant graft dysfunction or graft loss if not treated aggressively. These include focal segmental glomerulosclerosis (FSGS) and hemolytic uremic syndrome.

FSGS is the commonest glomerulonephritis that can recur in the immediate postoperative period (Artero et al. 1994). The diagnosis is established by the development of nephrotic-range proteinuria in a patient with a pretransplant diagnosis of FSGS and is confirmed by biopsy. Electron microscopy shows diffuse foot process effacement, which is diagnostic in this setting. Various strategies have been employed to treat recurrent FSGS, including high-dose calcineurin inhibitors, prednisone, and plasmapheresis.

Hemolytic uremic syndrome can recur in the imme-

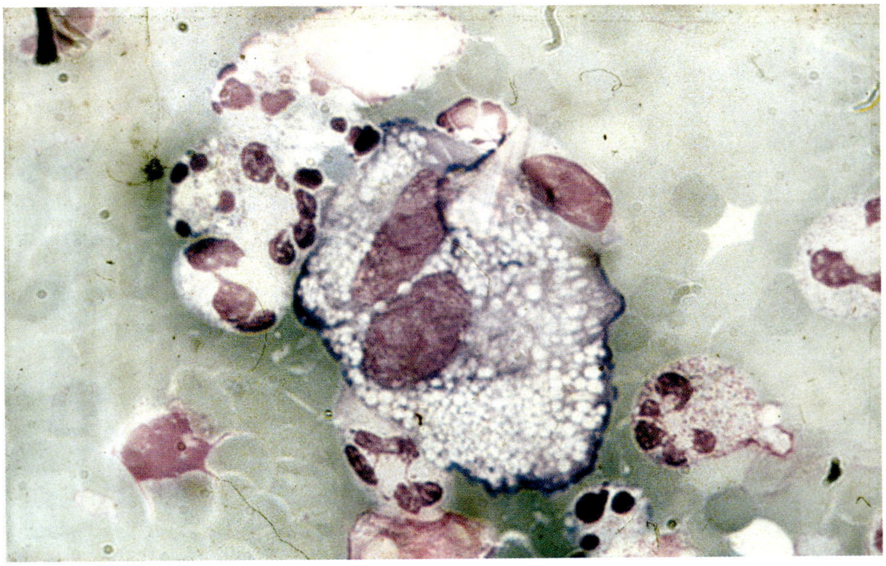

Fig. 18.4.8. Fine needle aspiration cytology showing cyclosporine nephrotoxicity with the characteristic fine vacuoles in the renal tubules

diate postoperative period (Kaplan et al. 1998). It is characterized clinically by a fall in hematocrit and/or platelet count with evidence of a microangiopathic process on peripheral blood smear, increased lactate dehydrogenase and transplant allograft dysfunction. Kidney biopsy shows fibrin clot in the small arterioles of the kidney. Hemolytic uremic syndrome has been noted to be induced by cyclosporine or tacrolimus. Discontinuation of the calcineurin inhibitor and plasmapheresis have been beneficial in some series (Kaplan 1999, 2003). The use of anticoagulants and aspirin is of uncertain benefit.

18.4.3.3 Late Graft Dysfunction

Late graft dysfunction is defined as gradual and progressive deterioration of the renal function after at least 2 months of stable function. This could be due to renal artery stenosis, ureteral obstruction, lymphocele, or chronic rejection.

Renal Artery Stenosis

Transplant renal artery stenosis is a primary and potentially reversible cause of hypertension and graft loss. The reported incidence is 1%–16% (Lo et al. 1996; Halimi et al. 1999) and 0.4% in our series (Osman et al. 2003), with a mean incidence of around 6% for live-donor and cadaveric transplantations (Sutherland et al. 1993). Zaontz et al. (1988) summarized the etiological factors of renal artery stenosis as faulty surgical technique, trauma to the donor kidney from the perfusion cannula or intimal tears from overstretching the artery, intimal injury during end-to-end anastomosis, or artery angulation secondary to excessive length from end-to-end anastomosis with the hypogastric artery. The disease usually manifests late after transplantation by severe persistent hypertension. Diagnosis is confirmed by intraarterial angiography (Fig. 18.4.9). The role of Doppler US and magnetic resonance angiography is still controversial. The disease can be managed by percutaneous angioplasty or surgical correction.

Ureteric Obstruction

The reported incidence of intrinsic ureteric obstruction is 1.3% (Ghasemian et al. 1996) to 10.2% (Rigg et al. 1994) and 1.9% in our series (El-Mekresh et al. 2001). Ureteric obstruction may occur in either the early or the late postoperative period. Most of the obstructions involve the distal ureter or the ureterovesical junction. Various causes are possible in the pathogenesis of this complication, among which ischemia of the ureter is the most common (Rigg et al. 1994; Shokeir et al. 1993a). Other causes including technical problems (Ghasemian et al. 1996), urinary leaks with periureteric

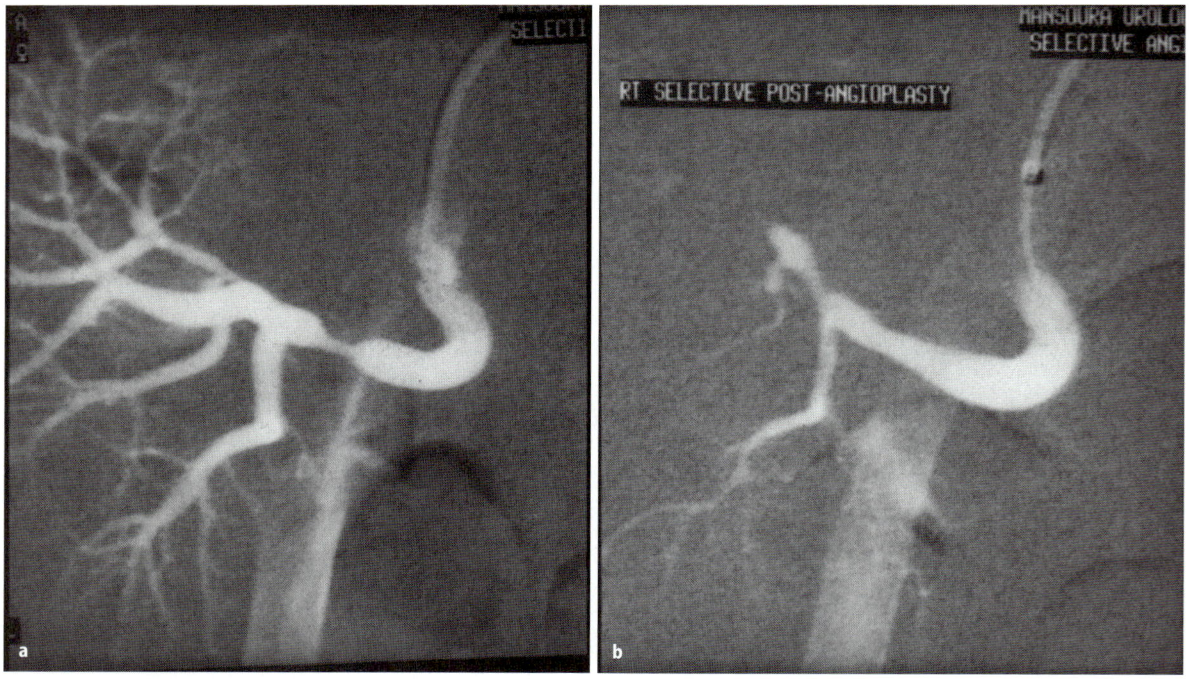

Fig. 18.4.9a, b. Renal artery stenosis (RAS). **a** Intraarterial angiography showing RAS before treatment. **b** Intraarterial angiography of the same patient after percutaneous angioplasty showing resolution of the stenosed segment

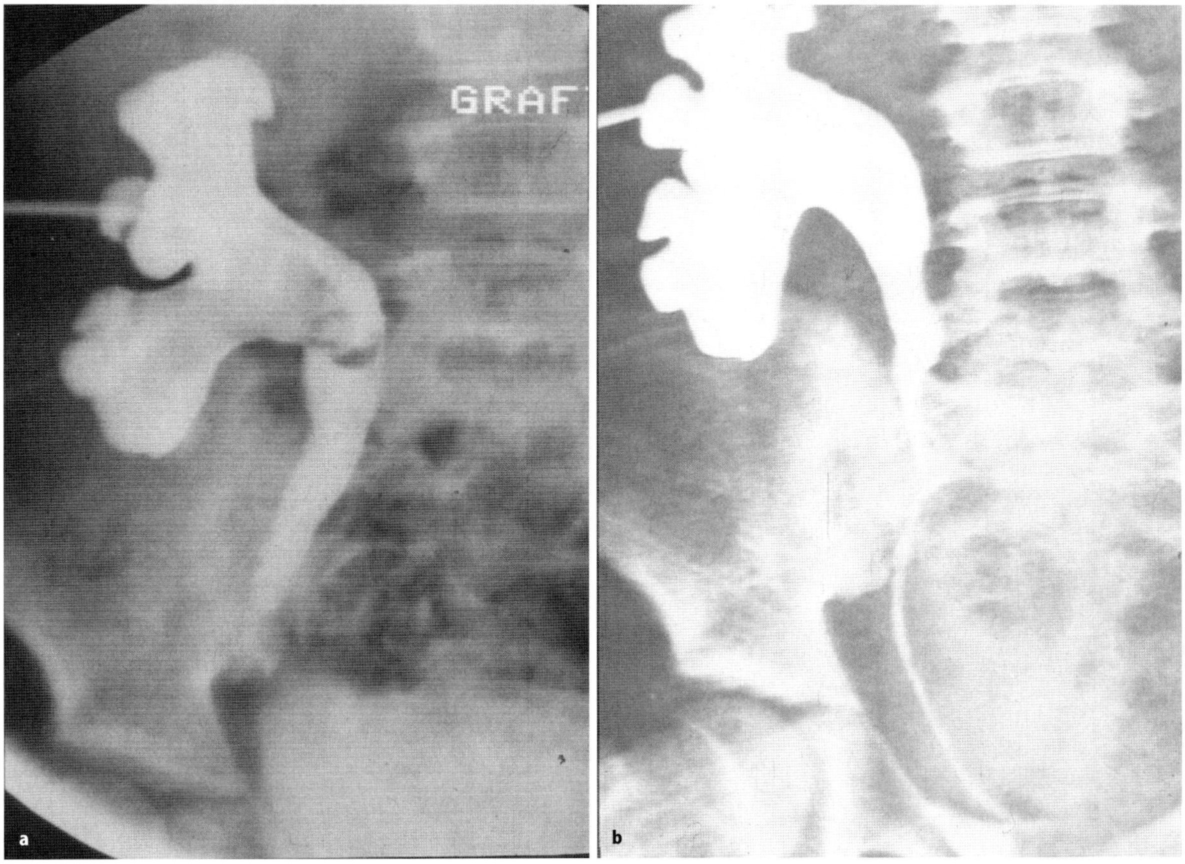

Fig. 18.4.10a, b. Ureteric obstruction. **a** Antegrade study showing distal ureteric obstruction. **b** Antegrade study of the same patient after ureterovesical reimplantation showing resolution of the ureteric obstruction

fibrosis (Rigg et al. 1994), and ureteritis resulting from acute rejection episodes (Katz et al. 1988; Schweizer 1977) were all implicated.

The diagnosis of ureteric obstruction is usually suspected by a progressive increase in the serum creatinine level and dilatation of the graft pelvicaliceal system by routine ultrasonography. Further investigations include diuretic radioisotope renography and magnetic resonance urography. The diagnosis is confirmed by antegrade pyelography after fixation of a graft percutaneous nephrostomy (PCN) tube (Fig. 18.4.10).

Percutaneous drainage with antegrade dilatation and stenting can be attempted as initial management of ureteric obstruction. For failures, open surgical revision is necessary and should involve the use of a healthy, well-vascularized proximal segment. Ureteroureteric, pelviureteric, and pyelovesical anastomosis can all be used. The replacement of the ureter by an isolated ileal segment was successfully used in three patients in our series in whom there was extensive ischemic damage of the ureter (Shokeir et al. 1993c) (Fig. 18.4.11).

Prolonged use of azathioprine may result in formation of uric acid stones, which may obstruct the ureter (Fig. 18.4.12a). In this situation, the stone could be removed through antegrade ureteroscopy (Fig. 18.4.12b).

Lymphocele

Lymphocele may be an asymptomatic incidental finding, but when it becomes large enough to compress adjacent structures it may cause a variety of clinical manifestations, some of which may result in serious morbidity. The incidence of lymphocele is 0.6%–41% (Boedker et al. 1990; Stephenian et al. 1992) and 1.4% in our series (El-Mekresh et al. 2001). The cause of lymphocele is not fully recognized, but most authors believe it emanates either from unligated lymphatics from the iliac dissection in the recipient or from interrupted channels of the donor kidney itself (Stephenian et al. 1992).

In clinical practice, a lymphocele usually presents later than a urinary leak. The former may be recognized as early as the 18th posttransplantation day or as late as the 17th month after surgery (Meyers et al. 1977). In our series, the earliest lymphocele was ob-

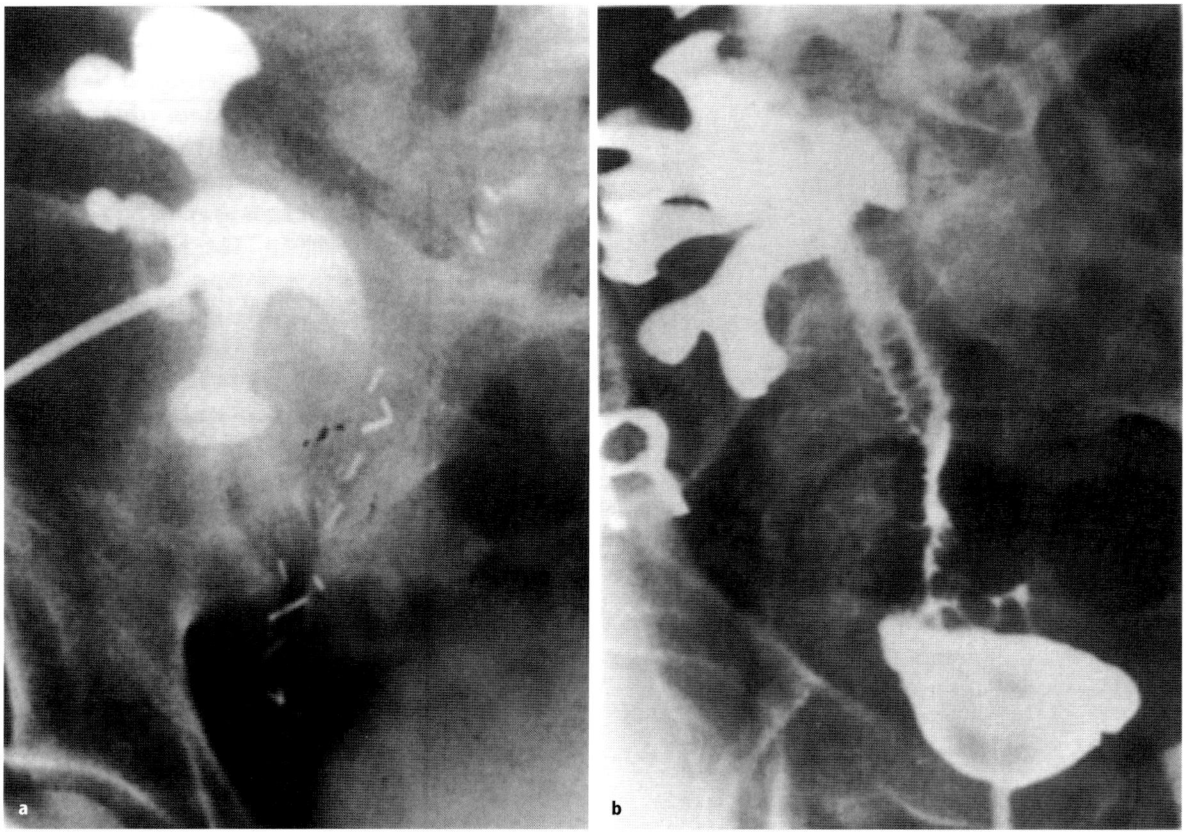

Fig. 18.4.11. **a** Antegrade study showing arrest of dye at the site of pelviureteric junction due to extensive fibrosis of the ureter. **b** Antegrade study after ileal replacement of the transplanted ureter

served after 3 weeks and the majority during the 3rd month (Shokeir et al. 1993b).

Ultrasonography is the method of choice for the diagnosis and follow-up of lymphoceles. The technique is noninvasive and can be performed without difficulty even when renal function is seriously impaired. Other investigations that complement US include IVU and CT (Fig. 18.4.13) (when the renal function permits) and MRU. An analysis of the chemical composition of a fluid collection is also useful, because lymph constituents are similar to those of plasma, whereas urinary creatinine, potassium, and urea nitrogen concentrations are higher than in lymph.

Single percutaneous needle aspiration is ineffective in the treatment of symptomatic lymphocele and should be done only for diagnostic purposes. Percutaneous catheter drainage with the use of a sclerosant (tetracyeline, providone-iodine, ampicillin, and fibrin) may be a safe and successful alternative (Shokeir et al. 1993b) (Fig. 18.4.14). Should catheter drainage fail or the lymphocele recurs, surgical marsupialization by laparoscopic or open techniques usually be effective.

Chronic Rejection

Chronic rejection is currently referred to as chronic allograft nephropathy because the etiology includes factors that can be considered both immune, or alloantigen-dependent, and nonimmune, or alloantigen-independent. An example of the former factor is previous acute rejection and examples of the latter factors are chronic ischemia and use of cyclosporine. Chronic allograft nephropathy is an important cause of graft failure in the late posttransplantation period. Clinically, it usually presents as a finding in patients undergoing biopsy for gradually declining renal function or proteinuria. Chronic rejection is characterized by stenosis of the peripheral arteries with magnetic resonance angiography. No effective treatment is currently available. Nevertheless, some measures could be used for prophylaxis against chronic rejection such as prevention of attacks of acute rejection by induction therapy and use of potent immunosuppressive drugs, early detection of rejection by protocol biopsy and avoidance of calcineurin inhibitor nephrotoxicity.

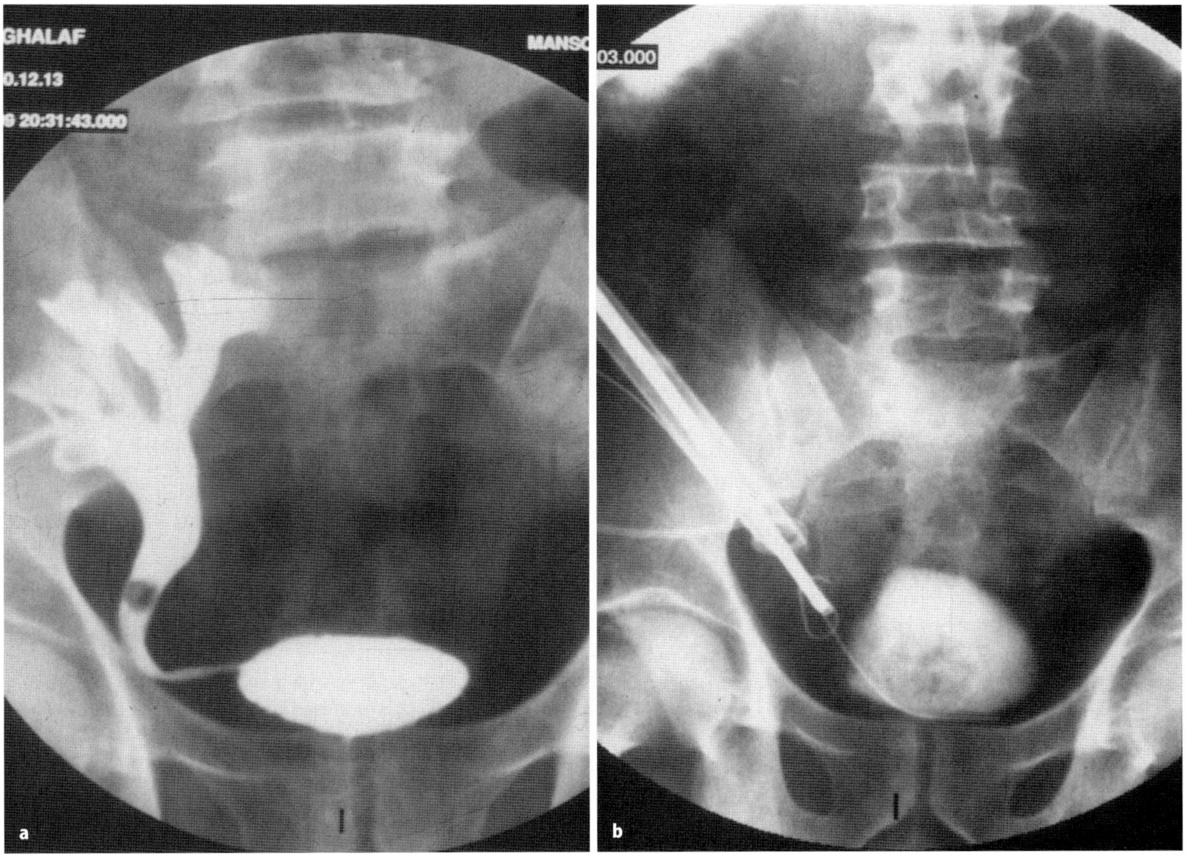

Fig. 18.4.12a, b. Ureteric stones. **a** Antegrade study showing a filling defect of a stone in the ureter of a transplanted kidney. **b** Antegrade ureteroscopy for removal of the ureteric stone

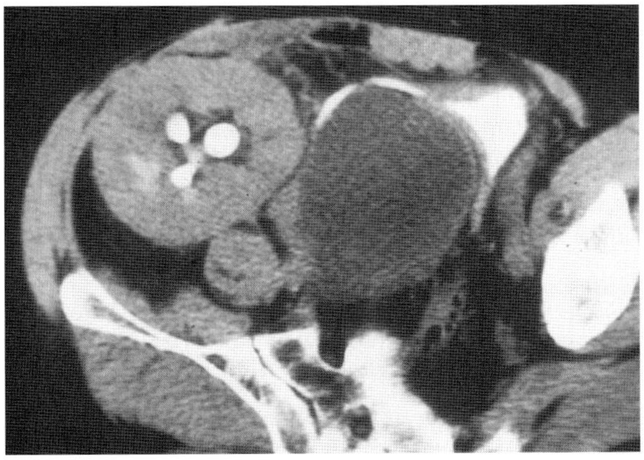

Fig. 18.4.13. CT showing large lymphocele displacing the urinary bladder and obstructing the ureter of a transplanted kidney

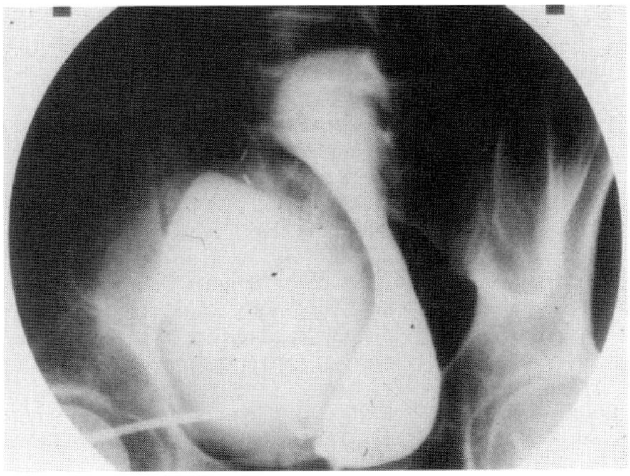

Fig. 18.4.14. Percutaneous drainage of lymphocele

18.4.3.4 Surgical Complications Related to Immunosuppressive Drugs

Some recent kidney transplantation prospective randomized trials have demonstrated higher surgical wound complication rates with sirolimus immunosuppression in comparison to other types of immunosuppressive drugs (Dean et al. 2004; Troppmann et al. 2003). A surgical wound complication is defined as any complication directly related to the surgical transplant wound that needs reintervention, such as hematoma and lymphocele requiring relaparotomy, seroma requiring repeated aspirations, delayed healing requiring serial wound debridement, and incisional hernia requiring surgical repair.

Mycophenolate mofetil (MMF) has been used successfully since 1995 as an adjunct immunosuppressive agent for the prevention of acute rejection in renal transplantation. However, hematologic and GI side effects are a concern with MMF-containing immunosuppressive regimens. Diarrhea, abdominal pain, nausea, vomiting, intestinal bleeding, and perforation occurred more frequently in the MMF-treated group than in placebo or azathioprine-treated groups in phase III clinical trials (Sollinger et al. 1995; European Study Group 1995; MMF Study Group 1996; Hardinger et al. 2004).

Hemorrhagic cystitis is one of the complications of prolonged use of cyclophosphamide. Sometimes the hematuria is so severe that it causes clot retention. Improvement usually occurs with discontinuation of the drug.

In conclusion, emergencies following live-donor renal transplantation need integration of urologists, nephrologists, radiologists, and pathologists for proper diagnosis and treatment. Early diagnosis and prompt management can save the graft as well as the patient. Improper diagnosis will result in mismanagement that may aggravate the condition. Therefore, the key to success is to start the proper treatment in the optimal time.

References

Artero ML, Sharma R, Savin VJ, Vincenti F (1994) Plasmapheresis reduces proteinuria and serum capacity to injure glomeruli in patients with recurrent focal glomerulosclerosis. Am J Kidney Dis 25:574

Baghossian T, Henri M, Dube S, Bendavid Y, Morin M (2005) Laparoscopic nephrectomy donor death due to cerebral gas embolism in a specialized transplant center; risk zero does not exist. Transplantation 79:258

Bakir N, Sluiter WJ, Ploeg RJ, van San WJ, Tegzess AM (1996) Primary renal graft thrombosis. Nephrol Dial Transplant 11:140

Benoit G, Jaber N, Moukarzel M, Douguet D, Bensadoun D, Bensadoun H, Blanchet P et al (1994) Incidence of vascular complications in kidney transplantation: is there any interference with the nature of the perfusion solution? Clin Transplant 8:485

Blohme I, Fehrman I, Norden (1992) Living donor nephrectomy complication rates in 490 consecutive cases. Scand J Urol Nephrol 26:149

Boedker A, Roikjaer O, Rasmussen F, Loekkegaard H (1990) Lymphocele following renal transplantation: a clinical study. Transplant Proc 22:54

Broyer M, Gognadoux MF, Sierro A, Fischer AH, Niaudet P (1991) Preventive treatment of vascular thrombosis after kidney transplantation in children with low molecular weight heparin. Transplant Proc 23:1384

Cimic J, Meuleman EJH, Oosterhof GON, Hoitsma AJ (1997) Urological Complications in renal transplantation: a comparison between living-related and cadaveric grafts. Eur Urol 31:433

Dean PG, Lund WJ, Larson TS, Prieto M, Nyberg SL, Ishitani MB et al (2004) Wound-healing complication after kidney transplantation: a prospective randomized comparison of sirolimus and tacrolimus. Transplantation 77:1555

El-Mekresh M, Osman Y, Ali-El-Dein B, El-Diasty T, Ghoneim MA (2001) Urological complications after living-donor renal transplantation. BJU Int 87:295

European Mycophenolate Mofetil Study Group (1995) Placebo-controlled study of mycophenolate mofetil combined with cyclosporine and corticosteroids for prevention of acute rejection. Lancet 345:1321

Garret ED Jr, Groshart K, Duvall-Seaman D, Combs D, Stuggs R (2002) Treatment of humoral rejection with rituximab. Ann Thorac Surg 74:1240

Ghasemian SMR, Guleria AS, Khawand NY, Light JA (1996) Diagnosis and management of the urologic complications of renal transplantation. Clin Transplant 10:218:23

Groggel GC (1991) Acute thrombosis of the renal transplant artery: a case report and review of the literature. Clin Nephrol 36:42

Halimi JM, Al-Najjar A, Buchler M, Birmele B, Tranquart F, Alison D et al (1999) Transplant renal artery stenosis: potential role of ischemia renal reperfusion injury and long-term outcome following angioplasty. J Urol 161:28

Hardinger KL, Brennan DC, Lowell J, Schnitzer MA (2004) Long-term outcome of gastrointestinal complications in renal transplant patients treated with mycophenolate mofetil. Transpl Int 17:609

Huynth PN, Hollander JB (2005) Trends toward laparoscopic nephrectomy at a community hospital. J Urol 173:547

Jacobs SC, Cho E, Foster C, Liao P, Bartlett ST (2004) Laparoscopic donor nephrectomy: the university of Maryland 6-year experience. J Urol 171:47

Kaplan AA (1999) Therapeutic apheresis for renal disorders. Ther Apher 3:25

Kaplan AA (2003) The use of apheresis in immune renal disorders. Ther Apher 7:165

Kaplan BS, Meyers KE, Schulman SL (1998) The pathogenesis and treatment of hemolytic uremic syndrome. J Am Soc Nephrol 9:1126

Katz JP, Greensstein M, Hakki A, Miller A, Katz SM, Simonian S (1988) Transitional epithelial lesions of the ureter in renal transplant rejection. Transplantation 45:710

Kyriakides GK, Simmons RL, Najarian JS (1979) Mycotic aneurysms in transplant patients. Arch Surg 111:472

Land W (1998) Postischemic reperfusion injury and kidney transplantation: prologue. Transplant Proc 30:4210

Lo CY, Chang IK, Tso WK, Mak KO (1996) Percutaneous transluminal angioplasty for transplant renal artery stenosis. Transplant Proc 28:1468

Loauad I, Buchler M, Noel C, Sadek T, Maazouz H, Westeel PF, Lebranchu Y (2005) Renal artery aneurysm secondary to Candida albicans in four kidney allograft recipients. Transplant Proc 37:2834

Loughlin KR, Tilney NL, Richie JP (1984) Urologic complications in 718 renal transplant patients. Surgery 95:296

Makisalo H, Eklund B, Salmela K et al (1997) Urological complications after 2084 consecutive kidney transplantation. Transplant Proc 29:152

Matas AJ, Bartlett ST, Leichtman AB, Delmonico FL (2003) Morbidity and mortality after living kidney donation, 1999 survey of United States transplant centers. Am J Transplant 3:830

Meyers AM, Levine E, Myburgh JA, Goudie E (1977) Diagnosis and management of lymphoceles after renal transplantation. Urology 10:497

Mohan P, Murphy DM, Counihan A, Cunningham P, Hickey DP (1999) The role of intraoperative heparin in cyclosporine

treated cadaveric renal transplant recipients. J Urol 162:682
Murphy BG, Hill C, Middleton D, Deherty CC, Brown JH, Nelson WE et al (1994) Increased renal allograft thrombosis in CAPD patients. Nephrol Dial Transplant 9:1166
Najarian JS, Chavers BM, McHugh LE, Matas AJ (1992) 20 years or more of follow-up of living kidney donors. Lancet 340:807
Osman Y, Shokeir A, Ali El-Dein B, Tantawy M, Wafa EW, Shehab El-Dein AB, Ghoneim MA (2003) Vascular complications after live donor renal transplantation: study of risk factors and effects on graft and patient survival. J Urol 169:859
Pescovitz MD (2004) The use of rituximab, anti-CD_{20} monoclonal antibody, in pediatric transplantation. Pediatr Transplant 8:9
Pirsch JD, Friedman R (1994) Primary care of the renal transplant patient. J Gen Intern Med 9:29
Ratner LE, Montgomery RA, Kavoussi LR (1999) Laparoscopic live donor nephrectomy: the four years John Hopkins University experience. Nephrol Dial Transplant 14:2090
Rawlins MC, Hefty TL, Brown SL, Biehl TR (2002) Learning laparoscopic donor nephrectomy safety: a report on 100 cases. Arch Surg 137:531
Rigg KM, Proud G, Taylor RM (1994) Urological complications following renal transplantation: a study of 1016 consecutive transplants from a single center. Transplant Int 7:120
Sanchez de la Nieta MD, Sanchez-Fructuoso AI, Alcazar R, Perez-Contin MJ, Prats D, Grimalt J, Blanco J (2004) Higher graft salvage rate in renal allograft rupture associated with acute tubular necrosis. Transplant Proc 36:3016
Schweizer RT, Bartus SA, Kahn CS (1977) Fibrosis of a renal transplant ureter. J Urol 117:125
Shahrokh H, Rasouli H, Zargar MA, Karimi K, Zargar K (2005) Spontaneous kidney allograft rupture. Transplant Proc 37:3079
Shokeir AA, El-Diasty TA, Ghoneim MA (1993a) Endouroligic management of ureteric complications after live-donor kidney transplantation. J Endourol 7:487
Shokeir AA, El-Diasty TA, Ghoneim MA (1993b) Percutanous treatment of lymphocele in renal transplant recipients. J Endourol 7:481
Shokeir AA, Shamaa MA, Bakr MA, El-Diast TA, Ghoneim MA (1993c) Salvage of difficult transplant urinary fistulae by ileal substitution of the ureter. Scand J Urol Nephrol 27:537
Shoskes DA, Cecka JM (1997) Effect of delayed graft function on short and long-term kidney graft survival In: Clinical Transplant (JM Cecka and PL Terasaki, eds) P 297, UCLA Tissue Typing Laboratory. Los Angeles
Sollinger HW (1995) for the US Renal Transplant Mycophenolate Mofetil Study Group. Mycophenolate mofetil for the prevention of acute rejection in primary cadaveric renal allograft recipients. Transplantation 60:225
Stephenian E, Matas AJ, Gores P (1992) Sutherland DER, Najarian JS Retransplantation as a risk factor for lymphocele formation. Transplantation 53:676
Sutherland RS, Spees EK, Jones JW, Fink DW (1993) Renal artery stenosis after renal transplantation: The impact of the hypogastric artery anastomosis. J Urol 149:980
The Tricontinental Mycophenolate Mofetil Renal Transplantation Study Group (1996) A blinded, randomized clinical trial of mycophenolate mofetil for the prevention of acute rejection on cadaveric renal transplantation. Transplantation 61:1029
Troppmann C, Pierce JL, Gandhi MM, Gallay BJ, McVicar JP, Perez RV (2003) Higher surgical wound complication rates with sirolimus immunosuppression after kidney transplantation: A matched-pair pilot study. Transplantation 76:426
Ubhi CS, Lam FT, Mavor AI, Giles GR (1989) Subcutaneous heparin therapy for cyclosporine-immunosupprised renal allograft recipients. Transplantation 48:886
Van Lieburg AF, de Jong MC, Hoitsma AJ, Buskens FG, Schroder CH, Monnens LA (1995) Renal transplant thrombosis in children. J Pediatr Surg 30:615
Vastag B (2003) Living-donor transplants reexamined: Experts cite growing concerns about safety of donors. JAMA 290:181
Veroux M, Veroux P, Puliatti C, Fiamingo P, Macarone M, Cappello D (2003) Renal allograft rupture caused by acute tubular necrosis. Chir Ital 55:753
Zaontz MR, Hatch DA, Firlit CF (1988) Urological complications in pediatric renal transplantation: Management and prevention. J Urol 140:1123

18.5 Open Salvage Surgery

C. Wotkowicz, M.A. Jacobs, J.A. Libertino

18.5.1 Introduction

There are limited reports of open salvage procedures in the urological literature. Surgical outcome reports from institutions across the world are readily available; however, in-depth discussion about associated complications is sparse. Many reports simply list complications in table format. This stems from the reluctance to discuss complications and associated failures. Although failed operations due to technical error may be difficult to accept, the documentation and recognition of predisposing factors will limit further mishaps. Some outcomes are unavoidable due to the condition of the patient and these cases should serve as reminders that surgery cannot cure every ailment. Being open to sharing our failures and heeding the warnings of others will allow surgeons and patients to gain something positive from these complicated situations.

This chapter will look at the complications urologists and some general surgeons may encounter when dealing with surgical disease of the genitourinary tract. It will discuss the role of relaparotomy during the postoperative period and techniques for managing some of these complications.

18.5.2 Indications

There have been several reviews in the field of general surgery addressing the indications and outcomes of relaparotomy. Although the indications for initial laparotomy differ between general surgeons and urologists, the reasons for reexploration are quite similar. In a review by Harbrecht et al., these included infection, anastomotic leak, dehiscence, bleeding, obstruction, and ischemia (Harbrecht et al. 1984). The mortality rate associated with relaparotomy has been previously reported to range from 20% to 71% for all indications (Bunt 1985). Subgroup analysis demonstrated increased mortality in older patients and those with peritonitis, sepsis, or associated multiorgan failure (Harbrecht et al. 1984; Bunt 1985).

Severity scoring systems may be useful in these critically ill patients. A commonly used system used by American Surgeons is the APACHE II (Acute Physiology and Clinical Health Evaluation) system (Table 18.5.1) (Knaus et al. 1985; Stein 2001). Points are assigned based on multiple clinical parameters in conjunction with the GCS (Glasgow Coma Score) and chronic health conditions. The APACHE II system is helpful in stratifying patient outcomes; however, the severity of illness should not be dismissed simply due to a low APACHE II score.

The relaparotomy rate is lower after urological procedures owing to limited bowel, hepatic, and pancreatic manipulation. Even so, the incidence of relaparotomy will no doubt increase as the bowel becomes more integrated into reconstructive procedures. In addition, advances in perioperative care have enabled urologists to operate on more advanced disease in an older patient population. It is not uncommon to operate on individuals over 75 years of age. This increase in age predisposes patients to complications due to the inherent co-morbid factors associated with an older population.

Table 18.5.1. APACHE II Score Calculation

1. Age in years	
Under 44	0 Points
45–54	2 Points
55–64	3 Points
65–74	5 Points
over 74	6 Points
2. History of severe organ insufficiency or immuno-compromised?	
Yes, and nonoperative or emergency post-operative patient	5 Points
Yes, and elective postoperative patient	2 Points
No	0 Points
3. Rectal Temperature	
Over 40.9	4 Points
39–40.9	3 Points
38.5–38.9	1 Points
36–38.4	0 Points
34–35.9	1 Points
32–33.9	2 Points
30–31.9	3 Points
Below 30	4 Points
4. Mean arterial pressure (mm Hg)	
Over 159	4 Points
130–159	3 Points
110–129	2 Points
70–109	0 Points
50–69	2 Points
Below 50	4 Points
5. Heart rate (ventricular response)	
Over 179	4 Points
140–179	3 Points
110–139	2 Points
70–109	0 Points
55–69	2 Points
40–54	3 Points
Below 40	4 Points
6. Respiratory rate	
Over 49	4 Points
35–49	3 Points
25–34	1 Points
12–24	0 Points
10–11	1 Points
6–9	2 Points
Below 6	4 Points
7. Oxygenation (use PaO_2 if $FiO_2 < 50\%$, otherwise use A-a gradient)	
A-a gradient over 499	4 Points
A-a gradient 350–499	3 Points
A-a gradient 200–349	2 Points
A-a below 200 (if FiO_2 over 49%) or pO_2 more than 70 (if FiO_2 less than 50%)	0 Points
pO_2 = 61–70	1 Points
pO_2 = 55–60	3 Points
pO_2 below 55	4 Points
8. Arterial pH	
Over 7.69	4 Points
7.60–7.69	3 Points
7.50–7.59	1 Points
7.33–7.49	0 Points
7.25–7.32	2 Points
7.15–7.24	3 Points
Below 7.15	4 Points
9. Serum sodium (mmol/l)	
Over 179	4 Points
160–179	3 Points
155–159	2 Points
150–154	1 Points
130–149	0 Points
120–129	2 Points
111–119	3 Points
Below 111	4 Points
10. Serum potassium (mmol/l)	
Over 6.9	4 Points
6–6.9	3 Points
5.5–5.9	1 Points
3.5–5.4	0 Points
3–3.4	1 Points
2.5–2.9	2 Points
Below 2.5	4 Points
11. Serum creatinine (mg/100 ml)	
Over 3.4 and acute renal failure	8 Points
2.0–3.4 And acute renal failure	6 Points
Over 3.4 and chronic renal failure	4 Points
1.5–1.9 And acute renal failure	4 Points
2.0–3.4 And chronic	3 Points
1.5–1.9 And chronic	2 Points
0.6–1.4	0 Points
Below 0.6	2 Points
12. Hematocrit	
Over 59.9	4 Points
50–59.9	2 Points
46–49.9	1 Points
30–45.9	0 Points
20–29.9	2 Points
Below 20	4 Points
13. White blood count	
Over 39	4 Points
20–39.9	2 Points
15–19.9	1 Points
3.0–14.9	0 Points
1.0–2.9	2 Points
Below 1.0	4 Points

14. Minus the Glasgow Coma Score (maximum GCS =15)

Eye opening	*Verbal*	*Motor response*
4: Spontaneously	5: Alert and oriented	6: Obeys commands
3: To command	4: Confused	5: Localizes to pain
2: To pain	3: Inappropriate	4: Withdraws to pain
1: No response	2: Incomprehensible	3: Flexion to pain
	1: No response	2: Extension to pain
		1: No response

Total points	
0–4	4% Death rate
5–9	8% Death rate
10–14	15% Death rate
15–19	25% Death rate
20–24	40% Death rate
25–29	55% Death rate
30–34	75% Death rate
over 34	85% Death rate

This trend toward the higher-risk patient and more complicated procedure requires that urologists be more attuned to undesired outcomes than ever before. Problematic outcomes must be recognized early and treated immediately. Management of these complicated patients should be conservative if possible, but more invasive measures must be instituted immediately when they are necessary. In a retrospective review by Lamme et al., mortality associated with relaparotomy on demand (ROD) was 69% of that associated with patients with planned relaparotomies (PR) (Lamme et al. 2004). When comparing patients with similar clinical severity profiles (APACHE II scores 10.8 vs 11.7) ROD was associated with significantly lower in-hospital mortality rates (21.8% vs 36%) and longer 2-year survival (65.8% vs 55.5%) than PR. Indications for ROD received further support from Haut et al., who found the incidence of postoperative multiorgan system failure (MOF) to be higher in PR than ROD patients (Haut et al. 1995). Relaparotomy on demand was defined in a generic manner to include patients who deteriorated rapidly or failed to improve clinically (Lamme et al. 2004).

The most common indications for emergent relaparotomy are hemorrhage, infection, and elevated intraabdominal pressure (Lamme et al. 2004; Haut et al. 1995; Martin and Rossi 1997). These diagnoses and treatment of these complications as well as other common reasons for returning to the operating room are outlined below.

18.5.3 Infectious Peritonitis

Recognition and control of abdominal sepsis is critical, as failure to do so will result in MOF and mortality rates approaching 100% (Bohnen et al. 1983; Anderson et al. 1996; Koperna and Schultz 2000; Hutchins et al. 2004; Hindsdale and Jaffe 1984; Pusajo 1993). Infections in the postoperative period result in significant morbidity and health care costs with intraabdominal infections being the most costly. Sepsis has been estimated to develop in over 750,000 patients yearly in the United States, with over 200,000 associated deaths (Angus et al. 2001; Hotchkiss and Karl 2003). Some of the contributing causes include: (1) widespread use of antibiotics, (2) concentrations of multidrug-resistant organisms in hospitals, (3) older patient populations with associated co-morbidities, and (4) increased use of steroids and other immunosuppressive agents (Hunt and Mueller 1994). Outcomes of postoperative infections depend on the balance between the host's immune response and bacterial virulence (Hunt and Mueller 1994; Wittman et al. 1996). Even with great advances in critical care and antibiotic therapy, mortality is high.

The terms "peritonitis" and "intraabdominal infection" are often used interchangeably, however; the latter has numerous etiologies. A review by Marcello has helped better define peritonitis (Table 18.5.2) (Marcello 2001). Type II peritonitis remains the most common in the surgical population with polymicrobial contamination from aerobic and anaerobic bacteria. Concentration and variability increase as the surgical site moves toward the colon. Devitalized tissue, foreign bodies, and blood will promote bacterial growth leading to a more virulent form of peritonitis (Martin and Rossi 1997). Type III peritonitis has an extremely poor prognosis as the infection is technically cleared; however, the immune system continues to function as if it is still present. The end result is MOF, which is outlined in Table 18.5.3, adapted from Clarke (Clarke 2001). Many of the criteria are not specific to septic patients and may be found in postoperative patients without bacteremia. Differentiating these patients from those who are septic is critical.

Systemic inflammatory response syndrome (SIRS) is a transition to sepsis and is linked to a complex cascade of inflammatory mediators and cytokines. The most widely studied pro-inflammatory cytokines include tumor necrosis factor (TNF), interleukin-1 (IL-1), and interleukin-8 (IL-8). The anti-inflammatory cytokines are interleukin-6 (IL-6) and interleukin-10 (IL-10) (Clarke 2001; Christman et al. 1991). Patients with poor nutritional status and compromised immune systems are often incapable of mounting an appropriate response because of high metabolic demands. Efforts to supplement their response with extrinsic means are promising, as discussed below.

Septic patients may present with a spectrum of clinical manifestations. Classically, patients with intraabdominal sepsis have fluid sequestration and systemic vasodilatation resulting in tachycardia, hypotension, and

Table 18.5.2. Peritonitis classification

Type	Examples
I. Primary peritonitis: diffuse bacterial infection without abdominal viscus injury	Spontaneous pediatric peritonitis Peritoneal dialysis peritonitis Tuberculosis and granulomatous peritonitis
II. Secondary peritonitis: localized or diffuse peritonitis from an abdominal viscus injury	Intraperitoneal inflammation Gastrointestinal perforation Intestinal ischemia Retroperitoneal inflammation Postoperative peritonitis Anastomotic leak or perforation Posttraumatic perforation Blunt and penetrating injury
III. Tertiary peritonitis: abnormal host immune response	Sterile peritonitis Fungal peritonitis Peritonitis with low-grade bacterial infection

oliguria. The physical exam should provide insight if there is injury to the bowel. Palpation and percussion of the abdomen may manifest frank peritonitis. In some instances, there may be drainage from the incision site, which often precedes dehiscence. In other instances, frank stool can be documented in the surgical wound. When drains have been left in place, their volume and content should be evaluated and sent for Gram stain and culture. In particular, elevated BUN and creatinine content can suggest a urine leak.

Table 18.5.3. Sepsis progression

Infection	Microbial phenomenon characterized by an inflammatory response to the presence of microorganisms or the invasion of normally sterile host tissue by those organisms
Bacteremia	The presence of viable bacteria in the blood
SIRS	The systemic inflammatory response to a variety of severe clinical insults. The response is characterized by two or more or the following conditions: Temperature >38 °C or <36 °C Heart rate >90 beats/min Respiratory rate >20 breaths/min or $PaCO_2$ <32 torr WBC >12,000 cells/mm^3, <4,000 cells/mm^3 =, or >10 % bands
Sepsis	The systemic response to infection characterized by two or more of the above conditions. Differs from SIRS, which can be noninfectious in nature.
Severe sepsis	Sepsis associated with organ dysfunction, hypoperfusion, or hypotension. Examples include lactic acidosis, oliguria, or change in mental status
Septic shock	Sepsis with hypotension, despite adequate fluid resuscitation, along with the presence of perfusion abnormalities
Multiple organ dysfunction syndrome	Presence of altered organ function in an acutely ill patient such that homeostasis cannot be maintained without organ system support. Examples include mechanical ventilation, hemodialysis, or inotropic support

Broad-spectrum antibiotics should be started when an infectious source is being considered. Patients with chronic illnesses are often infected with multidrug-resistant bacteria because of prior antibiotic usage (Marcello 2001; Clarke 2001; Gold and Moellering 1996. There are several patient populations that should have a low threshold for medical or surgical intervention when sepsis is suspected. These include patients with a history of multiple prior abdominal surgeries, complicated primary surgery, poor nutritional status, and chronic immunosuppression.

Antibiotics remain the mainstay of treating postoperative infections. Broad-spectrum coverage should be initiated at the first sign of infection. Studies estimate that approximately 10 % of patients do not receive prompt antibiotic coverage. This same group of patients demonstrated a 10 %–15 % increase in mortality when compared to those receiving immediate antibiotic treatment for intraabdominal infections (Pittet et al. 1996). Antimicrobial therapy should be tailored to bacterial sensitivities when they become available. The use of continuous broad-spectrum triple-antibiotic therapy, (ampicillin, gentamycin, and metronidazole), has been replaced with dual-agent antibiotics such as Unasyn (ampicillin/sulbactam) and Zosyn (piperacillin/tazobactam) (Hotchkiss and Karl 2003). Infectious disease specialists should be consulted in all cases of intraabdominal infections.

New concepts in treating sepsis are targeted at enhancing the host immune response while minimizing the deleterious side effects of hyperinflammation commonly seen in ill patients (Table 18.5.4) (Marcello 2001; Clarke 2001; Marshall 2003; Zielger et al. 1991; Alejandria et al. 2002; Bernard et al. 2001; Root et al. 2003; Makita et al. 1998). Wheeler and Bernard (1999) advocate infection prevention in high-risk individuals with preoperative antibiotics complemented with the use of brief, targeted immunosuppressive therapy in the presence of sepsis. Although the concepts associated with these investigations seem promising, the clinical trials have shown limited effect. It is also important to remember that an overzealous inflammatory reaction

Table 18.5.4. Immunomodulation therapies

Agent	Example	Mechanism	Clinical outcomes
Nitric oxide antagonists	Methylated arginine analogues (l-NMMA and l-NAME)	Minimize vascular dysregulation and associated hypoperfusion	No clinical benefit in human studies
Endotoxin inhibitors, complement antibodies & IL-1 inhibitors	Polyvalent antibodies	Limit inflammation cascade	Mortality benefit in human trials
Anticoagulants	Activated protein C (Xigris)	Limit microvascular thrombosis and associated ischemia	Mortality reduction in human trials
Granulocyte colony stimulating factor	G-CSF	Promote host defense mechanisms	Limited clinical benefit in human studies
Macrophage inhibitory migration antibodies	MIF	Allows macrophage localization to site of infection	Preclinical trials in human studies

may tax an already ill patient, doing more harm than good.

When possible, imaging studies should be obtained to help locate the source of infection. Studies of the upper and lower gastrointestinal tracts help to determine the presence and location of a leak. The integrity of the urinary tract may need to be evaluated as well, especially when drain output is consistent with urine. Retrograde studies and loopograms may be used to evaluate urinary diversions and ureteroenteric anastomoses. In many cases, these studies can direct percutaneous drainage.

In the case of a urine leak, percutaneous nephrostomy tubes should be placed after a leak is confirmed by loopography or cystography. Ureteral stents should be in place from the time of surgery. These should remain for a minimum of 3 weeks before open repair is considered. During that period of time, nutritional support should be maximized.

If the infectious process is not amenable to percutaneous intervention, limited options exist other than surgery. One should have a low threshold for reoperation, as 40% of patients with loculated collections require reexploration (Boey 1994). The decision to operate should not be prolonged unless the patient is too hemodynamically unstable for transfer to the operating room. In 2004, Koperna and Schulz reviewed their relaparotomy experience and found that patients explored within 48 h had a statistically significant decrease in mortality, when stratified for APACHE II scores less than 26 (Table 18.5.1). Patients with scores greater than 26 have such profound physiological compromise that reexploration may be viewed as futile (Koperna and Schultz 2000).

Therefore, as soon as there is adequate resuscitation through a central venous line, initial administration of antibiotics and placement of appropriate monitoring devices (e.g., a Swan-Ganz catheter and arterial line), the patient can be mobilized to the operating room. The goals of surgical intervention include: (1) controlling the source of infection, (2) evacuating bacterial inoculum (peritoneal washout), (3) treating and preventing abdominal compartment syndrome, and (4) preventing or treating recurrent or persistent infection (Marcello 2001).

Prior to any planned exploration, the surgeon must address the need for diverting intestinal conduits. Ostomy marking can be performed by an enterostomal therapist if one is available (Fig. 18.5.1). The operating room should be prepared for a complicated surgery and should include supplies to leave an open abdomen. Reexploration should be thorough enough to locate and remove infectious sources; however, operative time should be minimized to prevent unnecessary and insensible fluid loss in an already sick patient.

One method for eliminating infection is by staged abdominal repair (STAR). STAR is a surgical treatment policy consisting of scheduled multiple laparotomies every 24–48 h until the peritoneum is clear. This form of intervention should be used with caution if the source of infection is from an upper gastrointestinal injury in close proximity of the pancreas (Agalar et al. 2005).

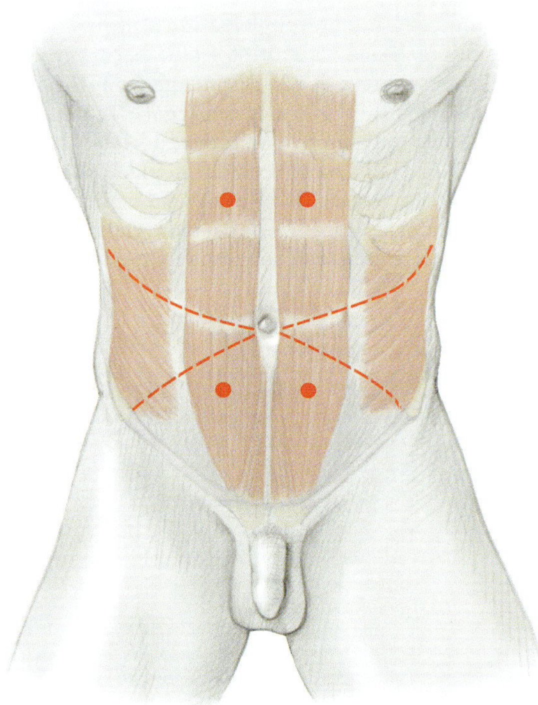

Fig. 18.5.1. Preoperative stomal marking utilizing the rectus muscle anatomy. Consider using the upper rectus in patients whose anatomy limits catheterization (e.g., obese or wheelchair-bound). Adapted from Libertino 1998 (© Hohenfellner 2007)

18.5.3.1 Intraabdominal Abscess

Abscess development can be linked to many etiologies and presents with a variety of symptoms. Bacteria become localized under the influence of peritoneal fluid movement and gravity (Fry and Clevenger 1991). In addition, the presence of foreign bodies and dead tissue promote bacterial growth. Hematomas are high in iron content and act as excellent media for bacteria growth. The end result is a walled-off collection of bacteria protected from the host immune response and antibiotics (Fig. 18.5.2).

Because of the focal nature of an abscess, these patients have a different presentation than those with generalized peritonitis. They have low-grade fevers or an irregular pattern of temperature spikes with negative culture work-up. The physical exam is often compromised by incisional pain and the use of narcotics. A

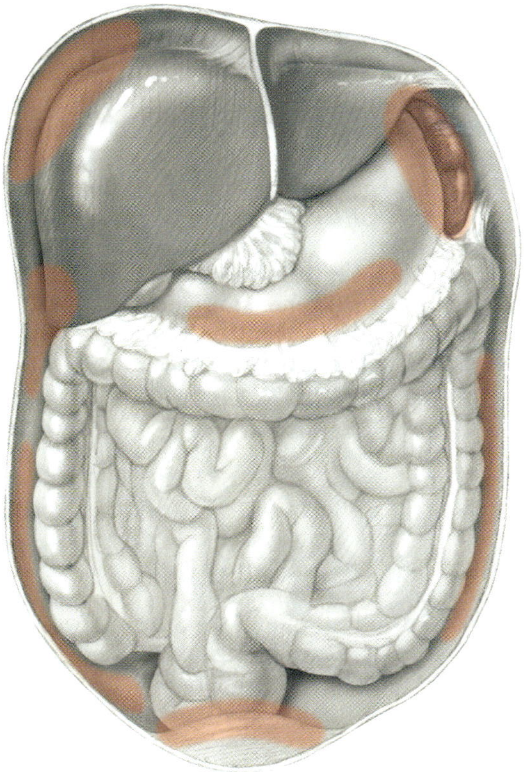

Fig. 18.5.2. Peritoneal fluid patterns and abscess locations (© Hohenfellner 2007)

CT scan is the best imaging study for evaluation of a mature abscess. Early stages of abscess formation are difficult to discern from routine postoperative fluid and inflammatory changes. A bedside ultrasound can also be used in the critically ill patients; however, the sensitivity is marginal.

When an abscess is identified, the surgeon needs to determine if a second surgery is warranted. Percutaneous drainage is an ideal option when the precise anatomical location can be identified and there is no bowel at risk during the drainage. An abscess that forms in the retroperitoneum is more amenable to percutaneous drainage because there is limited interference with intraabdominal contents. Retroperitoneal collections track along tissue planes and often involve the psoas muscle (Boey 1994). Loculated pockets can persist after percutaneous drain placement. Many surgeons and interventional radiologists agree that if there is no resolution within 3 days the drain should be repositioned or surgical drainage performed.

When surgery must be performed on high-risk patients, a limited approach may be a more prudent course of action. Fluid collections along the paracolic gutters may be managed with a lateral abdominal incision that utilizes extraperitoneal access routes to avoid recontamination of the peritoneum (Fry and Clevenger 1991). Deep pelvic collections that are not amenable to percutaneous drainage may require exploration through the original incision.

The operation for abdominal abscess can worsen a patient's condition if care is not taken when handling inflamed tissues that are prone to tearing. Upon entering the abdomen, there is likely to be a moderate number of thin adhesions between the bowel, omentum, and surrounding organs. Bleeding should be managed with compression since electrocautery leaves necrotic tissue behind, promoting bacterial growth. The surgical site is examined first. If an anastomosis is completely compromised, then a resection and reanastomosis should be performed (see Sect. 18.5.3.2). In those cases where abscess formation is not secondary to perforated bowel, the abscess cavity should be evacuated and regional tissue debrided. The area should then be copiously irrigated and reinspected. Closed-system drains may be placed prior to closing. These should exit at sites separate from the incision. The use of synthetic materials is discouraged because of the increased morbidity associated with removal of infected mesh.

Surgical drainage for postoperative abscesses carries a high degree of morbidity. Success is based on locating the source and repairing it appropriately. In critically ill patients, the immune response is often dampened and the peritoneum provides an ideal environment for bacterial proliferation. Even with aggressive irrigation there are bound to be minute foci of bacteria that remain. Broad-spectrum antibiotics should be started and then tailored to organism and sensitivity as appropriate. Efforts should be made to maximize nutritional status to reduce catabolic effects. Patients should be encouraged to ambulate if possible, to reduce the fluid from becoming stagnant. ICU patients should be turned frequently.

18.5.3.2 Anastomotic Leaks

Bowel has proven useful in the creation of reliable urinary reservoirs and conduits. A thorough description has been afforded to us by Dr. Hendren who elaborates on the historical use of bowel in adult and pediatric reconstructive surgery (Hendron 1997). The incorporation of ileal and colonic segments for urinary diversion has evolved into catheterizable stomas derived from the ileum, ureter, stomach, fallopian tube, and appendix. Despite refinements in technique that have produced astounding cosmetic and functional results, there are still certain complications requiring surgical intervention. Reoperation rates for early complications are 3% for continent catheterizable reservoirs and up to 7% in orthotopic bladder substitution, with long-term complications requiring surgical intervention in 30% and 13%, respectively (Hautman 2003). Early

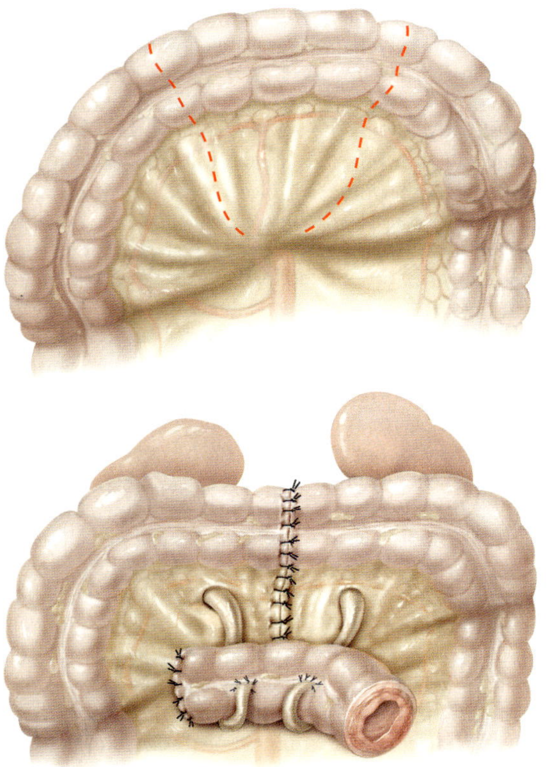

a

b

Fig. 18.5.3. a The transverse colon is mobilized and the blood supply (middle colic artery) preserved prior to creation of the colon conduit. **b** Following implantation of the ureters (antirefluxing technique) into the taenia coli, an end urostomy is created. Adapted from Libertino 1998 (© Hohenfellner 2007)

complications necessitating urgent relaparotomy include bowel wall necrosis and perforation, bleeding, obstruction, and urinary leakage (Hautman 2003; Killeen and Libertino 1988). Prompt recognition and immediate repair can limit the morbidity associated with these complications.

Anastomotic leaks can be the result of technical error; however, other factors make them more common. Poor preoperative nutritional status and chronic steroid use predispose patients to anastomotic breakdown. In addition, patients with bladder cancer are often older with multiple cardiac and pulmonary risk factors often in the setting of recent weight loss associated with their malignancy. Prior abdominal surgery or radiation therapy may complicate matters further. A transverse colon conduit is often a more acceptable form of urinary diversion in these patients (Fig. 18.5.3a) (Mattos and Libertino 1998). Efforts should be made to maximize the nutritional status of these patients prior to surgery while obtaining the appropriate preoperative clearance.

The disruption of a bowel anastomosis may have a myriad of clinical presentations depending on the bowel segment used. Small-bowel leaks may present in the first 48 h compared to colonic leaks, which may take 3–5 days to present. The spectrum can range from localized abscess to frank fecal peritonitis, as described in Sect. 18.5.3. In select case, a conservative approach with antibiotics and percutaneous drainage may be taken or the patient may need to have a laparotomy.

Although cosmetically alarming, a well-controlled fistula may resolve without surgery. They can be managed conservatively with parenteral nutrition and proximal decompression for 4–6 weeks. After this period of time, surgical intervention is indicated. A second surgery is also warranted in those with progressive deterioration despite broad-spectrum antibiotics.
Surgical intervention with enteroenterostomy can be performed, although proximal diversion with a terminal ileostomy, colostomy, or fistula bypass may need to be performed in the presence of extensive adhesions, which limit the ability to perform a primary repair. An attempt to restore fecal continuity is dependent on the resolution of adhesions. These patients may also be at risk for developing a dehiscence.

At the time of laparotomy, the original surgical site is inspected. Depending on the severity and status of the patient, a hand-sewn primary repair may be performed at the leak site. Using a standard two-layer closure for enterotomies is recommended, with interposition of omentum where appropriate. Compromised tissue from inflammatory reactions may need to be resected and a second anastomosis performed. A proximal diversion may be required in critically ill patients with florid sepsis or those with gross fecal peritonitis in whom the anastomosis is unlikely to heal. In some cases, one may opt to prepare the patient for exploration at a later time. Techniques for leaving a patient with an open abdomen are described in Sect. 18.5.8.

For surgical repair of urine leaks, primary revision of the ureteroenteric anastomosis is appropriate when the distal ureter segment is healthy. When a segment of ureter needs resection, an ileal interposition (Fig. 18.5.4a) or ileal add-on can be used (Fig. 18.5.4b). The transverse colon can be used as a conduit in patients with prior radiation. Transureteroureterostomy is another alternative (Fig. 18.5.4c). A unilateral nephrectomy can be performed with good contralateral function.

In extreme cases, ureteroenteric anastomosis may not be feasible and distal urinary control needs to be addressed with planned delayed definitive repair. Although urine leakage does not produce the same reaction as fecal contamination, the inflammatory reaction associated with extravasated urine will further complicate matters. Temporary urinary diversion can be accomplished by intubating the distal ureter with a single-J stent, which will then be externalized through separate stab incisions (Coburn 1997). Alternative techniques include ureter ligation with nephrostomy tube placement; however, attempts should be made to

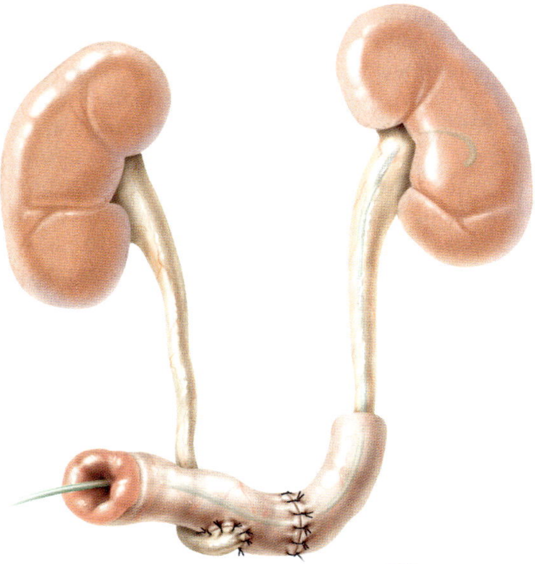

a

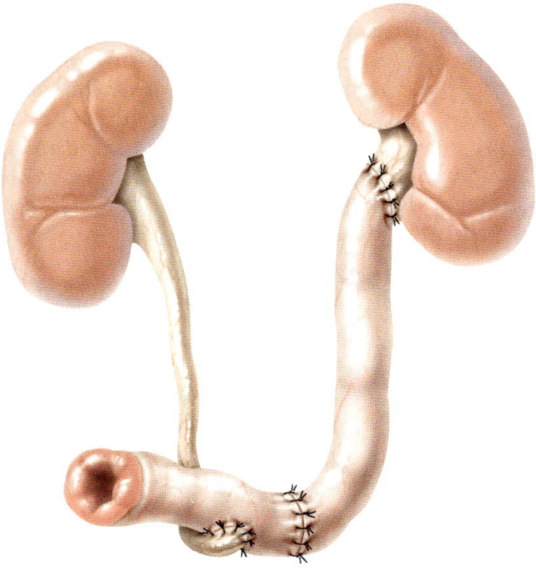

b

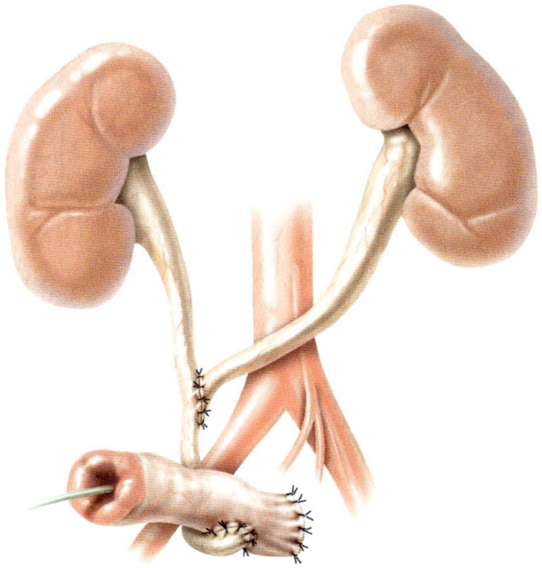

c

Fig. 18.5.4a–c. Ureterointestinal revisions. An ileal interposition graft (**a**), ileal add-on (**b**) or transureterostomy (**c**) are safe alternatives for revision of ureteroenteric anastomosis. Adapted from Libertino 1998 (© Hohenfellner 2007)

conserve as much of the ureter as possible for reimplantation. Cutaneous ureterostomy following transureteroureterostomy can also be performed.

If there is no evidence of a leak at the surgical site, all four quadrants should be explored, ruling out missed enterotomies or sequestered fluid collections. Common findings at relaparotomy include abscess, suture line leak, necrotic bowel, technical error, or a negative finding. In the select cases, where a urine and bowel leak are present, the surgeon must repair the bowel leak with drainage of the urine to prevent urinoma formation. Only in rare instances should both injuries be simultaneously repaired.

18.5.3.3
Injury to the Colon and Rectum

Iatrogenic injury to the colon or rectum is an inherent risk in urological surgery given their close proximity to the prostate, bladder, and urethra. These warrant special mention given the chronic problems, such as fistulas, associated with occurrence. In addition, patients will not only have a prolonged hospital stay, but will likely require another surgery or intervention due to sepsis or abscess. Cases not amenable to primary repair or conservative management will require temporary diversion of urine and or stool. For these reasons, surgeons need to be very direct when describing potential complications and should include injury to the colon and rectum in almost all urological procedures from prostatectomies to percutaneous nephrostolithotomy.

Studies report that incidence of injury to colon or rectum is 0.5%–3.0% (Morse et al. 1988; Dillioglugil et al. 1997; Lepor et al. 2001; Leandri et al. 1992). This often occurs as the prostate is dissected off of Denonvilliers fascia, which can be compromised by inflammation or malignancy. Morse et al. (1988) described their experience with 14 patients who sustained such injuries. Presentation was often delayed and manifested with fecaluria or stool at the incision. In the acute setting, the patient needs prompt wound management. Urine should be diverted with a Foley catheter and suprapubic tube. Because the peritoneum is not violated during standard prostatectomy, there is limited risk for the development of peritonitis. A well-controlled fistula may be treated with elective surgery and spontaneous closure may occur with catheter drainage and meticulous wound care.

Rectal injury identified in the operating room should be repaired primarily only when the bowel has been prepped. The procedure should be stopped and the rectum assessed with digital exam if there is a concern for rectal injury. Following aggressive wound irrigation, a standard two-layered closure should be performed. In the presence of frank stool or compromised tissue from prior surgery or radiation, the surgeon should elect for diverting colostomy with delayed repair.

Surgeons may consider a separate laparotomy incision with creation of a double-lumen colostomy using the transverse colon with delayed injuries to the rectum. The left colonic flexure should also be mobilized in anticipation of future reconstruction for continuity. Once the transverse colon is mobilized through a separate incision, the laparotomy is closed, thus limiting peritoneal contamination. A double-lumen colostomy is then created in standard fashion (Fig. 18.5.5). Once proximal diversion is achieved, the prior prostatectomy incision is reopened and the surgical site is copiously irrigated with warm normal saline. Two drains should be placed alongside the bladder and the incision closed. With time and antibiotics, the rectal fistula should heal in 4–6 weeks. The urethral catheter remains in place for 6 weeks and is only removed following a negative cystogram. The colostomy may be reversed after 3 months following a negative barium enema study.

Colonic injury during nephrectomy is uncommon unless the vascular supply has been compromised (Fry and Clevenger 1991). Unintended ligation of anatomically variant vessels unrecognized during the procedure may compromise perfusion to the colon with resultant ischemia. Like most ischemic injuries, the clinical presentation should be promptly recognized and the appropriate management undertaken. A formal colectomy may need to be performed. In patients with vascular and cardiac disease, suspicion for ischemia must be high as low flow states can easily precipitate these types of injuries in such patient populations.

The anatomic relationship between the colon and kidney varies greatly, with one study reporting the incidence of a posterolateral colon in 3%–19% and retrorenal colon in 2% of patients studied (Clayman 1985). The latter position is at high risk for perforation during percutaneous procedures, making preoperative imaging crucial. Prompt recognition of stool in nephrostomy tubes will minimize morbidity and fistula formation. If iatrogenic injury does occur one may remove

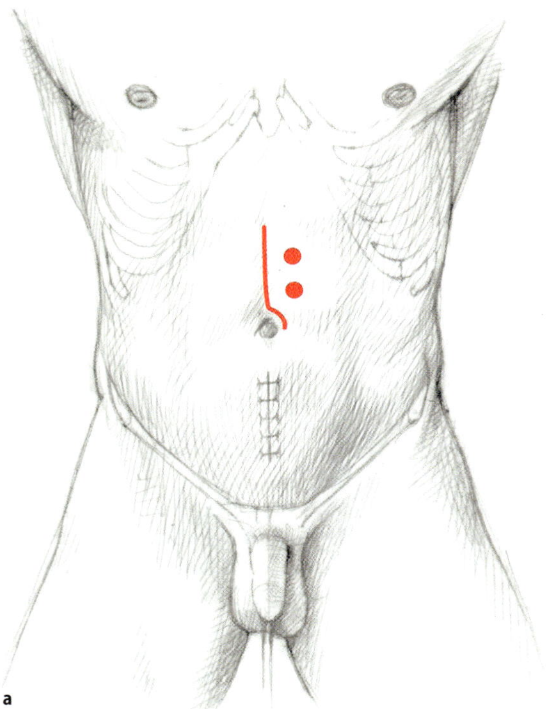

a

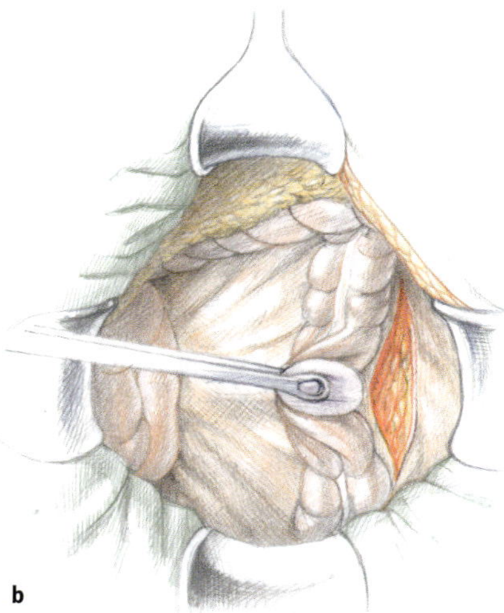

b

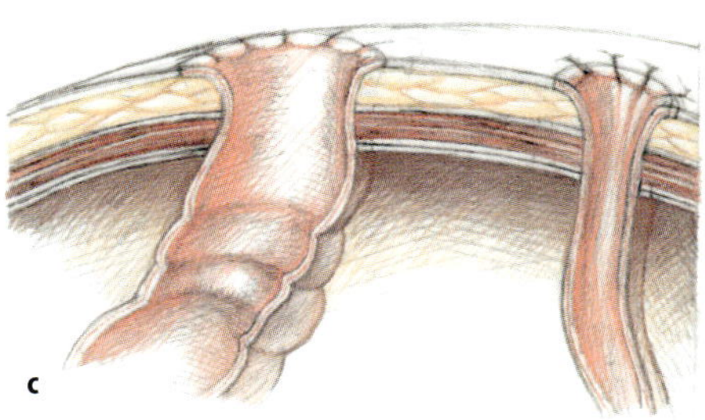

c

Fig. 18.5.5. a Planned site of second incision separate from prior lower abdominal incision for radical retropubic prostatectomy (RRP). Enterostomal therapy should be consulted for upper abdominal urostomy marking. **b** Following a midline incision, the descending colon is mobilized along the white line of Toldt. **c** At the level of the skin, a double-lumen colostomy is created with the distal portion left as a mucus fistula

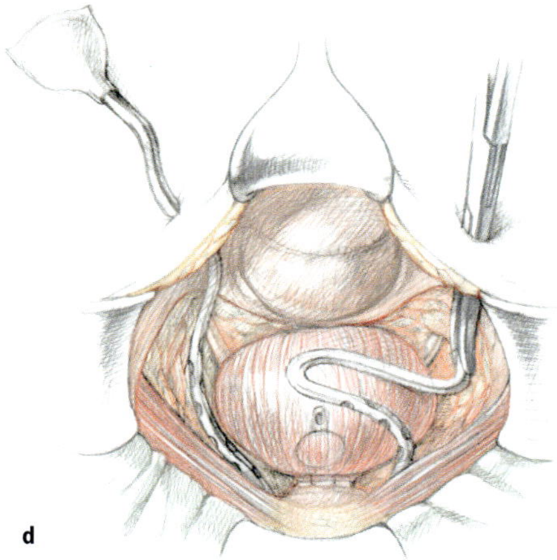

d

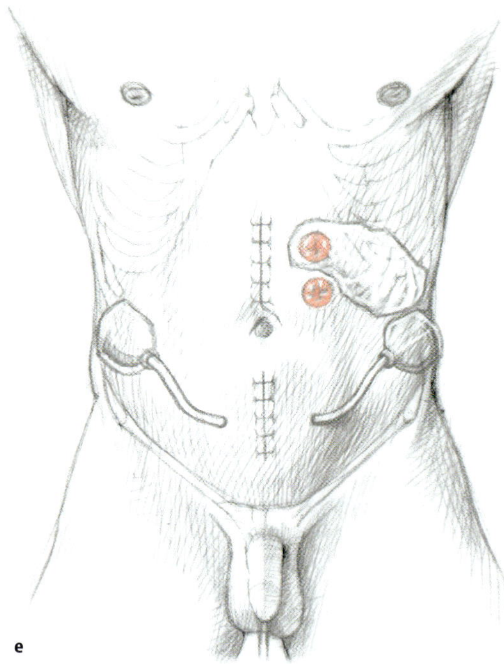

e

Fig. 18.5.5. d Following creation of the colostomy and mucus fistula, the superior incision is closed and the prior lower incision is reexplored with placement of closed drains on both sides of the prostatourethral anastomosis. Efforts to repair the anastomosis should be limited at this time because of the high likelihood of breakdown **e** Final appearence

the nephrostomy tube completely or retract it into the colon with a staged removal, hoping to limit fecal contamination of the retroperitoneum. Double-J ureteral stents are placed prior to removal. Experienced colorectal surgeons should be involved when managing patients with difficult fistulas.

18.5.3.4 Laparoscopic Bowel Injury

The incidence of bowel injury in laparoscopic surgery is reported less than open surgery. Bishoff et al. from Johns Hopkins reviewed their experience with eight bowel injuries associated with laparoscopic urological procedures (Bishoff et al. 1999). A Medline review by this group demonstrated that bowel perforation occurred in 1.3/1,000 cases, with the majority of injuries not recognized at the time of surgery. In instances where bowel injury is identified, immediate repair is essential, as delayed intervention usually necessitates open laparotomy for repair.

Laparoscopic patients may actually present with leukopenia, diarrhea, and often complain of extreme trocar site pain. When these symptoms are overlooked, the outcome can be devastating. Two patients in the above study experienced colon injuries during pelvic lymph node dissection and died in 4 days from overwhelming sepsis. Therefore, postoperative laparoscopic patients with nonspecific abdominal complaints should trigger a thorough exam and review of the operative record to determine the need for imaging studies. Venous bleeding may be underestimated or unrecognized during laparoscopy secondary to compression from pneumoperitoneum.

Laparoscopy limits the view of the abdomen and instruments. It is estimated that the surgeon only sees 10%–15% of the instrument within the surgical viewing field. Faulty equipment and lack of attention will contribute to thermal injury, given the high-energy state associated with electrocautery. These oversights contribute to the incidence of bowel injury. As reported by Bishoff et al. (1999), the small bowel is injured 58% of the time, with colon and stomach injury reported in 32% and 7%, respectively. Trocar placement can also lead to bowel injury when performed carelessly or not under direct visualization. Of the total number of injuries observed in 12 series, 32% were attributed to Veress needle punctures or trocar insertion. Multiple adhesions also predispose patients to thermal and trocar injuries.

Upper gastrointestinal tract injuries will present before colon injury. The choice of repair and need for a proximal diversion will be determined by the injury. Most gastric and small-bowel injuries can be repaired primarily due to early presentation. Good outcomes have been reported for bowel perforations managed laparoscopically. Percutaneous drainage and parenteral nutrition may be more appropriate in critically ill patients.

An interesting hypothesis regarding the etiology of sepsis after laparoscopy comes from studies with IL-6 by Cruikshank et al., who theorize that the minimal trauma associated with laparoscopic surgery leads to lower immune and metabolic responses (Cruickshank et al. 1990; Harmon et al. 1994). These authors postulate lower levels of IL-6 may dampen the acute-phase response associated with the initiation of the inflammatory cascade and the ability to fight infection. Additional studies will need to be conducted to confirm this work.

18.5.4 Postoperative Bleeding

Surgeries of the upper urinary tract and retroperitoneum are inherently associated with a risk of serious bleeding from major vessels for many reasons. Renal and adrenal masses commonly have extensive venous and arterial collaterals involving the inferior vena cava and aorta. Retroperitoneal masses may encase regional vasculature in desmoplastic reactions following chemotherapy or radiation (Zinman and Libertino 1988). Surgery of the lower urinary tract and prostate may be complicated by inadequate exposure secondary to pelvic anatomy. In addition, the vascular framework deep within the pelvis is prone to vascular accidents during mobilization.

Patients with ongoing blood loss usually present within the first 24 h (Zinman and Libertino 1988; Hirshberg et al. 1997; Thompson et al. 2003). Bleeding in the hemodynamically unstable patient may be difficult to distinguish from other postoperative processes. Hematocrit values can be misleading in the setting of large-volume resuscitation because of dilutional effects. Tachycardia, although helpful in the setting of adequate pain control, and oliguria, a reliable indicator of organ perfusion, are nonspecific. Sepsis may also produce hypotension resulting from systemic vasodilation. Exacerbation of underlying pulmonary and cardiac disease may also present similarly. Pulmonary artery catheterization may help distinguish these underlying causes of hemodynamic instability (Table 18.5.5) (Takhar and Rosenthal 2001).

Imaging studies benefit the management of these patients greatly. A CT scan may help differentiate between blood and fluid collections with the use of Hounsfield Units (HU). Angiography may be both diagnostic and therapeutic in dealing with arterial bleeding in the hands of a skilled interventional radiologist. One should be wary of contrast nephropathy when performing angiography in patients with limited renal function and institute appropriate pretreatment protocols in high-risk individuals (Table 18.5.6) (Rezkella 2003). Although helpful, imaging should never take precedence in an emergent case where time is critical.

In preparation for relaparotomy, it is essential to establish adequate venous access and arterial monitoring when possible. Blood and related blood products should be readied by the blood bank. The coagulation profile should be assessed and any clotting abnormalities treated appropriately. In 50 % of cases, the cause of postoperative bleeding is inadequate hemostasis during surgery. The other causes include liver failure, acquired deficiency of clotting factors, and shock-related disseminated intravascular coagulation (DIC) (Hirshberg et al. 1997; Mulvihill and Pellegrini 1994; Schell and Barbul 1998). One should make a strong effort to rule out nonsurgical causes, given the morbidity and mortality associated with relaparotomies, especially when unwarranted.

Restoration of the clotting cascade with blood and blood products is a more suitable approach in dealing with this subgroup of patients. In addition, the surgeon's recognition of DIC is critical. DIC is characterized by intravascular coagulation and diffuse thrombosis, resulting in consumption of clotting factors. Several factors precipitating DIC are inherent outcomes of surgical treatment. These include release of tissue debris into the bloodstream, introduction of intravascular platelet aggregates, which is commonplace in sepsis, and extensive endothelial injury. Treatment includes removal of the precipitating factor along with platelet and fresh frozen plasma transfusions (Schell and Barbul 1998). In patients requiring emergent relaparotomy there may not be time to fix all coagulopathies.

In select cases, the need for a second surgery may have already been made prior to closing. This latter group of patients tends to be hypothermic and coagulopathic with minimal reserve to withstand a lengthy procedure. Often packing provides an interim for stabilization and patient survival (Hirshberg et al. 1997).

18.5.4.1 Delayed Bleeding

The two main indications for urgent unplanned relaparotomy include ongoing hemorrhage and elevated intraabdominal pressure (Flint 1988). When the decision is made to proceed to surgery, blood products need to

Table 18.5.5. Shock classification

	CO[a]	SVR[a]	CVP[a]
Cardiogenic shock	Decreases	Increased	Increases
Septic shock	Increased	Decreased	Decreased
Hypovolemic shock	Decreased	Increased	Decreased

[a] Appearance of shock by several components of the pulmonary artery catheter reading

Table 18.5.6. Topical hemostatic agents

Baseline creatinine	Treatment
Less then 2.6	Hydration with 0.9 % normal saline N-acetylcysteine 600 mg BID Theophylline 200 mg Replete magnesium Limit dye exposure
2.5 – 3.0 With diabetes or Above 3.0	Hydration with 0.9 % normal saline N-acetylcysteine 600 mg BID Theophylline 200 mg Replete magnesium Fenoldapam (dopamine agonist) Limit dye exposure Prophylactic hemodialysis

be immediately available and the anesthesiologist needs to be prepared for an unstable patient. There must be constant communication between the surgeon and anesthesia staff, as bleeding and associated fluid shifts are unavoidable. Unlike planned reoperation, the coagulopathies of many patients have not been corrected. Autotransfusion should be available with the use of a Cell Saver (Haemonetics, Inc, Braintree, MA, USA). A surgeon needs a broad spectrum of instruments in managing arterial bleeding. These should include vascular forceps and needle holders, 5-0 and 6-0 sutures, bulldog clamps, partial and total occlusion clamps for the aorta and inferior vena cava, in addition to umbilical and silastic loops for arterial control (Zinman and Libertino 1988).

Following adequate anesthesia, the prior incision should be opened and extended for exposure. There will likely be a large amount of clot that needs to be evacuated. Caution must be used to prevent damage to adjacent structures. Generous irrigation of the field will help facilitate clot removal (Hirshberg et al. 1997). The source of bleeding will likely be in the vicinity of the primary surgery; however, all aspects of the cavity – abdominal, retroperitoneal, or pelvic – need to be explored.

In some cases, a suture knot may have slipped or a clip fallen off, and treatment may be as simple as suture ligature. However, in other instances a bleeding vessel may have retracted, requiring more definitive exposure to gain proximal control. After hemostasis is attained, the field should be copiously irrigated with warm saline and again inspected. When operating in deep confined spaces, packing laparotomy pads into the site makes examination for bleeding easier. In some circumstances there may be extensive venous bleeding that will require packing with plans to return later. All components of reconstructive cases should be inspected for ischemia, because ongoing blood loss may lead to bowel ischemia, especially in patients with cardiac and vascular disease.

Iatrogenic injury to the liver and spleen need to remain in the differential, as these organs may be damaged during retraction (Leandri et al. 1992). Bleeding from liver trauma is often very difficult to control, especially in an ill patient with coagulopathy. The mobilization required to expose the retrohepatic inferior vena cava (IVC) can lead to liver trauma and extensive bleeding associated with generous venous collateralization from chronic venous obstruction (Libertino et al. 1987). One cannot be cavalier about extensive liver damage given the risk of massive bleeding and associated coagulation dysfunction.

There should be no need for arterial reconstruction during a second surgery, assuming that arterial bleeding during the primary surgery was controlled at that time. An exception warranting reconstruction may occur in bypass surgery for renovascular hypertension. However, in most circumstances the original graft anastomosis can be revised after gaining proximal and distal control. Vein patch angioplasty is a safe alternative for difficult revisions.

18.5.4.2 Planned Reoperation

Compressive techniques are useful in dealing with troublesome bleeding during prolonged cases. Packing laparotomy pads may be prudent in patients with persistent bleeding that does not come from a major arterial source, namely the renal artery or aorta. A known or suspected source of arterial bleeding needs to be resolved before closing. Bleeding from the retroperitoneum, perirenal space, and prostatic fossa have been adequately controlled with packing techniques (Zinman and Libertino 1988).

Bleeding may also be secondary to coagulopathy, which may be associated with malignancy or related to the procedure itself. Massive transfusions, greater than one total blood volume, lead to dilutional thrombocytopenia with coagulopathy. Studies estimate clotting factors are decreased by 30% for each total volume of blood replaced (Schell and Barbul 1998). Platelets, fresh frozen plasma (FFP), and calcium should supplement blood replacements. With extensive blood loss there is often a need for massive transfusion. When large-volume blood replacement is accomplished solely by packed red blood cells, coagulopathies are inevitable. This is due to the lack of platelets and clotting factors in packed cells. In this setting, replacement with other blood products is necessary.

Until recently, algorithms for the administration of FFP and platelets were rather prevalent in anesthesia literature and can still be found in many texts. These formulas use measured blood loss, either in liters or body volumes, as the determining factor for replacement of all blood products. Recently, however, these formulaic guidelines have fallen out of favor. For this reason, none will be presented here.

Instead, it is important to underscore other, more critical determinants in providing exogenous clotting factors and platelets. In particular, physical signs of coagulopathy, such as bleeding or uncontrollable oozing should direct prompt administration of complimentary blood products. Similarly, abnormal lab values such as an elevated INR or low platelets direct more specific treatment with constituents such as FFP and platelets (Ho et al. 2005a, b; Hardy et al. 2004).

Laparotomy pads should be removed in a timely manner, as foreign body packing may promote bacterial proliferation in contaminated cases with associated sepsis. In addition to limiting ongoing blood loss, packing requires a second surgery, at which time debridement can take place and appropriate drains placed. In the interim, the patient can be resuscitated in the intensive care unit and any coagulation issues attended to prior to a second surgery.

During the second look operation, there must be an organized approach and plan to deal with any hemostatic complications. In critically ill patients, one may elect for bedside relaparotomy in the intensive care unit. After adequate prepping and draping, the laparotomy pads should be removed one by one. Inflammation reactions produce adhesions between laparotomy pads and tissues. Underwater approaches using warm saline are utilized to help tease apart the gauze pads. Hirshberg et al. (1997) recommend using a constant jet of water from a 100-ml syringe during pack removal. The surgical bed is explored and bleeding sources may be ligated or dealt with by electrocautery. Bleeding is managed at the time of encounter, not when all lap pads are removed. In some cases, a surgeon will have to admit defeat, repack the wound cavity, provide a temporary closure and return at a later date.

Often times, the bleeding arises from raw surfaces. Hemostasis will never be complete in these select cases; however, additional options are available. The argon beam laser is a good resource for raw oozing surfaces such as the liver bed. Topically applied hemostatic agents may assist in these situations (Table 18.5.7) (Kelleher et al. 2005). These agents provide great benefit during the primary cases. In the presence of elevated intraabdominal pressure, closure may need to be delayed until postoperative days 4–6, when the majority of interstitial fluid has mobilized.

Table 18.5.7. Limiting contrast nephrotoxicity

Agent	Mechanism
Gelatin sponge (Gelfoam)	Can absorb many times its weight of whole blood via capillary action and provides a platform for coagulation.
Oxidized cellulose (Surgicel)	Cellulose in knitted form that promotes clotting via absorption of blood with associated swelling. Swelling forms scaffold for coagulation
Collagen sponge (Helistat)	Derivative of bovine collagen tendon, which promotes platelet adhesion.
Microfibrillar collagen (Avitene)	Stimulates platelet adhesion promoting thrombus formation
Topical thrombin	Powder derived from bovine source that may be applied to wound directly or dissolved in saline and applied to wound to form fibrin-rich hemostatic plug
Fibrin sealant (Tisseel)	Concentrated fibrinogen and factor XIII combined with thrombin and calcium to form fibrin clot stimulating the final stage of the clotting cascade.
Topical thrombin and collagen (Floseal)	Synergistic interaction of gelatin granules, thrombin, and the patient's fibrinogen to promote hemostasis
Recombinant activated factor VII (NovoSeven)	Recombinant DNA preparation of activated blood coagulation factor VII

18.5.5 Stomal Complications

According to the literature, it has been estimated that 1%–10% of colostomies and 1%–5% of ileostomies will need surgical revision, with increased incidence in obese patients and emergent cases. The most common causes include stomal stenosis and parastomal herniation (Luck and Bokey 2003; Carroll and Barbour 2000)).

18.5.5.1 Necrosis

One of the most devastating complications of a stoma is acute postoperative necrosis. Necrosis is the unfortunate result of ischemia that may result from excess tension related to inadequate bowel length or inadvertent ligation of the blood supply. It may also be caused by excessive mesentery stripping to accommodate the fascial opening. In most instances, necrosis presents within 48 h as dark black slough, vs venous congestion, which has a more dark purple hue. When the question of viability is raised, the appliance should be taken down and the stoma examined by intubation with a sterile glass tube and adequate lighting or endoscopy.

The degree of necrosis dictates the need for surgery. Simple clearing of the sloughed tissue with a moist lap pad may be sufficient for superficial cases (Luck and Bokey 2003). When there is evidence of full-thickness necrosis, the patient must be prepped for relaparotomy. The abdomen is entered through the prior midline incision. An inflated Foley catheter will help identify the appropriate bowel segment. During the procedure, special attention must be given to the ureteroenteric anastomosis to rule out compromise secondary to necrosis. In cases of incontinent urinary diversion, the distal portion may be stapled off and a revision performed (Carroll and Barbour 2000). The necrotic segment is resected and an appropriate length for a tension-free stoma is made. In obese individuals, this may necessitate widening the fascial defect up to four fingerbreadths. Another option may be the formation of a loop ostomy that provides less tension. The loop end ileostomy has a lower incidence of stomal stenosis; however, parastomal herniation is higher. Individuals with evidence of superficial and partial thickness necrosis who do not undergo revision are at increased risk for stomal stenosis as a long-term complication (Rowbotham and Eyre 1998).

18.5.5.2
Stenosis

Stricture and stenosis of a stoma are often the result of chronic ischemia with a component of chronic inflammation secondary to alkaline urine, leading to fibrous tissue build-up. Stenosis has been reported to occur in up to 24% of patients with ileal conduits and 20% of colon conduits (Fitzgerald et al. 1997). Inability to pass a catheter should be followed by an IVP or loopogram study to estimate the degree of stricture. Digital manipulation is discouraged to avoid mucosal trauma and increased risk for infection. Conservative measures such as urine acidification may be used for treatment of hyperplasia and encrustation (Rowbotham and Eyre 1998).

A limited surgical approach for repair starts with a circumferential incision at the mucocutaneous border to identify the bowel serosa. The conduit is then mobilized with sharp dissection, avoiding injury to the mesentery and associated blood supply. This technique can provide a few centimeters of additional length. With the added length, the stoma is matured and the conduit fixed to the fascia. A Turnball loop stoma is a better option for patients with significant abdominal wall inversion (Bloom et al. 1983). A 16-F rubber catheter should be left in place to reduce risk of urinary retention from postoperative edema.

A small midline incision should be used when a greater length of bowel is needed. In many cases, resection of a small segment of the distal bowel is necessary, as blood supply may be compromised during mobilization. Ileal conduits often need revision for stricture disease. Following the midline incision, the conduit is identified and the degree of stricture determined. Multiple or lengthy strictures are best treated with add-on ileal segments and creation of a new stoma.

18.5.5.3
Parastomal Hernias

Patients who experience parastomal pain secondary to herniation of abdominal contents or peristomal leakage are best suited for surgical revision. Large hernias, although cosmetically a concern, should be left alone if asymptomatic (Ho et al. 2004). Colonic stomas are more prone to herniation because of larger fascial defects during creation. Inadequate fascial fixation, large fascial windows, and passing a conduit lateral to the rectus muscle are additional risk factors for parastomal herniation (Rubin et al. 1994).

If available, enterostomal nursing can mark the site of possible translocation. A Foley catheter is placed to help identify the conduit after making the midline incision. Adhesions are taken down to identify the conduit and fascial edges. Meticulous attention to detail will help avoid unnecessary enterotomies that can lead to troublesome fistulas at a later date. With the fascial edges identified, one may opt for repair with interrupted figure-of-eight 1-0 Prolene stitches. A conduit that will remain in situ should be sewn to healthy fascial edges. In cases with larger defects or a when translocation is not possible secondary to adhesions, a piece of polypropylene mash or polytetrafluoroethylene (PTFE) can bridge the defect (Rowbotham and Eyre 1998). One must weigh the benefits of prosthetic materials with their risks, namely infection requiring prosthetic removal, erosion, and urinary leakage.

18.5.6
Bowel Obstruction

Intestinal adhesions are and will likely remain the most common cause of obstruction in our surgical population. A high-grade obstruction with a definitive transition point needs immediate attention. Another concern is an internal herniation with the formation of a closed loop obstruction, which also needs immediate attention. Partial small-bowel obstructions may be treated with nasogastric drainage. When the pattern of obstruction is complete, immediate intervention is required.

In a report by Liauw et al. (2005) the laparoscopic approach has shown diagnostic and therapeutic utility. Caution is emphasized when placing the trocars to prevent iatrogenic perforation of grossly distended small bowel. In cases where incarceration is questionable, a mini-laparotomy may be more beneficial. Laparoscopy minimizes tissue trauma and associated release of inflammatory mediators, which may lead to a decrease in future adhesions. Studies evaluating the relationship between laparoscopy and postoperative bowel obstructions are underway at many centers, and preliminary data suggest that the incidence is reduced when matched with an open surgery cohort (Vrijland et al. 2002; Becker et al. 1996).

The technical approach for these cases can vary depending on the degree of adhesions encountered. At one end of the spectrum are patients with multiple adhesions and a matted appearance to the bowel. The most important aspect of this surgery is the technique used to lyse adhesions. Avoiding enterotomies limits the formation of future fistulas and contamination of the wound. There is an art to performing this procedure and one should be cautious when using a finger for blunt dissection. Instead, the surgeon should use a combination of sharp dissection with minimal traction and counter traction. When the procedure seems to be going nowhere, moving to a different area may enhance exposure of more difficult tissue planes when completed. All enterotomies and serosal tears need to be addressed as they occur. Full-thickness enterotomies are closed in two layers, while serosal tears can be treated with simple 4-0 nylon stitches.

In some obstruction cases, a single adhesive band may be responsible. In these instances, a collapsed portion of bowel is identified and worked in a retrograde fashion to the point of obstruction, therefore limiting handling of the edematous segment. In a similar fashion, the laparoscopic surgeon should use atraumatic graspers when handling the bowel. The band should be excised and bowel viability assessed.

Intraoperative assessment of bowel viability is a critical part of the repair. We recommend wrapping the involved portion of bowel in warm saline-soaked gauze and reassessing in 10–20 min. Another option involves intravenous fluorescein dye followed by fluorescent illumination (Holmes et al. 1993). Any areas with a patchy distribution are worrisome and should be resected. A Doppler ultrasound can also be used to determine the borders of resection; however, the sensitivity and specificity are limited. Once the obstruction has been relieved, the entire length of bowel should be examined as well as any other areas of concern. An end-to-end anastomosis should be performed whenever possible. Prior to closure, one may choose to place Seprafilm (Genzyme Corp., Cambridge, MA, USA) over the bowel, which acts to prevent future adhesions (Fazio et al. 2006). Seprafilm is a sterile, bioabsorbable, translucent adhesion barrier that separates adhesiogenic tissue for 24–48 h after placement.

An exception to the rule of resection is the patient who may develop short gut syndrome from prior resection or who has an extensive length of affected bowel. In these cases, the surgeon may opt to return the bowel to the abdominal cavity in the absence of frank necrosis and plan to return for a second look surgery in 24–48 h. Fluorescein can also help in these situations. Rarely will there be a need for ileostomy in these patients, who tend to present before overt sepsis, indicating bowel perforation.

18.5.7 Dehiscence

By definition a dehiscence is a partial or total disruption of any or all layers of the operative wound. (Fig. 18.5.6) The incidence is 1%–4 % in abdominal procedures and dehiscence tends to occur between postoperative days 6–8, at which time tensile strength is low. The major systemic factors contributing to occurrence include diabetes, sepsis, malnutrition, and immunosuppression (Mulvihill and Pellegrini 1994; Riou et al. 1992; Angood et al. 2001). Improper closure techniques in association with increased abdominal pressure from third spacing or abdominal pathology will predispose to dehiscence. Unraveled knots or 'scored' monofilament sutures will lead to dehiscence as well.

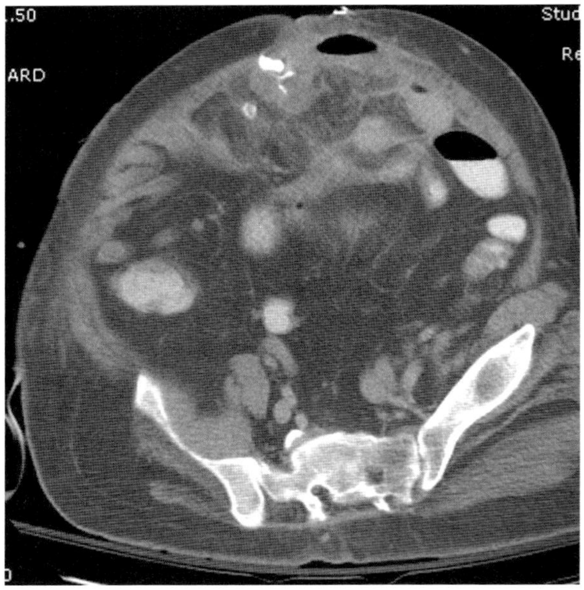

Fig. 18.5.6. Abdominopelvic CT scan in a patient with a post-augmentation cystoplasty dehiscence. The patient developed a small dehiscence at the lower pole of the wound. Interrupted 2-0 nylon sutures were used during the initial closure. The patient was in grave critical condition secondary to acute respiratory distress syndrome and could not be transferred to the operating room. Following resolution of the pulmonary issues, the patient was taken to the operating room for repair

Any patient with a suspected wound dehiscence needs immediate evaluation. Often the event is preceded by a popping sensation while straining. All dressings should be removed and the wound thoroughly inspected. One investigative approach utilizes a cotton swab to evaluate the integrity of the fascia and rule out a localized wound infection or seroma. Interrogation of the wound should be limited when a dehiscence has been diagnosed to minimize the incidence of bedside evisceration. Exposed bowel is covered with moist towels and evaluated in the operating room. There is no need for an imaging study in this situation. Critically ill patients may be explored within the surgical intensive care unit.

The best treatment for dehiscence is prevention with sound surgical technique. Following a well-placed incision, the surgeon should limit devitalization of fascia. When closing, interrupted figure-of-eight stitches with heavy synthetic suture placed 2–3 cm apart 1 cm from the wound edge are recommended. One advantage over a running suture is that a localized dehiscence in a critically ill patient can be managed with minimal intervention. A running fascial repair will undoubtedly lead to complete separation as the suture pulls through. Excess sutures tend to compromise the structural integrity of fascia and will pull through the fascial edges.

During reexploration, prior suture should be removed and bowel briefly evaluated if there are concerns for ischemia or infection. If there are concerns about elevated intraabdominal pressure, a temporary abdominal closure can be considered as described in Sect. 18.5.8. Healthy fascia is reapproximated as above and retention sutures are placed. Drains exit through separate incisions, as do ostomies if there is a need to create one. An abdominal binder should be firmly applied prior to patient extubation.

No surgeon will complete a career without having to deal with a wound dehiscence. In some instances technical error may be the culprit, while other wounds will fall apart in the presence of severe intraabdominal or wound infections. When the integrity of the fascia is questionable upon closure of a primary laparotomy, one may consider using synthetic mesh to add structural support to the fascia. One disadvantage to consider, however, is the development of an infection in the presence of synthetic mesh and the subsequent need for excision, leaving the surgeon with an even greater deficit at the time of the second closure.

18.5.8 Abdominal Compartment Syndrome

Patients requiring relaparotomy secondary to intraabdominal catastrophes will be at increased risk to experience abdominal compartment syndrome (ACS) if incisions are closed primarily. Although common in trauma patients, ACS has multiple etiologies and can occur in various clinical conditions (Table 18.5.8) (Emerson 1911; Schein and Ivatury 1998; Wagner 1926; Overhold 1931; Saggi et al. 1999b).

Because of the vast size of the abdominal cavity, large volumes can be accommodated during resuscitation; however, there is limited if any room after a critical threshold is reached. Resultant abdominal hypertension impairs intraabdominal and adjacent extraabdominal organs. Wittmann et al. (2000) have graded

Table 18.5.8. Abdominal compartment syndrome

Anatomical location	Causes
Retroperitoneal	Pancreatitis, hemorrhage, abdominal aneurysm rupture, abscess
Intraperitoneal	Hemorrhage, bowel obstruction, abdominal aneurysm, ileus, pneumoperitoneum, abscess, visceral edema
Abdominal wall	Hernia reduction, gastroschisis or lymphocele repair, eschar

Table 18.5.9. ACS grading system

Grade	Characteristics and recommendations
Mild	Sustained acute elevation of 10–20 cm H_2O, compensation of physiological effects, limits need for surgical intervention
Moderate	Sustained acute elevation of 21–35 cm H_2O, surgical intervention is strongly suggested
Severe	Sustained acute elevation over 35 cm H_2O, operative decompression indicated.

Table 18.5.10. Organ dysfunction associated with abdominal compartment syndrome

Cardiac	Low cardiac output and stroke volume from IVC and SVC compression and decreased venous return. Left-side heart failure associated with right ventricular dysfunction from elevated intrathoracic pressures (elevated PEEP).
Respiratory	Hypoxia refractory to increased $Fi0_2$/PEEP and hypercarbia secondary to elevated intraabdominal pressure and decreased thoracic compliance with elevated peak inspiratory pressures.
Renal	Oliguria unresponsive to fluid resuscitation secondary to arterial hypoperfusion. Venous outflow obstruction from elevated intraabdominal pressure, "renal compartment syndrome"
Gastrointestinal	Ischemia secondary to venous outflow obstruction and arteriolar compression can lead to bacterial translocation.
Neurological	Decreased cerebral perfusion pressure from decreased venous (jugular) outflow secondary to elevated intrathoracic pressures.

abdominal hypertension (Table 18.5.9) (Wittmann and Iskander 2000).

Pressures greater than 25 cm H_2O (normal, 1–5 cm H_2O) with dysfunction in one organ system should prompt reexploration. The most common method of obtaining intraabdominal pressure (IAP) is through the bladder. One should keep in mind that obese individuals may have resting pressures of 30–40 cm H_2O. When resuscitation commences following surgery, the degree of edema may be so massive that intraabdominal pressure will rapidly rise therefore affecting multiple systems (Table 18.5.10) (Ivatury et al. 1998; Ridings et al. 1995; Richardson and Trinkle 1976; Cullen et al. 1989; Saggi et al. 1999a).

Dehiscences are more likely to occur when tissue anastomoses are under elevated strain with resultant ischemia. Abdominal binders are discouraged because of further decreases in abdominal wall perfusion.

Whenever the risk of abdominal compartment syndrome presents itself, the surgeon should err on the side of leaving the patient open with planned relaparotomy under more stable conditions. The disadvantages of an open abdomen are exposed bowel and difficulty

Table 18.5.11. Temporary closures in the management of ACS

1. Simple closure (moist lap pads or surgical towels)
2. Towel clip skin reapproximation
3. Repeated entry (Whitmann Velcro patch – Star Surgical)
4. Synthetic mesh
5. Sterile transparent bags (Bogota bag)

in closure secondary to huge incisional hernias from fascial retraction.

Surgical decompression will improve end-organ perfusion if performed in a timely manner, as reported in several series. Nonoperative management has been utilized in cirrhotic patients with massive ascites. In this case, intravascular volume should be maximized and coagulopathies corrected to prevent circulatory embarrassment and minimize the risk of developing reperfusion syndrome. The latter is believed to occur after venous decompression with a subsequent washout of toxic potassium and byproducts of anaerobic metabolism. The high blood concentrations may impair cardiac performance by limiting contractility.

General indications to leave the abdomen open include: (1) hemodynamic and pulmonary compromise, (2) suspected bowel edema, (3) tight fascial closure, and (4) planned reoperation with or without packing. Intraoperative measurements of urinary bladder pressure can be helpful during the decision-making. The options for temporary closure are listed in Table 18.5.11 (Cipolla et al. 2005; Hedderich et al. 1986; Alfici et al. 2004; Garcia-Sabrido et al. 1988).

The simple closure technique leaves moist lap pads or surgical towels in the wound with an occlusive dressing in place. Surgeons may choose to place nonadherent material between the bowel and surgical towels along with a drain to prevent adhesion between towel and bowel, which prevents deserosalization when removed. Prior to reexploration, the cavity should be copiously irrigated to minimize the aforementioned. Towel clips provide a very loose approximation and also call for an occlusive dressing to minimize insensible fluid losses. These two techniques are much more commonplace in trauma surgery for damage control in which patients are extremely unstable.

Synthetic mesh may be used to extend the fascial edges and provide a means for primary closure. Mesh may be outfitted with zippers, zip-lock devices, and Velcro to facilitate laparostomies. These devices are invaluable, as they not only provide a means to expedite surgery, but also allow bedside inspection of the abdomen. In the unfortunate circumstance that compartment syndrome should recur, these mesh devices provide immediate venting. Goretex mesh provides a sound barrier at an effective cost if one plans on repeat laparotomy.

Sterile translucent bags can be used to store abdominal viscera and minimize fluid losses. The Bogota bag, so named for the Colombian surgeon who discovered it, is a sterile 3-l cystoscopy fluid irrigation bag that accommodates viscera (Alfici et al. 2004). The bag is layered out over the exposed abdomen and sutured into the fascia. Some trauma reports advocate the incorporation of zippers and zip locks to the Bogota bag for improved visualization. The Bogota bag can also be modified to accept diverting stomas, so-called Hadera stomas (Alfici et al. 2004). Once the bag is sewn into the fascia, an opening sufficient in size to accommodate bowel is made. A 3-mm or 6-mm soft rubber tube drain is opened lengthwise and transfixed to the Bogota bag with 3-0 nylon sutures. With the ostomy ready, at least 5 cm of bowel with associated mesentery are brought out and sutured in using 3-0 absorbable sutures. Similar techniques have been described by Subramaniam et al. (2002) in dealing with abdominal trauma.

Abdominal closure may often be precluded secondary to persistently elevated intraabdominal pressure and fascial retraction and or necrosis. Granulation tissue will need to bridge the gap in these patients. Enterocutaneous fistulae can be limited by using absorbable mesh over the exposed viscera. Split-thickness skin grafts have also been shown to work well. The postoperative course for many of these patients is often markedly improved after decompression in the absence of peritonitis and sepsis.

18.5.9 Cutaneous Ureterostomy

Cutaneous ureterostomy with nephropexy is primarily a palliative surgery for critically ill individuals with urinary obstruction secondary to neoplastic obstruction (Mahoney et al. 1998). Patients will often present with clinical signs and symptoms consistent with uremia. Individuals who have received pelvic radiation may develop a variety of fistulae after having been cured of their primary malignancy. These patients may not be amenable to ureteral drainage with stents and require low-stress surgical intervention. Patients with slow-growing tumors, which are amenable to hormonal or systemic therapy, can benefit greatly from the procedure.

The principle steps include (1) mobilization of the kidney with limited devascularization of the renal pelvis and ureter, (2) nephropexy to the anterior or lateral abdominal wall creating a short, straight course for urine drainage, and (3) creation of a pedicle flap and ureterostomy (Fig. 18.5.7). Lusuardi et al. (2005) recently published a technical review describing their success with ureteroureterocutaneostomy using an omental wrap.

Extensive trauma to the urinary tract may also be treated with a temporary ureterocutaneostomy. The aforementioned procedure will likely acquire revision depending on the severity of the trauma. Bowel seg-

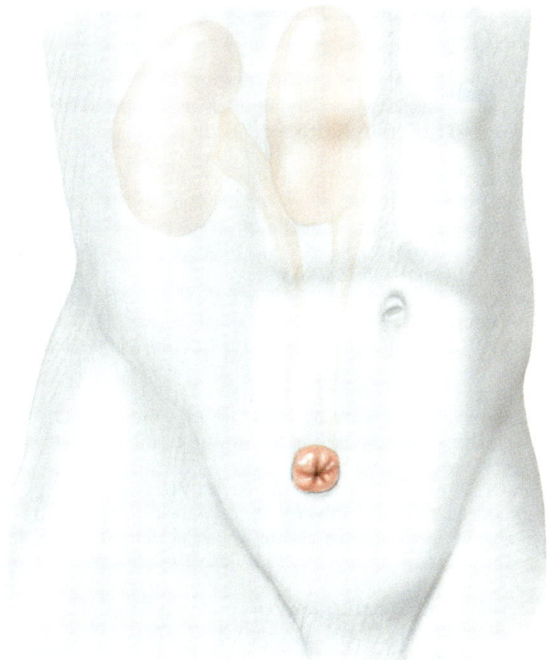

a

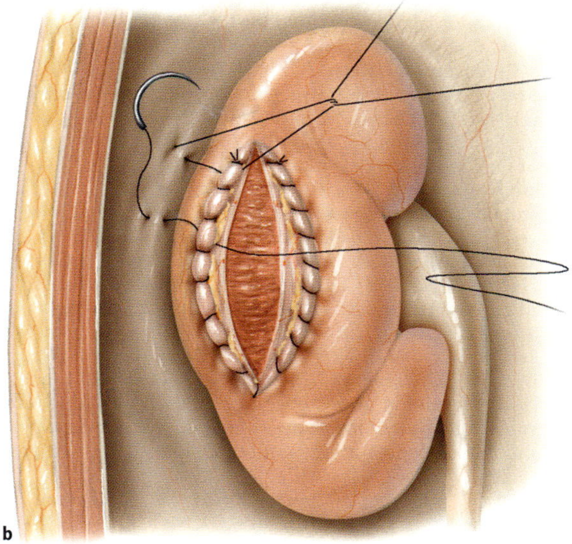

b

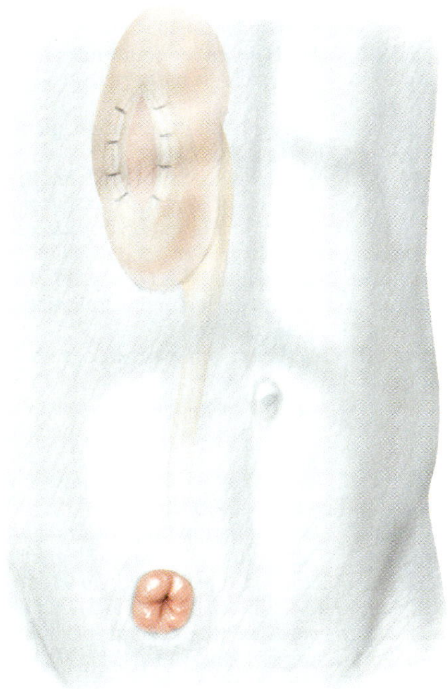

c

Fig. 18.5.7a–c. Mobilization of the right kidney with associated nephropexy suture technique and associated cutaneous ureterostomy

ments can provide adequate conduits during restoration of continuity if one is unable to perform a primary reanastomosis or Boari flap procedure. Please refer to Chaps. 15.1 – 15.9 for further management of ureteral trauma.

Cutaneous ureterostomy is not typically classified as an emergent open salvage procedure; however, the need for a semiurgent procedure may present itself. In addition, although percutaneous nephrostomy tubes may be used for urinary obstruction, there are long-term complications to consider.

18.5.10 Conclusions

Advances in technology and critical care have pushed the limits of all surgical specialties. With more aggressive monitoring and improved anesthesia, the patient population continues to age. Operations on the geriatric patient are not only accepted but also expected. In addition, our surgical techniques have become increasingly complicated because of better outcomes with lengthy procedures and anesthesia time. For this reason, complications involve a whole host of anatomical considerations that once were not a concern.

Emergency surgery is associated with increased morbidity and mortality across all surgical specialties. It is hoped that this discussion of surgical complications and the techniques to manage them will serve as a resource when confronted by these complex situations.

References

Agalar F, Eroglu MD, Bulbul M, Agalar A Tarhan OR, Sari M (2005) Staged abdominal repair for treatment of moderate to severe secondary peritonitis. World J Surg 29:240

Alejandria MM, Lansang MA, Dans LF, Mantaring JB (2002) Intravenous immunoglobulin for treating sepsis and septic shock. Cochrane Database Syst Rev CD001090
Alfici R, Ashkenazi I, Kessel B, Zut N, Sternberg A (2004) Temporary bowel diversion using the Bogota bag (hadera stoma): technical details. J Am Coll Surg 199:344
Anderson ID, Fearon KC, Grant IS (1996) Laparotomy for Abdominal sepsis in the critically ill. Br J Surg 83:535
Angood PB, Gingalewski CA, Andersen DK (2001) Surgical complications. In: Townsend CM (ed) Sabiston textbook of surgery, 16th edn. WB Saunders, Philadelphia, p 198
Angus DC, Linde-Zwirble WT, Lidicker J, Clermont G, Carcillo J, Pinsky MR (2001) Epidemiology of severe sepsis in the united states: analysis of incidence, outcome, and associated costs of care. Crit Care Med 29:1303
Becker JM, Dayton MT, Fazio VW, Beck DE, Stryker SJ, Wexner SD, Wolff BG, Roberts PL, Smith LE, Sweeney SA Moore M (1996) Prevention of postoperative adhesions by a sodium hyaluronate-bases bioresorbable membrane: a prospective. randomized double-blind multicenter study. J Am Coll Surg 183:297
Bernard GR, Vincent JL, Laterre PF, LaRosa SP, Dhainaut JF, Lopez-Rodriguex S, Steingrub JS, Garber GE, Helterbrand JD, Ely EW, Fisher CJ (2001) Efficacy and safety of recombinant human activated protein C for severe sepsis. N Eng J Med 344:699
Bishoff JT, Allaf Mohamad ME, Kirkels W, Moore RG, Kavoussi LR Schroder F (1999) Laparoscopic bowel injury: incidence and clinical presentation. J Urol 161:887
Bloom DA, Lieskovsky G, Rainwater G (1983) The Turnball loop stoma. J Urol 129:715
Boey JH (1994) Peritoneal cavity. In: Way LW (ed) Current surgical diagnosis treatment, 10th edn. Appleton Lange,Norwalk, p 453
Bohnen J, Bonlanger M, Meakins JL, Mclean AP (1983) Prognosis and generalized peritonitis. Arch Surg 118:285
Bunt TJ (1985) Urgent relaparotomy: the high-risk no-choice operation. Surgery 98:555
Carroll PR, Barbour S (2000) Urinary diversion and bladder substitution. In: Tanagho EA, McAninch JW (eds) Smith's general urology, 15th edn. McGraw Hill, New York, p 346
Christman JW, Wheeler AP, Bernard GR (1991) Cytokines and sepsis: what are the therapeutic implications? J Intens Care 6:172
Cipolla J, Stawicki SP, Hoff WS, Mcquay N, Hoey BA Wainwright G, Grossman MD (2005) A proposed algorithm for managing the open abdomen. Am Surg 71:202
Clarke GM (2001) Sepsis. In: O'Donnell JM, Nacul FE (eds) Surgical intensive care medicineKluwer Academic, Boston, p 411
Clayman RV (1985) Editorial comment. Radiology 166:83
Coburn M (1997) Damage control of urologic injuries. Surg Clin North Am 77:821
Cruickshank AM, Fraser WD, Burns HJ, Van Damme J, Shenkin A (1990) Response of serum interleukin-6 in patients undergoing surgery of varying severity. Clin Sci (London) 79:161
Cullen DJ, Coyle JP, Teplick R, Long MC (1989) Cardiovascular, pulmonary, and renal effects of massively increases abdominal pressure in critically ill patients. Crit Care Med 17:118
Dillioglugil O, Leibman BD, Leibman NS, Kattan MW, Rosas AL, Scardino (1997) Risk factors for complications and morbidity after radical retropubic prostatectomy. J Urol 157:1760
Emerson H (1911) Intra-abdominal pressures. Arch Intern Med 7:754
Fazio VW, Cohen Z., Fleshman JW, Goor H, Bauer JJ (2006) Reduction in adhesive small-bowel obstruction by Seprafilm adhesion barrier after intestinal resection. Dis Colon Rectum 49:1
Fitzgerald J, Malone MJ, Gaertner RA Zinman LN (1997) Stomal construction complications, and reconstruction. Urol Clin North Am 24:729
Flint LM (1988) Early postoperative acute abdominal complications. Surg Clin North Am 68:445
Fry DE, Clevenger FW (1991) Reoperation for intra-abdominal abscess. Surg Clin North Am 71:159
Garcia-Sabrido JL, Tallado JM, Christou NV, Polo JR, Valdecantos E (1988) Treatment of severe intra-abdominal sepsis and/or necrotic foci by an "open-abdomen" approach. Zipper and Zipper-Mesh Techniques. Arch Surg 123:152
Gold HS, Moellering RC (1996) Antimicrobial-drug resistance. N Engl J Med 335:1445
Harbrecht PJ, Garrision RN, Fry DE (1984) Early urgent relaparotomy. Arch Surg 119:369
Hardy JF, De Moerloose P, Samama M (2004) Massive transfusion and coagulopathy: pathophysiology ad implications for clinical management. Can J Anaes 51:293
Harmon GD, Senagore AJ, Kilbride MJ Warzynski MJ (1994) Interleukin-6 response to laparoscopic and open colectomy. Dis Colon Rectum 37:754
Haut T, Ohmann C, Wolmershauser A, Wacha H, Yang Q (1995) Planned relaparotomy versus relaparotomy on demand in the treatment of intra-abdominal infections. The Peritonitis Study Group of the Surgical Infection Society – Europe. Arch Surg 130:1193
Hautman RE, (2003) Urinary diversion: ileal conduit to neobladder. J Urol 169:834
Hedderich GS, Wexler MJ, McLean AP, Meakins JL (1986) The septic abdomen: open Management with Marlex mesh with a zipper. Surgery 99:399
Hendron WH (1997) Historical perspective of the use of bowel in urology. Urol Clin North Am 24:703
Hinsdale JG, Jaffe BM (1984) Reoperation for intra-abdominal sepsis: indications and results in modern critical care setting. Ann Surg 199:31
Hirshberg A, Stein M, Adar R (1997) Reoperation: planned and unplanned. Surg Clin North Am 77:897
Ho AM, Dion PW, Cheng CA, Karmakar MK, Cheng G, Peng Z, Ng YW (2005a) A mathematical model for fresh frozen plasma transfusion strategies during major trauma resuscitation with ongoing hemorrhage. Can J Surg 48:470
Ho AM, Karmakar MK, Dion PW (2005b) Are we giving enough coagulation factors during major trauma resuscitation? Am J Surg 190:479
Ho RMT, Fawcett DP (2004) Parastomal hernia repair using the lateral approach. BJU Int 94:598
Holmes NJ, Cazi G, Redell MT, Gorman JH, Fedorciw B, Semmlow JL Brolin RE (1993) Intraoperative assessment of bowel viability. J Invest Surg 6:211
Hotchkiss RS, Karl IE (2003) The pathophysiology and treatment of sepsis. N Eng J Med 348:138
Hunt TK, Mueller RV (1994) Inflammation infection and antibiotics. In: Way LW (ed) Current surgical diagnosis treatment, 10th edn. Appleton & Lange Norwalk, p 95
Hutchins RR, Gunning MP, Lucas DN, Allen-Mersh TG, Soni NC (2004) Relaparotomy for suspected intraperitioneal sepsis after abdominal surgery. World J Surg 28:137
Ivatury RR, Porter JM, Simon RJ, Islam S, John R, Stahl WM (1998) Intra-abdominal hypertension after life-threatening penetrating abdominal trauma: prophylaxis incidence and clinical relevance of gastric mucosal pH, abdominal compartment syndrome. J Trauma 44:1016
Kelleher CM, Curci JA, Blinder MA (2005) Hemostasis and transfusion therapy. In: Klingensmith ME, Amos KD, Green DW, Halpin VJ, Hunt SR (eds) The Washington manual of surgery, 4th edn. Lippincott Williams and Wilkins, Philadelphia, p 108

Killeen KP, Libertino JA (1988) Management of bowel and urinary tract complications after urinary diversion. Urol Clin North Am 15:183
Knaus WA, Draper EA, Wagner DP, Zimmerman JE (1985) APACHE II. A severity of disease classification system. Crit Care Med 13:818
Koperna T, Schultz F (2000) Relaparotmoy in peritonitis: prognosis and treatment of patients with persisting intraabdominal infection. World J Surg 24:32
Lamme B, Boermeester MA, Belt JWO, Gouma DJ Obertop H (2004) Mortality and morbidity of planned relaparotomy versus relaparotomy on demand for secondary peritonitis. Br J Surg 91:1046
Leandri P, Rossignol G, Gautier JR, Ramon J (1992) Radical retropubic prostatectomy: morbidity and quality of life. Experience with 620 consecutive cases. J Urol 147:883
Lepor H, Nieder AM, Ferrandino MN (2001) Intraoperative and postoperative complications of radical retropubic prostatectomy in a consecutive series of 1,000 cases. J Urol 166:1729
Liauw JJY, Cheah WK (2005) Laparoscopic management of acute small bowel obstruction. Asian J Surg 28:185
Libertino JA (ed) (1998) Reconstructive urology, 3rd edn.Mosby, New York
Libertino JA, Zinman L, Watkins E Jr (1987) Long-term results of resection of renal cell cancer with extension in to the inferior vena cava. J Urol 137:21
Luck AJ, Bokey EL (2003) Reoperative surgery for stomal complications and closure. In: Longo WE, Dunitz JM (eds) Reoperative colon and rectal surgery Taylor and Francis, London, p 78
Lusuardi L, Lodde M, Pycha A (2005) Surgical atlas. Cutaneous ureterostomy. BJU Int 96:1149
Mahoney EM, Kearney GP, Tarabulcy JG (1998) Cutaneous ureterostomy. In: Libertino JA (ed) Reconstructive urology, 3rd edn.Mosby, New York, p 325
Makita H, Nishimura M, Miyamoto K, Nakano T, Tanino Y, Hirokawa J, Nishihira J Kawakami (1998) Effect of anti-macrophage migration inhibitory factor antibody on lipopolysaccharide-induced pulmonary neutrophil accumulation. Am J Respir Crit Care Med158:573
Marcello PW (2001) Intra-abdominal sepsis. In: O'Donnell JM, Nacul FE (eds) Surgical intensive care medicine. Kluwer Academic, Boston, p 461
Marshall JC (2003) Such stuff as dreams are made on: mediator-directed therapy in sepsis. Nat Rev Drug Discov 2:391
Martin RF, Rossi RL (1997) The acute abdomen: an overview and algorithms. Surg Clin North Am 77:1227
Mattos RM, Libertino JA (1998) Complications associated with urinary diversions, continent reservoirs, and neobladders. In: Libertino JA (ed) Reconstructive urologic surgery, 3rd edn. Mosby, Saint Louis, p 423
Morse RM, Spirnak JP, Resnick MI (1988) Iatrogenic colon and rectal injuries associated with urological intervention: report of 14 patients. J Urol 140:101
Mulvihill SJ, Pellegrini CA (1994) Postoperative complications. In: Way LW (ed) Current surgical diagnosis treatment, 10th edn. Appleton Lange, Norwalk, p 24
Mulvihill SJ, Pellegrini CA (1994) Postoperative Complications. In: Way LW (ed) Current surgical diagnosis treatment, 10th edn. Appleton Lange, Norwalk, p 441
Overholt RH (1931) Intraperitoneal pressure. Arch Surg 22:691
Pittet D, Thievent B, Wenzel RP, Li N, Auckenthaler R Suter PM (1996) Bedside prediction of mortality from bacteremic sepsis: a dynamic analysis of ICU patients. Am J Respir Crit Care Med 153:684
Pusajo JF, Bumaschny EB, Doglio GR, Cherjovsky MR, Lipinszki AI, Hernandez MS, Egurrola MA (1993) Postoperative intra-abdominal sepsis requiring reoperation. Arch Surg 128:218
Rezkella SH (2003) Contrast nephropathy. Clin Med Res 1:301
Richardson JD, Trinkle JK (1976) Hemodynamics and respiratory alterations with increased intra-abdominal pressure. J Surg Res 20:401
Ridings PC, Bloomfield GL, Blocher CR, Sugerman HJ (1995) Cardiopulmonary effects of raised intra-abdominal pressure before and after intravascular volume expansion. J Trauma 39:1071
Riou JP, Cohen JR, Johnson J (1992) Factors influencing wound dehiscence. Am J Surg 163:324
Root RK, Lodato RF, Cade JF, Fotheringham N, Milwee S, Vincernt JL, Torres S, Rello J, Nelson S (2003) Multicenter, double-blind, placebo-controlled study of the use of filgrastim in patients hospitalized with pneumonia and sever sepsis. Crit Care Med 31:367
Rowbotham JL, Eyre RC (1998) Urinary stoma. In: Libertino JA (ed) Recontructive urologic surgery, 3rd edn. Mosby, St. Louis, p 433
Rubin MS, Schoetz DJ, Matthews JB (1994) Parastomal hernia. Is stoma relocation superior to fascial repair? Arch Surg 129:413
Saggi BH, Bloomfield GK, Sugerman HJ, Blocher CR, Hull JP, Maramarou AP, Bullock MR (1999a) Treatment of intracranial hypertension using nonsurgical abdominal decompression. J Trauma 46:646
Saggi BH, Sugerman HJ, Bloomfield GL (1999b) Multisystem organ failure secondary to increased intraabdominal pressure. 27:61
Schein M, Ivatury R (1998) Intra-abdominal hypertension and the abdominal compartment syndrome. Br J Surg 85: 1027
Schell SR, Barbul A (1998) Coagulopathy. In: Cameron JL (ed) Current Surgical Therapy, 6th edn. Mosby, St. Louis, p 1146
Stein KL (2001) Scoring systems and outcome prediction. In: O'Donnell JM, Nacul FE (eds) Surgical intensive care medicine. Kluwer, Boston, p 853
Subramaniam MH, Liscum KR, Hirshberg A (2002) The floating stoma: a new technique for controlling exposed fistulae in abdominal trauma. J Trauma 53:386
Takhar S, Rosenthal MH (2001) Shock. In: O'Donnell JM, Nacul FE (eds) Surgical intensive care medicine. Kluwer, Boston, p 71
Thompson JS, Baxter T, Allison JG, Johnson FE, Lee KK, Park WY (2003) Temporal patterns of postoperative complications. Arch Surg 138:596
Vrijland W, Tseng LN, Eijkman HJ, Hop WC, Jakimowicz JJ, Leguit P, Stassem LP, Swank DJ, Haverlag R, Bonjer HJ, Jeekel H (2002) Fewer intraperitoneal adhesions with the use of hyaluronic acid-carboxymethycellulose membrane: a randomized clinical trial. Ann Surg 235:193
Wagner GW (1926) Studies on intra-abdominal pressure. Am J Med 171:697
Wheeler AP, Bernard GR (1999) Treating patients with severe sepsis. N Engl J Med 340:207
Wittmann DH, Schein M, Condon RE (1996) Management of secondary peritonitis. Ann Surg 224:10
Wittmann DH, Iskander GA (2000) The compartment syndrome of the abdominal cavity: a state of the art review. J Inten Care Med 15:201
Zielger EJ, Fisher CJ, Sprung CL, Straube RC, Sadoff JC, Foulke GE, Wortel CH, Fink MP, Teng NN (1991) Treatment of Gram-negative bacteremia and septic shock with HA-1A human monoclonal antibody against endotoxin. A randomized, double-blind, placebo controlled trial. The HA-1A Sepsis Study Group. N Engl J Med 324:429
Zinman L, Libertino JA (1988) Control of bleeding in upper urinary tract and retroperitoneal surgery. Urol Clin North Am 15:139

19 Surgical Techniques: Endoscopic and Percutaneous Procedures

J.S. Wolf Jr.

Owing to the nature of the urinary tract, the urologist is afforded the opportunity to address many urgent or emergency procedures using endoscopic and percutaneous access. Such procedures are often less physiologically stressful to the patient and can be performed with less intensive preparation than their open counterparts. A large part of urological practice is endoscopic or percutaneous in nature, but this chapter is limited to those procedures that are frequently performed in the urgent or emergent setting.

19.1 Lower Urinary Tract

19.1.1 Urethral Catheterization

19.1.1.1 Blind Urethral Catheterization

Indications

Blind urethral catheterization (i.e., visual guidance at the urethral meatus, but none beyond that) is performed in the urgent or emergent setting to collect a specimen of urine (if a midstream specimen cannot be obtained, or if contamination [especially in women] is suspected), to measure the volume of urine in the bladder (if ultrasonography is not available or is suspected of being inaccurate), or to drain the bladder. A request for assistance with urethral catheterization is a common urological consultation, typically in an emergency department or inpatient unit when the primary care team has attempted but failed to place the catheter. Failure of catheter insertion may be due to poor technique or obstruction below the level of the bladder, including urethral stricture, prostatic enlargement, or bladder neck obstruction.

Equipment

Various urethral catheters are available to facilitate blind catheter placement. The two basic tip designs are a conical tip (Fig. 19.1) and a curved, or coudé, tip (Fig. 19.2). The conical tip is the standard one, generally useful in most situations. In cases of prostatic or bladder neck obstruction (in men), a coudé tip guides the catheter anteriorly to get over the obstructing lesion, in cases when a standard catheter might dig into the obstruction and either fail to pass or create a false passage. Catheter diameters are provided using the French (F) scale, in which 1 F = 0.33 mm in diameter (or, more easily remembered, 1 mm = 3 F). For example, an 18-F catheter is 6 mm in diameter. This is the outer diameter. The inner diameter of a catheter depends not only on the outer diameter but also on the material the catheter is made of and the configuration of lumen(s) within the catheter.

If the catheter is to be inserted and then removed, rather than left indwelling, then a simple catheter with-

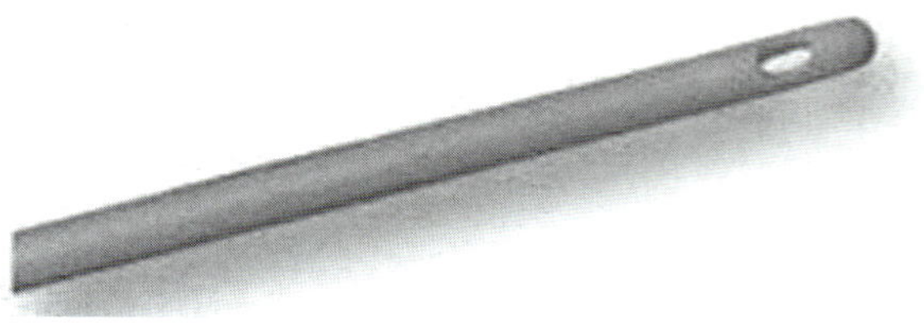

Fig. 19.1. Conical tip urethral catheter

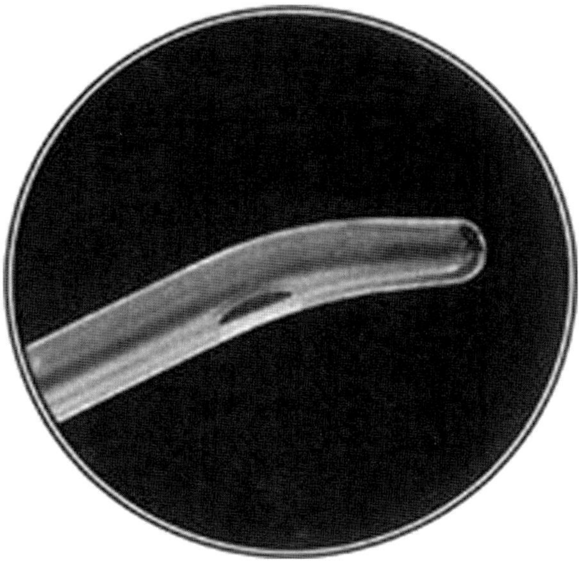

Fig. 19.2. Curved (coudé) tip urethral catheter

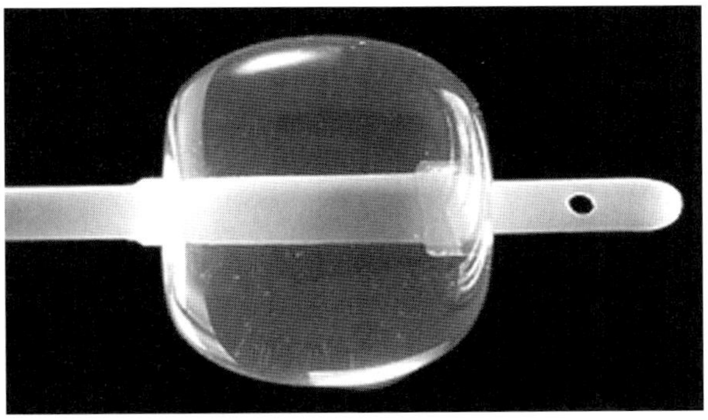

Fig. 19.3. Foley balloon retention mechanism

out a retention mechanism (see below) is used. When made of rubber or latex, these are commonly called Robinson catheters. Catheters made from other materials, often with a lubricious coating to ease passage and reduce trauma, are available with the options of a standard conical tip or a curved (coudé) tip. Catheters intended to be left indwelling most commonly have a Foley balloon on the end (Fig. 19.3) and are usually referred to as Foley catheters. The balloon, located proximal to the drainage holes on the distal tip of the catheter, is filled with fluid via a separate port that accepts a standard syringe. When inflated with 5 – 10 cc of fluid, the balloon is larger than the bladder outlet and therefore keeps the catheter tip within the bladder.

Catheters for one time use (straight catheterization) are often made of relatively hard material such as polyurethane to allow use of a small-diameter catheter (12 – 16 F) that nonetheless has an adequate lumen for drainage and adequate stiffness for insertion. Indwelling catheters are made of softer, more biocompatible material such as latex or silicone. Although the inner diameter of such catheters is smaller for a given outer diameter than stiff ones, a 16- to 20-F catheter provides adequate drainage in an adult in the absence of urinary clots, debris, etc. The smallest catheter that provides adequate drainage should be used not only to reduce discomfort of passage, but also to allow drainage of urethral secretions alongside the catheter, which reduces the inflammatory response to the catheter.

Technique

In order to prevent introduction of infectious organisms, prepare the urethral meatus in a sterile fashion, and apply proper sterile draping. Use water-soluble lubricant to ease catheter passage and reduce trauma. For women, apply a small amount of lubricant to the tip of the catheter. For men, in whom the longer and more tortuous urethra means a correspondingly more difficult and painful insertion, instill 10 – 15 ml of a lubricant containing 2 % lidocaine into the urethra and then place a urethral clamp for 5 – 10 min to provide mucosal anesthesia.

To expose the external urethral meatus in women, spread the labia. In obese women, assistance is sometimes needed, as better exposure can be obtained by the assistant grasping the labia and gently retracting outward. After inserting the catheter tip into the urethra, advancement of the catheter into the bladder is only a few more centimeters. For men, stretch the penis perpendicular to the body without compressing the urethra and insert the catheter tip into the urethral meatus. Gently advance the catheter to reach its tip into the bladder. Apply continuous, gentle pressure in case of resistance, which is most commonly at the urethral sphincter.

Difficulties and Complications

Once the urethral meatus is successfully identified in women, catheter placement is usually simple. Any difficulty usually stems from the inability to visualize the urethral meatus, either due to obesity or anatomical retraction of the meatus. Optimizing patient position (including placement in dorsal lithotomy position, if required), improving the lighting, and obtaining assistance will typically solve the problem. Use of a vaginal speculum may be helpful. Occasionally, the urethral meatus can be palpated but not visualized; in such cases, sterile preparation of the entire vaginal introitus and manually guided catheter placement may be necessary.

Difficult catheterization is more commonly encountered in men, owing to the S-shaped bulbar urethra, the resistance of the external sphincter, urethral strictures, prostatic enlargement, or postsurgical bladder neck contractures. Most commonly, it is simply the normal anatomy of the urethra and external sphincter, with or without prostatic enlargement, that challenges catheterization. Instillation of 10–15 ml of 2% lidocaine lubricant, a 16-F curved (coudé) tip catheter with the tip pointing up, and continuous, gentle pressure will be successful in such cases. If a urethral stricture is suspected, then use of a smaller catheter (10–14 F) may be successful. In cases of suspected bladder neck contracture, a 12- or 14-F curved (coudé) tip catheter is best. If these maneuvers fail, then cystoscopy usually is the next step (see Sect. 19.1.1.2).

Most complications of urethral catheterization relate to failed attempts. If undue force is applied, then false passages (perforations) of the urethra or under the bladder neck can preclude any retrograde catheter placement, even with cystoscopy. Even brief periods of catheterization can result in bacterial colonization of the urine, and long-term urethral catheterization can results in urethral erosion.

19.1.1.2
Cystoscopically Directed Urethral Catheterization

Indications

When urethral catheterization cannot be performed with the steps outlined in Sect. 19.1.1.1.3, then additional methods are needed. Filiform catheters can be used for this purpose, and are likely still in use in expert hands, but flexible cystoscopic inspection of the urethra to place a guidewire is safer and more reliable. The wide availability of flexible cystoscopy makes this the procedure of choice when routine methods fail.

Equipment

Cystoscopically directed urethral catheterization utilizes a cystoscope, a guidewire, and a urethral catheter with an end hole (Council catheter). In the urgent or emergent setting, a flexible cystoscope is more versatile than a rigid one because it can be used in supine (men) or frog-leg (women) position without requiring a lithotomy position. For the guidewire, a hydrophilic wire, preferably one with a stiff shaft (e.g., Stiff Glidewire, Microvasive, Natick, MA, USA) is best. An end hole can be made in any urethral catheter with a urethral catheter tip punch (Fig. 19.4). This device provides a hole with smooth edges, which will not catch in the urethra, much better than what can be made with scalpel or scissors. An alternative to the urethral catheter tip punch is to place an angiocatheter with its needle through the tip of the urethral catheter, remove the needle leaving the angiocatheter in place, thread the wire through the angiocatheter, and remove the angiocatheter. In some cases, a 5- or 6-F ureteral catheter is useful as well, as explained in the next section.

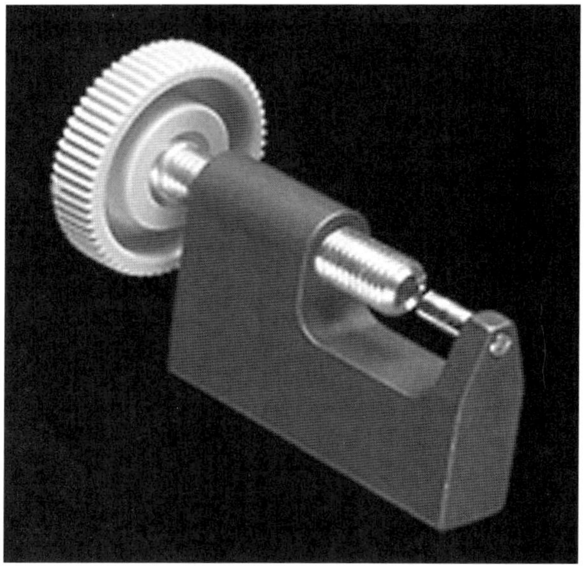

Fig. 19.4. Urethral catheter tip punch

Technique

After sterile preparation and draping, slowly advance a flexible cystoscope into the urethra until the bladder is entered or the obstructing lesion is seen. Pass a wire beyond the obstruction under vision and advance it into the bladder. If there is concern that the wire may not be in the bladder, then use fluoroscopy to verify proper coiling of the wire. Alternatively, pass a 5- or 6-F ureteral catheter over the wire, and after withdrawing the wire, aspirate urine out of the ureteral catheter to confirm proper placement. Replace the wire into the bladder through the ureteral catheter. If it appears that the obstruction can be bypassed without formal dilation, then remove the cystoscope and thread the end-hole urethral catheter over the wire into the bladder.

Difficulties and Complications

In cases of false passage (urethral perforation or bladder neck undermining) or a high but otherwise nonobstructing bladder neck, cystoscopically directed urethral catheterization is usually successful. If the obstruction is secondary to a narrow urethral stricture or bladder neck contracture, then dilation will be required if retrograde urethral access is desired (see Sect. 19.1.1.3)

19.1.1.3
Urethral Catheterization with Dilation of Stricture

Indications

Dilation of an otherwise normally functioning external urethral meatus or fossa navicularis is not uncommonly required for transurethral surgery, since the diameter of the instruments often exceeds that of the urethral lumen at these sites. In the absence of pathological narrowing, however, simple catheter placement usually does not require dilation. Stricture disease compromising the urethra, anywhere along its length from the external urethral meatus to the bladder neck, can make blind urethral catheterization or even cystoscopically directed urethral catheterization impossible without formal urethral dilation.

Equipment

Straight metal sounds (Fig. 19.5) are used to dilate the urethra of a woman or the external urethral meatus or fossa navicularis in a man. Curved metal sounds (Fig. 19.6) can be used for dilation of the entire urethra in men, but are best used in the elective setting of transurethral surgery; in the urgent or emergent setting, where a urethral stricture proximal to the fossa navicularis has been found cystoscopically (see Sect. 19.1.1.2), they are not advised. For such cases, access into the bladder should first be obtained and then Goodwin sounds (curved metal sounds with lumen), rigid plastic dilators (Fig. 19.7), or a urethral balloon dilation catheter (Fig. 19.8) can be passed.

Technique

In cases of urethral obstruction in women, or external urethral meatus or fossa navicularis stricture in men, insert straight metal sounds. Start with a sound narrow enough that it passes with minimal force, and if it is certain that the lumen is maintaining integrity, then use sequentially larger sounds up to a caliber of 2 F more than the catheter to be used has been passed. Insert the urethral catheter into the bladder. If this does not meet with success, either because the dilation cannot be performed without great force or the catheter does not subsequently pass easily, then use flexible cystoscopy. In such cases, or when a more proximal urethral stricture is the problem, visualize the obstruction cystoscopically, pass a wire into the bladder and confirm the wire placement (see Sect. 19.1.1.2). For rigid dilation, first pass the 8-F introducer catheter (Fig. 19.7) over the wire and then sequentially pass the larger dilators into the bladder. A less traumatic method is to use a urethral balloon catheter, by passing it over a wire into the bladder and inflating to full circumference. For this method, fluoroscopic monitoring is recommended.

Difficulties and Complications

In cases of solitary strictures, urethral dilation is usually successful in gaining retrograde access to the bladder. In cases of multiple and/or dense obstruction(s) however, persistence can lead to significant urethral injury with resulting extravasation and (albeit usually self-limited) hemorrhage. Percutaneous cystostomy (see Sect. 19.1.2) may be preferred or required.

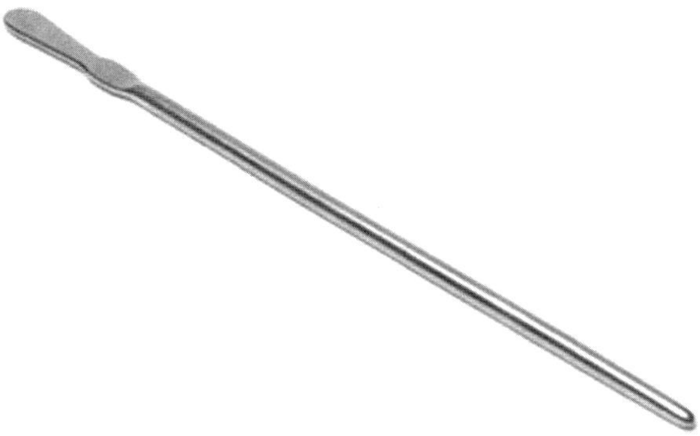

Fig. 19.5. Straight metal urethral sound

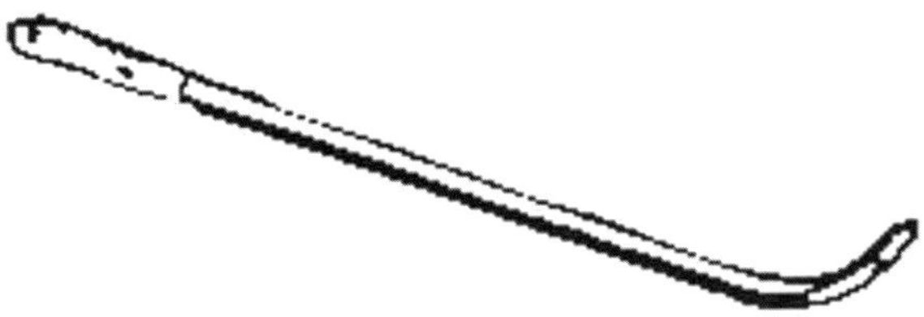

Fig. 19.6. Curved metal urethral sound

Fig. 19.7. Rigid plastic dilator (*top*) and introducer catheter (*bottom*)

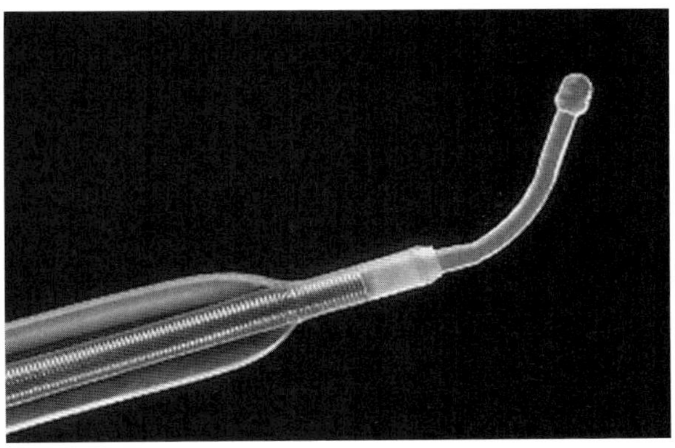

Fig. 19.8. Urethral balloon dilation catheter

19.1.2 Percutaneous Cystostomy

19.1.2.1 Indications

When retrograde urethral catheterization using the aforementioned techniques either fails or is contraindicated, then a cystostomy should be placed in the bladder. In cases of suspected bladder trauma, open surgical placement is preferred (see Chap. 15). In the setting where the bladder simply needs to be drained, percutaneous cystostomy can be performed in the operating room or at the bedside.

19.1.2.2 Equipment

There are two types of dedicated percutaneous cystostomy sets available. One set includes a sharp obturator that fits inside a catheter (10- to 14-F) with a self-retaining mechanism (Cope-type loop, Fig. 19.9, or extruding wings). Another set uses a sharp obturator that fits inside a peel-away sheath, through which a Foley catheter can be placed after removal of the obturator. Other catheters that can be placed through the sheath include Malecot (Fig. 19.10) and Pezzer catheters, which have self-retaining wings or solid cuffs, respectively. The self-retaining portions of the catheter are stretched out with an obturator during insertion through the sheath and then are released with removal of the obturator to allow expansion of the self-retaining mechanism. Because there is no balloon port, these catheters have a larger internal diameter for a given external diameter than do Foley catheters. In addition, a catheter can be placed over a wire after proper dilation of fascia, similar to the technique for a nephrostomy tube (see Sect. 19.2.2).

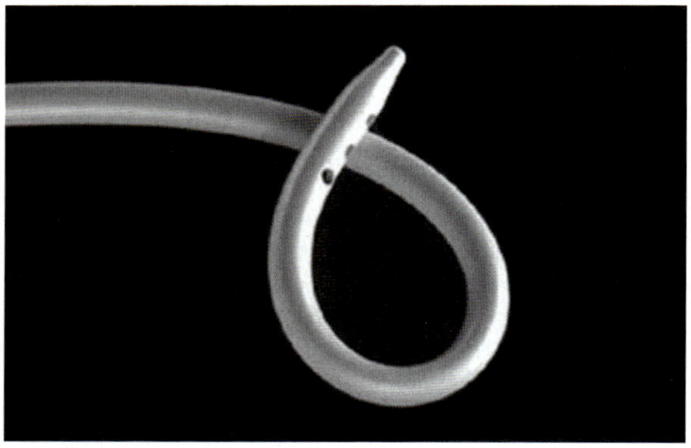

Fig. 19.9. Cope-loop retention mechanism

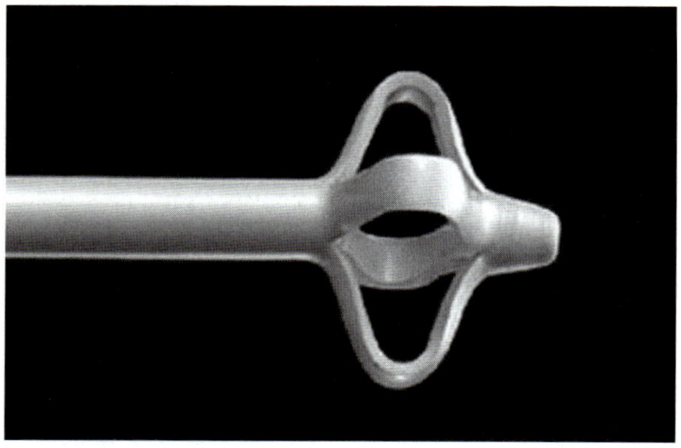

Fig. 19.10. Malecot retention mechanism

19.1.2.3 Technique

With the patient supine, prepare and drape the suprapubic area sterilely. Inject a local anesthetic agent into the skin and fascia in the intended suprapubic tract, two fingerbreadths above the symphysis pubis. Insert a long thin needle (e.g., 21-G spinal needle) with attached syringe in the direction of the intended tract, drawing back on the syringe such that aspiration of urine confirms correct trajectory and depth. Alterna-

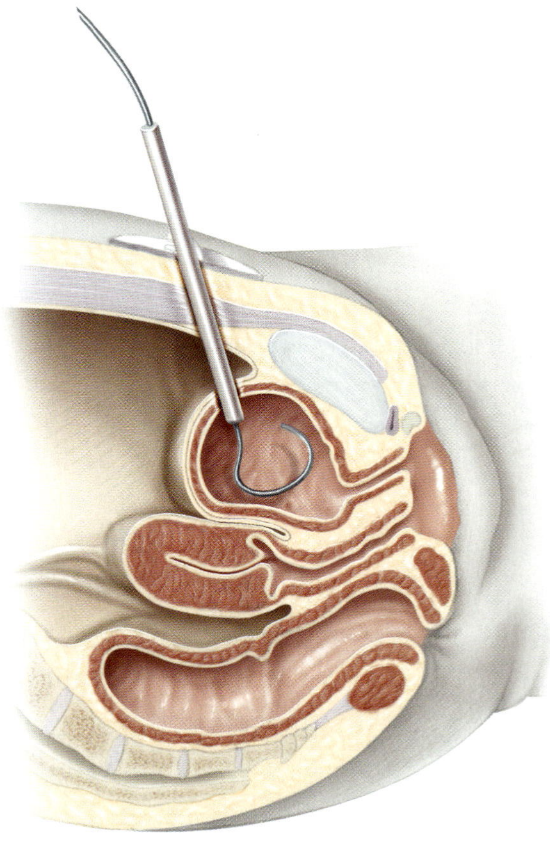

Fig. 19.11. Suprapubic catheter, placed over a guidewire, demonstrating proper orientation of catheter to pubis and bladder (© Hohenfellner 2007)

tively, in patients with a history of abdominal or pelvic surgery, surface ultrasonography can be used to localize a path to the bladder that avoids bowel.

Insert the catheter or sheath, containing the sharp obturator, at the same trajectory. Efflux of urine out of the hollow obturator again confirms placement. For kits with a catheter, advance the catheter, remove the obturator, activate the self-retaining mechanism, and suture the catheter in place. For sets with a peel-away sheath, insert the appropriately sized Foley catheter after removing the obturator, remove the sheath, and suture the catheter into place. Apply a sterile dressing and hook the catheter to dependent drainage (Fig. 19.11).

19.1.2.4
Difficulties and Complications

In obese patients, or those with altered anatomy, localization of the bladder can be difficult. Complications of percutaneous cystostomy include hemorrhage, bowel injury, or injury to the posterior bladder wall or rectum.

19.2
Upper Urinary Tract

19.2.1
Ureteral Catheterization

19.2.1.1
Cystoscopy with Blind Ureteral Catheterization

Indications

When performing urgent or emergent open surgical procedures on the abdomen or pelvis, the surgeon might request that a catheter be placed into one or both ureters to aid in their identification during surgery. If the ureter is anatomically normal, this can usually be performed blind, meaning that the ureteral orifice is visualized cystoscopically but the catheter is passed up the ureter by feel and by examining the markings on the catheter, rather than by following the catheter advancement fluoroscopically.

Equipment

Stiff closed-tip ureteral catheters (5-F) are available with a variety of tip configurations, including whistle, olive, and spiral (Fig. 19.12). The stiffness of these catheters facilitates their insertion. An alternative is to insert a softer 5- or 6-F open-ended ureteral catheter (Fig. 19.13) with the tip of guidewire protruding 1 cm out the end. This apparatus has a more flexible tip, enabling navigation of a more tortuous ureter.

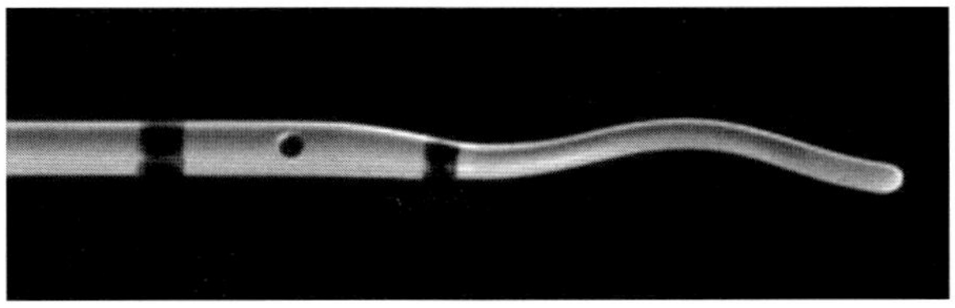

Fig. 19.12. Spiral tip of closed-ended ureteral catheter

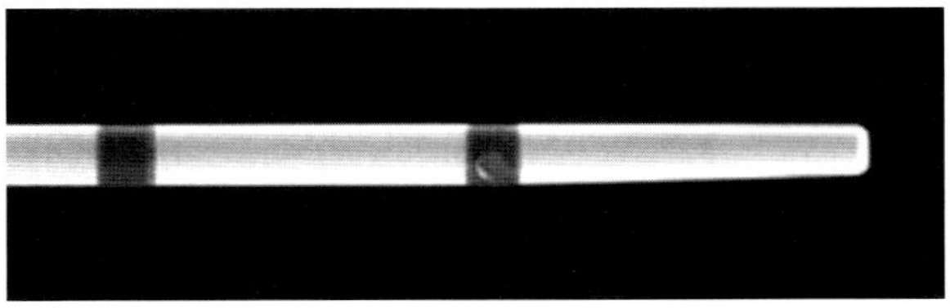

Fig. 19.13. Five-F open-ended ureteral catheter

Technique

With the patient in dorsal lithotomy position, and after sterile preparation and draping, insert the cystoscope via the urethra into the bladder. After inspecting for abnormalities that might interfere with ureteral catheterization, insert the tip of the ureteral catheter into the ureteral orifice, watching the markings on the catheter as it is advanced, and pass it upward into the ureter to the desired distance (15–20 cm into the adult ureter, depending on the height of the patient). If a single-port cystoscope bridge has been used, and catheterization is requested on both sides, then remove the cystoscope, leaving the catheter in place, and then reinsert the cystoscope alongside the catheter to address the other side. A dual-port cystoscope can be used to insert bilateral catheters without removing the cystoscope for the second side, taking care not to dislodge the first catheter when inserting the second. Insert a urethral Foley catheter and tape the ureteral catheters securely to it. Drain the ureteral catheters separately, and instruct the surgeons on sequential catheter removal after the open surgical procedure.

Difficulties and Complications

Identification of the ureteral orifice can be challenging in the face of inflammation, altered bladder anatomy, bladder neck elevation, or median lobe prostatic hypertrophy. Careful inspection of the trigone and attempts with varying degrees of bladder filling will help. Intravenous injection of one ampule of indigo carmine will stain the ureteral jet of urine to assist in identification of the ureteral orifice. Complications include inability to identify the ureteral orifice, difficulty passing the catheter, or perforation of the ureter. In cases of difficult passage, the decision is made as to abort the ureteral catheterization or to bring in a fluoroscopy unit to assist in catheterization (see Sect. 19.2.1.2).

19.2.1.2 *Cystoscopy with Fluoroscopically Directed Ureteral Catheterization*

Indications

Fluoroscopically directed ureteral catheterization might be indicated in the urgent or emergent setting when blind ureteral catheterization fails, or more commonly when retrograde ureteropyelography is needed to assess the ureter and renal pelvis for obstruction, injury, fistula, source of bleeding, etc.

Equipment

A variety of catheters and techniques are used in this situation, with the choice depending on the urologist's preference and the examination's purpose. Whistle-, olive-, and spiral-tip (closed-tip) catheters, and open-ended straight ureteral catheters are placed into the upper tract before injection of contrast material. A guidewire can be placed through the open-ended catheter. The most useful guidewire in this setting is an angled tip stiff hydrophilic wire. A torque device, which locks onto the wire, provides wire rotation under active control to guide the angled tip of the wire to the desired location. Cone-tip catheters with 8- to 12-F-wide cones (Fig. 19.14) are used to occlude the ureteral orifice as contrast material is injected, thereby filling the upper tract with contrast material with the cone preventing back-flow of contrast material into the bladder.

Technique

Identify the ureteral orifice cystoscopically as above. Although closed-ended catheters can be used, our preference is to place an open-ended catheter into the ureteral orifice and advance it slowly up the ureter under fluoroscopic guidance, injecting contrast material periodically to obtain the ureteropyelogram. Especially in the urgent or emergent setting, where the indication is usually obstruction or injury, this allows careful delineation of the problem and allows for wire manipulation through the open-ended catheter to bypass the site of abnormality. If this catheter does not pass easily, however, then a guidewire should be inserted such that the floppy tip of the wire exits the upper end of the catheter and provides a smoother passage up the ureter. An angled stiff hydrophilic wire with attached torque device, placed through a 5-F ureteral catheter and guided by continuous fluoroscopy, are the best tools to gain retrograde access to the intrarenal collecting system in challenging situations.

Difficulties and Complications

The same problems are encountered here as in Sect. 19.2.1.1.4. Failure to access the upper tract in a retrograde fashion necessitates antegrade, percutaneous access (Sect. 19.2.2).

19.2.1.3 Cystoscopy with Ureteral Stent Placement

Indications

The purpose of a ureteral stent in the urgent or emergent setting is to drain the upper urinary tract in cases of ureteral or intrarenal collecting system injury (obstruction, extravasation, fistula, etc.). Stents can be externalized, with the distal end exiting the body and draining into a receptacle, or internalized, draining into the bladder. Externalized stents are useful when separate control or assessment of ureteral drainage is desired. More commonly, internal stents are used, such that the urethral catheter captures the urine from both upper tracts.

Equipment

Ureteral stents are composed of polyurethane, silicone, or a variety of proprietary polymers. Any ureteral catheter can serve as an externalized ureteral stent, although most commonly a single-pigtail catheter is used, which has a retention coil on the proximal end (placed into the renal pelvis) and an open-ended straight distal end which is left external and hooked to a drainage bag. Internal ureteral stents have a retention coil on both ends (Fig. 19.15), with one end placed in the renal pelvis and the other in the bladder. There are multiple side holes along the pigtail and the shaft of the catheter to improve drainage. Stents for routine situations vary in diameter from 4.8 F (the smallest that will fit over a standard 0.035-inch guidewire) to 8 F, with 6 or 7 F being most commonly used. The length of the stent is selected based on measurements from an abdominal radiograph or after measuring the length of

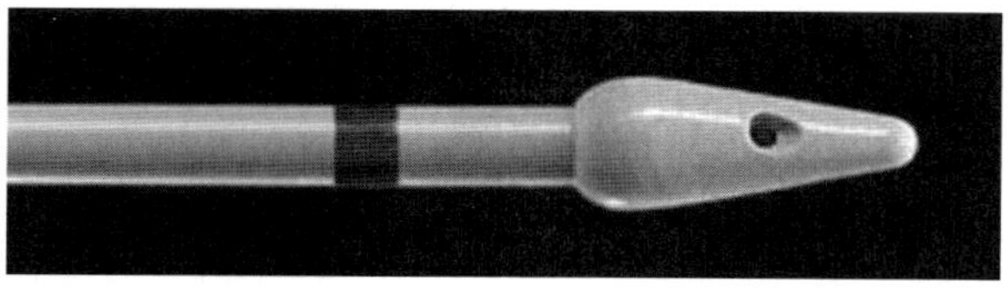

Fig. 19.14. Cone-tip ureteral catheter

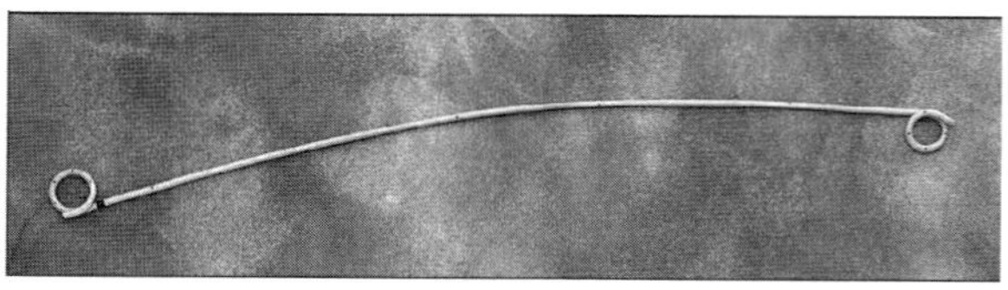

Fig. 19.15. Internal ureteral stent

the ureter using a (marked) straight ureteral catheter, but more commonly a length is simply estimated based up the height of the patient. Various formulae are used, and the stent length is varied based upon other considerations as well, but a general scheme is: 74 in. or taller, 30-cm stent; 70–73 in., 28-cm stent; 67–69 in., 26-cm stent; 64–66 in., 24-cm stent; 61–63 in., 22-cm stent; 60 in. or shorter, 20-cm stent.

Technique

Identify the ureteral orifice cystoscopically as above. Pass a guidewire within a straight ureteral catheter up the ureter into the renal pelvis, and after removing the wire obtain a retrograde ureteropyelogram to confirm anatomy. Replace the guidewire. Place the ureteral stent either through the cystoscope, or after removing the cystoscope and using fluoroscopic guidance. For the cystoscopic method, advance the stent over the guidewire until the marker on the lower end of the shaft is seen, and then withdraw the cystoscope to outside the bladder neck while maintaining the position of the stent, visualize the end of the positioning catheter (pusher), and remove the wire. For the fluoroscopic method, remove the cystoscope, leaving the wire in place, and pass the stent and pusher over the wire. Advance the pusher until its end (marked with a radiopaque metal band) is fluoroscopically visualized at the top of symphysis pubis in men, or the bottom of the symphysis pubis in women, and then withdraw the wire. Confirm the appropriate curls of the ends of the stent fluoroscopically.

Difficulties and Complications

In most cases, if a guidewire can be placed into the intrarenal collecting system, then a stent can be passed as well. A 0.035-inch guidewire is 2.7 F in diameter, so a 6-F stent is only about 1 mm wider. In some situations, however, especially in the setting of extrinsic compression, even this small increase in diameter is problematic. In this case, use of a stiff hydrophilic wire and stent placement under cystoscopic rather than fluoroscopic control will increase the chances of success. Backing the rigid cystoscope up 1 cm at a time and advancing the pusher and cystoscope together toward the ureteral orifice will often give just the extra bit of rigidity to enable stent placement. Of course, if the stent is very hard to pass up the ureter, then one must consider that the stent will not drain well (flow of urine in the typical situation occurs around as well as through a stent). If this proves to be the case, or if stent or even wire passage retrograde up the ureter cannot be obtained, then percutaneous nephrostomy placement is required (see Sect. 19.2.2). In addition to the complications of any retrograde manipulation as outlined above, indwelling ureteral stents can be associated with infection, dislodgement, erosion (rarely), and encrustation with subsequent secondary ureteral obstruction. Broad-spectrum antibiotics are usually indicated prior to upper tract manipulation.

19.2.2 Percutaneous Nephrostomy

19.2.2.1 Indications

A percutaneous nephrostomy tube has the same indications as a ureteral stent, to drain the upper urinary tract in cases of ureteral or intrarenal collecting system injury or obstruction. A stent has the advantage of being completely internalized, while the percutaneous nephrostomy tube requires an external drainage bag. In terms of discomfort, a stent produces more bladder symptoms while the nephrostomy tube can be associated with irritation at the skin exit site. The percutaneous nephrostomy tube does have a few definite advantages over the retrograde passage of an internal stent, however: it diverts much of the urine away from the ureter or bladder (useful in some cases of extravasation or fistula), it is more readily placed under local rather than regional or general anesthesia (advantageous in an ill patient), and successful placement is more likely in the setting of significant ureteral obstruction (especially in cases of distal obstruction that might involve the ureteral orifice).

19.2.2.2 Equipment

Although a variety of catheters can be used as a nephrostomy tube, in the urgent or emergent setting where simple drainage is all that is required, the most commonly used are 8- to 14-F catheters with a Cope-loop mechanism (Fig. 19.9) to retain the catheter in the intrarenal collecting system. A string is pulled at the external end of the catheter to fix the loop into place. The catheter is generally inserted with the aid of an inner stylet that fits over the guidewire to stiffen the catheter to facilitate its passage through the flank into the kidney.

19.2.2.3 Technique

Both radiologists and urologists place nephrostomy tubes, with the expertise in a given locale based upon practice and referral patterns. The antegrade approach, from the skin of the flank into the kidney, is preferred by most and is the applicable technique in the urgent or emergent setting. When percutaneous access is gained as the initial step in percutaneous nephrostolithotomy, the process can be aided by retrograde placement of a ureteral catheter to inject contrast material and air to define the collecting system and a posterior calyx under fluoroscopy. In the urgent or emergent setting this is usually not done, and as such ultrasonographic rather fluoroscopic guidance is used to guide the initial puncture.

With the patient in a prone position, prepare and drape the flank sterilely. Use an ultrasound probe in sterile wrap to examine the kidney. In the presence of hydronephrosis, the dilated calyces can be visualized easily. Pass an 18- to 21-gauge needle directly into a posterior calyx. If the tube is to be used for drainage only, then use a lower pole calyx, through a subcostal approach, as it is safest. If the patient has a calculus or other indication for subsequent percutaneous surgery, then an upper calyx might provide better access for that eventuality. The 21-gauge needle is safer to use if access is uncertain, as it is less traumatic to the kidney with multiple attempts. This needle can accept only a 0.018-in. guidewire, which subsequently needs to be upsized to a 0.035-in. wire using a tapered exchange catheter to guide the nephrostomy tube. If access appears to be straightforward, then use an 18-gauge needle, which will accept the 0.035-in. guidewire.

If the calyces cannot be defined ultrasonographically, then pass the 21-gauge needle into the renal pelvis, which even in the absence of hydronephrosis can usually be seen as a small hypoechoic region surrounded by the hyperechoic renal sinus fat. Inject dilute contrast material through this needle to confirm entry into the collecting system fluoroscopically, and once confirmed inject a small amount of air to delineate the posterior calyces. Then proceed with needle placement into an appropriate posterior calyx and remove the first needle. With fluoroscopy, use a triangulation technique to direct the needle into the proper calyx. With the C-arm tilted laterally approximately 30° from vertical, the needle is directed like a bulls eye straight toward the selected calyx (Fig. 19.16a). Once the needle is fixed, rotate the C-arm 90° medially and then advance the needle, which is now seen along its length, into the calyx (Fig. 19.16b).

Once needle access has been gained and appropriate entry confirmed with injection of contrast material and fluoroscopic inspection, insert a wire down the needle, either coiling it in the kidney or preferentially passing it down the ureter. Pass a fascial dilator (made of stiff plastic or a sharp metal) over the guidewire to dilate the fascia so that it will accept the nephrostomy tube. Finally, insert the nephrostomy tube loaded with the stylet over the wire. Once the tip of the catheter is in the calyx, push the catheter over the stylet to advance the flexible

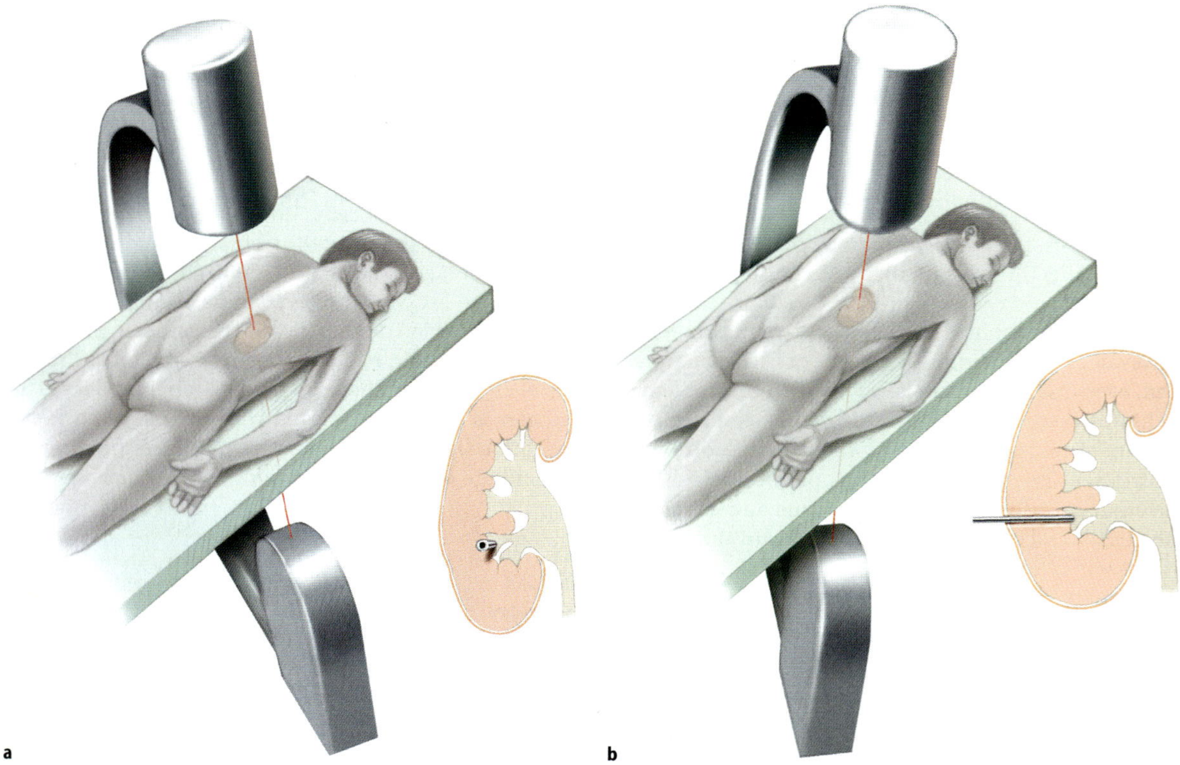
a b

Fig. 19.16. Triangulation technique for fluoroscopic percutaneous needle placement into the kidney. *Top* C-Arm is tilted laterally 30°, and the needle is directed like a bulls eye toward the selected calyx. *Bottom* With C-arm rotated 90° medially, the needle is seen along its length and is directed into the calyx (© Hohenfellner 2007) catheter tip further into the collecting system. Pull the drawstring on the external end of the catheter to create the loop on the end of the tube, monitoring fluoroscopically the entire time. Fix the string in place by lokking or wrapping it, depending on the design of the catheter. Obtain a final nephrostogram, suture the tube into place, and apply sterile dressing and a drainage bag.

19.2.2.4
Difficulties and Complications

Obesity, altered body habitus, prior flank scars or previous retroperitoneal processes including surgery and infection, and lack of hydronephrosis can all conspire to make percutaneous nephrostomy tube placement difficult. Careful persistence and knowledge of anatomy are the best tools in these situations. In rare cases, percutaneous access cannot be obtained and, if the indication is strong enough, open surgical drainage might be required. Complications of percutaneous nephrostomy tube placement include hemorrhage, infection, tube dislodgement, damage to other organs, and, if supracostal access is used, hydro- or pneumothorax. Many cases of hemorrhage can be avoided with proper technique. A tube placed into the infundibulum or pelvis, rather than a calyx, poses a greater risk to intrarenal arteries with subsequent hemorrhage (Fig. 19.17). As with any upper tract manipulation, prophylactic broad-spectrum antibiotics are indicated for percutaneous nephrostomy placement.

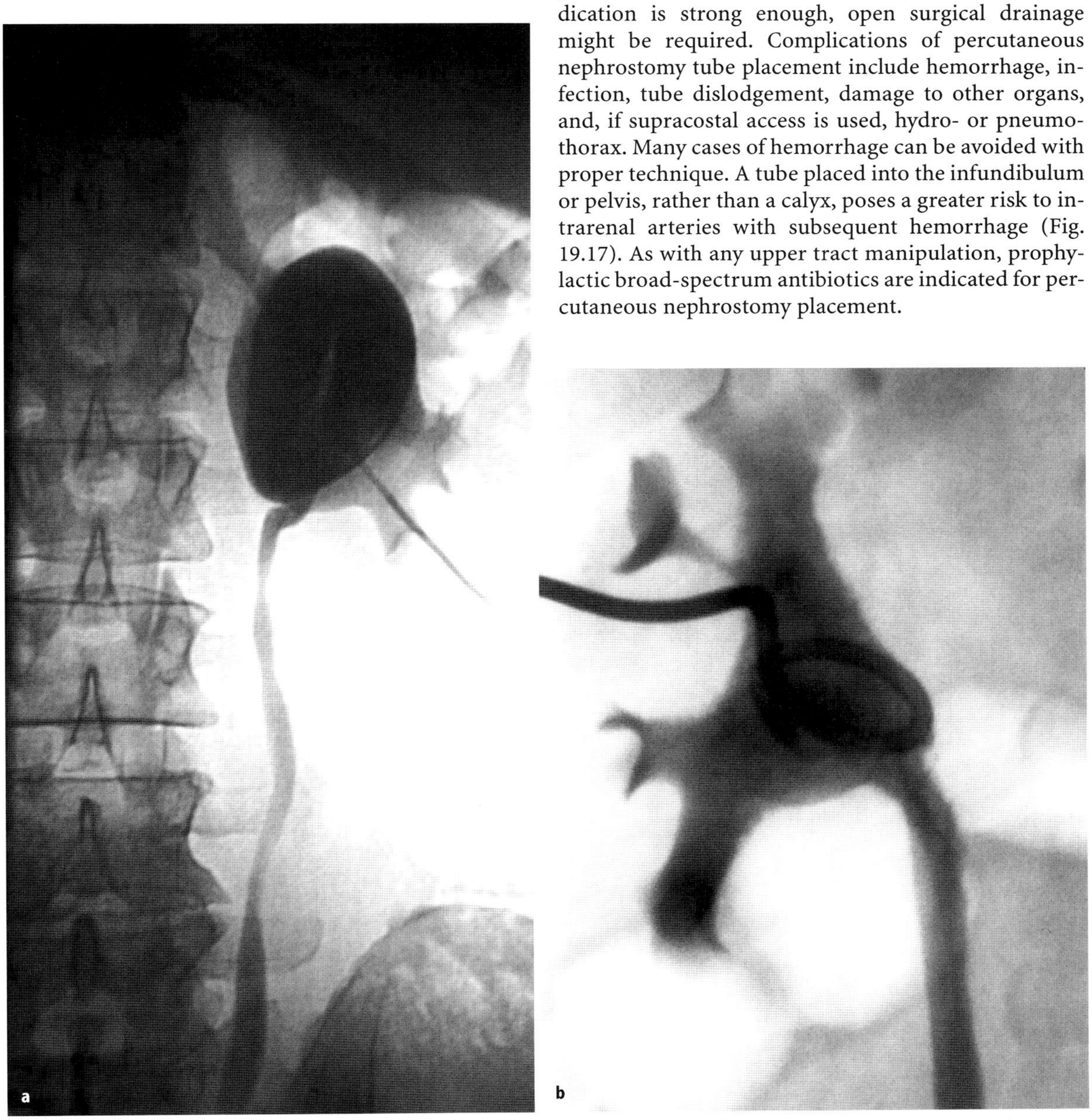

Fig. 19.17. a Proper percutaneous nephrostomy placement, entering a (lower pole) calyx. **b** Improper percutaneous nephrostomy placement (which increases the risk of hemorrhage), entering the base of an infundibulum

20 Interventional Radiology in Emergencies in Urology

J.E. Wildberger, R.W. Günther

20.1 Transcatheter Embolization

Percutaneous transcatheter embolization is defined as the intravascular deposition of autologous blood clots or alternatively particulate, liquid, or solid agents to produce intentional vessel occlusion.

Transcatheter embolization is a well-established technique for the management of bleeding in benign and malignant lesions of the urogenital tract (kidney, retroperitoneum, pelvis). It can either be performed as total occlusion in bleeding tumors as well as for defunctionalization of the kidney or as pin-pointed superselective occlusion of a bleeding vessel without collateral damage to the surrounding normal tissue.

Embolic vascular occlusion may be performed at any level from large arteries or veins to the capillary bed, and it may be temporary or permanent in nature (Drooz et al. 2003).

Liquid materials include absolute ethanol, tissue glue (*N*-butyl cyanoacrylate [N-BCA]; histoacryl) and ethylene vinyl alcohol polymer (Onyx). Ethanol is nonradiopaque and its spread is difficult to assess. N-BCA mixed with lipiodol is radiopaque and suitable for high-flow lesions such as arteriovenous malformations. Early polymerization within the catheter makes this material less easy to handle. Prior to injection, the catheter should be flushed with 40 % glucose in order to prevent early polymerization within the catheter. The use of a coaxial catheter system is a prerequisite for superselective embolization therapy, e.g., 3-F microcatheter within a 4-F to 5-F guiding catheter system. Onyx is rather costly and mostly used for intracranial embolization, while oily contrast-labeled amino acids such as Ethibloc were initially used to treat pancreatic disease and also for embolization of kidney tumors.

Solid materials comprise coils (e.g., metal, steal, mini, or Gianturco coils), detachable balloons, microspheres, hydroxylated polyvinyl acetal (PVAc, e.g., ivalon), and gelatin sponge particles. Regarding safety and radiopacity, macro- and microcoils are the most suitable embolization materials. Particles are nonradiopaque, but also practical to work with.

20.1.1 Kidney and Urinary Tract

20.1.1.1 Benign Lesions

Bleeding caused by different entities may be an emergency indication for embolization of the kidney (Uflakker et al. 1984; Vorwerk et al. 1993; Lovaria et al. 1999; Hagiwara et al. 2001; Dinkel et al. 2002; Goffette and Laterre 2002; Vignali et al. 2004; Heye et al. 2005). Benign causes of renal bleeding include trauma, previous biopsy, surgical operation, or benign tumors (such as hemangioma or arteriovenous malformations). Superselective embolization with pin-pointed occlusion of the lesion avoids damage to the noninvolved renal parenchyma. It is usually painless, free from complications, and can be performed under local anesthesia. The choice of

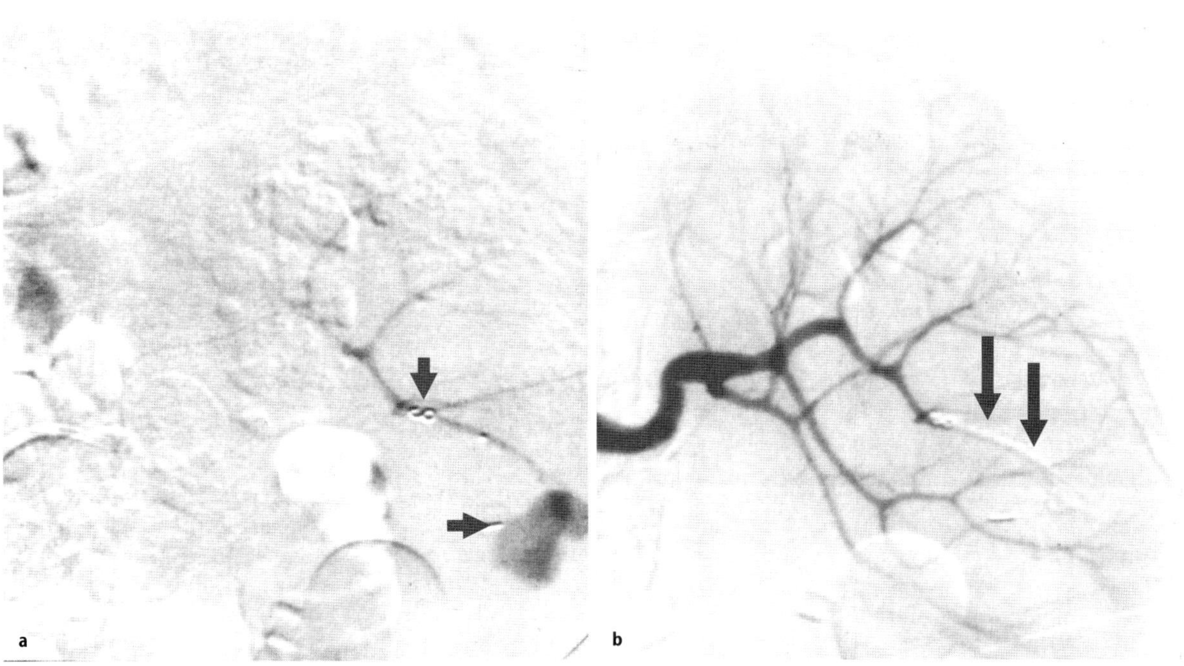

Fig. 20.1. Kidney. Superselective transcatheter embolization of renal bleeding due to false aneurysms following percutaneous litholapaxy (*left, horizontal arrow*). Initial therapy was performed using a microcoil (*left, vertical arrow*) in an outside hospital. After recurrent bleeding, definitive occlusion was achieved by superselective embolization with *N*-butyl cyanoacrylate mixed with lipiodol (*right, arrows*)

the embolization material depends on the type of lesion. Microcoils are often sufficient. However, in arteriovenous malformations we prefer N-BCA mixed with lipiodol, which provides a cast of the lesion.

Superselective embolization of symptomatic large renal angiomyolipomas has also been described. The treatment is minimally invasive, preserves renal function, and can be performed multiple times if necessary (Ewalt et al. 2005; Kothary et al. 2005; Williams et al. 2006) (Fig. 20.1).

Complete defunctionalization of the kidney by transcatheter embolization may serve as an alternative to operative nephrectomy in end-stage kidney disease associated with severe proteinuria, in therapy-resistant hypertension or as a measure of last resort for the management of inoperable urinary fistulas in far advanced pelvic malignancies and previous radiation therapy (Günther et al. 1979; Gaylord and Johnsrude 1989; Farrell et al. 1997; De Baere et al. 2000). For the management of inoperable urinary fistulas, unilateral total embolization of the kidney combined with contralateral percutaneous nephrostomy (PN) and transrenal ureteral occlusion may be an option. This can effectively interrupt urinary flow toward the urinary bladder (Schild et al. 1994; Farrell et al. 1997). Materials for ureteral occlusion with proximal urinary diversion can be Gianturco coils, gelatin sponge pledgets, detachable balloons or N-BCA as well as a combination of solid and liquid agents (Fig. 20.2).

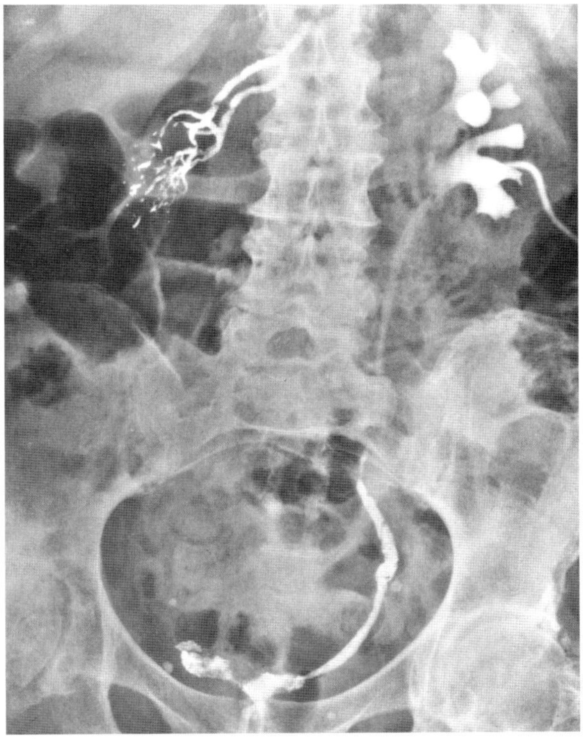

Fig. 20.2. Urinary tract. Chronic urinary fistula in a patient with inoperable cervical cancer. As a measure of last resort, the right kidney was defunctionalized by transcatheter embolization combined with transrenal embolization of the left ureter (*N*-butyl cyanoacrylate mixed with lipiodol). Additional external drainage of the left kidney via percutaneous nephrostomy

20.1.1.2
Malignant Tumors

Upper Urinary Tract

Catheter angiography has basically been abandoned for the diagnosis of renal tumors, as staging is nowadays performed with computed tomography (CT) and magnetic resonance imaging (MRI). Angiography plays, however, a certain role in preoperative embolization of large tumors in order to reduce intraoperative blood loss, and in palliation of bleeding due to renal cell cancer not amenable to surgery (stage IV) (Heidenreich and Ravery 2004; Hallscheidt et al. 2006). Since its first description in 1973 by Almgard et al., several thousand patients have been treated by transcatheter embolization (Kalman and Varenhorst 1999). In contrast to superselective embolization, a total tumor embolization may additionally result in pain, fever and nausea causing a postembolization syndrome (Bergreen et al. 1997). Other complications are relatively rare and occur in the range of 0%–20% with a mortality of up to 3.3% (Neuerburg and Lehrmann 2004).

Capillary embolization is required to safely achieve a reliable breakdown of the peritumor vasculature to meet the surgical requirements for excision of large tumor burden (Kauffmann et al. 1992). Nowadays, preoperative embolization has mostly been abandoned (Munro et al. 2003). However, there is a lack of good-quality evidence to determine the efficacy of embolization nephrectomy.

Palliative embolization in nonoperable tumors with serious hemorrhage seems to have been successful in most cases to stop bleeding (Marx et al 1982; Kalman and Varenhorst 1999). The procedure is usually performed under general or peridural anesthesia and is supported by additional analgesia thereafter. Especially in elderly patients or those with severe comorbidity, palliative embolization is a reasonable and safe option (Lamb et al. 2004) (Fig. 20.3).

Lower Urinary Tract

Transcatheter arterial embolization was first applied to the urinary bladder for the management of intractable bleeding accompanying radiation cystitis (Hald and Mygind 1974). Bleeding control can be achieved by embolization of the anterior division of the internal iliac artery also in patients with intractable bladder hemorrhage due to bladder cancer or advanced carcinomas of the prostate (Pisco et al. 1989; Nabi et al. 2003). Pisco et al. reported an initial complete bleeding control in 83 of 108 patients with various malignant pelvic tumors.

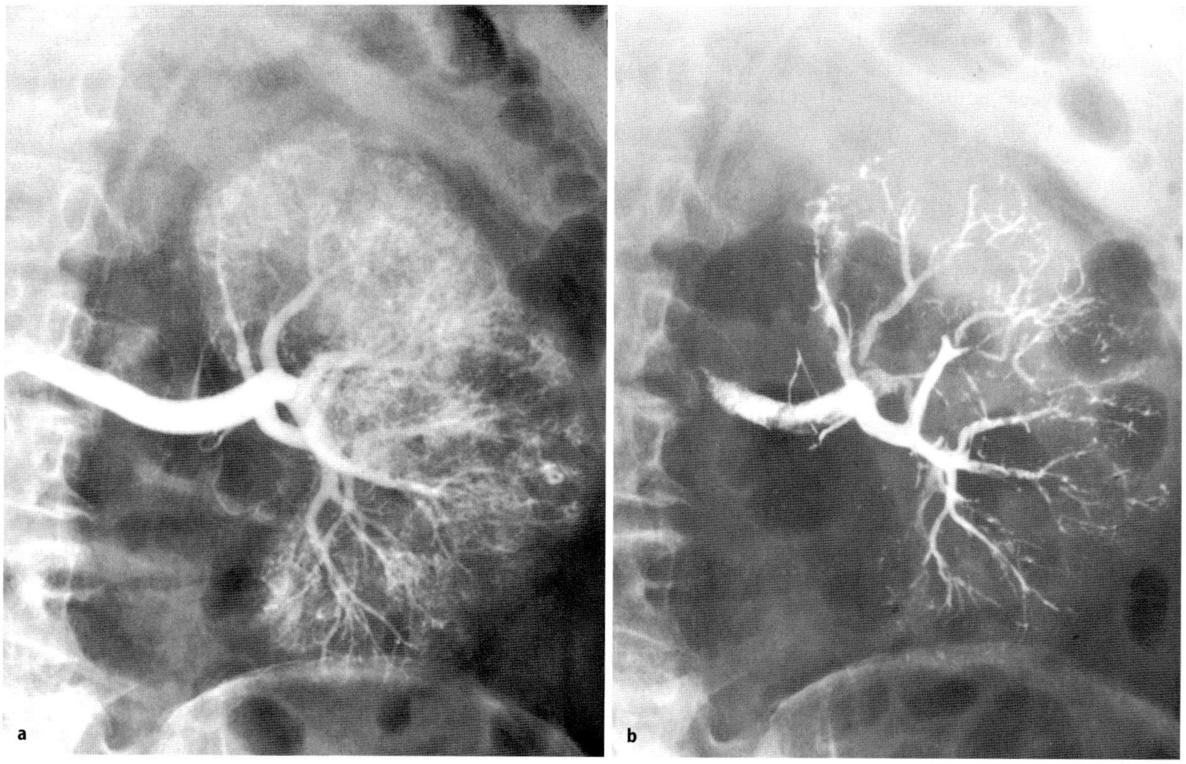

Fig. 20.3. Malignant tumors in the upper urinary tract. Nonresectable bleeding renal cancer. Palliative transcatheter embolization of the left kidney with *N*-butyl cyanoacrylate mixed with lipiodol for treatment of recurrent hematuria

Several authors have stressed that these palliative measures should be performed bilaterally and should be permanent, irrespective of whether the bleeding point is detectable or not (Carmignani et al. 1980; Nabi et al. 2003). If superselective catheterization and localization of the bleeding site is technically feasible, unilateral embolization may be adequate as well. Embolization of the superior and inferior gluteal arteries should be avoided in any case. Embolization materials include tissue glue (Ethibloc; histoacryl) (Textor et al. 2000) as well as tungsten/platinum coils (Nabi et al. 2003) and contour microspheres (155–500 μm) (Hayes et al. 1996). Typical minor complications after the intervention include nausea, vomiting, fever, and pain.

In non life-threatening cases, intraarterial mitoxantrone chemoperfusion (20 mg/m^2 body surface area) has been reported as a therapeutic alternative with low postprocedural complication rates. However, only short-term hemostasis (up to 15 days; mean, 10 days) was achieved (Textor et al. 2000).

20.1.2 Retroperitoneal Non-organ-Related Bleeding (Post-traumatic)

Trauma patients are quickly and accurately diagnosed with helical CT. Potentially life-threatening complications (hemorrhage or organ rupture, displaced bone fractures) can be diagnosed directly on the scanogram and thick axial sections, respectively. Direct monitoring of the pathologic findings can guide further imaging and therapy. Posttraumatic retroperitoneal and pelvic bleeding is a primary indication for angiographic hemostasis. Angiography should be carried out rapidly, before the patient decompensates from considerable blood loss. The intervention also contributes to changing hierarchy of injuries to be treated surgically (Dondelinger et al. 2002). However, a transcatheter approach can even be performed in hemorrhagic hypotension. In these patients, the hemodynamics have to be improved by resuscitation of fluid prior to the intervention (Hagiwara et al. 2004). In selected patients with blunt pelvic trauma and unsuccessful bleeding control (e.g., previous laparotomy), bilateral embolization of internal iliac arteries may also be a safe and effective alternative in controlling retroperitoneal bleeding (Velhamos et al. 2000) (Fig. 20.4).

20.1.3 High-Flow Priapism

Priapism is a pathological condition of a penile erection that persists beyond or is unrelated to sexual stimulation (Berger et al. 2001). This entity can be subdivided into two general subgroups. Based on pathophysiology, low-flow priapism is defined as a venous outflow obstruction. High-flow priapism often occurs after blunt trauma to the perineum resulting in a pathological increased arterial influx into the cavernosal bodies. Cavernosal blood–gas analysis, color Doppler ultrasound and angiography are the most effective diagnostic tools to distinguish high-flow from low-flow

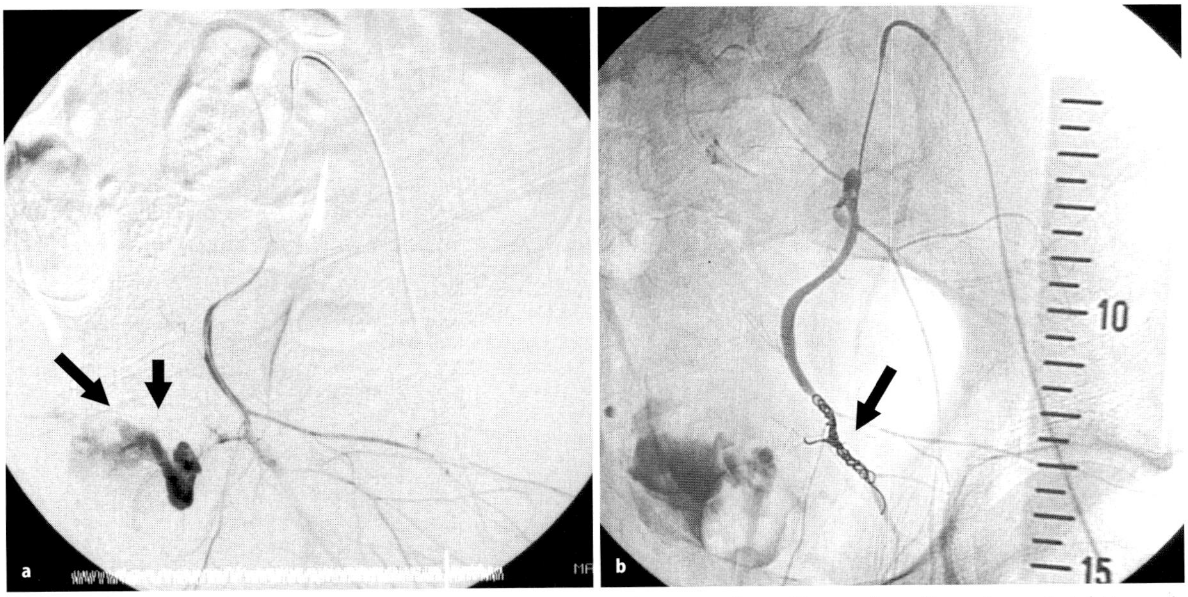

Fig. 20.4. Retroperitoneal non-organ-related bleeding. **a** Posttraumatic retroperitoneal hemorrhage (jump from a height in a suicide attempt) (*left, arrows*). **b, c** Superselective embolization of the left inferior gluteal artery with ten microcoils (*right, arrow*). **d–g** Initial emergency CT of the pelvis delineates fractures of the sacral bone and surrounding hematoma (*arrows*). Primary indication for angiographic hemostasis. This facilitates surgical intervention for additional fixation of fractures of the lower limbs

priapism. The blood supply of the penis usually derives from the internal pudendal artery. Angiographic features are arteriovenous/arterial-sinusoidal fistulas and pseudoaneurysms of the cavernosal arteries. Selective catheterization of the internal iliac and/or pudendal arteries is necessary to demonstrate contrast extravasation and the communication between the cavernosal artery and the corpora cavernosa with delayed clearing. Superselective coaxial embolization using 2-F or 3-F microcatheters is the treatment of choice in patients with high-flow priapism (Colombo et al. 1999; Pieri et al. 2005).

Interventional therapy provides equivalent rates of detumescence when compared to surgical techniques (O'Sullivan et al. 2006). Prognosis is good with high probability of preserving the erectile function (Savoca et al. 2004). According to a retrospective analysis of 202 published cases for the treatment of high-flow priapism, the overall success rate with restored erectile function without recurrent priapism was 89 % for arterial embolization, while the outcome of shunt surgery was quite poor (20 %) (Kuefer et al. 2005).

A review of the literature has suggested that unilateral embolization is usually sufficient and that bilateral embolization is indicated when unilateral treatment does not result in detumescence of the penis (Langenhuijsen et al. 2001). A variety of agents has been proposed for embolotherapy, including autologous clot material (Crummy et al. 1979; Walker et al. 1990), gelatin sponge pledgets (Cohen et al. 1996; Ji et al. 1994), *N*-butyl cyanoacrylate (N-BCA) (Alvarez Gonzalez et al. 1994; Numan et al. 1996) as well as microcoils (Kerlan et al. 1998; Kress et al. 2002). Autologous clots as well as Gelfoam are temporary occlusive agents without per-

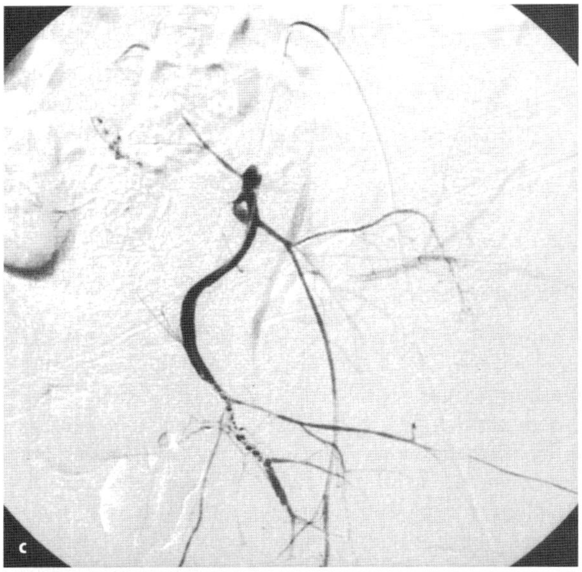

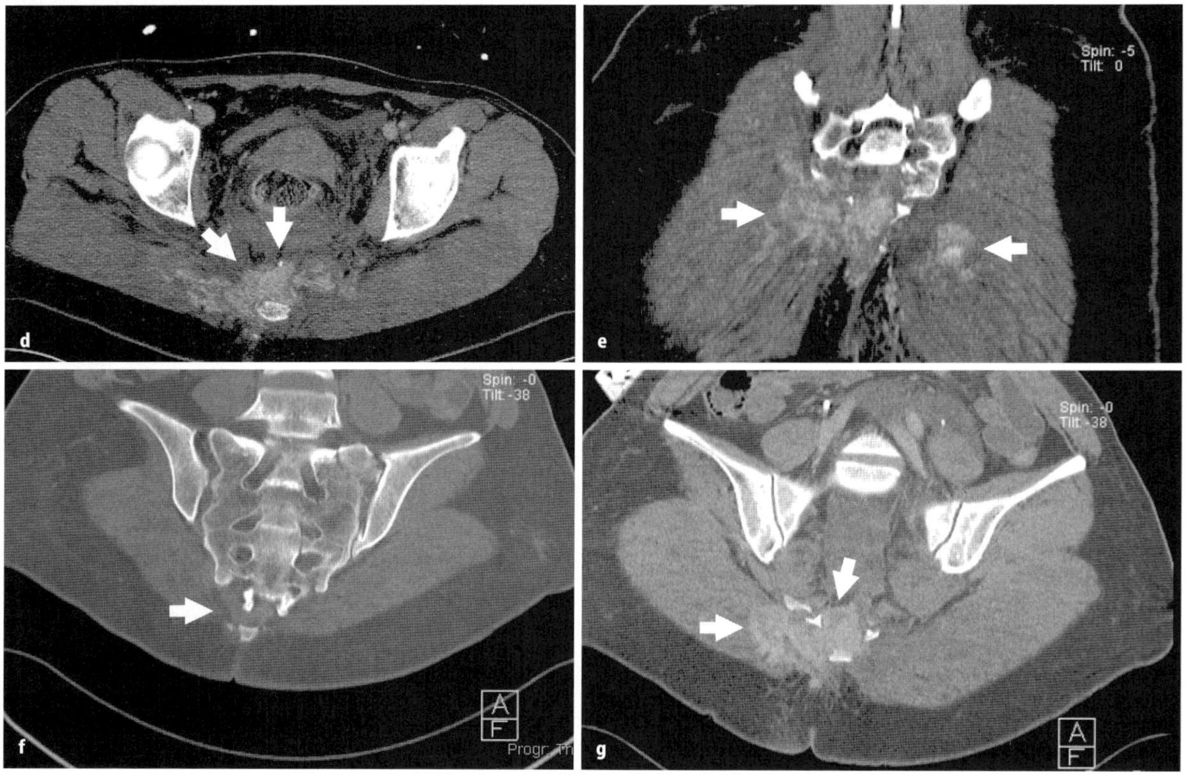

Fig. 20.4c–g

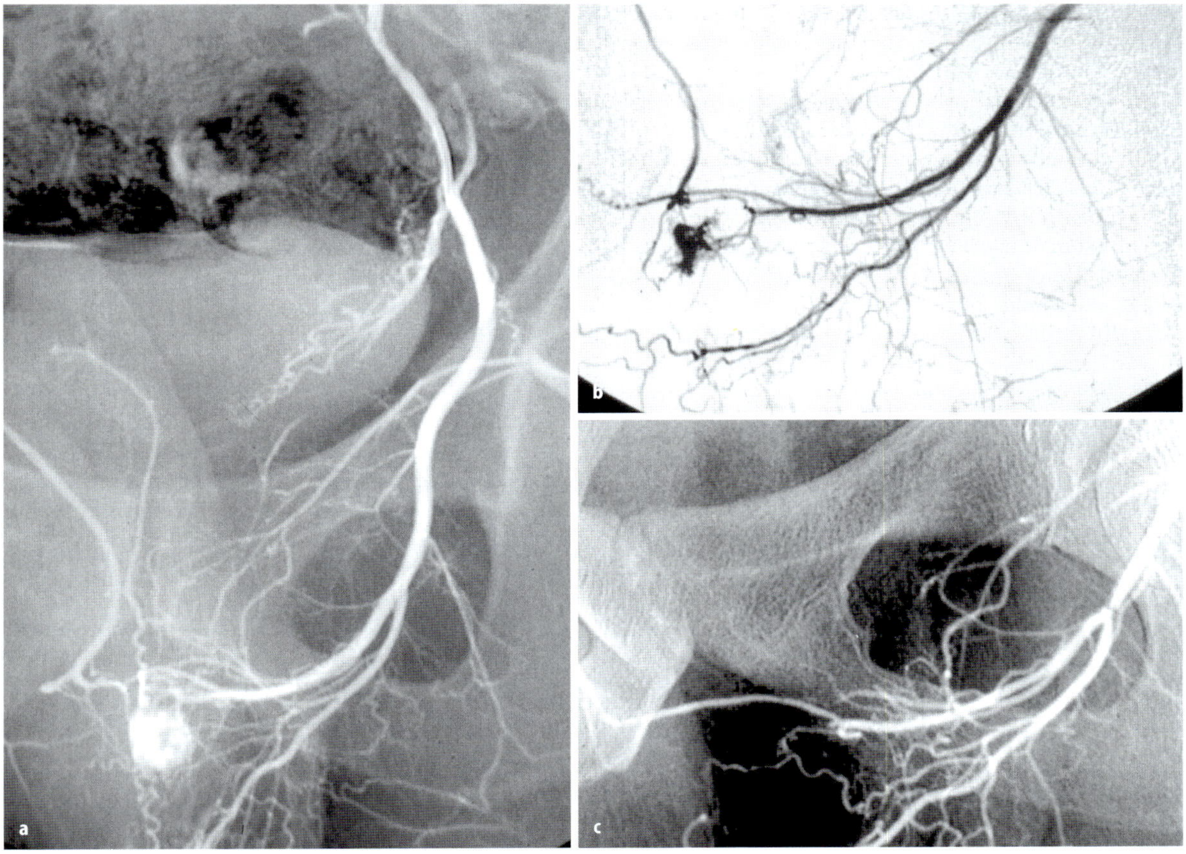

Fig. 20.5. High-flow priapism. Superselective transcatheter embolization of the proximal pudendal artery supplying an arterial-sinusoidal fistula using gelatin sponge pledgets in high-flow priapism after perineal trauma (Courtesy of H.P. Busch, Trier, Germany)

manent vascular ablation, while N-BCA and microcoils are permanent occlusive agents. There is a theoretical increased risk of subsequent erectile dysfunction for permanent embolization materials. Therefore, we prefer temporary agents (blood clot, Gelfoam particles) for the treatment of high-flow priapism (Fig. 20.5).

20.2 Transcatheter Lysis and Thrombectomy in Renal Artery Occlusion

There are two forms of renal artery occlusion: acute and chronic. Acute renal artery occlusion may result from thromboembolism, thrombosis of a stenosed vessel, or trauma. Systemic emboli commonly originate in the heart. Among contributing cardiac disorders, atrial fibrillation, myocardial infarction (postinfarction thrombi), and rheumatic mitral stenosis are the most important ones (Lessman et al. 1978). Irrespective of the underlying cause of obstruction, prognosis is determined by the duration of ischemia. Acute occlusion requires immediate reaction since warm ischemia time of the kidney is roughly 90 min (Blum et al. 1993). After that, it is usually inlikely that complete restitution of renal function is obtained (Schunk et al. 1990).

Since patients with acute renal artery occlusion arrive mostly too late for treatment, there are no large series in the literature; neither are there any dedicated protocols regarding lysis therapy. However, thrombolysis and mechanical thrombectomy have been described in isolated cases.

Generally speaking, the standard contraindications to lysis therapy should be considered, such as history of hemorrhagic stroke, active intracranial neoplasm, recent surgery, as well as active and recent internal bleeding in the prior 6 months (UpToDate 2006). Also, there is no indication to provide lysis therapy if angiography shows complete occlusion of the vessel (no stump left of the renal artery) once the ischemic tolerance of the kidney has been exceeded. Patients with partial occlusion and residual flow in the renal artery are suitable candidates for an attempt at lysis therapy, particularly if salvage of the kidney is crucial (e.g., solitary kidney).

The risk of systemic bleeding can be minimized by local intraarterial infusion of the thrombolytic agent, rather than intravenous administration (Rose 2006). Thrombolytic agents used include streptokinase (Cronan and Dorfman 1983; Pilmore et al. 1995; Gluck et al. 2000), urokinase (Hirota et al. 1997), tissue plasminogen activator (tPA) (Mugge et al. 1990), as well as a combination of these agents (Klein et al. 1992). Urokinase (4,000 IU/h) or tPA (5 mg bolus) can be administered directly into the thrombus followed by renal artery infusion (2 mg/h for 10 h). It is important to establish some flow beyond the embolic obstruction rapidly. Sole or additional PTA may be helpful in order to displace the thrombus slightly to the vessel wall (Kadir et al. 1987; Salam et al. 1993). During thrombolysis, 1,000 IU/h of heparin should be administered intravenously. Hydrodynamic catheter thrombectomy (e.g., Hydrolyser [Siezenga et al. 2005] or AngioJet [Sternbergh et al. 2000; Siablis et al. 2005]) may also be considered if available. For percutaneous thrombectomy, however, there is a risk of thrombus dislocation into the aorta. In acute renal artery occlusion, the combination of balloon angioplasty, arterial stenting, and additional lysis may be considered to salvage the kidney as well. The results in the literature dealing with selective lysis are very limited and restricted to case reports or series of only a few cases.

Astonishingly, successful thrombolysis initiated much later after the embolic event may still result in improvement of renal function. This is probably because minimal perfusion of the kidney may be preserved via collaterals (Zuckerman et al. 1993).

In summary, there are no general rules or existing guidelines regarding percutaneous revascularization for acute embolic occlusion of the renal arteries. Lysis therapy can be successful even if the embolic event has occurred more than 2 h before angiography in partial occlusion with reduced but maintained blood flow. However, no realistic salvage of the kidney can be expected by lysis therapy or hydrodynamic thrombectomy in patients with complete embolic occlusion of the renal artery approximately 2 h after the embolic event. Apart from the embolic occlusion of the renal artery, missing collaterals on angiography as well as lack of enhancement of the renal parenchyma in CT and MRI are prognostically unfavorable signs.

There are also isolated reports of renal vein thrombosis treated by selective catheter lysis via the renal artery combined with selective venous lysis (Stella et al. 2001) and percutaneous catheter-directed thrombectomy with or without thrombolysis (Kim et al. 2006). Particularly if deterioration of renal function is seen, catheter-directed thrombectomy or thrombolysis of native and allograft veins may improve creatine levels and glomerular filtration rates rapidly (Fig. 20.6).

20.3 PTA and Stenting

Percutaneous transluminal angioplasty (PTA) and stent implantation have become an established therapy for selected patients with renovascular occlusive disease (Spies et al. 2003). These interventional procedures should be carried out in accordance with existing guidelines (Levy et al. 2000; Martin et al. 2003).

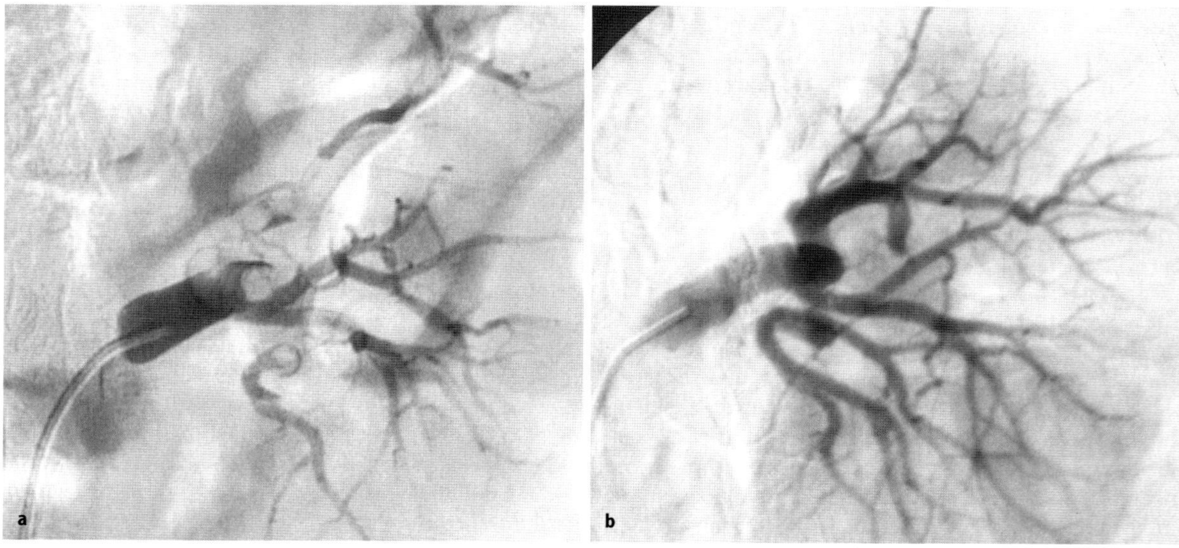

Fig. 20.6. Transcatheter lysis and thrombectomy in renal artery occlusion. Embolization due to atrial fibrillation into the left renal artery in a 78-year-old patient with a solitary kidney. Selective transcatheter lysis with tPA (bolus application, 5 mg; followed by 2 mg/h for a total of 25 mg). During follow-up, relief of flank pain. Initial anuria was followed by polyuria

20.3.1 Aortic Dissection with Involvement of the Renal Arteries

The distal type B lesion is generally associated with a favorable outcome as compared with the proximal type A aortic dissection. In contrast to a type A lesion, which usually requires immediate surgical attention (Miller et al. 1979), medical management (e.g., antihypertensive, cardiac output suppressive) is the preferred method of treatment for uncomplicated type B lesions (Fann and Miller 1995). Complicated type B lesions may require at times emergent (e.g., rupture, enlargement) surgical management, whereas others (e.g., intractable pain, visceral malperfusion) may allow more time for medical or interventional management (Suzuki et al. 2003). Patients experiencing any in-hospital complications (hypotension, mesenteric ischemia or infarction, coma or altered consciousness, limb ischemia, and acute renal failure) are at the greatest risk of in-hospital mortality (up to 13%).

Hypertension and increasing serum creatinine levels are suggestive of renal artery involvement in type B dissection. Percutaneous stent placement may be a therapeutic option (Lacombe et al. 1992; Behrendt et al. 2000; Hausegger et al. 2001). To relieve renal ischemia and restore renal function, percutaneous balloon fenestration of the aorta was also performed successfully (Park et al. 1997; Williams et al. 1997; Manke et al. 1999).

Renal artery angioplasty and stenting from above using a craniocaudal approach may serve as an attractive alternative technique in patients with unfavorable vessel anatomy (Scheinert et al. 2001). A transbrachial access can be performed in patients suffering from chronic aortic occlusion (chronic Leriche syndrome) and dissections with renal artery involvement as well (Dimitrios et al. 2004; Shiraishi et al. 2005) (Fig. 20.7).

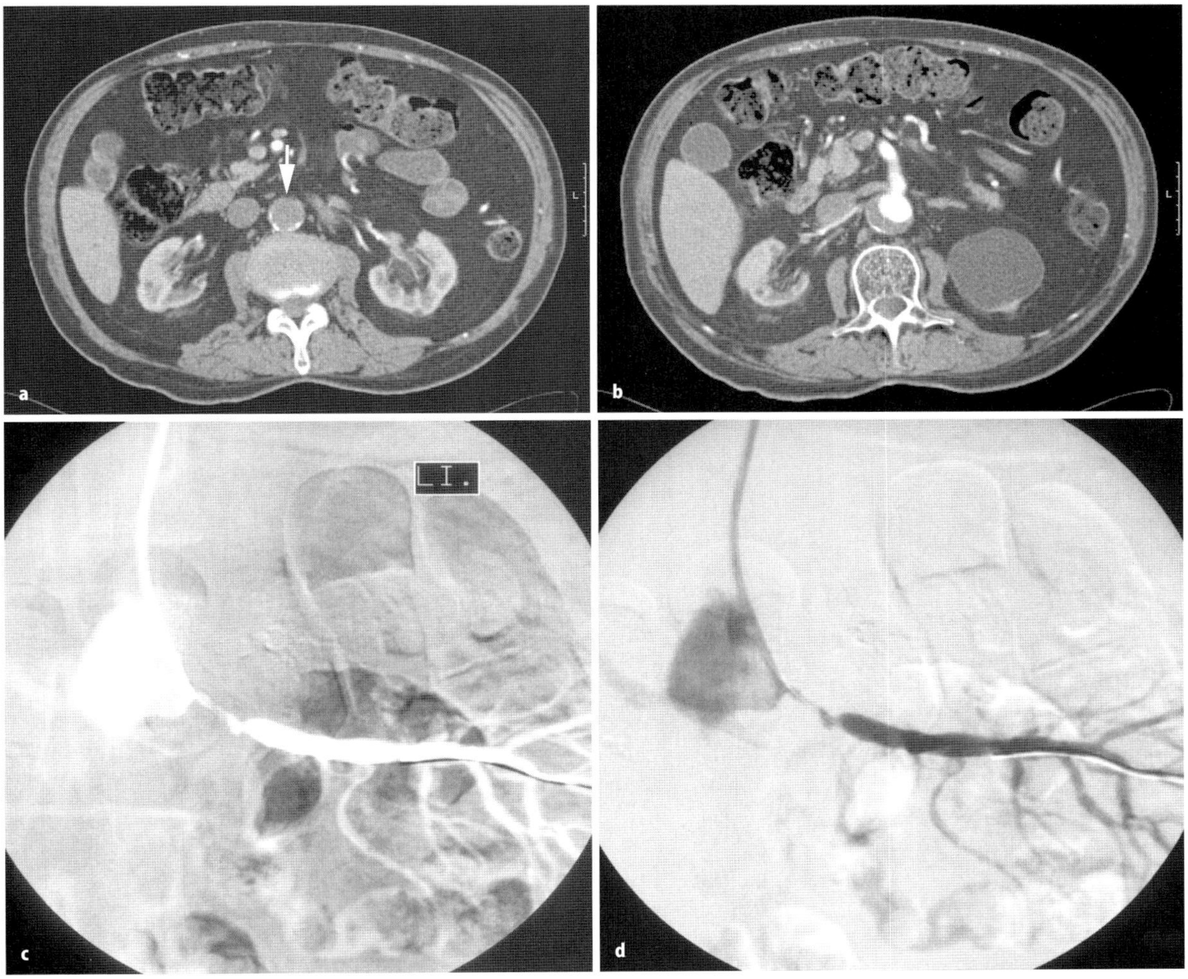

Fig. 20.7. Aortic dissection with involvement of the renal arteries. **a, b** Type B aortic dissection with involvement of the left renal artery. **c–f** Percutaneous stent placement in the left renal artery (stent diameter, 5 mm; length, 18 mm) using a transbrachial access leading to significant improvement of renal function (decline of serum creatinine from 3 mg/dl to 1.5 mg/dl). **g–h** Concomitant chronic Leriche syndrome (*arrowhead*)

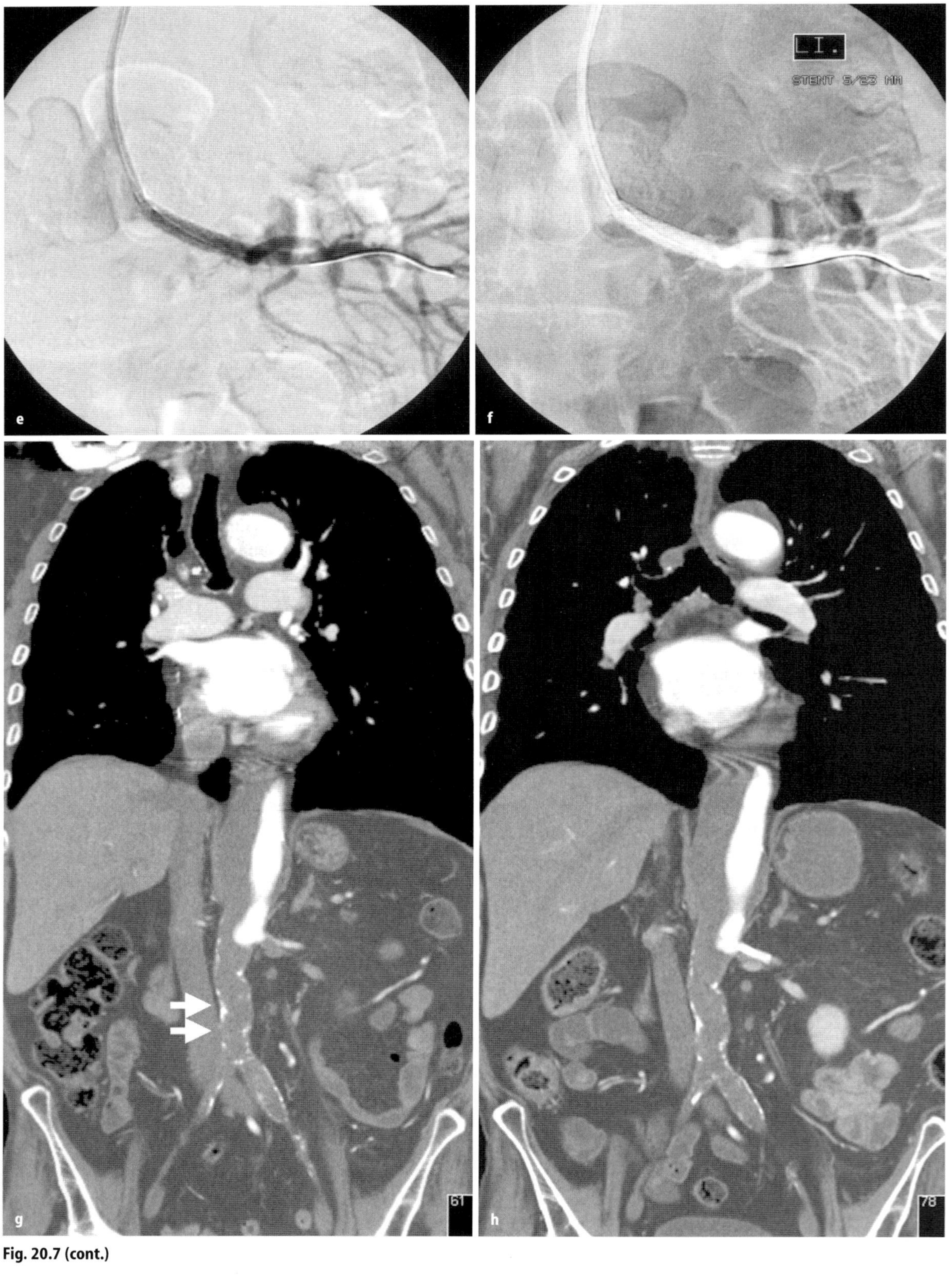

Fig. 20.7 (cont.)

Renal artery dissection, occlusion of the renal artery as well as a rupture of the vessel during renal percutaneous transluminal angioplasty (PTA) and stenting are major complications. However, in most cases, these can be solved by interventional procedures as well.

20.3.2 Renal Artery Dissection Following Renal PTA and Stenting

PTA and stent placement is a suitable technique, particularly for the treatment of ostial and eccentric lesions of the renal artery (Van de Ven et al. 1999). Complications such as dissection, occlusion, and rupture of the renal artery are rare, but can be treated percutaneously as well. Patients with renal insufficiency seem to be at higher risk for peri-interventional complications (Martin et al. 1988).

20.3.3 Occlusion of the Renal Artery Following Renal PTA and Stenting

It should be kept in mind that thrombolytic therapy does not fundamentally restore renal function. For renal artery thrombosis, thrombolysis with urokinase and tissue plasminogen activator (tPA) has been recommended (Morris et al. 2001) (see Sect. 20.2). Since most thromboses are associated with an intimal flap, additional stabilization by stenting may be considered as well. Thromboembolic complications can also be treated rapidly and successfully by combined measures, such as catheter thrombus extraction and pharmacological strategies (e.g., urokinase and abciximab) (Di Valentino et al. 2004). Mechanical thrombectomy has been successfully performed using hydrodynamic catheters such as the Hydrolyser (Siezenga et al. 2005) and the AngioJet system (Greenberg et al. 2002; Siablis et al. 2005). An overview on the different devices and their mechanisms of action was given in review articles by Sharafuddin and Hicks in 1997 and 1998 (Sharafuddin and Hicks 1997, 1998a, b). Selection of the most suitable technique depends on the personal preferences and the local availability of devices in this emergency setting.

There are no general rules or existing guidelines regarding percutaneous revascularization for occluded renal arteries. Thrombolysis might not be indicated once the ischemic tolerance of the kidney (approximately 90 min) has been exceeded (Blum et al. 1993). After that time, percutaneous intervention will be unsuccessful in complete embolic occlusion of the renal artery. Missing collaterals on angiography as well as lack of enhancement of the renal parenchyma in CT and MRI are prognostically unfavorable signs. However, thrombolysis is worth an attempt even after the time in patients with reduced but maintained blood flow with partial occlusion of the main renal artery (see Sect. 20.2).

20.3.4 Rupture of the Renal Artery Following PTA and Stenting

Iatrogenic renal artery perforation or rupture is a very rare, but well-described complication of percutaneous renal artery intervention. In a larger patient series, five ruptures of the main renal artery were reported in 212 consecutive patients (308 treated arteries; 117 PTA, 191 stent procedures) (Morris et al. 2001). Perforation can occur from guidewires (especially hydrophilic wires), angioplasty balloons, stents, and even from the guiding catheter itself. Management of iatrogenic renal artery perforation or rupture includes temporary balloon tamponade and/or deployment of a covered stent (Friedel et al. 2005). The size of the balloon chosen for tamponade should be 1 mm smaller than the diameter of the balloon catheter or stent that caused the rupture. Figure 20.8 illustrates a successful interventional therapy including emergency balloon occlusion at the perforation site with stent placement after previous rupture of the right renal artery during PTA.

20.3.5 Ureteroarterial Fistula

Prior pelvic and vascular surgery, prolonged ureteral stenting, radiation therapy, and periureteral inflammation in the immediate neighborhood of an artery may explain the extremely rare occurrence of an ureteroarterial fistula. Ureteral ischemia and subsequent necrosis promote the formation of these fistulae.

Percutaneous treatment options include the implantation of a covered stent into the ureter (Bilbao et al. 2005), transcatheter embolization of the bleeding branch (Siablis et al. 2002), and a hybrid procedure with transcatheter embolization of the iliac artery proximal and distal to the site of the defect followed by femoral-to-femoral bypass operation immediately thereafter (Keller et al. 1990; Quillin et al. 1994).

20.4 Percutaneous Drainage

Ultrasound is a fast and inexpensive imaging modality for guidance of many interventional procedures. Advantages of this technique are the ability to provide three-dimensional orientation and the avoidance of any radiation exposure. As a real-time modality, this technique is especially suitable for application at structures that move when the patient breathes. However, for more challenging interventions such as complex abscess drainage procedures and drainage of renal and

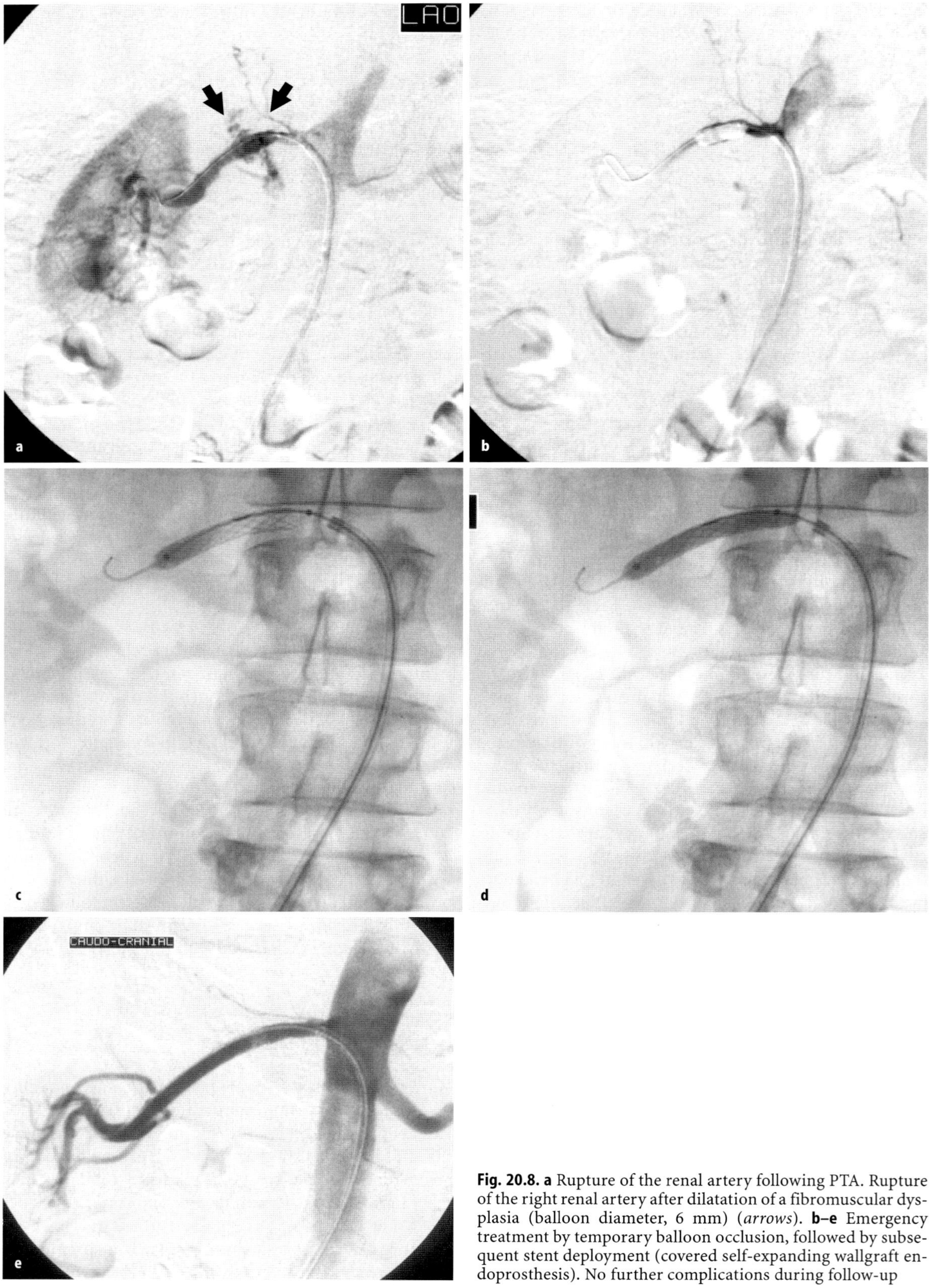

Fig. 20.8. a Rupture of the renal artery following PTA. Rupture of the right renal artery after dilatation of a fibromuscular dysplasia (balloon diameter, 6 mm) (*arrows*). **b–e** Emergency treatment by temporary balloon occlusion, followed by subsequent stent deployment (covered self-expanding wallgraft endoprosthesis). No further complications during follow-up

perirenal fluid collections, CT guidance, or even magnetic resonance (MR) guidance are preferable.

Abdominal abscess formation should be drained percutaneously either by the Seldinger or trocar technique because of high success and low morbidity, mortality, and recurrence rates (Akinci et al. 2005). Retroperitoneal CT- and MR-guided percutaneous drainage procedures are usually done with a standard Seldinger approach (Fig. 20.9). First, the abscess formation is localized by a diagnostic, contrast-enhanced series (**a**) and an external localizer (e.g., radiopaque grid) is placed on the skin of the patient (**b**).

In the next step, the different landmarks, such as distance between cutis and retroperitoneum, cutis and lesion, as well as the angle needed are calculated (**c**). A 18- to 22-gauge needle is then advanced into the abscess formation (**d**), exchanged against a guidewire and, after dilatation of the access tract, a drainage catheter is placed in the target region (**e**). A final series with dilute contrast material applied into the abscess cavity reveals the effect of the percutaneous drainage and depicts potential extravasation (**f**).

Generally speaking, percutaneous abscess and fluid drainage has resulted in reduced morbidity and mor-

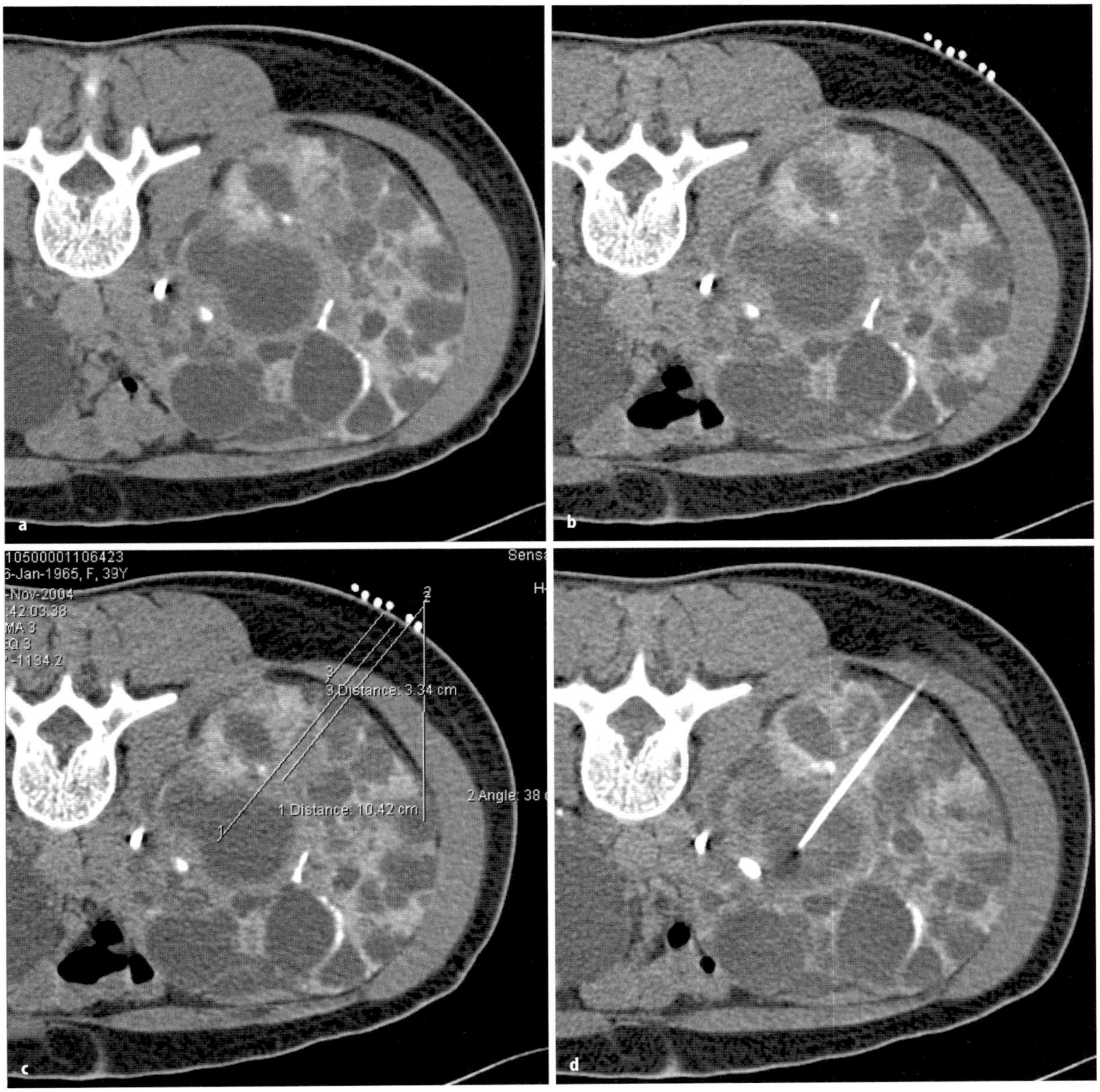

Fig. 20.9a–d. Percutaneous drainage. Polycystic kidney disease in a 40-year-old woman presenting with sepsis. Contrast-enhanced CT revealed superinfection of a centrally located cyst. Previous ureteral stone removal 1 week before. CT-guided percutaneous drainage of the superinfected cyst using the Seldinger technique

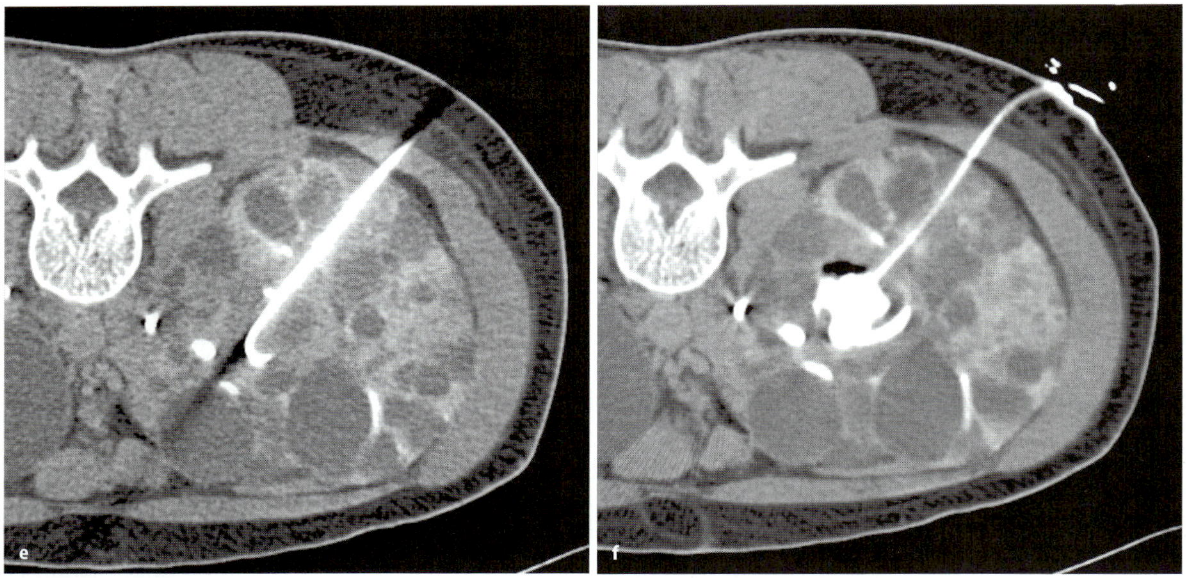

Fig. 20.9e, f

tality and has helped reduce length of the hospital stay and hospital costs (Bakal et al. 2003).

20.4.1 Renal Abscess

Current percutaneous drainage techniques are usually curative in the majority of cases of renal and perirenal abscesses. Many patients can be treated safely, and if necessary, on an outpatient basis (Deyoe et al. 1990). Several aspects have to be considered prior to a renal drainage procedure (adapted from Salvatierra et al. 1967; Caldamone and Frank 1980; Siegel et al. 1996; Shu et al. 2004):

- A small abscess (less than 3 cm) can be successfully managed with long-term (up to 6 weeks) antimicrobial therapy alone.
- In addition to antibiotics, percutaneous abscess aspiration and drainage is appropriate therapy for medium and large abscesses (greater than 3 cm), while larger abscesses (greater than 5 cm) may need multiple drainage procedures.
- Regardless of abscess size, immunocompromised patients should strongly be considered for percutaneous drainage.

In principle, MR has been shown to be a safe and effective guidance method (Adam et al. 1999; Buecker et al. 2001). For the routine clinical setting, however, MR-guided drainage procedures are limited to anatomic locations difficult to achieve, such as the subdiaphragmatic region, and in patients with absolute contraindications for CT (Fig. 20.10).

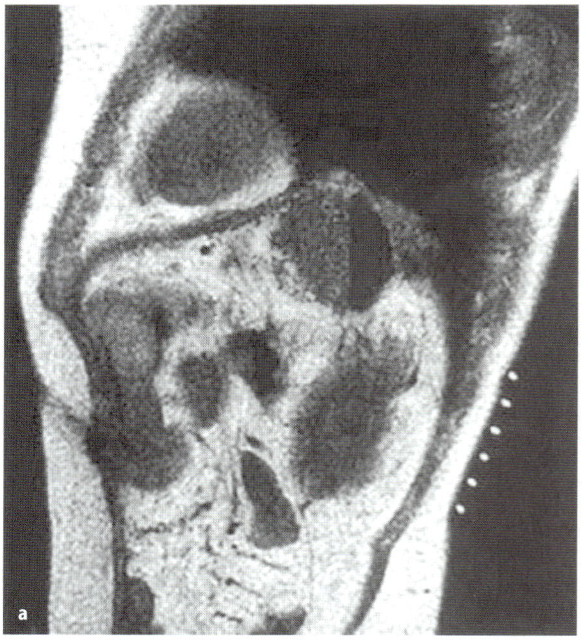

Fig. 20.10. Retroperitoneal abscess formation. A sagittally oriented T1-weighted gradient-echo sequence shows subphrenic abscess formation with fluid-fluid levels. The patient is placed in supine position for the intervention. An external grid is placed on the patient's back (**a**)

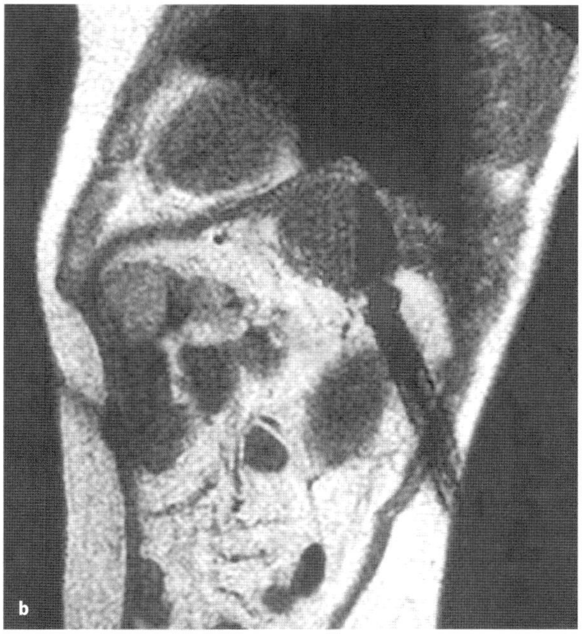

Fig. 20.10. An 18-gauge needle is advanced in an angulated fashion protecting the dorsal pulmonary recess and the kidney parenchyma (**b**). (Courtesy of Arno Buecker, Homburg, Germany. From Buecker et al. 2001)

20.5 Percutaneous Nephrostomy

Percutaneous nephrostomy (PN), initially introduced in 1955, has become a commonplace since its reappraisal in the 1970s of the last century (Goodwin et al. 1955; Günther et al. 1978; Pfister and Newhouse 1979). Nowadays, it is usually performed under ultrasound or fluoroscopic guidance. CT- and MR-guided PN are restricted to more complex cases when conventional guidance techniques fail, particularly in obese patients and in the absence of pelvicalyceal dilatation. The feasibility of CT-guidance for percutaneous antegrade pyelography and PN was first described by Haaga et al. in 1977. CT is capable of detecting subtle density differences within the tissue so that even the nonopacified or nondilated renal pelvis can be punctured accurately. In addition, CT precisely displays the perinephric space so that assessment of complications is feasible. CT fluoroscopic guidance allows routine nephrostomy tube placement with patients in the supine or the supine-oblique position and is associated with the lowest complication rate (Barbaric et al. 1997). In complicated cases, such as drainage of the nondilated pelvicalyceal system, (multislice) spiral CT as well as MR imaging may acquire volumetric (3D) data sets, which display the anatomical region not only in a standard axial orientation, but also from any requested perspective, for example in the coronal and sagittal projection.

A selected group of patients will benefit from CT- and MR-guided percutaneous access. This group includes certain patients with ectopic kidneys, a retrorenal colon or any form of megacolon, severe spinal dysraphism, and other causes of an abnormal body habitus as well as selected individuals with hepatomegaly, splenomegaly, or renal angiomyolipoma (Matlaga et al. 2003).

The technique used for puncture of the pelvicalyceal system depends on the personal preference and experience and the degree of dilatation. Applying a Seldinger technique (see Sect. 20.4) with puncture along the Brödel relatively avascular line into the lower pole calyx with an 18-gauge sheath needle, followed by a 0.035-in. guidewire and fascial track dilatation to accommodate nephrostomy catheters, is the most commonly employed method. Finally, 8-F- to 12-F self-retaining nephrostomy drainage catheters are placed. All variations based on personal practical experience are acceptable as long as they are in accordance with published guidelines and patently are effective (Rickards 2002; Ramchandani et al. 2003; Brountzos 2006).

MR-guided percutaneous nephrostomy of the nondilated upper urinary tract has been performed successfully in animal experiments using low field (0.2 T) magnets (Merkle et al. 1999) as well as high-field (1.5 T) MR imaging (Nolte-Ernsting et al. 1999). The first case of a successful percutaneous nephrostomy tube placement in humans with MR guidance was published by Hagspiel et al. in 1998.

However, neither CT nor MR will replace the current standard. Fluoroscopy and ultrasound guidance will be sufficient in most cases to monitor access into the renal collecting system (Fig. 20.11).

20.5.1 Urinary Obstruction and Infection

Percutaneous decompression may be life-saving in the presence of pyonephrosis with urosepsis. The trocar-cannula technique can be applied if the pelvicalyceal system is dilated, for example from urinary obstruction. It allows faster placement of drainage catheters, as intermediate steps such as dilating the nephrostomy tract are not necessary. If CT fluoroscopy is used in obstructed kidneys, the mean time needed for placement will be in the range of 10–45 min (mean, 25 min), with an average fluoroscopy duration of 49 s (7–110 s) (Le Maitre et al. 2000). Again, the standard procedure will be ultrasound guidance and fluoroscopy.

20.5.2 Postoperative Urinary Leakage and Urinoma

A urinoma is an encapsulated collection of chronically extravasated urine. Obstructive and nonobstructive

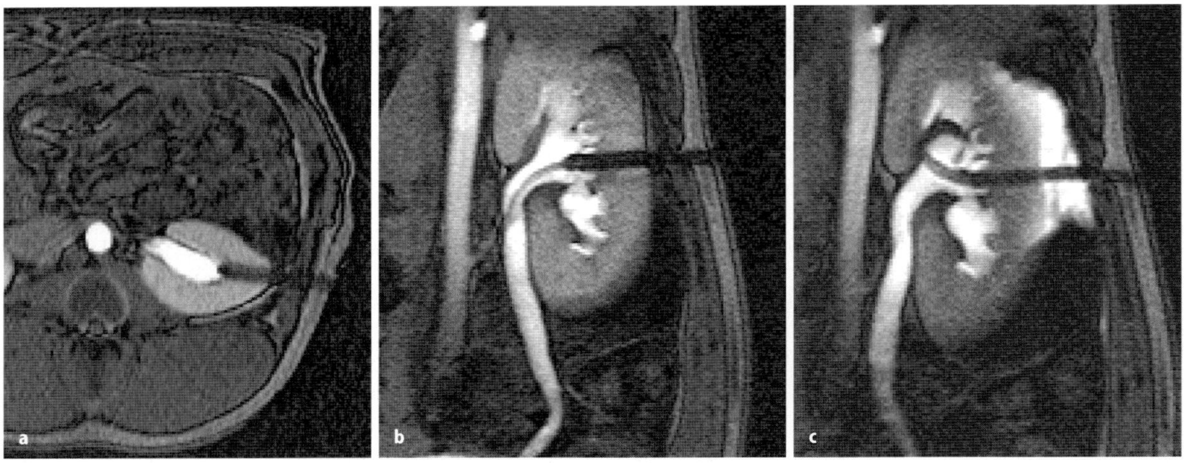

Fig. 20.11. Percutaneous nephrostomy. MR-guided nephrostomy of the nondilated urinary tract after previous MR urography. The puncture procedure is performed with MR-compatible equipment using dynamic T1-weighted dual-stack gradient echo sequences in the coronal and axial plane. (Courtesy of C. Nolte-Ernsting, Hamburg, Germany. See also Nolte-Ernsting et al. 1999)

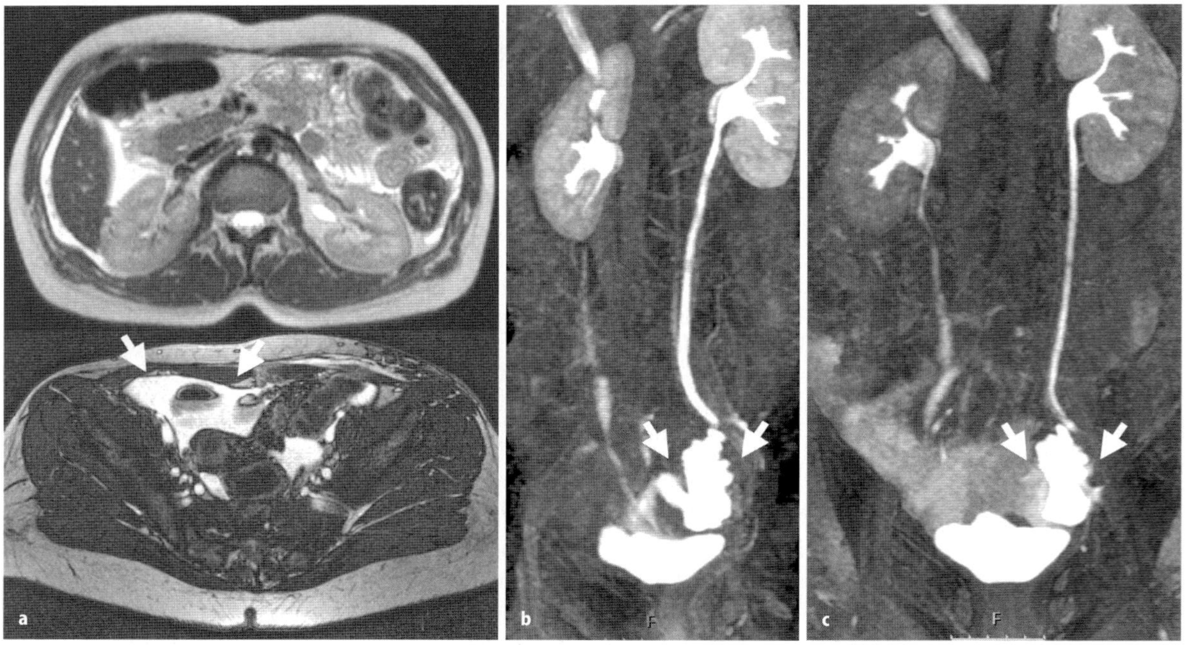

Fig. 20.12. Postoperative urinary leakage: urinoma. MR imaging reveals urinoma due to iatrogenic injury of the left ureter during gynecological surgery (*left, arrows*). Nondilated upper urinary tract, no urinary obstruction. MR urography nicely depicts the leakage of the ureter and the local urinoma as well as urine in the abdominal cavity (*right, arrows*)

causes (including abdominal trauma and injury to the collecting system during surgery or diagnostic instrumentation) can both lead to urinary extravasation (Healy et al. 1984). Although urinoma is typically located in the perirenal space, it may be seen in other locations as well. Moderate or severe hydronephrosis is present in most patients. At unenhanced CT, urinoma usually manifests as a fluid collection with water attenuation values. However, the attenuation can increase progressively after intravenous administration of contrast material because contrast-enhanced urine enters the urinoma. Additional late-phase scanning is recommended for CT. Postoperative urinary leakage and urinoma can also be confirmed and treated successfully by percutaneous aspiration and drainage (Yang et al. 2004). For noninvasive diagnosis, MR urography may serve as a valuable alternative (Nolte-Ernsting et al. 1998). Especially in postoperative urinary leakage, diverting operations (pyelostomy, nephrostomy) are desirable (Ihse et al. 1975). In patients with a nondilated upper

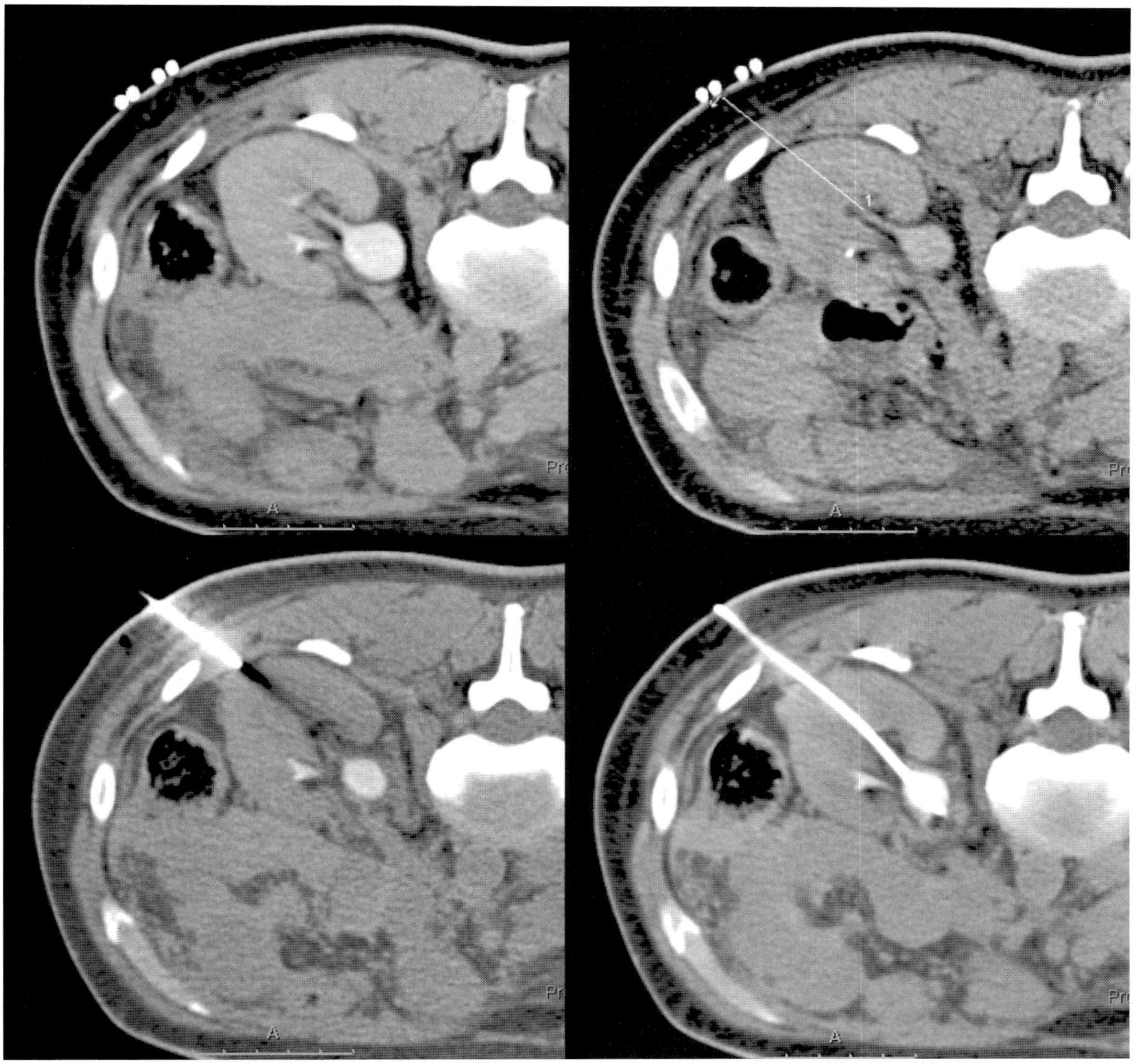

Fig. 20.13. Postoperative urinary leakage: urinoma. Percutaneous nephrostomy is performed under CT guidance from a dorsolateral approach using the Seldinger technique

urinary tract, CT guidance can be a valuable alternative to ultrasound and fluoroscopic guidance for PN (Figs. 20.12, 20.13).

20.6 Failure of Transplant Kidney

Apart from acute rejection or cyclosporine toxicity, vascular and nonvascular complications may lead to renal allograft dysfunction.

Bleeding, ureteral obstruction, urinary leak, venous thrombosis, hemodynamically relevant stenosis and occlusion of the renal transplant artery are causes for failure of a transplant kidney. Transplant renal artery stenosis is a common complication after transplantation and an important cause of graft dysfunction (Rengel et al. 1998). It occurs in 1%–12% of transplanted renal arteries and is a potentially curable cause of hypertension following transplantation and/or renal dysfunction (Surlan and Popovic 2003).

Treatment with PTA alone or in combination with a stent has been technically successful in 82%–92% of cases, and the graft salvage rate has ranged from 80% to 100% (Surlan and Popovic 2003). According to a recently published Italian retrospective study, 34 complications on 288 transplantation patients were observed (Carrafiello et al. 2005), 27 of which were treated by in-

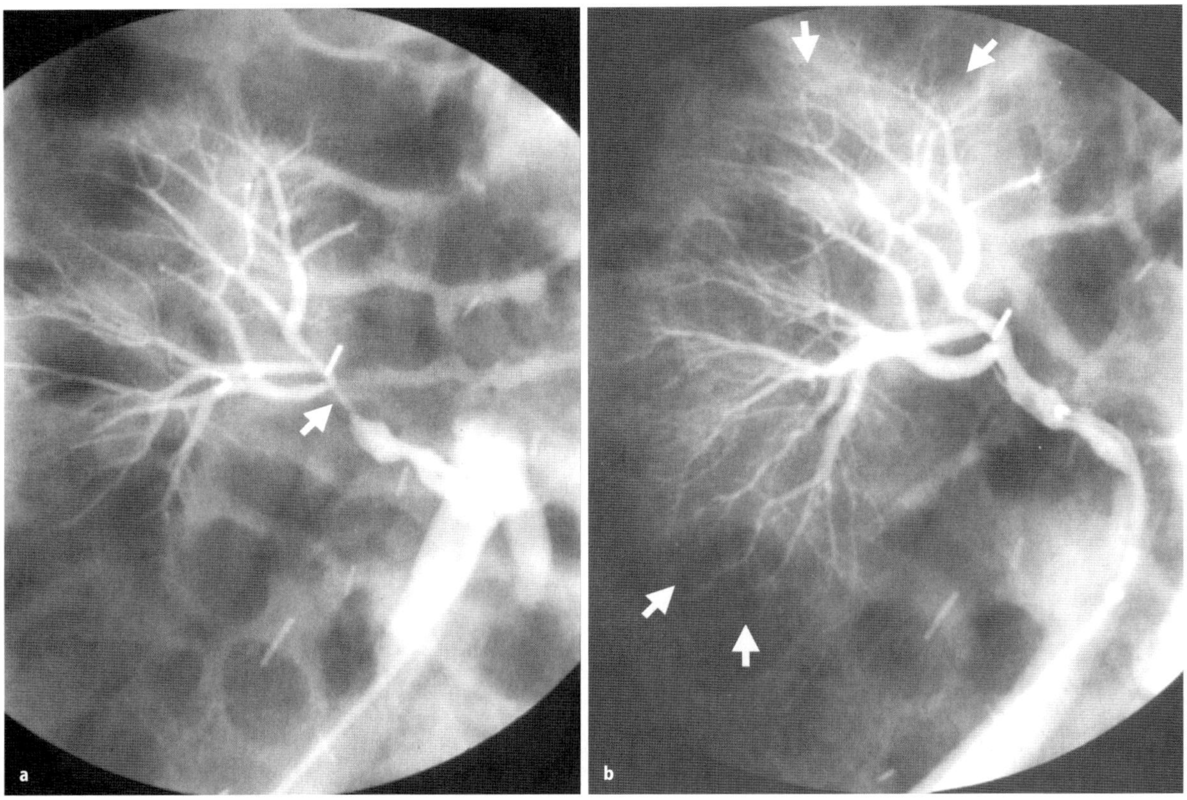

Fig. 20.14. Failure of a transplant kidney. Renal transplant kidney in the right iliac fossa. High-grade stenosis in the renal artery (*left, arrow*). Small peripheral arteries can be depicted after successful balloon dilatation via a transfemoral approach (*right, arrows*)

terventional radiology. The primary success rate was 85.2% (23/27 interventions), including therapy of renal artery stenoses, ureteral obstructions, ureteral leaks, and lymphoceles.

Renal vein thrombosis is an unusual complication of transplantation; it occurs in less than 5% of patients and usually in the first postoperative week. Renal vein thrombosis is heralded by an abrupt cessation of urinary function and swelling and tenderness over the graft (Akbar et al. 2005). Immediate surgical thrombectomy is warranted.

Biopsy-related vascular injuries in renal transplants are another dramatic situation prompting immediate treatment. Several studies evaluated the potential of superselective transcatheter embolization in iatrogenic biopsy-related vascular lesions of renal allografts (Perini et al. 1998; Dorffner et al. 1998; Maleux et al. 2003). Dorffner et al. reported four major complications out of seven patients treated with infarction of 30%–50% of the renal parenchyma (two cases) and nephrectomy after embolization because of renal artery occlusion (one case) or acute hemorrhage at the renal artery anastomosis (one case). Perini et al. achieved a technical success in 95% of cases and an eradication of the clinical signs or symptoms prompting referral in 15 of 17 patients (88%). According to Maleux et al., clinical symptoms disappeared in all 13 patients. Therefore, immediate clinical success and significant benefit in renal function can be achieved in the vast majority of cases by endovascular transcatheter embolization. The longevity of the allograft after successful embolization mainly depends on the natural (medical) outcome.

Other complications, such as postoperative hematomas, urinomas, or lymphoceles may jeopardize renal function in renal transplants due to an obstruction of the pelvicalyceal system. Here, catheter drainage offers a means of percutaneous treatment (see Sect. 20.5) (Fig. 20.14).

References

Adam G, Bücker A, Nolte-Ernsting C, Tacke J, Günther RW (1999) Interventional MR imaging: percutaneous abdominal and skeletal biopsies and drainages of the abdomen. Eur Radiol 9:1471

Akbar SA, Jafri SZ, Amendola MA, Madrazo BL, Salem R, Bis KG (2005) Complications of renal transplantation. Radiographics 25:1335

Akinci D, Akhan O, Ozmen MN, Karabulut N, Ozkan O, Cil BE, Karcaaltincaba M (2005) Percutaneous drainage of 300 in-

traperitoneal abscesses with long-term follow-up. Cardiovasc Intervent Radiol 28:744
Almgard LE, Fernstrom I, Haverling M, Ljungqvist A (1973) Treatment of renal adenocarcinoma by embolic occlusion of the renal circulation. Br J Urol 45:474
Alvarez Gonzalez E, Pamplona M, Rodriguez A, Garcia-Hidalgo E, Nunez V, Leiva O (1994) High flow priapism after blunt perineal trauma: resolution with bucrylate embolization. J Urol 151:426
Bakal CW, Sacks D, Burke DR, Cardella JF, Chopra PS, Dawson SL, Drooz AT, Freeman N, Meranze SG, Van Moore A Jr, Palestrant AM, Roberts AC, Spies JB, Stein EJ, Towbin R; Society of Interventional Radiology Standards of Practice Committee (2003) Quality improvement guidelines for adult percutaneous abscess and fluid drainage. J Vasc Interv Radiol 14:S223
Barbaric ZL, Hall T, Cochran ST, Heitz DR, Schwartz RA, Krasny RM, Deseran MW (1997) Percutaneous nephrostomy: placement under CT and fluoroscopy guidance. Am J Roentgenol 169:151
Behrendt P, Do D, Baumgartner I, Triller J, Kniemeyer H, Mahler F (2000) Renal artery stenting following acute aortic dissection: implantation and follow-up. Vasa 29:138
Berger R, Billups K, Brock G, Broderick GA, Dhabuwala CB, Goldstein I, Hakim LS, Hellstrom W, Honig S, Levine LA, Lue T, Munarriz R, Montague DK, Mulcahy JJ, Nehra A, Rogers ZR, Rosen R, Seftel AD, Shabsigh R, Steers W; AFUD Thought Leader Panel on Evaluation and Treatment of Priapism (2001) Report of the American Foundation for Urologic Disease (AFUD) Thought Leader Panel for evaluation and treatment of priapism. Int J Impot Res 13 [Suppl 5]:S39
Bergreen PW, Woodside J, Paster SB (1997) Therapeutic renal infarction. J Urol 118:372
Bilbao JI, Cosin O, Bastarrika G, Rosell D, Zudaire J, Martinez-Cuesta A (2005) Treatment of ureteroarterial fistulae with covered vascular endoprostheses and ureteral occlusion. Cardiovasc Intervent Radiol 28:159
Blum U, Billmann P, Krause T, Gabelmann A, Keller E, Moser E, Langer M (1993) Effect of local low-dose thrombolysis on clinical outcome in acute embolic renal artery occlusion. Radiology 189:549
Brountzos EN (2006) Quality improvement guidelines for percutaneous nephrostomies. http://www.cirse.org/_files/contentmanagement/05_qig.pdf. Cited 9 April 2006
Buecker A, Neuerburg JM, Adam GB, Nolte-Ernsting CC, Hunter DW, Glowinski A, van Vaals JJ, Günther RW (2001) MR-guided percutaneous drainage of abdominal fluid collections in combination with X-ray fluoroscopy: initial clinical experience. Eur Radiol 11:670
Caldamone AA, Frank IN (1980) Percutaneous aspiration in the treatment of renal abscess. J Urol 123:92
Carmignani G, Belgrano E, Puppo P, Cichero A, Giuliani L (1980) Transcatheter embolization of the hypogastric arteries in cases of bladder hemorrhage from advanced pelvic cancers: follow-up in 9 cases. J Urol 124:196
Carrafiello G, Lagana D, Mangini M, Cuffari S, Cafaro T, Recaldini C, Genovese E, Fugazzola C (2005) The role of interventional radiology in the management of kidney transplant complications. Radiol Med (Torino) 110:249
Cohen GS, Braunstein L, Ball DS, Roberto PJ, Reich J, Hanno P (1996) Selective arterial embolization of idiopathic priapism. Cardiovasc Intervent Radiol 19:47
Colombo F, Lovaria A, Saccheri S, Pozzoni F, Montanaris E (1999) Arterial embolization in the treatment of post-traumatic priapism. Ann Urol (Paris) 33:210
Cronan JJ Jr, Dorfman GS (1983) Low dose thrombolysis: a nonoperative approach to renal artery occlusion. J Urol 130:757
Crummy AB, Ishizuka J, Madsen PO (1979) Posttraumatic priapism: successful treatment with autologous clot embolization. Am J Roentgenol 133:329
De Baere T, Lagrange C, Kuoch V, Morice P, Court B, Roche A (2000) Transcatheter ethanol renal ablation in 20 patients with persistent urine leaks: an alternative to surgical nephrectomy. J Urol 164:1148
Deyoe LA, Cronan JJ, Lambiase RE, Dorfman GS (1990) Percutaneous drainage of renal and perirenal abscesses: results in 30 patients. Am J Roentgenol 155:81
Di Valentino M, Alerci M, Tutta P, Sartori F, Marone C, Vandoni R, Mahler F, Gallino A (2004) Thrombus aspiration as a bail-out procedure during percutaneous renal angioplasty. J Endovasc Ther 11:522
Dimitrios M, Achilles C, Andrew K, Charalampos L, Katsenis K, Vlachos L (2004) Bilateral renal artery stenting in a patient with Leriche syndrome. Urol Int 73:283
Dinkel HP, Danuser H, Triller J (2002) Blunt renal trauma: minimally invasive management with microcatheter embolization experience in nine patients. Radiology 223:723
Dondelinger RF, Trotteur G, Ghaye B, Szapiro D (2002) Traumatic injuries: radiological hemostatic intervention at admission. Eur Radiol 12:979
Dorffner R, Thurnher S, Prokesch R, Bankier A, Turetschek K, Schmidt A, Lammer J (1998) Embolization of iatrogenic vascular injuries of renal transplants: immediate and follow-up results. Cardiovasc Intervent Radiol 21:129
Drooz AT, Lewis CA, Allen TE, Citron SJ, Cole PE, Freeman NJ, Husted JW, Malloy PC, Martin LG, Van Moore A, Neithamer CD, Roberts AC, Sacks D, Sanchez O, Venbrux AC, Bakal CW; Society of interventional radiology standards of practice committee (2003) Quality Improvement Guidelines for Percutaneous Transcatheter Embolization. J Vasc Interv Radiol 14: S237-S242
Ewalt DH, Diamond N, Rees C, Sparagana SP, Delgado M, Batchelor L, Roach ES (2005) Long-term outcome of transcatheter embolization of renal angiomyolipomas due to tuberous sclerosis complex. J Urol 174:1764
Fann JI, Miller DC (1995) Aortic dissection. Ann Vasc Surg 9:311
Farrell TA, Wallace M, Hicks ME (1997) Long-term results of transrenal ureteral occlusion with use of Gianturco coils and gelatin sponge pledgets. J Vasc Interv Radiol 8:449
Friedel JM, Khalil R, Lasorda D (2005) Treatment of iatrogenic renal artery perforation with a covered stent and subsequent rheolytic thrombectomy. J Invasive Cardiol 17:374
Gaylord GM, Johnsrude IS (1989) Transrenal ureteral occlusion with Gianturco coils and gelatin sponge. Radiology 172:1047
Gluck G, Croitoru M, Deleanu D, Platon P (2000) Local thrombolytic treatment for renal arterial embolism. Eur Urol 38:339
Goffette PP, Laterre PF (2002) Traumatic injuries: imaging and intervention in post-traumatic complications (delayed intervention) Eur Radiol 12:994
Goodwin WE, Casey WC, Woolf W (1955) Percutaneous trocar (needle) nephrostomy in hydronephrosis. J Am Med Assoc 157:891
Greenberg JM, Steiner MA, Marshall JJ (2002) Acute renal artery thrombosis treated by percutaneous rheolytic thrombectomy. Catheter Cardiovasc Interv 56:66
Günther R, Alken P, Altwein JE (1978) Percutaneous nephropyelostomy applications and results. Rofo 128:720
Günther R, Marberger M, Klose K (1979) Transrenal ureteral embolization. Radiology 132:317
Haaga JR, Zelch MG, Alfidi RJ, Stewart BH, Daugherty JD (1977) CT-guided antegrade pyelography and percutaneous nephrostomy. Am J Roentgenol 128:621

Hagiwara A, Sakaki S, Goto H, Takenega K, Fukushima H, Matuda H, Shimazaki S (2001) The role of interventional radiology in the management of blunt renal injury: a practical protocol. J Trauma 51:526
Hagiwara A, Murata A, Matsuda T, Matsuda H, Shimazaki S (2004) The usefulness of transcatheter arterial embolization for patients with blunt polytrauma showing transient response to fluid resuscitation. J Trauma 57:271
Hagspiel KD, Kandarpa K, Silverman SG (1998) Interactive MR-guided percutaneous nephrostomy. J Magn Reson Imaging 8:1319
Hald T, Mygind T (1974) Control of life-threatening vesical hemorrhage by unilateral hypogastric artery muscle embolization. J Urol 112:60
Hallscheidt P, Besharati S, Noeldge G, Haferkamp A, Lopez R, Kauffmann GW (2006) Preoperative and palliative embolization of renal cell carcinomas: follow-up of 49 patients. Rofo 178:391
Hausegger KA, Tiesenhausen K, Schedlbauer P, Oberwalder P, Tauss J, Rigler B (2001) Treatment of acute aortic type B dissection with stent-grafts. Cardiovasc Intervent Radiol 24:306
Hayes MC, Wilson NM, Page A, Harrison GS (1996) Selective embolization of bladder tumours. Br J Urol 78:311
Healy ME, Teng SS, Moss AA (1984) Uriniferous pseudocyst: computed tomographic findings. Radiology 153:757
Heidenreich A, Ravery V; European Society of Oncological Urology (2004) Preoperative imaging in renal cell cancer. World J Urol 22:307
Heye S, Maleux G, Van Poppel H, Oyen R, Wilms G (2005) Hemorrhagic complications after nephron-sparing surgery: angiographic diagnosis and management by transcatheter embolization. Am J Roentgenol 184:1661
Hirota S, Matsumoto S, Yoshikawa T, Ichikawa S, Sako M, Kono M (1997) Simultaneous thrombolysis of superior mesenteric artery and bilateral renal artery thromboembolisms with three transfemoral catheters. Cardiovasc Intervent Radiol 20:397
Ihse I, Arnesjo B, Jonsson G (1975) Surgical injuries of the ureter. A review of 42 cases. Scand J Urol Nephrol 9:39
Ji MX, He NS, Wang P, Chen G (1994) Use of selective embolization of the bilateral cavernous arteries for posttraumatic arterial priapism. J Urol 151:1641
Kadir S, Watson A, Burrow C (1987) Percutaneous transcatheter recanalization in the management of acute renal failure due to sudden occlusion of the renal artery to a solitary kidney. Am J Nephrol 7:445
Kalman D, Varenhorst E (1999) The role of arterial embolization in renal cell carcinoma. Scand J Urol Nephrol 33:162
Kauffmann GW, Richter GM, Roeren TK (1992) Renal tumor embolization. Radiologe 32:127
Keller FS, Barton RE, Routh WD, Gross GM (1990) Gross hematuria in two patients with ureteral-ileal conduits and double-J stents. J Vasc Interv Radiol 1:69
Kerlan RK, Gordon RL, LaBerge JM, Ring EJ (1998) Superselective microcoil embolization in the management of high-flow priapism. J Vasc Interv Radiol 9:85
Kim HS, Fine DM, Atta MG (2006) Catheter-directed thrombectomy and thrombolysis for acute renal vein thrombosis. J Vasc Interv Radiol 17:815
Klein RM, Niehues R, Hollenbeck M, Horstkotte D, Furst G, Strauer BE (1992) The local lysis therapy of spontaneous renal artery dissection with arterial thrombosis. Dtsch Med Wochenschr 117:1185
Kothary N, Soulen MC, Clark TW, Wein AJ, Shlansky-Goldberg RD, Crino PB, Stavropoulos SW (2005) Renal angiomyolipoma: long-term results after arterial embolization. J Vasc Interv Radiol 16:45
Kress O, Heidenreich A, Klose KJ, Wagner HJ, Alfke H (2002) Superselective embolization with coils in high-flow priapism.Cardiovasc Intervent Radiol 25:326
Kuefer R, Bartsch G, Herkommer K, Kramer SC, Kleinschmidt K, Volkmer BG (2005) Changing diagnostic and therapeutic concepts in high-flow priapism. Int J Impot Res 17:109
Lacombe P, Mulot R, Labedan F, Jondeau G, Barre O, Chagnon S, Judet O, Tcherdakoff P (1992) Percutaneous recanalization of a renal artery in aortic dissection. Radiology 185:829
Lamb GW, Bromwich EJ, Vasey P, Aitchison M (2004) Management of renal masses in patients medically unsuitable for nephrectomy–natural history, complications, and outcome. Urology 64:909
Langenhuijsen JF, Reisman Y, Reekers JA, de Reijke TM (2001) Highly selective embolization of bilateral cavernous arteries for post-traumatic penile arterial priapism. Int J Impot Res 13:354
LeMaitre L, Mestdagh P, Marecaux-Delomez J, Valtille P, Dubrulle F, Biserte J (2000) Percutaneous nephrostomy: placement under laser guidance and real-time CT fluoroscopy. Eur Radiol 10:892
Lessman RK, Jhonson SF, Coburn JW, Kaufman JJ (1978) Renal artery embolism, clinical features and long-term follow-up of 17 cases. Ann Intern Med 89:477
Levy JM, Duszak RL Jr, Akins EW, Bakal CW, Denny DF Jr, Martin LG, Van Moore A Jr, Pentecost MJ, Roberts AC, Vogelzang RL, Kent KC, Perler BA, Resnick MI, Richie J (2000) Percutaneous transluminal renal angioplasty. American College of Radiology. ACR Appropriateness Criteria. Radiology 215 [Suppl]:1015
Lovaria A, Nicolini A, Meregaglia D, Saccheri S, Rivolta R, Rampoldi A, Rossi P, Montanari E (1999) Interventional radiology in the treatment of urological vascular complications. Ann Urol (Paris) 33:156
Maleux G, Messiaen T, Stockx L, Vanrenterghem Y, Wilms G (2003) Transcatheter embolization of biopsy-related vascular injuries in renal allografts. Long-term technical, clinical and biochemical results. Acta Radiol 44:13
Manke C, Strotzer M, Seitz J, Lenhart M, Aebert H, Kasprzak P, Kaiser B, Feuerbach S (1999) Ischemic complications in aortic dissection–percutaneous treatment with balloon fenestration and stent implantation. Rofo 170:198
Martin LG, Casarella WJ, Gaylord GM (1988) Azotemia caused by renal artery stenosis: treatment by percutaneous angioplasty. Am J Roentgenol 150:839
Martin LG, Rundback JH, Sacks D, Cardella JF, Rees CR, Matsumoto AH, Meranze SG, Schwartzberg MS, Silverstein MI, Lewis CA; Society of Interventional Radiology Standards of Practice Committee (2003) Quality improvement guidelines for angiography angioplasty, and stent placement in the diagnosis and treatment of renal artery stenosis in adults. J Vasc Interv Radiol 14:S297
Marx FJ, Chaussy C, Moser E (1982) Limitations and hazards of palliative renal tumor embolization. Urologe A 21:206
Matlaga BR, Shah OD, Zagoria RJ, Dyer RB, Streem SB, Assimos DG (2003) Computerized tomography guided access for percutaneous nephrostolithotomy. J Urol 170:45
Merkle EM, Hashim M, Wendt M, Lewin JS (1999) MR-guided percutaneous nephrostomy of the nondilated upper urinary tract in a porcine model. Am J Roentgenol 172:1221
Miller DC, Stinson EB, Oyer PE, Rossiter SJ, Reitz BA, Griepp RB, Shumway NE (1979) Operative treatment of aortic dissections. Experience with 125 patients over a sixteen-year period. J Thorac Cardiovasc Surg 78:365
Morris CS, Bonnevie GJ, Najarian KE (2001) Nonsurgical treatment of acute iatrogenic renal artery injuries occurring after renal artery angioplasty and stenting. Am J Roentgenol 177:1353

Mugge A, Gulba DC, Frei U, Wagenbreth I, Grote R, Daniel WG, Lichtlen PR (1990) Renal artery embolism: thrombolysis with recombinant tissue-type plasminogen activator. J Intern Med 228:279

Munro NP, Woodhams S, Nawrocki JD, Fletcher MS, Thomas PJ (2003) The role of transarterial embolization in the treatment of renal cell carcinoma. BJU Int 92:240

Nabi G, Sheikh N, Greene D, Marsh R (2003) Therapeutic transcatheter arterial embolization in the management of intractable haemorrhage from pelvic urological malignancies: preliminary experience and long-term follow-up. BJU Int 92:245

Neuerburg JM, Lehrmann K (2004) Transarterial embolization of the kidney: review of the literature. Rofo 176:809

Nolte-Ernsting CC, Bücker A, Adam GB, Neuerburg JM, Jung P, Hunter DW, Jakse G, Günther RW (1998) Gadolinium-enhanced excretory MR urography after low-dose diuretic injection: comparison with conventional excretory urography. Radiology 209:147

Nolte-Ernsting CC, Bücker A, Neuerburg JM, Glowinski A, Adam GB, Günther RW (1999) MR imaging-guided percutaneous nephrostomy and use of MR-compatible catheters in the nondilated porcine urinary tract. J Vasc Interv Radiol 10:1305

Numan F, Cakirer S, Islak C, Ogut G, Kadioglu A, Cayan S, Tellaloglu S (1996) Posttraumatic high-flow priapism treated by N-butyl-cyanoacrylate embolisation. Cardiovasc Intervent Radiol 19:278

O'Sullivan P, Browne R, McEniff N, Lee MJ (2006) Treatment of "high-flow" priapism with superselective transcatheter embolization: a useful alternative to surgery. Cardiovasc Intervent Radiol 29:198–201

Park JH, Chung JW, Cho YK, Kim SH, Ahn H, Oh BH (1997) Percutaneous fenestration of aortic dissection: salvage of an ischemic solitary left kidney. Cardiovasc Intervent Radiol 20:146

Perini S, Gordon RL, LaBerge JM, Kerlan RK Jr, Wilson MW, Feng S, Ring EJ (1998) Transcatheter embolization of biopsy-related vascular injury in the transplant kidney: immediate and long-term outcome. J Vasc Interv Radiol 9:1011

Pieri S, Agresti P, La Pera G, Atzori M, Ialongo P (2005) Posttraumatic high flow priapism percutaneously treated with transcatheter embolisation. Radiol Med (Torino) 110:370

Pfister RC, Newhouse JH (1979) Interventional percutaneous pyeloureteral techniques. II. Percutaneous nephrostomy and other procedures. Radiol Clin North Am 17:351

Pilmore HL, Walker RJ, Solomon C, Packer S, Wood D (1995) Acute bilateral renal artery occlusion: successful revascularization with streptokinase. Am J Nephrol 15:90

Pisco JM, Martins JM, Correia MG (1989) Internal iliac artery: embolization to control hemorrhage from pelvic neoplasms. Radiology 172:337

Quillin SP, Darcy MD, Picus D (1994) Angiographic evaluation and therapy of ureteroarterial fistulas. Am J Roentgenol 162:873

Ramchandani P, Cardella JF, Grassi CJ, Roberts AC, Sacks D, Schwartzberg MS, Lewis CA; SCVIR Standards of Practice Committee (2003) Quality improvement guidelines for percutaneous nephrostomy. J Vasc Interv Radiol 14:S277

Rengel M, Gomes-Da-Silva G, Inchaustegui L, Lampreave JL, Robledo R, Echenagusia A, Vallejo JL, Valderrabano F (1998) Renal artery stenosis after kidney transplantation: diagnostic and therapeutic approach. Kidney Int Suppl 68:S99

Rickards D (2002) Non-traumatic abdominal emergencies: imaging and intervention in acute urinary conditions. Eur Radiol 12:2435

Rose BD (2006) Diagnosis and treatment of thromboembolic renal infarction. http://www.uptodateonline.com/utd/content/topic.do?topicKey=renldis/17093&type=A&selectedTitle=1~18 Cited 13 April 2006

Salam TA, Lumsden AB, Martin LG (1993) Local infusion of fibrinolytic agents for acute renal artery thromboembolism: report of ten cases.Ann Vasc Surg 7:21

Salvatierra O, Bucklew WB, Morrow JW (1967) Perinephric abscess: a report of 71 cases. J Urol 98:296

Savoca G, Pietropaolo F, Scieri F, Bertolotto M, Mucelli FP, Belgrano E (2004) Sexual function after highly selective embolization of cavernous artery in patients with high flow priapism: long-term follow up. J Urol 172:644

Scheinert D, Braunlich S, Nonnast-Daniel B, Schroeder M, Schmidt A, Biamino G, Daniel WG, Ludwig J (2001) Transradial approach for renal artery stenting. Catheter Cardiovasc Interv 54:442

Schild HH, Günther R, Thelen M (1994) Transrenal ureteral occlusion: results and problems. J Vasc Interv Radiol 5:321

Schunk K, Schild H, Wandel E, Schinzel H, Weingartner K (1990) Local fibrinolysis in renal artery occlusion. Rofo 152:147

Sharafuddin MJ, Hicks ME (1997) Current status of percutaneous mechanical thrombectomy. Part I. General principles. J Vasc Interv Radiol 8:911

Sharafuddin MJ, Hicks ME (1998a) Current status of percutaneous mechanical thrombectomy. Part II. Devices and mechanisms of action. J Vasc Interv Radiol 9:15

Sharafuddin MJ, Hicks ME (1998b) Current status of percutaneous mechanical thrombectomy. Part III. Present and future applications. J Vasc Interv Radiol 9:209

Shiraishi J, Higaki Y, Oguni A, Inoue M, Tatsumi T, Azuma A, Matsubara H (2005) Transradial renal artery angioplasty and stenting in a patient with Leriche syndrome. Int Heart J 46:557

Shu T, Green JM, Orihuela E (2004) Renal and perirenal abscesses in patients with otherwise anatomically normal urinary tracts. J Urol 172:148

Siablis D, Liatsikos EN, Kalogeropoulou CP, Zabakis P, Tsota I, Karnabatidis D, Fokaefs E, Barbalias GA (2002) Arterioureteral fistula – a rare complication of ureterolithotomy: treatment with embolization. J Endourol 16:97

Siablis D, Liatsikos EN, Goumenos D, Karnabatidis D, Voudoukis T, Barbalias G, Vlahogiannis J (2005) Percutaneous rheolytic thrombectomy for treatment of acute renal-artery thrombosis. J Endourol 19:68

Siegel JF, Smith A, Moldwin R (1996) Minimally invasive treatment of renal abscess. J Urol 155:52

Siezenga MA, van Overhagen H, van Buren M (2005) Acute occlusion of the renal artery treated by means of rheolytic thrombectomy. Ned Tijdschr Geneeskd 149:2413

Spies JB, Bakal CW, Burke DR, Cardella JF, Drooz A, Edwards ME, Husted JW, Palestrant AM, Pentecost MJ, Roberts AC, Rogers WF, Spencer MC, Weyman PJ; Society of Interventional Radiology Standards of Practice Committee (2003) Angioplasty standard of practice. J Vasc Interv Radiol 14:S219

Stella N, Rolli A, Catalano A, Udini M (2001) Simultaneous urokinase perfusion in renal artery and vein in a case of renal vein thrombosis. Minerva Cardioangiol 49:273

Sternbergh WC 3rd, Ramee SR, DeVun DA, Money SR (2000) Endovascular treatment of multiple visceral artery paradoxical emboli with mechanical and pharmacological thrombolysis. J Endovasc Ther 7:155

Surlan M, Popovic P (2003) The role of interventional radiology in management of patients with end-stage renal disease. Eur J Radiol 46:96

Suzuki T, Mehta RH, Ince H, Nagai R, Sakomura Y, Weber F, Sumiyoshi T, Bossone E, Trimarchi S, Cooper JV, Smith DE, Isselbacher EM, Eagle KA, Nienaber CA; International Registry of Aortic Dissection (2003) Clinical profiles and outcomes of acute type B aortic dissection in the current era: lessons from the International Registry of Aortic Dissection (IRAD). Circulation 108 [Suppl 1]:II312

Textor HJ, Wilhelm K, Strunk H, Layer G, Dolitzsch C, Schild HH (2000) Locoregional chemoperfusion with mitoxantrone for palliative therapy in bleeding bladder cancer compared with embolization. Rofo 172:462

Uflacker R, Paolini RM, Lima S (1984) Management of traumatic hematuria by selective renal artery embolization. J Urol 132:662

UpToDate (2006) Contraindications to thrombolytic therapy in pulmonary embolism. http://www.uptodateonline.com/utd/content/image.do?imageKey=pulm_pix/contra15.gif. Cited 13 April 13 2006

Van de Ven PJ, Kaatee R, Beutler JJ, Beek FJ, Woittiez AJ, Buskens E, Koomans HA, Mali WP (1999) Arterial stenting and balloon angioplasty in ostial atherosclerotic renovascular disease: a randomised trial. Lancet 353:282

Velmahos GC, Chahwan S, Hanks SE, Murray JA, Berne TV, Asensio J, Demetriades D (2000) Angiographic embolization of bilateral internal iliac arteries to control life-threatening hemorrhage after blunt trauma to the pelvis. Am Surg 66:858

Vignali C, Lonzi S, Bargellini I, Cioni R, Petruzzi P, Caramella D, Bartolozzi C (2004) Vascular injuries after percutaneous renal procedures: treatment by transcatheter embolization. Eur Radiol 14:723

Vorwerk D, Günther RW, Keulers P, Jakse G (1993) Superselective kidney artery embolization as therapy of choice in bleeding of benign origin. Dtsch Med Wochenschr 118:325

Walker TG, Grant PW, Goldstein I, Krane RJ, Greenfield AJ (1990) "High-flow" priapism: treatment with superselective transcatheter embolization. Radiology 174:1053

Williams DM, Lee DY, Hamilton BH, Marx MV, Narasimham DL, Kazanjian SN, Prince MR, Andrews JC, Cho KJ, Deeb GM (1997) The dissected aorta: percutaneous treatment of ischemic complications–principles and results. J Vasc Interv Radiol 8:605

Williams JM, Racadio JM, Johnson ND, Donnelly LF, Bissler JJ (2006) Embolization of renal angiomyolipomata in patients with tuberous sclerosis complex. Am J Kidney Dis 47:95

Yang DM, Jung DH, Kim H, Kang JH, Kim SH, Kim JH, Hwang HY (2004) Retroperitoneal cystic masses: CT, clinical, and pathologic findings and literature review. Radiographics 24:1353

Zuckerman AM, Martin LG, Silverstein MI (1993) Emergent renal artery revascularization for acute anuria. J Vasc Interv Radiol 4:489

Selected Case Reports and Personal Experience 21

Percutaneous Approach for Difficult Stones

S. Arap, M.A. Arap

We would like to present the case of a 65-year-old man who underwent a radical cystoprostatectomy plus ureterosigmoidostomy (Mainz Pouch II) in 1996, due to a high-grade invasive transitional cell carcinoma of the bladder. He had an uneventful postoperative period and was free of disease in his 2-year follow-up visit (1998). Clinically, he had total control over his anal voiding, with no diurnal or nocturnal urine leakage. However, 2 years after surgery his intravenous pyelogram showed a stenosis of the left ureterosigmoidal anastomosis, and sonography revealed mild to moderate ureterohydronephrosis. He also had an obstructive 1-cm left renal pelvic stone.

This is one of the interesting aspects of this case. We were facing a unilateral ureterointestinal stenosis in a patient with a previous extensive abdominal procedure. In addition, he had a symptomatic renal stone. After the evaluation, we decided to treat both pathologies at the same time using a left percutaneous approach. Contrast was instilled in the collecting system using a fine needle, followed by percutaneous access to the left inferior calyx. The stone was easily removed and the ureterointestinal stenosis was incised over a guidewire using an Acucise catheter. An 8.5-F double-J stent was left in place for 3 weeks and antibiotics were used preemptively, as the ureter drained to the bowel.

In regard to this procedure, we believe that the percutaneous approach allowed us to treat the calculus and to treat the ureteral stenosis. The patient's follow-up evidenced a normal nondilated ureter and good drainage was confirmed by intravenous pyelogram.

The patient had an uneventful oncological follow-up, and all laboratory and radiological studies were normal until 2002. At this time, he presented a mild ureteral dilation and a 0.5-cm left renal calculus. As it was a mild dilatation, we decided to keep a close follow-up. In 2004, he presented with the same radiological findings except for the stone, which was 0.6 cm at this time.

In March 2005, he underwent a myocardial revascularization due to four arterial obstructions and started on prophylactic aspirin. In December 2005, 9 years after cystoprostatectomy, 7 years after the Acucise incision of the ureterointestinal stenosis, and 6 months after the myocardial revascularization, his uro-oncological follow-up revealed normal thoracic CT scan and no signs of recurrent transitional cell carcinoma of the bladder. However, his abdominal CT scan showed a moderate left hydronephrosis, a redundant dilated ureter, three 2.5- to 3-cm renal stones and two 2-cm lower ureteral stones (Fig. 21.1.1). Interestingly, he was asymptomatic except from two self-limited episodes of

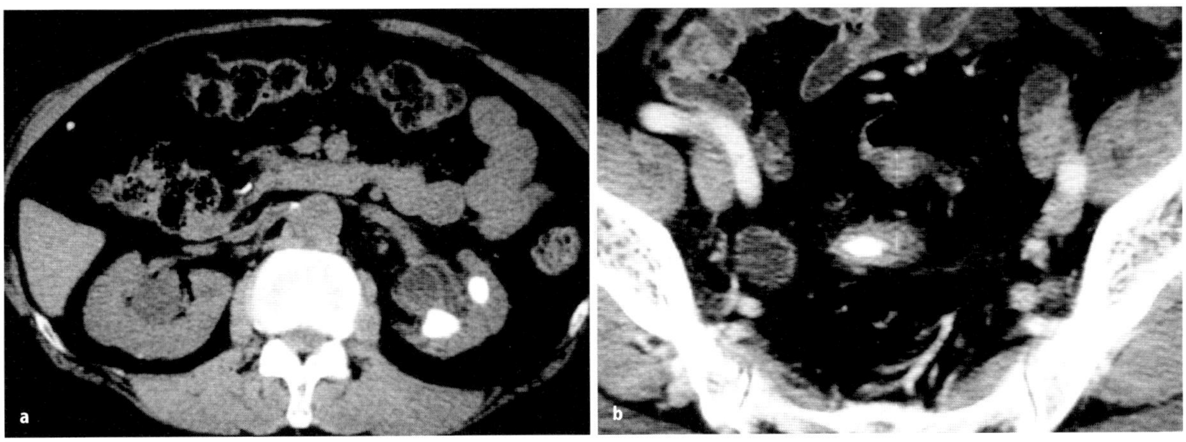

Fig. 21.1.1a, b. Preoperative CT scan. **a** Renal stones in the left inferior calyx. **b** Left lower ureteral stone visualized just above the ureterointestinal anastomosis

macroscopic hematuria. He did not have fever, weight loss, lack of appetite, or any other symptoms or signs of urinary infection.

This is the second very interesting situation we faced in this case. First, he had significant renal and ureteral lithiasis, which might be either cause or consequence of the hydronephrosis. Second, we could not run urine cultures before the certainly necessary surgical procedure. Third, we would probably face a challenging surgery in a cardiologically impaired patient. We had an extensive discussion with the patient in regard to the risks, benefits, and success rates of what we believed would be a complex surgery. All possible techniques were described in detail to the patient and finally we agreed he should be submitted to a new percutaneous procedure.

He was started on preemptive antibiotic prophylaxis, the urinary tract was accessed using a fine needle, and contrast was instilled into the collecting system. The inferior left calyx was accessed percutaneously and we initiated the procedure by navigating in all renal calyces using rigid and flexible nephroscopes. All renal stones were soft enough to be easily removed with forceps and baskets and we did not need ballistic or laser devices. The first part of the surgery was completed in 40 min and we then proceeded to the ureteral stones.

The left pyeloureteral junction was accessed and dilated using two guidewires and a flexible ureteroscope. The proximal ureter was explored and no signs of lithiasis or obstruction were found. In the distal third of the ureter, a thick layer of debris was found, and the procedure was slightly more difficult because of the ureteral kinks and poor irrigant flow. When we reached the distal third of the ureter, the stones were found directly above the anastomosis, apparently causing the obstruction. We then proceeded to an exhaustive laser ureterolithotripsy and when finished, a ureteral catheter was easily inserted into the sigmoid over the previously placed guidewire. The flexible ureteroscope was also inserted into the sigmoid with no difficulty. Finally, we placed a nephrostomy, and an antegrade pyelography confirmed a patent ureterointestinal anastomosis.

We believe several lessons can be learned from this case. First, the Mainz Pouch II is a very good urinary diversion in patients who are anally continent for liquids. Second, the percutaneous access allowed us to treat the ureterointestinal stenosis most easily. Third, the patient rapidly developed a significant mass of calculi both in the ureter and kidney, probably due to an asymptomatic urinary infection. Fourth, percutaneous nephroscopy, antegrade flexible ureteroscopy and modern guidewires, laser fibers, and good imaging allowed us to remove endoscopically all calculi in a patient who would probably need an extensive open procedure if treated only a decade ago. Finally, percutaneous approaches and expertise in endourological procedures are essential for all urology services, especially in the university context.

The Relaxing Incision for Priapism

C.F. Donatucci

Urological emergencies are rare for the andrologist. However, a patient with priapism can challenge any urological surgeon. Early in my career, I followed the normal paradigm for relief of priapism, but each successive step met with less than spectacular results. Initially at least, my efforts appeared successful, a distal glanular shunt would lead to rapid detumescence, but within hours the penis would again be rigid, and the patient would again be crying in pain. The standard of care would next be to perform a more proximal surgical shunt such as a shunt between the corpus spongiosum and the corpus cavernosum. This was done diligently, as I had learned during residency. Yet within hours I would receive a call from the nurses on the floor that the penis was again rigid and the patient in pain. After cavernosal blood gases would demonstrate ongoing anoxia, off I would go to the operating room for yet a third attempt at surgical relief, now utilizing a saphenous vein to corpus cavernosum shunt. I was not alone in this experience, for as the local andrologist I would receive calls from private practice urological surgeons in my locale with questions about patients with priapism whose medical course followed a similar track.

Vexed by these episodes, I determined to try to do better. I reviewed the classic article by Frank Hinman on the pathophysiology of priapism and considered analogous clinical scenarios. I came to the conclusion that my efforts were not aggressive enough and that the surgical shunts I created were inadequate to take care of the physiologic changes that occurred after I had relieved the priapism. Initial efforts using distal glanular shunts, whether percutaneous or open, do relieve the anoxic state, but relief of anoxia is followed by vascular hyperperfusion, because the normal control mechanisms (arteriolar and venous) have been compromised by the anoxic state of the tissue. Hyperperfusion leads to increased edema in the trabecular tissue. Confined within the tunica albuginea of the penis, a compartment syndrome is created that leads again to anoxia and triggers a circular pathophysiologic event: relief of hypoxia leads to hyperperfusion, which leads to trabecular edema, which leads to compression of arterial inflow, which leads to hypoxia. The solution is to follow the techniques of orthopedic surgeons faced with compartment syndromes in the limbs, or neurosurgeons faced with closed head trauma. Relieve the anoxia, but create defects in the closed system that will allow the edema of hyperperfusion to expand without further compromise of the already injured tissue. So now I am much more aggressive in my surgical treatment of priapism. I create larger defects in the tunica, whether by amputation of the distal corporal tips through the glans penis, or by large bilateral proximal spongeosal–cavernosal shunts. This more aggressive initial surgical approach has broken the cycle of successive trips to the operating room for unrelieved priapism, which I believe has improved surgical outcomes for my patients.

References

Hinman F Jr (1960) Priapism: reasons for failure of therapy. J Urol 83:420

Priapism Redux

W.O. Brant

A 31-year-old male was evaluated in the emergency department. He complained of a painful erection that had been present for 48 h. He had been at a party where he used intranasal cocaine and methamphetamine as well as oral sildenafil. His erection was not coincident with any erotic stimulus. He denied any similar past episodes, as well as recent or remote perineal trauma. His erectile function had always been good. His past medical history was unremarkable except for frequent alcohol and tobacco use. His family history was unremarkable for sickle cell anemia, hematologic malignancies, or bleeding dyscrasias.

Physical examination was unremarkable for a Caucasian male in moderate distress. Chest, abdominal, and neurologic exams were all within normal limits and there was no evidence of lymphadenopathy. His penis was rigid except for a soft glans penis and was tender to manipulation.

Given the history and physical exam, he was given a preliminary diagnosis of ischemic priapism. We discussed the risk of future erectile dysfunction that might result from tissue changes within the corpora due to the length of time he had had the erection. The patient was given parenteral narcotic analgesics, as well as a penile block with 0.25% Marcaine without epinephrine, and the skin was sterilely prepped. A blood gas was sent: it revealed pH 6.95, PO2 10, PCO2 80. A 19-gauge scalp needle was placed into the left corpus cavernosum and dark blood was slowly evacuated. A diluted solution of phenylephrine, 500 μg, was injected into the corpus cavernosum. After 3 min, aspiration and injection were repeated. With each cycle, there was slight detumescence but no significant change. After over 1 h, we had used 10 mg of phenylephrine and had aspirated 500 cc of blood. The patient's vital signs remained stable.

The patient agreed to a more aggressive intervention. He still had excellent anesthesia from the penile block. He was reprepped and a 10-blade was introduced through the glans penis into the corpus, twisted 90° laterally, and withdrawn. This was repeated on the opposite side. The penis immediately detumesced. The glans incisions were closed using 5-0 chromic gut sutures. The patient was admitted to the hospital for observation.

The following day, the patient had very little pain and his penis was full but not rigid. A duplex ultrasound was performed, revealing peak systolic velocities of 36 cm/s in the cavernous arteries. He was discharged to home.

The following week, he returned to the clinic. He had been pain-free and some of the postprocedural swelling had dissipated. His penis still had a full-appearance but was softer than previously. Duplex ultrasound was repeated, with peak systolic velocities of 25 cm/s in the corporal arteries.

Six months later, the patient had not had any further episodes of priapism. He had moderate erectile dysfunction controlled with oral phosphodiesterase inhibitors.

Iatrogenic Pathology, Undiversion, Contralateral Renal Autotransplantation

J.M. GIL-VERNET

The technological advancements in this last quarter of a century have been a great help to both patients and doctors, but their constant evolution brings home to us that we are still a long way from achieving perfection.

However, these advancements also lead us to the painful reality of illnesses created by the surgeon who is encouraged by this fabulous modern-day technology to perform interventions of great daring, which may result in the development of an iatrogenic pathology if he fails to consider the consequences of his interventions.

We often feel that we will be overtaken by our own work, a perennial topic of humanity, from Prometheus to Disney's Sorcerer's Apprentice.

Extracorporeal lithotripsy and endourological methods have greatly advanced the treatment of urinary lithiasis, but they are subject to their indications and have their limitations. To stretch these limitations, because the surgeon lacks the capacity or sufficient surgical experience, constitutes a risk for the patient and sometimes a violation of medical ethics.

The inherent complications of such methods, their learning curve, together with gynecological iatrogenic damage and laparoscopy, among others, make up an important chapter in the plastic and reconstructive surgery of the urinary apparatus. Urgent complications can be solved by placement of a pigtail, by nephrostomy, by drainage of the substantial subcapsular or perirenal hematomas, by nephrectomy when there is serious rupture, or by selective embolization of the pre- or retropyelic arteries, etc.

It is the late complications that, at any given moment, can create emergency situations, particularly urinary sepsis, renal deterioration, or mental instability.

These complications, represented by extensive stenoses or fistulae of the excretory tract, demand imagination and highly diverse solutions. Complications of the pelvic ureter are better solved by means of the cross-ureterostomy than with the Boari flap or the psoas hitch, as long as the anastomosis is performed by microsurgery using the surgical microscope and the surgeon observes very strict rules as regards its technical execution. The segmental lesions of the pyeloureteral junction or the lumboiliac ureter are treated by lowering the right renal vein or by ipsilateral autotransplantation. Multiple lesions of the ureter are treated by means of contralateral autotransplantation.

Perirenal fibrosis (Page kidney) requires decortication and omentoplasty or peripheral revascularization with a patch of small intestine from which the mucosa has been removed. The substitution of the ureter with the ileum is a recourse that has been practically abandoned since experience with renal transplantation has shown that the best substitute for the ureter is the ureter itself, and this concept applies just as much to autotransplantation as to homotransplantation. In 1963, Hardy performed the first renal autotransplantation to resolve an extensive ureteral lesion.

Case report: A 40-year-old woman with a history of urinary lithiasis mentioned that she had been hospitalized 1 year before because of right lumbar pain and urinary sepsis. She was diagnosed with a stone impacted in the iliac ureter. She had been treated with antibiotics and immediately thereafter with extracorporeal shock wave lithotripsy (ESWL), but without success. Thereafter she had undergone endoscopic procedures resulting in serious complications, probably perforation and tearing of the ureter. In view of the extent of the lesion, urinary derivation of the right cutaneous ureterostomy type was decided on (Fig. 21.4.1a).

Changing the catheter every 15 days caused her pain and the chronic urinary infections caused the patient to have increasingly frequent and increasingly severe depressive crises.

She presented to my hospital department in search of an urgent solution to her problem, which was causing her serious disability in her family and social environment. Her depression was the main reason that brought her to me.

IVU and angiographic exploration were performed. After a lumbotomy incision, the ureter was dissected and removed with its cutaneous stoma, revealing profound anatomical and functional alteration with highly thickened walls due to decubitus from the catheter and the infection. Reconstruction of urinary continuity with a Boari-type flap or a psoas hitch was therefore out of the question since the thickness of the conduit

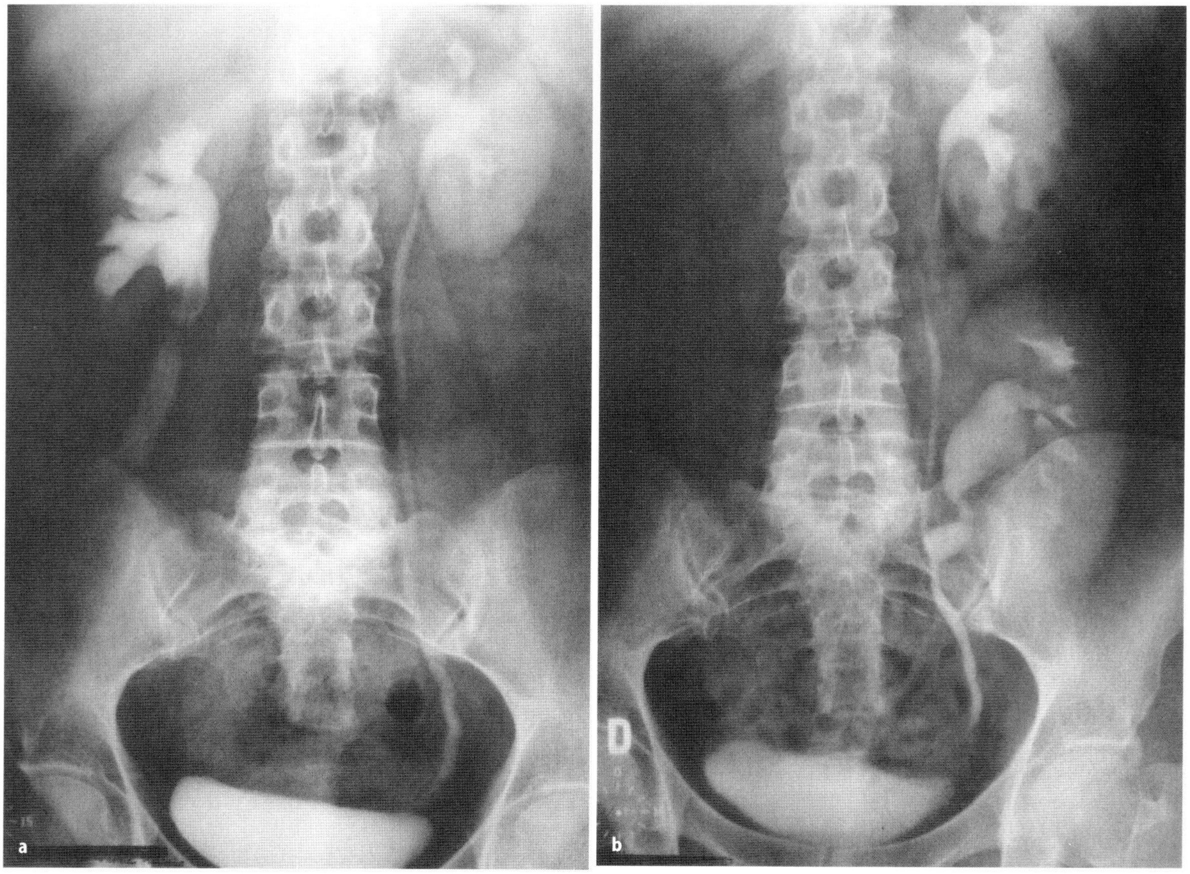

Fig. 21.4.1. a Iatrogenic damage resulting from endoscopic procedures, impaction of a stone in the right ureter. Serious lesion of the iliac and pelvic ureter. Cutaneous ureterostomy. **b** Undiversion. Contralateral renal autotransplantation and ureteroureteral anastomosis after 10 years

would not have permitted a submucosal antireflux tunnel and its precarious vascularization would have led to stenosis. The poor locoregional state of the tissues showed such procedures to be inadvisable.

I decided on temporary nephroureterectomy, contralateral autotransplantation, and ureteroureteral derivation (Higgins operation). After the kidney had been transferred to the bench it was perfused with Collins solution at 4 °C, remaining submerged in a basin in constant hypothermia. There the ureter was resected to within 2 cm of the pyelic junction. The intraoperative biopsy showed that there was no irrecuperable degradation at this level.

Meanwhile, the lumbotomy was closed and the patient repositioned. Via a left paramedial, pararectal, extraperitoneal incision, the primitive iliac vessels to which the graft vessels were to be anastomosed were dissected.

The kidney was autotransplanted into the contralateral iliac fossa. While its vessels were being anastomosed, the organ was maintained in hypothermia by placing it between two compresses containing crushed ice. The clamps were removed and the kidney regained its normal color. Section of the sliding sleeve of the ureter of the contralateral kidney was followed by careful dissection of the iliac segment of the ureter, avoiding injury to Feitel's artery which, as is frequently the case, originated from the trunk of the internal iliac artery, forming one of the most important lower pedicles of the ureter.

Finally, using the surgical microscope at 4-6× and microsurgical instruments with 6-0 sutures, I performed the ureteroureteral anastomosis. The first two sutures of the anastomosis were made in the proximal and distal extremes of the two anastomotic orifices and from there on the suture was continuous, avoiding the eversion of the mucosa. The suture was watertight, because no catheter was to be inserted.

The postoperative phase was without complications. The undiversion restored the woman's urinary apparatus to normal – both anatomically and functionally – and, above all, she regained her mental stability. The psychological benefit of the procedure has been enormous (Fig. 21.4.1b).

The ureteroureteral derivation, or the Higgins operation, has been the subject of much discussion and has even been considered reckless. The risk of this operation lies in the technical imperfection of the anastomosis, but since the introduction of the surgical microscope and the development of microsurgery, and provided that the operation is performed meticulously using microsurgical techniques within a perfectionist mindset, it has every chance of success. Without a doubt, this operation must be included in the framework of microsurgery.

This surgery is subject to certain methodological rules:

- Use magnification systems (surgical microscope or magnifying glasses).
- When exposing the receiving ureter, identify and preserve its vascular and nerve pedicles.
- In the iliac segment of the receiving ureter, make the longitudinal incision on the lateroexternal side.
- At the beginning, make the incision on the receiving ureter small so that it can be enlarged afterward as necessary.
- Never make the perimeter of the longitudinal incision of the receiving ureter larger than the orifice of the other ureter.
- Choose resistant 6-0 suture material, above all with good gliding capacity.
- Make the two knots outside of the ureteral lumen.
- Avoid eversion, tension, and kinking of the mucosa.
- The continuous suture from the two cardinal sutures is preferable since it is tighter, is less likely to cause ischemia, and diminishes the risk of cutting the tissues.
- When making the side-to-end anastomosis, there are two main sutures: the upper-angle suture and the lower-angle suture, which must be placed with rigorous precision and perfection so that they do not diminish the diameters of the proximal and distal orifices of the receiving ureter, since they are decisive for the permeability of the anastomosis. To achieve this, both in the distal extreme as well as in the proximal extreme of the receiving ureter, the suturing must be located at no more than 1 mm from the edge of the incision.
- Remember that the result depends on the quality of the anastomosis.

It will be precisely in this type of small-suture surgery that the surgeon will have to aim to achieve maximum perfection and master the surgical technique, so as to make a work of art out of every operation. These are the surgeon's principal qualities and raison d'être.

Deferred Emergency Surgery of Total Rupture of the Posterior Urethra

J.M. Gil-Vernet

Total rupture of the posterior urethra is a topic that interests all surgeons: general surgeons, orthopedic surgeons, and urological surgeons, because it is a serious trauma occurring with ever greater frequency and presenting with severe pathology since the urinary and sexual dysfunction of the patient, who is generally young, interferes with his family and social environment.

Its treatment is difficult and it is one of the most controversial chapters in urology. This emergency surgery, whether of the urethra, the bladder, or the kidneys, presupposes a change in our usual approach since it requires that urologists involve themselves more in emergency surgery, participate in the progression of the trauma patient, and be familiar with the general lines of management of the multiple-injury patient. The course of the serious lesion of the urethra essentially depends on the immediate initial treatment, and therefore emergency departments receiving accident victims must have an integrated strategy for the treatment of multiple-injury patients in which the emergency rooms and the urology departments collaborate on the basis of a protocol agreed upon with traumatologists and orthopedic surgeons.

This protocol takes into account that, upon arrival in the emergency room, a trauma patient with signs of suspected fractured pelvis and consequently suspected urological injury must, if the x-ray examination of the skeleton confirms the fracture and if the patient's hemodynamic condition permits, be given an IVU, which will permit elimination of a renal lesion or rupture of the bladder, or will reveal the elevated position of the bladder due to a substantial pelvic hematoma, this latter being a *pathognomonic sign* of total rupture of the membranous urethra. An overwhelming desire to urinate, discrete urethrorrhagia, and retention of urine are *signs of suspected* urethral rupture.

As soon as bladder distention starts, the minimal cystotomy will be performed prior to checking the location of the bladder by means of sonography.

Toward the 4th or 5th day, the patient's general orthopedic and urological condition will be evaluated and, if the patient's condition permits, the following explorations will be performed immediately before surgical repair of the urethra: (1) transrectal sonography, (2) cystography in optimal aseptic conditions and antibiotic cover, (3) voiding cystourethrography attempted through the suprapubic catheter, and (4) retrograde urethrography with a small quantity of contrast medium with fluoroscopic monitoring.

These explorations can confirm the clinical diagnosis of complete rupture of the urethra, the degree of diastasis, and the prostatourethral dislocation marked by the elevation of the bladder.

From this point on, the urologist must meet with the traumatologist in order to evaluate all the information compiled concerning the urethral rupture and the pelvic fracture and to decide the time and type of urethral and pelvic repair.

There can be two basic scenarios as regards pelvic fractures: the fracture can be stable or unstable. In the case of unstable fractures of the pelvic girdle, the current attitude of orthopedic surgeons is becoming more and more interventionist, an attitude that is very positive for reducing urethral shift.

Orthopedic surgeons prefer osteosynthetic procedures for stabilizing the pelvic ring, using the external fixator for its reduction and fixation, or internal fixation with nails or plates, which requires open surgery.

If the urethral rupture is accompanied by unstable pelvic fracture, the urologist and the orthopedic surgeon must operate simultaneously, starting with urethral repair and continuing with osteosynthesis.

For the urologist, the fracture of pubic branches or diastasis facilitates urethral repair extraordinarily.

In cases of stable fracture of the pelvis, the orthopedic surgeon will advise rest, and will not intervene; it will therefore be the urologist who must decide what treatment to pursue.

This is where an old controversy emerges. When to operate? Must one operate immediately or later?

There are two possible therapeutic attitudes: one is to perform end-to-end anastomosis of the urethral edges during deferred emergency surgery between the 4th and the 8th day, and the other is to leave the drainage of the cystostomy for 3–6 months and then treat the existing complex stricture. These are two different concepts. The objective of the first is to repair the acute lesion in order to avoid stenosis, while the second attempts to provoke stenosis.

Operating at 3–6 months is a strategy whose objective is to avoid medicolegal problems as regards impotence.

Apart from great loss of time for the patient, a long period of incapacity for work, expense, and prolonged hospitalization, intervention between 3 and 6 months makes the relatively simple treatment of the injury tract – end-to-end anastomosis – the complicated treatment – posttraumatic stenosis.

The repair of these stenoses at 3–6 months is always a difficult operation, since the membranous urethra and the external striated sphincter are encased and infiltrated by hard scar tissue, and in these conditions, irrespective of the approach route and the type of reconstruction that one uses, it is always a highly aggressive operation, since one has to extirpate the scar tissue enclosing the urethra and its sphincter and, even if the reconstruction of urinary continuity is successful, the loss of the voluntary urinary control mechanism of stress incontinence due to cervicourethral insufficiency and alterations in ejaculation due to absence of the energetic contractions of the external sphincter in orgasm. It jeopardizes the patient's future since, with increasing age, hyperplasia or cancer of the prostate may develop, and surgery will leave the patient completely incontinent.

The other position is that of reestablishing urinary continuity in deferred emergency treatment within the 1st week after the accident, before pelvic fibrosis rigidifies the anatomical structures.

There are two treatment methods for this: one limits itself to bringing the extremes of the urethral rupture closer together, the other involves suturing the urethral extremes edge to edge.

The first involves the urethral splint, which aligns the urethra by means of a permanent catheter placed with open surgery or endoscopy.

Others attempt to reduce the separation between the edges by placing a Foley catheter and with permanent traction, bringing the prostate closer to the urogenital diaphragm, tying the prostatic apex with transfixion sutures. These methods result in a very high percentage of stenosis.

In the rare case of partial ruptures with little shift, these procedures can achieve acceptable results, but not in the case of total ruptures where the shift does not permit the coalescence of the urethral segments.

Other procedures such as urethrorrhaphy suture the edges of the urethral extremes without tension. This is the ideal treatment. Its objective is to ensure healing all at once and to avoid stenosis. It is the preferred method since the results are better both from the urinary and sexual point of view as well as with respect to the patient's future.

The main problem in urethrorrhaphy is finding the edges of the rupture, identifying them, and exposing them in order to achieve a good anastomosis without tension.

There are three approach routes for this: the perineal, the transpubic or transsymphysial, and the retropubic route.

The perineal route is often contraindicated in the case of fractures of the ischiopubic rami, since the positioning of the patient in the peritoneotomy position is not advisable. This route demands dissection of the bulbar urethra and ligation of the bulbar arteries, which supply most of the vascularization of the urethra; longitudinal section of the striated sphincter is obligatory. The hematic infiltration makes identification of neurovascular structures located in the diaphragm impossible.

The transpubic route with resection of the symphysis is highly aggressive, jeopardizes the stability of the pelvic girdle, and must therefore be avoided.

Pubic symphysiotomy using the cold knife technique is an excellent approach route, but it obliges the surgeon to perform the longitudinal incision of the anterior side of the striated sphincter in its middle line in order to look for the distal extreme of the sectioned urethra and to perform the urethrorrhaphy. The surgical aggression causes injury to the walls, vessels, and nerves of the striated sphincter and the other structures contained in the urogenital diaphragm, and therefore the surgical iatrogenic damage is similar to that of late repair of the stenosis.

The retropubic route is less aggressive. It does not require changing the position of the patient, and it permits simultaneous treatment of the osseous and urinary lesions as well as evacuation of the hematoma. The disadvantage is the narrowness and depth of the surgical field, which makes anatomical repair difficult since the distal extreme of the urethra is retracted below the upper leaf of the middle perineal aponeurosis, which becomes difficult to find and clearly expose for good anastomosis between the two urethral ends. Therefore, this route was abandoned in favor of the transsymphysial and perineal route.

This was the situation until 1988, when we described the urogenital diaphragm-raising maneuver, which marked a new surgical focus of the problem, making it less aggressive, easier, and providing better results by facilitating suturing of the edges, which improved the prognosis of this serious trauma while preserving the sphincter mechanism. In traumatic ruptures of the posterior urethra, the central perineal musculature and the membranous urethra have greater mobility due to the tearing of the middle perineal aponeurosis, thus facilitating the maneuver.

Raising the urogenital diaphragm pulls the distal membranous urethra situated in a deep plane toward

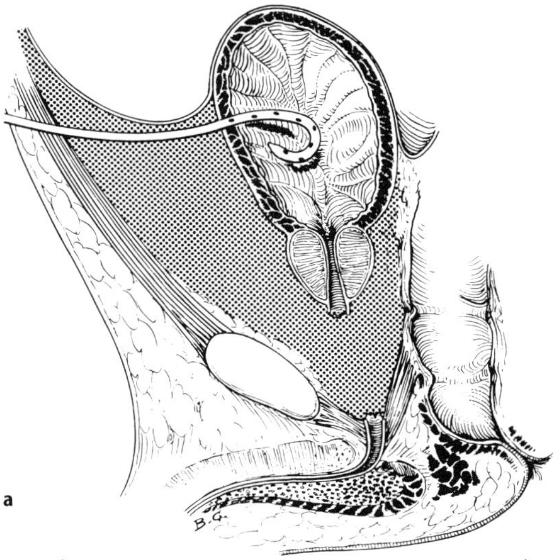

a

the surgeon, achieving greater superficial exposure, making an anastomosis of a high technical quality and thus preserving the vascularization of the urethra without the risk of injuring the external sphincter, thus explaining the excellent anatomical and functional results in reestablishing the urinary continuity (Figs. 21.5.1–21.5.3).

Case Report: A 44-year-old man was brought to the emergency room following a traffic accident presenting signs of a pelvic fracture that was confirmed by x-ray as a fracture of the left ischiopubic rami. The patient presented signs of hypovolemic shock, thus impeding the IVU, an overwhelming desire to urinate, and discrete urethrorrhagia. Fortunately, no urethral catheterization was attempted. Bladder distention appeared and sonography revealed major pelvic hematoma, so minimum cystostomy was performed. On rectal palpation,

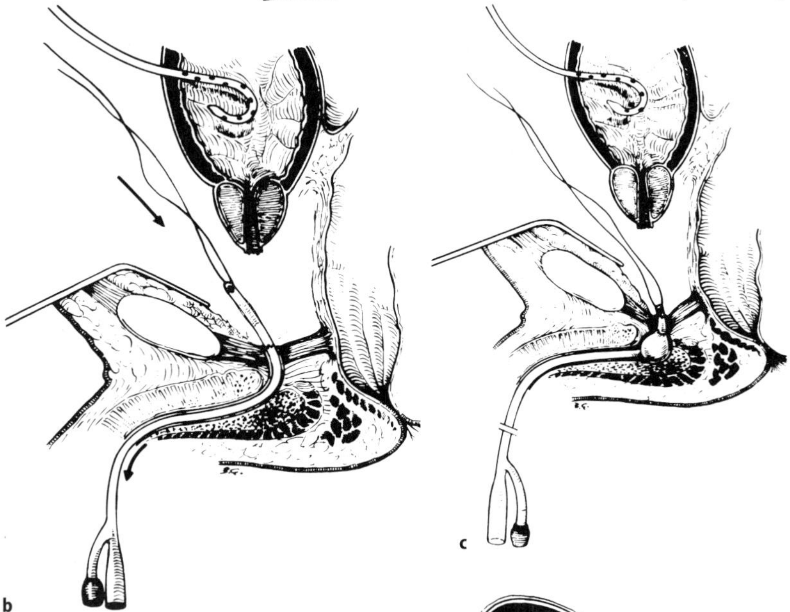

b c

Fig. 21.5.1. **a** Pelvic hematoma elevating the prostate and bladder. Retracted distal urethral edge. **b** Foley catheter in the pelvic cavity, thread knotted at its extreme. **c** Foley balloon inflated with 4.5 cc situated in the bulbar urethra

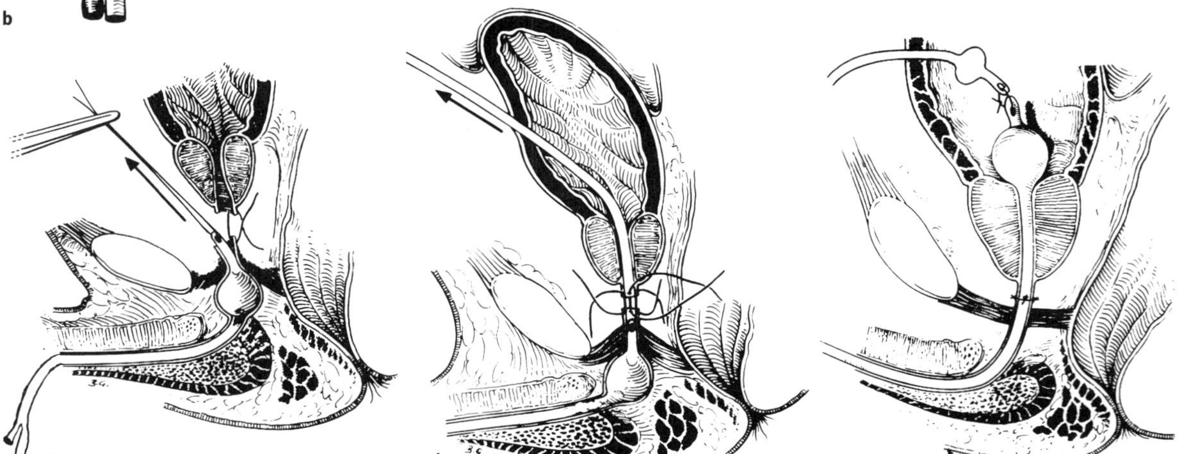

a b c

Fig. 21.5.2. **a** Upward traction of the catheter raising the urogenital diaphragm, raising of the distal end of the urethra. **b, c** Good exposure of the edges, easy placement of the four to five 5-0 Dexon sutures. End-to-end anastomosis without tension

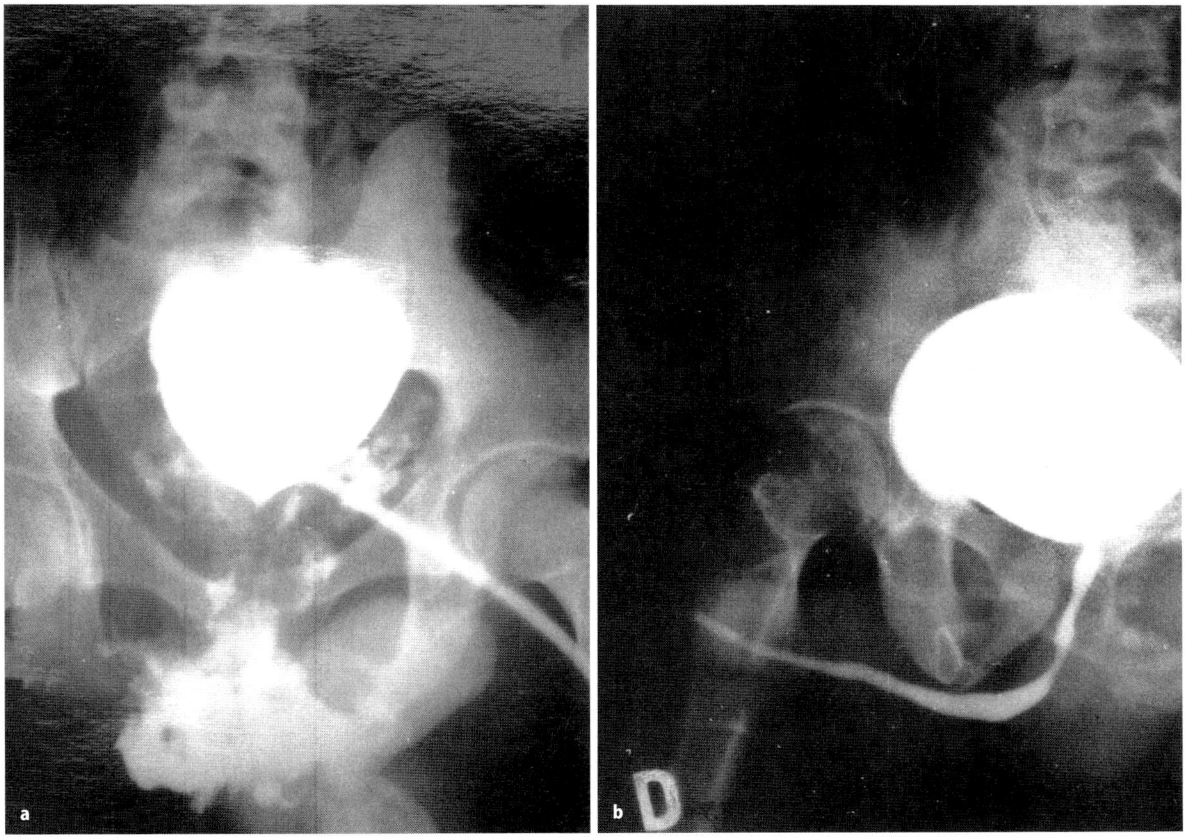

Fig. 21.5.3. a Cystography through a suprapubic catheter, prostatourethral dislocation, marked by elevation of the bladder. Simultaneous retrograde urethrography, pelviperineal extravasation of contrast medium. **b** Voiding cystourethrography 1 year after surgery. No stenosis, good continence. Excellent result

the prostate was not palpable, only bulging of the anterior surface of the rectum and pain at the level of the membranous urethra. On the 4th day, the patient was evaluated with the orthopedic surgeon who confirmed that the pelvic ring was stable and only required bed rest. The urologist took charge of the case and intervened on the 5th day after the accident. Retrograde urethrography and cystography were performed in the same operation. A puboumbilical incision and symphysiotomy using the cold knife method achieved a separation of 4-5 cm between the pubes. The Retzius cavity and iliac fossas contained large clots, which were extracted from the same; thereafter careful hemostasis was achieved. A puboprostatic ligament and one of the endopelvic fascias of the prostate were torn, the other fascia and the puboprostatic ligament, which were undamaged, were cut, achieving mobilization of the prostate and thus facilitating the realignment of the urethra.

The prostatic apex maintained the proximal extreme of the membranous urethra some 3–4 mm in length. The ischemic and torn edges were resected.

The large hematic infiltration of the pelvic tissues made it impossible to identify the retracted urethral edge at the bottom of the pelvic excavation. In these conditions, it was considered impossible to complete the urethrorrhaphy. However, it occurred to me to catheterize the urethra with a 14-F Foley catheter, and when it emerged in the pelvic excavation, I tied a thread to its end, pulling it back until it was situated in the bulbar urethra. I inflated the balloon with 5 cc, pulled the thread in the cephalic direction, and when raising the urogenital diaphragm, which, as usual, was torn, the urethral edge appeared, allowing an easy and good end-to-end anastomosis, yielding a perfect anatomical and functional result.

In cases with narrow and deep pelvises or in obese patients, it is preferable to perform symphysiotomy using the cold knife method and to finalize the operation reestablishing the pubic symphysis with two or three sutures.

The total rupture of the posterior urethra is the principal indication for this maneuver, which has shown itself to be successful in the treatment of this serious accident and in radical prostatectomy and intestinal bladder replacement.

Surgery of Complicated Horseshoe Kidney

J.M. GIL-VERNET

The horseshoe kidney must be regarded as a clinical entity because of the importance of its pathology and its incidence (1/200 pyelograms), even though it has no pathognomonic signs or symptoms.

The renal anomalies, be they of rotation, position, but above all fusion, are very frequently associated with urinary anomalies of the upper excretory tract and are the cause of hydronephrosis, pyelonephritis, and lithiasis resulting from urinary obstruction.

The multiple etiopathogenetic factors responsible are high and ventral position of the pelvis, high insertion and angulation of the pyeloureteral junction, and the ureter riding above the isthmus. But the most important pathologies are the structural lesions of the proximal ureter such as segmental aplasia or hypoplasia of the muscular stratum, or orientational anomaly of its muscular fibers. In a histological study conducted with W. Gregoir, the most frequent type of structural alteration observed was collagenous hypertrophy, which is the aspect frequently encountered in congenital hydronephrosis where the obstacle is essentially functional, constituted by achalasia, and is not a true stenosis, which in the case of the horseshoe kidney (Fig. 21.6.1) even reaches 3–5 cm below the pyeloureteral junction.

The conventional techniques for the treatment of these types of hydronephrosis in horseshoe kidney are not suitable for correcting this anomaly since they are not capable of eliminating the multiple etiopathogenetic factors responsible for this complication, thus explaining the poor results.

However, the horseshoe kidney has a pathology of its own, resulting from its topographic characteristics, in which the pain caused by the pressure exerted by the prevertebral isthmus on the solar plexus and its visceral rami, on the aorta and the lymphatic circulation, is the dominant clinical element. It is the nonpathological, but painful, horseshoe kidney, resulting in the division of the symphysis followed by the displacement of each kidney toward the corresponding lumbar fossa and nephropexy by suturing the leaves of the renal capsule to the adventitia of the lateral wall of the aorta, thus liberating all these structures from the compression caused by the isthmus.

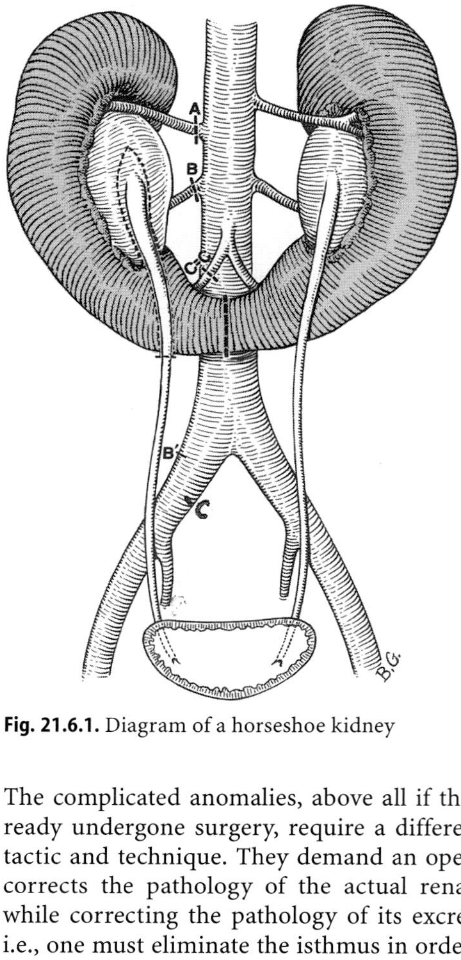

Fig. 21.6.1. Diagram of a horseshoe kidney

The complicated anomalies, above all if they have already undergone surgery, require a different surgical tactic and technique. They demand an operation that corrects the pathology of the actual renal anomaly while correcting the pathology of its excretory tract, i.e., one must eliminate the isthmus in order to relieve the compression on nerves and vascular structures, resect the entire dysplastic segment of the ureter, giving the kidney a normal anatomical orientation so that its ventral pelvis remains in the posterior or dorsal position, achieving downward drainage of the urine and preserving all of the renal parenchyma.

This is achieved by means of uni- or bilateral autotransplantation and bench surgery. This surgery is not particularly complicated, but it solves the problem.

Case Report: A 10-year-old boy, with no relevant family history and presenting at the age of 7 with undefined abdominal pain with gastrointestinal upsets. He underwent appendectomy without benefit. After that, he presented with episodes of pain in the upper abdomen, particularly in the periumbilical region, radiating toward the bilateral lumbar region. Analysis revealed slowly progressive albuminuria. The diagnosis of bilateral hydronephrosis was established by sonography, but it was the IVP that defined the existence of a horseshoe kidney complicated by substantial dilation of the pelvis, infundibula, and renal calyces on both sides. With this diagnosis, he was admitted at the age of 9 to another hospital department where a left nephrostomy was performed. On the 30th day, a ureteropyeloplasty of the left kidney was performed.

In 1981, he was admitted to my urology department with painful symptoms, urinary infection, and recurrence of the obstruction of the half of the kidney that had undergone surgery. It is well known that the renal lesion associated with a malformation is all the more serious the smaller the child is, requiring a rapid solution.

In the surgical sessions of the 8th International Course of Urology in Barcelona in 1981, I performed ex situ horseshoe kidney surgery in a child with autotransplantation of the right kidney (Fig. 21.6.2).

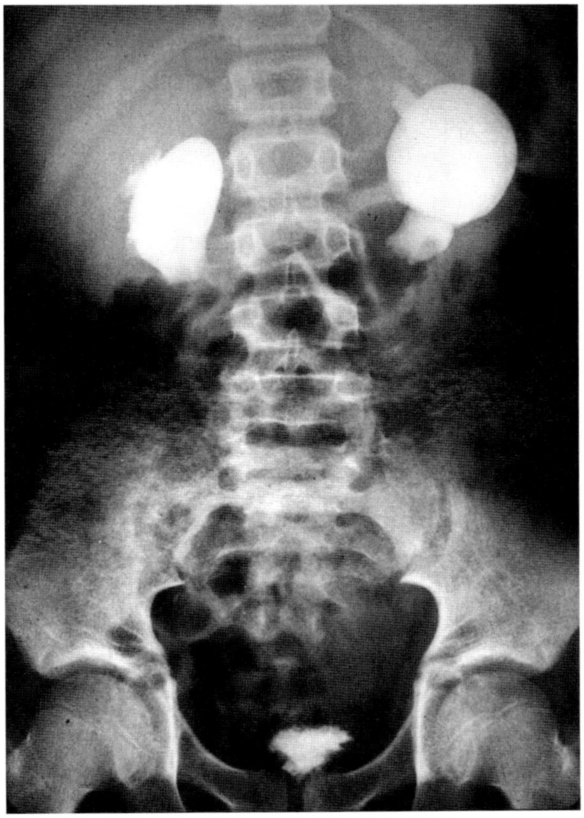

Fig. 21.6.2. IVP of a complicated horseshoe kidney. Bilateral congenital hydronephrosis

Among other preliminary explorations, the most important is arteriography to clarify the vascular map of the horseshoe kidney; it is particularly useful to visualize the isthmic artery, which comes out of the anterior side of the aorta and divides into two branches (Figs. 21.6.3, 21.6.4), each of which irrigates the lower third of each half of the kidney. It is very important to know their length and caliber, since when half of the kidney is extracted, the branch of the isthmic bifurcation that corresponds to it should not be ligated. Only a small bulldog-type clamp is placed because when the kidney is transplanted it will be inverted so that its inferior pole will be at the cephalic position to facilitate the end-to-end anastomosis of the edges of the branch of the isthmic artery, because its small caliber requires that the surgical microscope or magnifying glasses be used.

The kidney was extracted through a paramedial, pararectal, extraperitoneal incision, the ureter having been cut below the parenchymatous edge, and placed in a vessel where the three arteries were cannulated and simultaneously perfused with Collins 3 solution at 4 °C. The organ remained constantly immersed in controlled hypothermia and we proceeded to prepare the renal vessels. Two veins were anastomosed to one another, the other very small one was ligated (sometimes it is also possible to join two arteries), all using microsurgical

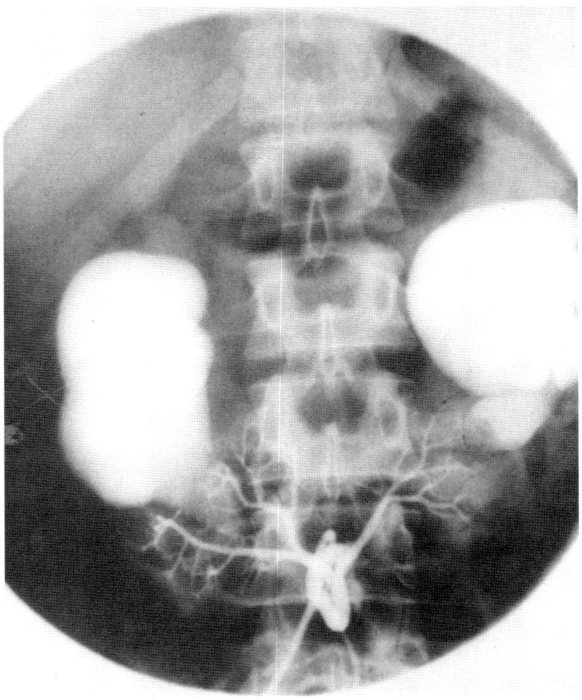

Fig. 21.6.3. Selective arteriography of the isthmic artery irrigating the lower third of each kidney

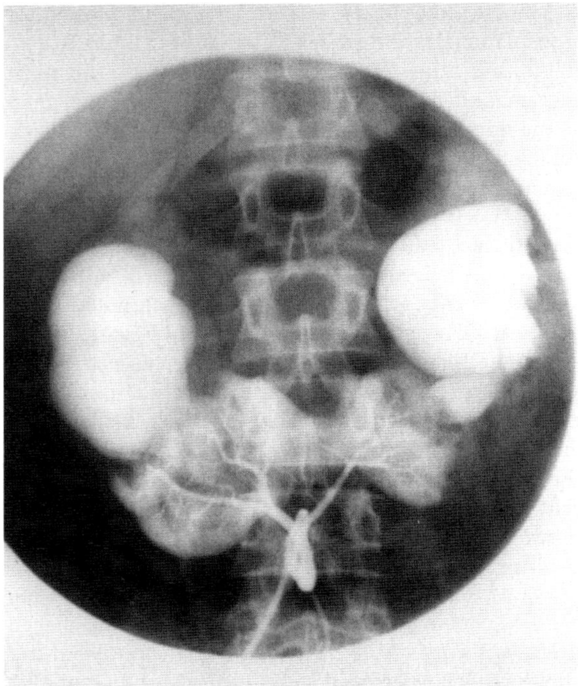

Fig. 21.6.4. The trunk and the two dividing branches of the isthmic artery in the inverted renal autotransplantation must be conserved

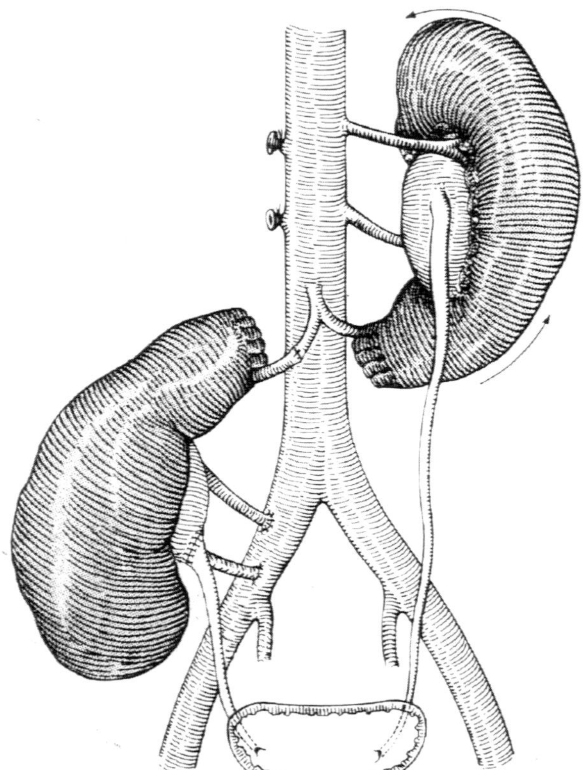

Fig. 21.6.5. Diagram of the transplanted kidney half

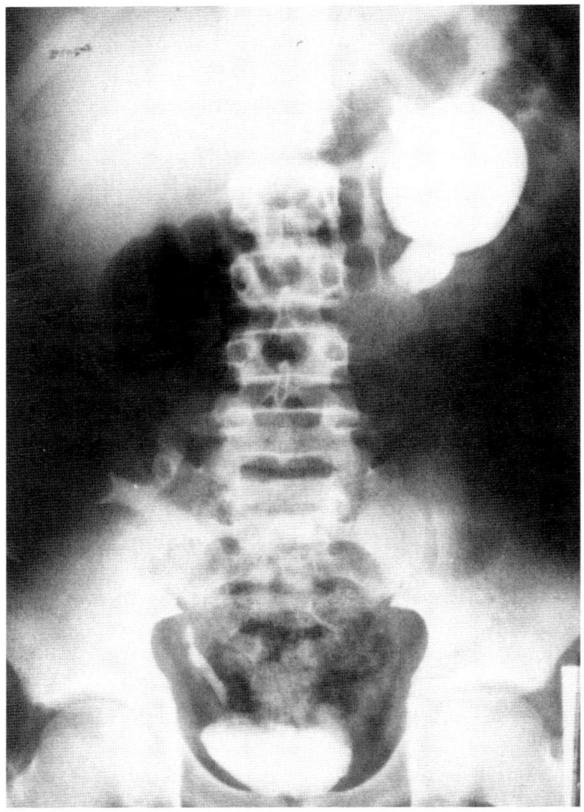

Fig. 21.6.6. IVP of the right kidney after inverted renal autotransplantation into the iliac fossa

techniques. The edge of the branch of the isthmic artery was exposed, the ureter and the pyeloureteral junction resected, the pyelic sac reduced, and a place for implantation of the ureter prepared. After completion of the bench surgery, the kidney was transferred to the patient's iliac fossa where it was placed in an inverted position, that is to say, the superior pole was placed in the inferior location, thus facilitating the vascular anastomoses (Fig. 21.6.5). The iliac ureter was anastomosed to the inferior renal pelvis (Fig. 21.6.6, 21.6.7). During the course of the transplantation and in order to prevent the organ from warming up again during the long period of ischemia, the kidney was kept in hypothermia between two cushions of cold compresses. This method of cooling does not obstruct the surgeon, it protects the kidney effectively, and the surgeon has sufficient time to make the multiple vascular anastomoses without having to hurry, using the best technique. The kidney recovered its function immediately and no postoperative problems occurred.

Two months later, I performed the autotransplantation of the left kidney (Fig. 21.6.7) following the same surgical strategy. Figure 21.6.8 shows the IVP 25 years after the result.

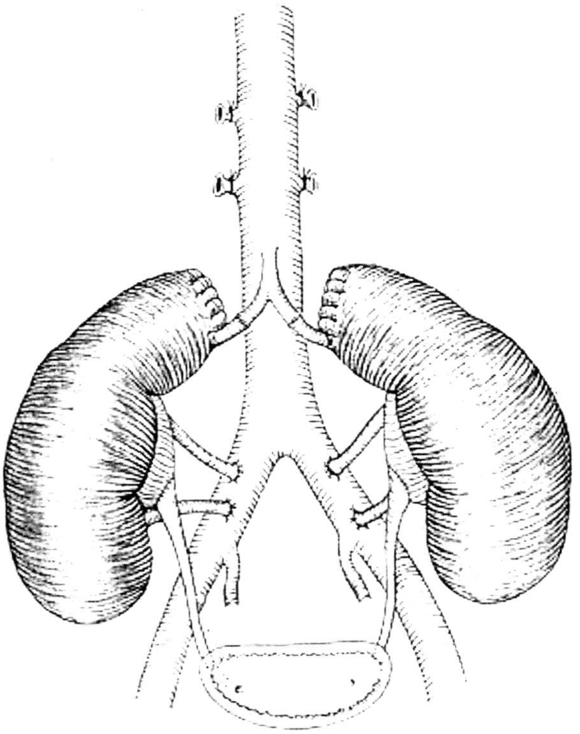

Fig. 21.6.7. Diagram of the transplant of the inverted horseshoe kidney

It is the only surgical technique that can correct this renal anomaly and the associated lesions.

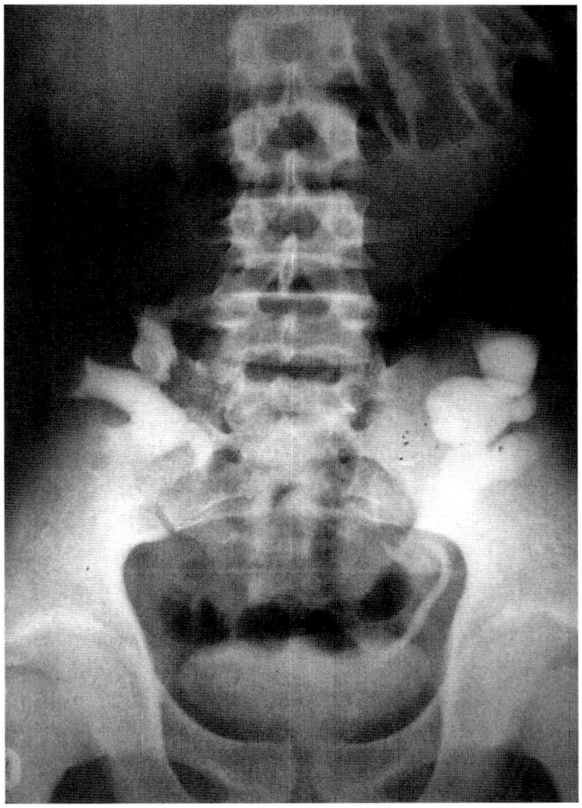

Fig. 21.6.8. IVP 25 years after inverted renal autotransplantation of the horseshoe kidney. Both kidneys have normal function, and the pain, infection, and proteinuria have disappeared.

Cold Fire

Ch.F. Heyns

The word for gangrene in my home language, Afrikaans, is *kouevuur*, literally "cold fire": to the patient a gangrenous limb "burns like fire," yet it feels cold. Unlike ordinary fire, which reveals itself by light, heat, and smoke, "cold fire" is an insidious threat, which can be more dangerous than searing flames.

One

When I was a houseman (intern) doing medicine, I worked with a registrar (resident) who had a rather high opinion of his own medical knowledge and an equal disdain for the ignorance displayed by "stupid" surgeons who just "cut everything" and then referred their patients to medicine because they lacked the clinical acumen to diagnose or treat simple cardiac failure. The registrar always carried a hugely impressive stethoscope around his neck, and never failed to meticulously auscultate the chest of every patient we encountered on ward rounds (which consequently lasted all day).

One day a known diabetic patient was admitted in a state of confusion. As usual, innumerable blood tests and special investigations were requested, and the registrar wrote his usual meticulous orders for insulin to be given according to a glucose sliding scale. Every morning on the ward round, he would carefully examine the patient's chest with his stethoscope, pore endlessly over the results of blood tests, ECGs, and x-rays, and berate the nursing staff for not adhering to his insulin sliding scale.

This continued for 2 or 3 days, but the patient's condition did not improve and the blood glucose remained out of control. Then one morning, the ward sister said "Look at this, doctor" and pulled up the bed sheets, showing us the extensive gangrene of the patient's feet. I would have liked to conclude this anecdote by saying that it had made the registrar a little more tolerant toward "stupid" surgeons, but sadly this did not occur.

Two

About 30 years ago, I was involved in the following drama that occurred at a referral hospital about 1,500 km from the medical school where I had graduated. Although I prefer not to reveal which role I personally played during the drama, it will be clear that there were no heroes.

The patient, a 50-year-old female with diabetes mellitus on oral medication, was admitted to the surgery ward late on a Friday night with a referral letter simply stating "Ischio-rectal abscess, please see and treat." The patient was somewhat confused and vaguely complained of pain "down below."

The houseman did not really want to examine the obese and rather malodorous patient, so he simply did his job, clerking (filling in forms) and sending blood samples away. However, because the patient continued moaning as if in severe pain, he telephoned his immediate superior, the medical officer (MO) on call.

The MO, in his second posthouseman year, had only worked in surgery for a few months and his clinical experience was limited. Despite being on call, he had gone to a party, had drunk too much, and got to bed very late. At 3 a.m. the phone rang and he was told about the patient. He advised giving her an opiate i.m. and said he would come to see her in the morning. Unfortunately, he overslept and did not see the patient before the ward round with the consultant surgeon at 8 o'clock.

The surgeon was a very experienced and energetic man, but not very communicative. The moment he saw the patient, he ordered that she be taken to the operating room immediately, but did not bother to explain why. The houseman reported that the laboratory results showed not only a very high glucose level, but also an elevated urea and creatinine, low sodium and high potassium. The irate surgeon only repeated his command that the patient should be taken to the operating room immediately.

The anesthesiologist was very experienced and proud of his reputation for being quick, but his knowledge was rather outdated. He set up a peripheral line and put the patient "under" with a bolus of pentothal and mask anesthesia on spontaneous breathing of nitrous oxide and halothane, thinking that it would merely be an incision and drainage of an ischiorectal abscess.

Only when the massively obese patient was put into lithotomy did the area of perineal gangrene become apparent. The taciturn surgeon, a very slick operator, excised the gangrenous tissues in a flash and, to the horror of his assistants, rapidly extended the debridement until the patient's whole left buttock was denuded. The odor was intolerable, bleeding was profuse, the assistants struggled to keep up with the surgeon's flying hands, the anesthesiologist eventually discovered that the blood pressure was zero, and then it turned out that no crossmatch had been ordered.

While the houseman rushed off to get blood, the surgeon proceeded with his radical debridement, the anesthesiologist strapped the mask to the patient's face and started pumping in i.v. fluids. Halfway through the debridement, the patient had a cardiac arrest and, despite vigorous CPR, she died on the table.

The most powerful diagnostic instrument in all of medicine is the retrospectoscope. Unfortunately it can only be used when it is too late to be of real use to the patient. It has been said that doctors bury their mistakes. However, the truth is that most of our mistakes live on in memory to haunt us for the rest of our lives.

Three

A 21-year-old man had undergone ritual circumcision and was brought to hospital about 1 week later with gangrene of his entire penis (Fig. 21.7.1). The patient also had bruises and abrasions on his arms and legs, consistent with being beaten and tied up, but refused to provide any information about his injuries.

Among certain African tribes, circumcision has for centuries formed part of an initiation ceremony led by elders, lasting several days and constituting an essential rite of passage from boyhood to manhood. Traditionally, circumcision was performed in early puberty, but nowadays it is often performed on adults who are already sexually active and who may, in some cases, be unwilling to undergo the procedure. Those who develop complications are sometimes prohibited from seeking medical help, which was probably the case in our patient.

Traditionally, hemostasis was obtained using non-compressive dressings made from the leaves of certain plants, possibly with antiseptic properties, but these are not available in urban areas, so materials such as paper or even plastic are sometimes used. The most dangerous is when a string in the form of a small noose is placed around the base of the penis to control bleeding. Ischemia and infection act synergistically to form a deadly combination. Circumcision subjects are not allowed to eat or drink during the period of initiation, therefore septicemia is usually compounded with dehydration.

The patient in question was admitted to hospital on a weekend, given intravenous fluids and antibiotics, but not taken to the operating room immediately, because the registrar thought that the gangrene had demarcated and that the penis would slough spontaneously. When the patient was first seen by the urologist on Monday, he appeared generally well and pain-free, and did not have an elevated temperature. However, the tell-tale sign was that he had slight tachypnea and flaring nostrils, indicating early respiratory distress.

He was taken to the intensive care unit for intubation and aggressive resuscitation, then to the operating room for urgent penectomy (Fig. 21.7.2). However, he developed septicemia and multiorgan failure and, despite full ICU support, died a few days later.

Clinical experience cannot be learned from books, it must be learned in the school of life. But without books to impart the knowledge distilled from clinical experience, we would be forever condemned to learn only from our own mistakes – at our patients' expense .

The simple lesson to be learned from these anecdotes is clear: gangrene may be an insidious *kouevuur* (cold fire), but it can consume the patient's life just as rapidly as open flames.

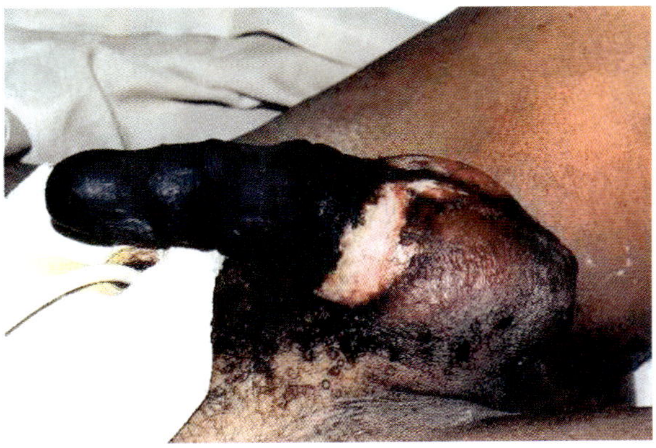

Fig. 21.7.1. Gangrene of the penile shaft as a complication of ritual circumcision

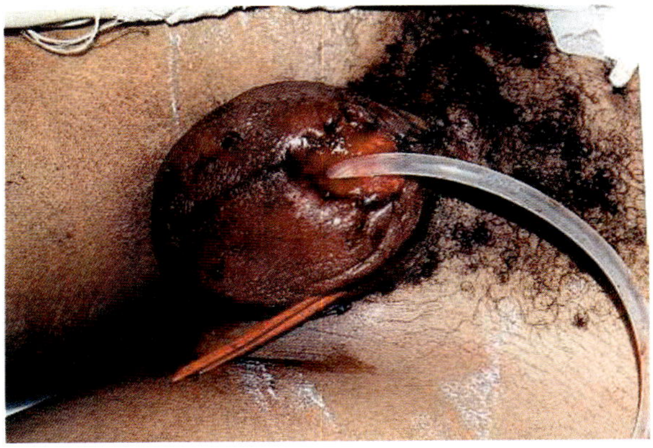

Fig. 21.7.2. Amputation of the penile shaft for gangrene after ritual circumcision

Lost in the Kidney

M. Hohenfellner

The general surgeons once presented a patient to us who had had a hemicolectomy for large bowel cancer more than 1 year before. The patient's immediate problem was that he had developed secondary bilateral renal metastases.

The therapeutic strategy was to remove the metastases in a single surgical session to allow adjuvant chemotherapy as soon as possible. A median laparotomy was performed. First the right kidney was exposed. However, the metastases seen clearly in the MRI could not be located, neither visually nor by palpation. So the next step was to employ intraoperative ultrasound, but even this tool and a significant number of investigators, including urologists and radiologists, could not clarify the whereabouts of the metastasis.

It was clear that any consideration to nephrectomize the patient simply for not being able to find the tumor was unacceptable. As a last attempt, I incised the fibrous capsule and, very carefully, stripped the kidney nearly completely of its capsule, leaving it just attached at the lower pole. After removing the capsule, repeated palpation immediately identified the exact location of the metastasis, which subsequently was easily removed with free margins. Surgical hemostasis included reposition of the kidney capsule.

With this experience behind us, the removal of the contralateral metastasis was a straightforward procedure. The postoperative course was uneventful.

Summary

1. The fibrous capsule of the kidney is a strong filter for any haptic sensations. Its removal allows even the smallest nodules to be detected by careful palpation.
2. A relaxed overview in a complex situation can facilitate simple and effective solutions by preserving the creativity of the surgeon in charge.

A Rare Accident

R. Hohenfellner

Background

In 1964, I moved from Vienna to Homburg/Saar to take an Associate Professor position in one of the most recognized departments of urology headed by Prof. C.E. Alken. Still on duty at 4 p.m., I received a call from the chief of the surgical department to join him immediately in the emergency room.

History

At 3 p.m. a 60-year-old gynecologist had a rather exceptional accident in his office in a small town nearby. When he tried to take a seat on his swivel chair in front of his patient, the chair turned over and the metal thread went through his anus high up into his rectum. The emergency team arrived immediately and transferred him, with the iron thread still in place, to the surgical department of the university hospital.

The Situation at Arrival

The patient was stable and fully conscious and was placed in a Trendelenburg position on the operating table; the anesthesiologist started with general anesthesia.

Diagnosis and Therapy

The chief of the surgical department accompanied by his senior resident looked at me:

"What is your diagnosis, Mr. Hohenfellner?"

It was a critical question. He was an experienced abdominal surgeon, had served many years during the Second World War in different army hospitals, and had certainly encountered similar stab wound injuries before. He had already placed the patient on the operating table, making it impossible to take an x-ray.

With the iron post still in his rectum, moving him was highly risky.

"Well," I said, "the patient is stable, the emergency lab will arrive soon, the length of the post is unknown, an x-ray cannot be taken, but I want to insert a Foley, Sir."

I inserted an 18-French Foley with no difficulty and 150 ml of hemorrhagic urine passed.

"What does it tell you?"

"The thread went through the rectum and there is some sort of a bladder injury, maybe a penetrating one, but it is proximal of the prostate, Sir."

"So what will be the first step?"

Again it was a difficult question for a urologist with almost no experience in rectal and bladder stab wound injuries. However, from my residency in general surgery I remembered a case of severe bleeding during a so-called synchronous rectum resection from the perineal wound performed by two teams. A Mikulicz tampon solved the problem in the end. So, I thought, removing the post may cause severe bleeding.

"The first step, Sir, should be a median laparotomy from the sternum down to the symphysis with inspection of the abdomen. At that time, the anesthesiologist will have enough blood transfusion supplies to keep him stable, when a second team removes the post from below."

"Let's scrub!"

The Operation

He opened the abdomen and there was not much blood inside. The top of the post had perforated the rectum and the bladder above the trigone and then went out through the bladder dome in the rectus muscle. The second team was ready and removed the post. The severe bleeding was immediately stopped by about 2 m of the transrectally inserted Mikulicz tampon.

"It is your turn," he said and moved to the other side of the table. I opened the back side of the bladder from the dome down to the perforation as in a vesicovaginal fistula. Fortunately, the orifices could be identified within the hemorrhagic edematous bladder mucosa and intubated with ureter catheters. He helped me close the rectal wound with two layers of interrupted catgut and silk sutures. I took a peritoneal graft from the left abdominal wall and fixed it between the rectum and the bladder to secure the overlying suture lines from the rectum and the bladder. Then three layers of a running mucosa, interrupted detrusor suture line, and an extra row of peritoneal sutures closed the bladder. A cystostomy tube was inserted.

"Why this?" he asked.

"Well, Sir, the running mucosa suture line is the hemostatic one. Postoperatively, if the small bowel and the peritoneal cavity become distended the peritoneum overlying the bladder will also distend and the bladder suture line will probably be disrupted if it was closed by a single-layer suture line."

"Have you seen this before?"

"Yes, Sir, in a young lady with a bladder rupture following a car accident. On day 5, the abdomen distended and suture insufficiency ensued, and she had to be operated again."

"And what is the next step?"

"Well, Sir, I have not much experience but a right-side colostomy may protect the rectal suture line."

Outcome

He performed the colostomy and the postoperative course was uneventful. The Mikulicz tampon was removed with the patient under general anesthesia on the 5th day and the bladder catheter 10 days later.

The voiding cystourethrogram was normal, the cystostomy was removed and the patient went home for 3 months, when finally the colostomy was closed.

Remarks

Today a CT would probably be the first diagnostic step but with the same therapeutic strategy.

Still today the gynecologist's present is on my desk: a small silver dish with the engraving "Thank you".

But one question remains. How does one cross the ocean with no navigational equipment? With lots of luck.

Appendectomy

R. Hohenfellner

Introduction

Homburg/Saar 1965. I received the emergency call on Saturday, 11 p.m. during a birthday party and went in the surgical department's operating room. The senior resident said, "Thank you for coming and please have a look inside."

I climbed on a step behind him.

History and Situation

"This is an 8-year-old girl, admitted by her mother, a pediatrician, 2 hours ago with the symptoms of acute appendicitis. So we performed a standard suprainguinal incision and found a normal appendix. However, behind the appendix in the retroperitoneum – here you can see it – there is a strange structure, maybe a tumor, but we aren't sure what it is. Since it's located in the retroperitoneum, it may be arising from the urogenital system, which is why I called you."

Diagnosis

The cylinder-like bulging structure, 2–3 cm in size, was located behind the cecum reaching down into the pelvis and I had absolutely no idea what it could be. I washed my hands longer than necessary.

The skin incision along the Langer line was rather short and the exposure was limited. By palpation I had the impression of elasticity, possibly with fluid inside.

In the early 1960s, pediatric urology was still a young discipline. The diagnosis concerning the upper tract was made exclusively based on an IVP. Quite often reflux studies performed preoperatively were compared with postoperative IVPs to demonstrate the excellent results in grade 4 antireflux surgery. The same was true for so-called tailoring in obstructive megaureters. Extensive tailoring of the upper and lower ureter was done in a single session with still unknown late results.

"Maybe it is a megaureter," I murmured. "Have you done a urine analysis?"

"I don't know if this was done. She was admitted by her mother with an acute abdomen, high temperature, and 14,000 white cells, a clear indication to operate on her immediately."

Treatment

"So let's do a puncture." With a rather thin needle, I punctured the structure and aspirated roughly 80 ml of putrid fluid, obviously infected urine. The structure collapsed and a second normal ureter could be identified lying close to the wall of the dilated one.

"It's a double system," I said, "and one is obstructed and infected. The problem is we don't know if the dilated ureter is only obstructive and drains the better part of the kidney or if it is dilated and infected because it is obstructed and refluxing. Furthermore, we have no information on the contralateral side. Is there a healthy kidney or almost none at all?"

"So you have to reimplant the obstructed and dilated orifice, and also the refluxing one in the bladder."

"But she has a severe infection!"

"So what would you like to do?"

"First of all, the nurse can insert a bladder catheter because it's easier to prepare the ureter if the bladder is empty."

I started to separate the normal ureter from the dilated one, anxious not to disturb the common blood supply. By chance I found a cleavage plane between the dense fibrous tissue with the longitudinally running vessels and the adventitia of the normal ureter. It took a long time, but finally the megaureter was separated down to the bladder, so I clamped and dissected it. I left the distal stump open due to the risk of ureteral stump empyema. It became easier to prepare in the proximal direction and we inserted a hook. The normal ureter showed good peristalsis, and when the separation was finished the dilated megaureter was long enough to perform a ureterocutaneostomy.

Postoperative Course

The patient's temperature dropped immediately and the postoperative course was uneventful. There was only a small amount of urine in the cutaneostomy bag.

Ten days later, the IVP showed a normal kidney on the left side and a normal lower system on the right side with a small nonfunctioning upper pole. Fortunately, there was no reflux in the right lower system.

Dr. Oberhausen from the Institute for Radioisotopes took an interest in the case. Later recognized worldwide for the Oberhausen Clearance Curve, he performed one of the first split renal function tests with regions of interest on the right side. The right upper pole region showed less then 10 % but the total right function was still 40 % of the total renal function.

The girl went home and was readmitted 2 months later. She was asymptomatic and the stoma looked perfect. The cystoscopy showed a normal left orifice and two on the right side with a small ureterocele on the lower one. A right supracostal incision was made and 3–4 cm of the upper pole, showing severe pyelonephritic scars, was resected. The lower part of the kidney looked normal and the ureter was carefully dissected free from the dilated one. A Foley catheter was inserted in the stoma and fixed with sutures at the upper pole. The "pull through and out maneuver" was performed easily and thereafter the stoma was excised and closed.

Remarks

The discussion concerning the nomenclature and classification of the dilated ureter continued for many years until the Philadelphia Consensus was reached in 1974. Until that time, primary obstructed megaureter had been classified as a reflux or nonreflux megaureter. Parkulainen's Reflux Grading was accepted at the same time, as was Emmet's Grading for dilatation.

However, the discussion concerning the treatment of megaureters and double systems persisted.

In the early 1980s, looking at the long-term follow-up in adults with obstructive megaureters, we found that the majority of gross dilated ureters in childhood ended up as asymptomatic, low segmental dilated ureters.

For duplex systems, Woodard's Strategy, developed in 1996, was accepted worldwide. In symptomatic double systems:

1. Start from below, resect the ureterocele, and implant both ureters with an antireflux method.
2. Wait and see and approach the upper tract only if it becomes necessary.

In children with a pyelocutaneostomy and ureterocutaneostomy, stomal obstruction is an extremely rare finding. If the greater omentum is wrapped around the ureter (Roth 1967; Lodde 2004), stomal obstruction also significantly reduced in adults later on.

References

Roth A (1967) Transabdominal transperitoneal bilateral omento-ureterostomy. Annual meeting of North Central section, AUA, Cleveland Ohio Sept. 27–30:196

Winter CC (1972) Cutaneous ureterostomy: clinical application. J Urol 1o7:233–239

Winter CC (1976) Long term results of cutaneous omento-ureterostomy. J Urol 116:311–315

Lodde M et al. (2004) Uretero-ureterocutaneostomy wrapped by Omentum. BJU International 953:371–373

Posterior Sagittal Approach in Pediatric Urology

F. Ikoma

What is the best route to surgically treat an iatrogenic high-grade female hypospadias in a 2-year-old girl with subsequent, almost total urinary incontinence? Is the posterior sagittal approach the best to treat such a difficult emergency? Or are other treatments more appropriate?

Some years ago, a small 2-year-old girl had received a surgical treatment by a pediatric surgeon for her congenital urethral diverticulum. The pediatric surgeon had cut with scissors both the anterior wall of vagina and the posterior wall of urethra from the urethral meatus to the bladder neck. After the procedure for the urethral diverticulum, it was impossible for the surgeon to make sutures to close the opened urethra, even with large bilateral perineal incisions, and her urethra remained with high-grade female hypospadias after surgery. This pediatric surgeon soon afterward introduced me to this unfortunate child who had subtotal urinary incontinence after surgery.

At this time, I tried to redo the interrupted sutures with absorbable sutures to close the posterior urethral wall and the anterior vaginal wall separately in layers. However, because of very small field of view and very difficult manipulation of instruments in the small vagina, my surgical repair disappointingly failed and her urinary incontinence continued. I thought it was better to wait until puberty for the next radical treatment. Perhaps a sufficient field of view would be possible at that time, via the vaginal approach, but a good or poor result after surgery could not be guaranteed. I chose not to reconstruct the bladder neck (Young-Dees-Leadbetter) because the child was too young. Ureterosigmoidostomy was, I thought, only the last-resort treatment. Now she has a cystostomy and is awaiting future surgery at puberty.

However, I am afraid that I will no longer be able do such detailed and difficult surgery when she reaches puberty, because I have already retired. The surgical solutions she needs should come in the near future.

Now I would like to emphasize the importance of the posterior approach (Kraske 1885) in pediatric and adult urology. If I had been able to use the posterior approach at that time, we could have celebrated a successful surgical result for this child.

The posterior approach consists of three main routes: pararectal routes, transanorectal routes, and perianorectal routes (Fig. 21.11.1).

Pararectal routes (posterior pararectal routes) involve lateral displacement of rectum and are suitable for reaching the bladder neck and prostate. Pararectal routes (Fig. 21.11.2) are classified into several routes depending on the site of incision: the ischiorectal route (Voelcker 1919) through the fossa ischiorectalis; the coccygoperineal route (Couvelaire 1951); the sacral route (Thiermann 1952); and the sagittal route (deVries and Peña 1982). Since 1993, I have used this posterior sagittal pararectal route for minimization (plication) and/or denudation of enlarged Müllerian duct cysts (prostatic utricle), which are handled easily in this manner. Seminal vesicles and seminal ducts are also easily viewed.

Transanorectal routes (posterior sagittal transanorectal routes) (Fig. 21.11.3) involve a longitudinal incision of the anorectal wall and reach not only the bladder neck and prostate, but also the posterior urethra and caudal vagina. Transanorectal routes are also classified into several routes depending on the site of the anorectal wall incision: the posterior and anterior transrectal route (Kraske 1885); the posterior and anterior transanorectal route (York Mason 1969; Peña and deVries 1982), involving a longitudinal incision of both the posterior and anterior anorectal wall; the anterior transanorectal route (Young 1913), with a longitudinal incision of only the anterior anorectal wall; the anterior transrectal route (Saposhkoff 1922), with a transverse incision of anterior rectal wall; and the anterior perineal transanorectal route (Cukier1985), entailing a perineal incision and longitudinal incision of the anterior anorectal wall. These transanorectal routes require a temporal colostomy.

Another route, the posterior sagittal perianorectal route (Boeckel 1908; Pintér 1996) (Fig. 21.11.4) entails temporal mobilization and cranial displacement of the entire rectum and anus and does not require temporal colostomy.

The perianorectal route followed by the transvaginal route or anterior perineal transanorectal route followed by the transvaginal route is, I believe, an optimal route to treat the iatrogenic expansive high-grade fe-

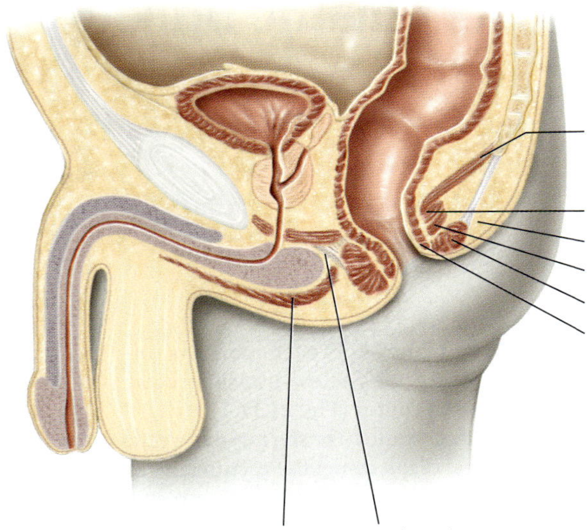

Fig. 21.11.1a

Posterior Approach: 1. Para-rectal route
2. Trans-anorectal route
3. Peri-anorectal route

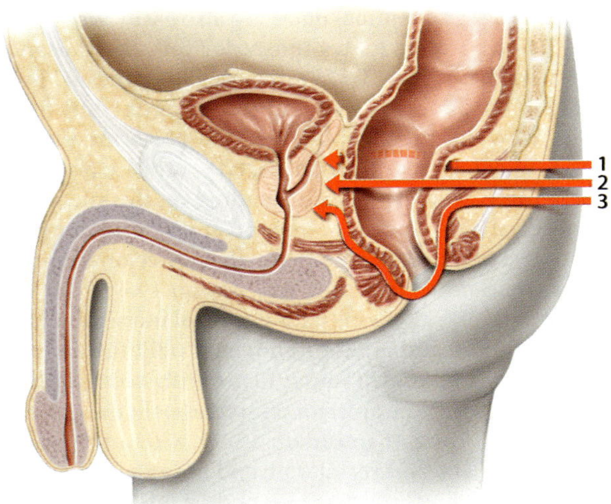

Fig. 21.11.1b

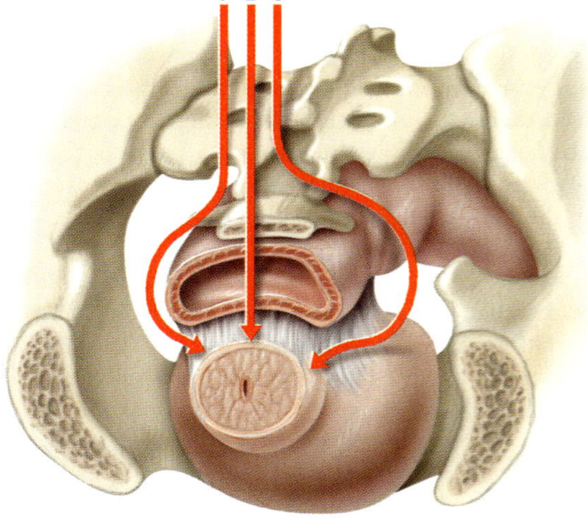

(© Hohenfellner 2007)

Fig. 21.11.1c

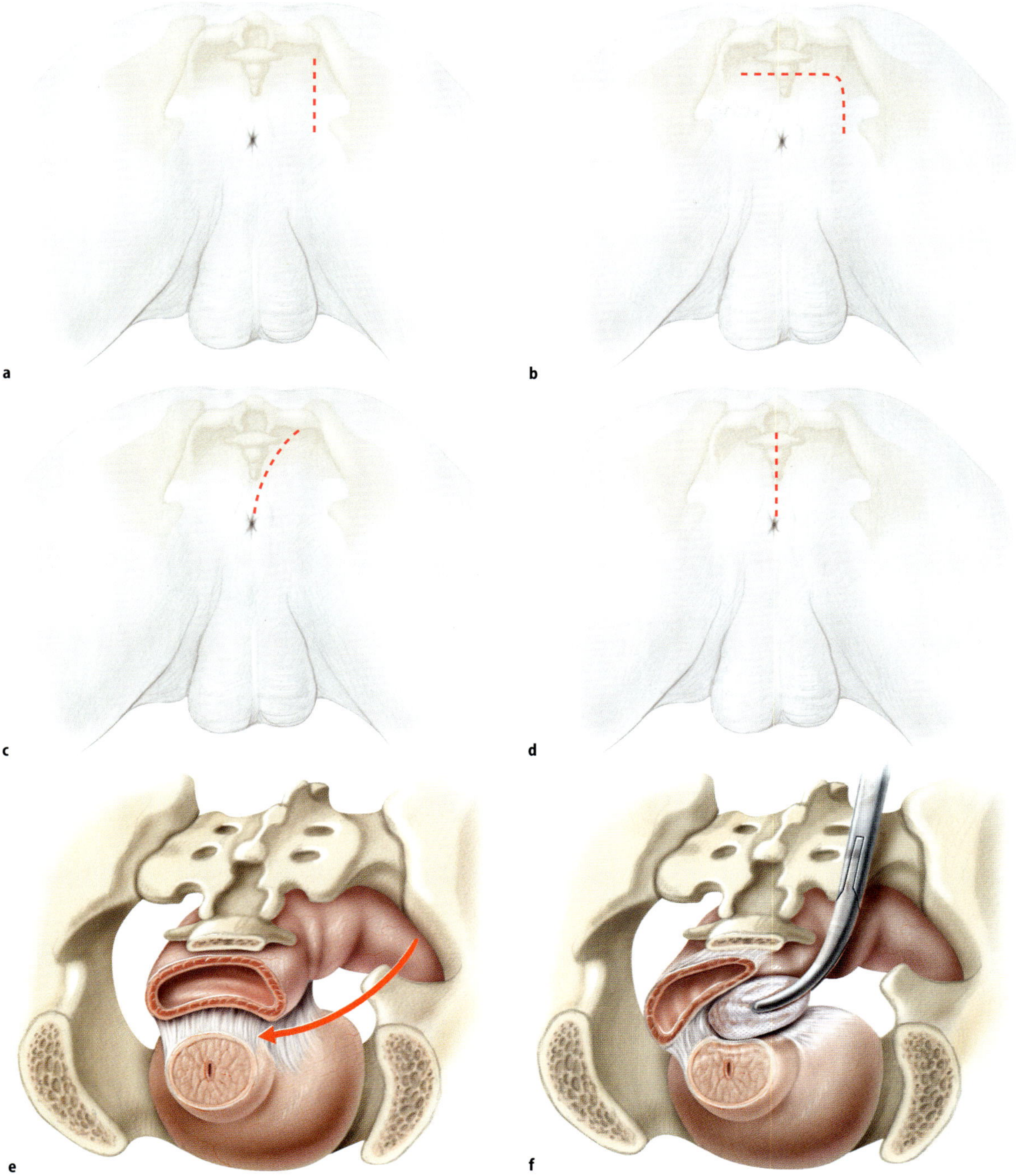

Fig. 21.11.2a–f. Para-rectal route. **a** Ischiorectal route (Voelker, 1919), **b** Coccygo-perineal route (Couvelaire, 1951), **c** Sacral route (Thiermann, 1952), **d** Sagittal route (deVries and Peña, 1982), **e, f** Blunt dissection of rectum from prostate and lateral displacement of rectum (© Hohenfellner 2007)

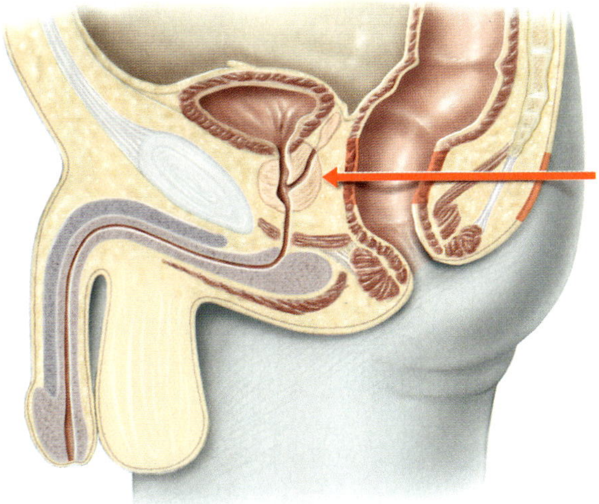

a

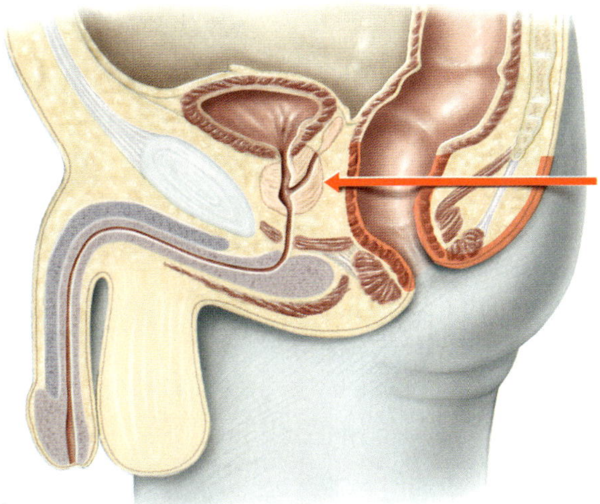

b

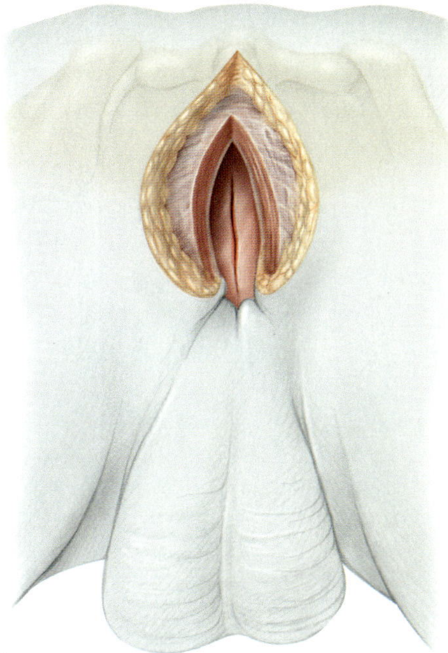

c

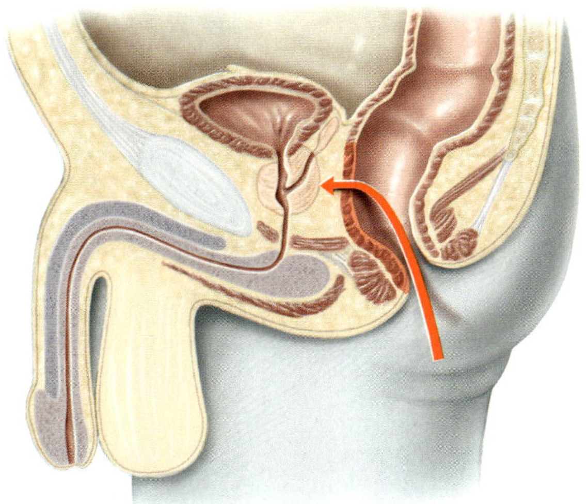

d

Fig. 21.11.3a–i. Trans-anorectal route (porterior sagittal trans-anorectal route). **a** Posterior and anterior transrectal route prone position (Kraske, 1885), **b, c** Posterior and anterior transanorectal route (York Mason, 1969; Peña and deVries, 1982), **d** Anterior transanorectal route supine position (Young, 1913) (© Hohenfellner 2007)

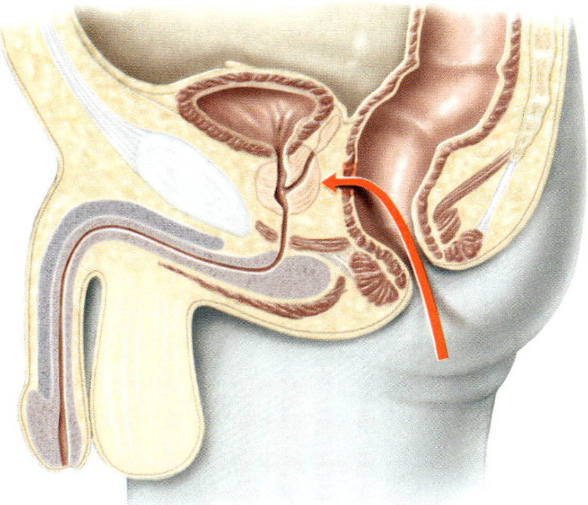

e

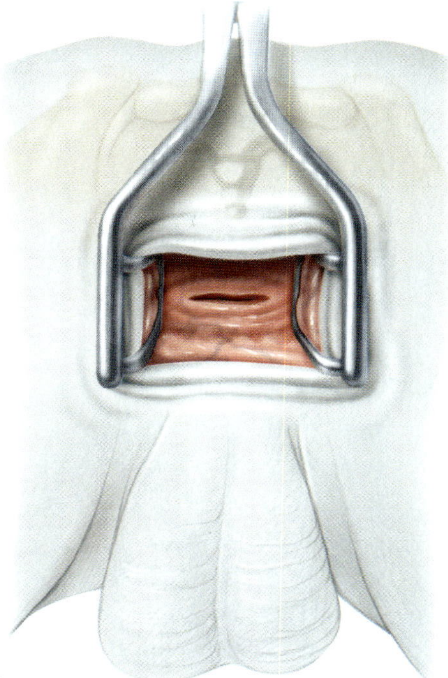

f

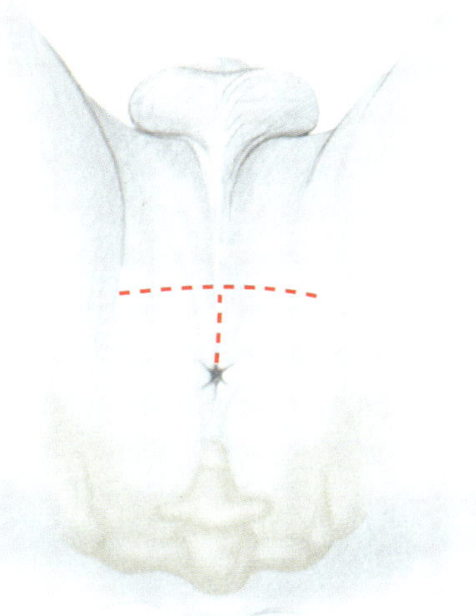

g

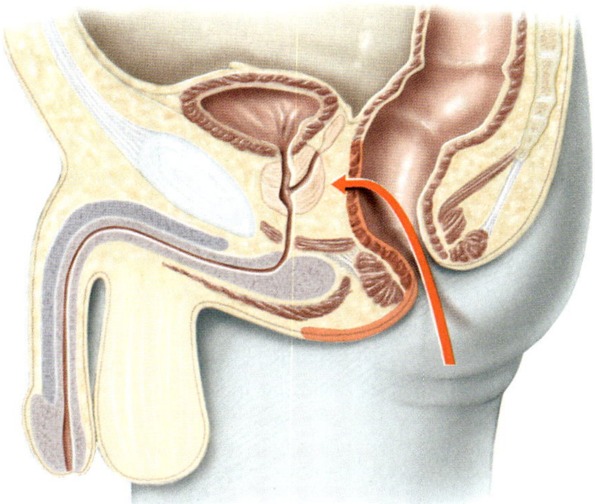

h

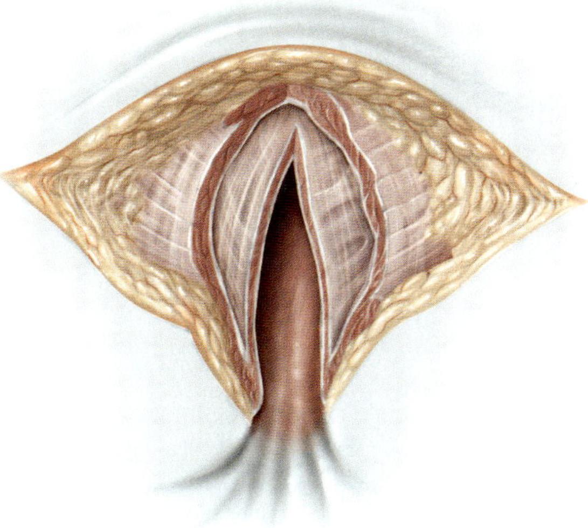

i

Fig. 21.11.3. e, f Anterior transrectal route (transverse incision of anterior rectal wall between bilateral tuber ischii) (Saposhkoff, 1922), **g, h, i** Anterior perineal transanorectal route (Cukier, 1985)

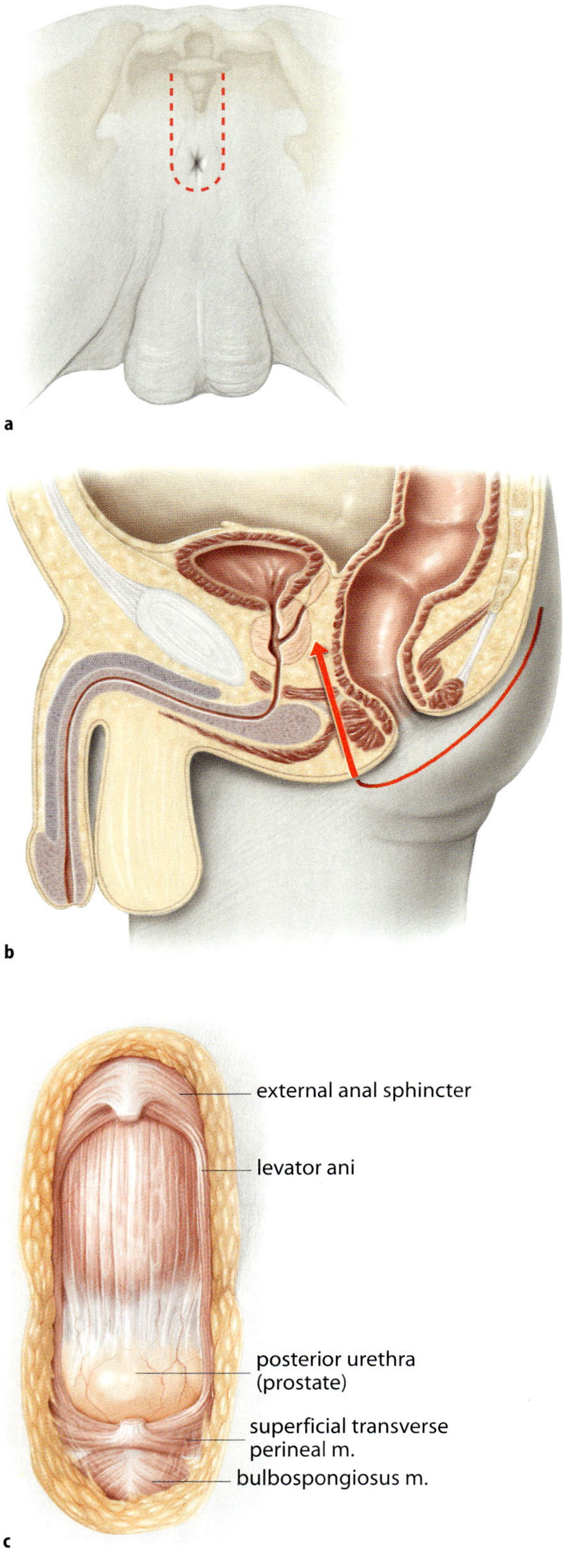

Fig. 21.11.4 a–c. Peri-anorectal route. **a–c** Dissection and mobilisation of anus and rectum after dividing of both distal and proximal sphincter mechanisms (Pintér, 1996)

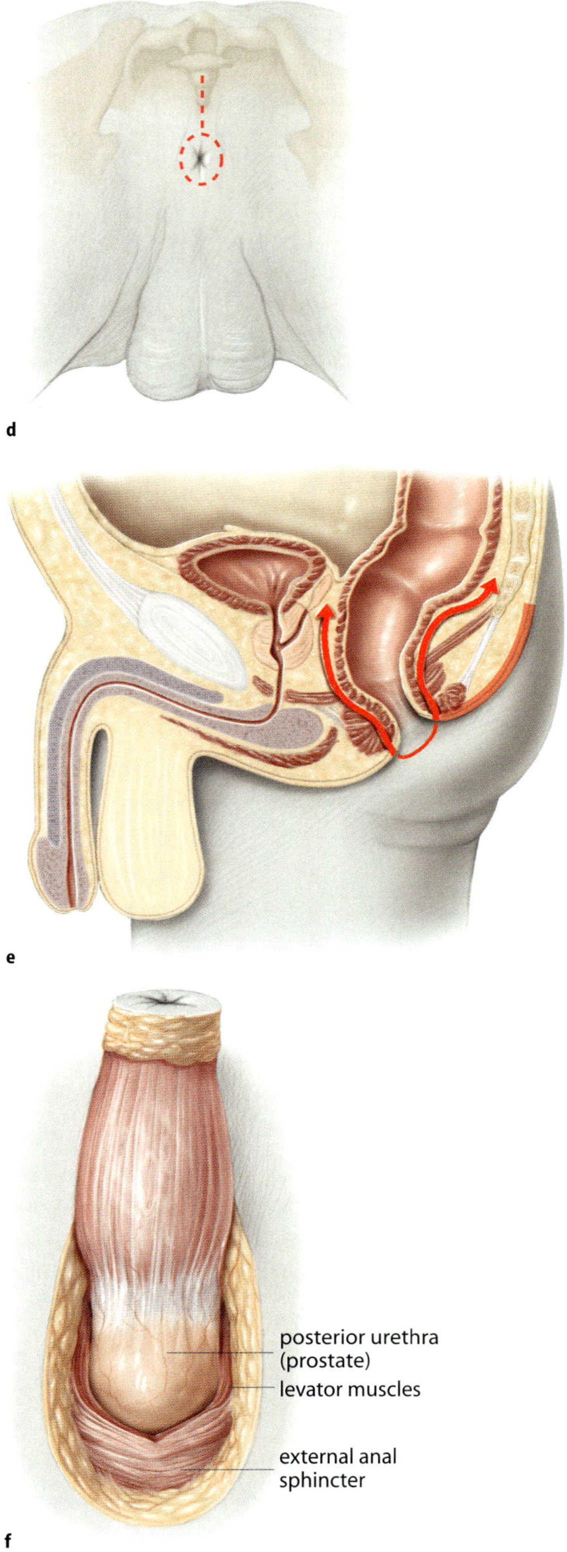

Fig. 21.11.4 d–f. Dissection and mobilisation of anus and rectum together with all sphincter mechanisms (Boeckel, 1908) (© Hohenfellner 2007)

male hypospadias of my young female patient. But until now I have had no experience with these routes.

The posterior sagittal approaches have recently been used in pediatric surgery (Peña and deVries 1982) for anorectal anomalies, but in urology, especially in pediatric urology, they are very seldom used.

For the radical surgery of high-grade adrenogenital syndrome, hydrometrocolpos, cloacal anomaly, enlarged Müllerian duct cyst, vesico- and/or urethrorectal fistula, trauma and stenosis of posterior urethra, and iatrogenic female urethral trauma, as in the case presented herein, these posterior sagittal approaches are very useful. I would like to see a young urologist now learn to use these routes routinely so that they can be available for emergency treatment in pediatric and adult urology.

References

Boeckel J (1908) Nouveau procédé de prostatectomie par mobilisation temporaire du segment ano-rectal. Rev Chirurg 3:386

Couvelaire R, Bouffard J-R (1951) L'adénomectomie prostatique par voie coccypérinéale droite. J Urol 57:362

DeVries PA, Peña A (1982) Posterior sagittal anorectoplasty. J Ped Surg 17:638

Kilpatrick FR, Mason AY (1969) Post-operative recto-urethral fistula. J Urol 41:649

Kraske P (1885) Zur Exstirpation hochsitzender Mastdarmkrebse. Verhand Deutsch Gesell Chir 14:464

Peña A, deVries PA (1982) Posterior sagittal anorectoplasty: important technical considerations and new applications. J Ped Surg 17:796

Pintér AB, Hock A, Vástyán A, Farkas A (1996) Does the posterior sagittal approach with the perirectal dissection impair fecal continence in a normal rectum? J Ped Surg 31:1349

Saposhkoff KJ (1922) Über den Zutritt zur Prostata und Samenblasen. Verhand. d. XV Kongr Russ Chir St Petersburg Sept. br.

Thiermann E (1952) Sakrale Prostatektomie bei Hypertrophie der Vorsteherdrüse. Z Urol 45:742

Voelcker F (1919) Die Prostatektomie als gut übersichtliche Operation. Z Urol. Chir 4:253

Young HH, Stone HB (1913) An operation for urethro-rectal fistula. report of three cases. Trans Am Assoc Genito Urin Surg 8:270

Zimmern PE, Cukier J (1985) Prostatic and membranous urethrorectal fistulas: a new technique of surgical closure. J Urol 134:355

Postoperative Urinary Retention After Hypospadias Repair

F. Ikoma

If complete urinary retention occurs just after removing an indwelling catheter for hypospadias repair, what is the best course of action?

Some young boys can experience urinary retention after removing an indwelling catheter placed for hypospadias repair on the 2nd or 3rd postoperative day because of edema, pain, or simply fear. Manipulating the formed urethra and inserting catheters are strongly discouraged. If this is done, the urethra will form a fistula. It is better to make a temporary cystostomy immediately and to await diminishing of local edema for a few days so that the boy can urinate independently.

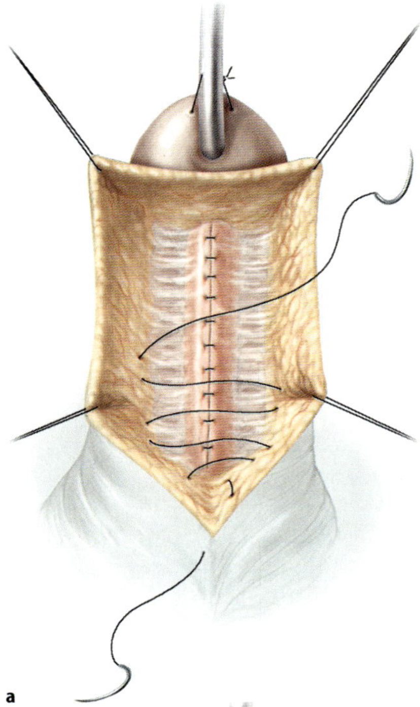

a

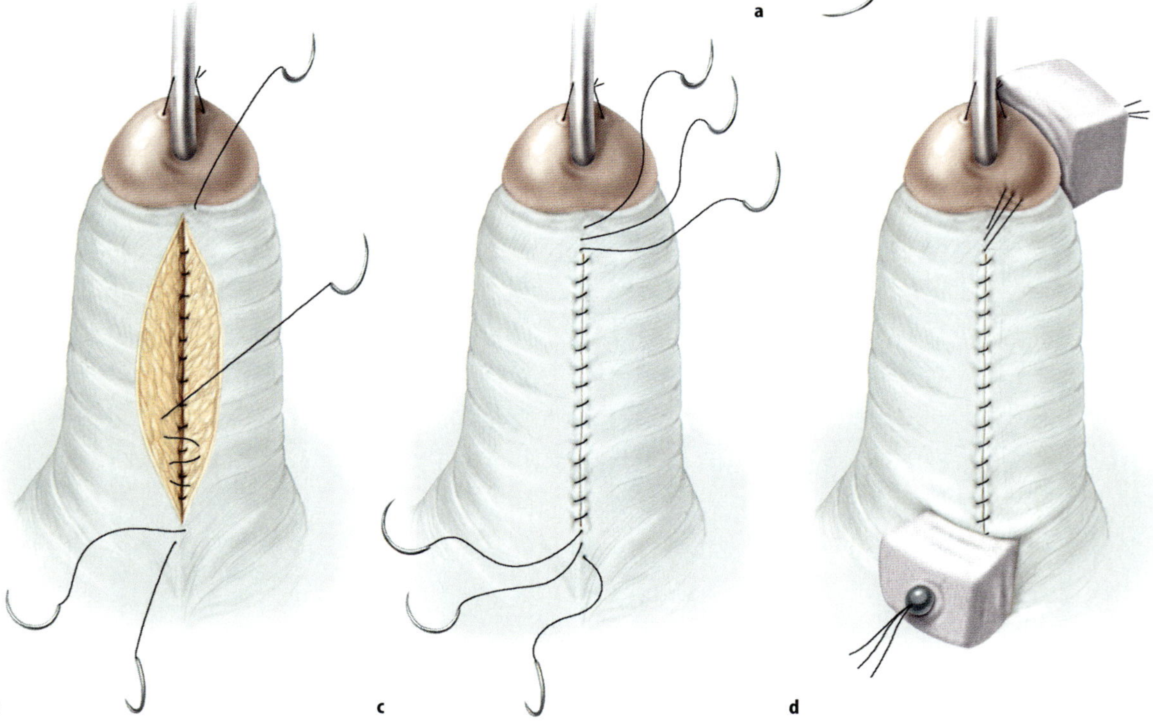

b c d

Fig. 21.12.1. a–g The use of a fishing lead sinker for the double stop suture
a–d The second stage of hypospadias repairs (© Hohenfellner 2007)

Hairs in the Urethra of a Hypospadias Patient

F. Ikoma

When at puberty hairs are found in the skin–urethra formed in a hypospadias patient who has received urethroplasty using penoscrotal skin as a child, what is the best course to follow?

Occasionally, urethroscopy shows hair growth in the formed skin–urethra in high-grade hypospadias patients. Optic electric coagulation of hair roots is sometimes possible, but most often it is difficult and incomplete. I believe that it is better to surgically open the skin–urethra at the site where hairs are found from the ventral side with careful, complete electric coagulation of every hair root directly in situ. This procedure is followed by placing an indwelling catheter through the entire urethra into the bladder, closing the window of skin–urethra using interrupted sutures with absorbable threads such Vicryl 6-0, covering the closed window with bilateral penile skin by three layers of subcutaneous continuous sutures with nonabsorbable threads such as nylon or Prolene(6-0) (the first layer, deep dartos; the second layer, superficial subcutaneous dartos; the third layer, edge of penile skin for adaptation), and fixing these three threads with double stops at both ends using sponge fragments and small lead sinkers (Fig. 21.12.1) (see Ikoma 1994). If these three covering layers of subcutaneous continuous sutures can be made securely, we can leave the skin-urethral window open. Postoperative fistula formation is very rare. A few days after the surgery, the indwelling catheter is removed and the patient can urinate by himself. At the 10th postoperative day, the three layers of sutures are removed.

If we are afraid of too much scarring of the skin–urethra at the site of hairs after electric coagulation, the Johannson procedure is better. After 6 months, we can close the urethral Johannson window using the same method as mentioned above.

References

Ikoma F (1994) Hypospadiekorrektur nach Denis Browne. In: Hohenfellner R (ed) Ausgewählte urologische OP-Techniken. Georg Thieme Verlag, p 477

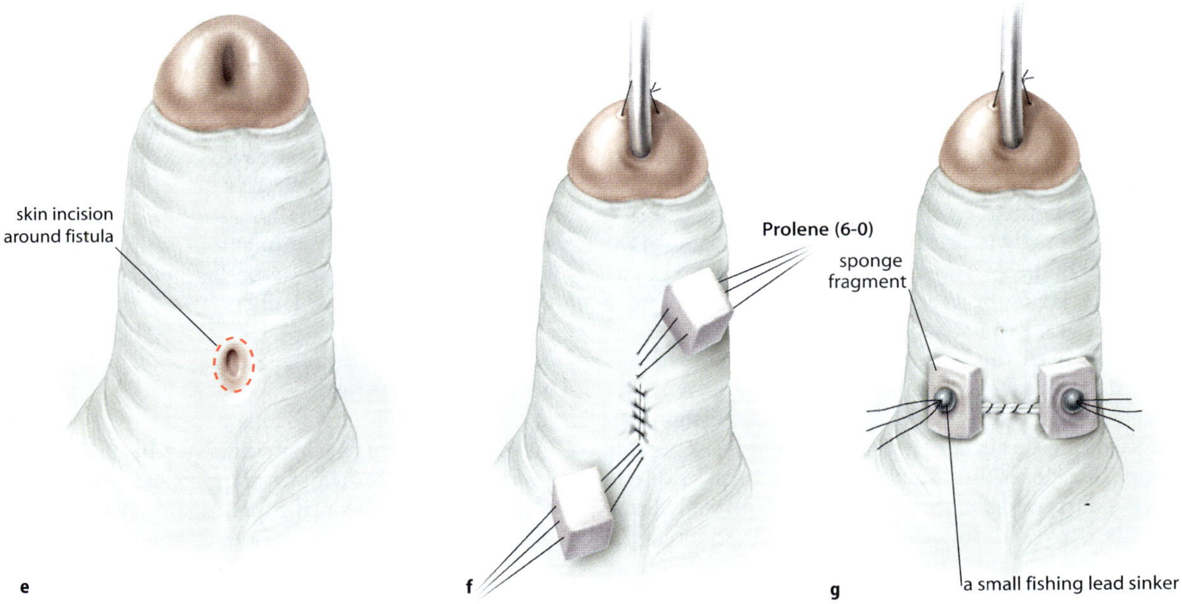

Fig. 21.12.1. e–f Closure of urethral fistula (© Hohenfellner 2007)

A Tale of Two Brothers

W. Månsson

Reconstruction of the urinary tract using intestinal segments is associated with the risk of numerous side effects, most of which develop gradually after surgery. This case report of two brothers, now 36 and 34 years of age, illustrates an acute emergency situation that requires immediate evaluation and treatment. Both brothers suffered from the same type of life-threatening complication, and different treatment options were applied.

The Elder Brother

This man suffered from urge incontinence, refractory to conservative treatment. Cystometry showed detrusor instability. He had no abnormal neurological findings. He underwent urinary diversion in October of 1997. Based on previous psychiatric history, we initially recommended an ileal conduit, but testing the appliances available caused allergic skin problems, hence the dermatologist advised against conduit diversion.

Continent diversion with construction of a Lundiana pouch (Davidsson et al. 1996; Månsson et al. 2003) was performed. Briefly, in this procedure the distal 10 cm of the ileum and the right colonic segment are isolated. The colonic segment is opened along the anterior taenia down to the level of the ileocecal valve, and from there a transverse incision is made to the base of the valve. The ileal segment is tapered snugly over a 10-F catheter with a GIA stapler. The first cartridge is placed obliquely to preserve as much as possible of the diameter of the ileal opening, as this will create the stoma. The edges of the cecal wall incision are then grasped with two Babcock clamps and a third Babcock clamp is used to grasp the ileocecal valve, which is pulled out between the previous two clamps. A TA 55-stapler with 4.8-mm staples is placed to incorporate the edges of the cecal wall and part of the valve. The fired staple line closes the cecum, tapers the valve, and tethers the narrowed ileocecal valve to the cecal wall. A uniformly narrowed diameter is thus achieved along the entire length of the outlet and a small flap valve created at the junction with the pouch. The ileocecal segment is rotated 180° counter-clockwise, the ureters are implanted with the LeDuc technique, and the pouch is detubularized and closed. The stoma is in the right lower quadrant or in the umbilicus. Catheterization is usually done with a 16-F Foley catheter.

After the continent diversion, the patient had a well-functioning reservoir and was continent with convenient catheterization intervals. Nonetheless, over the following 4 years, he presented at the emergency room several times with epididymitis and symptoms of pyelonephritis and abdominal pain, but the symptoms disappeared and several workups were uneventful. He also developed epilepsy.

He was admitted to our department in October 2001 with a history of a fall and trauma to the abdomen 2 days previously, possibly in conjunction with an epileptic fit. He initially felt no pain, but great discomfort gradually developed. He was febrile with a temperature of 39 °C and had an increase in WBC, and his abdomen was tender with clinical signs of peritonitis. A CT scan showed fluid around the reservoir.

The patient was taken to the OR with a tentative diagnosis of perforation/rupture of the pouch. There was foul-smelling fluid in the pelvic cavity. A 1×1-cm hole in the reservoir wall was observed, initially covered by small bowel loops. Inflammatory reactions were noted on the reservoir wall and the small bowel loops. The defect in the reservoir wall was revised and closed in two layers, and the abdominal cavity was irrigated and drained, as was the pouch. The postoperative course was uneventful, and the patient was able to resume intermittent self-catheterization after 4 weeks. In August 2005, IVP was normal, as was endoscopic control of the reservoir and the native bladder.

The Younger Brother

This man also had a psychiatric history. In 1995, he sustained a spinal cord injury after a fall, and became paraplegic and developed a neurogenic bladder with urine leakage due to severe hyperreflexia. Conservative treatment measures were unsuccessful. In November 1999, he underwent continent urinary diversion with construction of a Lundiana pouch, as described above.

Except for a few episodes of pyocystitis, the course at follow-up was uneventful with a well-functioning, easily catheterized pouch. However, he eventually developed fecal incontinence and a colostomy was performed in 2001. The following year, he underwent acute laparotomy due to small-bowel obstruction caused by adhesions, and he later developed a large incisional hernia that was repaired with a preperitoneal synthetic net. His psychiatric problems recurred, and he was placed on lithium medication. There was a suspicion of renal tubular damage, probably due to the lithium medication. Nevertheless, he was able to care for his two stomas.

In August 2005, he sustained trauma to his right leg when it was jammed in a closing bus door. A week later, he was admitted to the emergency room of the orthopedic department due to swelling of the leg, and he was diagnosed with a deep venous thrombosis up to the level of the inguinal ligament. He was referred to the department of internal medicine, and full-dose heparinization was instituted along with warfarin therapy.

On the 2nd day, the patient started to complain of abdominal pain. He had no trouble emptying his reservoir. In the evening, he took himself by wheelchair to the designated smoking area to have a cigarette. The following day he had a temperature of 39 °C. The general surgeon found his abdomen distended and tense and believed that the problem was constipation. When it was noted that serum creatinine had risen to 190 μmol/l, a catheter was reintroduced in the pouch but yielded only 220 ml of urine, after which a bladder scan revealed a remaining volume of 850 ml. At that point, the urologist on call was notified, and he found the patient febrile and mentally confused. The abdominal findings were difficult to interpret, but due to suspected perforation, a wide-bore catheter was introduced into the pouch, which yielded 1,500 ml of urine. The patient was taken to the x-ray department, contrast medium was introduced into the pouch, and a CT was performed, which showed large amounts of fluid with contrast medium in the abdominal cavity. By that time, the patient was septic with disturbed electrolytes and circulation, and he was tachypneic. He was intubated and ventilated with a respirator.

In this case we chose a conservative approach, because the patient was fully heparinized and in poor circulatory and respiratory condition. He was placed on broad-spectrum antibiotics, and he was ventilated for 3 days. He had an indwelling catheter, and a drainage tube was inserted to drain abdominal fluid. Over the course of time, two more tubes had to be inserted under guidance of ultrasound due to recurring fever and raised C-reactive protein caused by the remaining infected urine. The course was protracted, and it was not until 6 weeks after admission that all drainage tubes could be removed and the patient could resume intermittent self-catheterization.

Two weeks after this patient was discharged, his elder brother underwent emergency laparotomy at another hospital due to a second perforation of the pouch! A small hole was closed.

Perforation or Rupture of Continent Urinary Pouch

The urological histories of these two brothers illustrate the most serious acute complication after continent reconstruction of the urinary tract. The etiology of the perforation or rupture may differ, although overdistension, blunt trauma, and trauma from catheterization have been suggested (Månsson et al. 1997; Singh and Choong 2004). The complication seems to be more common after continent cutaneous diversion than after neobladder construction, because in the latter the external sphincter can yield to high pressure in the pouch and function as a pop-off valve to allow the escape of urine. This might not happen in a reservoir that has an outlet with a competent closure mechanism. Treatment may be achieved through laparotomy with closure of the hole, which is usually rather small, or simply by drainage of the pouch, the latter of which requires careful observation of the patient.

Lessons Learned

- Continent urinary tract reconstruction should not be performed in patients with a psychiatric history.
- Acute abdominal pain in a patient with continent cutaneous diversion or an orthotopic neobladder should be regarded as a perforation or rupture of the pouch until proven otherwise.
- Symptoms and signs of this complication may be obscured in patients with a spinal cord injury.

References

Davidsson T, Hedlund H, Månsson W (1996) Detubularized right colonic reservoir with intussuscepted ileal nipple valve or stapled ("Lundiana") outlet. Clinical and urodynamic results in a prospective randomized study. World J Urol 14:78

Månsson W, Bakke A, Bergman B, Brekkan E, Jonsson O, Kihl B, Nurmi M, Pedersen J, Schultz A, Sörensen B, Urnes T, Wolf H (1997) Perforation of continent urinary reservoirs. Scandinavian experience. Scand J Urol Nephrol 31:529

Månsson W, Davidsson T, Könyves J, Liedberg F, Månsson Å, Wullt B (2003) Continent urinary tract reconstruction – the Lund experience. BJU Int 92:271

Singh S, Choong S (2004) Rupture and perforation of urinary reservoirs made from bowel. World J Urol 22:222

Unfortunate Honeymoon Under the Palm Trees

J.A. Martínez-Piñeiro

In February 1989, a 31-year-old Spanish man and his young wife went to Santo Domingo on honeymoon to enjoy the balmy climate and beaches of the Caribbean island, while Europe was freezing.

One windy day, when the couple was lying on the sand, a nearly palm tree fell, killing the wife instantly and crushing the man's pelvis. As a result of the pelvic fracture, the membranous urethra, bladder neck, and rectum were severely ruptured. In the local hospital, a suprapubic catheter was placed, but no surgery was undertaken. A few days later, Fournier's gangrene developed, which prompted the evacuation of the patient to a Florida hospital, where a life-saving, wide excision of the necrotic scrotal skin and a colostomy were performed.

Two months later, the patient was flown to Avilés, Spain, his home city. At the local hospital, posttransfusional hepatitis was detected and the colostomy closed, leaving the cystostomy in place.

Six months after the trauma, the patient was sent to the urological department of La Paz University Hospital of Madrid. He still bore the cystostomy catheter, the right testis was palpable underneath the skin of the inner face of the thigh, and the left one remained in a small scrotal remnant. He complained of impotence, the hepatic enzymes were elevated, and x-rays showed a severe pelvic deformity and large bony callus in both ischiopubic rami (Fig. 21.15.1); the antegrade cystourethrogram revealed a gaping and distorted bladder neck as well as obstruction of the prostatic urethra at the level of the verumontanum and faint contrast images, suggesting the existence of several fistulous tracts (Fig. 21.15.2); the retrograde urethrogram confirmed the occlusion of the bulbar urethra and faint fistulous tracts within the perineum (Fig. 21.15.3).

With diagnosis of a complex posterior urethral distraction defect, a bulboprostatic end-to-end anastomosis was undertaken via a perineal route. The operation succeeded in restoring urethral continuity (Fig. 21.15.4),

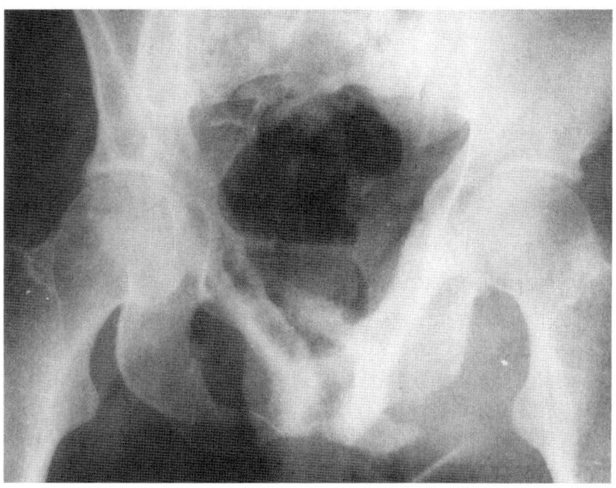

Fig. 21.15.1. X-ray of the pelvis, showing severe deformity

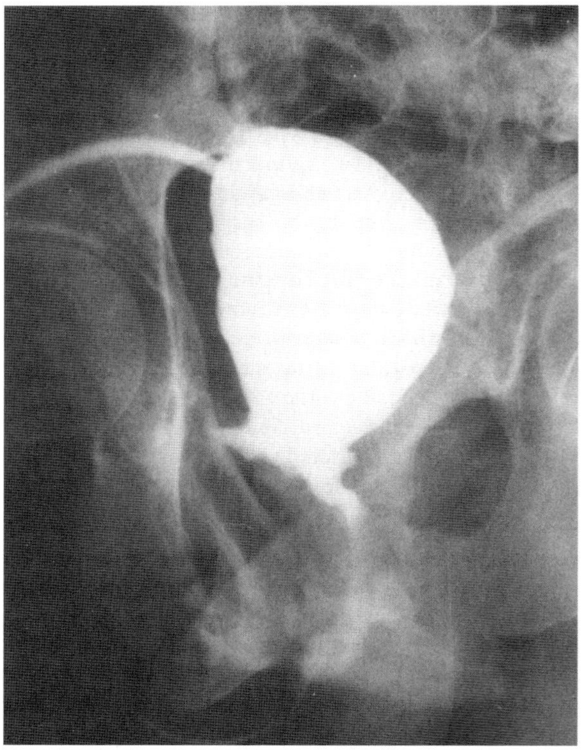

Fig. 21.15.2. Cystourethrogram through the cystostomy catheter. Open and distorted bladder neck. Urethral disruption at the level of verumontanum and faintly contrasted tracts in the perineum

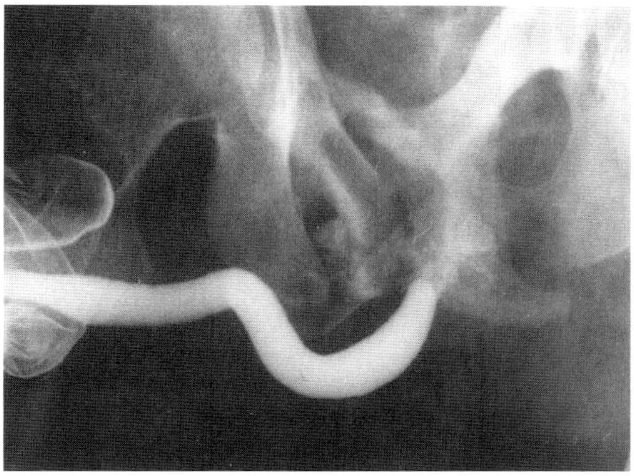

Fig. 21.15.3. Retrograde urethrogram showing an occluded bulbar urethra and fistulous tracts in the perineum

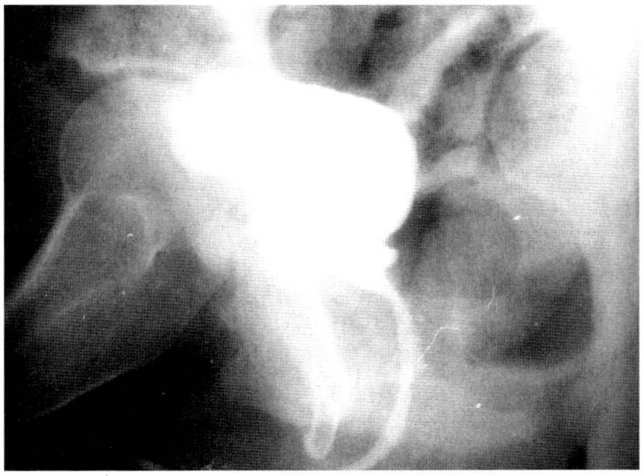

Fig. 21.15.4. Cystourethrogram after end-to-end anastomotic urethroplasty. Urethral continuity restored, but bladder neck wide open

but total urinary incontinence was a disturbing sequel for the patient, although it was foreseen by us in view of the cystogram image, suggestive of bladder neck injury and adhesions to the pubic rami. Usually, this condition moves the urologist to perform a bladder neck plasty in the same stage as the urethroplasty in order to spare the patient another operation. In this case, we left the bladder neck surgery for a second stage, which was performed 1 month later. Then the bladder neck was liberated from firm adherences to the pubic bone and tubularized; an omental flap was also interposed between the neck and bones.

Despite a good anatomic result (Fig. 21.15.5), the patient still complained of stress incontinence and nocturnal enuresis, suggestive of a lesion of the external sphincter. Because the patient also suffered from a loss

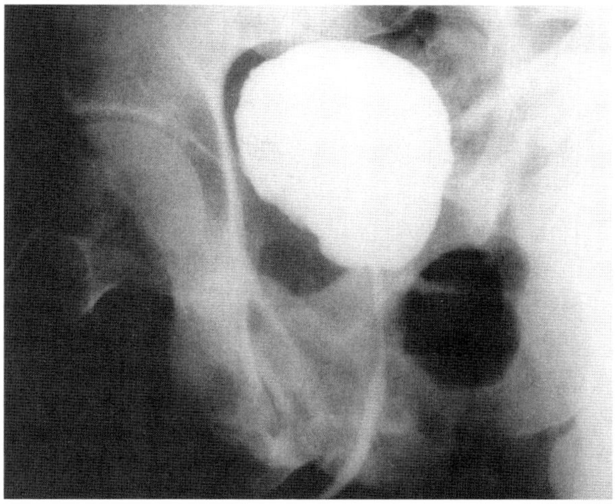

Fig. 21.15.5. Cystourethrogram after bladder neck tubularization. Morphology restored

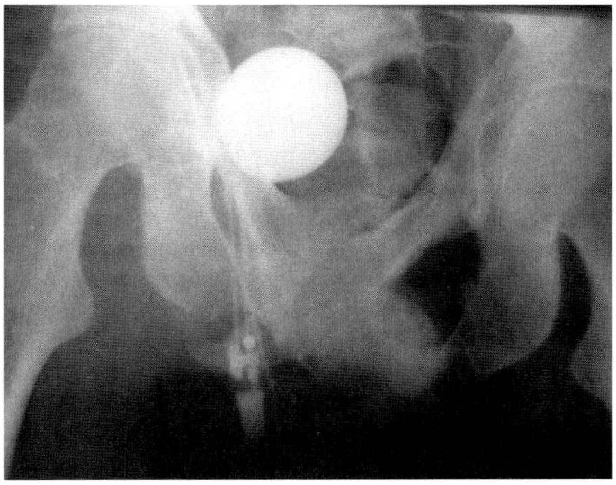

Fig. 21.15.6. Plain film showing the AMS urinary artificial sphincter components

of erection, we proposed the simultaneous implantation of two prosthetic devices, a Scott-AMS artificial sphincter and a Dynaflex impotence intracavernous prosthesis. The latter model was chosen in view of the small size of the scrotum, which would not admit two intrascrotal pumps. The implantation took place in January 1991 and the success was impressive, with high patient satisfaction for 4 years (Fig. 21.15.6). Then recurrent incontinence due to malfunction of the cuff occurred, requiring replacement of the 4.5-cm cuff with a close-fitting 4-cm cuff.

Seven years and eight operations after the honeymoon casualty, the young man was enjoying a dry and potent life, but at what price!

Intravenous Uroperitoneogram

J.A. Martínez-Piñeiro

In April 1979, a 68-year-old woman underwent a hysterectomy for a huge myoma. Anuria ensued immediately, which proved resistant to diuretics and aggressive hydration. Three days later, a urologic consultation was requested by the gynecologists and she was referred to the urological department of La Paz University Hospital in Madrid. The exam revealed an obese patient with severely distended abdomen, signs of ascites, arterial hypertension (190/100 mm Hg), moderate acidosis (pH 7.25), blood creatinine 2.80 mg/dl, K 5.5 nmol/l, Na 130 nmol/l, and mild hypocalcemia (7.9 mg/dl). Ultrasound revealed a left dilated upper urinary tract and intraperitoneal fluid. An IVU showed bilateral nephrogram in early films, but very poor concentration of the contrast medium in the excretory phase prevented an accurate diagnosis. In delayed films, the entire peritoneal cavity appeared to be filled with contrast, which outlined a distended stomach and some intestinal loops, but hindered the visualization of the urinary tract (Fig. 21.16.1). A section of one of the ureters, with intraperitoneal urine leakage, was suspected, and to confirm the suspicion a bilateral retrograde ureteral catheterization was undertaken. The right catheter did not pass beyond the 10-cm mark, the left catheter passed only 5 cm; contrast injection revealed complete obstruction on both sides.

Given the left upper tract dilatation, together with radiopaque ascites (uroperitoneogram), a tentative diagnosis of left ureteric ligation and right ureteric section with ligation of the distal stump was made. An urgent laparotomy was undertaken, in which more than 6 l of peritoneal fluid were aspirated before damage was assessed. The right pelvic ureter appeared completely severed with the proximal stump draining urine freely, while the distal stump was ligated. The left juxtavesical ureter appeared only ligated (with silk). A right spatulated end-to-end anastomosis was performed and the left ureter simply deligated.

The patient's recovery was uneventful, but 7 months afterward she complained of pain in the left lumbar fossa and a left obstructive uropathy was detected on ultrasound scan and IVU. The right urinary tract was normal. A left ureteroneocystostomy with psoas hitch was performed; the last 5 cm of the ureter were surrounded by severe fibrosis, and the ureter itself showed a 5-mm-long stricture. The pathologist reported intense fibrosis of the wall, unspecific inflammation, and granulomatous reaction to a foreign body. One year later, both upper tracts looked normal on IVU.

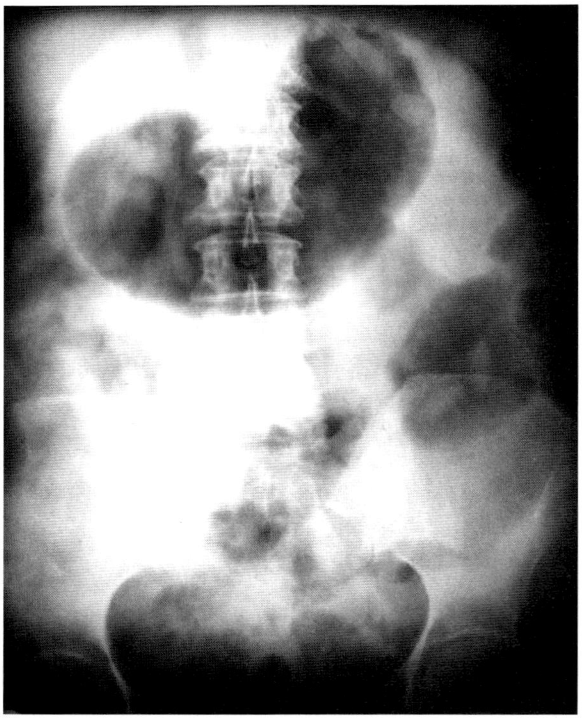

Fig. 21.16.1. Delayed IVU shows right kidney nephrogram and contrast medium filling the entire peritoneal cavity and outlining a gas-distended stomach and some intestinal loops

The intravenous urogram is usually diagnostic when an intraoperative ureteral trauma is suspected. In this particular case, the curious and as yet undescribed peritoneal uroperitoneogram aroused the suspicion of a ureteral section with intraperitoneal urine leakage. Another lesson is that the removal of a ureteral nonabsorbable suture standing for 3 days may entail the risk of stricture, even when the assessment of ureteral viability seems positive, contradicting the general feeling that simple deligation gives satisfactory restoration of the ureter, particularly if the interval of ligation is less than 1 week.

Coitus Interruptus

J.A. Martínez-Piñeiro

In the evening of February 26, 1991, a 25-year-old man presented at the emergency unit of La Paz University Hospital of Madrid with swelling and subcutaneous ecchymoses of the penis and scrotum (Fig. 21.17.1). He said that in the heat of sexual intercourse he had hit the mons pubis of his partner with his erect penis, then heard an audible crack and experienced pain and immediate detumescence.

Ultrasound revealed a lateral tear in the right corpus cavernosum, near the penoscrotal junction. Surgical exploration made it possible to evacuate a hematoma and close the tunica albuginea tear with a running suture of an absorbable 3-0 monofilament. A pressure dressing was applied and cyproterone acetate prescribed for 3 weeks to avoid erections.

The patient regained spontaneous erections 1 month later and full sexual activity shortly afterward.

Fracture of the penis is a relatively uncommon trauma that occurs during erection, usually caused by a sudden bending during intercourse. More uncommon is the association with partial or total urethral disruption, that when left unrepaired leads to stricture.

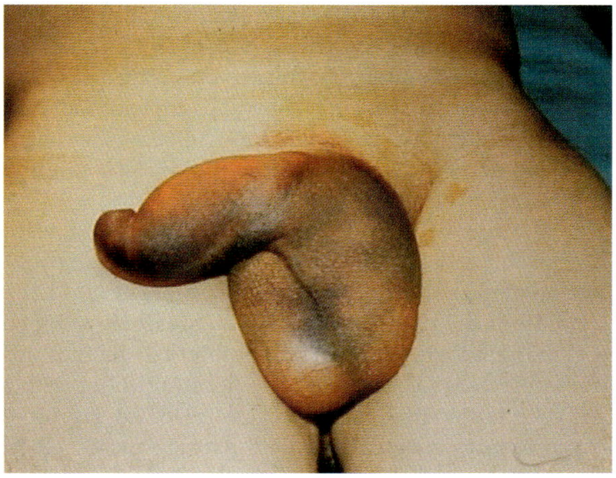

Fig. 21.17.1. Sight of the genitalia with swelling and ecchymoses.

Early surgical repair of the corpora (and urethra if involved) offers the best chance for healing and preservation of erectile function.

Exploding Bladder

J. Motsch, Ch. Schramm

A 64-year-old Jehovah's Witness with initially no coagulation defect and no anemia suffered from severe hematuria from a bladder tumor, so that a transurethral monopolar electrocoagulation and insertion of an irrigation Foley catheter was performed under general anesthesia. After the procedure, the irrigational solution showed no further bleeding.

A few hours later, a drop of the hemoglobin concentration to 6 g% and unstable vital signs were encountered and the patient was transferred to the ICU. The irrigation of the bladder via infusion suddenly stopped and manual irrigation was impossible. The patient was immediately transferred to the operating room with a suspected tamponade of the bladder. During the 4 h of transurethral coagulation and extraction of blood clots, a noise like a dog's bark was heard.

Upon returning to the ICU, a drop in the oxygen saturation occurred. Breathing sounds were attenuated. The chest x-ray showed a bilateral (double-sided) pneumothorax and retroperitoneal air bubbles. For treatment, chest tubes were inserted in both pleural cavities.

Two main reasons may explain this dramatic event. First, during the long electrocoagulation of the bladder, a significant amount of hydrolysis with a consecutive production of a small amount of detonating gas (oxyhydrogen) occurred. This mini-explosion caused the introduction of air retroperitoneally up to the interpleural space and the double-sided pneumothorax. Second, the shock-wave caused by the explosion in the bladder induced a barotrauma by direct rupture of alveoli on the surface of the lungs.

Education by Humiliation

By Far the Best Way of Learning!

A.R. Mundy

Roughly 10 years ago, I was invited to operate in Iran to treat a number of urological problems relating to war wounds during the Iran–Iraq war. On the first day, I was taken on a ward round and the first patient I saw was standing smartly to the side of his bed holding a urine drainage bag on the end of a suprapubic catheter. I was told that he had a prostatorectal fistula as a result of a gunshot wound and was shown an x-ray with a bullet perfectly in place between his rectum and bladder. Contrast studies confirmed that the bullet was in a cavity that communicated with the rectum and the prostate. I was told that everything else was normal. He told me he had feces in his urine and he was very glad that I had come over from England to fix it, as he had had three failed operations over the previous 4 years.

We went to the operating room that afternoon and I did a transperineal excision of the cavity and closure of the fistula, removing the bullet and interposing a gracilis flap between the two closure lines. The following day, I went to see him to see how he was and he said he was very well indeed and that he was very grateful to me for doing his operation but why was he still passing feces in his urine. We obtained another contrast study and I was told that there was another fistula slightly higher up, this one into the bladder, presumably from one of the previous attempts to close his fistula; and so we took him back to the operating room later that same day and closed that fistula, transperineally as before.

The following day, I went back to see him again and was again pleased to see him standing by his bed, although not quite as robust as the previous day. "Thank you so much," he said, "I am very grateful to you for doing the operation but why am I still passing feces in my urine?" A further contrast study showed a second vesicocolic fistula higher up than the other. We went back to the operating room and this time did a transabdominal closure of that fistula. The following morning I went back to see him. This time he was unable to stand by his bed, not surprisingly, and when he said "Thank you very much for doing the operation," I was terrified he was going to tell me about feces in his urine again, but on that third occasion we had finally dealt with the problem – at last.

I learned two lessons from that experience. Firstly, if somebody has had an injury and has one problem as a consequence of it he may well have a second or third problem as well: I have come across this situation several times. The second lesson I learned was never to trust other people's results or reports of x-ray studies without the images. I have experienced this type of problem many times. An investigator, when he is a surgeon, and particularly when he is not, never has quite the same attitude toward an investigation and its interpretation, if he himself is not going to be doing the surgery. Get your own investigations and review them carefully yourself.

Vena Caval Injury

C.A. Olsson

I have encountered vena caval problems on two different occasions during my lifetime. Fortunately, all caval injury cases were successfully managed. In this brief presentation, I will explain how I was able to secure the caval injury without losing the patient.

On two separate occasions, I was urgently called to the operating room because of a caval injury. The first instance was when I was hosting a visiting professor who was carrying out a nephrectomy with our resident staff. The second occasion was when one of my junior faculty was carrying out a radical nephrectomy whereupon I was called urgently to the OR for consultation.

In both instances, the persons in the OR took the appropriate initial stance. Obviously, whenever a caval injury occurs, there is a considerable amount of blood loss and the individuals in the operating room have to make the appropriate initial responses. The initial responses are simply to use sponge sticks to occlude the area of blood leakage from the cava and have the anesthesia team vigorously replenish the rapid loss of blood.

What should be done then? Obviously, as soon as the sponge sticks are removed from the area of vena cava laceration, considerable blood loss will again ensue. What I have found useful in the these circumstances is to have the scrub nurse supply me with a set of long Allis clamps.

By gravitating the sponge sticks either upward from the caval defect or downward, the defect can be identified serially, and be pinched off by grasping the defect in the long Allis forceps. Once the entire defect has been clamped by Allis clamps, the suturing of the caval defect can be achieved without the intrusive presence of sponge sticks, which would prevent appropriate suturing. As the suturing proceeds from either cephalad-caudad or vice versa, the Allis clamps can be serially removed with no further bleeding. I generally ask for a double-armed 5-0 Prolene for this maneuver. I generally have the 5-0 Prolene placed roughly equidistantly at one end or the other of the defect and tie three or four knots at that end. Thereafter, I sew each suture down to the end of the defect, removing the Allis clamps along the way as I secure the defects held by the clamps. I then "baseball" the stitch with the opposite limb, taking care not to disturb the first suture line, but placing new sutures equidistantly between the previously sewn sutures. At the conclusion of the procedure, six or seven rows of knots are sufficient and the Prolene ends can be cut, removing the needles from the OR field.

As mentioned above, this is a circumstance in which there is an impressive amount of calamity in the operating room. The surgeons responsible for the caval laceration or loss of the ligature around the renal vein have the greatest responsibility for the lifesaving procedure. Immediate pressure on the cava in the region of the defect is mandatory. However, if you are called to salvage the situation, you must keep in mind that as soon as the emergent techniques are removed, there is considerable additional blood loss. By sliding downward or upward from the point of the defect, the serial application of the long Allis clamps will stop the bleeding and allow sufficient freedom to oversew any defect that might be present.

False Sepsis and Advanced TCC

C.A. Olsson

I have seen two circumstances in my lifetime where a patient with transitional cell cancer (usually well advanced) has presented with significant leukocytosis and fever. The very presence of these two findings would keep your medical consultants from allowing you to intervene surgically in such cases for fear of engendering urosepsis. However, after seeing that both blood and urine cultures are negative, and instituting a raft of antibiotic support, there comes a time when one should respect the fact that leukocytosis and febrile reactions are common in advanced TCC.

I first learned this about 5 years ago when a single article appeared in the Japanese literature reviewing a case of a patient with metastatic TCC syndrome, fevers of unknown origin, and aggressive leukocytosis (in the mid-20,000 range). Having struggled with the patients that I was caring for and deferring resectional biopsies repeatedly because of the fear of urosepsis, we finally had to bite the bullet and respect the concept that this was "tumor fever" and "tumor leukocytosis" as well. I should mention that in the Japanese report and in the two cases that I have experienced over the years, the outcome was not good. In all three instances, the patient expired in the very near future after exhibiting these two findings.

Laparoscopic Vascular Emergency

V. Pansadoro

In the majority of cases, bleeding during a laparoscopic procedure can be managed conservatively. Initial compression and subsequent suture are the best way to handle the problem. The situation is different when there is substantial bleeding from major vessels, most frequently venous vessels. These are true vascular emergencies, when the surgical team must work as a unit and everything needed has to be readily available.

The main problem is in the delay needed to prepare the surgical instruments and to convert the procedure to open surgery. The first goal is to reduce blood loss during the few minutes necessary to have access to the surgical instruments and to open the patient. In the case of arterial bleeding, compression is the best option.

If a major vein has been opened the gas pressure inside the abdominal cavity can be raised to 20 mm Hg until the abdomen is opened.

I would like to describe a rare experience in a 72-year-old gentlemen with a right upper pole renal cell carcinoma that was responsible for causing a huge hematoma. Because of the presence of the hematoma, which surrounded the upper pole and the vena cava, a retroperitoneal approach was chosen to provide easy access to the renal artery. With the patient in a straightforward flank position, the retroperitoneal space was created, first manually and then with a balloon, in the usual way. After opening Gerota's fascia, the artery was prepared with no problems, double-clipped with Hem-o-lock, and severed. The renal vein was then prepared accordingly. A right-angle clamp was passed around the vein and a space created. At this time, the entire renal vein suddenly broke and the limited retroperitoneal space was filled with blood. Conversion was clearly inevitable. The surgeon moved to the other side of the operating table and a very quick and appropriate flank incision was performed. The tear in the cava was largely due to the damaged tissue and it was not possible to apply a vascular clamp of appropriate size and angle.

In the early 1980s, I attended a session of "clinical weekends" in Bern, at Insel Spital, organized by Prof. Ernst Zingg. During this meeting, a vascular surgeon demonstrated a series of vascular emergencies and their repair on pigs.

One of the vascular accidents was a large hole in the vena cava and the simple management was the introduction of a finger, inside the hole, to stop the blood loss.

At the time, I greatly appreciated the surgical tip but luckily I had never needed to use it.

At that very moment, I realized it was time to use the almost forgotten trick: after introducing the left index finger inside the hole in the cava, the bleeding stopped almost immediately. Once visibility was obtained, it was easy to perform a running suture with a Prolene 4-0 and obtain complete hemostasis.

Lessons to be learned:

1. Don't stretch the indications for laparoscopic surgery.
2. Always have a conversion kit, ready for use, in the operating room.

Percutaneous Nephrolithotomy

E. Perez-Castro E.

After visiting several university hospitals in Germany to watch the percutaneous nephrolithotomy (PCNL) procedures, a colleague and I planned to return to Madrid with the desire to start this technique in our university hospital.

My colleague and friend would perform the percutaneous access and dilation of the tract and I would do the endoscopic part.

We carefully selected the case: a slim female patient with a solitary 1.5-cm stone in the renal pelvis and moderate dilation.

Everything went fine: perfect renal access on the third try and dilation without problems. We changed positions and I passed the nephroscope into the kidney. There was the calculus! Right in front of me! Looking at me! After such encouragement I took the forceps, strongly grasped the stone (which was hard and did not break) and, thinking I was in the bladder, pulled out everything – nephroscope, forceps and stone – but obviously there was no urethra to go back in easily.

The patient went back to her room with neither stone nor nephrostomy tube, with only a ureteral catheter and a Foley, and was very well escorted by both of us, who kept our eyes on her and prayed for an outcome with no complications.

Only many months later did we read publications about this innovative (not for us), tubeless, technical option for percutaneous surgery. Because the patient had a perfect recovery and was discharged home in record time in comparison to standard surgery, we have been using this procedure ever since.

Bladder Tumor

E. Perez-Castro E.

We describe a singular experience that I had not seen before nor since. I have not read a similar case report in the urologic literature.

This case was a patient with an infiltrative bladder tumor that we had diagnosed by TURBT. He was treated with definitive radiotherapy with sensitizing chemotherapy.

A few months later, we performed an endoscopic bladder biopsy and we found a very irregular urethral stenosis, which we thought was secondary to the radiotherapy. In subsequent endoscopies, the stenosis was worsening despite a Sachse urethrotomy.

During one of the cystoscopies, we made several urethral incisions in different areas, but vision was almost null because of multiple areas of stenosis. One of my colleagues was helping me by compressing the saline irrigation bags to increase flow. In time, we realized there was some extravasation to the genital area (penis and scrotum), but it was moderate. I tried to see to be able to cut, and we continued to apply pressure to the irrigant bag.

All of a sudden, we heard a terrifying explosion, very loud, louder than the sound made by the rubber tube exploding off the O2 line, louder than the explosion I have also heard (fortunately only a few times) when you have a gas explosion within the bladder during a TUR of a dome tumor.

We stopped the procedure to explore the origin of the sound and we found the scrotum had exploded. There was a neat opening along the raphe, as if done with a scalpel, with copious serous drainage. A very unpleasant sight.

The procedure was completed, eventually accessing the bladder with the Sachse and performing a bladder biopsy. We sutured the scrotum with very good clinical and cosmetic results, and the only problem we had was several millimeters narrowing of . . . our own coronary arteries

Frenulum

E. Perez-Castro E.

Twenty-five years ago, open discussion of sex in our country (Spain) was taboo; nobody talked about it and there were no office visits for impotence.

One night, while I was on call at the ward of the Hospital Universitario La Paz in Madrid, a young man came to the emergency room at 3:00 a.m. with severe bleeding from the penile frenulum, with an almost complete rupture of the penile skin.

Once the wound was cleaned and prepared for surgical repair under local anesthesia, I asked the patient several innocuous questions to calm him down. One of the questions (although already obvious to me), was "how had this injury occurred?"

Very seriously, he explained that he was walking on the street and suddenly, he did not know how, he lost his footing and fell on the curb of the street, unfortunately hitting his penis!

I answered, also very seriously, that it was an interesting etiology – new for me – and I advised him to warn his friends about the risks of walking alone at night in Madrid.

Penile Fracture Associated with Urethral Rupture and Its Complex Repair

S.V. Perovic

Sexual activity provides great enjoyment and is very important for quality of life, but sometimes can be disastrous for a man. This occurred to our patient who fractured his penis during sexual intercourse when his extremely rigid penis slipped out of the vagina hitting the pubis of his female partner. The result of this accident was penile fracture with concomitant complete urethral rupture.

The patient was admitted to our institution 6 h after the accident. He reported he had heard a cracking sound followed by immediate loss of erection, onset of severe pain, and penile deformity with discoloration due to a huge hematoma; he also had bleeding from the urethra and could not urinate.

The patient immediately underwent surgery with no further investigation because signs of complex penile trauma were obvious. Surgery was performed via circumferential subcoronal incision. After evacuation of the huge hematoma, a very large ventral albuginea tear and complete urethral rapture were identified. The patient was very lucky: the surgeon who performed the surgery was experienced in penile and urethral recon-

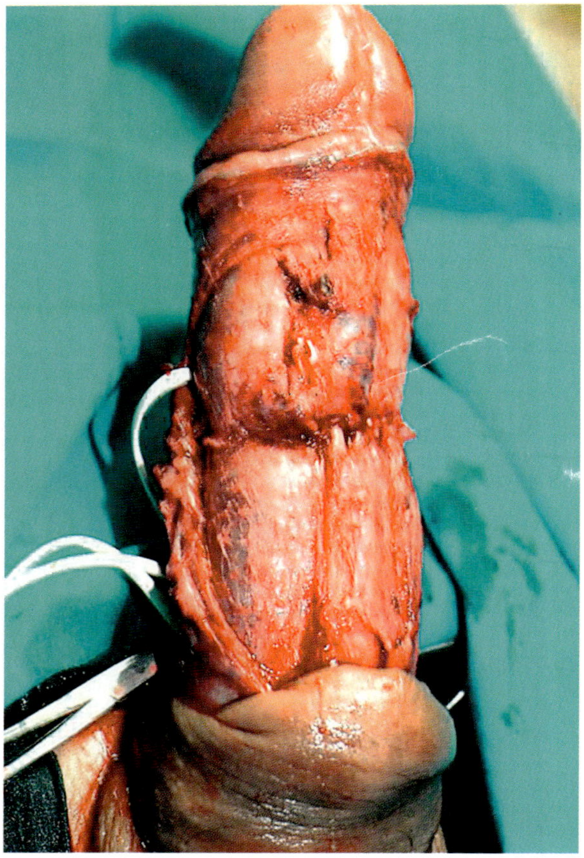

Fig. 21.26.1. After penile degloving and NVB mobilization, a very large ventral albuginea tear involving both cavernosal bodies with urethral rupture is seen

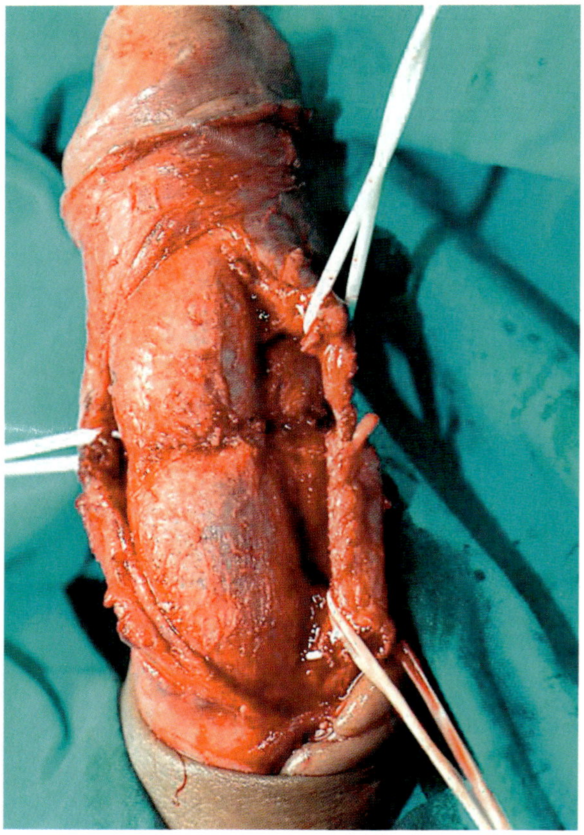

Fig. 21.26.2. After urethral mobilization, complete urethral rupture is obvious

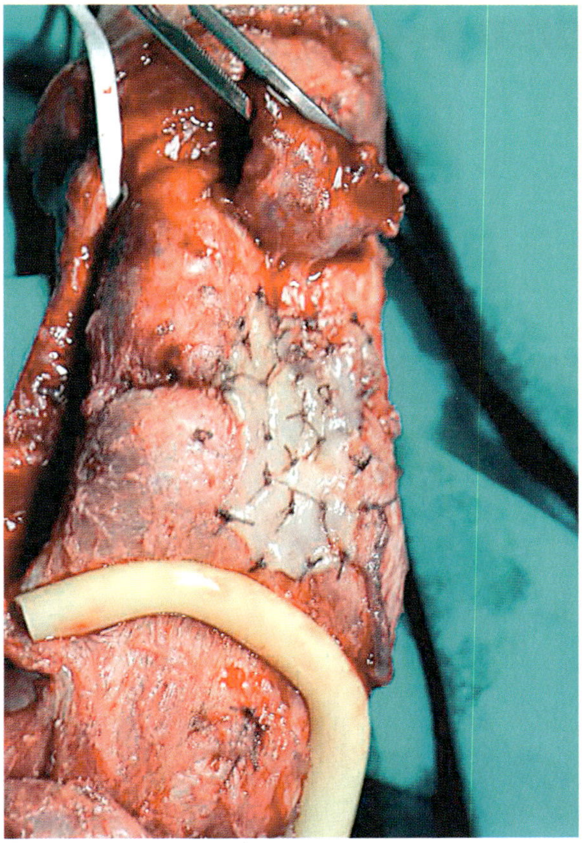

Fig. 21.26.3. Buccal mucosa graft is used both to cover the cavernosal defect and to augment urethral anastomotic repair as a dorsal roof

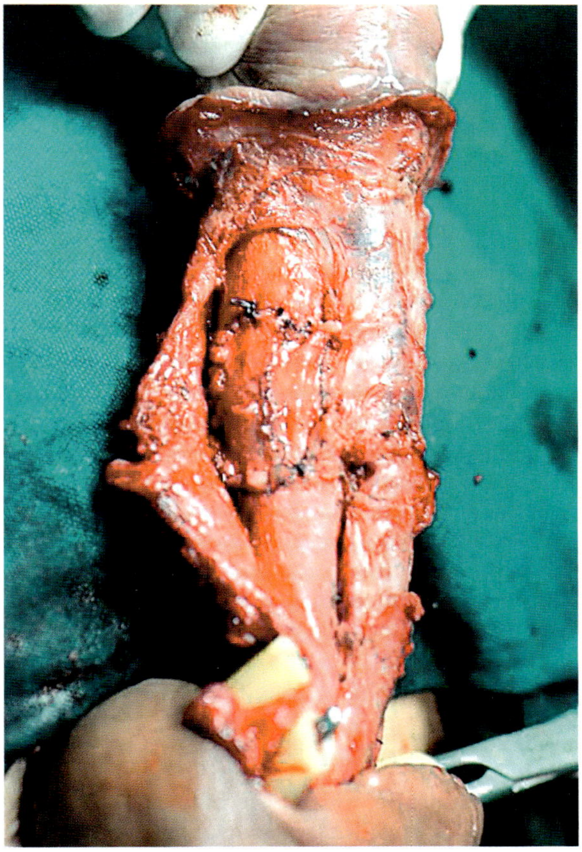

Fig. 21.26.4. Remaining cavernosal defect is grafted with saphenous vein

structive surgery. Augmented anastomotic urethral repair with dorsal buccal mucosa roofing and reconstruction of the corpora by saphenous graft was carried out. A 12-F Foley catheter was placed for 7 days as a stent as well as suprapubic urinary drainage for 3 weeks to prevent formation of a urethrocavernosal fistula. Follow-up 1 year after surgery by urethrography and flexible urethroscopy demonstrated excellent urethral patency and normal penile contour with full rigid erection (Figs. 21.26.1 – 21.26.4).

Fracture of the penis is considered a rare trauma, but we believe it is an underreported one. Details of proper treatment remain uncertain; some authors recommend conservative management or delayed surgical repair, while others advocate immediate surgery. In the complex penile fracture associated with urethral rupture, only prompt surgery can provide good functional and aesthetic results. Experience with penile and urethral surgery is crucial to avoid postoperative complications such as penile curvature, corporeal narrowing, and urethral strictures.

Low-Flow Priapism in Children

S.V. Perovic

As with many surgical emergencies, the saying “time is tissue” holds true for priapism. This condition is a true urological emergency and early intervention provides the best chance of functional recovery. It has been described at nearly all ages. Idiopathic low-flow ischemic priapism in the pediatric population is extremely rare.

A 7-year-old boy was admitted to our emergency department 5 days after the onset of painful rigid erection. He underwent thorough examination and no predisposing condition was found. Because of the long duration of the priapism, we decided to start with immediate surgical, instead of conservative treatment. Cavernosal bodies were punctured with two 19-gauge needles through the glans and dark blood was aspirated; blood gas analysis showed pH 6.8, PCO_2 68 mm Hg, and PO2 24 mm Hg, which clearly indicated severe ischemic priapism. Since this was not sufficient for penile detumescence, a small lateral corporotomy was performed and blood with some clots was aspirated. Cavernosal bodies were irrigated with phenylephrine solution (10 mg phenylephrine in 1,000 ml of 9% saline) (Figs. 21.27.1 – 21.27.4).

After thorough irrigation and appearance of bright red blood, the tunica albuginea and skin were closed with loose sutures to allow postoperative drainage. Immediately after surgery, the penis was in incomplete detumescence and 24 h later in complete detumescence. Biopsy of cavernosal muscle showed beginning of muscle necrosis. One year after surgery, the parents reported that the child had spontaneous erections and the PGE1 test showed almost full erection.

Despite long-lasting priapism, children have a higher recovery potential than adults and aggressive surgical approach may preserve erectile function.

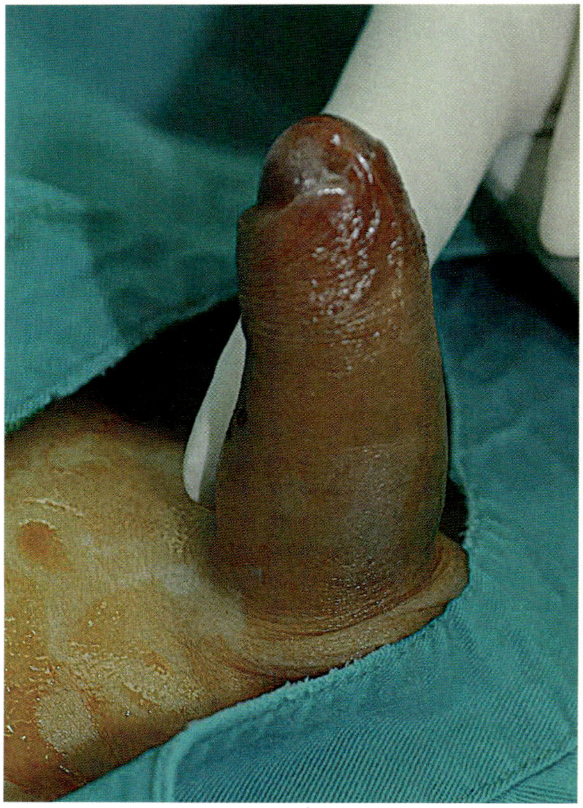

Fig. 21.27.1. Full rigid erection in a 7-year-old boy

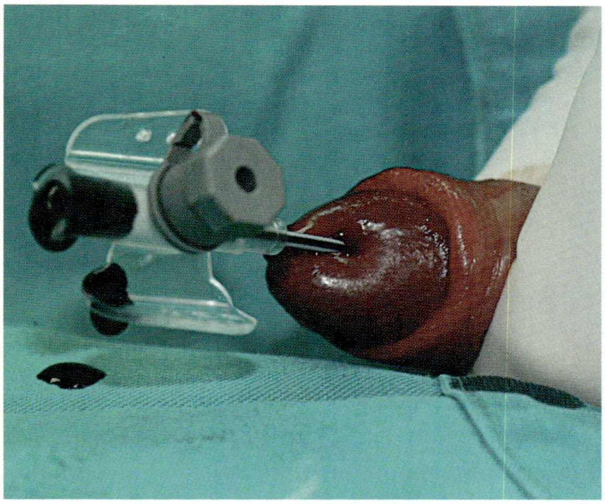

Fig. 21.27.2. Transglanular puncture of the cavernosal body showed dark blood, a sign of ischemic priapism

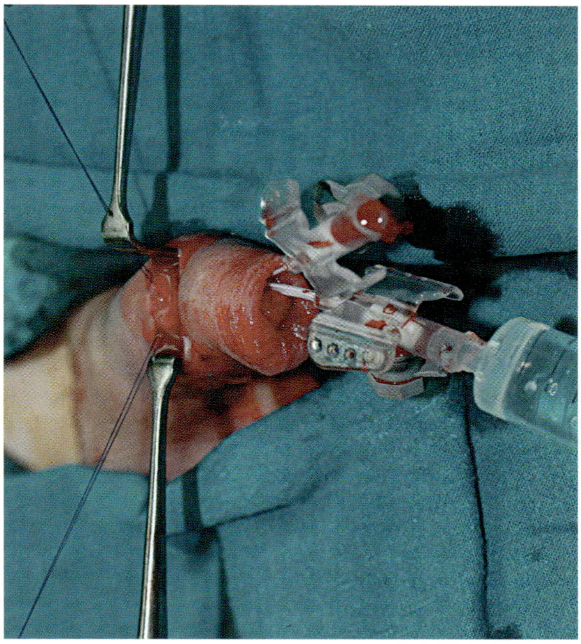

Fig. 21.27.3. Irrigation through a needle combined with lateral corporotomy resulted in red blood appearing

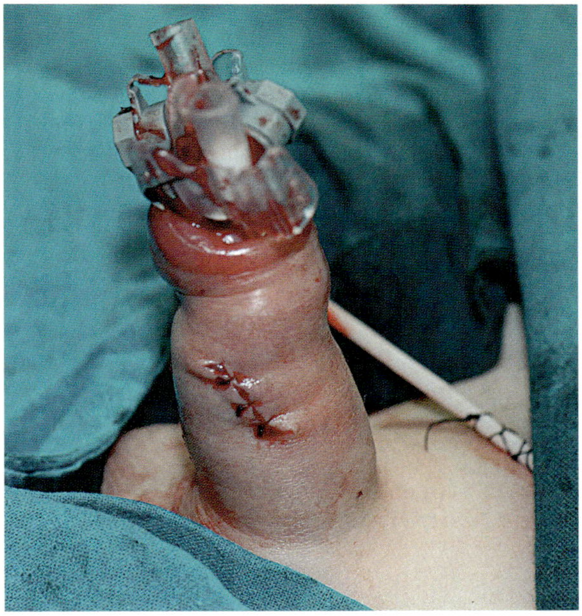

Fig. 21.27.4. Cavernosal bodies and skin closed with rare sutures, punctured needles left for irrigation and suprapubic urinary drainage is placed

Tragic Complications of Missed Urethral Injury

E. Pontes

A 21-year-old African-American male was brought to the emergency room of a suburban community hospital following a motorcycle accident. The patient had sustained severe injuries, including a fracture of the right femur and a pelvic fracture. In the emergency room, a Foley catheter was placed without any evaluation of a possible urologic injury. The patient was taken to the operating room and the fracture of the femur repaired. On the third postoperative day, the Foley was removed but the patient experienced difficulty in voiding, at which time the catheter was reinserted. Another attempt at voiding was attempted 1 day later with similar results. At that point, it was noticed that the patient was septic and had severe perineal and lower abdominal swelling.

He was then transferred to the Detroit Receiving Hospital where a urethrogram reviewed a rupture of the prostate-membranous urethra with extravasation and urinary phlegmon. During this surgical exploration, debridement of the scrotum, the perineum, and the lower abdominal wall up to the level of umbilicus was performed. A suprapubic cystostomy was placed. After several weeks of care and multiple skin grafts, the patient was sent home in good condition (Fig. 21.28.1).

The moral of the story is that missed GU injuries can have devastating effects on the patient!

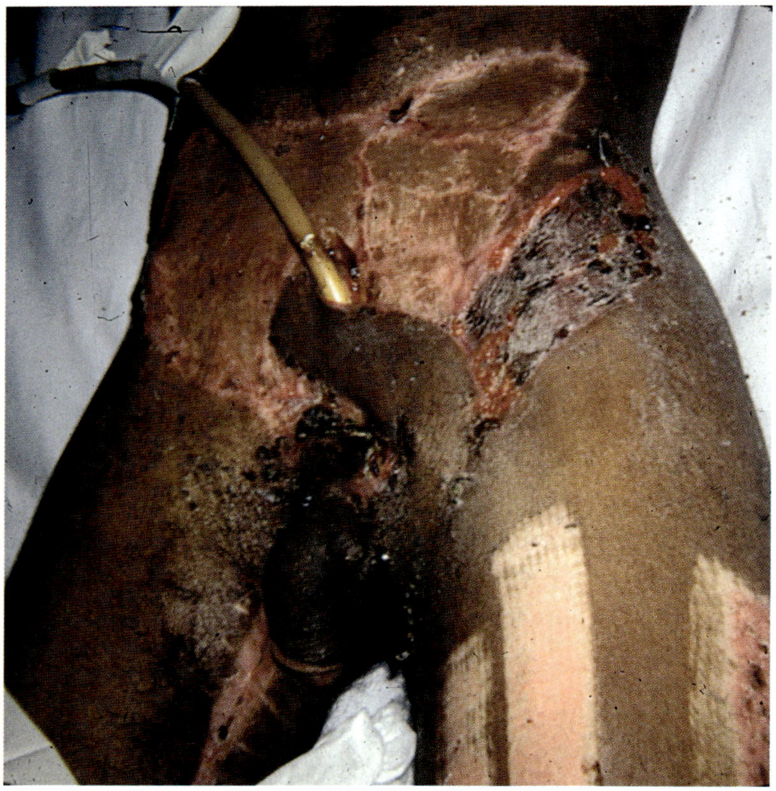

Fig. 21.28.1. After split thickness skin graft for Fournier's gangrene caused by missed urethral injury resulting from pelvic fracture

Keep Looking

R. Santucci

I recently treated an unconscious male who had suffered a small-caliber handgun gunshot wound to the pelvis and immediately had gross blood per urethra and inability to void. A retrograde urethrogram was obtained, which showed posterior urethral disruption. Per our protocol, we made a single unsuccessful attempt at gentle placement of a Foley catheter. Also per our usual protocol, the patient was then brought to the operating room for an attempt at endoscopic placement of a Foley catheter, or failing that, a suprapubic tube. During flexible cystoscopy, a large defect in the posterior urethra was seen, a defect that seemed much more than would be seen by a small-caliber bullet wound. While attempting to find the proximal urethra with the scope, a glint of shiny metal was seen (Fig. 21.29.1). Closer examination revealed the broken off tip of a knife! This explained why instead of a small, neat bullet hole in the urethral we found a completely divided urethra, cut in half by a thin knife that left little sign of skin entry.

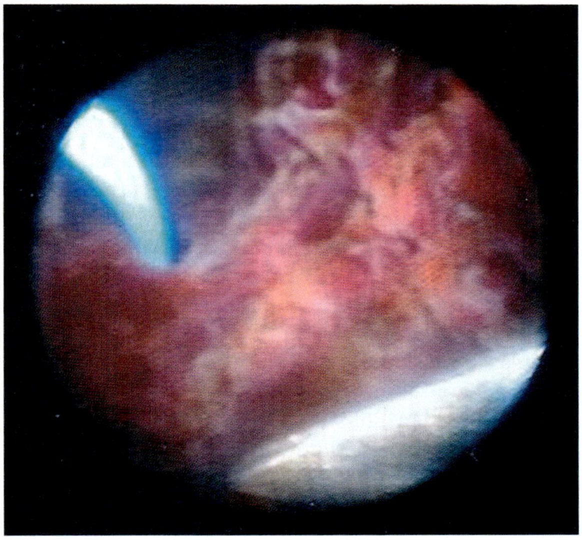

Fig. 21.29.1

We realized that his gunshot wound was incidental, and later discovered, when we spoke to the patient after he awakened, that he had indeed been viciously stabbed in the perineum. The knife had lodged in his pubic bone and the tip had broken off. We were eventually able to retrieve the knife tip with a cystoscopic grasper, and were also able to gain entry into the bladder for Foley placement. In trauma, one must keep one's mind open. The injury you are treating may not be the injury the patient actually has.

What Goes in Must Come Out

R. Santucci

Everyone knows that extraperitoneal bladder lacerations are usually benign. They most often heal spontaneously with a period of catheter drainage. However, they are not, I have found, always completely benign.

I once had an elderly female patient with neurogenic bladder who was managed with the placement of a suprapubic tube. The tube was placed uneventfully, using an endoscopic approach with a Lowsley retractor. In the subsequent days, she had persistent hematuria, presumably from a lacerated bladder vessel. She developed clot retention and we brought her back to the operating room for clot evacuation and cystoscopic examination to ensure that nothing else was amiss. During routine clot evacuation, a large amount of fluid was irrigated into the bladder, both during cystoscopy and during aggressive clot evacuation with an Ellik evacuator. The bladder was eventually emptied of blood, and as is common with these cases, after the blood was removed and the bladder decompressed, the bladder bleeding stopped.

In the recovery room, the patient could not be extubated. She had poor inspiratory effort and she was eventually sent to the intensive care unit, intubated. A plain film of the chest showed a bilaterally elevated diaphragm. A CT scan of the abdomen and chest were obtained and they showed massive *extraperitoneal* extravasation of saline from our cystoscopy. The entire retroperitoneum was ballooned out and upward, but the intraperitoneal space was dry. The massively inflated retroperitoneum put upward pressure on the diaphragm, and in this elderly, compromised patient led to respiratory failure. In 24 h, the fluid resorbed and she could be extubated.

Not all extraperitoneal lacerations are benign.

Metabolic Dangers of the Neobladder

M. Schumacher, U.E. Studer

In a 63-year-old male, a cystectomy and continent urinary diversion were performed for muscle-invasive transitional cell carcinoma of the bladder. The postoperative course was uneventful and the patient was discharged from the hospital with a base excess of –0.5 mmol/l. He was instructed to drink at least 2 l of fluid per day and to increase his salt intake. Additionally, he received sodium bicarbonate 3 g orally per day.

Five days later, he had to be rehospitalized because of severe dehydration associated with vomiting and weight loss (3 kg). The skin color was grayish and he was increasingly disorientated. The venous blood gas analysis showed a base excess of –9.7 mmol/l. Emergency treatment consisted of fluid substitution with 3 l of Ringer's lactate and increased sodium bicarbonate dosage to 6 g per day. The reservoir was catheterized with a 20-F indwelling catheter to empty the neobladder and therefore reduce the contact time of urine with the intestine.

The next day, venous blood gas analysis showed a base excess of –3.4 mmol/l and the patient was feeling well. After a few days of observation, he left the hospital and was supplemented with 6 g sodium bicarbonate orally per day until his next visit at our outpatient clinic.

After cystectomy and continent urinary diversion with an ileal neobladder, most patients have to be supplemented with sodium bicarbonate for a period of 4–6 weeks. In case of severe dehydration, generous fluid and sodium bicarbonate substitution, together with continuous drainage of the neobladder with an indwelling catheter have a dramatic effect in resuscitation of these patients.

Torsion After Minor Insult

E. Serafetinides

A 21-year-old soldier was working out in his company's gym. While practicing some wrestling techniques, he felt a sharp pain in the left testis. He completed his session and at the end of the session he reported his problem to his company's paramedic. The latter warned him that he might lose his position on the wrestling team and gave him a non-steroid anti-inflammatory tablet. The pain eased for a few hours and the soldier returned to duty. During the night he awoke with great scrotal discomfort. When he presented to the infirmary, he had a large painful swelling in the left scrotum. The testis could not be palpated. He was transferred to the hospital and a Doppler ultrasound revealed a nonfunctioning left testis. Later the same night, exploration revealed torsion and a small hematoma of the left testis. Orchiectomy was carried out at the same time.

A minor injury of a testis during sports may incite torsion. Physical examination and adequate evaluation is mandatory in young men complaining of testis pain.

Fleas *and* Lice at the Same Time

E. SERAFETINIDES

A 27-year-old resident in radiology presented in the urology department complaining of renal colic. He had a family history of renal lithiasis and reported frequent incidents of renal colic and spontaneous hematuria during the last 6 months. Anti-inflammatory medication had occasionally been given to him. He was advised to have an ultrasound examination. The ultrasound findings showed a medium dilatation of the left ureter and renal pelvis, several stones in the left kidney, 0.5–0.8 mm in size, and a 3.5×2.5-cm lesion on the bladder wall. A cystoscopy revealed a TCC close to the left ureteric orifice. The young radiologist had a TUR bladder 2 days later. Histopathologic examination confirmed the presence of a Grade 1, pTa TCC.

A previously known disease does not exclude a patient from investigation if signs and symptoms are suggestive.

Continent Urinary Diversion for the Treatment of Urinary Fistulae Through a Sacral Scar in a Paraplegic Patient

F. Trigo-Rocha

A 53-year-old male initially suffering from spinal cord injury was referred from another unit. He had a T8–T9 complete lesion due to a car accident dating from September 1996. Since then he had complete paraplegia. The urological management consisted in the use of an indwelling catheter followed by a condom collector. During rehabilitation, he had adapted well to the wheel chair. However, during progression of his condition he presented several symptomatic urinary tract infections and sacral scars. He was referred to our department 2 years later.

In the initial evaluation in our department in 1999, the main complaints were urinary and fecal incontinence, urinary tract infections, and sacral scarring from decubiti. Physical examination showed complete absence of movement in the legs and absence of sensitivity bellow the umbilicus. Bulbocavernous reflex was present and the anal sphincter had normal tonus. There was a superficial sacral scar extending to the perineum.

The blood analyses showed normal levels of creatinine. However, an ultrasound showed bilateral upper urinary tract dilation. A urodynamic test showed significant reduction in bladder capacity due to detrusor hyperactivity, low compliance, and a high detrusor leak point pressure (DLPP = 90 cm H_2O). A voiding cystourethrogram was performed and showed bilateral grade IV vesicoureteral reflux. The therapeutic alternatives were discussed and the patient was treated by sphincterotomy.

He had good recovery with no symptomatic infections for 1 year and partial remission of upper urinary tract dilation. After 1 year, he was admitted in the general surgery emergency unit with a severe perineal infection, with fever and urethral erosion. There was urine drainage through the perineum. He received general support measures and antibiotics. After general conditions had improved, he underwent surgery to clean the perineal wound and a colostomy was made in the right angle of the colon to avoid contact of stool with the perineum.

After being discharged, he returned to the urological unit with a large perineal lesion, significant urethral erosion, and urinary drainage through the perineum (Fig. 21.34.1). We decided to treat him by bladder neck closure, bladder augmentation, and a continent stoma. As he had an excluded left colon, our option was to use this segment to perform bladder augmentation and also to create the continent stoma using the Monti technique (Fig. 21.34.2). He had a good postoperative recovery and was discharged with a cystostomy after 1 week. One month later, he was able to perform intermittent self-catheterization, was dry, and the cystostomy tube was removed. After removing the urine drainage, the perineal decubitus healed very well and after

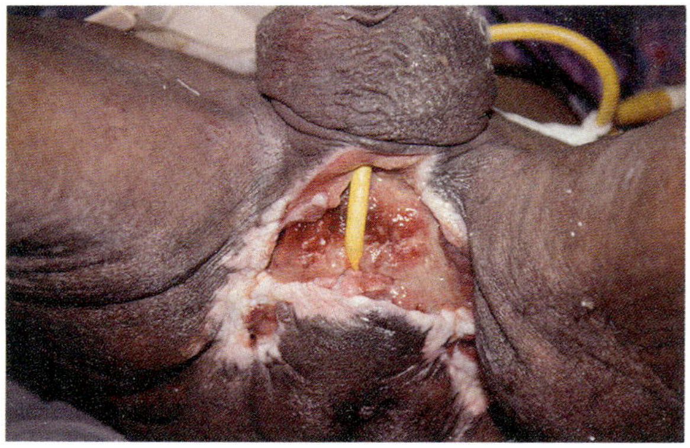

Fig. 21.34.1. Patient after the colostomy with a large perineal scar and urethral erosion

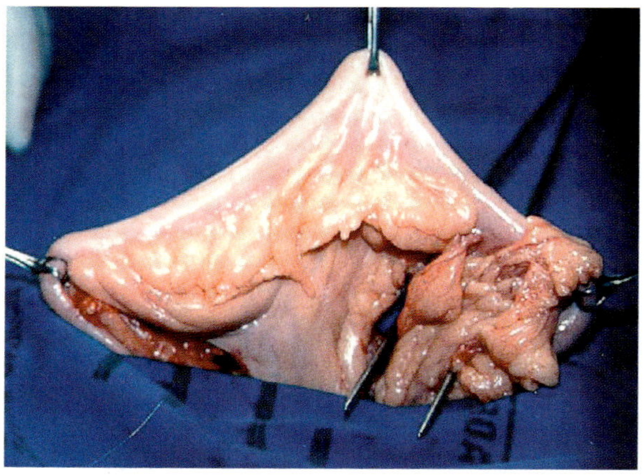

Fig. 21.34.2. A 20-cm sigma segment utilized for bladder augmentation together with a 3-cm segment utilized for stoma creation

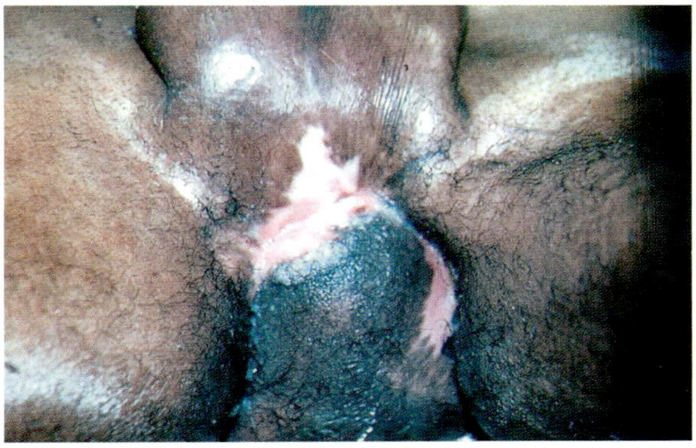

Fig. 21.34.3. Final result showing complete resolution of the perineal scar

3 months plastic surgeons treated him with a skin flap rotation with no complications and complete closure of the scar (Fig. 21.34.3). Six months later, ultrasound showed only mild renal dilation, urodynamics showed good bladder capacity (400 cc), normal compliance, and a continent stoma, even during high-pressure Valsalva maneuvers.

Currently, at the 5-year follow-up, the patient remains continent, performing catheterism through the stoma four times a day. He has not presented with symptomatic urinary tract infections or new decubiti. He has adapted well to colostomy and he declined to have it closed.

We conclude that continent urinary diversion could be a good solution for paraplegic patients with large perineal decubitus. The use of an excluded bowel segment in patients with colostomy may reduce surgical morbidity.

Entrapped Foley Catheter After Radical Prostatectomy

N.L. TÜRKERI

A 62-year-old male patient was diagnosed with prostate cancer after TRUS-guided biopsy prompted by a PSA level of 5.6 ng/ml. Pathological examination revealed adenocarcinoma of the prostate, a Gleason score of 3+3=6, and five out of 12 cores were positive for cancer. A baseline bone scintigraphy was negative for metastatic disease and abdominal ultrasonography revealed normal kidneys and bladder. After discussion of possible treatment options, he decided for radical retropubic prostatectomy, which was performed 6 weeks after the biopsy. The surgery and postoperative period were uneventful and his drain came out on postoperative day 3. Retrograde cystography was performed on day 7 and showed no extravasation and catheter removal was planned. However, after deflation of the Foley catheter balloon, it was not possible to withdraw the catheter. Further tension on the catheter produced significant pain and a small amount of bleeding per urethra. The catheter was then twisted 720° around itself to set it free, with no success. A repeat cystography confirmed the watertight anastomosis and complete deflation of the catheter balloon. A few hours later, another attempt to withdraw the catheter was again unsuccessful. The patient was then taken to the OR and under general anesthesia his entire urethra and the site of urethrovesical anastomosis was examined using a 7-F. A semirigid ureteroscope passed alongside the catheter. At the site of anastomosis, it was noted that the Foley was entrapped by left lower quadrant anastomotic suture, which had formed a tight loop around the catheter and tightened further when pulled back. Since it was not possible to release the catheter by further maneuvers applied on the catheter, a 200-μm holmium laser probe was inserted through the ureteroscope and the suture was cut using a low-power setting, which immediately released the catheter. The patient had no further problems, voided spontaneously with no difficulty, and had minimal stress incontinence with complete urinary control within 2 weeks of the operation.

Unexpected Inferior Vena Caval Thrombus

E.D. Vaughan, Jr.

The Problem

The patient was undergoing a routine left radical nephrectomy through an 11th rib flank approach. Preoperative CT revealed a 7-cm central solid renal mass without renal vein or nodal involvement. MRI confirmed the CT and the inferior vena cava (IVC) was normal without tumor involvement.

Upon exposure of the renal vein, a freely movable thrombus was palpated. The distal extent could not be palpated. Further dissection to the IVC revealed that the thrombus had entered the IVC and continued as high as could be palpated.

The Solution

The anesthesia team was asked to obtain an intraesophageal ultrasound device; using this technique the entire vena cava could be visualized to the right atria. The thrombus extended just below the hepatic veins, but was thin and it could be seen to move freely in the IVC. The kidney was totally mobilized, the renal artery ligated so that the renal vein with the thrombus was the last structure to be divided. With a vascular clamp in place but not applied and manual compression of the renal vein, the anterior wall of the vein was opened, the tumor thrombus extracted, the clamp applied, and the remaining vein divided and suture ligated. Blood loss was minimal and the patient recovered fully.

Comment

Mobile IVC tumor extensions from renal tumors can be missed on MRI because of the motion of the tumor. If there is any suspicion of IVC involvement a preoperative transesophageal sonographic study will avoid the problem encountered in this case. As illustrated, if an unexpected thrombosis is encountered, the emergency use of transesophageal ultrasound can give information to help plan corrective action. In this case, the thrombus was freely movable and easily extractable. If this had not been the case we would have extended the incision and handled the IVC in a standard fashion for a level three thrombus.

The Lord of the Rings – Fournier's Gangrene as a Consequence of Strangulating Testicular Rings

N. Zantl, R. Hartung

Fournier's gangrene is a rare but life-threatening, special form of dermal necrosis located in the genitourinary region. Mortality rates range from 4% to 43% in actual series (Dahm et al. 2000; Mindrup et al. 2005; Yeniyol et al. 2004; Korkut et al. 2003; Burdal et al. 2003; Chawla et al. 2003; Asci et al. 1998; Nisbet and Tompson 2002; Corman et al. 1999; Korhonen et al. 1998; Hollabaugh et al. 1998; Benizri et al. 1996; Palmer et al. 1995). The main treatment principle is an immediate, extensive debridement of the entire necrotic tissue under concurrent broad-spectrum antibiotic therapy. Reconstruction can be performed only when the wound is free from infection. In this chapter, we report a case of Fournier's gangrene caused by the deterioration of the blood supply caused by scrotal rings and discuss etiology, symptoms, and treatment of Fournier's gangrene.

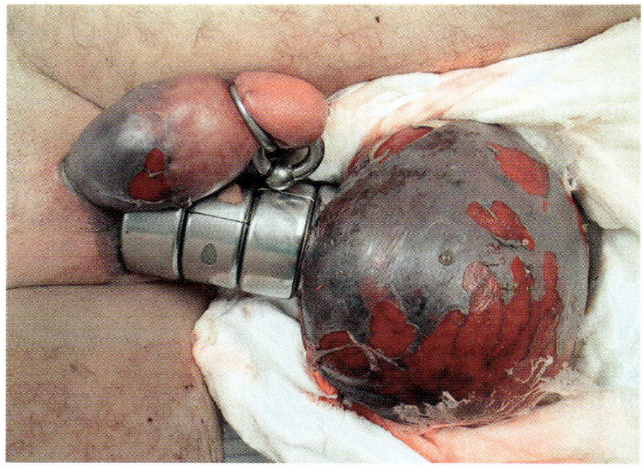

Fig. 21.37.1. Three scrotal rings were put around the scrotal base over 2 years. The third ring had deteriorated the blood supply to such an extent that necrosis of the scrotal skin resulted. Typical for Fournier's gangrene is the overlapping of the gangrene to healthy tissue, not affected by the ischemia. Note also the penile piercings

Report of the Case

A 42-year-old man was admitted to our department in a highly compromised condition. The temperature was 39.8 °C, the heart rate was 120 bpm, and his blood pressure was 100/60 mm Hg. He presented a leukocytosis of 19.60×109 cells/l (normal, 4.0 – 9.0), fibrinogen of 624 µg/l (normal, < 192), C-reactive protein of 7.4 mg/dl (normal, 0.5) (74 mg/l; normal, 5). Figure 21.37.1 shows the initial condition of his genital region. Over the previous 2 years he had put three metal rings around the base of his scrotum, the last ring obviously intensely deteriorating the blood supply and thus resulting in necrosis of the scrotal skin. Interestingly, the gangrenous delineation exceeded the proximal border of the most proximal ring, which is a typical property of Fournier's gangrene.

After initial assessment of physical and medical findings, after clinical stabilization, fluid resuscitation and application of broad-spectrum antibiotics, we immediately brought the patient into the operating room where we removed the foreign bodies with the help of the fire department, using their heavy equipment (the metal rings were fixed with some kind of "super glue," which made it impossible to disassemble them). Figure 21.37.2a shows this procedure. Note the ice cooling during the usage of the angle grinder. Figure 21.37.2b shows the remnants of the three rings; Fig. 21.37.3 shows the patients genitalia freed of the metal rings.

We then proceeded with the debridement of the entire necrotic skin, including a resection of approximately 0.5 cm in macroscopically healthy tissue. The right testicle was also necrotic, resulting in the indication of right-sided orchiectomy. Figure 21.37.4 shows the extent of the resection 1 week later. The spermatic cord is elongated due to the chronic overexpansion caused by the scrotal rings. We provided daily changes of the wound dressings, including wound cleaning and flushing, and performed two additional wound debridements during the course of treatment.

After 16 days, the denuded tissue showed no more signs of inflammation and appeared clean. Only then was plastic coverage performed in the lithotomy position with a Foley catheter inserted. Granulation tissue was completely removed. The dorsal part of the perineal wound was directly sutured. The penile skin defect was covered with a split-thickness skin graft without meshing in order to give it as much resistibility for potential mechanical exposure in the future, whereas all

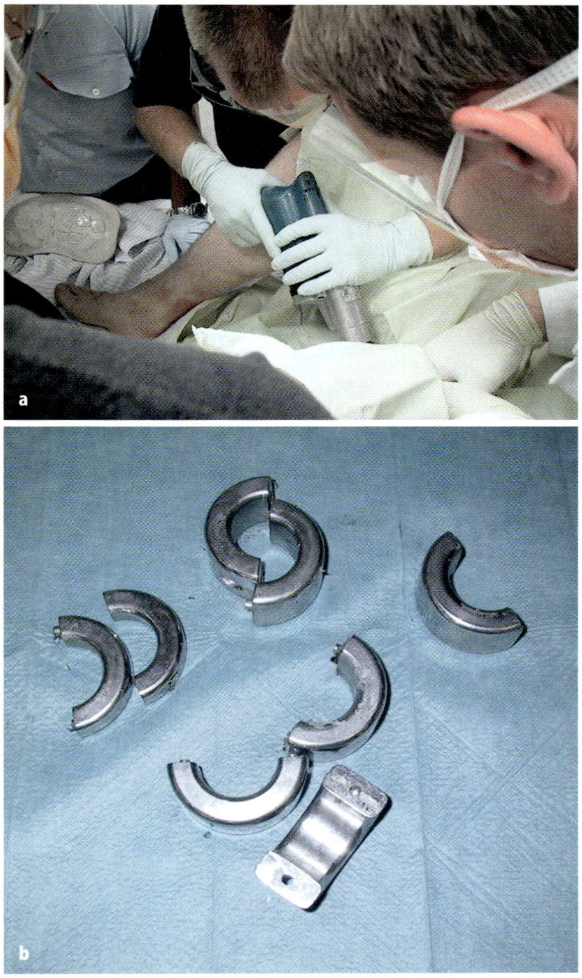

Fig. 21.37.2. a A firefighter is detaching the scrotal rings using an angle grinder. Note the imperatively required cooling with ice cubes. **b** The detached scrotal rings

other skin defects and especially the left testicle were covered with meshed split-thickness skin to allow exact molding of the skin onto the underlying tissue. Because of its elongation, the left spermatic cord was pulled up underneath the groin skin and fixed there with mounting sutures before plastic coverage. Split-thickness skin grafts and mesh grafts were covered with gentle pressure dressing for the first 5 days to ensure a tight adhesion of the grafts to the underlying tissue, which facilitates neovascularization.

Figure 5a–d depicts the findings after surgery. Figure 21.37.5a – still in the operating room – shows the penile split-thickness skin graft with insular puncture holes to allow wound fluid drainage. Furthermore, the molding of the mesh graft is clearly visible. Figure 21.37.5b, 2 weeks later, shows that the apertures of the mesh graft are already in the process of sealing, with the patient one last time in the operating room to

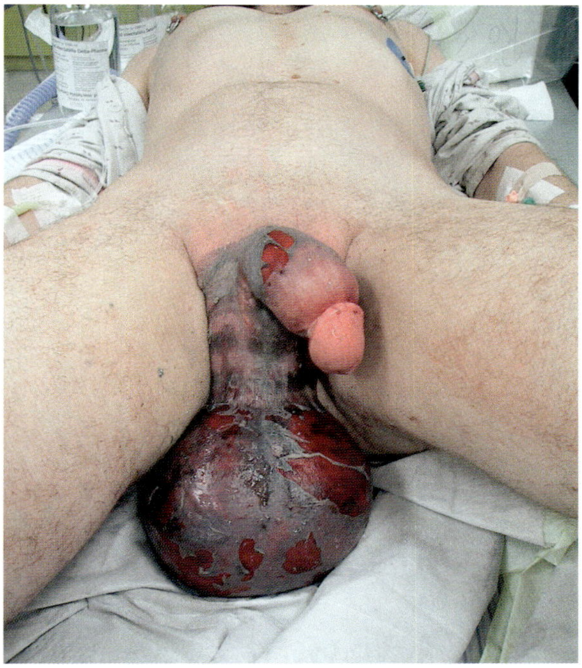

Fig. 21.37.3. The genitalia freed from the metal rings

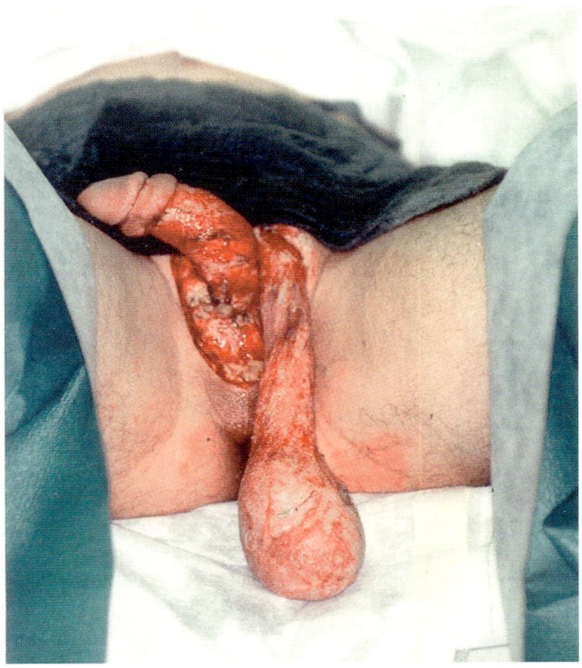

Fig. 21.37.4. The genitalia after right-sided orchiectomy and after skin debridement

resect the nonviable overlapping margins. Figure 21.37.5c, 1 year later, shows that the patient is very satisfied with the aesthetic and functional results of plastic coverage. Erectile function resembles the state before onset of the disease; the penis is furnished with

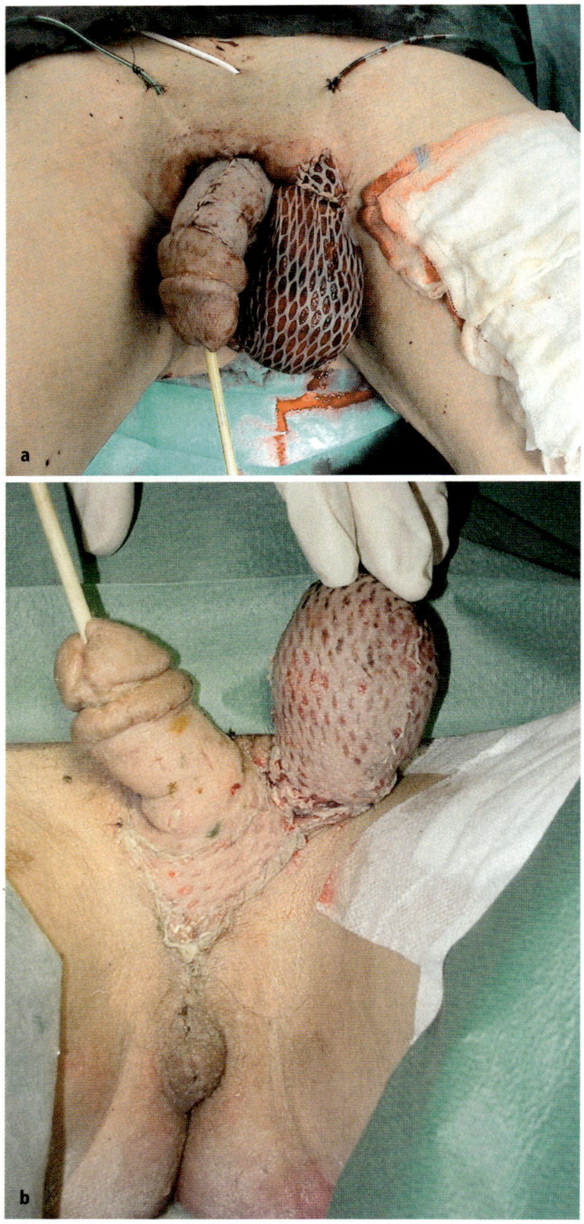

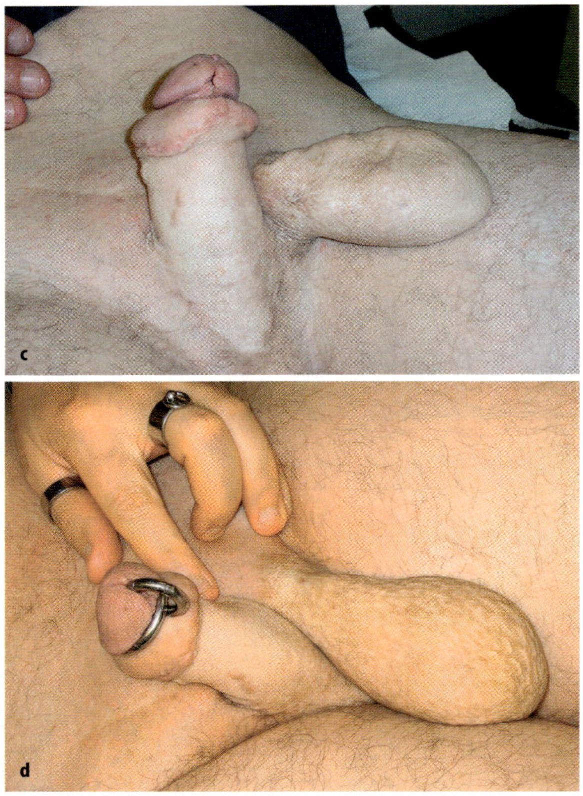

Fig. 21.37.5a–d. The intraoperative (**a**) and postoperative course (**b–d**) of the plastic surgical coverage of the genital skin defects. More detailed information is given in the text

bathyesthesia (deep sensation) albeit lacking normal sensation. The neoscrotum is comfortable while wearing normal underwear. Figure 21.37.5d shows that despite clear explanation of the risk of recurrence of Fournier's gangrene, the patient could not resist piercing his penis anew 2 years after treatment in our department.

Discussion

Fournier's gangrene has no clear-cut definition. Different terms have been proposed since the first descriptions by Baurienne in 1764 (Baurienne 1764) and Jean Alfred Fournier in 1883 (Fournier 1883), including "streptococcus gangrene," "necrotizing fasciitis," "periurethral phlegmon," and "synergistic necrotizing cellulitis." Today, most authors agree that Fournier's gangrene is "an infective necrotizing fasciitis of the perineal, genital or perianal regions." According to this definition, children, women, and older men are also included. Some authors do not accept Fournier's gangrene diagnosis if pathologic bacteria cannot be cultured from wound smears, e.g., in patients with arteriolosclerosis due to diabetes mellitus. However, from a clinical point of view, all patients fitting into the above-cited definition should be considered, because neither gender, age, nor culture positivity seem to have any relevance regarding treatment.

Three differential diagnoses are important: genital gangrene in association with pyoderma gangrenosum, vasculitis (Sohn et al. 1989; Schultz et al. 1995), and polyarteritis nodosa (Downing and Black 1985) are not necessarily treated by surgery. Pyoderma gangrenosum must initially be treated with systemic corticosteroids at high doses, because further tissue destruction may appear in spite of sufficient surgical debridement. Gangrene in association with polyarteritis nodosa or vasculitis may be diagnosed after surgical debridement, because it has not been reported that surgery deteriorates outcome. Vasculitis must be treated by azathioprine, cyclophosphamide, and thalidomide (Sohn et al. 1989; Schultz et al. 1995). Other causes of purulent ulceration such as neoplasia and artifact must be excluded (Farrell et al. 1998).

Fournier's gangrene is a diagnosis at first glance, although a variety of different macroscopic pictures are described (dry or wet gangrene, the surface still covered with a gangrenous layer or already free-lying testicles, only hanging suspended by their cords, like bell clappers [Eke 2000]). Every gangrenous alteration of the genitoanal region is suspicious for Fournier's gangrene. Most patients with Fournier's gangrene are admitted as emergency cases, often with signs of sepsis, and therefore must immediately be treated at the intensive care unit.

X-ray and ultrasound are reported to be helpful in determining the margins of necrosis, but their true usefulness has never been proven. CT or MRI can be helpful in determining intraabdominal or intrapelvic infectious foci in cases suspicious for such conditions (Benizri et al. 1996; Amendola et al. 1994; Okizuka et al. 1992).

Many presenting features of Fournier's gangrene have been described. In early stages, diagnosis may be difficult because patients present only minimal cutaneous manifestations such as cutaneous cellulitis, cyanosis, blistering, or bronzing of the skin as features of subcutaneous infection. Approximately 50% of patients present crepitus (Smith et al. 1998). Early diagnosis is very important in order to achieve a good clinical outcome.

A number of medical conditions are associated with Fournier's gangrene, including diabetes mellitus, alcohol abuse, obesity, HIV, chronic consuming diseases, immunosuppression, and arterial occlusive disease (Eke 2000). However, a pathophysiologic explanation has never been proven. Another suggested etiological factor is a focus of infection.

Management of Fournier's gangrene consists in the management of sepsis of hemodynamic stabilization, parenteral broad-spectrum antibiotic therapy, and urgent surgical removal of the infectious focus (Eke 2000). Most published recommendations do not rely on cultured germs or antibiograms, but they do try to cover all likely bacteria, targeting streptococcal species, Gram-positive and anaerobic organisms with penicillin combined with an inhibitor of beta-lactamase, and Gram-negative aerobes with a third-generation cephalosporin or aminoglycoside.

The spread of Fournier's gangrene is caused by microvascular thrombosis leading to necrosis of uninfected tissue, which in turn becomes infested by the bacteria. Therefore, the subcutaneous extent of the disease is larger than the visible borders of cutaneous necrosis. This makes radical resection of the entire affected tissue including healthy tissue margins mandatory to prevent further spread of the disease. Several techniques have been recommended to define the adequate resection margins, but none has proven to be effective. We define resection margins by clinical assessment and include at least 5 mm of viable and macroscopic healthy tissue. According to the pathophysiological theory, the testicles should not be affected by Fournier's gangrene because of their independent blood supply. However, unilateral or bilateral orchiectomy can be necessary if the testicles are the nidus of bacterial infection (epididymoorchitis or scrotal abscess [Eke 2000]) or if the testicular blood supply is deteriorated.

Urinary or fecal diversion may be necessary to avoid wound contamination or to treat underlying conditions such as intestinal or urethral fistulas (Eke 2000). In some cases, the creation of a protecting colostomy may therefore become necessary. In contrast, suprapubic catheters or at least transurethral catheters are inescapable in all cases.

Topical therapy is utilized to accelerate wound healing. Different substances are recommended (sodium hypochloride, hydrogen peroxide). In the 1990s, unprocessed honey was reported to stimulate growth and multiplication of epithelial cells at the wound edges and to exert antimicrobial effects (Eke 2000). However, flushings with provodone-iodine and isotonic NaCl-solutions are effective and easy to handle.

Data from several series provide evidence that hyperbaric oxygen therapy may improve survival by increasing tissue oxygen tension to a level that inhibits bacterial growth and kills bacteria (Korhonen et al. 1998). However, another retrospective study did not reproduce these beneficial effects (Shupak et al. 1995).

In order to further reduce the mortality of Fournier's gangrene, it is most important to identify factors associated with mortality. These factors could be related to the patient or the disease, but also to the management by the treating physician, e.g., diagnostic or therapeutic procedures, or the time course of these procedures. Fournier's gangrene is problematic in that it is a very rare disease and therefore only a small number of patients are investigated in single studies. In the literature, Fournier's gangrene is referred to as a special form of necrotizing soft tissue infection (NSTI). Therefore NSTI, with its larger patient numbers, can contribute conclusions on the treatment of Fournier's gangrene. Mortality rates are comparable between Fournier's gangrene (mean 19%) (Dahm et al. 2000; Mindrup et al. 2005; Yeniyol et al. 2004; Korkut et al. 2003; Burdal et al. 2003; Chawla et al. 2003; Asci et al. 1998; Nisbet and Tompson 2002; Corman et al. 1999; Korhonen et al. 1998; Hollabaugh et al. 1998; Benizri et al. 1996; Palmer et al. 1995) and NSTI (mean 20%) (Elliott et al. 2000; Endorf et al. 2005; Anaya et al. 2005; Wilkinson and Doolette 2004; McHenry et al. 1995). Management modalities and treatment course (i.e., diagnostics, medical therapy, type, and frequency of surgery) are also comparable. In our opinion, the most striking point is that in three of five studies on NSTI, time to surgery was identified as an independent risk factor for mortality. In Fournier's gangrene, most authors emphasize the importance of fast and extensive surgery, but only two of 13 studies could identify time to surgery as a risk factor for mortality (Dahm et al. 2000; Mindrup et al. 2005; Yeniyol et al. 2004; Korkut et al. 2003; Burdal et al. 2003; Chawla et al. 2003; Asci et al. 1998; Nisbet and Tompson 2002; Corman et al. 1999; Korhonen et al. 1998; Hollabaugh et al. 1998; Benizri et al. 1996; Palmer et al. 1995).

Given the mortality rates from 0%–80% (Stephens et al. 1993) in historic series and 0%–43% in recent series (Dahm et al. 2000; Mindrup et al. 2005; Yeniyol et al. 2004; Korkut et al. 2003; Burdal et al. 2003; Chawla et al. 2003; Asci et al. 1998; Nisbet and Tompson 2002; Corman et al. 1999; Korhonen et al. 1998; Hollabaugh et al. 1998; Benizri et al. 1996; Palmer et al. 1995), every case of Fournier's gangrene must be taken seriously. Especially those patients presenting clinical signs of sepsis suffer from immediate risk of death. However, the overall mortality rate in Eke's review of 1,726 published cases was 16% (Eke 2000). Thirteen recent publications (from 1990 to 2003) with 24–57 patients show mortality rates between 1% and 43%, which results in a combined mortality rate of 15% (44/301) (Dahm et al. 2000; Mindrup et al. 2005; Yeniyol et al. 2004; Korkut et al. 2003; Burdal et al. 2003; Chawla et al. 2003; Asci et al. 1998; Nisbet and Tompson 2002; Corman et al. 1999; Korhonen et al. 1998; Hollabaugh et al. 1998; Benizri et al. 1996; Palmer et al. 1995). This may represent the objective risk rather than mortality rates found in smaller series. In our opinion, the most important measure to reduce mortality is to perform surgery as soon as possible, provide rapid resuscitation, and start antibiotics immediately. This rapid and aggressive approach is common sense (Korhonen et al. 1998; Benizri et al. 1996; Stephens et al. 1993) and reflects the general approach to treatment of sepsis with a known focus of infection.

References

Amendola MA, Casillas J, Joseph R et al (1994) Fournier's gangrene: CT findings. Abdom Imaging 19:471

Anaya DA, McMahon K, Nathens AB et al (2005) Predictors of mortality and limb loss in necrotizing soft tissue infections. Arch Surg 140:151; discussion 158

Asci R, Sarikaya S, Buyukalpelli R et al (1998) Fournier's gangrene: risk assessment and enzymatic debridement with lyophilized collagenase application. Eur Urol 34:411

Baurienne H (1764) Sur une plaie contuse qui s'est terminée par le sphacèle du scrotum. J Med Chir Pharm 20:251

Benizri E, Fabiani P, Migliori G et al (1996) Gangrene of the perineum. Urology 47:935

Chawla SN, Gallop C, Mydlo JH (2003) Fournier's gangrene: an analysis of repeated surgical debridement. Eur Urol 43:572

Corman JM, Moody JA, Aronson WJ (1999) Fournier's gangrene in a modern surgical setting: improved survival with aggressive management. BJU Int 84:85

Dahm P, Roland FH, Vaslef SN et al (2000) Outcome analysis in patients with primary necrotizing fasciitis of the male genitalia. Urology 56:31; discussion 35

Downing R, Black J (1985) Polyarteritis nodosa: an unrecognised cause of Fournier's gangrene. Br J Urol 57:355

Eke N (2000) Fournier's gangrene: a review of 1726 cases. Br J Surg 87:718

Elliott D, Kufera JA, Myers RA (2000) The microbiology of necrotizing soft tissue infections. Am J Surg 179:361

Endorf FW, Supple KG, Gamelli RL (2005) The evolving characteristics and care of necrotizing soft-tissue infections. Burns 31:269

Farrell AM, Black MM, Bracka A et al (1998) Pyoderma gangrenosum of the penis. Br J Dermatol 138:337

Fournier JA (1883) Gangrène foudroyante de la verge. Medecin Practique 4:589

Gurdal M, Yucebas E, Tekin A et al (2003) Predisposing factors and treatment outcome in Fournier's gangrene. Analysis of 28 cases. Urol Int 70:286

Hollabaugh RS Jr, Dmochowski RR, Hickerson WL et al (1998) Fournier's gangrene: therapeutic impact of hyperbaric oxygen. Plast Reconstr Surg 101:94

Korhonen K, Hirn M, Niinikoski J (1998) Hyperbaric oxygen in the treatment of Fournier's gangrene. Eur J Surg 164:251

Korkut M, Icoz G, Dayangac M et al (2003) Outcome analysis in patients with Fournier's gangrene: report of 45 cases. Dis Colon Rectum 46:649

McHenry CR, Piotrowski JJ, Petrinic D et al (1995) Determinants of mortality for necrotizing soft-tissue infections. Ann Surg 221:558; discussion 563

Mindrup SR, Kealey GP, Fallon B (2005) Hyperbaric oxygen for the treatment of Fournier's gangrene. J Urol 173:1975

Nisbet AA, Thompson IM (2002) Impact of diabetes mellitus on the presentation and outcomes of Fournier's gangrene. Urology 60:775

Okizuka H, Sugimura K, Yoshizako T (1992) Fournier's gangrene: diagnosis based on MR findings. AJR Am J Roentgenol 158:1173

Palmer LS, Winter HI, Tolia BM et al (1995) The limited impact of involved surface area and surgical debridement on survival in Fournier's gangrene. Br J Urol 76:208

Schultz ES, Diepgen TL, von den Driesch P et al (1995) Systemic corticosteroids are important in the treatment of Fournier's gangrene: a case report. Br J Dermatol 133:633

Shupak A, Shoshani O, Goldenberg I et al (1995) Necrotizing fasciitis: an indication for hyperbaric oxygenation therapy? Surgery 118:873

Smith GL, Bunker CB, Dinneen MD (1998) Fournier's gangrene. Br J Urol 81:347

Sohn M, Kistler D, Kindler J et al (1989) Fournier's gangrene in hypersensitivity vasculitis. J Urol 142:823

Stephens BJ, Lathrop JC, Rice WT et al (1993) Fournier's gangrene: historic (1764) versus contemporary (1979) differences in etiology and clinical importance. Am Surg 59:149

Wilkinson D, Doolette D (2004) Hyperbaric oxygen treatment and survival from necrotizing soft tissue infection. Arch Surg 139:1339

Yeniyol CO, Suelozgen T, Arslan M et al (2004) Fournier's gangrene: experience with 25 patients and use of Fournier's gangrene severity index score. Urology 64:218

Overall Reference List

Aalami OO, Allen DB, Organ CH Jr (2000) Chylous ascites: a collective review. Surgery 128:761

Abdalati H, Bulas DI et al (1994) Blunt renal trauma in children: healing of renal injuries and recommendations for imaging follow-up. Pediatr Radiol 24:573

Abdel-Meguid TA, Gomella LG (1996) Prevention and management of complications. In: Smith AD, Badlani GH, Bagley DH, Clayman RV, Jordan GH, Kavoussi LR, Lingeman JE, Preminger GM, Segura JW (eds) Smith's textbook of endourology. Quality Medical, St. Louis, p 851

Aberer W, Bircher A, Romano A, Blanca M, Campi P, Fernandez J, Brockow K, Pichler WJ, Demoly P (2003) European Network for Drug Allergy (ENDA); EAACI interest group on drug hypersenitivity. Drug provocation testing in the diagnosis of drug hypersensitivity reactions:general considerations. Allergy 58:854

Abol-Enein H, Ghoneim MA (2001) Functional results of orthotopic ileal neobladder with serous-lined extramural ureteral reimplantation: experience with 450 patients. J Urol 165:1427

Abol-Enein H, Salem M, Mesbah A, Abdel-Latif M, Kamal M, Shabaan A et al (2004) Continent cutaneous ileal pouch using the serous lined extramural valves. The Mansoura experience in more than 100 patients. J Urol 172:588

Aboloyosr A, Moneim AE, Abdelatif AM, Abdalla MA, Imam HM (2005) The management of penile fracture based on clinical and magnetic resonance imaging findings. BJU Int 96:373

Aboseif S, Gomez R, McAninch JW (1983) Genital self-mutilation. J Urol 150:1143

Abou-Jaoude WA et al (1996) Indicators of genitourinary tract injury or anomaly in cases of pediatric blunt trauma. J Pediatr Surg 31:86; discussion 90

Abraham E, Laterre PF, Garg R et al (2005) Drotrecogin alfa (activated) for adults with severe sepsis and a low risk of death. N Engl J Med 353:1322

Abrams P (1997) Urodynamics. Springer, Berlin New York Heidelberg

Abrams P, Cardozo L, Fall M et al (2002) The standardisation of terminology of lower urinary tract function: report from the Standardisation Sub-committee of the International Continence Society. Neurourol Urodyn 21:167

Abu-Zidan FM, Al-Tawheed A et al (1999) Urologic injuries in the Gulf War. Int Urol Nephrol 31:577

ACCP/SCCM (1992) Consensus conference of the American College of Chest Physicians/Society of Critical Care Medicine (ACCP/SCCM). Des Plains, IL, August 1991

Acheson, AG, Graham AN et al (1998) Prospective study on factors delaying surgery in ruptured abdominal aortic aneurysms. J R Coll Surg Edinb 43:182

Adam C, Hofstetter A, Deubner J, Zaak D, Weitkunat R, Seitz M, Schneede P (2004) Retropubic transvesical prostatectomy for significant prostatic enlargement must remain a standard part of urology training. Scand J Urol Nephrol 38:472

Adam G, Bücker A, Nolte-Ernsting C, Tacke J, Günther RW (1999) Interventional MR imaging: percutaneous abdominal and skeletal biopsies and drainages of the abdomen. Eur Radiol 9:1471

Adams JE et al (2002) Analysis of the incidence of pelvic trauma in fatal automobile accidents. Am J Forensic Med Pathol 23:132

Adams JR Jr, Mata JA, Culkin DJ et al (1992) Ureteral injury in abdominal vascular reconstructive surgery. Urology 39:77

Addison WA, Livengood CH 3rd, Hill GB, Sutton GP, Fortier KJ (1984) Necrotizing fasciitis of vulval origin in diabetic patients. Obstet Gynecol 63:473

Addiss DG, Shaffer N, Fowler BS, Tauxe RV (1990) The epidemiology of appendicitis and appendectomy in the United States. Am J Epidemiol 132:910

Adeyoju AB, Olujohunabe AG, Morris J et al (2002) Priapism in sickle-cell disease; incidence, risk factors and complications – an international multicentre study. BJU Int 90:898

Adovasio R, Griselli F (2003) An unusual complication of open aortic surgery: hemorrhage due to the iatrogenic rupture of a renal cyst. Vasa 32:167

Aethman PLD (ed) (1974) Biology data book, vol 3. Federation of the American Society of Experimental Biology, Bethesda MD

Agalar F, Eroglu MD, Bulbul M, Agalar A Tarhan OR, Sari M (2005) Staged abdominal repair for treatment of moderate to severe secondary peritonitis. World J Surg 29:240

Agostini A et al (2006) Immediate complications of tension-free vaginal tape (TVT): results of a French Survey. Eur J Obstet Gynecol Reprod Biol 124:237

Agramunt Lerma M, Lonjedo Vicent E et al (2003) Selective embolization in the treatment of severe renal injury. Arch Esp Urol 56:83

Aharonson-Daniel L, Waisman Y, Dannon YL et al (2003) Epidemiology of terror-related versus non-terror-related traumatic injury in children. Pediatrics 112:280

Ahlering TE, Skinner DG (1989) Vena caval resection resection in bulky metastatic germ cell tumors. J Urol 142:1497

Ahmed I, Shaikh NA (1997) Treatment of intermittent idiopathic priapism with oral terbutaline. Br J Urol 80:341

Ahmed S, Batiuk TD (2001) Broken kidney: traumatic fracture of a renal allograft. Am J Kidney Dis 37:e33

Aihara R et al (2002) Fracture locations influence the likelihood of rectal and lower urinary tract injuries in patients sustaining pelvic fractures. J Trauma 52:205; discussion 208

Akabane S, Ushiyama T et al (2001) A case of traumatic renal graft rupture with salvage of renal function. Clin Transplant 15:289

Akashi T, Fuse H, Muraishi Y et al (2002) Parathyroid hormone related protein producing penile cancer. J Urol 167:249

Akbar SA, Jafri SZ, Amendola MA, Madrazo BL, Salem R, Bis

KG (2005) Complications of renal transplantation. Radiographics 25:1335
Akgun Y, Yilmaz G (2005) Factors affecting mortality in Fournier's gangrene (in Turkish). Ulus Travma Derg 11:49
Akinci D, Akhan O, Ozmen MN, Karabulut N, Ozkan O, Cil BE, Karcaaltincaba M (2005) Percutaneous drainage of 300 intraperitoneal abscesses with long-term follow-up. Cardiovasc Intervent Radiol 28:744
Al Ali M, Haddad LF (1996) The late treatment of 63 overlooked or complicated ureteral missile injuries: the promise of nephrostomy and role of autotransplantation. J Urol 156:1918
Alapont Alacreu JM, Broseta Rico E et al (2003) Complications of uretero-renoscopy. Actas Urol Esp 27:692
Albani JM, Novick AC (2003) Renal artery pseudoaneurysm after partial nephrectomy: three case reports and a literature review. Urology 62:227
Albqami N, Janetschek G (2005) Laparoscopic partial nephrectomy. Curr Opin Urol 15:306
Albright F (1941) Case records of the Massachusetts general Hospital-Case 390N. Eng J Med 225:789
Aldana JP, Lee BR et al (2003) Residual air persists in the renal collecting system following percutaneous nephrolithotomy. J Laparoendosc Adv Surg Tech A 13:317
Alejandria MM, Lansang MA, Dans LF, Mantaring JB (2002) Intravenous immunoglobulin for treating sepsis and septic shock. Cochrane Database Syst Rev CD001090
Alexander JW, Fischer JE, Boyajian M, Palmquist J, Morris MJ (1983) The influence of hair-removal methods on wound infections. Arch Surg 118:347
Alfici R, Ashkenazi I, Kessel B, Zut N, Sternberg A (2004) Temporary bowel diversion using the Bogota bag (hadera stoma): technical details. J Am Coll Surg 199:344
Ali MZ (2004) Fournier's gangrene – a rare complication of hydrocele aspiration. J Coll Physicians Surg Pak 14:304
Al-Janabi MA, Ahmad R et al (1995) Case report: renal scintigraphy in the diagnosis of urinary extravasation. Br J Radiol 68:12513
Alkibay T, Karaoglan U, Gundogdu S, Bozkirli I (1992) An unusual complication of extracorporeal shock wave lithotripsy: urinoma due to rupture of the renal pelvis. Int Urol Nephrol 24:11
Allen GA, Hoffman M, Roberts HR, Monroe DM 3rd (2002) Recombinant activated factor VII its mechanism of action and role in the control of hemorrhage. Can J Anaesth 49:S7
Allen ZA, Merrick GS, Butler WM et al (2005) Detailed urethral dosimetry in the evaluation of prostate brachytherapy-related urinary morbidity. Int J Radiat Oncol Biol Phys 62:981
Allgood RJ, Cook JH, Weedn RJ et al (1970) Prospective analysis of pulmonary embolism in the postoperative patient. Surgery 68:116
Almakdisi T, Massoud S, Makdisi G (2005) Lymphomas and chylous ascites: review of the literature. Oncologist 10:632
Almgard LE, Fernstrom I, Haverling M, Ljungqvist A (1973) Treatment of renal adenocarcinoma by embolic occlusion of the renal circulation. Br J Urol 45:474
Almogy G, Belzberg H, Mintz Y et al (2004) Suicide bombing attacks: update and modifications to the protocol. Ann Surg 239:295
Alonso-Perez M, Segura RJ et al (1999) Surgical treatment of ruptured abdominal aortic aneurysms in the elderly. Ann Vasc Surg 13:592
Alschibaja M, May F, Treiber U, Paul R, Hartung R (2005) Transurethral resection for benign prostatic hyperplasia. current developments. Urologe A 44:499
Altarac S (1993) A case of testicle replantation. J Urol 150:1507
Altarac S (1994) Management of 53 cases of testicular trauma. Eur Urol 25:119
Altman AL, Seftel AD, Brown SL et al (1999) Cocaine associated priapism. J Urol 161:1817
Altman AL, Haas C et al (2000) Selective nonoperative management of blunt grade 5 renal injury. J Urol 164:27; discussion 30
Alvarez Gonzalez E, Pamplona M, Rodriguez A, Garcia-Hidalgo E, Nunez V, Leiva O (1994) High flow priapism after blunt perineal trauma: resolution with bucrylate embolization. J Urol 151:426
Alvi A, Doherty T et al (2003) Facial fractures and concomitant injuries in trauma patients. Laryngoscope 113:102
Amaral, JF (1997) Thoracoabdominal injuries in the athlete. Clin Sports Med 16:739
Ameh EA, Sabo SY, Muhammad I (1997) Amputation of the penis during traditional circumcision. Trop Doct 27:117
Amendola MA, Casillas J, Joseph R et al (1994) Fournier's gangrene: CT findings. Abdom Imaging 19:471
American College of Surgeons. Committee on T (1997) Advanced trauma life support program for doctors: ATLS. American College of Surgeons, Chicago
American Urological Association; American Academy of Orthopaedic Surgeons (2003) Antibiotic prophylaxis for urological patients with total joint replacements. J Urol 169:1796
Ames D (1987) Autocastration and biblical delusions in schizophrenia (letter) Br J Psychiatry 150:407
Amin R (2002) Chylous ascites from prostatic adenocarcinoma. Urology 59:773
Amir LD, Aharonson-Daniel L, Peleg K et al (2005) The severity of injury in children resulting from acts against civilian population. Ann Surg 241:666
Anaya DA, McMahon K, Nathens AB et al (2005) Predictors of mortality and limb loss in necrotizing soft tissue infections. Arch Surg 140:151; discussion 158
Anderson CR (1992) Animal bites. Guidelines to current management. Postgrad Med 92:134
Anderson ID, Fearon KC, Grant IS (1996) Laparotomy for Abdominal sepsis in the critically ill. Br J Surg 83:535
Anderson JB, Grant JB (1991) Postoperative retention of urine: a prospective urodynamic study. BMJ 302:894
Anderson JB, Williamson RC (1988) Testicular torsion in Bristol: a 25-year review. Br J Surg 75:988
Anderson JB, Roehrborn CG, Schalken JA et al (2001) The progression of benign prostatic hyperplasia: examining the evidence and determining the risk. Eur Urol 39:390
Anderson RW, Vaslef SN (1997) Shock. Causes and management of circulatory collapse. In: Sabiston DC, Lyerly HK (eds) Sabiston textbook of surgery – the biological basis of modern surgical practice, 15th edn. WB Saunders Company, Philadelphia, p 68
Andersson KE, Chapple CR, Hofner K (2002) Future drugs for the treatment of benign prostatic hyperplasia. World J Urol 19:436
Andersson L (1980) Antifibrinolytic therapy in genitourinary tract surgery. J Clin Pathol Suppl (R Coll Pathol) 14:60
Andriole G, Bruchovsky N, Chung LW et al (2004) Dihydrotestosterone and the prostate: the scientific rationale for 5-alpha-reductase inhibitors in the treatment of benign prostatic hyperplasia. J Urol 172:1399
Andriole GL, Sandlund JT, Miser JS et al (1987) The efficacy of mesna (2-mercaptoethane sodium sulfonate) as a uroprotectant in patients with hemorrhagic cystitis receiving further oxazaphosphorine chemotherapy. J Clin Oncol 5:799
Andriole GL, Yuan JJ, Catalona WJ (1990) Cystotomy, temporary urinary diversion and bladder packing in the management of severe cyclophosphamide-induced hemorrhagic cystitis. J Urol 143:1006
Andronikou S, Bertelsmann J (2002) CT scanning–essential for

conservative management of paediatric blunt abdominal trauma. S Afr Med J 92:35
Anema JG, Morey AF et al (2001) Potential uses of absorbable fibrin adhesive bandage for genitourinary trauma. World J Surg 25:15737
Angelis M, Augenstein JS et al (2003) Ex vivo repair and renal autotransplantation after penetrating trauma: is there an upper limit of ischemic/traumatic injury beyond which a kidney is unsalvageable? J Trauma 54:606; discussion 609
Anger JT, Raj GV, Delvecchio FC et al (2005) Anastomotic contracture and incontinence after radical prostatectomy: a graded approach to management. J Urol 173:1143
Angood PB, Gingalewski CA, Andersen DK (2001) Surgical complications. In: Townsend CM (ed) Sabiston textbook of surgery, 16th edn. WB Saunders, Philadelphia, p 198
Angus DC, Linde-Zwirble WT, Lidicker J, Clermont G, Carcillo J, Pinsky MR (2001) Epidemiology of severe sepsis in the United States: analysis of incidence, outcome, and associated costs of care. Crit Care Med 29:1303
Angus LD, Tachmes L et al (1993) Surgical management of pediatric renal trauma: an urban experience. Am Surg 59:388
Anjum I, Ahmed M, Azzopardi A et al (1998) Prostatic infarction/infection in acute urinary retention secondary to benign prostatic hyperplasia. J Urol 160:792
Anonymous (1996) Fracture and dislocation compendium. Orthopaedic Trauma Association Committee for Coding and Classification. J Orthop Trauma 10 [Suppl 1]:v, 1
Anonymous (2004) National Nosocomial Infections Surveillance (NNIS) System Report, data summary from January 1992 through June 2004, issued October 2. Am J Infect Control 32:470
Anonymous (2004) Advanced trauma life support for doctors, 7th edn. American College of Surgeons, Chicago, pp 18, 76
Anonymous (2004) Advanced trauma life support for doctors, 7th edn. American College of Surgeons, Chicago, p 80
Anonymous (2006) Definition of Terrorism. Wikipedia. http://en.wikipedia.org/wiki/ Definition_of_terrorism. Cited 27 January 2006
Anonymous (2006) Terrorism. Wikipedia. http://en.wikipedia.org/wiki/Terrorism. Cited 27 January 2006
Anson KM, Barnes DG, Briggs TP et al (1993) Temporary prostatic stenting and androgen suppression: a new minimally invasive approach to malignant prostatic retention. J R Soc Med 86:634
Ansong K (1995) Re: outcome after temporary vascular occlusion for the management of renal trauma. J Urol 153:440
Antoci JP, Schiff MJ (1982) Bladder and urethral injuries in patients with pelvic fractures. J Urol 128:25
Antonipillai I (1993) Epidermal growth factor is a potent inhibitor of renin secretion. Hypertension 21:654
Antonipillai I, Le TH, Soceneantu L, Horton R (1993) Transforming growth factor-beta is a renin secretagogue at picomolar concentrations. Am J Physiol 265:F537
Anwar YA, Sullivan ED et al (1997) Abrupt, severe hypertension associated with dissection of a renal artery during selective catheterization. J Hum Hypertens 11:533
Apaydin R, Gul U, Bahadir S, Siviloglu C, Ofluoglu I (2002) Dermatomyositis without muscle weakness associated with transitional cell carcinoma of the bladder. J Eur Acad Dermatol Venereol 16:172
Apfel CC, Roewer N (2004) Postoperative Nausea and Vomiting. Anaesthesist 53:377
Apfel CC, Laara F, Koivurante M et al (1999) A simplified risk score for predicting postoperative nausea and vomiting: conclusions from cross validations between two centers. Anesthesiology 91:693
Arai Y, Egawa S, Terachi T, Suzuki K, Gotoh M, Kawakita M, Tanaka M, Terada N, Baba S, Okumura K, Hayami S, Ono Y, Matsuda T, Naito S (2003) Morbidity of laparoscopic radical prostatectomy: summary of early multi-institutional experience in Japan. Int J Urol 10:430
Araujo CE, Tessler J (1983) Treatment of ifosfamide-induced urothelial toxicity by oral administration of sodium 2-mercaptoethane sulphonate (MESNA) to patients with inoperable lung cancer. Eur J Cancer Clin Oncol 19:195
Archbold JA, Barros d'sa AA, Morrison E (1981) Genito-urinary tract injuries of civil hostilities. Br J Surg 68:625
Arena F, Peracchia G et al (1997) The role of echotomography in minor renal traumatology. Acta Biomed Ateneo Parmense 68:53
Arensman RM, Belman AB (1980) Ruptured congenital mesoblastic nephroma: chemotherapy and irradiation as adjuvants to nephrectomy. Urology 15:394
Armenakas NA (1999) Current methods of diagnosis and management of ureteral injuries. World J Urol 17:78
Armenakas NA, McAninch JW, Lue TF, Dixon CM (1993) Posttraumatic impotence: MRI and duplex ultrasound in diagnosis and management. J Urol 149:1272
Armenakas NA, McAninch JW (1994) A uniform approach to urethroplasty. Prob Urology 8:254
Armenakas NA, McAninch JW (1996) Acute anterior urethral injuries. In: McAninch JW (ed) Traumatic and reconstructive urology. WB Saunders Philadelphia, p 543
Armenakas NA, Duckett CP et al (1999) Indications for nonoperative management of renal stab wounds. J Urol 161:768
Armenakas NA et al (2004) Iatrogenic bladder perforations: longterm followup of 65 patients. J Am Coll Surg 198:78
Armstrong AL, Birch BR et al (1994) Renal arteriovenous fistula following blunt trauma. Br J Urol 73:321
Arnold JL, Tsai MC, Halpern P et al (2003) Mass-casualty, terrorist bombings: epidemiological outcomes, resource utilization, and time course of emergency needs (part I). Prehospital Disaster Med 18:220
Arnold JL, Halpern P, Tsai MC et al (2004) Mass casualty terrorist bombings: a comparison of outcomes by bombing type. Ann Emerg Med 43:263
Aron M, Rajeev TP, Gupta NP (2000) Antibiotic prophylaxis for transrectal needle biopsy of the prostate: a randomized controlled study. BJU Int 85:682
Aroney RS, Dalley DN, Levi JA (1980) Haemorrhagic cystitis treated with epsilon-aminocaproic acid. Med J Aust 2:92
Arozullah AM, Daley J, Henderson WG, Khuri SF (2000) Multifactorial risk index for predicting postoperative respiratory failure in men after major noncardiac surgery. The National Veterans Administration Surgical Quality Improvement Program. Ann Surg 232:242
Arrizabalaga M, Extramiana J, Parra JL et al (1987) Treatment of massive haematuria with aluminous salts. Br J Urol 60:223
Artero ML, Sharma R, Savin VJ, Vincenti F (1994) Plasmapheresis reduces proteinuria and serum capacity to injure glomeruli in patients with recurrent focal glomerulosclerosis. Am J Kidney Dis 25:574
Asayama K, Tsuda H et al (2005) Bilateral posterior ischemic optic neuropathy following subdural hematoma drainage. Nippon Ganka Gakkai Zasshi 109:26
Ascher E, Scheinman M et al (1999) Ruptured versus elective abdominal aortic aneurysm repair: outcome and cost. Ann Vasc Surg 13:613
Asci R, Sarikaya S, Buyukalpelli R et al (1998) Fournier's gangrene: risk assessment and enzymatic debridement with lyophilized collagenase application. Eur Urol 34:411
Asci R, Sarikaya S, Buyukalpelli R, Saylik A, Yilmaz AF, Yildiz S (1999) Voiding and sexual dysfunctions after pelvic fracture urethra injuries treated with either initial cystostomy and delayed urethroplasty or immediate primary urethral realignment. Scand J Urol Nephrol 33:228

Asensio A, Ramos A, Munez E, Vilanova JL, Torrijos P, Garcia FJ (2005) Preoperative low molecular weight heparin as venous thromboembolism prophylaxis in patients at risk for prosthetic infection after knee arthroplasty. Infect Control Hosp Epidemiol 26:903
Asensio JA, Chahwan S et al (2000) Operative management and outcome of 302 abdominal vascular injuries. Am J Surg 180:528; discussion 533
Asgari MA, Safarinejad MA, Hosseini SY, Dadhkah F (1999) Extracorporeal shock wave lithotripsy of renal calculi during early pregnancy. BJU Int 84:615
Ashebu SD, Dahniya MH et al (2004) Rupture of the renal pelvis of a ureteropelvic junction hydronephrosis after blunt abdominal trauma. Australas Radiol 48:256
Assenza M, Romagnoli F et al (2003) Conservative approach to IV grade renal trauma. Chir Ital 55:445
Atala A, Miller FB et al (1991) Preliminary vascular control for renal trauma. Surg Gynecol Obstet 172:386
Ather MH, Noor MA (2002) Role of imaging in the evaluation of renal trauma. J Pak Med Assoc 52:423
Ather MH, Memon W, Rees JR (2005) Clinical impact of incidental diagnosis of disease on non-contrast-enhanced helical CT for acute ureteral colic. Semin Ultrasound CT MRI 26:20
Atikeler MK, Gecit I, Yuzgec V, Yalcin O (2005) Complications of circumcision performed within and outside the hospital. Int Urol Nephrol 37:97
Attah CA (1992) New approach to the management of Fournier's gangrene. Br J Urol 70:78
Avisrror MU, Fernandez IA, Sanchez AS et al (2000) Doxazosin and priapism. J Urol 163:238
Aydin, MD, Akcay F et al (2005) Cerebral fat embolism: pulmonary contusion is a more important etiology than long bone fractures. Clin Neuropathol 24:86
Azam Uet al (2001) The tension-free vaginal tape procedure in women with previous failed stress incontinence surgery. J Urol 166:554
Azimuddin K, Milanesa D, Ivatury R et al (1998) Penetrating ureteric injuries. Injury 29:363
Baba H, Maezawa Y, Furusawa N et al (1995) Lumbar spinal stenosis causing intermittent priapism. Paraplegia 33:338
Baba K, Yajima M et al (2001) Clinical study on renal trauma. Hinyokika Kiyo 47:159
Badalament RA, Bahn DK, Kim H, Kumar A, Bahn JM, Lee F (2000) Patient-reported complications after cryoablation therapy for prostate cancer. Arch Ital Urol Androl 72:305
Badani KK, Hemal AK, Menon M (2004) Autosomal dominant polycystic kidney disease and pain – a review of the disease from aetiology, evaluation, past surgical treatment options to current practice. J Postgrad Med 50:222
Baddour LM, Wilson WR, Bayer AS, Fowler VG Jr, Bolger AF, Levison ME, Ferrieri P, Gerber MA, Tani LY, Gewitz MH, Tong DC, Steckelberg JM, Baltimore RS, Shulman ST, Burns JC, Falace DA, Newburger JW, Pallasch TJ, Takahashi M, Taubert KA (2005) Infective endocarditis: diagnosis, antimicrobial therapy, and management of complications: a statement for healthcare professionals from the Committee on Rheumatic Fever Endocarditis, and Kawasaki Disease Council on Cardiovascular Disease in the Young, and the Councils on Clinical Cardiology Stroke, and Cardiovascular Surgery and Anesthesia American Heart Association: endorsed by the Infectious Diseases Society of America. Circulation 111:e394
Badenoch DF, Murdoch DA, Tiptaft RC (1990)Microbiological study of bladder tumors, their histology and infective complications. Urology 35:5
Baehring JM (2005) Oncologic emergencies. In: DeVita VT Jr, Hellman S, Rosenberg SA (eds) Cancer principles and practice of oncology. Lippincott Williams and Wilkins, Philadelphia
Baert L, Verhamme L, Poppel Hv Vandeursen H, Baert J (1993) Long term consequences of urethral stents. J Urol 150:853
Baeten JM, Richardson BA, Lavreys L, Rakwar JP, Mandaliya K, Bwayo JJ et al (2005) Female-to-male infectivity of HIV-1 among circumcised and uncircumcised Kenyan men. J Infect Dis 191:546
Baeza-Herrera C, Dominguez-Perez ST et al (2002) Renal trauma in childhood. Second-level hospital experience. Gac Med Mex 138:313
Baghossian T, Henri M, Dube S, Bendavid Y, Morin M (2005) Laparoscopic nephrectomy donor death due to cerebral gas embolism in a specialized transplant center; risk zero does not exist. Transplantation 79:258
Bahlmann JC, Fourie IJ, Arndt TC (1983) Fournier's gangrene: necrotising fasciitis of the male genitalia. Br J Urol 55:85
Bahloul A, Krid M et al (1997) Contusions to the pathologic kidney. A retrospective study, apropos of 34 cases. Ann Urol (Paris) 31:253
Bailey SH, Mone MC, Holman JM, Nelson EW (2003) Laparoscopic treatment of post renal transplant lymphoceles. Surg Endosc 17:1896
Baka AG et al (2002) Current use and perceived utility of ultrasound for evaluation of pediatric compared with adult trauma patients. Pediatr Emerg Care 18:163
Bakal CW, Sacks D, Burke DR, Cardella JF, Chopra PS, Dawson SL, Drooz AT, Freeman N, Meranze SG, Van Moore A Jr, Palestrant AM, Roberts AC, Spies JB, Stein EJ, Towbin R; Society of Interventional Radiology Standards of Practice Committee (2003) Quality improvement guidelines for adult percutaneous abscess and fluid drainage. J Vasc Interv Radiol 14:S223
Baker HW (1998) Reproductive effects of nontesticular illness. Endocrinol Metab Clin North Am 27:831
Baker LA, Gearhart JP (1998) The staged approach to bladder exstrophy closure and the role of osteotomies. World J Urol 16:205
Baker SP, O'Neill B, Haddon W Jr et al (1974) The injury severity score: a method for describing patients with multiple injuries and evaluating emergency care. J Trauma 14:187
Bakir N, Sluiter WJ, Ploeg RJ, van San WJ, Tegzess AM (1996) Primary renal graft thrombosis. Nephrol Dial Transplant 11:140
Bakker AJ, Gorgels JP, van Vlies B, Koelemay MJ, Smits R, Tijssen JG, Haagen FD (1994) Contribution of creatine kinase MB mass concentration at admission to early diagnosis of acute myocardial infarction. Br Heart J 72:112
Bakker AJ, Koelemay MJ, Gorgels JP, van Vlies B, Smits R, Tijssen JG, Haagen FD (1994) Troponin T and myoglobin at admission: value of early diagnosis of acute myocardial infarction. Eur Heart J 15:45
Bakri YN et al (1993) Placenta percreta with bladder invasion: report of three cases. Am J Perinatol 10:468
Balkan E, Kilic N, Dogruygol (2005) Indirect computed tomography sign of renal artery injury: retrograde filling of the renal vein. Int J Urol 12:311
Balkan E, Kilic N, Dogruyol H (2005) The effectiveness of early primary realignment in children with posterior urethral injury. Int J Urol 12:62
Ballesteros Sampol JJ, Alameda Quitllet F et al (2002) 3 rare cases of textiloma after renal surgery. Review of the literature. Arch Esp Urol 55:25
Ballestri M, Baraldi A et al (2001) Liver and kidney foreign bodies granulomatosis in a patient with malocclusion, bruxism, and worn dental prostheses. Gastroenterology 121:12348
Ballinger S (2003) Henoch-Schonlein purpura. Curr Opin Rheumatol 15:591

Balthazar EJ (1994) For suspected small-bowel obstruction and an equivocal plain film, should we perform CT or a small-bowel series? AJR Am J Roentgenol 163:1260

Balthazar EJ, Birnbaum BA, Yee J, Megibow AJ, Roshkow J, Gray C (1994) Acute appendicitis: CT, US correlation in 100 patients. Radiology 190:31

Balzarro M, Ficarra V, Bartoloni A, Tallarigo C, Malossini G (2001) The pathophysiology, diagnosis and therapy of the transurethral resection of the prostate syndrome. Urol Int 66:121

Bandhauer K, Hassler H (1990) Injuries of the urogenital system. Urologe A 29:234

Baniel J, Schein M (1994) The management of penetrating trauma to the urinary tract. J Am Coll Surg 178:417

Baniel J, Sella A (1999) Complications of retroperitoneal lymph node dissection in testicular cancer: primary and post-chemotherapy. Semin Surg Oncol 17:263

Baniel J, Sella A (2001) Sperm extraction at orchiectomy for testis cancer. Fertil Steril 75:260

Baniel J, Foster RS, Rowland RG, Bihrle R, Donohue JP (1993) Management of chylous ascites after retroperitoneal lymph node dissection for testicular cancer. J Urol 150:1422

Banks DW, O'Brien DP 3rd, Amerson JR, Hester TR Jr (1986) Gracilis musculocutaneous flap reconstruction after Fournier gangrene. Urology 28:275

Bar K, Klijer R et al (2002) Ureter injury as a gynecologic surgery complication–prospects for conservative treatment. Ginekol Pol 73:50

Barbagli G, Selli C, Stomaci N, Delle-Rose A, Trippitelli A, Lenzi R (1987) Urethral trauma: radiological aspects and treatment options. J Trauma 27:256

Barbaric ZL, Hall T, Cochran ST, Heitz DR, Schwartz RA, Krasny RM, Deseran MW (1997) Percutaneous nephrostomy: placement under CT and fluoroscopy guidance. Am J Roentgenol 169:151

Barcena A, Lobato RD, Rivas JJ (1984) Spinal metastatic disease: analysis of factors determining functional prognosis and the choice of treatment. Neurosurgery 15:820

Bariol, SV, Stewart GD et al (2005) An analysis of urinary tract trauma in Scotland: imnpact on management and resource needs. Surgeon 3:27

Barker DE, Kaufman HJ, Smith LA, Ciraulo DL, Richart CL, Burns RP (2000) Vacuum pack technique of temporary abdominal closure: a 7-year experience with 112 patients. J Trauma 48:201; discussion 206

Barone GW, Sailors DM et al (1997) Trauma management in solid organ transplant recipients. J Emerg Med 15:169

Barone R, Borson-Chazot F et al (2005) Patient-specific dosimetry in predicting renal toxicity with (90)Y-DOTATOC: relevance of kidney volume and dose rate in finding a dose-effect relationship. J Nucl Med 46 [Suppl 1]:99SS

Barqawi A, de Valdenebro M, Furness PD 3rd, Koyle MA (2004) Lessons learned from stomal complications in children with cutaneous catheterizable continent stomas. BJU Int 94:1344

Barron WM (1985) Medical evaluation of the pregnant patient requiring non-obstetric surgery. Clin Perinatol 12:481

Barry JM (1976) Priapism: treatment with corpus cavernosum to dorsal vein of penis shunts. J Urol 116:754

Barry JM (1989) Visual urethrotomy in the management of the obliterated membranous urethra. Urol Clin North Am 16:319

Barsness KA, Bensard DD et al (2004) Renovascular injury: an argument for renal preservation. J Trauma 57:310

Base J, Navratilova J et al (1995) Blunt injury of the kidney–personal experience and present views on its therapy. Sb Ved Pr Lek Fak Karlovy Univerzity Hradci Kralove Suppl 38:81

Baskett PJ (1990) ABC of major trauma. Management of hypovolaemic shock. BMJ 300:1453

Baskin LS, McAninch JW (1993) Childhood urethral injuries: perspectives on outcome and treatment. Br J Urol 72:241

Baskin LS, Carroll PR, Cattolica EV, McAninch JW (1990) Necrotising soft tissue infections of the perineum and genitalia. Bacteriology, treatment and risk assessment. Br J Urol 65: 524

Bass DH, Semple PL et al (1991) Investigation and management of blunt renal injuries in children: a review of 11 years' experience. J Pediatr Surg 26:196

Bassiri A, Ahmadnia H et al (2002) Transureteral lithotripsy in pediatric practice. J Endourol 16:257

Bastuba MD, Saenz de Tejada I, Dinlenc CZ et al (1994) Arterial priapism: diagnosis, treatment and long-term followup. J Urol 151:1231

Basu D, Gallus A, Hirsh J, Cade J (1972) A prospective study of the value of monitoring heparin treatment with the activated partial thromboplastin time. N Engl J Med 287:324

Bateman BG, Kolp LA, Hoeger K (1996) Complications of laparoscopy–operative and diagnostic. Fertil Steril 66:30

Bates DW, Cook EF, Goldman L, Lee TH (1990) Predicting bacteremia in hospitalized patients. A prospectively validated model. Ann Intern Med 113:495

Bates MC, Shamsham FM et al (2002) Successful treatment of iatrogenic renal artery perforation with an autologous vein-covered stent. Catheter Cardiovasc Interv 57:39

Bates SM, Ginsberg JS (2004) Clinical practice. Treatment of deep-vein thrombosis. N Engl J Med 351:268

Baughman SM, Morey AF et al (2003) Percutaneous transrenal application of fibrin sealant for refractory urinary leak after gunshot wound. J Urol 170:522

Baumann L, Greenfield SP et al (1992) Nonoperative management of major blunt renal trauma in children: in- hospital morbidity and long-term followup. J Urol 148:691

Baurienne H (1764) Sur une plaie contuse qui s'est terminée par le sphacèle du scrotum. J Med Chir Pharm 20:251

Baverstock R, Simons R et al (2001) Severe blunt renal trauma: a 7-year retrospective review from a provincial trauma centre. Can J Urol 8:13726

Bechara A, Casabe A, Cheliz G et al (1997) Comparative study of papaverine plus phentolamine versus prostaglandin E1 in erectile dysfunction. J Urol 157:2132

Benjelloun S, el Mrini M, Aboutaieb R et al (1993) Priapism. A propos of 10 cases (translation). J Urol (Paris) 99:91

Becker CD, Mentha G et al (1998) Blunt abdominal trauma in adults: role of CT in the diagnosis and management of visceral injuries. Part 2: gastrointestinal tract and retroperitoneal organs. Eur Radiol 8(5):772

Becker F, Siemer S, Humke U, Hack M, Ziegler M, Stockle M (2005) Elective Nephron Sparing Surgery Should Become Standard Treatment for Small Unilateral Renal Cell Carcinoma: Long-term Survival Data of 216 Patients. Eur Urol 49:308

Becker JM, Dayton MT, Fazio VW, Beck DE, Stryker SJ, Wexner SD, Wolff BG, Roberts PL, Smith LE, Sweeney SA Moore M (1996) Prevention of postoperative adhesions by a sodium hyaluronate-bases bioresorbable membrane: a prospective. randomized double-blind multicenter study. J Am Coll Surg 183:297

Bedi A, Miller CB, Hanson JL et al (1995) Association of BK virus with failure of prophylaxis against hemorrhagic cystitis following bone marrow transplantation. J Clin Oncol 13: 1103

Beduschi R, Wolf JS Jr (1997) Fragment of a catheter as a foreign body in the kidney. Tech Urol 3:222

Behrendt P, Do D, Baumgartner I, Triller J, Kniemeyer H, Mahler F (2000) Renal artery stenting following acute aortic dissection: implantation and follow-up. Vasa 29:138

Bejanga BL (1979) Fournier's gangrene. Br J Urol 51:312

Bejany DE, Lockhart JL, Politano VA (1991) Ileal segment for ureteral substitution or for improvement of ureteral function. J Urol 146:302

Belda FJ, Aguilera L, Garcia de la Asuncion J et al (2005) Supplemental perioperative oxygen and the risk of surgical wound infection: a randomized controlled trial. JAMA 294:2035

Bell DM, Goldmann DA, Hopkins CC, Karchmer AW, Moellering RC Jr (1978) Unreliability of fever and leukocytosis in the diagnosis of infection after cardiac valve surgery. J Thorac Cardiovasc Surg 75:87

Bellanova G, Serao A et al (2003) Hepatic and renal trauma: importance of arteriography in diagnosis and treatment. Ann Ital Chir 74:31

Bellman GC (1996) Complications of endopyelotomy. J Endourol 10:177

Ben Meir D, Lask D, Koren R, Livne PM (2003) Intrarenal foreign body presenting as a solid tumor. Urology 61:1035

Benchekroun A, Lachkar A et al (1997) Kidney injuries. A propos of 30 cases. Ann Urol (Paris) 31:237

Benizri E, Fabiani P, Migliori G et al (1996) Gangrene of the perineum. Urology 47:935

Benizri E, Fabiani P, Migliori G, Chevallier D, Peyrottes A, Raucoules M, Amiel J, Mouiel J, Toubol J (1996) Gangrene of the perineum. Urology 47:935

Benjamin DK Jr, Fisher RG, McKinney RE Jr, Benjamin DK (1999) Candidal mycetoma in the neonatal kidney. Pediatrics 104:1126

Benjamin K (2002) Scrotal and inguinal masses in the newborn period. Adv Neonatal Care 2:140

Benjamin ME, Sandager GP et al (1999) Duplex ultrasound insertion of inferior vena cava filters in multitrauma patients. Am J Surg 178:92

Ben-Menachem Y (1988) Pelvic fractures: diagnostic and therapeutic angiography. Instr Course Lect 37:139

Ben-Menachem Y et al (1991) Hemorrhage associated with pelvic fractures: causes, diagnosis, and emergent management. AJR Am J Roentgenol 157:1005

Bennani S, Aboutaieb R et al (1995) Evaluation and treatment of closed traumas of the kidney. J Chir (Paris) 132:142

Benoit G, Jaber N, Moukarzel M, Douguet D, Bensadoun D, Bensadoun H, Blanchet P et al (1994) Incidence of vascular complications in kidney transplantation: is there any interference with the nature of the perfusion solution? Clin Transplant 8:485

Benson DA, Stockinger ZT et al (2005) Embolization of an acute renal arteriovenous fistula following a stab wound: case report and review of the literature. Am Surg 71:62

Benson MC, Ollson CA (2002) Cutaneous continent urinary diversion. In: Walsh PC et al (eds) Campbell's urology. Elsevier, Philadelphia, pp 3806

Benson MC, Ring KS, Olsson CA (1990) Ureteral reconstruction and bypass: experience with ileal interposition, the Boari flap-psoas hitch and renal autotransplantation. J Urol 143:20

Berbari EF, Osmon DR, Duffy MC et al (2006) Outcome of prosthetic joint infection in patients with rheumatoid arthritis: the impact of medical and surgical therapy in 200 episodes. Clin Infect Dis 42:216

Berger R, Billups K, Brock G, Broderick GA, Dhabuwala CB, Goldstein I, Hakim LS, Hellstrom W, Honig S, Levine LA, Lue T, Munarriz R, Montague DK, Mulcahy JJ, Nehra A, Rogers ZR, Rosen R, Seftel AD, Shabsigh R, Steers W; AFUD Thought Leader Panel on Evaluation and Treatment of Priapism (2001) Report of the American Foundation for Urologic Disease (AFUD) Thought Leader Panel for evaluation and treatment of priapism. Int J Impot Res 13 [Suppl 5]:S39

Berger RE (2005) Bacteria of preoperative urinary tract infections contaminate the surgical fields and develop surgical site infections in urological operations. J Urol 174:2244

Bergreen PW, Woodside J, Paster SB (1997) Therapeutic renal infarction. J Urol 118:372

Berkmen F, Peker AE et al (2000) Treatment of iatrogenic ureteral injuries during various operations for malignant conditions. J Exp Clin Cancer Res 19:441

Berkovich GY, Ramchandani P et al (2001) Renal vein thrombosis after martial arts trauma. J Trauma 50:144

Berman AT, Tom L (1974) Traumatic separation of the pubic symphysis with associated fatal rectal tear: A case report and analysis of mechanism of injury. J Trauma 14:1060

Bernard GR, Vincent JL, Laterre PF, LaRosa SP, Dhainaut JF, Lopez-Rodriguex S, Steingrub JS, Garber GE, Helterbrand JD, Ely EW, Fisher CJ (2001) Efficacy and safety of recombinant human activated protein C for severe sepsis. N Eng J Med 344:699

Bernath AS, Schutte H et al (1983) Stab wounds of the kidney: conservative management in flank penetration. J Urol 129:468

Bernhard PH, Reddy PK (1996) Retrograde ureteral intussusception: a rare complication. Endourology 10:349

Bernstein IL, Gruchalla RS, Lee RE et al (1999) Executive summary of disease management of drug hypersensitivity:a practice parameter. Joint task force on practice parameters, the American Academy of Allergy, Asthma and Immunology. Ann Allergy Asthma Immunol 83:665

Berry A, Barratt A (2002) Prophylatic antibiotic use in transurethral prostatic resection: a meta-analysis. J Urol 167:571

Bertini JE Jr, Corriere JN Jr (1988) The etiology and management of genital injuries. J Trauma 28:1278

Bertrand ME, Rupprecht HJ, Urban P, Gershlick AH; CLASSICS Investigators (2000) Double-blind study of safety of clopidogrel with and without a loading dose in combination with aspirin compared with ticlopidine in combination with aspirin after coronary stenting: the clopidogrel aspirin stent international cooperative study (CLASSICS). Circulation 102:624

Best CD, Petrone P, Buscarini M et al (2005) Traumatic ureteral injuries: a single institution experience validating the American Association for the Surgery of Trauma-Organ Injury Scale grading scale. J Urol 173:1202

Bevers RF, Bakker DJ, Kurth KH (1995) Hyperbaric oxygen treatment for haemorrhagic radiation cystitis. Lancet 346:803

Bhandari A, McIntire L, Kaul SA, Hemal AK, Peabody JO, Menon M (2005) Perioperative complications of robotic radical prostatectomy after the learning curve. J Urol 174:915

Bhanganada K, Chayavatana T, Pongnumkul C et al (1983) Surgical management of an epidemic of penis amputations in Siam. Am J Surg 146:376

Bhayani SB, Grubb RL 3rd et al (2002) Use of gelatin matrix to rapidly repair diaphragmatic injury during laparoscopy. Urology 60:514

Bialecki ES, Bridges KR (2002) Sildenafil relieves priapism in patients with sickle cell disease. Am J Med 113:252

Bianchi G, Lamazza A et al (1997) Diagnostic and therapeutic approach to kidney injuries. G Chir 18:308

Bigongiari LR et al (2000) Trauma to the bladder and urethra. American College of Radiology. ACR Appropriateness Criteria. Radiology 215:733

Bilbao JI, Cosin O, Bastarrika G, Rosell D, Zudaire J, Martinez-Cuesta A (2005) Treatment of ureteroarterial fistulae with covered vascular endoprostheses and ureteral occlusion. Cardiovasc Intervent Radiol 28:159

Bilen CY, Sahin A et al (1999) Nonoliguric renal failure after transurethral resection of prostate. J Endourol 13:751

Bilen CY, Inci K, Erkan I et al (2003) The predictive value of pu-

rified protein derivative results on complications and prognosis in patients with bladder cancer treated with bacillus Calmette-Guerin. J Urol 169:1702
Bircher M, Giannoudis PV (2004) Pelvic trauma management within the UK: a reflection of a failing trauma service. Injury 35:2
Birnbaum J, Porri F, Pradal M, Charpin D, Vervloet D (1994) Allergy during anaesthesia. Clin Exp Allergy 24:915
Bishoff JT, Allaf ME, Kirkels W, Moore RG, Kavoussi LR, Schroder F (1999) Laparoscopic bowel injury: incidence and clinical presentation. J Urol 161:887
Bittard H, Chaabouni MN et al (1995) Surgery for severe traumas of the kidney. Value of initial computed tomography, problem of surgical indication and use of a perirenal resorbable prosthesis of polyglactin 910. J Urol 101:209
Biyani CS, Joyce AD (2002a) Urolithiasis in pregnancy. I: pathophysiology, fetal considerations and diagnosis. BJU Int 89:811
Biyani CS, Joyce AD (2002b) Urolithiasis in pregnancy. II: management. BJU Int 89:819
Biyani CS, Powell CS (1998) Guidewire fragmentation during holmium: YAG laser endopyelotomy. Tech Urol 4:51
Bjornsson TD, Nash PV (1986) Variability in heparin sensitivity of APTT reagents. Am J Clin Pathol 86:199
Blacker KH, Wong N (1963) Four cases of autocastration. Arch Gen Psychiatry 8:189
Blackmer J (2003) Rehabilitation medicine: autonomic dysreflexia. CMAJ 28:169:931
Blake AM, Toker SI et al (2002) Trauma management in the end-stage renal disease patient. Am Surg 68:425
Blandy JP (1980) Urethral stricture. Postgrad Med 56:383
Blankenship B, Earls JP et al (1997) Renal vein thrombosis after vascular pedicle injuryclin conference. AJR Am J Roentgenol 168:1574
Blankenship JC, Gavant ML et al (2001) Importance of delayed imaging for blunt renal trauma. World J Surg 25:15614
Bleetman A, Dyer J (2000) Ultrasound assessment of the vulnerability of the internal organs to stabbing: determining safety standards for stab-resistant body armour. Injury 31:609
Bliem F, Lamche M, Janda R, Ilias W, Schramek P (2003) Blood loss and absorption in TURP vs. TUVRP under low pressure and high pressure conditions. Urologe A 42:1477
Blohme I, Fehrman I, Norden (1992) Living donor nephrectomy complication rates in 490 consecutive cases. Scand J Urol Nephrol 26:149
Bloom DA, Lieskovsky G, Rainwater G (1983) The Turnball loop stoma. J Urol 129:715
Bloomfield P, Hodson EM, Craig JC (2005) Antibiotics for acute pyelonephritis in children. Cochrane Database Syst Rev: CD003772
Bluebond-Langner R, Rha KH, Pinto PA et al (2004) Laparoscopic-assisted renal autotransplantation. Urology 63:853
Blum U, Billmann P, Krause T, Gabelmann A, Keller E, Moser E, Langer M (1993) Effect of local low-dose thrombolysis on clinical outcome in acute embolic renal artery occlusion. Radiology 189:549
Blumberg HM, Burman WJ, Chaisson RE et al (2003) American Thoracic Society/Centers for Disease Control and Prevention/Infectious Diseases Society of America: treatment of tuberculosis. Am J Respir Crit Care Med 167:603
Blute ML, Segura JW, Patterson DE (1988) Ureteroscopy. J Urol 139:510
Bochinski DJ, Dean RC, Lue TF (2004) Erectile dysfunction and priapism. Nat Clin Pract Urol 1:49
Bochud PY, Glauser MP, Calandra T (2001) Antibiotics in sepsis. Intensive Care Med 27 [Suppl 1]:S33
Bodey GP, Buckley M, Sathe YS et al (1966) Quantitative relationships between circulating leukocytes and infection in patients with acute leukemia. Ann Intern Med. 64:328
Bodey GP, Rodriguez V, Chang HY et al (1978) Fever and infection in leukemic patients: a study of 494 consecutive patients. Cancer 41:1610
Bodie B, Novick AC, Rose M et al (1986) Long-term results with renal autotransplantation for ureteral replacement. J Urol 136:1187
Bodmann KF, Vogel F (2001) Antimikrobielle Therapie der Sepsis. Chemother J 10:43
Boeckel J (1908) Nouveau procédé de prostatectomie par mobilisation temporaire du segment ano-rectal. Rev Chirurg 3:386
Boedker A, Roikjaer O, Rasmussen F, Loekkegaard H (1990) Lymphocele following renal transplantation: a clinical study. Transplant Proc 22:54
Boettiger BW, Motsch J, Teschendorf P et al (2004) Postoperative 12-lead ECG predicts perioperative myocardial ischaemia associated with myocardial cell damage. Anaesthesia 59:1083
Boey JH (1994) Peritoneal cavity. In: Way LW (ed) Current surgical diagnosis treatment, 10th edn. Appleton Lange,Norwalk, p 453
Bogdanovic J, Djozic J et al (2002) Successful surgical reconstruction of ruptured renal pelvis following blunt abdominal trauma. Urol Int 68:302
Boggi, U, R Berchiolli et al (1998) Renal hypertension due to giant perirenal haematoma: permanent resolution by percutaneous ultrasound-guided drainage. Scand J Urol Nephrol 32:64
Bohnen J, Boulanger M, Meakins JL, McLean AP (1983) Prognosis in generalized peritonitis. Relation to cause and risk factors. Arch Surg 118:285
Bohner H, Yang Q, Franke C et al (1998) Simple data from history and physical examination help to exclude bowel obstruction and to avoid radiographic studies in patients with acute abdominal pain. Eur J Surg 164:777
Bond SJ et al (1991) Predictors of abdominal injury in children with pelvic fracture. J Trauma 31:1169
Bone RC, Balk RA, Cerra FB et al (1992) Definitions for sepsis and organ failure and guidelines for the use of innovative therapies in sepsis. Chest 101:1644
Boone TB, Gilling PJ, Husmann DA (1993) Ureteropelvic junction disruption following blunt abdominal trauma. J Urol 150:33
Borboroglu PG, Kane CJ (2000) Current management of severely encrusted ureteral stents with a large associated stone burden. J Urol 164:648
Borboroglu PG, Kane CJ, Ward JF, Roberts JL, Sands JP (1999) Immediate and postoperative complications of transurethral prostatectomy in the 1990s. J Urol 162:1307
Borboroglu PG, Sands JP, Roberts JL et al (2000) Risk factors for vesicourethral anastomotic stricture after radical prostatectomy. Urology 56:96
Borer JG, Gargollo PC, Hendren WH, Diamond DA, Peters CA, Atala A et al (2005) Early outcome following complete primary repair of bladder exstrophy in the newborn. J Urol 174:1674
Borish L, Tamir R, Rosenwasser LJ (1987) Intravenous desensitization to beta-lactam antibiotics. J Allergy Clin Immunol 80:314
Bosl GJ, Bajorin DF, Sheinfeld J et al Cancer of the testis. In: DeVita VT Jr, Hellman S, Rosenberg SA (eds) Cancer principles and practice of oncology. Lippincott Williams and Wilkins, Philadelphia
Bosniak MA, Megibow AJ, Hulnick DH et al (1988) CT diagnosis of renal angiomyolipoma: the importance of detecting small amounts of fat. AJR Am J Roentgenol 151:497

Bothwell WN, Bleicher RJ, Dent TL (1994) Prophylactic ureteral catheterization in colon surgery. A five-year review. Dis Colon Rectum 37:330
Bousvaros A, Kirks DR, Grossman H (1986) Imaging of neuroblastoma: an overview. Pediatr Radiol 16:89
Bove KE (1999) Wilms' tumor and related abnormalities in the fetus and newborn. Semin Perinatol 23:310
Bow EJ, Schwarer AP, Laverdiere M et al (2003) Efficacy of piperacillin/tazobactam as initial therapy of febrile neutropenia in patients with hematologic malignancies. Paper presented at the 2003 Interscience Conference on Antimicrobial Agents and Chemotherapy, Chicago IL
Boxer RJ, Fritzsche P, Skinner DG et al (1979) Replacement of the ureter by small intestine: clinical application and results of the ileal ureter in 89 patients. J Urol 121:728
Bozeman C, Carver B et al (2004) Selective operative management of major blunt renal trauma. J Trauma 57:305
Bozzetti F, Braga M, Gianotti L, Gavazzi, C Mariani L (2001) Postoperative enteral versus parenteral nutrition in malnourished patients with gastrointestinal cancer: a randomised multicentre trial. Lancet 358:1487
Braams R, Vossen V et al (1999) Outcome in patients requiring renal replacement therapy after surgery for ruptured and non-ruptured aneurysm of the abdominal aorta. Eur J Vasc Endovasc Surg 18:323
Braasch WF (1952) End results following nephrectomy in patients with hypertension. J Urol 68:6
Braddom RL, RJ (1991) Autonomic dysreflexia. A survey of current treatment. Am J Phys Med Rehabil 70:234
Braf ZF, Koontz WW (1977) Gangrene of the bladder. Complication of hypogastric artery embolization. Urology 9:670
Brandes SB, McAninch JW (1999) Reconstructive surgery for trauma of the upper urinary tract. Urol Clin North Am 26:183
Brandes SB, McAninch JW (1999) Urban free falls and patterns of renal injury: a 20-year experience with 396 cases. J Trauma 47:643; discussion 649
Brandes SB, McAninch JW (2004) Renal trauma: a practical guide to evaluation and management. Sci World J 4[Suppl 1]:31
Brandes SB, Chelsky MJ, Buckman RF et al (1994) Ureteral injuries from penetrating trauma. J Trauma 36:766
Brandes SB, Chelsky MJ, Hanno PM (1994) Adult acute idiopathic scrotal edema. Urology 44:602
Brandes SB, Buckman RF, Chelsky MJ, Hanno PM (1995) External genitalia gunshot wounds: a ten-year experience with fifty-six cases. J Trauma 39:266
Brandes S, Coburn M, Armenakas N et al (2004) Diagnosis and management of ureteric injury: an evidence based analysis. BJU Int 94:277
Brandjes DP, Heijboer H, Buller HR, de Rijk M, Jagt H, ten Cate JW (1992) Acenocoumarol and heparin compared with acenocoumarol alone in the initial treatment of proximal-vein thrombosis. N Engl J Med 327:1485
Brandt B, Desroches A (1985) Echographie rénale chez la femme enceinte. In: Chatelain C et al (eds) Urologie : pathologie infectieuse et parasitaire, Masson, Paris, pp 400
Bratzler DW, Houck PM (2005) Antimicrobial prophylaxis for surgery: an advisory statement from the National Surgical Infection Prevention Project. Am J Surg 189:395
Braunschweig CL, Levy P, Sheean PM, Wang X (2001) Enteral compared with parenteral nutrition: a meta-analysis. Am J Clin Nutr 74:534
Brawn PN, Johnson EH, Speights VO et al (1994) Incidence, racial differences, and prognostic significance of prostate carcinomas diagnosed with obstructive symptoms. Cancer 74:1607
Breen DJ, Janzen DL et al (1997) Blunt bowel and mesenteric injury: diagnostic performance of CT signs. J Comput Assist Tomogr 21:706
Brennan PW, Everest ER et al (2002) Risk of death among cases attending South Australian major trauma services after severe trauma: the first 4 years of operation of a state trauma system. J Trauma 53:333
Brenneman FD et al (1997) Long-term outcomes in open pelvic fractures. J Trauma 42:773
Bretan PN Jr, McAninch JW et al (1986) Computerized tomographic staging of renal trauma:85 consecutive cases. J Urol 136:561
Bright TC III, Peters PC (1977) Ureteral injuries due to external violence:10 years' experience with 59 cases. J Trauma 17:616
Brill AI, Nezhat F, Nezhat CH, Nezhat C (1995) The incidence of adhesions after prior laparotomy: a laparoscopic appraisal. Obstet Gynecol 85:269
Brock G, Breza J, Lue TF et al (1993) High flow priapism: a spectrum of disease. J Urol 150:968
Brock N, Phol J, Stekar J (1981) Detoxification of urotoxic oxazaphosphorines by sulfhydryl compounds. J Cancer Res Clin Oncol 100:311
Brockow K (2005) Contrast media hypersensitivity – scope of the problem. Toxicology 209:189
Brockow K, Vieluf D, Puschel K, Grosch J, Ring J (1999) Increased postmortem serum mast cell tryptase in a fatal anaphylactoid reaction to nonionic radiocontrast medium. J Allergy Clin Immunol 104:237
Brockow K, Romano A, Blanca M, Ring J, Pichler W, Demoly P (2002) General considerations for skin test procedures in the diagnosis of drug hypersensitivity. Allergy 57:45
Brockow K, Christiansen C, Kanny G, Clément O, Barbaud A, Bircher A, DeWachter P, Guéant J-L, Guéant R-M R, Mouton-Faivre C, Ring J, Romano A, Sainte-Laudy J, Demoly P, Pichler WJ for ENDA and the EAACI interest group on drug hypersensitivity (2005) Management of hypersensitivity reactions to iodinated contrast media. Allergy 60:150
Broder LE, Weintraub BD, Rosen SW, Cohen MH, Tejada F (1977) Placental proteins and their subunits as tumor markers in prostatic carcinoma. Cancer 40:211
Broeders IA, Blankensteijn JD et al (1999) Mid-term fixation stability of the EndoVascular Technologies endograft. EVT Investigators. Eur J Vasc Endovasc Surg 18:300
Bronder CS, Cowey A, Hill J (2004) Delayed stoma formation in Fournier's gangrene. Colorectal Dis 6:518
Brountzos EN (2006) Quality improvement guidelines for percutaneous nephrostomies. http://www.cirse.org/_files/contentmanagement/05_qig.pdf. Cited 9 April 2006
Brown DF, Rosen CL et al (1997) Renal ultrasonography. Emerg Med Clin North Am 15:877
Brown KM, Borge MA et al (2002) Pelvic lymphocele following motor vehicle collision. Ann Vasc Surg 16:121
Brown MA, Sirlin CB et al (2005) Screening sonography in pregnant patients with blunt abdominal trauma. J Ultrasound Med 24:175; quiz 183
Brown RB (1969) A method of management of inoperable carcinoma of the bladder. Med J Aust 1:23
Brown SA, Munver R et al (2000) Microdialysis assessment of shock wave lithotripsy-induced renal injury. Urology 56:364
Brown SL, Elder JS et al (1998) Are pediatric patients more susceptible to major renal injury from blunt trauma? A comparative study. J Urol 160:138
Brown SL, Hoffman DM et al (1998) Limitations of routine spiral computerized tomography in the evaluation of blunt renal trauma. J Urol 160:19791
Brown SL, Haas C et al (2001) Radiologic evaluation of pediatric blunt renal trauma in patients with microscopic hematuria. World J Surg 25:15570
Browse NL, Wilson NM, Russo F, al-Hassan H, Allen DR (1992) Aetiology and treatment of chylous ascites. Br J Surg 79:1145
Broyer M, Gognadoux MF, Sierro A, Fischer AH, Niaudet P

(1991) Preventive treatment of vascular thrombosis after kidney transplantation in children with low molecular weight heparin. Transplant Proc 23:1384
Bruce AW, Reid G, Chan RC Costerton JW (1984) Bacterial adherence in the human ileal conduit: a morphological and bacteriological study. J Urol 132:184
Bruce LM, Croce MA et al (2001) Blunt renal artery injury: incidence, diagnosis, and management. Am Surg 67:550; discussion 555
Bruninx G, Wery D et al (1999) Emergency endovascular treatment of an acute traumatic rupture of the thoracic aorta complicated by a distal low-flow syndrome. Cardiovasc Intervent Radiol 22:515
Brunkwall J, Lanne T et al (1999) Acute renal impairment due to a primary aortocaval fistula is normalised after a successful operation. Eur J Vasc Endovasc Surg 17:191
Bryan DE, Mulcahy JJ, Simmons GR (2002) Salvage procedure for infected noneroded artificial urinary sphincters. J Urol 168:2464
Bryant K, Maxfield C, Rabalais G (1999) Renal candidiasis in neonates with candiduria. Pediatr Infect Dis J 18:959
Bschleipfer TH, Hauck EW, Diemer TH et al (2001) Heparin-induced priapism. Int J Impot Res 13:357
Bschleipfer T, Kallieris D et al (2002) Blunt renal trauma: biomechanics and origination of renal lesions. Eur Urol 42:614
Bschleipfer T, Kallieris D et al (2003) Validity of computerized tomography in blunt renal trauma. J Urol 170:24759
Bubley GJ (2001) Is the flare phenomenon clinically significant? Urology 58 [2 Suppl 1]:5
Buchberger W, Penz T et al (1993) Diagnosis and staging of blunt kidney trauma. A comparison of urinalysis, i.v. urography, sonography and computed tomography. Rofo Fortschr Geb Rontgenstr Neuen Bildgeb Verfahr 158:507
Buchholz HW, Elson RA, Engelbrecht E, Lodenkamper H, Rottger J, Siegel A (1981) Management of deep infection of total hip replacement. J Bone Joint Surg Br 63-B:342
Buckley JC, McAninch JW (2004) Pediatric renal injuries: management guidelines from a 25-year experience. J Urol 172:687; discussion 690
Buckman RF, AS Pathak, et al (2001) Injuries of the inferior vena cava. Surg Clin North Am 81:14317
Bucy JG (1968) Removal of strangulating objects from the penis. J Urol 99:194
Budman DR, Berry DA, Cirrincione CT et al (1998) Dose and dose intensity as determinants of outcome in the adjuvant treatment of breast cancer. The Cancer and Leukemia Group B. J Natl Cancer Inst 90:1205
Buecker A, Neuerburg JM, Adam GB, Nolte-Ernsting CC, Hunter DW, Glowinski A, van Vaals JJ, Günther RW (2001) MR-guided percutaneous drainage of abdominal fluid collections in combination with X-ray fluoroscopy: initial clinical experience. Eur Radiol 11:670
Bufalari A, Giustozzi G, Moggi L (1996) Postoperative intraabdominal abscesses: percutaneous versus surgical treatment. Acta Chir Belg 96:197
Buller HR, Lensing AW, Hirsh J, ten Cate JW (1991) Deep vein thrombosis: new non-invasive diagnostic tests. Thromb Haemost 66:133
Bunt TJ (1985) Urgent relaparotomy: the high-risk no-choice operation. Surgery 98:555
Burbridge BE, Groot G et al (1991) Emergency excretory urography in blunt abdominal trauma. Can Assoc Radiol J 42:326
Burke BJ, Washowich TL (1998) Ureteral jets in normal second and third trimester pregnancy. J Clin Ultrasound 26:423
Burkert H (1983) Clinical overview of mesna. Cancer Treat Rev 10 [Suppl A]:175
Burnett AL, Allen RP, Tempany CM et al (1995) Evaluation of erectile function in men with sickle cell disease. Urology 45:657
Burtis WJ, Brady TG, Orloff JJ et al (1990) Immunochemical characterization of circulating parathyroid hormone-related protein in patients with humoral hypercalcemia of cancer. N Engl J Med 322:1106
Busby JE, Pettaway CA (2005) What's new in the management of penile cancer? Curr Opin Urol 15:350
Buscarini et al (2000) Tube gastrostomy following radical cystectomy with urinary diversion: surgical technique and experience in 709 patients. Urology 56:150
Busch FM, Chenault OW Jr, Clarke BG et al (1967) Urological aspects of Vietnam War injuries. J Urol 97:763
Busch T, Lotfi S, Sirbu H, Aleksic I, Dalichau H (2000) Chyloperitoneum. A rare complication after abdominal aortic aneurysm repair. J Cardiovasc Surg 41:617
Bydder GM, Kreel L (1980) Computed tomography in the diagnosis of abdominal abscess. J Comput Tomogr 4:132
Byrne TN (1992) Spinal cord compression from epidural metastases. N Engl J Med 327:614
Cachecho R, Millham FH et al (1994) Management of the trauma patient with pre-existing renal disease. Crit Care Clin 10:523
Cadeddu JA, Regan F, Kavoussi LR, Moore RG (1997) The role of computerized tomography in the evaluation of complications after laparoscopic urological surgery. J Urol 158:1349
Cadeddu JA, Wolfe JS Jr, Nakada S, Chen R, Shalhav A, Bishoff JT, Hamilton B, Schulam PG, Dunn M, Hoenig D, Fabrizio M, Hedican S, Averch TD (2001) Complications of laparoscopic procedures after concentrated training in urological laparoscopy. J Urol 166:2109
Caine M, Raz S, Zeigler M (1975) Adrenergic and cholinergic receptors in the human prostate, prostatic capsule and bladder neck. Br J Urol 47:193
Cakir B, Cevik H et al (2005) Leptin ameliorates burn-induced multiple organ damage and modulates postburn immune response in rats. Regul Pept 125:135
Calandra T, Cohen J (1984) The international sepsis forum consensus conference on definitions of infection in the intensive care unit. Crit Care Med 33 1538
Caldamone AA, Frank IN (1980) Percutaneous aspiration in the treatment of renal abscess. J Urol 123:92
Callewaert PR, Van Poppel H, Vanderschueren D, Baert L (1999) Uncontrollable diabetes mellitus: a rare paraneoplastic manifestation of renal cell carcinoma. Nephrol Dial Transplant 14:2263
Cambria RP, Davison JK et al (1997) Thoracoabdominal aneurysm repair: perspectives over a decade with the clamp-and-sew technique. Ann Surg 226:294; discussion 303
Campbell EW Jr, Filderman PS, Jacobs SC (1992) Ureteral injury due to blunt and penetrating trauma. Urology 40:216
Camussi G, Albano E, Tetta C et al (1991) The molecular action of tumor necrosis factor-α. Eur J Biochem 202:3
Canby-Hagino ED, Morey AF, Jatoi I, Perahia B, Bishoff JT (2000) Fibrin sealant treatment of splenic injury during open and laparoscopic left radical nephrectomy. J Urol 164:2004
Cao P, P De Rango (1999) Abdominal aortic aneurysms: current management. Cardiologia 44:711
Capelli-Schellpfeffer M, Gerber GS (1999) The use of hyperbaric oxygen in urology. J Urol 162:647
Carcamo Valor PI, Hidalgo Togores L et al (1990) Kidney injuries in childhood: our experience in 64 cases. Arch Esp Urol 43:651; discussion 655
Carcamo Valor PI, Hidalgo Togores L et al (1991) Our experience with the diagnosis and treatment of 429 renal traumatisms. Arch Esp Urol 44:801
Carey JM, Korman HJ (2001) Transrectal ultrasound guided

biopsy of the prostate. Do enemas decrease clinically significant complications? J Urol 166:82
Carl P (1997) Diagnosis and therapy of kidney traumas. Urologe A 36:523
Carley ME, McIntire D, Carley JM et al (2002) Incidence, risk factors and morbidity of unintended bladder or ureter injury during hysterectomy. Int Urogynecol J Pelvic Floor Dysfunct 13:18
Carlin BI, Resnick MI (1995) Indications and techniques for urologic evaluation of the trauma patient with suspected urologic injury. Semin Urol 13:9
Carlton CE Jr, Scott R Jr, Goldman M (1968) The management of penetrating injuries of the kidney. J Trauma 8:1071
Carlton CE Jr, Guthrie AG, Scott R Jr (1969) Surgical correction of ureteral injury. J Trauma 9:457
Carlton CE Jr, Scott R Jr, Guthrie AG (1971) The initial management of ureteral injuries: a report of 78 cases. J Urol 105:335
Carmignani G, Belgrano E, Puppo P, Cichero A, Giuliani L (1980) Transcatheter embolization of the hypogastric arteries in cases of bladder hemorrhage from advanced pelvic cancers: follow-up in 9 cases. J Urol 124:196
Carmona Campos EC, Prieto Castro R et al (1998) Evaluation and treatment of closed renal trauma. Actas Urol Esp 22:23
Caro D (1974) Major disasters. Lancet 30:1309
Caro JJ, Trinidade E, McGregor M (1991) The risks of death and of severe nonfatal reactions with high- vs low-osmolality contrast media: a meta-analysis. AJR Am J Roentgenol 156:825
Carpio F, Morey AF (1999) Radiographic staging of renal injuries. World J Urol 17:66
Carr JA, Kralovich KA et al (2001) Primary venorraphy for traumatic inferior vena cava injuries. Am Surg 67:207; discussion 213
Carrafiello G, Lagana D, Mangini M, Cuffari S, Cafaro T, Recaldini C, Genovese E, Fugazzola C (2005) The role of interventional radiology in the management of kidney transplant complications. Radiol Med (Torino) 110:249
Carrel TP, Signer C (1999) Separate revascularization of the visceral arteries in thoracoabdominal aneurysm repair. Ann Thorac Surg 68:573
Carringer M et al (1996) Management of ureteric calculi during pregnancy by ureteroscopy and laser lithotripsy. Br J Urol 77:17
Carroll PR, Barbour S (2000) Urinary diversion and bladder substitution. In: Tanagho EA, McAninch JW (eds) Smith's general urology, 15th edn. McGraw Hill, New York, p 346
Carroll PR, McAninch JW (1984) Major bladder trauma: mechanisms of injury and a unified method of diagnosis and repair. J Urol 132:254
Carroll PR, McAninch JW (1985) Operative indications in penetrating renal trauma. J Trauma 25:587
Carroll PR, Leu TF, Schmidt RA et al (1985) Penile replantation: current concepts. J Urol 133:281
Carroll PR, McAninch JW et al (1990) Renovascular trauma: risk assessment, surgical management, and outcome. J Trauma 30:547; discussion 553
Carson CC 3rd (2004) Efficacy of antibiotic impregnation of inflatable penile prostheses in decreasing infection in original implants. J Urol 171:1611
Carson CC, Robertson CN (1988) Late hematogenous infection of penile prostheses. J Urol 139:50
Casati V, Bellotti F, Gerli C, Franco A, Oppizzi M, Calori G, Alfieri O, Torr G (2001) Tranexamic acid administration after cardiac surgery: a prospective, randomized, double-blind, placebo-controlled study. Anesthesiology 94:8
Cass AS (1984) False negative retrograde cystography with bladder rupture owing to external trauma. J Trauma 24:168
Cass AS (1989) Diagnostic studies in bladder rupture. Indications and techniques. Urol Clin North Am 16:267
Cass AS, Godec CJ (1978) Urethral injury due to external trauma. Urology 11:607
Cass AS, Luxenberg M (1987) Features of 164 bladder ruptures. J Urol 138:743
Cass AS, Luxenberg M (1988) Value of early operation in blunt testicular contusion with hematocele. J Urol 139:746
Cass AS, Luxenberg M (1989) Management of extraperitoneal ruptures of bladder caused by external trauma. Urology 33:179
Cass AS, Luxenberg M (1991) Testicular injuries. Urology 37:528
Cass AS, Luxenberg M et al (1987) Deaths from urologic injury due to external trauma. J Trauma 27:319
Cass AS, Ferrara L, Wolpert J, Lee J (1988) Bilateral testicular injury from external trauma. J Urol 140:1435
Cassar K, Munro A (2002) Iatrogenic splenic injury. J R Coll Surg Edinb 47:731
Castrucci M, D Ghio et al (1997) Embolization of iatrogenic renal vascular lesions with coaxial catheters and microcoils. Radiol Med (Torino) 93:576
Catalano O, Lobianco R et al (1999) Contrast media extravasation in upper abdominal injuries: detection with spiral computerized tomography. Radiol Med (Torino) 97:138
Catalano O, Nunziata A, Altei F et al (2002) Suspected ureteral colic: primary helical CT versus selective helical CT after unenhanced radiography and sonography. AJR Am J Roentgenol 178:379
Catalano O, Lobianco R et al (2004) Real-time, contrast-enhanced sonographic imaging in emergency radiology. Radiol Med (Torino) 108:454
Catto JW, Natarajan V, Tophill PR (2005) Simultaneous augmentation cystoplasty is associated with earlier rather than increased artificial urinary sphincter infection. J Urol 173:1237
Caumartin Y, Pouliot F, Sabbagh R, Dujardin T (2005) Chylous ascites as a complication of laparoscopic donor nephrectomy. Transpl Int 18:1378
Cayan S, Erdemir F, Ozbey I, Turek PJ, Kadioglu A, Tellaloglu S (2002) Can varicocelectomy significantly change the way couples use assisted reproductive technologies? J Urol 167:1749
Celli BR, Rodriguez KS, Snider GL (1984) A controlled trial of intermittent positive pressure breathing, incentive spirometry, and deep breathing exercises in preventing pulmonary complications after abdominal surgery. Am Rev Respir Dis 130:12
Centers for Disease Control and Prevention (2006) Explosions and blast injuries, a primer for clinicians. the Centers for Disease Control and Prevention, Atlanta. http://www.bt.cdc.gov/masstrauma/pdf/explosions-blast-injuries.pdf. Cited 27 January 2006
Cetti NE (2000) Blunt renal trauma: some personal thoughts. Scand J Urol Nephrol 34:5
Ceylan H, Gunsar C et al (2003) Blunt renal injuries in Turkish children: a review of 205 cases. Pediatr Surg Int 19:710
Chaabouni MN, Bittard M (1996) Application of a peri-renal prosthesis (Vicryl mesh) in the conservative treatment of multiple ruptured kidney fragments. Ann Urol (Paris) 30:61; discussion 64
Chaliha C, Stanton SL (2002) Urological problems in pregnancy. BJU 89:469
Challapalli H, Goldhaber SZ, Brown DF, Nadel ES (2004) Shortness of breath in the postoperative patient. J Emerg Med 27:171
Champault G, Cazacu F, Taffinder N (1996) Serious trocar accidents in laparoscopic surgery: a French survey of 103,852 operations. Surg Laparosc Endosc 6:367
Chan D, Bishoff JT, Ratner L, Kavoussi LR, Jarrett TW (2000)

Endovascular gastrointestinal stapler device malfunction during laparoscopic nephrectomy: early recognition and management. J Urol 164:319
Chan DY (2005) Stapler malfunction and management. In: Ramakumar S, Jarrett T (eds) Complications of urologic laparoscopic surgery. Taylor & Francis, Boca Raton, p 43
Chan RC, Reid G, Bruce AW, Costerton JW (2005) Microbial colonization of human ileal conduits. Appl Environ Microbiol 48:1159
Chan TC, Vilke GM, Pollack M, Brady WJ (2001) Electrocardiographic manifestations: pulmonary embolism. J Emerg Med 21:263
Chand B, Walsh RM, Ponsky J, Brody F (2001) Pancreatic complications following laparoscopic splenectomy. Surg Endosc 15:1273
Chandhoke PS, McAninch JW (1988) Detection and significance of microscopic hematuria in patients with blunt renal trauma. J Urol 140:16
Chandhoke PS, Albala DM, Clayman RV (1992) Long-term comparison of renal function in patients with solitary kidneys and/or moderate renal insufficiency undergoing extracorporeal shock wave lithotripsy or percutaneous nephrolithotomy. J Urol 147:1226
Chandler JC, Gauderer MW (2004) The neonate with an abdominal mass. Pediatr Clin North Am 51:979
Chandler JG, Corson SL, Way LW (2001) Three spectra of laparoscopic entry access injuries. J Am Coll Surg 192:478; discussion 490
Chang SS, Koch MO (1996) The use of an extended spiral bladder flap for treatment of upper ureteral loss. J Urol 156:1981
Chapple CR (2001) Alpha adrenoceptor antagonists in the year 2000: is there anything new? Curr Opin Urol 11:9
Chapple CR (2004) Pharmacological therapy of benign prostatic hyperplasia/lower urinary tract symptoms: an overview for the practising clinician. BJU Int 94:738
Chapple CR, MacDiarmid SA (2000) Urodynamics made easy. Churchill Livingstone, Edinburgh
Chapple CR, Png D (1999) Contemporary management of urethral trauma and the post-traumatic stricture. Curr Opin Urol 9:253
Chapple CR, Smith D (1994) The pathophysiological changes in the bladder obstructed by benign prostatic hyperplasia. Br J Urol 73:117
Chapron CM, Pierre F, Lacroix S, Querleu D, Lansac J, Dubuisson JB (1997) Major vascular injuries during gynecologic laparoscopy. J Am Coll Surg 185:461
Chatziioannou A, Brountzos E et al (2004) Effects of superselective embolization for renal vascular injuries on renal parenchyma and function. Eur J Vasc Endovasc Surg 28:201
Chaussy CG, Fuchs GJ (1989) Current state and future developments of noninvasive treatment of human urinary stones with extracorporeal shock wave lithotripsy. J Urol 141:782
Chawla SN, Gallop C, Mydlo JH (2003) Fournier's gangrene: an analysis of repeated surgical debridement. Eur Urol 43:572
Chazen MD, KS Miller (1997) Intrarenal pseudoaneurysm presenting 15 years after penetrating renal injury. Urology 49:774
Cheitlin MD, Armstrong WF, Aurigemma GP et al (2003) ACC/AHA/Ase 2003 Guidline update for the clinical application of echocardiography: summary article. Circulation 108:1146
Chen JL, O'Shea M (1998) Extravasation injury associated with low-dose dopamine. Ann Pharmacother 32:545
Chen X, Borsa JJ et al (2002) CT of a renal artery pseudoaneurysm caused by a stab wound. AJR Am J Roentgenol 178:736
Cheng DL, D Lazan et al (1994) Conservative treatment of type III renal trauma. J Trauma 36:491
Cherniavskii AM, Marchenko AV et al (2004) A case of surgical treatment of post-traumatic false arteriovenous aneurysm of the right kidney vessels. Angiol Sosud Khir 10:130
Cherr GS, Hansen KJ (2001) Renal complications with aortic surgery. Semin Vasc Surg 14:245
Cherullo EE, Hobart MG et al (1999) Caliceal injury during laparoscopic cyst decortication in adult polycystic kidney disease. J Urol 162:1367
Chicharro Molero JA, del Rosal Samaniego JM et al (1992) Diagnostic evaluation of closed renal trauma. Actas Urol Esp 16:192
Childs SJ (1986) Appropriate surgical prophylaxis in transurethral genitourinary surgery and potential reduction in nosocomial infections. Urology 27:415
Chintamani, Shankar M, Singhal V, Singh JP, Bansal A, Saxena S (2004) Squamous cell carcinoma developing in the scar of Fournier's gangrene – case report. BMC Cancer 4:16
Chiou RK, Gonzalez R, Ortlip S, Fraley EE (1988) Endoscopic treatment of posterior urethral obliteration: Long-term follow-up and comparison with transpubic urethroplasty. J Urol 140:508
Chitale SV, Scott-Barrett S, Ho ET et al (2002) The management of ureteric obstruction secondary to malignant pelvic disease. Clin Radiol 57:1118
Chiu AM, Kelly KJ (2005) Anaphylaxis: drug allergy, insect stings, and latex. Immunol Allergy Clin N Am 25:389
Choe JM, Battino BS, Benedict J, Bell TE (2001) Myositis and myonecrosis of the thigh: an unusual complication of a testicular thigh pouch. J Urol 165:1217
Choi MH, Kim B, Ryu JA, Lee SW, Lee KS (2000) MR imaging of acute penile fracture. Radiographics 20:1397
Chong KT, Hampson NB, Bostwick DG et al (2004) Hyperbaric oxygen does not accelerate latent in vivo prostate cancer: implications for the treatment of radiation-induced haemorrhagic cystitis. BJU Int 94:1275
Chong KT, Hampson NB, Corman JM (2005) Early hyperbaric oxygen therapy improves outcome for radiation-induced hemorrhagic cystitis. Urology 65:649
Choong S, Emberton M (2000) Acute urinary retention. BJU Int 85:186
Choong SK, Walkden M, Kirby R (2000) The management of intractable haematuria. BJU Int 86:951
Chopra P, St-Vil D, Yazbeck S (2002) Blunt renal trauma–blessing in disguise? J Pediatr Surg 37:779
Chorvat G, Kahn J, Camelot G, Henriet P, Gillet JY, Gillet M (1976) The fate of swabs forgotten in the abdomen (author's transl). Ann Chir 30:643
Chow GK (2005) Urinary leak complications of laparoscopy. In: S Ramakumar T Jarrett (eds) Complications of urologic laparoscopic surgery. Taylor & Francis, Boca Raton
Chowdhary SK, Pimpalwar A et al (2000) Blunt injury of the abdomen: a plea for CT Pediatr Radiol 30:798
Christensen R (2001) Invasive radiology for pediatric trauma. Semin Pediatr Surg 10:7
Christiansen C, Pichler WJ, Skotland T l (2000) Delayed allergy-like reactions to X-ray contrast media:mechanistic considerations. Eur Radio 10:1965
Christman JW, Wheeler AP, Bernard GR (1991) Cytokines and sepsis: what are the therapeutic implications? J Intens Care 6:172
Christou NV, Nohr CW, Meakins JL (1987) Assessing operative site infection in surgical patients. Arch Surg 122:165
Chu C, Chen K et al (2000) Delayed presentation of a posttraumatic perirenal urinoma in a 6-year-old boy. Pediatr Surg Int 16:140
Chung SY, Stein RJ, Landsittel D et al (2004) 15-year experience with the management of extrinsic ureteral obstruction with indwelling ureteral stents. J Urol 172:592
Chursin VK, Stetsenko MA et al (2000) Complete abruption of kidney off vascular pedicle. Urologiia 43
Chute CG, Stephenson WP, Guess HA et al (1991) Benign pros-

tatic hyperplasia: a population-based study. Eur Urol 20 [Suppl 1]:11
Ciftci AO, Bingol-Kologlu M, Senocak ME, Tanyel FC, Buyukpamukcu M, Buyukpamukcu N (2001) Testicular tumors in children. J Pediatr Surg, 36:1796
Cimic J, Meuleman EJH, Oosterhof GON, Hoitsma AJ (1997) Urological Complications in renal transplantation: a comparison between living-related and cadaveric grafts. Eur Urol 31:433
Cinman AC, Farrer J, Kaufman JJ (1985) Spontaneous perinephric hemorrhage in a 65-year-old man. J Urol 133:829
Cipolla J, Stawicki SP, Hoff WS, Mcquay N, Hoey BA Wainwright G, Grossman MD (2005) A proposed algorithm for managing the open abdomen. Am Surg 71:202
Citrin DL, Elson P, Kies MS, Lind R (1984) Decreased serum phosphate levels after high-dose estrogens in metastatic prostate cancer. Possible implications. Am J Med 76:787
Clancy TV et al (2001) A statewide analysis of level I and II trauma centers for patients with major injuries. J Trauma 51:346
Clark JY, Kearse WS Jr (1997) Extracorporeal shockwave lithotripsy for kidney stone on surgical clip. J Endourol 11:119
Clark RA (1981) Self-mutilation accompanying religious delusion: a case report and review. J Clin Psychiatry 42:243
Clark SS, Prudencio RF (1972) Lower urinary tract injuries associated with pelvic fractures. Surg Clin North Amer 52:183
Clarke GM (2001) Sepsis. In: O'Donnell JM, Nacul FE (eds) Surgical intensive care medicineKluwer Academic, Boston, p 411
Clarnette TD, Beasley SW (1997) Handlebar injuries in children: patterns and prevention. Aust N Z J Surg 67:338
Classen DC, Evans RS, Pestotnik SL, Horn SD, Menlove RL, Burke JP (1992) The timing of prophylactic administration of antibiotics and the risk of surgical-wound infection. N Engl J Med 326:281
Clayman RV (1985) Editorial comment. Radiology 166:83
Clayman RV, Elbers J, Miller RP, Williamson J, McKeel D, Wassynger W (1987) Percutaneous nephrostomy: assessment of renal damage associated with semi-rigid (24F) and balloon (36F) dilation. J Urol 138:203
Cleland JG, Swedberg K, Follath F et al (2003) The Euroheart failure survey programme – a survey on the quality of care among patients with heart failure in Europe. Part 1: patient characteristics and diagnostics. Eur Heart J 24:442
Cleveland RO, McAteer JA et al (1997) The effect of polypropylene vials on lithotripter shock waves. Ultrasound Med Biol 23:939
Cline KJ, Mata JA, Venable DD, Eastham JA (1998) Penetrating trauma to the male external genitalia. J Trauma 44:492
Close RJ, Sachs CJ, Dyne PL (2001) Reliability of bimanual pelvic examinations performed in emergency departments. West J Med 175:240
Coburn M (1997) Damage control for urologic injuries. Surg Clin N Am 77:821
Coffield KS, Weems WL (1977) Experience with management of posterior urethral injury associated with pelvic fractures. J Urol 117:722
Cohen BE, May JW, Daly JS et al (1977) Successful clinical replantation of an amputated penis by microneurovascular repair. Plast Reconstr Surg 59:276
Cohen GS, Braunstein L, Ball DS, Roberto PJ, Reich J, Hanno P (1996) Selective arterial embolization of idiopathic priapism. Cardiovasc Intervent Radiol 19:47
Cohen JK, Berg G, Carl GH, Diamond DD (1991) Primary endoscopic realignment following posterior urethral disruption. J Urol 146:1548
Cohen M, Morales R Jr et al (2001) Staged reconstruction after gunshot wounds to the abdomen. Plast Reconstr Surg 108:83
Cohen Z, Gabriel A et al (2000) Traumatic avulsion of kidney into the chest through a ruptured diaphragm in a boy. Pediatr Emerg Care 16:180
Colapinto V (1980) Trauma to the pelvis: urethral injury. Clin Ortho Rel Res 151:46
Colapinto V, McCallum RW (1977) Injury to the male posterior urethra in fractured pelvis: a new classification. J Urol 118:575
Colau A, Lucet JC, Rufat P, Botto H, Benoit G, Jardin A (2001) Incidence and risk factors of bacteriuria after transurethral resection of the prostate. Eur Urol 39:272
Cole BR, Conley SB, Stapleton FB (1987) Polycystic kidney disease in the first year of life. J Pediatr 111:693
Colegrove P, Ramakumar S, Hernia. In: Ramakumar S, Jarrett T (eds) Complications of urologic laparoscopic surgery. Taylor & Francis, Boca Raton, p 115
Coleman JA, Walther MM (2005) Urologic emergencies. In: DeVita VT Jr, Hellman S, Rosenberg SA (eds) Cancer principles and practice of oncology. Lippincott Williams and Wilkins, Philadelphia
Coleman RE (1997) Skeletal complications of malignancy. Cancer 80 [Suppl 8]:1588
Colistro R, Torreggiani WC, Lyburn ID et al (2002) Unenhanced helical CT in the investigation of acute flank pain. Clin Radiol 57:435
Collado A, Chechile GE, Salvador J, Vicente J (2000) Early complications of endoscopic treatment for superficial bladder tumors. J Urol 164:1529
Collinet P, Sabban F, Lucot JP, Boukerrou M, Stien L, Leroy JL (2004) Management of type III female genital mutilation. J Gynecol Obstet Biol Reprod 33:720
Collins JW, Macdermott S, Bradbrook RA, Keeley FX Jr, Timoney AG (2005) A comparison of the effect of 1.5% glycine and 5% glucose irrigants on plasma serum physiology and the incidence of transurethral resection syndrome during prostate resection. BJU Int 96:368
Collins R, Yusuf S, Peto R (1985) Overview of randomised trials of diuretics in pregnancy. BMJ 290:17
Colombo F, Lovaria A, Saccheri S, Pozzoni F, Montanaris E (1999) Arterial embolization in the treatment of post-traumatic priapism. Ann Urol (Paris) 33:210
Compton MT, Miller AH (2001) Priapism associated with conventional and atypical antipsychotic medications: a review. J Clin Psychiatry 62:362
Comstock CH et al (2004) Sonographic detection of placenta accreta in the second and third trimesters of pregnancy. Am J Obstet Gynecol 190:1135
Connolly A, Thorpe JM Jr (1999) Urinary tract infections in pregnancy. Urol Clin North Am 26:779
Conolly WB, Hedbert EA (1969) Observations on fractures of the pelvis. J Trauma 9:104
Consortium for Spinal Cord Medicine (2001) Acute management of autonomic dysreflexia: individuals with spinal cord injury presenting to health care facilities. Washington, DC, The Consortium of Paralyzed Veterans of America
Conway GS, MacConnell T, Wells G, Slater SD (1988) Importance of scrotal ultrasonography in gynaecomastia. BMJ 297:1176
Cook AJ, Farhat WA, Cartwright LM, Khoury AE, Pippi Salle JL (2005) Simplified mons plasty: a new technique to improve cosmesis in females with the exstrophy-epispadias complex. J Urol 173:2117
Cook DJ, Kollef MH (1998) Risk factors for ICU-acquired pneumonia. JAMA 279:1605
Cook DJ, Reeve BK, Guyatt GH, Heyland DK, Griffith LE, Buckingham L, Tryba M (1996) Stress ulcer prophylaxis in critically ill patients. Resolving discordant meta-analyses. JAMA 275:308

Coombs RRA, Gell PGH (1975) Classification of allergic reactions responsible for clinical hypersensitivity and disease. In: Gell PGH, Coombs RRA, Lachmann PJ (eds) Clinical aspects of immunology, 3rd edn. Blackwell, Oxford, pp 761

Cooper GJ, Maynard RL, Cross NL et al (1983) Casualties from terrorist bombings. J Trauma 23:955

Cooper MS, Stewart PM (2003) Current concepts: Corticosteroid insufficiency in acutely ill patients. N Engl J Med 348:727

Coppes MJ, Zandvoort SW, Sparling CR, Poon AO, Weitzman S, Blanchette VS (1992) Acquired von Willebrand disease in Wilms' tumor patients. J Clin Oncol 10:422

Coppes MJ, Haber DA, Grundy PE (1994) Genetic events in the development of Wilms' tumor. N Engl J Med 331:586

Coppola PT, Coppola M (2000) Emergency department evaluation and treatment of pelvic fractures. Emerg Med Clin North Am 18:1

Corman JM, Moody JA, Aronson WJ (1999) Fournier's gangrene in a modern surgical setting: improved survival with aggressive management. Br J Urol 84:85

Corrales JG, Corbel L, Cipolla B, Staerman F, Darnault P, Guille F, Lobel B (1993) Accuracy of ultrasound diagnosis after blunt testicular trauma. J Urol 150:1834

Corriere JN Jr (2001) 1-Stage delayed bulboprostatic anastomotic repair of posterior urethral rupture:60 patients with 1-year followup. J Urol 165:404

Corriere JN Jr, Harris JD (1981) The management of urological injuries in blunt pelvic trauma. Radiol Clin North Am 19:187

Corriere JN Jr, McAndrew JD et al (1991) Intraoperative decision-making in renal trauma surgery. J Trauma 31:1390

Corriere JN Jr, Rudy DC, Benson GS (1994) Voiding and erectile dysfunction after delayed one-stage repair of posterior urethral disruption in 50 men with fractured pelvis. J Trauma 37:587

Cortellini P, Ferretti S et al (1997) Major renal trauma. Therapeutic approaches and our experience. Minerva Urol Nefrol 49:183

Corvin S, Kuczyk M, Anastasiadis A, Stenzl A (2004) Laparoscopic retroperitoneal lymph node dissection for nonseminomatous testicular carcinoma. World J Urol 22:33

Couillard DR, Vapnek JM, Rentzepis MJ, Stone AR (1993) Fatal perforation of augmentation cystoplasty in an adult. Urology 42:585

Couvelaire R, Bouffard J-R (1951) L'adénomectomie prostatique par voie coccypérinéale droite. J Urol 57:362

Cowan NC, Traill ZC et al (1998) Direct percutaneous transrenal embolization for renal artery injury following percutaneous nephrostomy. Br J Radiol 71:1199

Cox JD, Stetz J, Pajak TF (1995) Toxicity criteria of the Radiation Therapy Oncology Group (RTOG) and the European Organization for Research and Treatment of Cancer (EORTC) Int J Radiat Oncol Biol Phys 31:1341

Cox PJ (1979) Cyclophosphamide cystitis: identification of acrolein as the causative agent. Biochem Pharmacol 28:2045

Cozar JM, Carcamo P et al (1990) Management of injury of the solitary kidney. Arch Esp Urol 43:15

Crain DS, Amling CL, Kane CJ (2004) Palliative transurethral prostate resection for bladder outlet obstruction in patients with locally advanced prostate cancer. J Urol 171:668

Crassweller PO, Farrow GA, Robson CJ, Russell JL, Colapinto V (1977) Traumatic rupture of the supramembranous urethra. 118:770

Crausman RS, Bravo K (1997) Ruptured abdominal aortic aneurysm masquerading as testicular pain. Am J Emerg Med 15:445

Craven DE, Steger KA (1995) Epidemiology of nosocomial pneumonia. New perspectives on an old disease. Chest 108:1S–16S

Craven JL, Evans GA, Davenport PJ, Williams RH (1974) The evaluation of the incentive spirometer in the management of postoperative pulmonary complications. Br J Surg 61:793

Cravens DD, Zweig S (2000) Urinary catheter management. Am Fam Physician 61:369

Crawford ED, Skinner DG (1980) Salvage cystectomy after radiation failure. J Urol 123:32

Crawford J, Dale DC, Lyman GH (2004) Chemotherapy-induced neutropenia: risks, consequences, and new directions for its management. Cancer 100:228

Creevy CD (1947) Haemolytic reactions during transurethral resection. J Urol 58:125

Crnich CJ, Maki DG (2002) The promise of novel technology for the prevention of intravascular device-related bloodstream infection. II Long-term devices. Clin Infect Dis 34:1362

Croft BY, Joyce JM, Parekh J et al (1996) Nuclide studies. In: Gillenwater et al (eds) Adult and pediatric urology, 3rd edn. Mosby, St Louis, pp 193

Cronan JJ Jr, Dorfman GS (1983) Low dose thrombolysis: a nonoperative approach to renal artery occlusion. J Urol 130:757

Crosson JT (1996) Massive transfusion. Clin Lab Med 16:873

Cruickshank AM, Fraser WD, Burns HJ, Van Damme J, Shenkin A (1990) Response of serum interleukin-6 in patients undergoing surgery of varying severity. Clin Sci (London) 79:161

Crummy AB, Ishizuka J, Madsen PO (1979) Posttraumatic priapism: successful treatment with autologous clot embolization. Am J Roentgenol 133:329

Cruse PJ, Foord R (1973) A five-year prospective study of 23,649 surgical wounds. Arch Surg 107:206

Cullen DJ, Coyle JP, Teplick R, Long MC (1989) Cardiovascular, pulmonary, and renal effects of massively increases abdominal pressure in critically ill patients. Crit Care Med 17:118

Culliford L (1987) Autocastration and biblical delusions in schizophrenia (letter) Br J Psychiatry 150:407

Culver DH, Horan TC, Gaynes RP et al (1991) Surgical wound infection rates by wound class, operative procedure, and patient risk index. National Nosocomial Infections Surveillance System. Am J Med 91:152S

Cummings JM, Boullier JA (2000) Scrotal dog bites. J Urol 164:57

Cummins RO, Hazinski MR (2000) The most important changes in the international ECC and CPR guidelines 2000. Circulation 102 [8 Suppl]:1371

Cywes S, Bass DH et al (1991) Blunt liver trauma in children. Injury 22:310

Da Silva JL, Lacombe C, Bruneval P, Casadevall N, Leporrier M, Camilleri JP, Bariety J, Tambourin P, Varet B (1990) Tumor cells are the site of erythropoietin synthesis in human renal cancers associated with polycythemia. Blood 75:577

Dacou-Voutetakis C, Maniati-Christidi M, Dracopoulou-Vabouli M (2001) Genetic aspects of congenital adrenal hyperplasia. J Pediatr Endocrinol Metab 14 [Suppl 5]:1303

Dafnis E, Sabatini S (1992) The effect of pregnancy on renal function: physiology and pathophysiology. Am J Med Sci 303:184

Dahm P, Roland FH, Vaslef SN et al (2000) Outcome analysis in patients with primary necrotizing fasciitis of the male genitalia. Urology 56:31; discussion 35

Dahm P, Rao DS, Donatucci CF (2002) Antiandrogens in the treatment of priapism. Urology 59:138

Dajani AS, Taubert KA, Wilson W et al (1997) Prevention of bacterial endocarditis: recommendations by the American Heart Association. Clin Infect Dis 25:1448

Dajani AS, Taubert KA, Wilson W et al (1997) Prevention of bacterial endocarditis. Recommendations by the American Heart Association. JAMA 277:1794

Dalbagni G, O'Donnell M (2006) Intravesical therapy. In: Vogelzang NJ, Scardino PT, Shipley WU, Debruyne FMJ, Linehan WM (eds) Comprehensive textbook of genitourinary oncology. Lippincott Williams and Wilkins, Philadelphia
Daling JR, Madeleine MM, Johnson LG, Schwartz SM, Shera KA, Wurscher MA et al (2005) Penile cancer: importance of circumcision, human papillomavirus and smoking in in situ and invasive disease. Int J Cancer 116:606
Dalla Palma L (2001) What is left of i.v. urography? Eur Radiol 11:931
Daly B, Sukumar SA, Krebs TL, Wong JJ, Flowers JL (1996) Nonbiliary laparoscopic gastrointestinal surgery: role of CT in diagnosis and management of complication. AJR Am J Roentgenol 167:455
Daly JW, Higgins KA (1988) Injury to the ureter during gynecologic surgical procedures. Surg Gynecol Obstet 167:19
Damaraju S, Krajcer Z (1999) Successful Wallstent implantation for extensive iatrogenic renal artery dissection in a patient with fibromuscular dysplasia. J Endovasc Surg 6:297
Danuser H, Wille S et al (2001) How to treat blunt kidney ruptures: primary open surgery or conservative treatment with deferred surgery when necessary? Eur Urol 39:9
Dare FO, Oboro VO, Fadiora SO, Orji EO, Sule-Odu AO, Olabode TO (2004) Female genital mutilation: an analysis of 522 cases in South-Western Nigeria. J Obstet Gynaecol. 24:281
Darewicz B, Galek L, Darewicz J, Kudelski J, Malczyk E (2001) Successful microsurgical replantation of an amputated penis. Int Urol Nephrol 33:385
Darouiche RO (2004) Treatment of infections associated with surgical implants. N Engl J Med 350:1422
Davenport M (1996) ABC of general surgery in children. Problems with the penis and prepuce. BMJ 312:299
Davidsson T, Hedlund H, Månsson W (1996) Detubularized right colonic reservoir with intussuscepted ileal nipple valve or stapled („Lundiana") outlet. Clinical and urodynamic results in a prospective randomized study. World J Urol 14:78
Davis JD (1999) Management of injuries to the urinary and gastrointestinal tract during cesarean section. Obstet Gynecol Clin North Am 26:469
Davis PM, Gloviczki P et al (1998) Aorto-caval and ilio-iliac arteriovenous fistulae. Am J Surg 176:115
Dawson C, H Whitfield (1996) ABC of urology. Urological trauma and bladder reconstruction. BMJ 312:1352
De Baere T, Lagrange C, Kuoch V, Morice P, Court B, Roche A (2000) Transcatheter ethanol renal ablation in 20 patients with persistent urine leaks: an alternative to surgical nephrectomy. J Urol 164:1148
De Berardinis E, Vicini P, Salvatori F et al (2005) Superselective embolization of bladder arteries in the treatment of intractable bladder haemorrhage. Int J Urol 12:503
De Boer EC, Steerenberg PA, van der Meijden AP et al (1992) Impaired immune response by isoniazid treatment during intravesical BCG administration in the guinea pig. Prog Clin Biol Res 378:81
De Ganck J, Everaert K, Van Laecke E, Oosterlinck W, Hoebeke P (2002) A high easy-to-treat complication rate is the price for a continent stoma. BJU Int 90:240
De la Fouchardiere C, Flechon A, Droz JP (2003) Coagulopathy in prostate cancer. Neth J Med 61:347
De Pablo Cardenas A, Jimenez Calvo JM, Grasa Lanau V et al (1999) High-flow priapism in the pediatric age: review (translation). Arch Esp Urol 52:862
De Pauw BE, Deresinski SC, Feld R et al (1994) Ceftazidime compared with piperacillin and tobramycin for the empiric treatment of fever in neutropenic patients with cancer. A multicenter randomized trial. Ann Intern Med 120:834
De Peretti F, Cambas PM, Veneau B, Argenson C (1993) Fuel tanks of motorcycles. Role in severe trauma of the pelvis. Presse Med 22:61
De Vries CR, Freiha FS (1990) Hemorrhagic cystitis: a review. J Urol 143:1
De Wit R, Roberts JT, Wilkinson PM et al (2001) Equivalence of three or four cycles of bleomycin, etoposide, and cisplatin chemotherapy and of a 3- or 5-day schedule in good-prognosis germ cell cancer. J Clin Oncol 19:1629
Dean PG, Lund WJ, Larson TS, Prieto M, Nyberg SL, Ishitani MB et al (2004) Wound-healing complication after kidney transplantation: a prospective randomized comparison of sirolimus and tacrolimus. Transplantation 77:1555
Dearnaley D, Khoo V, Normal A et al (1999) Comparison of radiation side-effects of conformal and conventional radiotherapy in prostate cancer: a randomized trial. Lancet 353:267
Deck AJ, Shaves S, Talner L et al (2000) Computerized tomography cystography for the diagnosis of traumatic bladder rupture. J Urol 164:43
Deck AJ, Shaves S, Talner L, Porter JR (2001) Current experience with computed tomographic cystography and blunt trauma. World J Surg 25:1592
Decousus H, Leizorovicz A, Parent F, Page Y, Tardy B, Girard P, Laporte S, Faivre R, Charbonnier B, Barral FG et al (1998) A clinical trial of vena caval filters in the prevention of pulmonary embolism in patients with proximal deep-vein thrombosis. Prevention du Risque d'EMBOlie Pulmonaire par Interruption Cave Study Group. N Engl J Med 338:409
DeHaven JI, Traynellis C, Riggs DR et al (1992) Antibiotic and steroid therapy of massive systemic bacillus Calmette-Guerin toxicity. J Urol 147:738
De La Pena A, Alcina E (1962) Suprapubic prostatectomy: a new technique to prevent bleeding. J Urol 88:86
Del Pizzo JJ (2005) Pleural injury during laparoscopic renal surgery. In: Ramakumar S, Jarrett T (eds) Complications of urologic laparoscopic surgery. Taylor & Francis, Boca Raton, p 83
Del Pizzo JJ, Jacobs SC et al (1998) Ureteroscopic evaluation in renal transplant recipients. J Endourol 12:135
Del Pizzo JJ, Jacobs SC, Bishoff JT, Kavoussi LR, Jarrett TW (2003) Pleural injury during laparoscopic renal surgery: early recognition and management. J Urol 169:41
Delattre JY, Arbit E, Rosenblum MK (1988) High dose versus low dose dexamethasone in experimental epidural spinal cord compression. Neurosurgery 22:1005
Delcroix M, Zone V, Cheront C et al (1994) L'infection urinaire de la femme enceinte. Rev Fr Gynécol Obstet 89:277
D'Elia G, Pahernik S, Fisch M, Hohenfellner R, Thuroff JW (2004) Mainz Pouch II technique:10 years' experience. BJU Int 93:1037
Dellabella M et al (2003) Efficacy of tamsulosine in the medical management of juxta vesical ureteral stones. J Urol 170:2202
Dellinger RP (2003) Inflammation and coagulation: implications for the septic patient. Clin Infect Dis 36:1259
Delorme E (2001) Transobturator urethral suspension: mini-invasive procedure in the treatment of stress urinary incontinence in women. Prog Urol 11:1306
Demetriades D et al (2002) Pelvic fractures: epidemiology and predictors of associated abdominal injuries and outcomes. J Am Coll Surg 195:1
Demoly P (2005) Anaphylactic reactions – value of skin and provocation tests. Toxicology 209:221
Dempfle CE (2005) Perioperative coagulation diagnostics. Anaesthesist 54:167
Deng DY, Meng MV, Nguyen HT, Bellman GC, Stoller ML (2002) Laparoscopic linear cutting stapler failure. Urology 60:415; discussion 419
Denstedt JD, Razvi H (1992) Management of urinary calculi during pregnancy. J Urol 148:1072

Denton AS, Clarke NW, Maher EJ (2002) Non-surgical interventions for late radiation cystitis in patients who have received radical radiotherapy to the pelvis. Cochrane Database Syst Rev (3):CD001773

DePalma RG, Burris DG, Champion HR et al (2005) Blast Injuries. N Engl J Med 352:1335

Desai MM, Aron M, Gill IS (2005) Laparoscopic partial nephrectomy versus laparoscopic cryoablation for the small renal tumor. Urology 66:23

Desai MM, Strzempkowski B, Matin SF, Steinberg AP, Ng C, Meraney AM, Kaouk JH, Gill IS (2005) Prospective randomized comparison of transperitoneal versus retroperitoneal laparoscopic radical nephrectomy. J Urol 173:38

Deshpande PV, Jones KV (2001) An audit of RCP guidelines on DMSA scanning after urinary tract infection. Arch Dis Child 84:324

Detweiler MB (2001) Penile incarceration with metal objects–a review of procedure choice based on penile trauma grade. Scand J Urol Nephrol 35:212

Devine PC, Devine CJ (1982) Posterior urethral injuries associated with pelvic fractures. Urology 20:467

DeVries CR, Anderson RU (1990) Endoscopic urethroplasty: An improved technique. J Urol 143:1225

DeVries PA, Peña A (1982) Posterior sagittal anorectoplasty. J Ped Surg 17:638

Dewan PA, Walton JK (1987) Spermatic cord torsion in the neonate. Aust N Z J Surg 57:331

Dewdney S, Sokoloff M, Yamada SD (2005) Conservative management of chylous ascites after removal of a symptomatic growing retroperitoneal teratoma. Gynecol Oncol 100:608

Dexeus FH, Logothetis CJ, Sella A et al (1991) Combination chemotherapy with methotrexate, bleomycin and cisplatin for advanced squamous cell carcinoma of the male genital tract. J Urol 146:1284

Deyoe LA (1995) New techniques of ultrasound and color Doppler in the prospective evaluation of acute renal obstruction: do they replace the intravenous urogram ? Abdom Imaging 20:58

Deyoe LA, Cronan JJ, Lambiase RE, Dorfman GS (1990) Percutaneous drainage of renal and perirenal abscesses: results in 30 patients. Am J Roentgenol 155:81

Deziel DJ, Millikan KW, Economou SG, Doolas A, Ko ST, Airan MC (1993) Complications of laparoscopic cholecystectomy: a national survey of 4,292 hospitals and an analysis of 77,604 cases. Am J Surg 165:9

Dhabuwala CB, Hamid S, Katsikas DM, Pierce J (1990) Impotence following delayed repair of prostate membranous urethral disruption. J Urol 144:677

Di Stasi SM, Poggi A, Giannantoni A, Zampa G (2000) Dermatomyositis associated with testicular germ cell cancer. J Urol 163:240

Di Tonno F, Fusaro V, Bertoldin R, Lavelli D (2003) Bladder explosion during transurethral resection of the prostate. Urol Int 71:108

Di Valentino M, Alerci M, Tutta P, Sartori F, Marone C, Vandoni R, Mahler F, Gallino A (2004) Thrombus aspiration as a bail-out procedure during percutaneous renal angioplasty. J Endovasc Ther 11:522

Diallo MB, Diallo AT, Sow KB, Guirassy S, Balde S, Balde A(2001) Early complications of transvesical prostatectomy for prostatic adenoma at the Conakry urologic department: report of 96 cases. Ann Urol 35:120

Diamond DA, Jeffs RD (1985) Cloacal exstrophy: a 22-year experience. J Urol 133:779

Diblasio CJ, Snyder ME, Kattan MW et al (2004) Ketorolac: safe and effective analgesia for the management of renal cortical tumors with partial nephrectomy. J Urol 171:1062

Dick A, Barnes R, Hadley H, Bergman RT, Ninan CA (1980) Complications of transurethral resection of bladder tumors: prevention, recognition and treatment. J Urol 124:810

Dietz (1996) Querschnittslähmung: Physiopathologie Klinik und Therapie von Blasenfunktion Bewegung und Vegetativum. Kohlhammer, Stuttgart

DiGiacomo JC, Rotondo MF et al (2001) The role of nephrectomy in the acutely injured. Arch Surg 136:1045

Dillioglugil O, Leibman BD, Leibman NS et al (1997) Risk factors for complications and morbidity after radical retropubic prostatectomy. J Urol 157:1760

Dillioglugil O, Leibman BD, Leibman NS, Kattan MW, Rosas AL, Scardino (1997) Risk factors for complications and morbidity after radical retropubic prostatectomy. J Urol 157:1760

Dimitrios M, Achilles C, Andrew K, Charalampos L, Katsenis K, Vlachos L (2004) Bilateral renal artery stenting in a patient with Leriche syndrome. Urol Int 73:283

Dinarello CA (1984) Interleukin-1 and the pathogenesis of the acute-phase response. N Engl J Med 311:1413

Dinkel HP, Danuser H, Triller J (2002) Blunt renal trauma: minimally invasive management with microcatheter embolization experience in nine patients. Radiology 223:723

Dixon CM, Hricak H, McAninch JW (1992) Magnetic resonance imaging of traumatic posterior urethral defects and pelvic crush injuries. J Urol 148:1162

Dixon MD (1996) Diagnosis and acute management of posterior urethral disruptions. In: McAninch JW (ed) Traumatic and reconstructive urology. WB Saunders Philadelphia

Djavan B, Chapple C, Milani S et al (2004) State of the art on the efficacy and tolerability of alpha1-adrenoceptor antagonists in patients with lower urinary tract symptoms suggestive of benign prostatic hyperplasia. Urology 64:1081

Dobrowolski Z, Kusionowicz J, Drewniak T et al (2002) Renal and ureteric trauma: diagnosis and management in Poland. BJU Int 89:748

Dobrowolski ZF, Lipczynsky W, Drewniak T et al (2002) External and iatrogenic trauma of the urinary bladder: a survey in Poland. BJU Int 89:755

Dodge HW Jr, Svien HJ, Camp JD et al (1951) Tumors of the spinal cord without neurologic manifestations, producing low back and sciatic pain. Mayo Clin Proc 26:88

Dogra PN, Nabi G (2002) Core-through urethrotomy using the neodynium yag laser for obliterative urethral strictures after traumatic urethral disruption and/or distraction defects: long-term outcome. J Urol 167:543

Dolin SJ, Cashman JN (2005) Tolerability of acute postoperative pain management: nausea, vomiting, sedation, pruritus, and urinary retention. Evidence from published data. Br J Anaesth 95:584

Doll R (1995) Hazards of ionising radiation: 100 years of observations on man. Br J Cancer 72:1339

Donahue LA, Frank IN (1989) Intravesical formalin for hemorrhagic cystitis: analysis of therapy. J Urol 141:809

Donat SM, Russo P (1996) Ureteral decompression in advanced nonurologic malignancies. Ann Surg Oncol 3:393

Dondelinger RF, Trotteur G, Ghaye B, Szapiro D (2002) Traumatic injuries: radiological hemostatic intervention at admission. Eur Radiol 12:979

Donohue JP (1989) Postchemotherapy retroperitoneal lymphadenectomy for bulky tumor including extended suprahilar posterior mediastinal dissection and/or major vessel resection. In: McDougal WS (ed) Difficult problems in urologic surgery. Year Book Medical Publishers

Donovan JF, Kaplan WE (1989) The therapy of genital trauma by dog bite. J Urol 141:1163

Donzella JG, Merrick GS, Lindert DJ, Andreini HJ, Jr Curtis RL, Luna IH, Allen Z, Butler WM (2004) Epididymitis after transrectal ultrasound-guided needle biopsy of prostate gland. Urology 63:306

Dorairajan G, Rani PR, Habeebullah S et al (2004) Urological injuries during hysterectomies: a 6-year review. J Obstet Gynaecol Res 30:430

Dore B (2004) La lithiase urinaire de la femme enceinte. In: Dore B (ed) Les lithiases rénales. Springer Berlin Heidelberg New York, pp 353

Dorffner R, Thurnher S, Prokesch R, Bankier A, Turetschek K, Schmidt A, Lammer J (1998) Embolization of iatrogenic vascular injuries of renal transplants: immediate and follow-up results. Cardiovasc Intervent Radiol 21:129

Dorfinger K, Maier U, Base W (1999) Parathyroid hormone related protein and carcinoma of the penis: paraneoplastic hypercalcemia. J Urol 161:1570

Dorosz P (2003) Guide pratique des médicaments. Maloine, Paris, pp 1460

Doublet JD, Tchala K, Tligui M et al (1997) In situ extracorporeal shock wave lithotripsy for acute colic due to obstructing ureteral stones. Scand J Urol Nephrol 31:137

Downing R, Black J (1985) Polyarteritis nodosa: an unrecognised cause of Fournier's gangrene. Br J Urol 57:355

Drachenberg D, Nguan C, Norman RW et al. (1999) Penile entrapment injury: a case report. Can J Urol 6:709

Dreesen DW, Hanlon CA (1998) Current recommendations for the prophylaxis and treatment of rabies. Drugs 56:801

Dreitlein DA et al (2001) Genitourinary trauma. Emerg Med Clin North Am 19:569

Drooz AT, Lewis CA, Allen TE, Citron SJ, Cole PE, Freeman NJ, Husted JW, Malloy PC, Martin LG, Van Moore A, Neithamer CD, Roberts AC, Sacks D, Sanchez O, Venbrux AC, Bakal CW; Society of Interventional Radiology Standards of Practice Committee (2003) Quality Improvement Guidelines for Percutaneous Transcatheter Embolization. J Vasc Interv Radiol 14: S237-S242

Dumarey N, Egrise D, Blocklet D, Stallenberg B, Remmelink M, del Marmol V, Van Simaeys G, Jacobs F, Goldman S (2006) Imaging infection with 18F-FDG-labeled leukocyte PET/CT initial experience in 21 patients. J Nucl Med 47:625

Duncan AO et al (1989) Management of transpelvic gunshot wounds. J Trauma 29:1335

Dunn CJ, Goa KL (1999) Tranexamic acid: a review of its use in surgery and other indications. Drugs 57:1005

Durek C, Rusch-Gerdes S, Jocham D et al (2000) Sensitivity of BCG to modern antibiotics. Eur Urol 37 [Suppl 1]:21

Dyer RB, Assimos DG, Regan JD (1997) Update on interventional uroradiology. Urol Clin North Am 24:623

Earle CM, Stuckey BG, Ching HL et al (2003) The incidence and management of priapism in Western Australia: a 16 year audit. Int J Impot Res 15:272

Eastham JA, Bennett CJ (1992) The occurrence of urologic injuries in patients with gunshot wounds to the spine. Semin Urol 10:112

Eastham JA, Wilson TG et al (1991) Radiographic assessment of blunt renal trauma. J Trauma 31:1527

Eastham JA, Wilson TG et al (1992) Angiographic embolization of renal stab wounds. J Urol 148:268

Eastham JA, Wilson TG et al (1993) Urological evaluation and management of renal-proximity stab wounds. J Urol 150:1771

Eastridge BJ, Burgess AR (1997) Pedestrian pelvic fractures:5-year experience of a major urban trauma center. J Trauma 42:695

Eaton SH, Cendron MA, Estrada CR, Bauer SB, Borer JG, Cilento BG et al (2005) Intermittent testicular torsion: diagnostic features and management outcomes. J Urol 174:1532

Edino ST, Yakubu AA, Obidiaso A (2005) Fournier's gangrene in a tertiary health facility in Nigeria. Afr J Urol 11:1

Edwards JE Jr, Bodey GP, Bowden RA, Buchner T, de Pauw BE, Filler SG, Ghannoum MA, Glauser M, Herbrecht R, Kauffman CA, Kohno S, Martino P, Meunier F, Mori T, Pfaller MA, Rex JH, Rogers TR, Rubin RH, Solomkin J, Viscoli C, Walsh TJ, White M (1997) International Conference for the Development of a Consensus on the Management and Prevention of Severe Candidal Infections. Clin Infect Dis 25:43

Edwards Life Sciences (2001) Protocol for Early Goal-Directed Therapy for Sepsis. Edwards Life Sciences, Irvine, CA, USA

Ehrich WS (1929) Two unusual penile injuries. J Urol 21:239

Eickenberg HU, Amin M (1976) Gunshot wounds to the ureter. J Trauma 16:562

Eickenberg HU, Amin M, Klompus W et al (1976) Urologic complications following abdominoperineal resection. J Urol 115:180

Einarsson G, Goldstein M, Laungani G (1983) Penile replantation. Urology 22:404

Einav S, Feigenberg Z, Weissman C et al (2004) Evacuation priorities in mass casualty terror-related events: implications for contingency planning. Ann Surg 239:304

Eke N (2000) Fournier's gangrene: a review of 1726 cases. Br J Surg 87:718

Ekengren J, Hahn RG (1994) Continuous versus intermittent flow irrigation in transurethral resection of the prostate. Urology 43:328

Ekman P, Sjogren L, Englund G et al (2000) Optimizing the therapeutic approach of transurethral alprostadil. BJU Int 86:68

El Khader K, Bouchot O et al (1998) Injuries of the renal pedicle: is renal revascularization justified? Prog Urol 8:995

El Khader K, Mhidia A et al (1998) Conservative treatment of stage III kidney injuries. Acta Urol Belg 66:25

El-Abd S (1995) Endoscopic treatment of posttraumatic urethral obliteration: experience in 396 patients. J Urol 153:67

El-Bahnasawy MS, Dawood A, Farouk A (2002) Low-flow priapism: risk factors for erectile dysfunction. BJU Int 89:285

El-Banna M, Abdel-Atty M, El-Meteini M, Aly S (2000) Management of laparoscopic-related bowel injuries. Surg Endosc 14:779

Elder JS, Snyder HM, Hulbert WC, Duckett JW (1988) Perforation of the augmented bladder in patients undergoing clean intermittent catheterization. J Urol 140:1159

Elem B, Ranjan P (1995) Impact of immunodeficiency virus (HIV) on Fournier's gangrene: observations in Zambia. Ann R Coll Surg Engl 77:283

El-Haddad G, Zhuang H, Gupta N, Alavi A (2004) Evolving role of positron emission tomography in the management of patients with inflammatory and other benign disorders. Semin Nucl Med 34:313

Elhilali M, Emberton M, Matzkin H et al (2006) Long-term efficacy and safety of alfuzosin 10 mg once daily: a 2-year experience in 'real-life' practice. BJU Int 97:513

Elias AN (2005) New-onset insulinopenic diabetes mellitus in a patient with an incidentally discovered renal cell carcinoma. Am J Med 118:1047

Elliott D, Kufera JA, Myers RA (2000) The microbiology of necrotizing soft tissue infections. Am J Surg 179:361

Elliott DS, Barret DM (1997) Long-term follow-up and evaluation of primary realignment of posterior urethral disruptions. J Urol 157:814

Elliott SP, McAninch JW (2003) Ureteral injuries from external violence: The 25-year experience at San Francisco general hospital. J Urol 170:1213

Elmajian DA, Stein JP, Esrig D, Freeman JA, Skinner EC, Boyd SD et al (1996) The Kock ileal neobladder: updated experience in 295 male patients. J Urol 156:920

El-Mekresh M, Osman Y, Ali-El-Dein B, El-Diasty T, Ghoneim MA (2001) Urological complications after living-donor renal transplantation. BJU Int 87:295

Elshaikh MA, Ulchaker JC, Reddy CA et al (2005) Prophylactic tamsulosin (Flomax) in patients undergoing prostate 125I brachytherapy for prostate carcinoma: final report of a double-blind placebo-controlled randomized study. Int J Radiat Oncol Biol Phys 62:164

Emberton M, Anson K (1999) Acute urinary retention in men: an age old problem. BMJ 318:921

Emerson H (1911) Intra-abdominal pressures. Arch Intern Med 7:754

Endorf FW, Supple KG, Gamelli RL (2005) The evolving characteristics and care of necrotizing soft-tissue infections. Burns 31:269

Engel RM (1974) Exstrophy of the bladder and associated anomalies. Birth Defects Orig Artic Ser 10:146

Enlund AL, Varenhorst E (1997) Morbidity of ultrasound-guided transrectal core biopsy of the prostate without prophylactic antibiotic therapy. A prospective study in 415 cases. Br J Urol 79:777

Erber WN (2002) Massive blood transfusion in the elective surgical setting. Transfus Apher Sci 27:83

Erickson LM, Nicholson SF, Lewel DB et al (1979) Ultrasound evaluation of hydronephrosis of pregnancy. J Clin Ultrasound 7:128

Eriksen MT, Wibe A, Norstein J, Haffner J, Wiig JN (2005) Anastomotic leakage following routine mesorectal excision for rectal cancer in a national cohort of patients. Colorectal Dis 7:51

Ersay A, Akgun Y (1999) Experience with renal gunshot injuries in a rural setting. Urology 54:972

Ertekin C, Akyildiz H et al (2001) Results of conservative treatment for solid abdominal organ trauma. Ulus Travma Derg 7:224

Esclarin de Ruz A, Leoni EG, Cabrera RH (2000) Epidemiology and risk factors for urinary tract infection in patients with spinal cord injury. J Urol 164:1285

Eskelinen M, Ikonen J, Lipponen P (1998) Usefulness of history-taking, physical examination and diagnostic scoring in acute renal colic. Eur Urol 34:467

Espinoza R, Rodriguez A (1997) Traumatic and nontraumatic perforation of hollow viscera. Surg Clin North Am 77:1291

European Mycophenolate Mofetil Study Group (1995) Placebo-controlled study of mycophenolate mofetil combined with cyclosporine and corticosteroids for prevention of acute rejection. Lancet 345:1321

Evan AP, Connors BA et al (1999) Renal disease potentiates the injury caused by SWLJ Endourol 13:619

Evans BK, Fagan C, Arnold T, Dropcho EJ, Oh SJ (1990) Paraneoplastic motor neuron disease and renal cell carcinoma: improvement after nephrectomy Neurology 40:960

Evans HJ, Wollin TA (2001) The management of urinary calculi in pregnancy. Curr Opin Urol 11:379

Evans TW (2001) Hemodynamic and metabolic therapy in critically ill patients. N Engl J Med 345:1417

Evins SC, Whittle T, Rous SN (1977) Self-emasculation: review of the literature, report of a case and outline of the objectives of management. J Urol 188:775

Evins SC (1989) Nonoperative management of iatrogenic prostatorectal fistula. Urology 33:418

Ewalt DH, Diamond N, Rees C, Sparagana SP, Delgado M, Batchelor L, Roach ES (2005) Long-term outcome of transcatheter embolization of renal angiomyolipomas due to tuberous sclerosis complex. J Urol 174:1764

Fabian TC (2002) Infection in penetrating abdominal trauma: risk factors and preventive antibiotics. Am Surg 68:29

Fabris F, Luzzatto G, Stefani PM, Girolami B, Cella G (2000) Heparin-induced thrombocytopenia. Haematologica 85:72

Fahlenkamp D, Rassweiler J, Fornara P, Frede T, Loening SA (1999) Complications of laparoscopic procedures in urology: experience with 2,407 procedures at 4 German centers. J Urol 162:765; discussion 770

Fahn HJ, Lee YH, Chen MT (1991) The incidence and prognostic significance of humoral hypercalcemia in renal cell carcinoma. J Urol 145:248

Failinger MS, McGanity PL (1992) Unstable fractures of the pelvic ring. J Bone Joint Surg Am 74:781

Falagas ME, Vergidis PI (2005) Urinary tract infections in patients with urinary diversion. Am J Kidney Dis 46:1030

Falcoz PE, Laluc F, Toubin MM et al (2005) Usefulness of procalcitonin in the early detection of infection after thoracic surgery. Eur J Cardiothorac Surg 27:1074

Fallick ML, Long JP (1996) Laparoscopic marsupialization of lymphocele after laparoscopic lymph node dissection. J Endourol 10:533

Fallon B et al (1984) Urological injury and assessment in patients with fractured pelvis. J Urol 131:712

Fann JI, Miller DC (1995) Aortic dissection. Ann Vasc Surg 9:311

Farah I, Tarabula P et al (1997) Traumatic and iatrogenic lesions of abdominal vessels. Chirurgie 122:572; discussion 578

Farid A, Sullivan TM (1996) Aortocaval fistula in ruptured inflammatory abdominal aortic aneurysm. A report of two cases and literature review. J Cardiovasc Surg (Torino) 37:561

Farrell AM, Black MM, Bracka A et al (1998) Pyoderma gangrenosum of the penis. Br J Dermatol 138:337

Farrell TA, Wallace M, Hicks ME (1997) Long-term results of transrenal ureteral occlusion with use of Gianturco coils and gelatin sponge pledgets. J Vasc Interv Radiol 8:449

Fatkenheuer G, Buchheidt D, Cornely OA, Fuhr HG, Karthaus M, Kisro J, Leithauser M, Salwender H, Sudhoff T, Szelenyi H, Weissinger F (2003) Central venous catheter (CVC)-related infections in neutropenic patients–guidelines of the Infectious Diseases Working Party (AGIHO) of the German Society of Hematology and Oncology (DGHO) Ann Hematol 82 [Suppl 2]:S149

Favorito LA, Lott FM et al (2004) Traumatic rupture of adrenal pseudocyst leading to massive hemorrhage in retroperitoneum. Int Braz J Urol 30:35

Fazio VW, Cohen Z., Fleshman JW, Goor H, Bauer JJ (2006) Reduction in adhesive small-bowel obstruction by Seprafilm adhesion barrier after intestinal resection. Dis Colon Rectum 49:1

Fedel M, Venz S, Andreessen R, Sudhoff F, Loening SA (1996) The value of magnetic resonance imaging in the diagnosis of suspected penile fracture with atypical clinical findings. J Urol 155:1924

Feigin E, Carmon M, Szold A, Seror D (1993) Acute stump appendicitis. Lancet 341:757

Feld LG, Waz WR et al (1997) Hematuria. An integrated medical and surgical approach. Pediatr Clin North Am 44:1191

Feldman NT, Huber GL (1976) Fiberoptic bronchoscopy in the intensive care unit. Int Anesthesiol Clin 14:31

Feldmeier J, Carl U, Hartmann K et al (2003) Hyperbaric oxygen: does it promote growth or recurrence of malignancy? Undersea Hyperb Med 30:1

Feldmeier JJ, Hampson NB (2002) A systematic review of the literature reporting the application of hyperbaric oxygen prevention and treatment of delayed radiation injuries: an evidence based approach. Undersea Hyperb Med 29:4

Feliciano DV, Moore EE, Mattox KL (2000) Trauma damage control. In: Mattox KL et al (eds) McGraw-Hill, New York, p 907

Feneley MR, Pal MK, Nockler IB, Hendry WF (1997) Retrograde embolization and causes of failure in the primary treatment of varicocele. Br J Urol 80:642

Fennerty MB (2002) Pathophysiology of the upper gastrointestinal tract in the critically ill patient: rationale for the therapeutic benefits of acid suppression. Crit Care Med 30:S351

Fernandez Arancibia MI, Martinez Portillo FJ, Musial A et al (2000) Diagnosis and therapeutic options for prolonged erection and priapism: up-date review (translation). Arch Esp Urol 53:919
Fernandez L et al (1998) Ultrasound in blunt abdominal trauma. J Trauma 45:841
Ferrara A, MacArthur JD, Wright HK, Modlin IM, McMillen MA (1990) Hypothermia and acidosis worsen coagulopathy in the patient requiring massive transfusion. Am J Surg 160:515
Ferrer J, Roldan J (2000) Clinical management of the patient with pleural effusion. Eur J Radiol 34:76
Ferrera PC, Hill DA (1999) Good outcomes of open pelvic fractures. Injury 30:187
Ferrozzi F, Bova D et al (1999) Foreign-body granuloma of the kidney: CT, MR and pathologic correlation. Eur Radiol 9: 1590
Fiala R, Zatura F, Vrtal R (2001) Personal experience with treatment of posttraumatic urethral distraction defects. Acta Chir Orthop Traumatol Cech 68:99
Fialkov JM, Watkins K, Fallon B Kealey GP (1998) Fournier's gangrene with an unusual urologic etiology. Urology 52:324
Ficarra BJ (1996) Diseases and injuries in athletes. A review. J Med 27:241
Fielding JR, Steele G, Fox LA et al (1997) Spiral computerized tomography in the evaluation of acute flank pain: a replacement for excretory urography. J Urol 157:2071
Fife RS, Williams S, Eyanson S (1984) Dermatomyositis associated with treated testicular carcinoma. J Rheumatol 11:397
Fisher BW, Majumdar SR, McAlister FA (2002) Predicting pulmonary complications after nonthoracic surgery: a systematic review of blinded studies. Am J Med 112:219
Fisher MM, Baldo BA (1998) Mast cell tryptase in anaesthetic anaphylactoid reactions. Br J Anaesth 80:26
Fisher MM, Bowey CJ (1997) Intradermal compared with prick testing in the diagnosis of anaesthetic allergy. Br J Anaesth 79:59
Fisher MM, Merefield D, Baldo BA (1999) Failure to prevent an anaphylactic reaction to a second neuromuscular blocking drug during anaesthesia. Br J Anaesth 82:770
Fisher RG, Ben-Menachem Y, Whigham C (1989) Stab wounds of the renal artery branches: angiographic diagnosis and treatment by embolization. AJR Am J Roentgenol 152:1231
Fitzgerald J, Malone MJ, Gaertner RA Zinman LN (1997) Stomal construction complications, and reconstruction. Urol Clin North Am 24:729
Fitzpatrick JM (2006) The natural history of benign prostatic hyperplasia. BJU Int 97:3
Fitzpatrick JM, Kirby RS (2006) Management of acute urinary retention. BJU Int 97:16
Flaherty JJ, Kelley R, Burnett B, Bucy J, Surian M, Schildkraut D, Clark BG (1968) Relationship of pelvic bone fracture patterns to injuries of urethra and bladder. J Urol 99:297
Flam TA, Malone MJ, Roth RA (1988) Complications of ureteroscopy. Urol Clin North Am 15:167
Flam TA, Peyromaure M, Chauveinc L et al (2004) Post-brachytherapy transurethral resection of the prostate in patients with localized prostate cancer. J Urol 172:108
Flancbaum L et al (1988) Blunt bladder trauma: manifestation of severe injury. Urology 31:220
Fleisch H (1991) Bisphosphonates. Pharmacology and use in the treatment of tumour-induced hypercalcaemic and metastatic bone disease. Drugs 42:919
Fleischmann JD, Catalona WJ (1985) Endocrine therapy for bladder outlet obstruction from carcinoma of the prostate. J Urol 134:498
Flint LM (1988) Early postoperative acute abdominal complications. Surg Clin North Am 68:445
Flombaum CD (2000) Metabolic emergencies in the cancer patient. Semin Oncol 27:322
Flynn DF, Shipley WU (1991) Management of spinal cord compression secondary to metastatic prostatic carcinoma. Urol Clin North Am 18:145
Fojo T (2005) Oncologic emergencies. In: DeVita VT Jr Hellman S, Rosenberg SA (eds) Cancer principles and practice of oncology. Lippincott Williams and Wilkins, Philadelphia
Földi M, Földi E, Kubik S (2005) Lehrbuch der Lymphologie. Anatomie des Lymphgefäßsystems. Urban Fischer Elsevier, München
Follis WH, Koch MO, McDougal WS (1992) Immediate management of prostatomembranous urethral disruptions. J Urol 147:1259
Fong YK, Milani S, Djavan B (2005) Natural history and clinical predictors of clinical progression in benign prostatic hyperplasia. Curr Opin Urol 15:35
Foote J, Yun S, Leach GE (1991) Postprostatectomy incontinence. Pathophysiology, evaluation, and management. Urol Clin North Am 18:229
Forest MG (2004) Recent advances in the diagnosis and management of congenital adrenal hyperplasia due to 21-hydroxylase deficiency. Hum Reprod Update 10:469
Forni AM, Koss LG, Geller W (1964) Cytological study of the effect of cyclophosphamide on the epithelium of the urinary bladder in man. Cancer 17:1348
Fourie CE (2003) The role of glycaemic control in preventing complications in the critically ill. South Afr J Crit Care 19:46
Fournier GR Jr, Laing FC, McAninch JW (1989) Scrotal ultrasonography and the management of testicular trauma. Urol Clin North Am 16:377
Fournier JA (1883) Gangrène foudroyante de la verge. Medecin Practique 4:589
Fowler AA 3rd, Scoggins WG, O'Donohue WJ Jr (1978) Positive end-expiratory pressure in the management of lobar atelectasis. Chest 74:497
Fowler CJ, Kirby RS (1985) Abnormal electromyographic activity (decelerating burst and complex repetitive discharges) in the striated muscle of the urethral sphincter in 5 women with persisting urinary retention. Br J Urol 57:67
Fowler CJ, Kirby RS, Harrison MJ et al (1984) Individual motor unit analysis in the diagnosis of disorders of urethral sphincter innervation. J Neurol Neurosurg Psychiatry 47:637
Fowler CJ, Kirby RS, Harrison MJ (1985) Decelerating burst and complex repetitive discharges in the striated muscle of the urethral sphincter, associated with urinary retention in women. J Neurol Neurosurg Psychiatry 48:1004
Fowler KA, Locken JA, Duchesne JH et al (2002) US for detecting renal calculi with nonenhanced CT as a reference standard. Radiology 222:109
Fraenkel DJ, Rickard C, Lipman J (2000) Can we achieve consensus on central venous catheter-related infections? Anaesth Intensive Care 28:475
Francis RB Jr, Johnson CS (1991) Vascular occlusion in sickle cell disease: current concepts and unanswered questions. Blood 77:1405
Franco de Castro A, Gibanel Garanto R et al (2001) Selective embolization of post-traumatic renal pseudoaneurysm in monorenal patient. Actas Urol Esp 25:64
Frank RG, Gerard PS et al (1992) Serial sonographic evaluation of buckshot colic following a penetrating gunshot wound. Urol Radiol 14:172
Frank SM, Kluger MJ, Kunkel SL (2000) Elevated thermostatic setpoint in postoperative patients. Anesthesiology 93:1426
Franke M, Lenk S, Petras T (1999) Genitalverletzung durch Hundebisse. Extr Urol 22:15
Frankenschmidt A, Sommerkamp H (1998) Shock wave litho-

tripsy during pregnancy: a successful clinical experiment. J Urol 159:501
Frassinelli P, Pasquale MD et al (1997) Bilateral renal artery thrombosis secondary to blunt trauma: case report and review of the literature. J Trauma 42:330
Frauscher F, Klauser A, Stenzl A, Helweg G, Amort B, zur Nedden D (2001) US findings in the scrotum of extreme mountain bikers. Radiology 219:427
Frazier HA, Robertson JE, Paulson DF (1992) Complications of radical cystectomy and urinary diversion: a retrospective review of 675 cases in 2 decades. J Urol 148:1401
Fresenius M, Heck M (2001) Repetitorium of Intensive Care. Springer, Berlin Heidelberg New York
Friedel JM, Khalil R, Lasorda D (2005) Treatment of iatrogenic renal artery perforation with a covered stent and subsequent rheolytic thrombectomy. J Invasive Cardiol 17:374
Friederich PW, Henny CP, Messelink EJ, Geerdink MG, Keller T, Kurth KH, Buller HR, Levi M (2003) Effect of recombinant activated factor VII on perioperative blood loss in patients undergoing retropubic prostatectomy: a double-blind placebo-controlled randomised trial. Lancet 361:201
Friedman SC, Sheynkin YR (1995) Acute scrotal symptoms due to perforated appendix in children: case report and review of literature. Pediatr Emerg Care 11:181
Fry DE, Clevenger FW (1991) Reoperation for intra-abdominal abscess. Surg Clin North Am 71:159
Frykberg ER (2002) Medical management of disasters and mass casualties from terrorist bombings: how can we cope? J Trauma 53:201
Frykberg ER (2004) Principles of Mass Casualty Management Following Terrorist Disasters. Ann Surg 239:319
Frykberg ER, Tepas JJ 3rd (1988) Terrorist bombings. Lessons learned from Belfast to Beirut. Ann Surg 208:569
Fuenfer MM, Olson GE, Polk HC Jr (1975) Effect of various corticosteroids upon the phagocytic bactericidal activity of neutrophils. Surgery 78:27
Fuhrman GM et al (1993) The single indication for cystography in blunt trauma. Am Surg 59:335
Fujiwara K, Kigawa J, Hasegawa K, Nishimura R, Umezaki N, Ando M, Itamochi H, Yamaguchi S, Oda T, Terakawa N, Kohshima I, Kohno I (2003) Effect of simple omentoplasty and omentopexy in the prevention of complications after pelvic lymphadenectomy. Int J Gynecol Cancer 13:61
Fukuoka M, Negoro S, Masuda N et al (1991) Placebo-controlled double-blind comparative study on the preventive efficacy of mesna against ifosfamide-induced urinary disorders. J Cancer Res Clin Oncol 117:473
Fukutani K, Libby JM, Panko WB, Scardino PT (1983) Human chorionic gonadotropin detected in urinary concentrates from patients with malignant tumors of the testis, prostate, bladder, ureter and kidney. J Urol 129:74
Fukuzumi M, Hamakawa H, Onishi A, Sumida T, TaniokaH (2000) Gene expression of GLUT isoforms and VHL in oral squamous cell carcinoma. Cancer Lett 161:133
Fulford SC, Vafidis JA et al (1998) An unusual neurological complication of a staghorn renal calculus. Br J Urol 81:322
Fumi L (1997) An unexpected complication of urinary stomata. Br J Urol 79:813
Furno P, Bucaneve G, Del Favero A (2002) Monotherpay or aminoglycoside-containing combinations for empirical antibiotic treatment of febrile neutropenic patients: a meta-analysis. Lancet Infect Dis 2:231
Furukawa K, Ohteki H et al (1997) A case of ruptured thoraco-abdominal aortic aneurysm with aortitis syndrome–operation with selective cold visceral arteries perfusion. Nippon Kyobu Geka Gakkai Zasshi 45:1747
Furuno JP, Perencevich EN, Johnson JA et al (2005) Methicillin-resistant Staphylococcus aureus and vancomycin-resistant Enterococci co-colonization. Emerg Infect Dis 11:1539
Gabal-Shehab L, Alagiri M (2005) Traumatic adrenal injuries. J Urol 173:1330
Gaeta M, Volta S, Minutoli A, Bartiromo A, Pandolfo I (1991) Fournier's gangrene caused by perforated retroperitoneal appendix. AJR Am J Roentgenol 156:341
Gagnadoux MF, Habib R, Levy M, Brunelle F, Broyer M (1989) Cystic renal diseases in children. Adv Nephrol Necker Hosp 18:33
Gale DW, Notley RG (1985) TURP without TURP syndrome. Br J Urol 57:708
Gallus A, Jackaman J, Tillett J, Mills W, Wycherley A (1986) Safety and efficacy of warfarin started early after submassive venous thrombosis or pulmonary embolism. Lancet 2:1293
Galvin DJ, Mulvin D, Quinlan DM (2004) Thromboprophylaxis for radical prostatectomy: a comparative analysis of present practice between the USA, the UK, and Ireland. Prostate 60:338
Gambone JC, Reiter RC, and Lench JB (1990) Quality assurance indicators and short-term outcome of hysterectomy. Obstet Gynecol 76:841
Gan TJ, Meyer T, Apfel CC, Chung F, Davis PJ, Eubanks S, Kovac A, Philip BK, Sessler DI, Temo J, Tramer MR, Watcha M (2003) Consensus guidelines for managing postoperative nausea and vomiting. Anesth Analg 97:62
Ganatra AM, Loughlin KR (2005) The management of malignant ureteral obstruction treated with ureteral stents. J Urol 174:2125
Ganesan GS, Nguyen DH, Adams MC et al (1993) Lower urinary tract reconstruction using stomach and the artificial sphincter. J Urol 149:1107
Garcia-Sabrido JL, Tallado JM, Christou NV, Polo JR, Valdecantos E (1988) Treatment of severe intra-abdominal sepsis and/or necrotic foci by an „open-abdomen" approach. Zipper and Zipper-Mesh Techniques. Arch Surg 123:152
Gargollo PC, Kozakewich HP, Bauer SB, Borer JG, Peters CA, Retik AB et al (2005) Balanitis xerotica obliterans in boys. J Urol 174:1409
Garibaldi RA, Mooney BR, Epstein BJ, Britt MR (1982) An evaluation of daily bacteriologic monitoring to identify preventable episodes of catheter-associated urinary tract infection. Infect Control 3:466
Garner WL, Reiss M (2005) Burn care in Los Angeles, California: LAC+USC experience 1994. Burns 31 [Suppl 1]:S32
Garret ED Jr, Groshart K, Duvall-Seaman D, Combs D, Stuggs R (2002) Treatment of humoral rejection with rituximab. Ann Thorac Surg 74:1240
Gasparini ME, Broderick GA, Narayan P (1993) The syndrome of inappropriate antidiuretic hormone secretion in a patient with adenocarcinoma of the prostate. J Urol 150:978
Gassner HL, Toppari J, Quinteiro Gonzalez S, Miller WL (2004) Near-miss apparent SIDS from adrenal crisis. J Pediatr 145:178
Gattegno B, Guillemenot F, Fiatte P et al (1990) Treatment of hemorrhagic cystitis caused by cyclophosphamide using intravesical instillation of potassium alum. Apropos of 5 cases. Ann Urol (Paris) 24:190
Gavant ML, Menke PG, Fabian T et al (1995) Blunt traumatic aortic rupture: detection with helical CT of the chest. Radiology 197:125
Gaylord GM, Johnsrude IS (1989) Transrenal ureteral occlusion with Gianturco coils and gelatin sponge. Radiology 172:1047
Gaynes RP, Culver DH, Horan TC, Edwards JR, Richards C, Tolson JS (2001) Surgical site infection (SSI) rates in the United States, 1992: the National Nosocomial Infections Surveil-

lance System basic SSI risk index. Clin Infect Dis 33 [Suppl 2]: S69
Gburek BM, Lieber MM, Blute ML (1998) Comparison of studer ileal neobladder and ileal conduit urinary diversion with respect to perioperative outcome and late complications. J Urol 160:721
Gearhart JP, Ben-Chaim J, Jeffs RD, Sanders RC (1995) Criteria for the prenatal diagnosis of classic bladder exstrophy. Obstet Gynecol 85:961
Geerts WII, Pieno GF, Heit JA et al (2004) Prevention of venous thromboembolism:the seventh ACCP conference on antithrombotic and thrombolytic therapy. Chest 126:338S
Geh JL, Curley P, Mayfield MP, Price JJ (1997) Small bowel perforation after extracorporeal shock wave lithotripsy. Br J Urol 79:648
Gelbard MK, Heyman AM, Weintraub P (1989) A technique for immediate realignment and catheterization of the disrupted prostatomembranous urethra. J Urol 142:52
Gelblum DY, Potters L, Ashley R et al (1999) Urinary morbidity following ultrasound-guided transperineal prostate seed implantation. Int J Radiat Oncol Biol Phys 45:59
Geller E, Smergel EM, Lowry PA (1997) Renal neoplasms of childhood. Radiol Clin North Am 35:1391
Geoghegan T, Benfayed W et al (2003) Rupture of ureteropelvic junction-obstructed kidney. AJR Am J Roentgenol 181:886
Georgi BA, Massad M, Obeid M (1991) Ballistic trauma to the abdomen: shell fragments versus bullets. J Trauma 31:711
Gerard C (2003) Complement C5a in the sepsis syndrome – too much of a good thing? N Engl J Med 348:167
Gerhardt W, Katus HA, Ravkilde J, Hamm CW (1992) S-troponin-T as a marker of ischemic myocardial injury. Clin Chem 38:1194
Gerharz EW, Kohl U, Weingartner K, Melekos MD, Bonfig R, Riedmiller H (1997) Complications related to different continence mechanisms in ileocecal reservoirs. J Urol 158:1709
Gerspach JM, Bellman GC et al (1997) Conservative management of colon injury following percutaneous renal surgery. Urology 49:831
Gerstenbluth RE, Spirnak JP et al (2002) Sports participation and high grade renal injuries in children. J Urol 168:2575
Gerstner GJ et al (1978) Amoxicillin in the treatment of asymptomatic bacteriura in pregnancy: a single dose of 3 g amoxicillin versus a 4-days of 3 doses 750 mg amoxicillin. Gynecol Obstet Invest 27:84
Gesundheit B, Smith CR, Gerstle JT, Weitzman SS, Chan HS (2004) Ataxia and secretory diarrhea: two unusual paraneoplastic syndromes occurring concurrently in the same patient with ganglioneuroblastoma. J Pediatr Hematol Oncol 26:549
Gettman MT (2005) Complications of laparoscopic access. In: Ramakumar S, Jarrett T (eds) Complications of urologic laparoscopic surgery. Taylor & Francis, Boca Raton, p 13
Ghai B, Dureja GP et al (2003) Massive intra-abdominal extravasation of fluid: a life threatening complication following percutaneous nephrolithotomy. Int Urol Nephrol 35:315
Ghali AM, El Malik EM et al (1999) Ureteric injuries: diagnosis, management, and outcome. J Trauma 46:150
Ghanem AN (2003) Validation of the ethanol breath test and on-table weighing to measure irrigation absorption during transurethral prostatectomy. BJU Int 92:154
Ghanem AN, Ward JP (1990) Osmotic and metabolic sequelae of volumetric overload in relation to the TUR syndrome. Br J Urol 66:71
Ghasemian SMR, Guleria AS, Khawand NY, Light JA (1996) Diagnosis and management of the urologic complications of renal transplantation. Clin Transplant 10:218:23
Gheiler EL, Frontera JR (1997) Immediate primary realignment of prostatomembranous urethral disruptions using endourologic techniques. Urology 49:596
Giannarini G, Grossetti B et al (2004) Post-traumatic ureteropelvic junction obstruction. Arch Ital Urol Androl 76:100
Giannitsis E, Katus HA (2002) Acute posterior myocardial infarct. A typical diagnostic error. Internist (Berl) 43:618
Giannopoulos A, Serafetinides E et al (1999) Urogenital lesions diagnosed incidentally during evaluation for blunt renal injuries. Prog Urol 9:464
Giannopoulos A, Manousakas T et al (2004) Delayed life-threatening haematuria from a renal pseudoaneurysm caused by blunt renal trauma treated with selective embolization. Urol Int 72:352
Gibson GR (1970) Impotence following fractured pelvis and ruptured urethra. Br J Urol 42:86
Gibson GR (1974) Urological management and complications of fractured pelvis and ruptures urethra. J Urol 111:353
Gilbert DN, Moellering RC, Eliopoulos GM, Sande MA (2006) The Sanford guide to antimicrobial therapy 2006, 36th edn. Antimicrobial Therapy Inc., Sperryville, VA, USA, p 44
Gilbert RW, Kim JH, Posner JB (1978) Epidural spinal cord compression from metastatic tumor: diagnosis and treatment. Ann Neurol 3:40
Gill IS, Hodge EE, Munch LC, Goldfarb DA, Novick AC, Lucas BA (1995) Transperitoneal marsupialization of lymphoceles: a comparison of laparoscopic and open techniques. J Urol 153:706
Gill IS, Kavoussi LR, Clayman RV, Ehrlich R, Evans R, Fuchs G, Gersham A, Hulbert JC, McDougall EM, Rosenthal T et al (1995) Complications of laparoscopic nephrectomy in 185 patients: a multi-institutional review. J Urol 154:479
Gill IS, Clayman RV, Albala DM, Aso Y, Chiu AW, Das S, Donovan JF, Fuchs GJ, Gaur DD, Go H, Gomella LG, Grune MT, Harewood LM, Janetschek G, Knapp PM, McDougall EM, Nakada SY, Preminger GM, Puppo P, Rassweiler JJ, Royce PL, Thomas R, Urban DA, Winfield HN (1998) Retroperitoneal and pelvic extraperitoneal laparoscopy: an international perspective. Urology 52:566
Gill IS, Kerbl K, Meraney AM, Clayman RV (2002) Basic principles techniques, and equipment of laparoscopic surgery. In: Walsh PC, Retik AB, Vaughan ED, Wein AJ (eds) Campbell's urology. Saunders, Philadelphia, p 3455
Gilligan TD, Steele GS, Zietman AL (2003) Bladder cancer. In: Kufe DW, Pollock RE, Weichselbaum RR, Bast RC, Gansler TS, Holland JF, Frei E (eds) Cancer medicine. BC Decker, Hamilton
Gilmartin JJ, Wright AJ, Gibson GJ (1985) Effects of pneumothorax or pleural effusion on pulmonary function. Thorax 40:60
Gilmour DT et al (1999) Lower urinary tract injury during gynecologic surgery and its detection by intraoperative cystoscopy. Obstet Gynecol 94:883
Gintautas J, Angus LD et al (1994) Pharmacological and surgical management of pediatric renal injuries. Proc West Pharmacol Soc 37:99
Giovannini I, Giuliante F, Chiarla C, Ardito F, Vellone M, Nuzzo G (2005) Non-surgical management of a lymphatic fistula, after laparoscopic colorectal surgery, with total parenteral nutrition, octreotide, and somatostatin. Nutrition 21:1065
Girman CJ, Jacobsen SJ, Rhodes T et al (1999) Association of health-related quality of life and benign prostatic enlargement. Eur Urol 35:277
Glassberg KI, Tolete-Velcek F, Ashley R, Waterhouse K (1979) Partial tears of prostatomembranous urethra in children. Urology 13:500
Gluck G, Croitoru M, Deleanu D, Platon P (2000) Local thrombolytic treatment for renal arterial embolism. Eur Urol 38: 339
Gnanapragasam VJ, Kumar V, Langton D et al (2006) Outcome of transurethral prostatectomy for the palliative manage-

ment of lower urinary tract symptoms in men with prostate cancer. Int J Urol 13:711
Godden J, Hiley C (1998) Managing the patient with a chest drain: a review. Nurs Stand 12:35
Godzinski J, Weirich A, Tournade MF, Gauthier F, Buerger D, Moorman-Voestermans CG et al (2001) Primary nephrectomy for emergency: a rare event in the International Society of Paediatric Oncology Nephroblastoma Trial and Study no 9. Eur J Pediatr Surg 11:36
Goel MC, Kumar M, Kapoor R (1997) Endoscopic management of traumatic posterior urethral stricture: early results and follow-up. J Urol 157:95
Goff CD, Collin GR (1998) Management of renal trauma at a rural, level I trauma center. Am Surg 64:226
Goffette PP, Laterre PF (2002) Traumatic injuries: imaging and intervention in post-traumatic complications (delayed intervention) Eur Radiol 12:994
Goffette PP, Laterre PF (2002) Traumatic injuries: imaging and intervention in post-traumatic complications (delayed intervention) Eur Radiol 12:994
Gogos CA, Drosou E, Bassaris HP et al (2000) Pro-versus anti-inflammatory cytokine profile in patients with severe sepsis: a marker for prognosis and future therapeutic options. J Infect Dis 181:176
Gokcen EC et al (1994) Pelvic fracture mechanism of injury in vehicular trauma patients. J Trauma 36:789; discussion 795
Gold HS, Moellering RC (1996) Antimicrobial-drug resistance. N Engl J Med 335:1445
Gold PJ, Fefer A, Thompson JA (1996) Paraneoplastic manifestations of renal cell carcinoma. Semin Urol Oncol 14:216
Goldberg PK, Kozinn PJ, Wise GJ, Nouri N (1979) Brooks RB Incidence and significance of candiduria. JAMA 241:582
Golde DW, Schambelan M, Weintraub BD, Rosen SW (1974) Gonadotropin-secreting renal carcinoma. Cancer 33:1048
Goldfarb DA (1999) Contemporary evaluation and management of Cushing's syndrome. World J Urol 17:22
Goldfarb RA, Neerhut GJ, Lederer E (1989) Management of acute hydronephrosis of pregnancy by ureteral stenting: risk of stone formation. J Urol 141:921
Goldhaber SZ (2002) Echocardiography in the management of pulmonary embolism. Ann Intern Med 136:691
Goldman HB, Zimmern PE (2006) The treatment of female bladder outlet obstruction. BJU Int 98 [Suppl 1]:17
Goldman HB, Dmochowski RR, Cox CE (1996) Penetrating trauma to the penis: functional results. J Urol 155:551
Goldman HB, Idom CB Jr, Dmochowski RR (1998) Traumatic injuries of the female external genitalia and their association with urological injuries. J Urol 159:956
Goldman SM, CM Sandler (2004) Urogenital trauma: imaging upper GU trauma. Eur J Radiol 50:84
Goldman SM, Sandler CM, Corriere-Jr, JN, McGuire EJ (1997) Blunt urethral trauma: a unified, anatomical mechanical classification. J Urol 157:85
Goldmeier D, Lamba H (2002) Drug points: prolonged erections produced by dihydrocodeine and sildenafil. BMJ 324:1555
Goldstein FW (2000) Histoire naturelle, évolution de la sensibilité, participation à la résistance bactérienne. In: Choutet P, Goldstein FW (eds) Escherichia coli. Phase 5. Editions Médicales, Paris, p 7
Goldstein M (1978) Microsurgical reimplantation of amputated penis. Urol 12:237
Golijanin D, Katz R, Verstandig A, Sasson T, Landau EH, Meretyk S (1998) The supracostal percutaneous nephrostomy for treatment of staghorn and complex kidney stones. J Endourol 12:403
Gomella LG, Raj GV, Moreno JG (1997) Reverse transcriptase polymerase chain reaction for prostate specific antigen in the management of prostate cancer. J Urol 158:326
Gomes Almeida F, Reis J et al (2000) Traumatic rupture of angiomyolipoma: a case report. Arch Esp Urol 53:286
Gomes CM, Ribeiro-Filho L, Giron AM, Mitre AI, Figueira ER, Arap S (2000) Genital trauma due to animal bites. J Urol 165:80
Gomes CM, Ribeiro-Filho L, Giron AM, Mitre AI, Figueira ER, Arap S (2001) Genital trauma due to animal bites. J Urol 165:80
Gomez RG, Ceballos L, Coburn M et al (2004) Consensus statement on bladder injuries. BJU Int 94:27
Gomez RG, Castanheira ACC, McAninch JW (1993) Gunshot wounds to the male genitalia. J Urol 150:1147
Gomez Pascual JA, Chicharro Molero JA et al (2002) Post-traumatic renal arteriovenous fistula. Conservative treatment with superselective embolization. Arch Esp Urol 55:949
Gomez Vegas A, Silmi Moyano A et al (1999) Ureteral iatrogenic disease of obstetric-gynecologic origin. Arch Esp Urol 52:923
Gomha MA, Boone TB (2002) Artificial urinary sphincter for post-prostatectomy incontinence in men who had prior radiotherapy: a risk and outcome analysis. J Urol 167:591
Gong M, Geary ES, Shortliffe LM (1996) Testicular torsion with contralateral vanishing testis. Urology 48:306
Gonzalez RP, Falimirski M et al (1999) Surgical management of renal trauma: is vascular control necessary? J Trauma 47:1039; discussion 1042
Goodman DN, Saibil EA et al (1998) Traumatic intimal tear of the renal artery treated by insertion of a Palmaz stent. Cardiovasc Intervent Radiol 21(1:69
Goodman JS, Schaffner W, Collins HA, Battersby EJ, Koenig MG (1968) Infection after cardiovascular surgery. Clinical study including examination of antimicrobial prophylaxis. N Engl J Med 278:117
Goodwin WE, Casey WC, Woolf W (1955) Percutaneous trocar (needle) nephrostomy in hydronephrosis. J Am Med Assoc 157:891
Gornicka G, Papierkowski A (2002) Foreign body in the kidney as a cause of erythruria in a 4-year old girl. Wiad Lek 55:338
Gorsline RT, Kaeding CC (2005) The use of NS AIDs and nutritional supplements in athletes with osteoarthritis: prevalence, benefits, and consequences. Clin Sports Med 24:71
Gorton E, Whitfield HN (1997) Renal calculi in pregnancy. Br J Urol 80 [Suppl 1]:4
Gosalbez R, Castellan M, Ibrahim E, DiSandro M, Labbie A (2005) New concepts in feminizing genitoplasty–is the Fortunoff flap obsolete? J Urol 174:2350
Gosling P (1998) The cellular, immune, and metabolic response to trauma. Crit Rev Clin Lab Sci 35:59
Goswami GK, Levin DQ (2001) Traumatic renal artery thrombosis. Am J Surg 181:187
Gottesman J, Ehrlich RM (1974) Preventing vesicoureteral reflux during intravesical formalin instillation. Urology 3:494
Gould MK, Dembitzer AD, Doyle RL, Hastie TJ, Garber AM (1999) Low-molecular-weight heparins compared with unfractionated heparin for treatment of acute deep venous thrombosis. A meta-analysis of randomized, controlled trials. Ann Intern Med 130:800
Govier FE, Jonsson E, Kramer-Levien DA (1994) Oral terbutaline for the treatment of priapism. J Urol 151:878
Grabe M (2001) Perioperative antibiotic prophylaxis in urology. Curr Opin Urol 11:81
Grady RW, Mitchell ME (1999) Complete primary repair of exstrophy. J Urol 162:1415
Grainger DA, Soderstrom RM, Schiff SF et al (1990) Ureteral injuries at laparoscopy: insights into diagnosis, management, and prevention. Obstet Gynecol 75:839
Grasso M (2000) Ureteropyeloscopic treatment of ureteral and intrarenal calculi. Urol Clin North Am 27:623

Grasso M (2001) Complications of ureteropyloscopy. In: Taneja SS, Smith RB, Ehrlich RM (eds) Complications of urologic surgery, 3rd edn. WB Saunders, Philadelphia, p 268
Gravenstein D (1997) Transurethral resection of the prostate (TURP) syndrome: a review of the pathophysiology and management. Anesth Analg 84:438
Gray LH, Conger AD, Ebert M et al (1953) The concentration of oxygen dissolved in tissues at the time of irradiation as a factor in radiotherapy. Br J Radiol 26:638
Green LS, Loughlin KR, Kavoussi LR (1992) Management of epigastric vessel injury during laparoscopy. J Endourol 2:99
Greenberg JM, Steiner MA, Marshall JJ (2002) Acute renal artery thrombosis treated by percutaneous rheolytic thrombectomy. Catheter Cardiovasc Interv 56:66
Greenberger PA, Halwig JM, Patterson R, Wallemark CB (1986) Emergency administration of radio contrast media in high-risk patients. J Allergy Clin Immunol 77:630
Greilsheimer H, Groves JE (1979) Male genital self-mutilation. Arch Gen Psychiatry 36:441
Gremmo E, Ballanger P, Dore B, Aubert J (1999) Hemorrhagic complications during percutaneous nephrolithotomy. Retrospective studies of 772 cases (in French). Prog Urol 9:460
Grenier N, Pariente JL, Trillaud H et al (2000) Dilatation of the collecting system during pregnancy: physiologic vs obstructive dilatation. Eur Radiol 10:271
Grey NJ, Perdrizet GA (2004) Reduction of nosocomial infections in the surgical intensive-care unit by strict glycemic control. Endocr Pract 10 [Suppl 2]:46
Griffet J, Bastiani-Griffet F et al (2002) Management of seat-belt syndrome in children. Gravity of 2-point seat-belt. Eur J Pediatr Surg 12:63
Griffith BC, Morey AF, Ali-Khan MM, Canby-Hagino E, Foley JP, Rozanski TA (2002) Single dose levofloxacin prophylaxis for prostate biopsy in patients at low risk. J Urol 168:1021
Griffith BC, Morey AF et al (2004) Central renal stab wounds: treatment with augmented fibrin sealant in a porcine model. J Urol 171:445
Griscom NT, Colodny AH, Rosenberg HK, Fliegel CP, Hardy BE (1977) Diagnostic aspects of neonatal ascites: report of 27 cases. AJR Am J Roentgenol 128:961
Grober ED, Chan PT, Zini A, Goldstein M (2004) Microsurgical treatment of persistent or recurrent varicocele. Fertil Steril 82:718
Groggel GC (1991) Acute thrombosis of the renal transplant artery: a case report and review of the literature. Clin Nephrol 36:42
Grosse A, Grosse CA, Mauermann J et al (2005) [Imaging techniques and their impact in treatment management of patients with acute flank pain]. Radiologe 45:871
Grossman MD, Miller D et al (2002) When is an elder old? Effect of preexisting conditions on mortality in geriatric trauma. J Trauma 52:242
Gruessner RW, Fasola C, Benedetti E, Foshager MC, Gruessner AC, Matas AJ, Najarian JS, Goodale RL (1995) Laparoscopic drainage of lymphoceles after kidney transplantation: indications and limitations. Surgery 117:288
Gschwend JE, Sauter TW et al (1995) Renal pelvis rupture after blunt abdominal trauma. Urol Int 55:108
Guazzoni G, Montorsi F, Bergamaschi F et al (1994) Prostatic UroLume Wallstent for urinary retention due to advanced prostate cancer: a 1-year follow-up study. J Urol 152:1530
Guerriero WG (1989) Ureteral injury. Urol Clin North Am 16:237
Guille F, Cipolla B, Leveque JM, Guirassy S, Olivo JF, Lobel B (1991) Early endoscopic realignment of complete traumatic rupture of the posterior urethra. Br J Urol 68:178
Guillonneau B, Rozet F, Cathelineau X, Lay F, Barret E, Doublet JD, Baumert H, Vallancien G (2002) Perioperative complications of laparoscopic radical prostatectomy: the Montsouris 3-year experience. J Urol 167:51
Guillonneau B, Bermudez H, Gholami S, El Fettouh H, Gupta R, Adorno Rosa J, Baumert H, Cathelineau X, Fromont G, Vallancien G (2003) Laparoscopic partial nephrectomy for renal tumor: single center experience comparing clamping and no clamping techniques of the renal vasculature. J Urol 169:483
Guillonneau B, el-Fettouh H, Baumert H, Cathelineau X, Doublet JD, Fromont G, Vallancien G (2003) Laparoscopic radical prostatectomy: oncological evaluation after 1,000 cases a Montsouris Institute. J Urol 169:1261
Guillonneau B, Gupta R, El Fettouh H, Cathelineau X, Baumert H, Vallancien G (2003) Laparoscopic [correction of laproscopic] management of rectal injury during laparoscopic [correction of laproscopic] radical prostatectomy. J Urol 169:1694
Guleria S, Ahmad N et al (1998) Transplant renal artery aneurysm following venous patch repair of a traction injury to the renal artery. Nephrol Dial Transplant 13:1577
Gulmi FA, Felsen D, Vaughan ED Jr (2002) Pathophysiology of upper tract obstruction. In: Walsh PC et al (eds) Campbell's urology, 8th edn. Saunders, Philadelphia, pp 411
Günther R, Alken P, Altwein JE (1978) Percutaneous nephropyelostomy applications and results. Rofo 128:720
Günther R, Marberger M, Klose K (1979) Transrenal ureteral embolization. Radiology 132:317
Gupta DK, Kataria R, Sharma MC (1999) Prepubertal testicular teratomas. Eur J Pediatr Surg 9:173
Gupta M, Bellman GC et al (1997) Massive hemorrhage from renal vein injury during percutaneous renal surgery: endourological management. J Urol 157:795
Gupta N, Kumar R, Dogra PN, Seth A (2006) Comparison of standard transurethral resection, transurethral vapour resection and holmium laser enucleation of the prostate for managing benign prostatic hyperplasia of >40 g. BJU Int 97:85
Gupta NP, Gill IS (1986) Core-through optical internal urethrotomy in management of impassable traumatic posterior urethral strictures. J Urol 136:1018
Gupta NP, Nabi G, Ansari MS (2002) Conservative management of spontaneous rupture of a sigmoid colon neobladder. Urol Int 69:325
Gupta NP, Nabi G, Hemal AK, Dogra PN, Seth A, Aron M (2002) Is incidental appendectomy necessary during radical cystectomy? Urol Int 69:181
Gurdal M, Yucebas E, Tekin A et al (2003) Predisposing factors and treatment outcome in Fournier's gangrene. Analysis of 28 cases. Urol Int 70:286
Guttmann L, Whitteridge D (1947) Effects of bladder distension on automatic mechanisms after spinal cord injury. Brain 70:361
Haaga JR, Zelch MG, Alfidi RJ, Stewart BH, Daugherty JD (1977) CT-guided antegrade pyelography and percutaneous nephrostomy. Am J Roentgenol 128:621
Haas CA, Spirnak JP (1998) Traumatic renal artery occlusion: a review of the literature. Tech Urol 4:1
Haas CA, Dinchman KH, Nasrallah PM et al (1998) Traumatic renal artery occlusion: a 15-year review. J Trauma 45:557
Haas CA, Reigle MD, Selzman AA et al (1998) Use of ureteral stents in the management of major renal trauma with urinary extravasation: is there a role? J Endourol 12:545
Haas CA, Brown SL, Spirnak JP (1999) Limitations of routine spiral computerized tomography in the evaluation of bladder trauma. J Urol 162:51
Haas CA, Brown SL, Spirnak JP (1999) Penile fracture and testicular rupture. World J Urol 17:101
Haas CA, Newman J, Spirnak JP (1999) Computed tomography

three-dimensional reconstruction in the diagnosis of traumatic renal artery thrombosis. Urology 54:559
Haas GP, Pittaluga S, Gomella L et al (1989) Clinically occult Leydig cell tumor presenting with gynecomastia. J Urol 142:1325
Haase GM, Perez C, Atkinson JB (1999) Current aspects of biology, risk assessment, and treatment of neuroblastoma. Semin Surg Oncol 16:91
Hackam DJ, Rotstein OD (1995) Stoma closure and wound infection: an evaluation of risk factors. Can J Surg 38:144
Hackam DJ, Rotstein OD (1995) Wound infection during stoma closure. Can J Surg 38:191
Haddad MC, Sharif HS, Shahed MS et al (1992) Renal colic: diagnosis and outcome. Radiology 184:83
Hader JE, Marzella L, Myers RA et al (1993) Hyperbaric oxygen treatment for experimental cyclophosphamide-induced hemorrhagic cystitis. J Urol 149:1617
Hadj-Abdelkader M, Perez N et al (1997) Post-traumatic arterial hypertension. Presse Med 26:1003
Hafez AT, El-Assmy A, Sarhan O, El-Hefnawy AS, Ghoneim MA (2005) Perineal anastomotic urethroplasty for managing post-traumatic urethral strictures in children: the long-term outcome. BJU Int 95:403
Hagiwara A, Sakaki S, Goto H, Takenega K, Fukushima H, Matuda H, Shimazaki S (2001) The role of interventional radiology in the management of blunt renal injury: a practical protocol. J Trauma 51:526
Hagiwara A, Murata A, Matsuda T, Matsuda H, Shimazaki S (2004) The usefulness of transcatheter arterial embolization for patients with blunt polytrauma showing transient response to fluid resuscitation. J Trauma 57:271
Hagspiel KD, Kandarpa K, Silverman SG (1998) Interactive MR-guided percutaneous nephrostomy. J Magn Reson Imaging 8:1319
Hahn RG (1990) Prevention of TUR syndrome by detection of trace ethanol in the expired breath. Anaesthesia 45:577
Hahn RG (1991a) Monitoring of TURP with ethanol. Lancet 338:1602
Hahn RG (1991b) The transurethral resection syndrome. Acta Anaesthesiol Scand 35:557
Hahn RG (1995) Transurethral resection syndrome after transurethral resection of bladder tumours. Can J Anaesth 42:69
Hahn RG (1997) Irrigating fluids in endoscopic surgery. Br J Urol 79:669
Hahn RG (2006) Fluid absorption in endoscopic surgery. Br J Anaesth 1:8
Hahn RG, Stalberg HP, Gustafsson SA (1989) Intravenous infusion of irrigating fluids containing glycine or mannitol with and without ethanol. J Urol 142:1102
Hahn RG, Algotsson LA, Tornebrandt K (1990) Comparison of ethanol absorption during continuous and intermittent flow irrigation in transurethral resection. Scand J Urol Nephrol 24:27
Hahn RG, Larsson H, Ribbe T (1995) Continuous monitoring of irrigating fluid absorption during transurethral surgery. Anaesthesia 50:327
Hahn-Pedersen J, Kvist N, Nielsen OH (1984) Hydrometrocolpos: current views on pathogenesis and management. J Urol 132:537
Hajivassiliou CA (1999) A review of the complications and results of implantation of the AMS artificial urinary sphincter. Eur Urol 35:36
Hald T, Mygind T (1974) Control of life-threatening vesical hemorrhage by unilateral hypogastric artery muscle embolization. J Urol 112:60
Halimi JM, Al-Najjar A, Buchler M, Birmele B, Tranquart F, Alison D et al (1999) Transplant renal artery stenosis: potential role of ischemia renal reperfusion injury and long-term outcome following angioplasty. J Urol 161:28
Hall DC, Lawson BX, Wilson LG (1981) Command hallucinations and self-amputation of the penis and hand during a first psychotic break. J Clin Psychiatry 42:322
Hall EJ (1991) Scientific view of low level radiation risks. Radiographics 11:509
Hallscheidt P, Besharati S, Noeldge G, Haferkamp A, Lopez R, Kauffmann GW (2006) Preoperative and palliative embolization of renal cell carcinomas: follow-up of 49 patients. Rofo 178:391
Hamasuna R, Betsunoh H, Sueyoshi T, Yakushiji K, Tsukino H, Nagano M, Takehara T, Osada Y (2004) Bacteria of preoperative urinary tract infections contaminate the surgical fields and develop surgical site infections in urological operations. Int J Urol 11:941
Hamm CW (2004) Guidelines: Acute coronary syndrome (ACS) II Acute coronary syndrome with ST-elevation. Z Kardiol 93:324
Hamm M, Knopfle E, Wartenberg S et al (2002) Low dose unenhanced helical computerized tomography for the evaluation of acute flank pain. J Urol 167:1687
Hammarskjold F, Wallen G, Malmvall BE (2006) Central venous catheter infections at a county hospital in Sweden: a prospective analysis of colonization, incidence of infection and risk factors. Acta Anaesthesiol Scand 50:451
Hammarstrom L, Vorechivsky I, Webster D. Selective IgA deficiency (SIgAD) and common variable immunodeficiency (CVID) (2000) Clin Exp Immunol 120:225
Hammer CC, Santucci RA (2003) Effect of an institutional policy of nonoperative treatment of grades I to IV renal injuries. J Urol 169:1751
Hamrahian AH, Oseni TS, Arafah BM (2004) Measurement of serum free cortisol in critically ill patients. N Engl J Med 350:1629
Hamza AF, Soliman HA, Abdel Hay SA, Kabesh AA, Elbehery MM (2001) Total urogenital sinus mobilization in the repair of cloacal anomalies and congenital adrenal hyperplasia. J Pediatr Surg 36:1656
Han Kr K, Goldstein DW et al (1998) Angiographic management of pseudoaneurysm and arteriocalyceal fistula following blunt trauma: case report and review of the literature. Can J Urol 5:654
Hanash KA (1982) The nonmetastatic hepatic dysfunction syndrome associated with renal cell carcinoma (hypernephroma): Stauffer's syndrome. Prog Clin Biol Res 100:301
Hanash KA, Utz DC, Ludwig J, Wakim KG, Ellefson RD, Kelalis PP (1971) Syndrome of reversible hepatic dysfunction associated with hypernephroma: an experimental study. Invest Urol 8:399
Hanazawa K, Higashi N, Kawachi Y, Suzuki F, Ishi K, Fujime M (2005) Small cell carcinoma of the prostate with hypercalcemia. Int J Urol 12:108
Hani MA, Sallami S et al (2004) Trauma of an ectopic kidney. A case report. Tunis Med 82:69
Hanstead B, John HT (1964) Idiopathic scrotal oedema of children. Br J Urol 36:110
Harbarth S, Ruef C, Francioli P, Widmer A, Pittet D (1999) Nosocomial infections in Swiss university hospitals: a multicentre survey and review of the published experience. Swiss-Noso Network. Schweiz Med Wochenschr 129:1521
Harbrecht PJ, Garrision RN, Fry DE (1984) Early urgent relaparotomy. Arch Surg 119:369
Hardeman SW, Husmann DA et al (1987) Blunt urinary tract trauma: identifying those patients who require radiological diagnostic studies. J Urol 138:99
Hardinger KL, Brennan DC, Lowell J, Schnitzer MA (2004) Long-term outcome of gastrointestinal complications in renal transplant patients treated with mycophenolate mofetil. Transpl Int 17:609

Hardy JF, De Moerloose P, Samama M (2004) Massive transfusion and coagulopathy: pathophysiology and implications for clinical management. Can J Anaesth 51:293
Harkki-Siren P et al (1998) Urinary tract injuries after hysterectomy. Obstet Gynecol 92:113
Harkki-Siren P, Sjoberg J, Kurki T (1999) Major complications of laparoscopy: a follow-up Finnish study. Obstet Gynecol 94:94
Harmon GD, Senagore AJ, Kilbride MJ Warzynski MJ (1994) Interleukin-6 response to laparoscopic and open colectomy. Dis Colon Rectum 37:754
Harrington KD (1984) Anterior cord decompression and spinal stabilization for patients with metastatic lesion of the spine. J Neurosurg 61:107
Harrington KD (1988) Anterior decompression and stabilization of the spine as a treatment for vertebral collapse and spinal cord compression from metastatic malignancy. Clin Orthop Relat Res 233:177
Harrington TG, Kandel LB (1997) Renal colic following a gunshot wound to the abdomen: the birdshot calculus. J Urol 157:1351
Harris AC, Zwirewich CV et al (2001) Ct findings in blunt renal trauma. Radiographics 21:S201
Harris RL et al (1997) The value of intraoperative cystoscopy in urogynecologic and reconstructive pelvic surgery. Am J Obstet Gynecol 177:1367; discussion 1369
Harrison RH 3rd, Boren JS, Robison JR (1956) Dilutional hyponatremic shock: another concept of the transurethral prostatic resection reaction. J Urol 75:95
Harvey EB, Boice JD Jr, Honeyman M, Flanner JT (1985) Prenatal x-ray exposure and childhood cancer in twins. N Engl J Med 312:541
Hashem FK, Ahmed S, al-Malaq AA, AbuDaia JM (1999) Successful replantation of penile amputation (post-circumcision) complicated by prolonged ischaemia. Br J Plast Surg. 52:308
Hashmi A, Klassen T (1995) Correlation between urinalysis and intravenous pyelography in pediatric abdominal trauma. J Emerg Med 13:255
Hasson HM (1971) A modified instrument and method for laparoscopy. Am J Obstet Gynecol 110:886
Hasson HM, Parker WH (1998) Prevention and management of urinary tract injury in laparoscopic surgery. J Am Assoc Gynecol Laparosc 5:99
Hastings MK, Sinacore DR et al (2005) Bone mineral density during total contact cast immobilization for a patient with neuropathic (Charcot) arthropathy. Phys Ther 85:249
Hattery RR, Williamson B Jr, Hartman GW et al (1988) Intravenous urographic technique. Radiology 167:593
Hatzichristou D, Salpiggidis G, Hatzimouratidis K et al (2002) Management strategy for arterial priapism: therapeutic dilemmas. J Urol 168:2074
Hau T, Ahrenholz DH, Simmons RL (1979) Secondary bacterial peritonitis: the biologic basis of treatment. Curr Probl Surg 16:1
Haukaas SA, Halvorsen OJ, Nygaard SJ, Paus E (1999) Cushing's syndrome in prostate cancer. An aggressive course of prostatic malignancy. Urol Int 63:126
Haupt G (2004) Re: safer transurethral resection of the prostate: coagulating intermittent cutting reduces hemostatic complications. J Urol 172:780
Haupt G, Pannek J, Knopf HJ, Schulze H, Senge T (1990) Rupture of ileal neobladder due to urethral obstruction by mucous plug. J Urol 144:740
Haupt MT (1995) Anaphylaxis and anaphylactic shock. In: Parillo JE, Bone RC (eds) Critical care medicine. Mosby Year Book, St. Louis, pp 433
Haupt G, Pannek J, Benkert S, Heinrich C, Schulze H, Senge T (1997) Transurethral resection of the prostate with microprocessor controlled electrosurgical unit. J Urol 158:497
Hausegger KA, Tiesenhausen K, Schedlbauer P, Oberwalder P, Tauss J, Rigler B (2001) Treatment of acute aortic type B dissection with stent-grafts. Cardiovasc Intervent Radiol 24: 306
Haut T, Ohmann C, Wolmershauser A, Wacha H, Yang Q (1995) Planned relaparotomy versus relaparotomy on demand in the treatment of intra-abdominal infections. The Peritonitis Study Group of the Surgical Infection Society – Europe. Arch Surg 130:1193
Hautman RE (2003) Urinary diversion: ileal conduit to neobladder. J Urol 169:834
Hautmann RE, de Petriconi R, Gottfried HW, Kleinschmidt K, Mattes R, Paiss T (1999) The ileal neobladder: complications and functional results in 363 patients after 11 years of followup. J Urol 161:422
Hayes MC, Wilson NM, Page A, Harrison GS (1996) Selective embolization of bladder tumours. Br J Urol 78:311
Hayes RJ (1977) Incidental appendectomies. Current teaching. JAMA 238:31
Hayhurst JW, O'Brien BM, Ishida H et al (1974) Experimental digital replantation after prolonged cooling. Hand 6:143
Head H, Riddoch G (1917) The autonomic bladder, excessive sweating and some other reflex conditions in gross injuries of the spinal cord. Brain 40:188
Healy ME, Teng SS, Moss AA (1984) Uriniferous pseudocyst: computed tomographic findings. Radiology 153:757
Hebuterne X, Frere AM, Bayle J et al (1992) Priapism in a patient treated with total parenteral nutrition. JPEN J Parenter Enteral Nutr 16:171
Heck M, Fresenius M (2004) Repetitorium Anaesthesiology. 4th edn. Springer, Berlin Heidelberg New York
Hedderich GS, Wexler MJ, McLean AP, Meakins JL (1986) The septic abdomen: open Management with Marlex mesh with a zipper. Surgery 99:399
Hedican SP (2004) Complications of hand-assisted laparoscopic urologic surgery. J Endourol 18:387
Hedican SP, Walsh PC (1994) Postoperative bleeding following radical retropubic prostatectomy. J Urol 152:1181
Hedlund PO (1969) Antifibrinolytic therapy with Cyklokapron in connection with prostatectomy. A double blind study. Scand J Urol Nephrol 3:177
Hedlund PO (1975) Postoperative venous thrombosis in benign prostatic disease. A study of 316 patients, using the 125I-fibrinogen uptake test. Scand J Urol Nephrol 27 [Suppl]:1
Heidelberger KP, Ritchey ML, Dauser RC, McKeever PE, Beckwith JB (1993) Congenital mesoblastic nephroma metastatic to the brain. Cancer 72:2499
Heidenreich A, Desgrandschamps F, Terrier F (2002) Modern approach of diagnosis and management of acute flank pain: review of all imaging modalities. Eur Urol 41:351
Heidenreich A, Ravery V; European Society of Oncological Urology (2004) Preoperative imaging in renal cell cancer. World J Urol 22:307
Heidenreich A, Ohlmann C, Hegele A, Beyer J (2005) Repeat retroperitoneal lymphadenectomy in advanced testicular cancer. Eur Urol 47:64
Heidler H (1999) Frequency and causes of fluid absorption: a comparison of three techniques for resection of the prostate under continuous pressure monitoring. BJU Int 83:619
Heimdal K, Hirschberg H, Slettebo H et al (1992) High incidence of serious side effects of high-dose dexamethasone treatment in patients with epidural spinal cord compression. J Neurooncol 12:141
Heinzelmann M, Scott M, Lam T (2002) Factors predisposing to bacterial invasion and infection. Am J Surg 183:179

Heinz-Peer G, Helbich T (2001) [Urological and nephrological emergency-value of diagnostic imaging]. Wien Med Wochenschr 151:560
Hejase MJ, Simonin JE, Bihrle R, Coogan CL (1996) Genital Fournier's gangrene: experience with 38 patients. Urology 47:734
Hellier WP, Higgs B (1996) Severe renal laceration from blunt trauma presenting with microhaematuria and a normal intravenous urogram. Br J Urol 78:309
Helweg-Larsen S (1996) Clinical outcome in metastatic spinal cord compression. A prospective study of 153 patients. Acta Neurol Scand 94:269
Helweg-Larsen S, Hansen SW, Sorensen PS (1995) Second occurrence of symptomatic metastatic spinal cord compression and findings of multiple spinal epidural metastases. Int J Radiat Oncol Biol Phys 33:595
Hemal AK, Dorairajan LN, Gupta NP (2000) Posttraumatic complete and partial loss of urethra with pelvic fracture in girls: an appraisal of management. J Urol 163:282
Hendrikx AJ, Strijbos WE, de Knijff DW, Kums JJ, Doesburg WH, Lemmens WA (1999) Treatment for extended-mid and distal ureteral stones: SWL or ureteroscopy? Results of a multicenter study. J Endourol 13:727
Hendron WH (1997) Historical perspective of the use of bowel in urology. Urol Clin North Am 24:703
Henriksson TG, Hahne B, Hakelius S et al (1982) Microsurgical replantation of an amputated penis. Scand J Plast Reconstr Surg Suppl 19:75
Henry GD, Wilson SK, Delk JR 2nd et al (2004) Penile prosthesis cultures during revision surgery: a multicenter study. J Urol 172:153
Henry GD, Wilson SK, Delk JR 2nd et al (2005) Revision washout decreases penile prosthesis infection in revision surgery: a multicenter study. J Urol 173:89
Henry PC, Chabannes E et al (2002) Management of severe renal trauma. Prog Urol 12:579
Henzi I, Walder B, Tramer MR (1999) Metoclopramide in the prevention of postoperative nausea and vomiting: a quantitative systematic review of randomized, placebo-controlled studies. Br J Anaesth 83:761
Herman TE, Shackelford GD, McAlister WH (1994) Acute idiopathic scrotal edema: role of scrotal sonography. J Ultrasound Med 13:53
Herndon CD, McKenna PH, Kolon TF, Gonzales ET, Baker LA, Docimo SG (1999) A multicenter outcomes analysis of patients with neonatal reflux presenting with prenatal hydronephrosis. J Urol 162:1203
Herold G et al (2006) Text of internal medicine. Gerd Herold, Cologne
Herrmann B, Crawford J (2002) Genital injuries in prepubertal girls from inline skating accidents. Pediatrics 110:e16
Herschorn S, Radomski SB et al (1991) Evaluation and treatment of blunt renal trauma. J Urol 146:274; discussion 276
Herschorn S, Thijssen A, Radomski SB (1992) The value of immediate or early catheterization of the traumatized posterior urethra. J Urol 148:1428
Hesselfeldt-Nielsen J, Bang-Jensen E, Riegels-Nielsen P (1986) Scrotal reconstruction after Fournier's gangrene. Ann Plast Surg 17:310
Hettenbach A, Tschada R, Hiltmann WD, Zimmermann T (1988) Untersuchungen zum Einfluss von beta-Stimulation and beta-1-Blockade auf die Motilitatt des oberen Harntraktes. Z Geburtshilfe Perinatol 192:273
Hewin DF, Campbell WB (1998) Ruptured aortic aneurysm: the decision not to operate. Ann R Coll Surg Engl 80:221
Heye S, Maleux G, Van Poppel H, Oyen R, Wilms G (2005) Hemorrhagic complications after nephron-sparing surgery: angiographic diagnosis and management by transcatheter embolization. AJR Am J Roentgenol 184:1661
Heymann AD, Bell-Thomson J, Rathod DM et al (1977) Successful reimplantation of the penis using microvascular techniques. J Urol 118:879
Heymans S, Verhaeghe R, Stockx L, Collen D (1998) Feasibility study of catheter-directed thrombolysis with recombinant staphylokinase in deep venous thrombosis. Thromb Haemost 79:517
Heyns CF, Fisher M (2005) The urological management of the patient with acquired immunodeficiency syndrome. BJU Int 95:709
Heyns CF, van Vollenhoven P (1992) Increasing role of angiography and segmental artery embolization in the management of renal stab wounds. J Urol 147:1231
Heyns CF, Van Vollenhoven P (1992) Selective surgical management of renal stab wounds. Br J Urol 69:351
Hiippala S (1998) Replacement of massive blood loss. Vox Sang 74 [Suppl 2]:399
Hiippala ST, Myllyla GJ, Vahtera EM (1995) Hemostatic factors and replacement of major blood loss with plasma-poor red cell concentrates. Anesth Analg 81:360
Hill JB, Sheffield JS, McIntire DD, Wendel GD Jr (2005) Acute pyelonephritis in pregnancy. Obstet Gynecol 105:18
Hinman F Jr (1960) Priapism: reasons for failure of therapy. J Urol 83:420
Hinsdale JG, Jaffe BM (1984) Reoperation for intra-abdominal sepsis: indications and results in modern critical care setting. Ann Surg 199:31
Hinz J, Hautzinger H, Stahl KW (1986) Rationale for and results from a randomised, double-blind trial of tetrachlorodecaoxygen anion complex in wound healing. Lancet 1:825
Hiramoto JS, Meng MV et al (2001) Successful transplantation of a donor kidney after penetrating grade 3 injury and renorrhaphy. J Urol 166:2299
Hirasawa K, Kitamura T, Oka T, Matsushita H (2002) Bladder tumor producing granulocyte colony-stimulating factor and parathyroid hormone related protein J Urol 167:2130
Hirota S, Matsumoto S, Yoshikawa T, Ichikawa S, Sako M, Kono M (1997) Simultaneous thrombolysis of superior mesenteric artery and bilateral renal artery thromboembolisms with three transfemoral catheters. Cardiovasc Intervent Radiol 20:397
Hirsch AT, Haskal ZJ, Hertzer NR et al (2006) ACC/AHA 2005 Practice Guidelines for the management of patients with peripheral arterial disease (lower extremity, renal, mesenteric, and abdominal aortic): a collaborative report from the American Association for Vascular Surgery/Society for Vascular Surgery, Society for Cardiovascular Angiography and Interventions, Society for Vascular Medicine and Biology, Society of Interventional Radiology, and the ACC/AHA Task Force on Practice Guidelines (Writing Committee to Develop Guidelines for the Management of Patients With Peripheral Arterial Disease): endorsed by the American Association of Cardiovascular and Pulmonary Rehabilitation; National Heart, Lung, and Blood Institute; Society for Vascular Nursing; TransAtlantic Inter-Society Consensus; and Vascular Disease Foundation. Circulation 113:e463
Hirsh J (1995) The optimal duration of anticoagulant therapy for venous thrombosis. N Engl J Med 332:1710
Hirsh J, Hoak J (1996) Management of deep vein thrombosis and pulmonary embolism. A statement for healthcare professionals. Council on Thrombosis (in consultation with the Council on Cardiovascular Radiology) American Heart Association. Circulation 93:2212
Hirsh J, Warkentin TE, Shaughnessy SG, Anand SS, Halperin JL, Raschke R, Granger C, Ohman EM, Dalen JE (2001) Heparin and low-molecular-weight heparin: mechanisms of action, pharmacokinetics, dosing, monitoring, efficacy, and safety. Chest 119:S64

Hirshberg A (2004) Multiple casualty incidents: lessons from the front line. Ann Surg 239:322
Hirshberg A, Mattox KL (1993) 'Damage control' in trauma surgery. Br J Surg 80:1501
Hirshberg A, Walden R (1997) Damage control for abdominal trauma. Surg Clin North Am 77:813
Hirshberg A, Wall MJ Jr, Mattox KL (1994) Planned reoperation for trauma: A two year experience with 124 consecutive patients. J Trauma 37:365
Hirshberg A, Stein M, Adar R (1997) Reoperation: planned and unplanned. Surg Clin North Am 77:897
Ho AM, Dion PW, Cheng CA, Karmakar MK, Cheng G, Peng Z, Ng YW (2005) A mathematical model for fresh frozen plasma transfusion strategies during major trauma resuscitation with ongoing hemorrhage. Can J Surg 48:470
Ho AM, Karmakar MK, Dion PW (2005) Are we giving enough coagulation factors during major trauma resuscitation? Am J Surg 190:479
Ho KY, Chiu JW (2005) Multimodal antiemetic therapy and emetic risk profiling. Ann Acad Med Singapore 34:196
Ho RMT, Fawcett DP (2004) Parastomal hernia repair using the lateral approach. BJU Int 94:598
Ho WK, Hankey GJ, Lee CH, Eikelboom JW (2005) Venous thromboembolism: diagnosis and management of deep venous thrombosis. Med J Aust 182:476
Hochberg E, Stone NN (1993) Bladder rupture associated with pelvic fracture due to blunt trauma. Urology 41:531
Hochmuth A, Fleck M et al (2000) First experiences in using a new ultrasound mode and ultrasound contrast agent in the diagnosis of blunt renal trauma: a feasibility study in an animal model. Invest Radiol 35:205
Hodge KK, McNeal JE, Terris MK, Stamey TA (1989) Random systematic versus directed ultrasound guided transrectal core biopsies of the prostate. J Urol 142:71
Hoeltl W, Hruby W, Aharinejad S (1990) Renal vein anatomy and its implications for retroperitoneal surgery. J Urol 143:1108
Hoffelt SC, Wallner K, Merrick G (2004) Epididymitis after prostate brachytherapy. Urology 63:293
Holcomb JB, Helling TS, Hirshberg A (2001) Military, civilian, and rural application of the damage control philosophy. Mil Med 166:490
Holden S, Hicks CC, O'Brien DP et al (1976) Gunshot wounds of the ureter: a 15-year review of 63 consecutive cases. J Urol 116:562
Holden S, McPhee M, Grabstald H (1979) The rationale of urinary diversion in cancer patients. J Urol 121:19
Hollabaugh RS Jr, Dmochowski RR, Hickerson WL et al (1998) Fournier's gangrene: therapeutic impact of hyperbaric oxygen. Plast Reconstr Surg 101:94
Hollenbeck BK, Miller DC, Taub D, Dunn RL, Khuri SF, Henderson WG, Montie JE, Underwood W 3rd, Wei JT (2005) Identifying risk factors for potentially avoidable complications following radical cystectomy. J Urol 174:1231; discussion 1237
Hollifield JW, Page DL, Smith C, Michelakis AM, Staab E, Rhamy R (1975) Renin-secreting clear cell carcinoma of the kidney. Arch Intern Med 135:859
Holman E et al (1992) Percutaneous nephrolithotomy in late pregnancy. J Endourol 6:421
Holmberg G, Spinnell S, Sjodin JG (1997) Perforation of the bowel during SWL in prone position. J Endourol 11:313
Holmes DG, Thrasher JB, Park GY, Kueker DC, Weigel JW (2002) Long-term complications related to the modified Indiana pouch. Urology 60:603
Holmes FC, Hunt JJ et al (2003) Renal injury in sport. Curr Sports Med Rep 2:103
Holmes JF et al (2001) Emergency department ultrasonography in the evaluation of hypotensive and normotensive children with blunt abdominal trauma. J Pediatr Surg 36:968
Holmes JF, Sokolove PE et al (2002) Identification of children with intra-abdominal injuries after blunt trauma. Ann Emerg Med 39:500
Holmes NJ, Cazi G, Redell MT, Gorman JH, Fedorciw B, Semmlow JL Brolin RE (1993) Intraoperative assessment of bowel viability. J Invest Surg 6:211
Holmes NM, Kogan BA, Baskin LS (2001) Placement of artificial urinary sphincter in children and simultaneous gastrocystoplasty. J Urol 165:2366
Holmgren H, Almroth L, Berggren V, Bergstrom S (2005) Genital mutilation of children is an offence. Do health services have a sufficient knowledge to see the problem? Lakartidningen 102:1637
Hora M, Hes O, Klecka J et al (2004) Rupture of papillary renal cell carcinoma. Scand J Urol Nephrol 38:481
Horger DC, Babanoury A (2004) Intravesical explosion during transurethral resection of bladder tumors. J Urol 172:1813
Horninger W, Unterlechner H, Strasser H, Bartsch G (1996) Transurethral prostatectomy: mortality and morbidity. Prostate 28:195
Horstman WG et al (1991) Comparison of computed tomography and conventional cystography for detection of traumatic bladder rupture. Urol Radiol 12:188
Hosking DJ, Cowley A, Bucknall CA (1981) Rehydration in the treatment of severe hypercalcemia. Q J Med 50:473
Hotchkiss RS, Karl IE (2003) The pathophysiology and treatment of sepsis. N Engl J Med 348:138
Hotchkiss RS, Karl IE (2003) The pathophysiology and treatment of sepsis. N Eng J Med 348:138
Hotker U, Rommens PM (1996) Postrenal anuria in pelvic or acetabular injury: a report of three cases. J Trauma 41:916
Hu K, Wallner K (1998) Urinary incontinence in patients who have a TURP/TUIP following prostate brachytherapy. Int J Radiat Oncol Biol Phys 40:783
Huang CR, Sun N, Wei P, Xie HW, Hwang AH, Hardy BE (2003) The management of old urethral injury in young girls: analysis of 44 cases. J Pediatr Surg 38:1329
Huang Q, Jiang ZW, Jiang J, Li N, Li JS (2004) Chylous ascites: treated with total parenteral nutrition and somatostatin. World J Gastroenterol 10:2588
Huang Y, Zhu Z (1997) Massive hydronephrosis associated with traumatic rupture. Injury 28:505
Hubert J, Cormier L, Gerbaud PF, Guillemin F, Pertek JP, Mangin P (1996) Computer-controlled monitoring of bladder pressure in the prevention of 'TUR syndrome': a randomized study of 53 cases. Br J Urol 78:228
Hudak SJ, Morey AF, Rozanski TA et al (2005) Battlefield urogenital injuries: changing patterns during the past century. Urology 65:1041
Hudolin T, Hudolin I (2003) Surgical management of urogenital injuries at a war hospital in Bosnia-Herzegovina, 1992 to 1995. J Urol 169:1357
Hudspeth AS (1975) Radical surgical debridement in the treatment of advanced generalized bacterial peritonitis. Arch Surg 110:1233
Huerta-Alardin AL, Varon J et al (2005) Bench-to-bedside review: Rhabdomyolysis – an overview for clinicians. Crit Care 9:158
Huffman JL (1989) Ureteroscopic injuries to the upper urinary tract. Urol Clin North Am 16:249
Hughes CR, Stewart PF Jr et al (1995) Renal cyst rupture following blunt abdominal trauma: case report. J Trauma 38:28
Hughes WT, Armstrong D, Bodey GP et al (2002) 2002 guidelines for the use of antimicrobial agents in neutropenic patients with cancer. Clin Infect Dis 34:730
Hull RD, Raskob GE, LeClerc JR, Jay RM, Hirsh J (1984) The di-

agnosis of clinically suspected venous thrombosis. Clin Chest Med 5:439
Hull RD, Raskob GE, Carter CJ (1990) Serial impedance plethysmography in pregnant patients with clinically suspected deep-vein thrombosis. Clinical validity of negative findings. Ann Intern Med 112:663
Hull RD, Raskob GE, Rosenbloom D, Panju AA, Brill-Edwards P, Ginsberg JS, Hirsh J, Martin GJ, Green D (1990) Heparin for 5 days as compared with 10 days in the initial treatment of proximal venous thrombosis. N Engl J Med 322:1260
Hull RD, Raskob GE, Pineo GF, Green D, Trowbridge AA, Elliott CG, Lerner RG, Hall J, Sparling T, Brettell HR et al (1992) Subcutaneous low-molecular-weight heparin compared with continuous intravenous heparin in the treatment of proximal-vein thrombosis. N Engl J Med 326:975
Huller T, Bazini Y (1970) Blast injuries of the chest and abdomen. Arch Surg 100:24
Hulten JO (2002) How to master absorption during transurethral resection of the prostate: basic measures guided by the ethanol method. BJU Int 90:244
Hunt TK, Mueller RV (1994) Inflammation infection and antibiotics. In: Way LW (ed) Current surgical diagnosis treatment, 10th edn. Appleton & Lange Norwalk, p 95
Hurd WW, Chee SS, Gallagher KL et al (2001) Location of the ureters in relation to the uterine cervix by computed tomography. Am J Obstet Gynecol 184:336
Husmann DA (1998) Editorial Comment. J Urol 159:959
Husmann DA, Morris JS (1990) Attempted nonoperative management of blunt renal lacerations extending through the corticomedullary junction: the short-term and long-term sequelae. J Urol 143:682
Husmann DA, Wilson WT, Boone TB, Allen TD (1990) Prostatomembranous urethral disruptions: Management by suprapubic cystostomy and delayed urethroplasty. J Urol 144:76
Husmann DA, Boone TB, Wilson WT (1993) Management of low velocity gunshot wounds to the anterior urethra: the role of primary repair versus urinary diversion alone. J Urol 150:70
Husmann DA, Gilling PJ et al (1993) Major renal lacerations with a devitalized fragment following blunt abdominal trauma: a comparison between nonoperative (expectant) versus surgical management. J Urol 150:1774
Hutchins RR, Gunning MP, Lucas DN, Allen-Mersh TG, Soni NC (2004) Relaparotomy for suspected intraperitioneal sepsis after abdominal surgery. World J Surg 28:137
Huynth PN, Hollander JB (2005) Trends toward laparoscopic nephrectomy at a community hospital. J Urol 173:547
Hyers TM, Agnelli G, Hull RD, Morris TA, Samama M, Tapson V, Weg JG (2001) Antithrombotic therapy for venous thromboembolic disease. Chest 119:176S–193S
Iacovou JW, Marks JC, Abrams PH et al (1985) Cord compression and carcinoma of the prostate: is laminectomy justified? Br J Urol 57:733
Ibanez Pradas V, Serrano Durba A et al (1999) Diagnostic attitude in a patient with kidney trauma. An Esp Pediatr 51:136
Ibarz Servio L, Perendreu Sans J et al (1997) Supraselective embolization of renal pseudoaneurysm caused by an abdominal stab wound. Arch Esp Urol 50:805
Ichigi Y, Takaki N et al (1999) Significance of hematoma size for evaluating the grade of blunt renal trauma. Int J Urol 6:502
Igel TC, Barrett DM, Segura JW et al (1987) Perioperative and postoperative complications from bilateral pelvic lymphadenectomy and radical retropubic prostatectomy. J Urol 137:1189
Igun GO, Nwadiaro HC et al (2001) Surgical experience with management of vascular injuries. West Afr J Med 20:102
Ihse I, Arnesjo B, Jonsson G (1975) Surgical injuries of the ureter. A review of 42 cases. Scand J Urol Nephrol 9:39
Ikoma F (1994) Hypospadiekorrektur nach Denis Browne. In: Hohenfellner R (ed) Ausgewaehlte urologische OP-Techniken. Georg Thieme Verlag, p 477
Ilkay AK, Levine LA (1995) Conservative management of high-flow priapism. Urology 46:419
Inaba K et al (2004) The increasing incidence of severe pelvic injury in motor vehicle collisions. Injury 35:759
Inenaga T, Takishita TS (2000) Hypertension following renal trauma. Nippon Rinsho 58 [Suppl 2]:483
Inoue S, Koizumi J et al (2004) Self-expanding metallic stent placement for renal artery dissection due to blunt trauma. J Urol 171:347
Inoue S, Sugitani A et al (2005) Effect of synthetic protease inhibitor gabexate mesilate on the attenuation of ischemia/reperfusion injury in canine kidney autotransplantation. Surgery 137:216
Ioannides AS, Turnock R (2001) An audit of the management of the acute scrotum in children with Henoch-Schonlein Purpura. J R Coll Surg Edinb 46:98
Iqbal N, Chughtai MN (2004) Management of blunt renal trauma: a profile of 65 patients. J Pak Med Assoc 54:516
Iregui M, Ward S, Sherman G, Fraser VJ, Kollef MH (2002) Clinical importance of delays in the initiation of appropriate antibiotic treatment for ventilator-associated pneumonia. Chest 122:262
Iselin CE, Webster GD (1999) The significance of the open bladder neck associated with pelvic fracture urethral distraction defects. J Urol 162:347
Ismail N et al (1996) Death from pelvic fracture: children are different. J Pediatr Surg 31:82
Issa MM, McNamara DE et al (1998) Surgical challenge of massive bilateral staghorn renal calculi in a spinal cord injury patient. Urol Int 61:247
Ivatury RR, Porter JM, Simon RJ, Islam S, John R, Stahl WM (1998) Intra-abdominal hypertension after life-threatening penetrating abdominal trauma: prophylaxis incidence and clinical relevance of gastric mucosal pH, abdominal compartment syndrome. J Trauma 44:1016
Ives E, Coffey R, Carter CO (1980) A family study of bladder exstrophy. J Med Genet 17:139
Ivy DD, Shaffer EM, Johnson AM, Kimberling WJ, Dobin A, Gabow PA (1995) Cardiovascular abnormalities in children with autosomal dominant polycystic kidney disease. J Am Soc Nephrol 5:2032
Izumi M, Yokoyama K et al (1997) A young man with acute renal failure and severe loin pain. Nephron 76:215
Izzidien AY (1981) Successful replantation of a traumatically amputated penis in a neonate. J Pediatr Surg 16:202
Jackson DH, Williams JL (1974) Urethral injury: a retrospective study. Br J Urol 46:665
Jackson MR, Taher MM et al (1998) Hemostatic efficacy of a fibrin sealant dressing in an animal model of kidney injury. J Trauma 45:662
Jacobellis U (2003) Modified radical inguinal lymphadenectomy for carcinoma of the penis: technique and results. J Urol 169:1349
Jacobi J, Fraser GL, Coursin DB et al (2002) Clinical practice guidelines for the sustained use of sedatives and analgetics in the critically ill adult. Crit Care Med 1:119
Jacobs LM Jr, Ramp JM, Breay JM (1979) An emergency medical system approach to disaster planning. J Trauma 19:157
Jacobs SC, Cho E, Foster C, Liao P, Bartlett ST (2004) Laparoscopic donor nephrectomy: the university of Maryland 6-year experience. J Urol 171:47
Jacobsen SJ, Girman CJ, Lieber MM (2001) Natural history of benign prostatic hyperplasia. Urology 58:5

Jakobi P, Neiger R, Merzbach D, Paldi E (1987) Single-dose antimicrobial therapy in the treatment of asymptomatic bacteriuria in pregnancy. Am J Obstet Gynecol 156:1148
Jan WA, Samad A et al (2004) Mortality and morbidity of abdominal inferior vena-caval injuries. J Coll Physicians Surg Pak 14:622
Janata K (2003) Managing pulmonary embolism. BMJ 326: 1341
Janetschek G, Hobisch A, Hittmair A, Holtl L, Peschel R, Bartsch G (1999) Laparoscopic retroperitoneal lymphadenectomy after chemotherapy for stage IIB nonseminomatous testicular carcinoma. J Urol 161:477
Janetschek G, Bagheri F, Abdelmaksoud A, Biyani CS, Leeb K, Jeschke S (2003) Ligation of the renal vein during laparoscopic nephrectomy: an effective and reliable method to replace vascular staplers. J Urol 170:1295
Janik JE, Sznol M, Urba WJ, Figlin R, Bukowski RM, Fyfe G, Pierce WC, Belldegrun A, Sharfman WH, Smith JW 2nd et al (1993) Erythropoietin production. A potential marker for interleukin-2/interferon-responsive tumors. Cancer 72:2656
Janzen DL, Zwirewich CV, Breen DJ et al (1998) Diagnostic accuracy of helical CT for detection of blunt bowel and mesenteric injuries. Clin Radiol 53:193
Jarow JP (1996) Risk factors for penile prosthetic infection. J Urol 156:402
Jarrard DJ, Gerber GS, Lyon ES (1993) Management of acute ureteral obstruction in pregnancy utilizing ultrasound-guided placement of ureteral stents. Urology 42:263
Jayanthi VR, Churchill BM, McLorie GA, Khoury AE (1995) Concomitant bladder neck closure and Mitrofanoff diversion for the management of intractable urinary incontinence. J Urol 154:886
Jayson M, Sanders H (1998) Increased incidence of serendipitously discovered renal cell carcinoma. Urology 51:203
Jebara VA, El Rassi I et al (1998) Renal artery pseudoaneurysm after blunt abdominal trauma. J Vasc Surg 27:362
Jeejeebhoy KN (2004) Enteral feeding. Curr Opin Gastroenterol 20:110
Jemal A, Murray T, Ward E et al (2005) Cancer statistics, 20CA. Cancer J Clin 55:10
Jeong HJ (2004) Fournier's gangrene associated with sparganosis in the scrotum. Urology 63:176
Jepsen S, Klaerke A, Nielsen PH, Nielsen ST, Simonsen O (1989) Systemic administration of N-acetylcysteine has no effect on postoperative lung function following elective upper laparotomy in lung healthy patients. Acta Anaesthesiol Scand 33:219
Jepsen S, Nielsen PH, Klaerke A, Nielsen ST, Simonsen O (1989) Peroral N-acetylcysteine as prophylaxis against bronchopulmonary complications of pulmonary surgery. Scand J Thorac Cardiovasc Surg 23:185
Jepson BR, Boullier JA, Moore RG, Parra RO (1999) Traumatic posterior urethral injury and early primary endoscopic realignment: evaluation of long-term follow-up. Urology 53: 1205
Jeromin L, Sosnowski M (1998) Ureteroscopy in the treatment of ureteral stones: over 10 years' experience. Eur Urol 34:344
Jezior JR, Brady JD, Schlossberg SM (2001) Management of penile amputation injuries. World J Surg 25:1602
Ji MX, He NS, Wang P, Chen G (1994) Use of selective embolization of the bilateral cavernous arteries for posttraumatic arterial priapism. J Urol 151:1641
Jimenez MF, Marshall JC (2001) Source control in the management of sepsis. Intensive Care Med 27 [Suppl 1]:S49
Jobe BA, Bierman MH, Mezzacappa FJ (1993) Hyperglycemia as a paraneoplastic endocrinopathy in renal cell carcinoma: a case report and review of the literature. Nebr Med J 78:349
Johansson JE, Andren O, Andersson SO et al (2004) Natural history of early, localized prostate cancer. JAMA 291:2713
Johansson SG, Hourihane JO, Bousquet J, Bruijnzeel-Koomen C, Dreborg S, Haahtela T, Kowalski ML, Mygind N, Ring J, van Cauwenberge P, van Hage-Hamsten M, Wuthrich B (2001) EAACI (the European Academy of Allergology and Clinical Immunology) nomenclature task force: a revised nomenclature for allergy. An EAACI position statement from the EAACI nomenclature task force. Allergy 56:813
Johnson DB, Pearle MS (2004) Complications of ureteroscopy. Urol Clin North Am 31:157
Johnson JE, Conlin M (2001) Calculus formation on a retained Acucise wire. Urology 57:168
Johnston WK 3rd, Patel BN et al (2005) Wireless teleradiology for renal colic and renal trauma. J Endourol 19:32
Jolly BB, Sharma SK, Vaidyanathan S, Mandal AK (1994) Gunshot wounds of the male external genitalia. Urol Int 53:92
Jonathan P, Wyatt RI, Clancy M, Munro PT, Robertson C (2005) Oxford handbook of accident and emergency medicine. Oxford University Press, Oxford
Jones AE et al (2003) Sonographic intraperitoneal fluid in patients with pelvic fracture: two cases of traumatic intraperitoneal bladder rupture. J Emerg Med 25:373
Jones CD, McGahan JP (1999) Computed tomographic evaluation and guided correction of malpositioned nephrostomy catheters. Abdom Imaging 24:422
Jones J, Shah J et al (1999) An unusual renal mass after partial nephrectomy for renal cell carcinoma. J Urol 161:913
Jones RB, Hirschmann JV, Brown GS, Tremann JA (1979) Fournier's syndrome: Necrotising subcutaneous infection of the male genitalia. J Urol 122:279
Joniau S, Benijts J, Van Kampen M, De Waele M, Ooms J, Van Cleynenbreugel B, Van Poppel H (2005) Clinical experience with the N-shaped ileal neobladder: assessment of complications, voiding patterns, and quality of life in our series of 58 patients. Eur Urol 47:666; discussion 672
Jordan GH (1996) Management of membranous urethral distraction injuries via the perineal approach. In: McAninch JW (ed) Traumatic and reconstructive urology. WB Saunders, Philadelphia, p 393
Jordan GH, Gilbert DA (1988) Male genital trauma. Clin Plast Surg 15:431
Jordan GH, Jezior JR et al (2001) Injury to the genitourinary tract and functional reconstruction of the urethra. Curr Opin Urol 11:257
Joseph JV, Turner KJ, Bramwell SP (2002) Dermatomyositis: a rare initial presentation of adenocarcinoma of the prostate. J Urol 168:637
Joshi HB, Obadeyi OO, Rao PN (1999) A comparative analysis of nephrostomy JJ stent and urgent in situ extracorporeal shock wave lithotripsy for obstructing ureteric stones. BJU Int 84:264
Jou WW, Powers RD (1998) Utility of dipstick urinalysis as a guide to management of adults with suspected infection or hematuria. South Med J 91:266
Kaartinen M, Imir T, Klockars M, Sandholm M, Makela O (1978) IgA in blood and thoracic duct lymph: concentration and degree of polymerization. Scand J Immunol 7:229
Kabalin JN, Kessler R (1988) Infectious complications of penile prosthesis surgery. J Urol 139:953
Kadir S, Watson A, Burrow C (1987) Percutaneous transcatheter recanalization in the management of acute renal failure due to sudden occlusion of the renal artery to a solitary kidney. Am J Nephrol 7:445
Kadish HA, Bolte RG (1998) A retrospective review of pediatric patients with epididymitis, testicular torsion, and torsion of testicular appendages. Pediatrics 102:73
Kahi CJ, Rex DK (2003) Bowel obstruction and pseudo-obstruction. Gastroenterol Clin North Am 32:1229

Kakkar VV, Cohen AT, Edmonson RA, Phillips MJ, Cooper DJ, Das SK, Maher KT, Sanderson RM, Ward VP, Kakkar S (1993) Low molecular weight versus standard heparin for prevention of venous thromboembolism after major abdominal surgery. The Thromboprophylaxis Collaborative Group. Lancet 341:259
Kakkar VV, Boeckl O, Boneu B, Bordenave L, Brehm OA, Brukke P, Coccheri S, Cohen AT, Galland F, Haas S et al (1997) Efficacy and safety of a low-molecular-weight heparin and standard unfractionated heparin for prophylaxis of postoperative venous thromboembolism: European multicenter trial. World J Surg 21:2; discussion 8
Kalman D, Varenhorst E (1999) The role of arterial embolization in renal cell carcinoma. Scand J Urol Nephrol 33:162
Kalyanakrishnan K, Scheid DC (2005) Diagnosis and management of acute pyelonephritis in adults. Am Fam Physician 71:933
Kamel IR, Berkowitz JF (1996) Assessment of the cortical rim sign in posttraumatic renal infarction. J Comput Assist Tomogr 20:803
Kane CJ, Nash P, McAninch JW (1996) Ultrasonographic appearance of necrotizing gangrene: aid in early diagnosis. Urology 48:142
Kane NM, Francis IR, Ellis JH (1989) The value of CT in the detection of bladder and posterior urethral injuries. AJR Am J Roentgenol 153:1243
Kansas BT, Eddy MJ, Mydlo JH, Uzzo RG (2004) Incidence and management of penetrating renal trauma in patients with multiorgan injury: extended experience at an inner city trauma center. J Urol 172:1355
Kao LS, Bulger EM et al (2003) Predictors of morbidity after traumatic pancreatic injury. J Trauma 55:898
Kaplan AA (1999) Therapeutic apheresis for renal disorders. Ther Apher 3:25
Kaplan AA (2003) The use of apheresis in immune renal disorders. Ther Apher 7:165
Kaplan BS, Meyers KE, Schulman SL (1998) The pathogenesis and treatment of hemolytic uremic syndrome. J Am Soc Nephrol 9:1126
Kaplan GW (1994) Major renal trauma in children. Urology 43:131
Kaplan SA, McConnell JD, Roehrborn CG et al (2006) Combination therapy with doxazosin and finasteride for benign prostatic hyperplasia in patients with lower urinary tract symptoms and a baseline total prostate volume of 25 ml or greater. J Urol 175:217
Kapoor DA, Klimberg IW, Malek GH et al (1998) Single-dose oral ciprofloxacin versus placebo for prophylaxis during transrectal prostate biopsy. Urology 52:552
Karabulut Z, Bostanoglu S et al (2002) Pancreatic injuries: analysis of 20 cases. Ulus Travma Derg 8:237
Karadeniz T, Topsakal M, Ariman A, Erton H, Basak D (1996) Penile fracture: differential diagnosis, management and outcome. Br J Urol 77:279
Karim MS (1984) Fournier gangrene following urethral necrosis by indwelling catheter. Urology 23:173
Karmazyn B, Steinberg R, Kornreich L et al (2005) Clinical and sonographic criteria of acute scrotum in children: a retrospective study of 172 boys. Pediatr Radiol 35:302
Karpenko LN, Driuk NF et al (2004) Surgical treatment of injured persons with the main blood vessels damage. Klin Khir:32
Kase H, Nagashima H et al (1995) Clinical analysis of 62 patients with blunt renal trauma. Hinyokika Kiyo 41:855
Kastelan Z, Derezic D et al (2004) Renal autotransplantation in management of bilateral ureteral mortar shell injuries: a case report. Mil Med 169:894
Katagiri H, Takahashi M, Inagaki J et al (1998) Clinical results of nonsurgical treatment for spinal metastases. Int J Radiat Oncol Biol Phys 42:1127
Katayama H, Yamaguchi K, Kozuka T, Takashima T, Seez P, Matsuura K (1990) Adverse reactions to ionic and nonionic contrast media. A report from the Japanese committee on the safety of contrast media. Radiology 175:621
Kats E, Venema PL, Kropman RF, Kieft GJ (1998) Diagnosis and treatment of osteitis pubis caused by a prostate-symphysis fistula: a rare complication after transurethral resection of the prostate. Br J Urol 81:927
Katus HA, Remppis A, Neumann FJ, Scheffold T, Diederich KW, Vinar G, Noe A, Matern G, Kuebler W (1991) Diagnostic efficiency of troponin T measurements in acute myocardial infarction. Circulation 83:902
Katz A, Epelman S, Anelli A et al (1995) A prospective randomized evaluation of three schedules of mesna administration in patients receiving an ifosfamide-containing chemotherapy regimen: sustained efficiency and simplified administration. J Cancer Res Clin Oncol 121:128
Katz JP, Greensstein M, Hakki A, Miller A, Katz SM, Simonian S (1988) Transitional epithelial lesions of the ureter in renal transplant rejection. Transplantation 45:710
Katz R, Meretyk S et al (1997) Abdominal compartment syndrome due to delayed identification of a ureteral perforation following abdomino-perineal resection for rectal carcinoma. Int J Urol 4:615
Kau E, Patel R et al (2004) Isolated renal vein thrombosis after blunt trauma. Urology 64:807
Kauffmann GW, Richter GM, Roeren TK (1992) Renal tumor embolization. Radiologe 32:127
Kaufman JD, Lepor H (2005) Reoperation versus observation in men with major bleeding after radical retropubic prostatectomy. Urology 66:561
Kaufman JJ, Lindner A, Raz S (1982) Complications of penile prosthesis surgery for impotence. J Urol 128:1192
Kaufman JM, Kaufman JL, Borges FD (1998) Immediate salvage procedure for infected penile prosthesis. J Urol 159:816
Kavia RB, Datta SN, Dasgupta R et al (2006) Urinary retention in women: its causes and management. BJU Int 97:281
Kavic SM, Atweh N et al (2002) Renal artery to inferior vena cava fistula following gunshot wound to the abdomen. Ann Vasc Surg 16:666
Kavoussi LR (2000) Complications of laparoscopic surgery. In: Bishoff JT, Kavoussi LR (eds) Atlas of laparoscopic retroperitoneal surgery. Saunders, Philadelphia, p 237
Kavoussi LR, Gelstein LD, Andriole GL (1986) Encephalopathy and an elevated serum aluminum level in a patient receiving intravesical alum irrigation for severe urinary hemorrhage. J Urol 136:665
Kavoussi LR, Albala DM, Basler JW et al (1992) Percutaneous management of urolithiasis during pregnancy. J Urol 148:1069
Kavoussi LR, Sosa E, Chandhoke P, Chodak G, Clayman RV, Hadley HR, Loughlin KR, Ruckle HC, Rukstalis D, Schuessler W et al (1993) Complications of laparoscopic pelvic lymph node dissection. J Urol 149:322
Kawai S, Hiroshima K, Tsukamoto Y, Tobe T, Suzuki H, Ito H, Ohwada H, Ito H (2003) Small cell carcinoma of the prostate expressing prostate-specific antigen and showing syndrome of inappropriate secretion of antidiuretic hormone: an autopsy case report. Pathol Int 53:892
Kawashima A, Sandler CM, Corriere JM Jr et al (1997) Ureteropelvic junction injuries secondary to blunt abdominal trauma. Radiology 205:487
Kawashima A, Sandler CM, Goldman SM et al (1997) CT of renal inflammatory disease. Radiographics 17:851
Kawashima A, Sandler CM, Corl FM et al (2001) Imaging of renal trauma: a comprehensive review. Radiographics 21:557

Kawashima A, Sandler CM et al (2002) Imaging evaluation of posttraumatic renal injuries. Abdom Imaging 27:199
Kawashima A, Vrtiska T, LeRoy AJ et al (2004) CT Urography. RadioGraphics 24:S35
Kayikcioglu A (2003) A new technique in scrotal reconstruction: short gracilis flap. Urology 61:1254
Kearon C (2001) Epidemiology of venous thromboembolism. Semin Vasc Med 1:7
Kearon C, Julian JA, Newman TE, Ginsberg JS (1998) Noninvasive diagnosis of deep venous thrombosis. McMaster Diagnostic Imaging Practice Guidelines Initiative. Ann Intern Med 128:663
Kelkar PS, Li JT (2001) Cephalosporin allergy. N Engl J Med 345:804
Kelleher CM, Curci JA, Blinder MA (2005) Hemostasis and transfusion therapy. In: Klingensmith ME, Amos KD, Green DW, Halpin VJ, Hunt SR (eds) The Washington manual of surgery, 4th edn. Lippincott Williams and Wilkins, Philadelphia, p 108
Keller FS, Barton RE, Routh WD, Gross GM (1990) Gross hematuria in two patients with ureteral-ileal conduits and double-J stents. J Vasc Interv Radiol 1:69
Keller MS, Eric Coln C, Garza JJ, Sartorelli KH, Christine Green M, Weber TR (2004) Functional outcome of nonoperatively managed renal injuries in children. J Trauma 57:108; discussion 110
Kelty CJ, Super PA, Stoddard CJ (2000) The driving force in trocar insertion: a comparison between disposable and reusable trocars. Surg Endosc 14:1045
Kemp SF, Lockey RF (2002) Anaphylaxis: a review of causes and mechanisms. J Allergy Clin Immunol 110:341
Kennedy C, Snell ME, Witherow RO (1984) Use of alum to control intractable vesical haemorrhage. Brit J Urol 56:673
Kenney PJ, Panicek DM, Witanowski LS (1987) Computed tomography of ureteral disruption. J Comput Assist Tomogr 11:480
Keoghane SR, Sullivan ME, Miller MA (2002) The aetiology, pathogenesis and management of priapism. BJU Int 90:149
Kerins M, Greene S, O'Connor N (2004) A human bite to the scrotum: a case report and review of the literature. Eur J Emerg Med 11:223
Kerlan RK, Gordon RL, LaBerge JM, Ring EJ (1998) Superselective microcoil embolization in the management of high-flow priapism. J Vasc Interv Radiol 9:85
Kern EO, Newman LN et al (2002) Abdominal catastrophe revisited: the risk and outcome of enteric peritoneal contamination. Perit Dial Int 22:323
Kernohan RM, Anwar KK, Johnston SR (1991) Complete urethral stricture of the membranous urethra: A different perspective. Br J Urol 65:51
Kessaris DN, Bellman GC, Pardalidis NP, Smith AG (1995) Management of hemorrhage after percutaneous renal surgery. J Urol 153:604
Kessler B, Albertsen P (2003) The natural history of prostate cancer. Urol Clin North Am 30:219
Khan AB, Reid AW (1994) Management of renal stab wounds by arteriographic embolisation. Scand J Urol Nephrol 28:109
Khan RM et al (2004) A survey of urinary bladder injuries in Abbottabad. J Ayub Med Coll Abbottabad 16:47
Khriakov AS, Esetov AK et al (2005) Perforating shotgun wound of the abdomen with injuries multiple visceral. Khirurgiia (Mosk) 1:65
Khurrum Baig M, Hua Zhao R, Batista O et al (2002) Percutaneous postoperative intra-abdominal abscess drainage after elective colorectal surgery. Tech Coloproctol 6:159
Kiberd B, Panek R et al (1999) The morbidity of prolonged wound drainage after kidney transplantation. J Urol 161: 1467
Kiddoo DA, Wollin TA, Mador DR (2004) A population based assessment of complications following outpatient hydrocelectomy and spermatocelectomy. J Urol 171:746
Kielb SJ, Voeltz ZL, Wolf JS (2001) Evaluation and management of traumatic posterior urethral disruption with flexible cystourethroscopy. J Trauma 50:36
Kilic A, Aksoy Y, Kilic L (2001) Fournier's gangrene: etiology, treatment, and complications. Ann Plast Surg 47:523
Killeen KP, Libertino JA (1988) Management of bowel and urinary tract complications after urinary diversion. Urol Clin North Am 15:183
Killion LT (1989) Management of intraoperative hemorrhage from open surgery of bladder and prostate. In: McDougal WS (ed) Difficult problems in urologic surgery. Year Book Medical Publishers
Kilpatrick FR, Mason AY (1969) Post-operative recto-urethral fistula. J Urol 41:649
Kim EK, Song TB (1996) A study on fetal urinary tract anomaly: antenatal ultrasonographic diagnosis and postnatal follow-up. J Obstet Gynaecol Res 22:569
Kim H, Xu M, Lin Y et al (1999) Renal dysfunction associated with the perioperative use of diclofenac. Anesth Analg 89:999
Kim HL, Belldegrun AS, Freitas DG, Bui MH, Han KR, Dorey FJ, Figlin RA (2003) Paraneoplastic signs and symptoms of renal cell carcinoma: implications for prognosis. J Urol 170:1742
Kim HS, Fine DM, Atta MG (2006) Catheter-directed thrombectomy and thrombolysis for acute renal vein thrombosis. J Vasc Interv Radiol 17:815
Kim JK, Jeong YY, Kim YH, Kim YC, Kang HK, Choi HS (1999) Postoperative pelvic lymphocele: treatment with simple percutaneous catheter drainage. Radiology 212:390
Kim JY, Lee SJ, Koo BN et al (2006) The effect of epidural sufentanil in ropivacaine on urinary retention in patients undergoing gastrectomy. Br J Anaesth 97:414
Kim SC, Oh CH, Moon YT, Kim KD (1991) Treatment of steinstrasse with repeat extracorporeal shock wave lithotripsy: experience with piezoelectric lithotriptor. J Urol 145:489
Kimber RM, Mellon JK (2004) The role of special cutting equipment and corporeal aspiration in the treatment of penile incarceration with a barbell retaining collar. J Urol 172:975
King J (1975) Impotence after fractures of the pelvis. J Bone Joint Surg 57:1107
King LR, Coughlin PW, Bloch EC, Bowie JD, Ansong K, Hanna MK (1984) The case for immediate pyeloplasty in the neonate with ureteropelvic junction obstruction. J Urol 132:725
King SH, Hallock M, Strote J et al (2005) Tadalafil-associated priapism. Urol 66:432
Kirby RS (2000) The natural history of benign prostatic hyperplasia: what have we learned in the last decade? Urology 56:3
Kirby RS, McConnell JD (2005) Fast facts: benign prostatic hyperplasia. Health Press, Oxford
Kirkland KB, Briggs JP, Trivette SL, Wilkinson WE, Sexton DJ (1999) The impact of surgical-site infections in the 1990 s: attributable mortality, excess length of hospitalization, and extra costs. Infect Control Hosp Epidemiol 20:725
Kirton OC, Jacobs JP et al (1994) Incidental finding of occult hydronephrosis after blunt abdominal trauma. Eur J Emerg Med 1:139
Kitrey ND, Peleg K, Givon A et al (2005) Terror-related urological injuries in Israel between 1997 and 2003. XXth EAU congress in Istanbul, Turkey
Klaric Custovic R, Krolo I et al (2004) Retained surgical textilomas occur more often during war. Croat Med J 45:422
Klastersky J (2003) Side effects of ifosfamide. Oncology 65 [Suppl 2]:7

Klastersky J, Paesmans M, Rubenstein EB et al (2000) The Multinational Association for Supportive Care in Cancer risk index: a multinational scoring system for identifying low-risk febrile neutropenic cancer patients. J Clin Oncol 18:3038

Klein AJ, Kozar RA et al (1999) Traumatic hematuria in patients with polycystic kidney disease. Am Surg 65:464

Klein EA (1984) Urologic problems of pregnancy. Obst Gynec Surv 39:605

Klein RM, Niehues R, Hollenbeck M, Horstkotte D, Furst G, Strauer BE (1992) The local lysis therapy of spontaneous renal artery dissection with arterial thrombosis. Dtsch Med Wochenschr 117:1185

Klimo P, Thompson CJ, Kestle JRW et al (2005) A meta-analysis of surgery versus conventional radiotherapy for the treatment of metastatic spinal epidural disease. Neuro-oncol 7:64

Klin B, Lotan G, Efrati Y, Zlotkevich L, Strauss S (2002) Acute idiopathic scrotal edema in children-revisited. J Pediatr Surg 37:1200

Klochkov ND, Sidorin VS (1998) Pathology of traumatic disease in wounded people. Arkh Patol 60:43

Klug R, Kurz F, Dunzinger M, Aufschnaiter M (2001) Small bowel perforation after extracorporeal shockwave lithotripsy of an ureter stone. Dig Surg 18:241

Kluger Y (2003) Bomb explosions in acts of terrorism – detonation, wound ballistics, triage and medical concerns. Isr Med Assoc J 5:235

Kluger Y, Soffer D, Sorkine P et al (1997) Blast injury: detonation and injury pattern. Harefuah 132:591

Kluger Y, Makarin V et al (1999) Absorbable mesh wrapping of injured kidney: a renal salvage technique. Harefuah 136:647

Kluger Y, Mayo A, Soffer D et al (2004) Functions and principles in the management of bombing mass casualty incidents: lessons learned at the Tel-Aviv Souraski Medical Center. Eur J Emerg Med 11:329

Kluger Y, Peleg K, Daniel-Aharonson L et al (2004) The special injury pattern in terrorist bombings. J Am Coll Surg 199:875

Knap MM, Lundbeck F, Overgaard J (2004) Early and late treatment-related morbidity following radical cystectomy. Scand J Urol Nephrol 38:153

Knaus WA, Draper EA, Wagner DP, Zimmerman JE (1985) APACHE II. A severity of disease classification system. Crit Care Med 13:818

Knight CD, Griffen FD (1983) Abdominal wound closure with a continuous monofilament polypropylene suture. Experience with 1,000 consecutive cases. Arch Surg 118:1305

Knight CG, Omert L (2004) Chylous ascites after nephrectomy for trauma. Am Surg 70:1083

Knockaert DC, Mortelmans LA, De Roo, MC Bobbaers HJ (1994) Clinical value of gallium-67 scintigraphy in evaluation of fever of unknown origin. Clin Infect Dis 18:601

Knopf HJ, Graff HJ, Schulze H (2003) Perioperative antibiotic prophylaxis in ureteroscopic stone removal. Eur Urol 44:115

Knudson MM, Maull KI (1999) Nonoperative management of solid organ injuries. Past, present, and future. Surg Clin North Am 79:1357

Knudson MM, McAninch JW et al (1992) Hematuria as a predictor of abdominal injury after blunt trauma. Am J Surg 164:482; discussion 485

Knudson MM, Harrison PB et al (2000) Outcome after major renovascular injuries: a Western trauma association multicenter report. J Trauma 49:1116

Kobayashi T, Nishizawa K, Watanabe J et al (2003) Clinical characteristics of ureteral calculi detected by nonenhanced computerized tomography after unclear results of plain radiography and ultrasonography. J Urol 170:799

Koch M, Steidle C, Brosman S et al (2003) An open-label study of abarelix in men with symptomatic prostate cancer at risk of treatment with LHRH agonists. Urology 62:877

Koch MO, Jr JS (1997) Low molecular weight heparin and radical prostatectomy: a prospective analysis of safety and side effects. Prostate Cancer Prostatic Dis 1:101

Koch MO, Smith JA Jr (1996) Blood loss during radical retropubic prostatectomy: is preoperative autologous blood donation indicated? J Urol 156:1077; discussion 1079

Kochakarn W, Tirapanich W, Kositchaiwat S (2000) Ileal interposition for the treatment of a long gap ureteral loss. J Med Assoc Thai 83:37

Kodos AB (1967) The vascular supply of the penis. Arkh Anat Embriol 43:525

Kokubo T, Itai Y, Ohtomo K, Yoshikawa K, Iio M, Atomi Y (1987) Retained surgical sponges: CT, US appearance. Radiology 165:415

Kollef MH (2004) Appropriate empiric antimicrobial therapy of nosocomial pneumonia: the role of the carbapenems. Respir Care 49:1530

Kollmeier MA, Stock RG, Cesaretti J et al (2005) Urinary morbidity and incontinence following transurethral resection of the prostate after brachytherapy. J Urol 173:808

Kondas J, Szentgyorgyi E (1992) Transurethral resection of 1250 bladder tumours. Int Urol Nephrol 24:35

Koopman MM, Prandoni P, Piovella F, Ockelford PA, Brandjes DP, van der Meer J, Gallus AS, Simonneau G, Chesterman CH, Prins MH (1996) Treatment of venous thrombosis with intravenous unfractionated heparin administered in the hospital as compared with subcutaneous low-molecular-weight heparin administered at home. The Tasman Study Group. N Engl J Med 334:682

Koperna T, Schultz F (2000) Relaparotmoy in peritonitis: prognosis and treatment of patients with persisting intraabdominal infection. World J Surg 24:32

Koraitim MM (1995) The lessons of 145 posttraumatic posterior urethral strictures treated in 17 years. J Urol 153:63

Koraitim MM (1996) Pelvic fracture urethral injuries: evaluation of various methods of management. J Urol 156:1288

Koraitim MM (1997) Post-traumatic posterior urethral strictures in children: A 20 year experience. J Urol 157:641

Koraitim MM (1999) Pelvic fracture urethral injuries: the unresolved controversy. J Urol 161:1433

Koraitim MM, Marzouk ME, Atta MA, Orabi SS (1996) Risk factors and mechanism of urethral injury in pelvic fractures. Br J Urol 77:876

Korhonen K, Hirn M, Niinikoski J (1998) Hyperbaric oxygen in the treatment of Fournier's gangrene. Eur J Surg 164:251

Korkut M, Icoz G, Dayangac M et al (2003) Outcome analysis in patients with Fournier's gangrene: report of 45 cases. Dis Colon Rectum 46:649

Kortmann BB, Sonke GS, D'Ancona F C, Floratos DL, Debruyne FM, De La Rosette JJ (1999) The tolerability of urodynamic studies and flexible cysto-urethroscopy used in the assessment of men with lower urinary tract symptoms. BJU Int 84:449

Kos X, Fanchamps JM et al (1999) Radiologic damage control: evaluation of a combined CT and angiography suite with a pivoting table. Cardiovasc Intervent Radiol 22:124

Koss LG (1967) A light and electron microscopic study of the effects of a single dose of cyclophosphamide on various organs in the rat. I. The urinary bladder. Lab Invest 16:44

Kothary N, Soulen MC, Clark TW, Wein AJ, Shlansky-Goldberg RD, Crino PB, Stavropoulos SW (2005) Renal angiomyolipoma: long-term results after arterial embolization. J Vasc Interv Radiol 16:45

Kotkin L, Koch MO (1995) Morbidity associated with nonoperative management of extraperitoneal bladder injuries. J Trauma 38:895

Kotkin L, Koch MO (1996) Impotence and incontinence after immediate realignment of posterior urethral trauma: results of injury or management? J Urol 155:1600

Kovacevic Z, Skataric V et al (1999) Complications of percutaneous transluminal renal angioplasty–case report. Vojnosanit Pregl 56:431
Koya MP, Manoharan M, Kim SS, Soloway MS (2005) Venous thromboembolism in radical prostatectomy: is heparinoid prophylaxis warranted? BJU Int 96:1019
Kracun MD, Wooten CL (1998) Crush injuries: a case of entrapment. Crit Care Nurs Q 21:81
Kraklau DM, Wolf JS Jr (1999) Review of antibiotic prophylaxis recommendations for office-based urologic procedures. Tech Urol 5:123
Kramer SC, Gorich J et al (1998) The percutaneous transarterial embolization therapy of traumatic kidney hemorrhages. ROFO 169:297
Kraske P (1885) Zur Exstirpation hochsitzender Mastdarmkrebse. Verhand Deutsch Gesell Chir 14:464
Kratzik C, Hainz A, Kuber W, Donner G, Lunglmayr G, Frick J, Schmoller HJ (1989) Has ultrasound influenced the therapy concept of blunt scrotal trauma? J Urol 142:1243
Kravchick S, Bunkin I, Stepnov E et al (2005) Emergency extracorporeal shockwave lithotripsy for acute renal colic caused by upper urinary tract stone. J Endourol 19:1
Kress O, Heidenreich A, Klose KJ, Wagner HJ, Alfke H (2002) Superselective embolization with coils in high-flow priapism.Cardiovasc Intervent Radiol 25:326
Krid M, Bahloul A et al (1997) Kidney injuries in children. Apropos of 65 cases. Ann Urol 31:259
Krieger JN (2002) Urinary tract infections: what's new? J Urol 168:2351
Krieger JN, Kaiser DL Wenzel RP (1983) Nosocomial urinary tract infections cause wound infections postoperatively in surgical patients. Surg Gynecol Obstet 156:313
Krieger JN, Algood CB, Mason JT et al (1984) Urological trauma in the Pacific Northwest: etiology, distribution, management and outcome. J Urol 132:70
Kristjansson A, Pedersen J (1993) Management of blunt renal trauma. Br J Urol 72:692
Kroovand RL (1992) Stones in pregnancy and children. J Urol 148:1076
Ku JH, Jeon YS et al (2001) Is there a role for magnetic resonance imaging in renal trauma? Int J Urol 8:261
Ku JH, Choi WJ, Lee KY et al (2005) Complications of the upper urinary tract in patients with spinal cord injury: a long-term follow-up study. Urol Res 33:435
Ku JH, Lee SW, Jeon HG et al (2004) Percutaneous nephrostomy versus indwelling ureteral stents in the management of extrinsic ureteral obstruction in advanced malignancies: are there differences? Urology 64:895
Kuefer R, Bartsch G, Herkommer K, Kramer SC, Kleinschmidt K, Volkmer BG (2005) Changing diagnostic and therapeutic concepts in high-flow priapism. Int J Impot Res 17:109
Kukreja RA, Desai MR, Sabnis RB, Patel SH (2002) Fluid absorption during percutaneous nephrolithotomy: does it matter? J Endourol 16:221
Kukreja R, Desai M, Patel S, Bapat S, Desai M (2004) Factors affecting blood loss during percutaneous nephrolithotomy: prospective study. J Endourol 18:715
Kulacoglu IH (2000) Regarding: small bowel obstruction and incisional hernia after laparoscopic surgery: should 5-mm trocar sites be sutured? J Laparoendosc Adv Surg Tech A 10:227
Kulmala R, Lehtonen T, Nieminen P et al (1995) Aetiology of priapism in 207 patients. Eur Urol 28:241
Kulmala RV, Lehtonen TA, Tammela TL (1996) Preservation of potency after treatment for priapism. Scan J Urol Nephrol 30:313
Kumar M, Aron M et al (1999) Stenturia: An unusual manifestation of spontaneous ureteral stent fragmentation. Urol Int 62:114
Kumar SM (2005) Photoselective vaporization of the prostate: a volume reduction analysis in patients with lower urinary tract symptoms secondary to benign prostatic hyperplasia and carcinoma of the prostate. J Urol 173:511
Kunin CM (1994) Guidelines for urinary tract infections. Rationale for a separate strata for patients with „low-count“ bacteriuria. Infection 22 Suppl 1:S38
Kunin CM (2001) Nosocomial urinary tract infections and the indwelling catheter: what is new and what is true? Chest 120:10
Kunin CM (2003) Definition of acute pyelonephritis vs the urosepsis syndrome. Arch Intern Med 163:2393
Kuno K, Menzin A, Kauder HH, Sison C, Gal D (1998) Prophylactic ureteral catheterization in gynecologic surgery. Urology 52:1004
Kuo RL, Eachempati SR et al (2002) Factors affecting management and outcome in blunt renal injury. World J Surg 26:416
Kuo YT, Wang CK et al (1999) Imaging features of simultaneous occurrence of renal and pancreatic foreign body granuloma due to chronically retained gauze: a case report. Kaohsiung J Med Sci 15:104
Kurasawa G, Kotani K, Kurasawa M et al (2005) Causes of chronic retention of urine in the primary care setting. Intern Med 44:761
Kurtz V, Muller-Sorg M, Federmann G (1999) Perforation of the small intestine after nephro-uretero-lithotripsy by ESWL–a rare complication. Chirurg 70:306
Kurz A, Sessler DI, Lenhardt R (1996) Perioperative normothermia to reduce the incidence of surgical-wound infection and shorten hospitalization. Study of Wound Infection and Temperature Group. N Engl J Med 334:1209
Kurz K, Katus HA, Giannitsis E (2005) Acute chest pain.. Internist (Berl) 46:957
Kuuva N, Nilsson CG (2002) A nationwide analysis of complications associated with the tension-free vaginal tape (TVT) procedure. Acta Obstet Gynecol Scand 81:72
Kuvezdic H, Tucak A, Grahovac B (1996) War injuries of the kidney. Injury 27:557
Kuwertz-Broeking E, Brinkmann OA, Von Lengerke HJ, Sciuk J, Fruend S, Bulla M et al (2004) Unilateral multicystic dysplastic kidney: experience in children. BJU Int 93:388
Kvarstein B (1996) Bladder cancer complicated with priapism. A case report. Scand J Urol Nephrol Suppl 179:155
Kyriakides GK, Simmons RL, Najarian JS (1979) Mycotic aneurysms in transplant patients. Arch Surg 111:472
Kyriakidis A, Karydis G, Yannopoulos P (1979) An unusual trauma of the glans penis. Br J Urol 51:161
Lachs MS, Nachamkin I, Edelstein PH et al (1992) Spectrum bias in the evaluation of diagnostic tests: lessons from the rapid dipstick test for urinary tract infection. Ann Intern Med 117:135
Lack EE, Cassady JR, Sallan SE (1985) Renal cell carcinoma in childhood and adolescence: a clinical and pathological study of 17 cases. J Urol 133:822
Lacombe P, Mulot R, Labedan F, Jondeau G, Barre O, Chagnon S, Judet O, Tcherdakoff P (1992) Percutaneous recanalization of a renal artery in aortic dissection. Radiology 185:829
Laguna MP, Brenninkmeier M, Belon JA, Marrero R, Wijkstra H, de la Rosette J et al (2005) Long-term functional and urodynamic results of 50 patients receiving a modified sigmoid neobladder created with a short distal segment. J Urol 174:963
Laing FC, Benson CB, DiSalvo DN et al (1994) Distal ureteral calculi: detection with vaginal US. Radiology 192:545
Lakhani A, Raptis A, Frame D et al (1999) Intravesicular instillation of E-aminocaproic acid for patients with adenovirus-induced hemorrhagic cystitis. Bone Marrow Transplant 24:1259

Lallas CD, Delvecchio FC, Evans BR, Silverstein AD, Preminger GM, Auge BK (2004) Management of nephropleural fistula after supracostal percutaneous nephrolithotomy. Urology 64:241

Lamb GW, Bromwich EJ, Vasey P, Aitchison M (2004) Management of renal masses in patients medically unsuitable for nephrectomy–natural history, complications, and outcome. Urology 64:909

Lambert AW, Nathan M et al (2001) A case of fatal tumor embolus following trauma in a patient with undiagnosed Wilms' tumor. Pediatr Emerg Care 17:356

Lamm DL (1992) Complications of bacillus Calmette-Guerin immunotherapy. Urol Clin North Am 19:565

Lamm DL, van der Meijden PM, Morales A et al (1992) Incidence and treatment of complications of bacillus Calmette-Guerin intravesical therapy in superficial bladder cancer. J Urol 147:596

Lamme B, Boermeester MA, Belt JWO, Gouma DJ Obertop H (2004) Mortality and morbidity of planned relaparotomy versus relaparotomy on demand for secondary peritonitis. Br J Surg 91:1046

Lammers RL, Gibson S, Kovacs D et al (2001) Comparison of test characteristics of urine dipstick and urinalysis at various test cutoff points. Ann Emerg Med 38:505

Lampel A, Fisch M, Stein R, Schultz-Lampel D, Hohenfellner M, Eggersmann C et al (1996) Continent diversion with the Mainz pouch. World J Urol 14:85

Land W (1998) Postischemic reperfusion injury and kidney transplantation: prologue. Transplant Proc 30:4210

Landing BH, Wells TR, Claireaux AE (1980) Morphometric analysis of liver lesions in cystic diseases of childhood. Hum Pathol 11:549

Langenhuijsen JF, Reisman Y, Reekers JA, de Reijke TM (2001) Highly selective embolization of bilateral cavernous arteries for post-traumatic penile arterial priapism. Int J Impot Res 13:354

Langer JE (2001) Computed tomography and ultrasonography of acute renal abnormalities. Semin Roentgenol 36:99

Lanoix R, Leak LV et al (2000) A preliminary evaluation of emergency ultrasound in the setting of an emergency medicine training program. Am J Emerg Med 18:41

Lantz PE, Smith JD (1994) Fatal carbon dioxide embolism complicating attempted laparoscopic cholecystectomy–case report and literature review. J Forensic Sci 39:1468

Laor E, Palmer LS, Tolia BM, Reid RE, Winter HI (1995) Outcome prediction in patients with Fournier's gangrene. J Urol 154:89

Lapides J, Diokno AC, Silber SJ et al (1972) Clean, intermittent self-catheterization in the treatment of urinary tract disease. J Urol 107:458

Larkin GL, Peacock WF 4th, Pearl SM et al (1999) Efficacy of ketorolac tromethamine versus meperidine in the ED treatment of acute renal colic. Am J Emerg Med 17:6

Larobina M, Nottle P (2005) Complete evidence regarding major vascular injuries during laparoscopic access. Surg Laparosc Endosc Percutan Tech 15:119

Laroche D, Aimone-Gastin I, Dubois F, Huet H, Gerard P, Vergnaud MC, Mouton-Faivre C, Gueant JL, Laxenaire MC, Bricard H (1998) Mechanisms of severe, immediate reactions to iodinated contrast material. Radiology 209:183

Laroche D, Dewachter P, Mouton-Faivre C, Clément O (2004) Immediate reactions to iodinated contrast media :the CIRTACI study (abstract no. 56). Allergologie 27:165

Larsen R (1999) Textbook of anaesthesia, 6th edn. Urban and Schwarzenberg, Munich

Larsen R, Lahme T, Wilhelm W et al. (2002) Manual of Anaesthesia, University Hospital of the Saarland, Homburg

Laski ME, Vugrin D (1987) Paraneoplastic syndromes in hypernephroma. Semin Nephrol 7:123

Laucks SS 2nd (1994) Fournier's gangrene. Surg Clin North Am 74:1339

Laupacis A, Fergusson D (1997) Drugs to minimize perioperative blood loss in cardiac surgery: meta-analysis using perioperative blood transfusion as the outcome. The International Study of Peri-operative Transfusion (ISPOT) Investigators. Anesth Analg 85:1258

Lauwers PR, Van Hee RH (2000) Intraperitoneal gossypibomas: the need to count sponges. World J Surg 24:521

Lawrentschuk N, Bolton DM (2005) Occult renal segmental arterial injury after trauma. Urology 65:386

Lawson JS, Rotem T, Wilson SF (1995) Catastrophic injuries to the eyes and testicles in footballers. Med J Aust 163:242

Lawton CA, Won M, Pilepich MV et al (1991) Long-term treatment sequelae following external beam irradiation for adenocarcinoma of the prostate: analysis of RTOG studies 7506 and 77. Int J Radiat Oncol Biol Phys 21:935

Laxenaire MC (1999) Again and always allergy. Ann Fr Anesth Reanim 18:831

Laxenaire MC, Charpentier C, Feldman L (1994) Anaphylactoid reactions to colloid plasma substitutes:incidence, risk factors, mechanisms. A French multicenter prospective study (in French). Ann Fr Anesth Reanim 13:301

Lazarides MK, Tsoupanos SS et al (1998) Incidence and patterns of iatrogenic arterial injuries. A decade's experience. J Cardiovasc Surg (Torino) 39:281

Le DT, Borgs P, Toneff TW, Witte MH (1998) Rapaport SI hemostatic factors in rabbit limb lymph: relationship to mechanisms regulating extravascular coagulation. Am J Physiol 274:H769

Le Neel JC, De Cussac JB, Dupas B, Letessier E, Borde L, Eloufir M, Armstrong O (1994) Textiloma. Apropos of 25 cases and review of the literature. Chirurgie 120:272; discussion 276

Leandri P, Rossignol G, Gautier JR et al (1992) Radical retropubic prostatectomy: morbidity and quality of life. Experience with 620 consecutive cases. J Urol 147:883

Leaphart WL et al (1997) Placenta previa percreta with bladder invasion. Obstet Gynecol 89:834

Leavitt JA (2000) Myasthenia gravis with a paraneoplastic marker. J Neuroophthalmol 20:102

Lebech A, HH Strange-Vognsen (1990) Hypertension following blunt kidney injury. Ugeskr Laeger 152:994

Lecuru F, Leonard F, Philippe Jais J, Rizk E, Robin F, Taurelle R (2001) Laparoscopy in patients with prior surgery: results of the blind approach. JSLS 5:13

Lee A, Cooper MC, Craig JC et al (2004) Effects of nonsteroidal anti-inflammatory drugs on post-operative renal function in adults with normal renal function. Cochrane Database Syst Rev 2:CD002765

Lee JM, Greenes DS (2000) Biphasic anaphylactic reactions in pediatrics. Pediatrics 106:762

Lee JT, White RA (2002) Endovascular management of blunt traumatic renal artery dissection. J Endovasc Ther 9:354

Lee JY, Cass AS, Streitz JM (1992) Traumatic dislocation of testes and bladder rupture. Urology 40:506

Lee MM, Donahoe PK (1997) The infant with ambiguous genitalia. Curr Ther Endocrinol Metab 6:216

Lee S, Thavaseelan J et al (2004) Renal trauma in Australian rules football: an institutional experience. Aust N Z J Surg 74:766

Lee TH, Rouan GW, Weisberg MC, Brand DA, Cook EF, Acampora D, Goldman L (1987) Sensitivity of routine clinical criteria for diagnosing myocardial infarction within 24 hours of hospitalization. Ann Intern Med 106:181

Lee TH, Marcantonio ER, Mangione CM et al (1999) Derivation and prospective validation of a simple index for prediction of cardiac risk of major noncardiac surgery. Circulation 100:1043

Leff EI, Groff W, Rubin RJ, Eisenstat TE, Salvati EP (1982) Use of ureteral catheters in colonic and rectal surgery. Dis Colon Rectum 25:457
Legg EA, Herbert FB et al (1998) Super-selective arterial embolization for blunt trauma in the horseshoe kidney. Urology 51:320
Lehtonen T, Tenhunen A (1973) Treatment of idiopathic priapism by Grayhack's caverno-saphenous shunt. Scand J Urol Nephrol 7:233
Leibovici D, Gofrit ON, Stein M et al (1996) Blast injuries: bus versus open-air bombings – a comparative study of injuries in survivors of open-air versus confined-space explosions. J Trauma 41:1030
Leibovitch I (2002) Postoperative chylous ascites–the urologist's view. Drugs Today (Barc) 38:687
Leibovitch I, Mor Y (2004) The vicious cycling: bicycling related urogenital disorders. Eur Urol Mar 47:277
Leibovitch I, Mor Y, Golomb J, Ramon J (2002)Chylous ascites after radical nephrectomy and inferior vena cava thrombectomy. Successful conservative management with somatostatin analogue. Eur Urol 41:220
Leissner J, Stein R, Hohenfellner R, Kohl U, Riedmiller H, Schroder A et al (1999) Radical cystoprostatectomy combined with Mainz pouch bladder substitution to the urethra: long-term results. BJU Int 83:964
Lemack GE, Poppas DP, Vaughan ED Jr (1995) Urologic causes of gynecomastia: approach to diagnosis and management. Urology 45:313
Lemaitre L, Gaillandre L et al (1996) Spiral scanners: the key to imaging of kidney injuries. Chirurgie 121:355
Lemaitre L, Claudon M, Dubrulle F et al (1997) Imaging of angiomyolipomas. Semin Ultrasound CT MR 18:100
LeMaitre L, Mestdagh P, Marecaux-Delomez J, Valtille P, Dubrulle F, Biserte J (2000) Percutaneous nephrostomy: placement under laser guidance and real-time CT fluoroscopy. Eur Radiol 10:892
Leman P (2002) Validity of urinalysis and microscopy for detecting urinary tract infection in the emergency department. Eur J Emerg Med 9:141
Lensing AW, Buller HR, Prandoni P, Batchelor D, Molenaar AH, Cogo A, Vigo M, Huisman PM, ten Cate JW (1992) Contrast venography, the gold standard for the diagnosis of deep-vein thrombosis: improvement in observer agreement. Thromb Haemost 67:8
Lent V (1995) What treatment in kidney trauma? A critical evaluation treatment reports up to now based on a new classification. Chirurg 66:708
Lent V (1996) What classification is appropriate in renal trauma? Eur Urol 30:327
Leonard MP, Emtaje J, Perez R, Morales A (1990) Endoscopic management of urethral stricture: Cut-to-the-light procedure. Urology 35:117
Leone M, Albanese J, Antonini F, Michel-Nguyen A, Blanc-Bimar MC, Martin C (2003) Long-term epidemiological survey of Candida species: comparison of isolates found in an intensive care unit and in conventional wards. J Hosp Infect 55:169
Leone M, Albanese J, Garnier F, Sapin C, Barrau K, Bimar MC, Martin C (2003) Risk factors of nosocomial catheter-associated urinary tract infection in a polyvalent intensive care unit. Intensive Care Med 29:929
Leone M, Garnier F, Avidan M, Martin C (2004) Catheter-associated urinary tract infections in intensive care units. Microbes Infect 6:1026
Leong C, McKenzie MR, Coupland DB, Gascoyne RD (1994) Disseminated intravascular coagulation in a patient with metastatic prostate cancer: fatal outcome following strontium-89 therapy. J Nucl Med 35:1662
Lepage E, Gisselbrecht C, Haioun C (1993) Prognostic significance of received relative dose intensity in non-Hodgkin's lymphoma patients: application to LNH-87 protocol. Ann Oncol 4:651
Lepor H, Kaci L (2003) Contemporary evaluation of operative parameters and complications related to open radical retropubic prostatectomy. Urology 62:702
Lepor H, Nieder AM, Ferrandino MN (2001) Intraoperative and postoperative complications of radical retropubic prostatectomy in a consecutive series of 1,000 cases. J Urol 166:1729
Leppaniemi AK, Kivisaari AO et al (1991) Role of magnetic resonance imaging in blunt renal parenchymal trauma. Br J Urol 68:355
Leppaniemi A, Lamminen A et al (1995) Comparison of high-field magnetic resonance imaging with computed tomography in the evaluation of blunt renal trauma. J Trauma 38:420
Leppaniemi A, Lamminen A et al (1997) MRI and CT in blunt renal trauma: an update. Semin Ultrasound CT MR 18:129
Lessman RK, Jhonson SF, Coburn JW, Kaufman JJ (1978) Renal artery embolism, clinical features and long-term follow-up of 17 cases. Ann Intern Med 89:477
Leveckis J, Boucher NR, Parys BT et al (1995) Bladder and erectile dysfunction before and after rectal surgery for cancer. Br J Urol 76:752
Level 1, Inc. 160 Weymouth Street, Rockland, MA, USA. http://www.smiths-medical.com. Cited 6 November 2006
Levine CD, Gonzales RN, Wachsberg RH, Ghanekar D (1997) CT findings of bowel and mesenteric injury. J Comput Assist Tomogr 21:974
Levine J, Wessells H (2001) Comparison of open and endoscopic treatment of posttraumatic posterior urethral strictures. World J Surg 25:1597
Levine JA, Neitlich J, Verga M et al (1997) Ureteral calculi in patients with flank pain: correlation of plain radiography with unenhanced helical CT. Radiology 204:27
Levine LA, Jarrard DF (1993) Treatment of cyclophosphamide-induced hemorrhagic cystitis with intravesical carboprost tromethamine. J Urol 149:719
Levine M, Gent M, Hirsh J, Leclerc J, Anderson D, Weitz J, Ginsberg J, Turpie AG, Demers C, Kovacs M (1996) A comparison of low-molecular-weight heparin administered primarily at home with unfractionated heparin administered in the hospital for proximal deep-vein thrombosis. N Engl J Med 334:677
Levine MN, Gent M, Hirsh J, Arnold A, Goodyear MD, Hryniuk W, De Pauw S (1988) The thrombogenic effect of anticancer drug therapy in women with stage II breast cancer. N Engl J Med 318:404
Leviov M, Dale J, Stein M et al (1993) The management of metastatic spinal cord compression: a radiotherapeutic success ceiling. Int J Radiat Oncol Biol Phys 27:231
Levy DA, Kay R, Elder JS (1994) Neonatal testis tumors: a review of the Prepubertal Testis Tumor Registry. J Urol 151:715
Levy JB, Baskin LS et al (1993) Nonoperative management of blunt pediatric major renal trauma. Urology 42:418
Levy JM, Duszak RL Jr, Akins EW, Bakal CW, Denny DF Jr, Martin LG, Van Moore A Jr, Pentecost MJ, Roberts AC, Vogelzang RL, Kent KC, Perler BA, Resnick MI, Richie J (2000) Percutaneous transluminal renal angioplasty. American College of Radiology. ACR Appropriateness Criteria. Radiology 215 [Suppl]:1015
Levy MJ, Seelig CB, Robinson NJ, Ranney JE (1997) Comparison of omeprazole and ranitidine for stress ulcer prophylaxis. Dig Dis Sci 42:1255
Lewis S, Patel U (2004) Major complications after percutaneous nephrostomy-lessons from a department audit. Clin Radiol 59:171

Li JS, Sexton DJ, Mick N, Nettles R, Fowler VG Jr, Ryan T, Bashore T, Corey GR (2000) Proposed modifications to the Duke criteria for the diagnosis of infective endocarditis. Clin Infect Dis 30:633

Li TC, Saravelos H, Richmond M, Cooke ID (1997) Complications of laparoscopic pelvic surgery: recognition, management and prevention. Hum Reprod Update 3:505

Liang MK, Lo HG, Marks JL (2006) Stump appendicitis: a comprehensive review of literature. Am Surg 72:162

Liapis A, Bakas P, Giannopoulos V et al (2001) Ureteral injuries during gynecological surgery. Int Urogynecol J Pelvic Floor Dysfunct 12:391

Liauw JJY, Cheah WK (2005) Laparoscopic management of acute small bowel obstruction. Asian J Surg 28:185

Libertino JA (ed) (1998) Reconstructive urology, 3rd edn.Mosby, New York

Libertino JA, Zinman L, Watkins E Jr (1987) Long-term results of resection of renal cell cancer with extension in to the inferior vena cava. J Urol 137:21

Lieberman P (2002) Anaphylactic reactions during surgical and medical procedures. J Allergy Clin Immunol 110:S64

Lieberman SF, Barry JM (1982) Retreat from transpubic urethroplasty for obliterated membranous urethral strictures. J Urol 128:379

Lifshitz DA, Lingeman JE (2002) Ureteroscopy as a first-line intervention for ureteral calculi in pregnancy. J Endourol 16:19

Light RW, George RB (1976) Incidence and significance of pleural effusion after abdominal surgery. Chest 69:621

Liles WC (1997) Apoptosis - role in infection and inflammation. Curr Opin Infect Dis 10:165

Lim JH, Kim B et al (1998) Anatomical communications of the perirenal space. Br J Radiol 71:450

Lim KB, Wong MY, Foo KT (2004) Transurethral resection of prostate (TURP) through the decades–a comparison of results over the last thirty years in a single institution in Asia. Ann Acad Med Singapore 33:775

Lim PHC, Chng HC (1989) Initial management of acute urethral injuries. Br J Urol 64:165

Lin JH (1996) Bisphosphonates: a review of their pharmacokinetic properties. Bone 18:75

Lind J, Mackay A, Withers SJ (2002) Henoch-Schönlein purpura and priapism. J Paediatr Child Health 38:526

Lindenauer PK, Pekow P, Wang K et al (2005) Perioperative beta-blocker therapy and mortality after major noncardiac surgery. N Engl J Med 4:349

Lindert KA, Kabalin JN, Terris MK (2000) Bacteremia and bacteriuria after transrectal ultrasound guided prostate biopsy. J Urol 164:76

Lindop GB, Fleming S (1984) Renin in renal cell carcinoma an immunocytochemical study using an antibody to pure human renin. J Clin Pathol 37:27

Linet OI, Neff LL (1994) Intracavernous prostaglandin E1 in erectile dysfunction. Clin Investig 72:139

Linet OI, Ogrinc FG (1996) Efficacy and safety of intracavernosal alprostadil in men with erectile dysfunction. The Alprostadil Study Group. N Engl J Med 334:873

Liroff SA, Pontes JE, Pierce JM Jr (1977) Gunshot wounds of the ureter:5 years of experience. J Urol 118:551

Little B, Ho KJ, Gawley S et al (2003) Use of nephrostomy tubes in ureteric obstruction from incurable malignancy. Int J Clin Pract 57:180

Little JR, Murray PR, Traynor PS, Spitznagel E (1999) A randomized trial of povidone-iodine compared with iodine tincture for venipuncture site disinfection: effects on rates of blood culture contamination. Am J Med 107:119

Liu W, Esler SJ, Kenny BJ et al (2000) Low-dose nonenhanced helical CT of renal colic: assessment of ureteric stone detection and measurement of effective dose equivalent. Radiology 215:51

Lo CY, Chang IK, Tso WK, Mak KO (1996) Percutaneous transluminal angioplasty for transplant renal artery stenosis. Transplant Proc 28:1468

Loauad I, Buchler M, Noel C, Sadek T, Maazouz H, Westeel PF, Lebranchu Y (2005) Renal artery aneurysm secondary to Candida albicans in four kidney allograft recipients. Transplant Proc 37:2834

Logothetis CJ, Assikis V, Sarriera JE (2003) Urologic complications. In: Kufe DW, Pollock RE, Weichselbaum RR, Bast RC, Gansler TS, Holland JF, Frei E (eds) Cancer medicine. BC Decker, Hamilton

Lojanapiwat B, Sripralakit S et al (1999) Ureteric obstruction by shotgun pellet pellet colic. J Med Assoc Thai 82:1048

Londergan TA, Gundersen LH, Every MJv (1997) Early fluoroscopic realignment for traumatic urethral injuries. Urology 49:101

Lone GN, Bhat AH, Tak MY, Garcoo SA (2005) Transdiaphragmatic migration of forgotten gauze sponge: an unreported entity of lung abscess. Eur J Cardiothorac Surg 28:355

Lonergan GJ, Martinez-Leon MI, Agrons GA, Montemarano H, Suarez ES (1998) Nephrogenic rests, nephroblastomatosis, and associated lesions of the kidney. Radiographics 18:947

Long JA, Descotes JL et al (2004) Endovascular aortic balloon catheter occlusion for severe renal trauma. Prog Urol 14:394; discussion 397

Long JP, Bahn D, Lee F, Shinohara K, Chinn DO, Macaluso JN Jr (2001) Five-year retrospective, multi-institutional pooled analysis of cancer-related outcomes after cryosurgical ablation of the prostate. Urology 57:518

Lont AP, Lamme B et al (2005) The aortocaval fistula, a rare complication of an aneurysm of the abdominal aorta. Ned Tijdschr Geneeskd 149:325

Loo GT et al (1996) Airbag protection versus compartment intrusion effect determines the pattern of injuries in multiple trauma motor vehicle crashes. J Trauma 41:935

Lopez Cubillana P, Rigabert Montiel M, Nicolas Torralba JA, Banon Perez V, Valdelvira Nadal P, Prieto Gonzalez A, Server Pastor G, Gomez Gomez G, Aguayo Albasino JA, Perez Albacete YM (1998) Ultrasonography and intravenous urography in the diagnosis of blunt renal trauma. Arch Esp Urol 51:669

Lorelli DR, Kralovich KA et al (2001) The impact of pre-existing end-stage renal disease on survival in acutely injured trauma patients. Am Surg 67:693

Lotte A, Wasz-Hockert O, Poisson N et al (1984) BCG complications. Estimates of the risks among vaccinated subjects and statistical analysis of their main characteristics. Adv Tuberc Res 21:107

Louca G (1999) MR urography in the diagnosis of urinary tract obstruction. Eur Urol 35:102

Loughlin K, Bailey R (1986) Internal ureteral stent for conservative management of ureteral calculi during pregnancy. N Engl J Med 315:1647

Loughlin KR (1994) Management of urologic problems during pregnancy. Urology 44:159

Loughlin KR (1997) Management of urologic problems in the pregnant patient. AUA Update Series 16:10

Loughlin KR, Lindsey AK (2002) The current management of urolithiasis during pregnancy. Urol Clin N Am 29:701

Loughlin KR, Tilney NL, Richie JP (1984) Urologic complications in 718 renal transplant patients. Surgery 95:296

Lovaria A, Nicolini A, Meregaglia D, Saccheri S, Rivolta R, Rampoldi A, Rossi P, Montanari E (1999) Interventional radiology in the treatment of urological vascular complications. Ann Urol (Paris) 33:156

Lowe FC, Jarow JP (1993) Placebo-controlled study of oral ter-

butaline and pseudoephedrine in management of prostaglandin E1-induced prolonged erections. Urology 42:51
Lowe LH, Isuani BH, Heller RM, Stein SM, Johnson JE, Navarro OM et al (2000) Pediatric renal masses: Wilms tumor and beyond. Radiographics 20:1585
Lowe MA, Mason JT, Luna GK, Maier RV, Copass MK, Berger RE (1988) Risk factors for urethral injuries in men with traumatic pelvic fractures. J Urol 140:506
Lowe PP, Roylance J (1976) Transitional cell carcinoma of the kidney. Clin Radiol 27:503
Lozen Y (1999) Intraabdominal hypertension and abdominal compartment syndrome in trauma: pathophysiology and interventions. AACN Clin Issues 10:104; quiz 135
Lu CY, Penfield JG et al (1999) Hypothesis: is renal allograft rejection initiated by the response to injury sustained during the transplant process? Kidney Int 55:2157
Luck AJ, Bokey EL (2003) Reoperative surgery for stomal complications and closure. In: Longo WE, Dunitz JM (eds) Reoperative colon and rectal surgery Taylor and Francis, London, p 78
Ludwig M, Beck A, Wickert L, Bolkenius U, Tittel B, Hinkel K et al (1998) Female pseudohermaphroditism associated with a novel homozygous G-to-A (V370-to-M) substitution in the P-450 aromatase gene. J Pediatr Endocrinol Metab 11:657
Luks FI, Lemire A et al (1993) Blunt abdominal trauma in children: the practical value of ultrasonography. J Trauma 34:607; discussion 610
Luna CM, Vujacich P, Niederman MS, Vay C, Gherardi C, Matera J, Jolly EC (1997) Impact of BAL data on the therapy and outcome of ventilator-associated pneumonia. Chest 111:676
Lundin C, Bersztel A, Wahlberg J, Wadstrom J (2002) Low molecular weight heparin prophylaxis increases the incidence of lymphocele after kidney transplantation. Ups J Med Sci 107:9
Lusuardi L, Lodde M, Pycha A (2005) Surgical atlas. Cutaneous ureterostomy. BJU Int 96:1149
Luther B, Sandmann W et al (1997) Aortic aneurysm in horseshoe kidney–special diagnosis and therapy. Chirurg 68:403
Lyman GH, Lyman CH, Agboola O (2005) Risk models for predicting chemotherapy-induced neutropenia. Oncologist 10:427
Lynch D, Martinez-Pineiro L, Plas E et al (2003) Ureteral trauma. EAU Guidelines on urological trauma, p 25
Lynch T, Martínez-Piñeiro L, Plas E, Serafetinides E, Türkeri L, Santucci RA, Hohenfellner M (2005) EAU Guidelines on urological trauma. Eur Urol 47:1
MacDiarmid S, Rosario D, Chapple CR (1995) The importance of accurate assessment and conservative management of the open bladder neck in patients with pelvic fracture membranous urethral distraction defects. Br J Urol 75:65
Machida T, Hanazaki K et al (1999) Snowboarding injuries of the abdomen: comparison with skiing injuries. Injury 30:47
MacNeily AE, Maizels M, Kaplan WE, Firlit CF, Conway JJ (1993) Does early pyeloplasty really avert loss of renal function? A retrospective review. J Urol 150:769
Madersbacher S, Schmidt J, Eberle JM, Thoeny HC, Burkhard F, Hochreiter W, Studer UE (2003) Long-term outcome of ileal conduit diversion. J Urol 169:985
Madhavan P, Sproule J et al (1999) Aorta–left renal vein fistula: an unusual complication of an abdominal aortic aneurysm. Eur J Vasc Endovasc Surg 17:87
Madiba TE, Haffejee AA (1999) Causes and outcome of bladder injuries in Durban. East Afr Med J 76:676
Madiba TE, Haffejee AA et al (2002) Renal trauma secondary to stab, blunt and firearm injuries–a 5-year study. S Afr J Surg 40:5; discussion 9
Madl C, Druml W (2003) Gastrointestinal disorders of the critically ill. Systemic consequences of ileus. Best Pract Res Clin Gastroenterol 17:445
Mahoney EM, Kearney GP, Tarabulcy JG (1998) Cutaneous ureterostomy. In: Libertino JA (ed) Reconstructive urology, 3rd edn.Mosby, New York, p 325
Maier U (2002)Autotransplantation der Niere bei Harnleiternekrose nach Ureteroskopie. In: Steffens J, Langen PH (eds) Komplikationen in der Urologie. Steinkopff Verlag, Darmstadt, p 108
Maikranz P (1994) Nephrolithiasis in pregnancy. Balliere's Clin Obstet Gynaecol 8:375
Mair J, Artner-Dworzak E, Dienstl A, Lechleitner P, Morass B, Smidt J, Wagner I, Wettach C, Puschendorf B (1991) Early detection of acute myocardial infarction by measurement of mass concentration of creatine kinase-MB. Am J Cardiol 68:1545
Major P, Lortholary A, Hon J et al (2001) Zoledronic acid is superior to pamidronate in the treatment of hypercalcemia of malignancy: a pooled analysis of two randomized, controlled clinical trials. J Clin Oncol 19:558
Makinen J et al (2001) Morbidity of 10 110 hysterectomies by type of approach. Hum Reprod 16:1473
Makisalo H, Eklund B, Salmela K et al (1997) Urological complications after 2084 consecutive kidney transplantation. Transplant Proc 29:152
Makita H, Nishimura M, Miyamoto K, Nakano T, Tanino Y, Hirokawa J, Nishihira J Kawakami (1998) Effect of anti-macrophage migration inhibitory factor antibody on lipopolysaccharide-induced pulmonary neutrophil accumulation. Am J Respir Crit Care Med158:573
Makoha FW et al (2004) Multiple cesarean section morbidity. Int J Gynaecol Obstet 87:227
Makoha FW et al (2005) Choice of abdominal incision and risk of trauma to the urinary bladder and bowel in multiple cesarean sections. Eur J Obstet Gynecol Reprod Biol
Malakoff AF, Schmidt JD (1975) Metastatic carcinoma of penis complicated by hypercalcemia. Urology 5:510
Malament M (1965) Maximal hemostasis in suprapubic prostatectomy. Surg Gynecol Obstet 120:1307
Malangoni MA (2005) Contributions to the management of intraabdominal infections. Am J Surg 190:255
Malek RS, OĎea MJ, Kelalis PP (1977) Management of ruptured posterior urethra in childhood. J Urol 117:105
Maleux G, Messiaen T, Stockx L, Vanrenterghem Y, Wilms G (2003) Transcatheter embolization of biopsy-related vascular injuries in renal allografts. Long-term technical, clinical and biochemical results. Acta Radiol 44:13
Mali V, Liu B et al (2005) Blunt renal trauma in occult congenital hydronephrosis. Singapore Med J 46:28
Malkowicz SB (2002) Management of superficial bladder cancer. In: Walsh PC, Retik AB, Vaughan ED Jr, Wein AJ (2002) Campbell's urology. Saunders, Philadelphia
Mallon E, Osborne G, Dinneen M, Lane RJ, Glaser M, Bunker CB (1999) Dermatomyositis in association with transitional cell carcinoma of the bladder. Clin Exp Dermatol 24:94
Mallonee S, Shariat S, Stennies G et al (1996) Physical injuries and fatalities resulting from the Oklahoma City bombing. JAMA 276:382
Mallow S, Rebuck JA, Osler T, Ahern J, Healey MA, Rogers FB (2004) Do proton pump inhibitors increase the incidence of nosocomial pneumonia and related infectious complications when compared with histamine-2 receptor antagonists in critically ill trauma patients? Curr Surg 61:452
Mancino P, Parlavecchio E, Melluso J, Monti M, Russo P (2003) Introducing colposcopy and vulvovaginoscopy as routine examinations for victims of sexual assault. Clin Exp Obstet Gynecol 30:40
Manglani HH, Marco RA, Picciolo A et al (2000) Orthopedic emergencies in cancer patients. Semin Oncol 27:299
Manke C, Strotzer M, Seitz J, Lenhart M, Aebert H, Kasprzak P,

Kaiser B, Feuerbach S (1999) Ischemic complications in aortic dissection–percutaneous treatment with balloon fenestration and stent implantation. Rofo 170:198
Mansi MK, Alkhudair WK (1997) Conservative management with percutaneous intervention of major blunt renal injuries. Am J Emerg Med 15:633
Manson AL (1988) Is antibiotic administration indicated after outpatient cystoscopy. J Urol 140:316
Månsson W, Bakke A, Bergman B, Brekkan E, Jonsson O, Kihl B, Nurmi M, Pedersen J, Schultz A, Sörensen B, Urnes T, Wolf H (1997) Perforation of continent urinary reservoirs. Scandinavian experience. Scand J Urol Nephrol 31:529
Månsson W, Davidsson T, Könyves J, Liedberg F, Månsson Å, Wullt B (2003) Continent urinary tract reconstruction – the Lund experience. BJU Int 92:271
Maranzano E, Latini P (1995) Effectiveness of radiation therapy without surgery in metastatic spinal cord compression: final results from a prospective trial. Int J Radiat Oncol Biol Phys 32:959
Marberger M, Hruby W (1981) Percutaneous litholapaxy of renal calculi with ultrasound. Scientific exhibit at annual meeting of American Urological Association, Boston, MA, May 10–14, 1981.
Marberger M, Stackl W, Hruby W (1982) Percutaneous litholapaxy of renal calculi with ultrasound. Eur Urol 8:236
Marberger M, Stackl W, Hruby W, Kroiss A (1985) Late sequelae of ultrasonic lithotripsy of renal calculi. J Urol 133:170
Marcello PW (2001) Intra-abdominal sepsis. In: O'Donnell JM, Nacul FE (eds) Surgical intensive care medicine. Kluwer Academic, Boston, p 461
Marchetti O, Calandra T (2004) Infections in the neutropenic cancer patient. In: Cohen J, Powderly WG (eds) Infectious diseases. Mosby, Philadelphia
Marcos HB, Noone TC et al (1998) MRI evaluation of acute renal trauma. J Magn Reson Imaging 8:989
Marekovic Z, Derezic D, Krhen I, Kastelan Z (1997) Urogenital war injuries. Mil Med 162:346
Margenthaler JA, Weber TR et al (2002) Blunt renal trauma in children: experience with conservative management at a pediatric trauma center. J Trauma 52:928
Mariappan P, Smith G, Bariol SV, Moussa SA, Tolley DA (2005) Stone and pelvic urine culture and sensitivity are better than bladder urine as predictors of urosepsis following percutaneous nephrolithotomy: a prospective clinical study. J Urol 173:1610
Marik PE (2000) Fever in the ICU. Chest 117:855
Marild S, Jodal U (1998) Incidence rate of first-time symptomatic urinary tract infection in children under 6 years of age. Acta Paediatr 87:549
Marini JJ, Pierson DJ, Hudson LD (1979) Acute lobar atelectasis: a prospective comparison of fiberoptic bronchoscopy and respiratory therapy. Am Rev Respir Dis 119:971
Mark SD, Webster GD (1996) Reconstruction of the failed repair of posterior urethral rupture. In: McAninch JW (ed) Traumatic and reconstructive urology. WB Saunders, Philadelphia
Mark SD, Keane TE, Vandemark RM, Webster GD (1995) Impotence following pelvic fracture urethral injury: incidence, aetiology and management. Br J Urol 75:62
Marr KA, Sexton DJ, Conlon PJ, Corey GR, Schwab SJ, Kirkland KB (1997) Catheter-related bacteremia and outcome of attempted catheter salvage in patients undergoing hemodialysis. Ann Intern Med 127:275
Marshall FF (1989) Endoscopic reconstruction of traumatic urethral transections. Urol Clin North Am 16:313
Marshall JC (2003) Such stuff as dreams are made on: mediator-directed therapy in sepsis. Nat Rev Drug Discov 2:391
Marshall JC (2004) Intra-abdominal infections. Microbes Infect 6:1015
Marshall JC, Maier RV, Jimenez M, Dellinger EP (2004) Source control in the management of severe sepsis and septic shock: an evidence-based review. Crit Care Med 32:S513
Martin J, Messelken M (1998) Sequential management of sedation and analgesia in the intensive care medicine. W. Zuckschwerdt, Munich
Martin J, Baesell K, Buerkle H et al (2005) Analgesia and sedation in the intensive care unit. S2: guidelines of the German society of anaesthesiology and intensive care medicine. Anaesth Intensivmed 1:S1
Martin LG, Casarella WJ, Gaylord GM (1988) Azotemia caused by renal artery stenosis: treatment by percutaneous angioplasty. Am J Roentgenol 150:839
Martin LG, Rundback JH, Sacks D, Cardella JF, Rees CR, Matsumoto AH, Meranze SG, Schwartzberg MS, Silverstein MI, Lewis CA; Society of Interventional Radiology Standards of Practice Committee (2003) Quality improvement guidelines for angiography angioplasty, and stent placement in the diagnosis and treatment of renal artery stenosis in adults. J Vasc Interv Radiol 14:S297
Martin RF, Rossi RL (1997) The acute abdomen: an overview and algorithms. Surg Clin North Am 77:1227
Martin X, Ndoye A, Konan PG, Feitosa Tajra LC, Gelet A, Dawahra M, Dubernard JM (1998) Hazards of lumbar ureteroscopy: apropos of 4 cases of avulsion of the ureter. Prog Urol 8:358
Martin X, Murat FJ, Feitosa LC, Rouviere O, Lyonnet D, Gelet A, Dubernard J (2000) Severe bleeding after nephrolithotomy: results of hyperselective embolization. Eur Urol 37:136
Martínez-Piñeiro JA, Carcamo P, García-Matres MJ, Martínez-Piñeiro L, Iglesias JR, Rodriguez-Ledesma JM (1997) Excision and anastomotic repair for urethral stricture disease: experience with 150 cases. Eur Urol 32:433
Martinez-Pineiro L Jr, Cerezo E, Cozar JM, Avellana JA, Moreno JA, Martinez-Pineiro JA (1992) Value of testicular ultrasound in the evaluation of blunt scrotal trauma without haematocele. Br J Urol 69:286
Martins FE, Boyd SD (1995) Post-operative risk factors associated with artificial urinary sphincter infection-erosion. Br J Urol 75:354
Marx FJ (1981) Therapy of priapism (translation). Urologe A 20:353
Marx FJ, Chaussy C, Moser E (1982) Limitations and hazards of palliative renal tumor embolization. Urologe A 21:206
Marx RE, Ehler WJ, Tayapongsak P et al (1990) Relationship of oxygen dose to angiogenesis induction in irradiated tissue. Am J Surg 160:519
Marzocco S, Di Paola R et al (2005) The cyclopentenone prostaglandin 15-deoxyDelta(12,14)-prostaglandin J(2) attenuates the development of zymosan-induced shock. Intensive Care Med 31:693
Master VA, Franks J et al (2002) Grade V renal injury: avulsion of the renal pedicle. J Am Coll Surg 195:425
Masumori N, Tsukamoto T, Rhodes T et al (2003) Natural history of lower urinary tract symptoms in men–result of a longitudinal community-based study in Japan. Urology 61:956
Matalon TS, Athanasoulis CA et al (1979) Hemorrhage with pelvic fractures: efficacy of transcatheter embolization. AJR Am J Roentgenol 133:859
Matas AJ, Bartlett ST, Leichtman AB, Delmonico FL (2003) Morbidity and mortality after living kidney donation, 1999 survey of United States transplant centers. Am J Transplant 3:830
Mateo E, Marin JP et al (1999) Perioperative morbidity and mortality in surgery for dissecting aneurysm of the ascending aorta. Rev Esp Anestesiol Reanim 46:333
Mathews R, Marshall FF (1997) Versatility of the adult psoas hitch ureteral reimplantation. J Urol 158:2078

Mathews R, Rajan N, Josefson L et al (1999) Hyperbaric oxygen therapy for radiation induced hemorrhagic cystitis. J Urol 161:435

Matlaga BR, Shah OD, Zagoria RJ, Dyer RB, Streem SB, Assimos DG (2003) Computerized tomography guided access for percutaneous nephrostolithotomy. J Urol 170:45

Matsumura M, Nishi T, Sasaki Y, Yamada R, Yamamoto H, Ohhama Y et al (1993) Prenatal diagnosis and treatment strategy for congenital mesoblastic nephroma. J Pediatr Surg 28:1607

Matsuura T, Nose K et al (2002) Evaluation of the management of blunt renal trauma and indication for surgery. Nippon Hinyokika Gakkai Zasshi 93:511

Matthay MA (2001) Severe sepsis – a new treatment with both anticoagulant and anti-inflammatory properties. N Engl J Med 344:759

Matthews LA, JP Spirnak (1995) The nonoperative approach to major blunt renal trauma. Semin Urol 13:77

Matthews LA, Smith EM et al (1997) Nonoperative treatment of major blunt renal lacerations with urinary extravasation. J Urol 157:2056

Matthiessen P, Hallbook O, Andersson M, Rutegard J, Sjodahl R (2004) Risk factors for anastomotic leakage after anterior resection of the rectum. Colorectal Dis 6:462

Mattila A, S Lundstedt et al (1999) Ureteropelvic rupture caused by a fall. Duodecim 115:1850

Mattos RM, Libertino JA (1998) Complications associated with urinary diversions, continent reservoirs, and neobladders. In: Libertino JA (ed) Reconstructive urologic surgery, 3rd edn. Mosby, Saint Louis, p 423

Matzkin H, Braf Z (1987) Paraneoplastic syndromes associated with prostatic carcinoma J Urol 138:1129

Maudgil DD, McHugh K (2002) The role of computed tomography in modern paediatric uroradiology. Eur J Radiol 43:129

Mauermayer W (1981) Transurethrale operationen, 1st edn. Springer, Berlin Heidelberg New York

Mauroy B, Beuscart C, Biserte J et al (1996) L'infection urinaire chez la femme enceinte. Prog Urol 6:607

May JW Jr, Chait LA, O'Brien BM et al (1978) The no-reflow phenomenon in experimental free flaps. Plast Reconstr Surg 61:256

May M, Gunia S et al (2004) An unusual complication of extracorporeal shock wave lithotripsy: rupture of the kidney with consecutive nephrectomy. Aktuelle Urol 35:316

Mayo ME, Halil T, Browse NL et al (1971) The incidence of deep vein thrombosis after prostatectomy. Br J Urol 43:738

Mayor B, Gudinchet F et al (1995) Imaging evaluation of blunt renal trauma in children: diagnostic accuracy of intravenous pyelography and ultrasonography. Pediatr Radiol 25:214

Mazur AW, Thompson IM (1991) Efficacy and morbidity of „channel" TURP. Urology 38:526

Mazuski JE, Sawyer RG, Nathens AB, DiPiro JT, Schein M, Kudsk KA, Yowler C (2002) The Surgical Infection Society guidelines on antimicrobial therapy for intra-abdominal infections: evidence for the recommendations. Surg Infect (Larchmt) 3:175

McAleer SJ, Loughlin KR (2004) Nephrolithiasis and pregnancy. Curr Opin Urol 14:123

McAleer IM, Kaplan GW, Scherz HC, Packer MG, Lynch FP (1993) Genitourinary trauma in the pediatric patient. Urology 42:563

McAleer IM, Kaplan GW, LoSasso BE (2002) Congenital urinary tract anomalies in pediatric renal trauma patients. J Urol 168:1808

McAleer IM, Kaplan GW, LoSasso BE (2002) Renal and testis injuries in team sports. J Urol 168:1805

McAllister M, Bhayani SB, Ong A, Jaffe W, Malkowicz SB, VanArsdalen K, Chow GK, Jarrett TW (2004) Vena caval transection during retroperitoneoscopic nephrectomy: report of the complication and review of the literature. J Urol 172:183

McAndrew JD, Corriere JN Jr (1994) Radiographic evaluation of renal trauma: evaluation of 1103 consecutive patients. Br J Urol 73:352

McAninch JW (1981) Traumatic injuries to the urethra. J Trauma 21:291

McAninch JW (1989) Pubectomy in repair of membranous urethral stricture. Urol Clin Norh Am 16:297

McAninch JW (1992) Urethral injuries in female subjects following pelvic fractures (Editorial Comment) J Urol 147:143

McAninch JW (1996) Pubectomy in repair of membranous urethral strictures. In: McAninch JW (ed) Traumatic and reconstructive urology. WB Saunders, Philadelphia

McAninch JW (1997) Editorial: Scars in the urinary system. J Urol 157:817

McAninch JW (2003) Editorial: New technology in renal trauma. J Urol 169: 1368

McAninch JW, Santucci RA (2002) Genitourinary trauma. In: Retik AB, Vaughan ED Jr, Wein AJ (eds) Campbell's urology, 8th edn. W.B. Saunders, Philadelphia, p 3707

McAninch JW, Kahn RI, Jeffrey RB, Laing FC, Krieger MJ (1984) Major traumatic and septic genital injuries. J Trauma 24:291

McAninch JW, Dixon CM et al (1990) The surgical treatment of renal trauma. Vestn Khir Im II Grek 145:64

McAninch JW, Carroll PR et al (1991) Renal reconstruction after injury. J Urol 145:932

McAninch JW, Carroll PR et al (1993) Renal gunshot wounds: methods of salvage and reconstruction. J Trauma 35:279; discussion 283

McAninch JW, Carroll PR, Jordan GH (1996) Traumatic and reconstructive urology. WB Saunders, Philadelphia

McClamrock HD, Adashi EY: Gestational hyperandrogenism. Fertil Steril 57:257

McCloskey BG, O'Connor FA (1982) Gonadotrophin secreting carcinoma of kidney. Ir J Med Sci 151:283

McConnell JD et al (1982) Rupture of the bladder. Urol Clin North Am 9:293

McConnell JD, Roehrborn CG, Bautista OM et al (2003) The long-term effect of doxazosin, finasteride, and combination therapy on the clinical progression of benign prostatic hyperplasia. N Engl J Med 349:2387

McCullough CS, Soper NJ, Clayman RV, So SS, Jendrisak MD, Hanto DW (1991) Laparoscopic drainage of a posttransplant lymphocele. Transplantation 51:725

McDougal WS, Kursh ED, Persky L (1975) Spontaneous rupture of the kidney with perirenal hematoma. J Urol 114:181

McGahan JP (1985) Aspiration and drainage procedures in the intensive care unit: percutaneous sonographic guidance. Radiology 154:531

McGahan JP, Richards JR et al (1999) Use of ultrasonography in the patient with acute renal trauma. J Ultrasound Med 18:207; quiz 215

McGahan PJ et al (2005) Ultrasound detection of blunt urological trauma: a 6-year study. Injury 36:762

McGee DC, Gould MK (2003) Preventing complications of central venous catheterization. N Engl J Med 348:1123

McGee SR (1993) Referred scrotal pain: case reports and review. J Gen Intern Med 8:694

McGinty DM, Mendez R(1977) Traumatic ureteral injuries with delayed recognition. Urology 10:115

McHenry CR, Piotrowski JJ, Petrinic D et al (1995) Determinants of mortality for necrotizing soft-tissue infections. Ann Surg 221:558; discussion 563

McIntyre JF, Eifel PJ, Levenmack C et al (1995) Ureteral stricture as a late complication of radiotherapy for stage IB carcinoma of the uterine cervix. Cancer 75:836

McIvor J, Williams G, Greswick Southcott RD (1982) Control of severe vesical haemorrhage by therapeutic embolisation. Clin Radiol 33:561
McKay TC, Waters WB (1994) Fournier's gangrene as the presenting sign of an undiagnosed human immunodeficiency virus infection. J Urol 152:1552
McLoud TC, Flower CD (1991) Imaging the pleura: sonography CT, and MR imaging. AJR Am J Roentgenol 156:1145
McMahon CG (2002) High flow priapism due to an arterial-lacunar fistula complicating initial veno-occlusive priapism. Int J Impot Res 14:195
McNeely SG Jr (1987) Treatment of urinary tract infections during pregnancy. Clin Obstet Gynecol 13:480
McNeill SA, Daruwala PD, Mitchell ID et al (1999) Sustained-release alfuzosin and trial without catheter after acute urinary retention: a prospective, placebo-controlled. BJU Int 84:622
McRoberts JW, Radge H (1970) The severed canine posterior urethra: a study of two distinct methods of repair. J Urol 104:724
McRoberts JW, Chapman WH, Ansell JS (1968) Primary anastomosis of the traumatically amputated penis: cast report and summary of literature. J Urol 100:751
Mebust WK, Holtgrewe HL, Cocked AT, Peters PC (1989) Transurethral prostatectomy: immediate and postoperative complications. A cooperative study of 13 participating institutions evaluating 3,885 patients. J Urol 141:243
Medica J, Caldamone A (1995) Pediatric renal trauma: special considerations. Semin Urol 13:73
Medina D, Lavery R, Ross SE et al (1998) Ureteral trauma: preoperative studies neither predict injury nor prevent missed injuries. J Am Coll Surg 186:641
Mee SL, McAninch JW (1989) Indications for radiographic assessment in suspected renal trauma. Urol Clin North Am 16:187
Mee SL et al (1987) Computerized tomography in bladder rupture: diagnostic limitations. J Urol 137:207
Mee SL, McAninch JW et al (1989) Radiographic assessment of renal trauma: a 10-year prospective study of patient selection. J Urol 141:1095
Megalli MR, Gursel EO, Demirag H et al (1974) External radiotherapy in ureteral obstruction secondary to locally invasive prostatic cancer. Urology 3:562
Mejean A, Vogt B et al (1999) Mortality and morbidity after nephrectomy for renal cell carcinoma using a transperitoneal anterior subcostal incision. Eur Urol 36:298
Melcher ML, Carter JT, Posselt A, Duh QY, Stoller M, Freise CE, Kang SM (2005) More than 500 consecutive laparoscopic donor nephrectomies without conversion or repeated surgery. Arch Surg 140:835; discussion 839
Meldrum DR, Moore FA et al (1997) Prospective characterization and selective management of the abdominal compartment syndrome. Am J Surg 174:667; discussion 672
Melekos MD (1988) Re: testicular torsion in a 62-year-old man. J Urol 140:387
Melekos MD, Pantazakos A, Daouaher H, Papatsoris G (1992) Primary endourologic re-establishment of urethral continuity after disruption of prostatomembranous urethra. Urology 39:135
Meller AE, Nesrallah LJ, Dall'Oglio MF, Srougi M (2002) Complications in radical cystectomy performed at a teaching hospital. Int Braz J Urol 28:522
Meller J, Altenvoerde G, Munzel U, Jauho A, Behe M, Gratz S, Luig H, Becker W (2000) Fever of unknown origin: prospective comparison of 18FFDG imaging with a double-head coincidence camera and gallium-67 citrate SPET. Eur J Nucl Med 27:1617
Melman A, Serels S (2000) Priapism. Int J Impot Res Suppl 12:S133
Menajovsky (2005) LB Heparin-induced thrombocytopenia: clinical manifestations and management strategies. Am J Med 118:21S
Mendez LE (2001) Iatrogenic injuries in gynecologic cancer surgery. Surg Clin North Am 81:897
Mendez Gallart R, Gomez Tellado M et al (1996) Blunt abdominal trauma. Nonoperative management. Cir Pediatr 9:60
Mendoza D, Newman RC, Albala D, Cohen MS, Tewari A, Lingeman J, Wong M, Kavoussi L, Adams J, Moore R, Winfield H, Glascock JM, Das S, Munch L, Grasso M, Dickinson M, Clayman R, Nakada S, McDougall EM, Wolf IS, Hulbert J, Leveillee RJ, Houshair A, Carson C (1996) Laparoscopic complications in markedly obese urologic patients (a multi-institutional review) Urology 48:562
Meng MV, Brandes SB, McAninch JW (1999) Renal trauma: indications and techniques for surgical exploration. World J Urol 17:71
Meraney AM, Samee AA, Gill IS (2002) Vascular and bowel complications during retroperitoneal laparoscopic surgery. J Urol 168:1941
Meria P, Mazeman E (2000) Immediate and delayed management of renal trauma. Eur Urol 37:121
Meria P, Anidjar M, Hermieu JF, Boccon-Gibod L (1993) Lithiase urinaire et grossesse. Prog Urol, 3:937
Merino E, Boix V, Portilla J, Reus S, Priego M (2001) Fournier's gangrene in HIV-infected patients. Eur J Clin Microbiol Infect Dis 20:910
Merkle EM, Hashim M, Wendt M, Lewin JS (1999) MR-guided percutaneous nephrostomy of the nondilated upper urinary tract in a porcine model. Am J Roentgenol 172:1221
Mermel LA, Maki DG (1993) Detection of bacteremia in adults: consequences of culturing an inadequate volume of blood. Ann Intern Med 119:270
Merrill DC (1988) Clinical experience with the Mentor inflatable penile prosthesis in 301 patients. J Urol 140:1424
Merrot T, Portier F et al (2000) Trauma of the renal pedicle in children. Report of 2 cases of late revascularization with endovascular prosthesis. Prog Urol 10:277
Meschia M et al (2001) Tension-Free vaginal tape: analysis of outcomes and complications in 404 stress incontinent women. Int Urogynecol J Pelvic Floor Dysfunct 12 [Suppl 2]: S24
Mesrobian HG, Balcom AH, Durkee CT (2004) Urologic problems of the neonate. Pediatr Clin North Am 51:1051
Messori A, Trippoli S, Vaiani M, Gorini M, Corrado A (2000) Bleeding and pneumonia in intensive care patients given ranitidine and sucralfate for prevention of stress ulcer: meta-analysis of randomised controlled trials. BMJ 321:1103
Meyer DM, Thal ER et al (1989) The role of abdominal CT in the evaluation of stab wounds to the back. J Trauma 29:1226; discussion 1228
Meyers AM, Levine E, Myburgh JA, Goudie E (1977) Diagnosis and management of lymphoceles after renal transplantation. Urology 10:497
Mhiri MN, Trifa M et al (1997) Kidney contusions and traffic accidents. Apropos of the Tunisian experience. Ann Urol (Paris) 31:243
Micallef M, Ahmad I, Ramesh N, Hurley M, McInerney D (2001) Ultrasound features of blunt testicular injury. Injury 32:23
Michel LA, Lacrosse M et al (1996) Blunt renal traumas: contribution of spiral CT with three dimensional reconstruction to the surgical decision process? Int Surg 81:377
Michigan S, Catalona WJ (1977) Ureteral obstruction from prostatic carcinoma: response to endocrine and radiation therapy. J Urol 118:733
Middleton AW Jr, Middleton GW, Dean LK (1980) Spontaneous renal rupture in pregnancy. Urology 15:60
Middleton RG (1980) Routine use of the psoas hitch in ureteral reimplantation. J Urol 123:352

Milas ZL, Dodson TF et al (2004) Pediatric blunt trauma resulting in major arterial injuries. Am Surg 70:443

Miley GB, Scheller AD, Jr Turner RH (1982) Medical and surgical treatment of the septic hip with one-stage revision arthroplasty. Clin Orthop Relat Res (170):76

Miller DC, Stinson EB, Oyer PE, Rossiter SJ, Reitz BA, Griepp RB, Shumway NE (1979) Operative treatment of aortic dissections. Experience with 125 patients over a sixteen-year period. J Thorac Cardiovasc Surg 78:365

Miller DC, Forauer A et al (2002) Successful angioembolization of renal artery pseudoaneurysms after blunt abdominal trauma. Urology 59:444

Miller DC, Rumohr JA, Dunn RL, Bloom DA, Park JM (2004) What is the fate of the refluxing contralateral kidney in children with multicystic dysplastic kidney? J Urol 172:1630

Miller EA, Mayo M, Kwan D, Mitchell M (1998) Simultaneous augmentation cystoplasty and artificial urinary sphincter placement: infection rates and voiding mechanisms. J Urol 160:750

Miller KS, McAninch JW (1995) Radiographic assessment of renal trauma: our 15-year experience. J Urol 154:352

Miller KS, Sahn SA (1987) Chest tubes. Indications, technique, management and complications. Chest 91:258

Miller LJ, Chandler SW, Ippoliti CM (1994) Treatment of cyclophosphamide-induced hemorrhagic cystitis with prostaglandins. Ann Pharmacother 28:590

Miller OF, Rineer SK, Reichard SR et al (1998) Prospective comparison of unenhanced spiral computed tomography and intravenous urogram in the evaluation of acute flank pain. Urology 52:982

Miller RA, May MW et al (1980) The prevention of secondary haemorrhage after prostatectomy: the value of antifibrinolytic therapy. Br J Urol 52:26

Miller RC, Sterioff S Jr, Drucker WR, Persky L, Wright HK, Davis JH (1966) The incidental discovery of occult abdominal tumors in children following blunt abdominal trauma. J Trauma 6:99

Miller RW (1995) Delayed effects of external radiation exposure: a brief history. Radiat Res 144:160

Milliner DS, Murphy ME (1993) Urolithiasis in pediatric patients. Mayo Clin Proc 68:241

Mills J, Utley J, Abbott J (1974) Heart failure in infective endocarditis: predisposing factors, course, and treatment. Chest 66:151

Mills JA, Michel BA, Bloch DA, Calabrese LH, Hunder GG, Arend WP et al (1990) The American College of Rheumatology: 1990 criteria for the classification of Henoch-Schönlein purpura. Arthritis Rheum 33:1114

Mills RD, Studer UE (1999) Metabolic consequences of continent urinary diversion. J Urol 161:1057

Mills RD, Studer UE (2000) Female orthotopic bladder substitution: a good operation in the right circumstances. J Urol 163:1501

Milroy EJG, Chapple CR, Eldrin A, Wallsen N (1989) A new treatment for urethral strictures – A permanently implanted stent. J Urol 141:1120

Milzman DP, Boulanger BR et al (1992) Pre-existing disease in trauma patients: a predictor of fate independent of age and injury severity score. J Trauma 32:236; discussion 243

Minaglia S et al (2004) Bladder injury during transobturator sling. Urology 64:376

Mindrup SR, Kealey GP, Fallon B (2005) Hyperbaric oxygen for the treatment of Fournier's gangrene. J Urol 173:1975

Minervini A, Ralph DJ, Pryor JP (2006) Outcome of penile prosthesis implantation for treating erectile dysfunction: experience with 504 procedures. BJU Int 97:129

Mintz Y, Shapira SC, Pikarsky AJ et al (2002) The experience of one institution dealing with terror: the El Aqsa Intifada riots. IMAJ 4:554

Mirvis SE (1996) Trauma. Radiol Clin North Am 34:1225

Mitchell JP (1981) Transurethral resection for neoplasm of the bladder. In: Mitchell JP (ed) Endoscopic Operative Urology. Wright & Sons, Bristol, p 341

Mizobata Y, Yokota J et al (2001) Successful evaluation of pseudoaneurysm formation after blunt renal injury with dual-phase contrast-enhanced helical CT. AJR Am J Roentgenol 177:136

Mizzi A, Shabani A et al (2002) The role of follow-up imaging in paediatric blunt abdominal trauma. Clin Radiol 57:908

Moberg AC, Montgomery A (2005) Primary access-related complications with laparoscopy: comparison of blind and open techniques. Surg Endosc 19:1196

Modi P, Goel R, Dodiya S (2005) Laparoscopic ureteroneocystostomy for distal ureteral injuries. Urology 66:751

Mohammad Naghi T, Kambiz K et al (2005) Musculoskeletal injuries associated with earthquake. A report of injuries of Iran's December 26, 2003 Bam earthquake casualties managed in tertiary referral centers. Injury 36:27

Mohan P, Murphy DM, Counihan A, Cunningham P, Hickey DP (1999) The role of intraoperative heparin in cyclosporine treated cadaveric renal transplant recipients. J Urol 162:682

Moiseienko VO, Krasiuk (IV 2001) Potential of current physical investigative methods in the diagnosis of injuries to organs of the abdominal cavity. Lik Sprava:189

Mokhmalji H, Braun PM, Martinez Portillo FJ et al (2001) Percutaneous nephrostomy versus ureteral stents for diversion of hydronephrosis caused by stones: a prospective, randomized clinical trial. J Urol 165:1088

Moller CM, Mommsen S et al (1995) The role of haematuria in the diagnosis of blunt renal trauma. Scand J Urol Nephrol Suppl 172:99

Monga M, Hellstrom WJ (2005) Testicular trauma. Adolesc Med 1996 7:141

Monga M, Klein E, Castaneda-Zuniga WR, Thomas R (1995) The forgotten indwelling ureteral stent: a urological dilemma. J Urol 153:1817

Monreal M, Montserrat E, Salvador R, Bechini J, Donoso L, MaCallejas J, Foz M (1989) Real-time ultrasound for diagnosis of symptomatic venous thrombosis and for screening of patients at risk: correlation with ascending conventional venography. Angiology 40:527

Monreal M, Lafoz E, Olive A, del Rio L, Vedia C (1994) Comparison of subcutaneous unfractionated heparin with a low molecular weight heparin (Fragmin) in patients with venous thromboembolism and contraindications to coumarin. Thromb Haemost 71:7

Monserrat Monfort JJ, Oliver Amoros F et al (1996) Renal traumatism: diagnostic protocol and therapeutic indications. Actas Urol Esp 20:534

Monstrey SJ, Beerthuizen GI et al (1989) Renal trauma and hypertension. J Trauma 29:65

Montague DK (1987) Periprosthetic infections. J Urol 138:68

Montague DK, Jarow J, Broderick GA et al (2003) American Urological Association guideline on the management of priapism. J Urol 170:1318

Montague DK, Jarow JP, Broderick GA et al (2005) Chapter 1: The management of erectile dysfunction: an AUA update. J Urol 174:230

Montana GS, Fowler WC (1989) Carcinoma of the cervix: analysis of bladder and rectal radiation dose and complications. Int J Radiat Oncol Biol Phys 16:95

Montgomery RC, JD Richardson et al (1998) Posttraumatic renovascular hypertension after occult renal injury. J Trauma 45:106

Montorsi F, Naspro R, Salonia A, Suardi N, Briganti A, Zanoni M, Valenti S, Vavassori I, Rigatti P (2004) Holmium laser enucleation versus transurethral resection of the prostate:

results from a 2-center, prospective, randomized trial in patients with obstructive benign prostatic hyperplasia. J Urol 172:1926
Montravers P, Villamizar J et al (2001) Superinfection of posttraumatic retroperitoneal hematoma secondary to ascending urinary tract infection. J Trauma 50:931
Mooney CJ, Dunphy EJ, Stone B, McNeel DG (2006) Identification of autoantibodies elicited in a patient with prostate cancer presenting as dermatomyositis. Int J Urol 13:211
Moore EE, Shackford SR, Pachter HL et al (1989) Organ injury scaling: spleen, liver, and kidney. J Trauma 29:1664
Moore EE, Cogbill TH, Jurkovich GJ, McAninch JW, Champion HR, Gennarelli TA, Malangoni MA, Shackford SR, Trafton PG (1992) Organ injury scaling III: chest wall, abdominal vascular, ureter, bladder, and urethra. J Trauma 33:337
Mor Y, Pinthus JH, Nadu A, Raviv G, Golomb J, Winkler H et al (2006) Testicular fixation following torsion of the spermatic cord–does it guarantee prevention of recurrent torsion events? J Urol 175:171
Morcos SK (2005) Review article: Acute serious and fatal reactions to contrast media: our current understanding. Br J Radiol 932:686
Morcos SK, Thomsen HS (2001) Adverse reactions to iodinated contrast media. Eur Radiol 11:1267
Morcos SK, Thomsen HS, Webb JA (2001) Contrast Media Safety Committee of the European Society of Urogenital Radiology. Prevention of generalized reactions to contrast media: a consensus report and guidelines. Eur Radiol 11:1720
Morehouse DD, Mackinnon KJ (1980) Management of prostatomembranous urethral disruption: a 13-year experience. J Urol 123:173
Morey AF (2005) Sonographic intraperitoneal fluid in patients with pelvic fracture: two cases of traumatic intraperitoneal bladder rupture. J Urol 174:2264
Morey AF, McAninch JW (1997) Reconstruction of posterior urethral disruption injuries: outcome analysis in 82 patients. J Urol 157:506
Morey AF, Bruce JE et al (1996) Efficacy of radiographic imaging in pediatric blunt renal trauma. J Urol 156:2014
Morey AF, Hernandez J, McAninch JW (1999) Reconstructive surgery for trauma of the lower urinary tract. Urol Clin North Am 26:49
Morey AF, McAninch JW, Tiller BK et al (1999) Single shot intraoperative excretory urography for the immediate evaluation of renal trauma. J Urol 161:1088
Morey AF, Anema JG, Harris R et al (2001) Treatment of grade 4 renal stab wounds with absorbable fibrin adhesive bandage in a porcine model. J Urol 165:955
Morey AF, Iverson AJ, Swan A et al (2001) Bladder rupture after blunt trauma: guidelines for diagnostic imaging. J Trauma 51:683
Morey AF, Metro MJ, Carney KJ, Miller KS, McAninch JW (2004) Consensus on genitourinary trauma: external genitalia. Br J of Urol Int 94:507
Morgan DE et al (2000) CT cystography: radiographic and clinical predictors of bladder rupture. AJR Am J Roentgenol 174:89
Moriarty KP, Lipkowitz GS e t al (1997) Capsulectomy: a cure for the page kidney. J Pediatr Surg 32:831
Morris CS, Bonnevie GJ, Najarian KE (2001) Nonsurgical treatment of acute iatrogenic renal artery injuries occurring after renal artery angioplasty and stenting. Am J Roentgenol 177:1353
Morrison D, Blaivas M, Lyon M (2005) Emergency diagnosis of Fournier's gangrene with bedside ultrasound. Am J Emerg Med 23:544
Morse RM, Spirnak JP, Resnick MI (1988) Iatrogenic colon and rectal injuries associated with urological intervention: report of 14 patients. J Urol 140:101
Morse TS (1975) Renal injuries. Pediatr Clin North Am 22:379
Mosahebi A, Butterworth M, Knight R, Berger L, Kaisary A, Butler PE (2001) Delayed penile replantation after prolonged warm ischemia. Microsurgery 21:52
Moscicki RA, Sockin SM, Corsello BF, Ostro MG, Bloch KJ (1990) Anaphylaxis during induction of general anesthesia: subsequent evaluation and management. J Allergy Clin Immunol 86:325
Mossner J (2005) Acute abdomen. Internist (Berl) 46:974
Motsch J, Walther A, Bock M, Boettiger BW (2006) Update in the prevention and treatment of deep vein thrombosis and pulmonary embolism. Curr Opin Anaesthesiol 19:52
Motzer RJ, Mazumdar M, Bacik J et al (1999) Survival and prognostic stratification of 670 patients with advanced renal cell carcinoma. J Clin Oncol 17:2530
Moudouni SM, Hadj Slimen M et al (2001) Management of major blunt renal lacerations: is a nonoperative approach indicated? Eur Urol 40:409
Moudouni SM, Patard JJ, Manunta A, Guiraud P, Guille F, Lobel B (2001) A conservative approach to major blunt renal lacerations with urinary extravasation and devitalized renal segments. BJU Int 87:290
Moudouni SM, Patard JJ, Manuta A, Guiraud P, Lobel B, Guille F (2001) Early endoscopic realignment of post-traumatic posterior urethral disruption. Urology 57:628
Mouraview V, Santucci R (2005) Cadaveric anatomy of pelvic fracture urethral distraction injury: most injuries are distal to the external urinary sphincter. J Urol 173:869
Mouraview V, Coburn M, Santucci R (2005) The treatment of posterior urethral disruption associated with pelvic fractures: comparative experience of early realignment versus delayed urethroplast. J Urol 173:873
Mugge A, Gulba DC, Frei U, Wagenbreth I, Grote R, Daniel WG, Lichtlen PR (1990) Renal artery embolism: thrombolysis with recombinant tissue-type plasminogen activator. J Intern Med 228:279
Muglia V, Tucci S Jr, Elias J Jr, Trad CS, Bilbey J, Cooperberg PL (2002) Magnetic resonance imaging of scrotal diseases: when it makes the difference. Urology 59:419
Muhlbauer S, Bard R (1980) Early definitive urologic management of patient with crush pelvic trauma and deep perineal laceration. Urology 15:56
Muir L et al (1996) The epidemiology of pelvic fractures in the Mersey Region. Injury 27:199
Mulcahy JJ (2000) Long-term experience with salvage of infected penile implants. J Urol 163:481
Mulcahy JJ, Brant MD, Ludlow JK (1995) Management of infected penile implants. Tech Urol 1:115
Mulhall JP, Gabram SG, Jacobs LM (1995) Emergency management of blunt testicular trauma. Acad Emerg Med 2:639
Muller-Suur R, Tyden O (1985) Evaluation of hydronephrosis in pregnancy using ultrasound and renography. Scand J Urol 19:267
Mulligan JM, Cagiannos I, Collins JP et al (1998) Ureteropelvic junction disruption secondary to blunt trauma: excretory phase imaging (delayed films) should help prevent a missed diagnosis. J Urol 159:67
Mulvihill SJ, Pellegrini CA (1994) Postoperative complications. In: Way LW (ed) Current surgical diagnosis treatment, 10th edn. Appleton Lange, Norwalk, p 24
Mulvihill SJ, Pellegrini CA (1994) Postoperative complications. In: Way LW (ed) Current surgical diagnosis treatment, 10th edn. Appleton Lange, Norwalk, p 441
Munarriz R, Talakoub L, Somekh NN, Lehrfeld T, Chudnovsky A, Flaherty E, Goldstein I (2002) Characteristics of female patients with sexual dysfunction who also had a history of blunt perineal trauma. J Sex Marital Ther 28 [Suppl 1]:175
Munden MM, Trautwein LM (2000) Scrotal pathology in pedi-

atrics with sonographic imaging. Curr Probl Diagn Radiol 29:185
Mundy AR (1991) The role of delayed primary repair in the acute management of pelvic fracture injuries to the urethra. Br J Urol 68:273
Mundy AR (1993) Results and complications of urethroplasty and its future. Br J Urol 71:322
Mundy AR (1996) Urethroplasty for posterior urethral strictures. Br J Urol 78:243
Mundy GR (1990) Pathophysiology of cancer-associated hypercalcemia. Semin Oncol 17 [2 Suppl 5]:10
Munk M, Hofmockel G et al (1997) Conservative therapy of blunt kidney injuries. Urologe A 36:531
Munoz D, Gutierrez C et al (1998) Traumatic renal artery thrombosis. Scand J Urol Nephrol 32:296
Munro NP, Woodhams S, Nawrocki JD, Fletcher MS, Thomas PJ (2003) The role of transarterial embolization in the treatment of renal cell carcinoma. BJU Int 92:240
Munver R, Delvecchio FC, Newman GE, Preminger GM (2001) Critical analysis of supracostal access for percutaneous renal surgery. J Urol 166:1242
Murkin JM (1994) Con: tranexamic acid is not better than aprotinin in decreasing bleeding after cardiac surgery. J Cardiothorac Vasc Anesth 8:474
Murphy BG, Hill C, Middleton D, Deherty CC, Brown JH, Nelson WE et al (1994) Increased renal allograft thrombosis in CAPD patients. Nephrol Dial Transplant 9:1166
Murphy JP, Holder TM, Ashcraft KW, Sharp RJ, Goodwin CD, Amoury RA (1984) Ureteropelvic junction obstruction in the newborn. J Pediatr Surg 19:642
Murphy JT, Borman KR et al (1996) Renal autotransplantation after horseshoe kidney injury: a case report and literature review. J Trauma 40:840
Murphy MF, Wallington TB, Kelsey P, Boulton F, Bruce M, Cohen H, Duguid J, Knowles SM, Poole G, Williamson LM (2001) Guidelines for the clinical use of red cell transfusions. Br J Haematol 113:24
Murray MJ, Cowen J, DeBlock H et al (2002) Clinical practice guidelines for sustained neuromuscular blockade in the adult critically ill patient. Crit Care Med 1:142
Murshidi MS (1988) Intraperitoneal rupture of the urinary bladder during transurethral resection of transitional cell carcinoma. Acta Urol Belg 56:68
Murthy LNS (1997) Urinary tract obstruction during pregnancy: recent developments in imaging. Br J Urol 80 [Suppl 1]:1
Muruve N, Hosking DH (1996) Intracorporeal phenylephrine in the treatment of priapism. J Urol 155:141
Musemeche CA et al (1987) Selective management of pediatric pelvic fractures: a conservative approach. J Pediatr Surg 22:538
Mutabagani KH, Coley BD et al (1999) Preliminary experience with focused abdominal sonography for trauma (FAST) in children: is it useful? J Pediatr Surg 34:48; discussion 52
Mutgi A, Williams JW, Nettleman M (1991) Renal colic. Utility of the plain abdominal roentgenogram. Arch Intern Med 151:1589
Muzzonigro G, Milanese G, Minardi D, Yehia M, Galosi AB, Dellabella M (2004) Safety and efficacy of transurethral resection of prostate glands up to 150 ml: a prospective comparative study with 1 year of followup. J Urol 172:611
Naber KG, Bergman B, Bishop MC, Bjerklund-Johansen TE, Botto H, Lobel B et al (2001) EAU guidelines for the management of urinary and male genital tract infections. Urinary Tract Infection (UTI) Working Group of the Health Care Office (HCO) of the European Association of Urology (EAU) Eur Urol 40:576
Nabi G, Mishriki SF (2005) Bite wounds of genitalia: clinical presentation and management. Hosp Med 66:112
Nabi G, Sheikh N, Greene D, Marsh R (2003) Therapeutic transcatheter arterial embolization in the management of intractable haemorrhage from pelvic urological malignancies: preliminary experience and long-term follow-up. BJU Int 92:245
Nadvi SS, Mokoena T et al (1996) Prognosis in posttraumatic acute renal failure is adversely influenced by hypotension and hyperkalaemia. Eur J Surg 162:121
Nagarajan VP, Pranikoff K, Imahori SC, Rabinowitz R (1983) Traumatic dislocation of testis. Urology 22:521
Nagel E, Jahne J et al (1997) Aspects relevant for abdominal surgery of attempted suicide. Langenbecks Arch Chir 382:29
Nagy KK, Brenneman FD et al (1997) Routine preoperative one-shot intravenous pyelography is not indicated in all patients with penetrating abdominal trauma. J Am Coll Surg 185:530
Najarian JS, Chavers BM, McHugh LE, Matas AJ (1992) 20 years or more of follow-up of living kidney donors. Lancet 340:807
Najmaldin A, Burge DM (1987) Acute idiopathic scrotal oedema: incidence, manifestations and aetiology. Br J Surg 74:634
Nakada I, Kawasaki S, Sonoda Y, Watanabe Y, Tabuchi T (2004) Abdominal stapled side-to-end anastomosis (Baker type) in low and high anterior resection: experiences and results in 69 consecutive patients at a regional general hospital in Japan. Colorectal Dis 6:165
Nance ML, Lutz N, Carr MC, Canning DA, Stafford PW (2004) Blunt renal injuries in children can be managed nonoperatively: outcome in a consecutive series of patients. J Trauma 57:474; discussion 478
Napal Lecumberri S, Pascual Piedrola I et al (1992) Kidney injuries: a review of 149 cases. A change in the diagnostic and therapeutic approaches. Arch Esp Urol 45:305
Nash PA, Bruce JE et al (1995) Nephrectomy for traumatic renal injuries. J Urol 153:609
Nasir GA, Baker KK (2001) Continuous double loop closure for midline laparotomy wounds. Saudi Med J 22:351
Nasser SM, Ewans PW (2001) Opiate-sensitivity: clinical characteristics and the role of skin prick testing. Clin Exp Allergy 31:1014
National Counterterrorism Center (2006) Worldwide Incidents Tracking System (WITS) of the National Counterterrorism Center. http://www.tkb.org/NCTC/Home.jsp. Cited 28 January 2006
National Guideline Clearinghouse (2002) 2002 National guidelines on the management of adult victims of sexual assault. http://www.guideline.gov/summary/summary.aspx?doc_id=3050. Cited 5 December 2006
Navarrete-Navarro P, Rodriguez A et al (2001) Adult respiratory distress syndrome among blunt and penetrating trauma patients: demographics, mortality, and resource utilization over 8 years. J Crit Care 16:47
Navascues del Rio JA, Arrojo Vila F et al (1997) Results of the conservative treatment of severe renal trauma in childhood. Actas Urol Esp 21:747
N'Dow J, Pearson, J Neal D (2004) Mucus production after transposition of intestinal segments into the urinary tract. World J Urol 22 178
Negri L, Albani E, Di Rocco M, Levi-Setti PE (2002) Aspermia and chronic testicular pain after imperforate anus correction. Cryopreservation of sperm cells extracted from whole orchiectomized testis: case report. Hum Reprod 17:2935
Neheman A, Nativ O, Moskovitz B et al (2005) Hyperbaric oxygen therapy for radiation-induced haemorrhagic cystitis. BJU Int 96:107
Nelson BA, Cookson MS, Smith JA Jr, Chang SS (2004) Complications of inguinal and pelvic lymphadenectomy for squamous cell carcinoma of the penis: a contemporary series. J Urol 172:494

Nelson CP, Dunn R, Wan J, Wei JT (2005) The increasing incidence of newborn circumcision: data from the nationwide inpatient sample. J Urol 173:978
Nelson JB, Chen RN, Bishoff JT, Oh WK, Kantoff PW, Donehower RC, Kavoussi LR (1999) Laparoscopic retroperitoneal lymph node dissection for clinical stage I nonseminomatous germ cell testicular tumors. Urology 54:1064
Nelson JH 3rd, Winter CC (1977) Priapism: evolution of management in 48 patients in a 22-year series. J Urol 117:455
Neuerburg JM, Lehrmann K (2004) Transarterial embolization of the kidney: review of the literature. Rofo 176:809
Neulander E, Walfisch S, Kaneti J (1996) Amputation of distal penile glans during neonatal ritual circumcision – a rate complication. Br J Urol. 77:924
Neulander EZ, Hawke CK, Soloway MS (2000) Incidental appendectomy during radical cystectomy: an interdepartmental survey and review of the literature. Urology 56:241
Nezhat C, Nezhat F, Ambroze W, Pennington E (1993) Laparoscopic repair of small bowel and colon. A report of 26 cases. Surg Endosc 7:88
Nguyen HT, PR Carroll (1995) Blunt renal trauma: renal preservation through careful staging and selective surgery. Semin Urol 13:83
Nguyen MM, Das S (2002) Pediatric renal trauma. Urology 59:762; discussion 766
Niall O, Russell J, MacGrego, R et al (1999) A comparison of noncontrast computerized tomography with excretory urography in the assessment of acute flank pain. J Urol 161:534
Nickel JC (2002) Acute pyelonephritis in adults. AUA Updates 21:306
Nickel JC, Heaton J, Morales A, Costerton JW (1986) Bacterial biofilm in persistent penile prosthesis-associated infection. J Urol 135:586
Nicol AJ, Theunissen D (2002) Renal salvage in penetrating kidney injuries: a prospective analysis. J Trauma 53:351
Nicolaides AN, Kakkar VV, Field ES, Renney JT (1971) The origin of deep vein thrombosis: a venographic study. Br J Radiol 44:653
Nicolaisen G, Melamud A, Williams RD, McAninch JW (1983) Rupture of the corpus cavernosum: surgical management. J Urol 130:917
Nicolaisen GS, McAninch JW, Marshall GA et al (1985) Renal trauma: re-evaluation of the indications for radiographic assessment. J Urol 133:183
Nieder AM, Meinbach DS, Kim SS, Soloway MS (2005) Transurethral bladder tumor resection: intraoperative and postoperative complications in a residency setting. J Urol 174:2307
Niel-Weise BS, Wille JC, van den Broek PJ (2005) Hair removal policies in clean surgery: systematic review of randomized, controlled trials. Infect Control Hosp Epidemiol 26:923
Nieminen MS, Boehm M, Cowie MR et al (2005) Executive summary of the guidelines on the diagnosis and treatment of acute heart failure: the Task Force on Acute Heart Failure of the European Society of Cardiology. Eur Heart J 26:384
Nijs E, Callahan MJ et al (2005) Disorders of the pediatric pancreas: imaging features. Pediatr Radiol 35:358
Ninomiya H, Kido M et al (1997) A surgical case of intrapericardial inferior vena cava injury complicating liver injury caused by a blunt trauma. Nippon Kyobu Geka Gakkai Zasshi 45:1616
Nippgen JB, Hakenberg OW, Manseck A, Wirth MP (2001) Spontaneous late rupture of orthotopic detubularized ileal neobladders: report of five cases. Urology 58:43
Nisbet AA, Thompson IM (2002) Impact of diabetes mellitus on the presentation and outcomes of Fournier's gangrene. Urology 60:775
Nisbeth U, Lindh E et al (1999) Increased fracture rate in diabetes mellitus and females after renal transplantation. Transplantation 67:1218
Nishikura T (1999) The clearance of procalcitonin (PCT) during continuous veno-venous hemodiafiltration (CVVHD) Intensive Care Med 25:1198
Nixon RG, O'Connor JL, Milam DF (2003) Efficacy of shunt surgery for refractory low flow priapism: a report on the incidence of failed detumescence and erectile dysfunction. J Urol 170:883
Noble JR, Mata JA, Humble RL, Culkin DJ (1990) Maxi-pouch: a new technique for ileal conduit conversion to continent urinary reservoir. J Urol 143:116
Noe HN (1996) Imaging in pediatric blunt renal trauma. J Urol 156:2019
Noh J, Kang TW, Heo T et al (2004) Penile strangulation treated with the modified string method. Urology 64:591
Nolte-Ernsting CC, Bücker A, Adam GB, Neuerburg JM, Jung P, Hunter DW, Jakse G, Günther RW (1998) Gadolinium-enhanced excretory MR urography after low-dose diuretic injection: comparison with conventional excretory urography. Radiology 209:147
Nolte-Ernsting CC, Bücker A, Neuerburg JM, Glowinski A, Adam GB, Günther RW (1999) MR imaging-guided percutaneous nephrostomy and use of MR-compatible catheters in the nondilated porcine urinary tract. J Vasc Interv Radiol 10:1305
Nolte-Ernsting CC, Tacke J, Adam GB et al (2001) Diuretic-enhanced gadolinium excretory MR urography: comparison of conventional gradient-echo sequences and echo-planar imaging. Eur Radiol 11:18
Nomura G (1996) Hypertension following renal trauma. Ryoikibetsu Shokogun Shirizu 12:83
Noone TC, Semelka RC, Worawattanakul S, Marcos HB (1998) Intraperitoneal abscesses: diagnostic accuracy of and appearances at MR imaging. Radiology 208:525
Noone TC, Semelka RC, Chaney DM, Reinhold C (2004) Abdominal imaging studies: comparison of diagnostic accuracies resulting from ultrasound, computed tomography, and magnetic resonance imaging in the same individual. Magn Reson Imaging 22:19
Noor MA, Ather MH (2003) Difference in the outcome of patients managed with isolated renal injury and co-existent abdominal organ injury. J Ayub Med Coll Abbottabad 15:29
Nordstrom M, Lindblad B, Bergqvist D, Kjellstrom T (1992) A prospective study of the incidence of deep-vein thrombosis within a defined urban population. J Intern Med 232:155
Norkool DM, Hampson NB, Gibbons RP et al (1993) Hyperbaric oxygen therapy for radiation-induced hemorrhagic cystitis. J Urol 150:332
Norlen H, Allgen LG (1993) A comparison between intermittent and continuous transurethral resection of the prostate. Scand J Urol Nephrol 27:21
Novak I (1996) Kidney injuries in childhood. Rozhl Chir 75:599
Novelline RA, Rhea JT et al (1999) Helical CT of abdominal trauma. Radiol Clin North Am 37:591:vi-vii
Novozhilova AP, Kuleshov VI et al (1999) Structural changes in the parenchymatous organs in animals in venous gas embolism of varying intensity and acute decompression disease. Morfologiia 115:41
Numan F, Cakirer S, Islak C, Ogut G, Kadioglu A, Cayan S, Tellaloglu S (1996) Posttraumatic high-flow priapism treated by N-butyl-cyanoacrylate embolisation. Cardiovasc Intervent Radiol 19:278
Nunes LW et al (2001) Diagnostic performance of trauma US in identifying abdominal or pelvic free fluid and serious abdominal or pelvic injury. Acad Radiol 8:128
Nunez D Jr, Becerra JL, Fuentes D et al (1996) Traumatic occlusion of the renal artery: helical CT diagnosis. AJR Am J Roentgenol 167:777

Nunez D Jr, Rivas L et al (1998) Helical CT of traumatic arterial injuries. AJR Am J Roentgenol 170:1621
Nurmohamed MT, Verhaeghe R, Haas S, Iriarte JA, Vogel G, van Rij AM, Prentice CR, ten Cate JW (1995) A comparative trial of a low molecular weight heparin (enoxaparin) versus standard heparin for the prophylaxis of postoperative deep vein thrombosis in general surgery. Am J Surg 169:567
Nuss R, Hays T, Manco-Johnson M (1994) Efficacy and safety of heparin anticoagulation for neonatal renal vein thrombosis. Am J Pediatr Hematol Oncol 16:127
Nussbaum SR, Younger J, Vandepol CJ et al (1993) Single-dose intravenous therapy with pamidronate for the treatment of hypercalcemia of malignancy: comparison of 30-, 60-, and 90-mg dosages. Am J Med 95:297
Nussbaum Blask AR, Nicholson HS et al (1999) Sonographic detection of uterine and ovarian abnormalities in female survivors of Wilms' tumor treated with radiotherapy. AJR Am J Roentgenol 172:759
Nussbaum Blask AR, Bulas D, Shalaby-Rana E, Rushton G, Shao C, Majd M (2002) Color Doppler sonography and scintigraphy of the testis: a prospective, comparative analysis in children with acute scrotal pain. Pediatr Emerg Care 18:67
Nygaard IE, Kreder KJ (1996) Spine update. Urological management in patients with spinal cord injuries. Spine 21:128
Obara W, Ohuchi A et al (2001) A case of congenital hydronephrosis suffering from rupture of the renal pelvis due to trauma. Hinyokika Kiyo 47:425
Ochsner MG Jr et al (1989) Pelvic fracture as an indicator of increased risk of thoracic aortic rupture. J Trauma 29:1376
O'Connor AR, Coakley FV, Meng MV, Eberhardt SC (2003) Imaging of retained surgical sponges in the abdomen and pelvis. AJR Am J Roentgenol 180:481
Oderich GS, Panneton JM et al (2004) Iatrogenic operative injuries of abdominal and pelvic veins: a potentially lethal complication. J Vasc Surg 39:931
Oelschlager BK, Boyle EM Jr et al (1997) Delayed abdominal closure in the management of ruptured abdominal aortic aneurysms. Am J Surg 173:411
Oesterling JE, Besinger RE, Brendler CB (1988) Spontaneous rupture of the renal collecting system during pregnancy: successful management with a temporary ureteral catheter. J Urol 140:588
Ogan K, Cadeddu JA (2005) Liver injury during urologic laparoscopy. In: Ramakumar S, Jarrett T (eds) Complications of urologic laparoscopic surgery. Taylor & Francis, Boca Raton, p 73
Oger E (2000) Incidence of venous thromboembolism: a community-based study in Western France. EPI-GETBP Study Group. Groupe d'Etude de la Thrombose de Bretagne Occidentale. Thromb Haemost 83:657
O'Grady NP, Barie PS, Bartlett J, Bleck T, Garvey G, Jacobi J, Linden P, Maki DG, Nam M, Pasculle W, Pasquale MD, Tribett DL, Masur H (1998) Practice parameters for evaluating new fever in critically ill adult patients. Task Force of the American College of Critical Care Medicine of the Society of Critical Care Medicine in collaboration with the Infectious Disease Society of America. Crit Care Med 26:392
O'Grady NP, Barie PS, Bartlett JG, Bleck T, Garvey G, Jacobi J, Linden P, Maki DG, Nam M, Pasculle W, Pasquale MD, Tribett DL, Masur H (1998) Practice guidelines for evaluating new fever in critically ill adult patients. Task Force of the Society of Critical Care Medicine and the Infectious Diseases Society of America. Clin Infect Dis 26:1042
O'Grady NP, Alexander M, Dellinger EP, Gerberding JL, Heard SO, Maki DG, Masur H, McCormick RD, Mermel LA, Pearson ML, Raad II, Randolph A, Weinstein RA (2002) Guidelines for the prevention of intravascular catheter-related infections. Am J Infect Control 30:476
Ohashi H, Oda H et al (1999) Predictors of survival in continuous ambulatory peritoneal dialysis patients: the importance of left ventricular hypertrophy and diabetic nephropathy. Adv Perit Dial 15:87
Ohman EM, Casey C, Bengtson JR, Pryor D, Tormey W, Horgan JH (1990) Early detection of acute myocardial infarction: additional diagnostic information from serum concentrations of myoglobin in patients without ST elevation. Br Heart J 63:335
Ok JH, Meyers FJ, Evans CP (2005) Medical and surgical palliative care of patients with urological malignancies. J Urol 174:1177
Okaneya T, Kontani K, Komiyama I et al (1993) Severe cyclophosphamide-induced hemorrhagic cystitis successfully treated by total cystectomy with ileal neobladder substitution: a case report. J Urol 150:1909
O'Keeffe NK, Mortimer AJ, Sambrook PA, Rao PN (1993) Severe sepsis following percutaneous or endoscopic procedures for urinary tract stones. Br J Urol 72:277
Okeke LI (2000) Fournier's gangrene in Ibadan. Afr J Med Sci 29:323
Okita Y, Ando M et al (1999) Early and long-term results of surgery for aneurysms of the thoracic aorta in septuagenarians and octogenarians. Eur J Cardiothorac Surg 16:317
Okizuka H, Sugimura K, Yoshizako T (1992) Fournier's gangrene: diagnosis based on MR findings. AJR Am J Roentgenol 158:1173
Okpala I, Westerdale N, Jegede T et al (2002) Etilefrine for the prevention of priapism in adult sickle cell disease. Br J Haematol 118:918
Oktar SÖ, Yucel C, Özdemir H, Karaosmanoglu D (2004) Doppler sonography of renal obstruction: value of venous impedance index measurements. J Ultrasound Med 23:929
Okur H, Kucikaydin M, Kazez A, Turan C, Bozkurt A (1996) Genitourinary tract injuries in girls. Br J Urol 78:446
Oldhafer KJ, Frerker M et al (1999) Complex inferior vena cava and renal vein reconstruction after abdominal gunshot injury. J Trauma 46:721
Oliveira EA, Diniz JS, Vilasboas AS, Rabelo EA, Silva JM, Filgueiras MT (2001) Multicystic dysplastic kidney detected by fetal sonography: conservative management and follow-up. Pediatr Surg Int 17:54
Olofsen-van Acht MJ, Quint S et al (1999) Three-dimensional treatment planning for postoperative radiotherapy in patients with node-positive cervical cancer. Comparison between a conventional and a conformal technique. Strahlenther Onkol 175:462
Olsson I, Kroon U (1999) A three-year postoperative evaluation of tension-free vaginal tape. Gynecol Obstet Invest 48:267
Olsson J, Nilsson A, Hahn RG (1995) Symptoms of the transurethral resection syndrome using glycine as the irrigant. J Urol 154:123
Olszewski WL (1991) Lymph stasis: pathophysiology diagnosis and treatment. In: Olszewski WL (ed) Lymphology and the lymphatic system. CRC Press, Boca Raton, p 3
Olszewski WL (2005) The innate reaction of the human skin lymphatic system to foreign and self-antigens. Lymphat Res Biol 3:50
Olszewski WL, Loe K, Engeset A (1978) Immune proteins and other biochemical constituents of peripheral lymph in patients with malignancy and postirradiation lymphedema. Lymphology 11:174
O'Moore PV, Mueller PR, Simeone JF, Saini S, Butch RJ, Hahn PF, Steiner E, Stark DD, Ferrucci JT Jr (1987) Sonographic guidance in diagnostic and therapeutic interventions in the pleural space. AJR Am J Roentgenol 149:1
Ondrus D, Hornak M, Breza J et al (2001) Delayed orchiectomy

after chemotherapy in patients with advanced testicular cancer. Int Urol Nephrol 32:665
O'Neill PJ, Feldman DR et al (1996) Trans-jugular extraction of bullet embolus to the heart. Mil Med 161:360
Onen A, Kaya M et al (2002) Blunt renal trauma in children with previously undiagnosed pre-existing renal lesions and guidelines for effective initial management of kidney injury. BJU Int 89:936
Onur R, Ozden M, Orhan I, Kalkan A, Semercioz A (2004) Incidence of bacteraemia after urodynamic study. J Hosp Infect 57:241
Opal SM, Garber GE, La Rosa SP et al (2003) Systemic host responses in severe sepsis analyzed by causative microorganism and treatment effects of drotrecogin alfa (activated). Clin Infect Dis 37:50
O'Reilly KJ, Hampson NB, Corman JM (2002) Hyperbaric oxygen in urology. AUA Update Series 21:26
Ortega AE, Tang E et al (1996) Laparoscopic evaluation of penetrating thoracoabdominal traumatic injuries. Surg Endosc 10:19
Orvis BR, McAninch JW (1989) Penile rupture. Urol Clin North Am 16:369
Osman Y, Shokeir A, Ali El-Dein B, Tantawy M, Wafa EW, Shehab El-Dein AB, Ghoneim MA (2003) Vascular complications after live donor renal transplantation: study of risk factors and effects on graft and patient survival. J Urol 169:859
Ostroff EB, Chenault Ow Jr (1982) Alum irrigation for the control of massive bladder hemorrhage. J Urol 128:929
Ostrzenski A, Ostrzenska KM (1998) Bladder injury during laparoscopic surgery. Obstet Gynecol Surv 53:175
Ostrzenski A, Radolinski B, Ostrzenska KM (2003) A review of laparoscopic ureteral injury in pelvic surgery. Obstet Gynecol Surv 58:794
Ostrzenski A, Radolinski B, Ostrzenska KM (2003) A review of laparoscopic ureteral injury in pelvic surgery. Obstet Gynecol Surv 58:794
O'Sullivan P, Browne R, McEniff N, Lee MJ (2006) Treatment of „high-flow" priapism with superselective transcatheter embolization: a useful alternative to surgery. Cardiovasc Intervent Radiol 29:198–201
Otte A, Herrmann R et al (1999) Yttrium 90 DOTATOC: a new somatostatin analog for cancer therapy of neuroendocrine tumors. Schweiz Rundsch Med Prax 88:1263
Oude Nijhuis CS, Gietema JA, Vellenga et al (2003) Routine radiography does not have a role in the diagnostic evaluation of ambulatory adult febrile neutropenic cancer patients. Eur J Cancer 39:2495
Ovalle A, Levancini M (2001) Urinary tract infections in pregnancy. Curr Opin Urol 11:55
Overby MC, Rothman AS (1985) Anterolateral decompression for metastatic epidural spinal cord tumors. J Neurosurg 62:344
Overholt RH (1931) Intraperitoneal pressure. Arch Surg 22:691
Ozdemir S, Cekirge S et al (1998) A rare complication of renal biopsy in a child with membranoproliferative glomerulonephritis. Int Urol Nephrol 30:689
Özer H, Armitage JO, Bennett CL et al (2000) 2000 update of recommendations for the use of hematopoietic colony-stimulating factors: evidence-based, clinical practice guidelines. J Clin Oncol 18:3558
Özer C, Yencilek E, Apaydin FD et al (2004) Diagnostic value of renal parenchyma density difference on unenhanced helical computed tomography scan in acutely obstructing ureteral stone disease. Urology 64:223
Ozkan S, Gurpinar T (1997) A serious circumcision complication: penile shaft amputation and a new reattachment technique with a successful outcome. J Urol 158:1946
Ozturk H, Otcu S et al (2003) Retroperitoneal organ injury caused by anterior penetrating abdominal injury in children. Eur J Emerg Med 10:164
Ozturk H, Dokucu AI et al (2004) Non-operative management of isolated solid organ injuries due to blunt abdominal trauma in children: a fifteen-year experience. Eur J Pediatr Surg 14:29
Ozucelik DN, Karcioglu O (1999) Kidney rupture following extracorporeal shock wave lithotripsy. Acad Emerg Med 6:664
Pagano S, Pachera F et al (1999) Complete pyelo-calyceal avulsion as a result of blunt abdominal trauma. Scand J Urol Nephrol 33:66
Palgon N, Greenstein F, Novetsky AD, Lichter SM, Rosen Y (1986) Hyperglycemia associated with renal cell carcinoma. Urology 28:516
Palmer KJ, Benson GS, Corriere JN Jr (1983) Diagnosis and initial management of urological injuries associated with 200 consecutive pelvis fracture. J Urol 130:712
Palmer LS, Winter HI, Tolia BM et al (1995) The limited impact of involved surface area and surgical debridement on survival in Fournier's gangrene. Br J Urol 76:208
Palmer LS, Rosenbaum RR, Gershbaum MD et al (1999) Penetrating ureteral trauma at an urban trauma center:10-year experience. Urology 54:34
Palou J, Angerri O, Segarra J et al (2003) Intravesical bacillus Calmette-Guerin for the treatment of superficial bladder cancer in renal transplant patients. Transplantation 76:1514
Pan American Health Organization (2000) Epidemiologic surveillance and disease control. In: Natural disasters: protecting the public health. World Health Organization, Pan American Health Organization, Washington, DC, p 43
Pansadoro A, Franco G, Laurenti C, Pansadoro V (2002) Conservative treatment of intraperitoneal bladder perforation during transurethral resection of bladder tumor. Urology 60:682
Pansadoro V, Emiliozzi P (1996) Internal urethrotomy in the management of anterior urethral strictures: long-term follow-up. J Urol 156:73
Pantanowitz L, Kruskall MS, Uhl L (2003) Cryoprecipitate. Patterns of use. Am J Clin Pathol 119:874
Papac RJ, Poo-Hwu WJ (1999) Renal cell carcinoma: a paradigm of lanthanic disease. Am J Clin Oncol 22:223
Papadopoulos I, Kelami A (1988) Priapus and priapism. From mythology to medicine. Urology 32:385
Papadopoulou D, Tsakiris D, Papadimitriou M (1999) The use of ultrasonography and linkage studies for early diagnosis of autosomal dominant polycystic kidney disease (ADPKD) Ren Fail 21:67
Paquette EL, Sun L, Paquette LR et al (2002) Improved prostate cancer-specific survival and other disease parameters: impact of prostate-specific antigen testing. Urology 60:756
Paragioudaki M, Stamouli V, Kolonitsiou F, Anastassiou ED, Dimitracopoulos G, Spiliopoulou I (2004) Intravenous catheter infections associated with bacteraemia: a 2-year study in a university hospital. Clin Microbiol Infect 10:431
Parikh AM, Milroy EJ (1995) Precautions and complications in the use of the UroLume wall stent. Eur Urol 27:1
Park DS, Park JH, Lee YT (2002) Percutaneous nephrostomy versus indwelling ureteral stents in patients with bilateral nongenitourinary malignant extrinsic obstruction. J Endourol 16:153
Park JH, Chung JW, Cho YK, Kim SH, Ahn H, Oh BH (1997) Percutaneous fenestration of aortic dissection: salvage of an ischemic solitary left kidney. Cardiovasc Intervent Radiol 20:146
Park JK, Yang SO et al (2001) Duodenal obstruction by retroperitoneal hematoma induced by severe blunt renal trauma. J Urol 165:1993
Parker CR, Freemont AJ et al (1999) Cross-sectional analysis of

renal transplantation osteoporosis. J Bone Miner Res 14: 1943
Parra RO, Hagood PG, Boullier JA, Cummings JM, Mehan DJ (1994) Complications of laparoscopic urological surgery: experience at St. Louis University. J Urol 151:681
Parrillo JE (2005) Severe sepsis and therapy with activated protein C. N Engl J Med 353:1398
Parsons CL, Benson G, Childs SJ et al (1993) A quantitatively controlled method to study prospectively interstitial cystitis and demonstrate the efficacy of pentosan polysulfate. J Urol 150:845
Parsons CL, Forrest J, Nickel JC et al (2002) Effect of pentosan polysulfate therapy on intravesical potassium sensitivity. Urology 59:329
Parsons JK, Schoenberg MP (2001) Successful conservative management of perforated ileal neobladder. J Urol 165:1214
Parsons JK, Jarrett TW, Lancini V, Kavoussi LR (2002) Infundibular stenosis after percutaneous nephrolithotomy. J Urol 167:35
Partrick DA, Bensard DD et al (1999) Nonoperative management of solid organ injuries in children results in decreased blood utilization. J Pediatr Surg 34:1695
Parvathy U, Saldanha R et al (2003) Blunt abdominal trauma resulting in urinothorax from a missed uretero-pelvic junction avulsion: case report. J Trauma 54:187
Pascual Samaniego M, Fernandez Dominguez L et al (2003) Traumatic intrathoracic herniation of the left kidney. Actas Urol Esp 27:229
Pasquier D, Hoelscher T, Schmutz J et al (2004) Hyperbaric oxygen therapy in the treatment of radio-induced lesions in normal tissues: a literature review. Radiother Oncol 72:1
Pastore LM, Savitz DA, Thorp JM Jr et al (1999) Predictors of symptomatic urinary tract infection after 20 weeks' gestation. J Perinatol 19:488
Pastore LM, Savitz DA, Thorp JM Jr (1999) Predictors of urinary tract infection at the first prenatal visit. Epidemiology 10:282
Paszkowski AL, Hewitt DJ, Taylor A Jr (1999) Disseminated intravascular coagulation in a patient treated with strontium-89 for metastatic carcinoma of the prostate. Clin Nucl Med 24:852
Patchell RA, Tibbs PA, Regine WF (2005) Direct decompressive surgical resection in the treatment of spinal cord compression caused by metastatic cancer: a randomised trial. Lancet 366:643
Patel AK, Chapple CR (2006) Female urethral diverticula. Curr Opin Urol 16:248
Patel HP, Bissler JJ (2001) Hematuria in children. Pediatr Clin North Am 48:1519
Patel R, Caruso RP et al (2003) Use of fibrin glue and gelfoam to repair collecting system injuries in a porcine model: implications for the technique of laparoscopic partial nephrectomy. J Endourol 17:799
Patel SS, Balfour JA, Bryson HM (1997) Fosfomycin tromethamine: a review of its antibacterial activity, pharmacokinetic properties and therapeutic efficacy as single-dose oral treatment for acute uncomplicated lower urinary tract infection. Drugs 53:637
Patel VG, Walker ML (1997) The role of one-shot intravenous pyelogram in evaluation of penetrating abdominal trauma. Am Surg 63:350
Paterson DL, Patel A (1998) Bacillus Calmette-Guerin (BCG) immunotherapy for bladder cancer: review of complications and their treatment. Aust N Z J Surg 68:340
Pathak AS, Chang JH, Parekh AR, Aboseif SR (2005) Use of rectus fascia graft for corporeal reconstruction during placement of penile implant. Urology 65:1198
Pathak IG, Williams DI (1964) Multicystic and cystic dysplastic kidneys. Br J Urol 36:318
Patil MG, Onuora VC (1994) The value of ultrasound in the evaluation of patients with blunt scrotal trauma. Injury 25:177
Paty R, Smith AD (1992) Gangrene and Fournier's gangrene. Urol Clin North Am 19:149
Paul LC (1999) Chronic allograft nephropathy: An update. Kidney Int 56:783
Pavlica P, Barozzi L (2001) Imaging of the acute scrotum. Eur Radiol 11:220
Payen JF, Bru O, Bosson JL et al (2001) Assessing pain in critically ill sedated patients by using a behavioral pain scale. Crit Care Med 12:2258
Peacock PR Jr, Souto HL et al (2001) What is gross hematuria? Correlation of subjective and objective assessment. J Trauma 50:1060
Pearle MS (2003) Pediatric staghorn calculi: the role of extracorporeal shock wave lithotripsy monotherapy with special reference to ureteral stenting. Int Braz J Urol 29:168
Pearle MS, Pierce HL, Miller GL et al (1998) Optimal method of urgent decompression of the collecting system for obstruction and infection due to ureteral calculi. J Urol 160:1260
Peclet MH, Newman KD et al (1990) Thoracic trauma in children: an indicator of increased mortality. J Pediatr Surg 25:961; discussion 965
Pedersen H, Finster M (1979) Anaesthetic risk in the pregnant surgical patient. Anaethesiology 51:439
Peleg K, Aharonson-Daniel L (2005) Blast injuries. New Engl J Med 352:2651
Peleg K, Aharonson-Daniel L, Michael M et al (2003) Patterns of injury in hospitalized terrorist victims. Am J Emerg Med 21:258
Peleg K, Aharonson-Daniel L, Stein M et al (2004) Gunshot and explosion injuries: characteristics, outcomes, and implications for care of terror-related injuries in Israel. Ann Surg 239:311
Pelger RC, Soerdjbalie-Maikoe V, Hamdy NA (2001) Strategies for management of prostate cancer-related bone pain. Drugs Aging 18:899
Peña A, deVries PA (1982) Posterior sagittal anorectoplasty: important technical considerations and new applications. J Ped Surg 17:796
Pena A, Levitt MA, Hong A, Midulla P (2004) Surgical management of cloacal malformations: a review of 339 patients. J Pediatr Surg 39:470
Pennal GF, Tile M, Waddell JP, Garside H (1980) Pelvic disruption: assessment and classification. Clin Orthop 151:12
Pepper RJ, Pati J, Kaisary AV (2005) The incidence and treatment of lymphoceles after radical retropubic prostatectomy. BJU Int 95:772
Perazella M, Brown E (1993) Acute aluminum toxicity and alum bladder irrigation in patients with renal failure. Am J Kidney Dis 21:44–46
Perdue PW, Watts DD et al (1998) Differences in mortality between elderly and younger adult trauma patients: geriatric status increases risk of delayed death. J Trauma 45:805
Pereverzev AS, Shchukin DV, Iliukhin IA et al (2005) Spontaneous ruptures of renal tumors. Urologiia 2:21
Perez CA (1998) Uterine cervix. In: Perez CA, Brady LW (eds) Principles and practice of radiation oncology. Lippincott-Raven, Philadelphia
Perez-Brayfield MR, Gatti JM et al (2002) Blunt traumatic hematuria in children. Is a simplified algorithm justified? J Urol 167:2543; discussion 2546
Perini S, Gordon RL, LaBerge JM, Kerlan RK Jr, Wilson MW, Feng S, Ring EJ (1998) Transcatheter embolization of biopsy-related vascular injury in the transplant kidney: immediate and long-term outcome. J Vasc Interv Radiol 9:1011
Perouansky M, Oppenheim A et al (1999) Effect of haemofil-

tration on pathological fibrinolysis due to severe sepsis: a case report. Resuscitation 40:53
Perrin LC, Goh J, Crandon AJ (1995) The treatment of recurrent pelvic lymphocysts with marsupialization and functioning omental flap. Aust N Z J Obstet Gynaecol 35:195
Perry MJ, Porte ME et al (1997) Limitations of ultrasound evaluation in acute closed renal trauma. J R Coll Surg Edinb 42:420
Perry MO, Husmann DA (1992) Urethral injuries in female subjects following pelvic fractures. J Urol 147:139
Perry R, Kecha O, Paquette J, Huot C, Van Vliet G, Deal C (2005) Primary adrenal insufficiency in children: twenty years experience at the Sainte-Justine Hospital Montreal. J Clin Endocrinol Metab 90:3243
Pershad J, Gilmore B (2000) Serial bedside emergency ultrasound in a case of pediatric blunt abdominal trauma with severe abdominal pain. Pediatr Emerg Care 16:375
Pescovitz MD (2004) The use of rituximab, anti-CD20 monoclonal antibody, in pediatric transplantation. Pediatr Transplant 8:9
Petero VG, Jr Diokno AC (2006) Comparison of the long-term outcomes between incontinent men and women treated with artificial urinary sphincter. J Urol 175:605
Peters AM (1998) The use of nuclear medicine in infections. Br J Radiol 71:252
Peters CA (1996) Complications in pediatric urological laparoscopy: results of a survey. J Urol 155:1070
Peterson NE (1991) Re: attempted nonoperative management of blunt renal lacerations extending through the corticomedullary junction: the short-term and long-term sequelae. J Urol 145:154
Peterson NE (1992) Repair of a traumatically amputated penis with return of erectile function. J Urol 147:1628
Peterson NE (2000) Genitourinary trauma. In: Mattox KL, Feliciano DV, Moore EE (eds) Trauma, 4th edn. McGraw-Hill, New York, p 839
Peterson NE, Moore EE (1997) Bilateral renal artery thrombosis secondary to blunt trauma. J Trauma 43:561
Petridis A, Pilavaki M et al (1999) CT of hemodynamically unstable abdominal trauma. Eur Radiol 9:250
Pettila V, Leinonen P, Markkola A, Hiilesmaa V, Kaaja R (2002) Postpartum bone mineral density in women treated for thromboprophylaxis with unfractionated heparin or LMW heparin. Thromb Haemost 87:182
Pfister RC, Newhouse JH (1979) Interventional percutaneous pyeloureteral techniques. II. Percutaneous nephrostomy and other procedures. Radiol Clin North Am 17:351
Pfitzenmaier J, Lotz J, Faldum A et al (2003) Metabolic evaluation of 94 patients 5 to 16 years after ileocecal pouch (Mainz pouch 1) continent urinary diversion. J Urol 170:1884
Phadke RV, Sawlani V et al (1997) Iatrogenic renal vascular injuries and their radiological management. Clin Radiol 52:119
Philips FS, Sternberg SS, Cronin AP (1961) Cyclophosphamide and urinary bladder toxicity. Cancer Res 21:1577
Philips TM, Bishoff JT (2005) Bowel injury. In: Ramakumar S, Jarrett T (eds) Complications of urologic laparoscopic surgery. Taylor & Francis, Boca Raton, p 49
Phillips JR, Karlowicz MG (1997) Prevalence of Candida species in hospital-acquired urinary tract infections in a neonatal intensive care unit. Pediatr Infect Dis J 16:190
Philpott JM, Nance ML et al (2003) Ureteral stenting in the management of urinoma after severe blunt renal trauma in children. J Pediatr Surg 38:1096
Pickenpack A, Lang B et al (1999) A 63-year-old patient with worsening general condition, bone demineralization, hypocalcemia and excess parathyroid hormone: late manifestations of pseudohypohyperparathyroidism. Dtsch Med Wochenschr 124:551
Pickhardt PJ, Shimony JS et al (1999) The abdominal compartment syndrome: CT findings. AJR Am J Roentgenol 173:575
Pickleman J, Lee RM (1989) The management of patients with suspected early postoperative small bowel obstruction. Ann Surg 210:216
Pieri S, Agresti P, La Pera G, Atzori M, Ialongo P (2005) Post-traumatic high flow priapism percutaneously treated with transcatheter embolisation. Radiol Med (Torino) 110:370
Pietrera P, Badachi Y et al (2001) Ultrasound for initial evaluation of post-traumatic renal lesions in children. J Radiol 82:833
Pigolkin Iu I, Denisova OP et al (1997) The forensic medical diagnosis of kidney trauma. Sud Med Ekspert 40:6
Pilmore HL, Walker RJ, Solomon C, Packer S, Wood D (1995) Acute bilateral renal artery occlusion: successful revascularization with streptokinase. Am J Nephrol 15:90
Ping AJ, Reeve AE, Law DJ, Young MR, Boehnke M, Feinberg AP (1989) Genetic linkage of Beckwith-Wiedemann syndrome to 11p. Am J Hum Genet, 44:720
Pintér AB, Hock A, Vástyán A, Farkas A (1996) Does the posterior sagittal approach with the perirectal dissection impair fecal continence in a normal rectum? J Ped Surg 31:1349
Pirsch JD, Friedman R (1994) Primary care of the renal transplant patient. J Gen Intern Med 9:29
Pisco JM, Martins JM, Correia MG (1989) Internal iliac artery: embolization to control hemorrhage from pelvic neoplasms. Radiology 172:337
Pisegna JR, Martindale RG (2005) Acid suppression in the perioperative period. J Clin Gastroenterol 39:10
Piso P, Dahlke MH, Mirena P, Schmidt U, Aselmann H, Schlitt HJ, Raab R, Klempnauer J (2004) Total mesorectal excision for middle and lower rectal cancer: a single institution experience with 337 consecutive patients. J Surg Oncol 86:115
Pittet D, Thievent B, Wenzel RP, Li N, Auckenthaler R Suter PM (1996) Bedside prediction of mortality from bacteremic sepsis: a dynamic analysis of ICU patients. Am J Respir Crit Care Med 153:684
Pittrow L, Penk A (1999) Special pharmacokinetics of fluconazole in septic, obese and burn patients. Mycoses 42 [Suppl 2]:87
Pitts JC III, Peterson NE (1981) Penetrating injuries of the ureter. J Trauma 21:978
Pizzorno R, Bonini F, Donelli A, Stubinski R, Medica M, Carmignani G (1997) Hyperbaric oxygen therapy in the treatment of Fournier's disease in 11 male patients. J Urol 158: 837
Platell C, Hall JC (1997) Atelectasis after abdominal surgery. J Am Coll Surg 185:584
Podesta A, Hafez A, El-Assmy A, Sarhan O, El-Hefnawy A, Ghoneim M (2005) Perineal anastomotic urethroplasty for managing post-traumatic urethral strictures in children: the long-term outcome. BJU Int 95:403
Pohl HG, Shukla AR, Metcalf PD, Cilento BG, Retik AB, Bagli DJ et al (2004) Prepubertal testis tumors: actual prevalence rate of histological types. J Urol 172:2370
Pokorny M, Pontes JE, Pierce JM Jr (1978) Urological injuries associated with pelvic trauma. J Urol 121:455
Polderman KH, Girbes AR (2002) Central venous catheter use. Part 2: infectious complications. Intensive Care Med 28:18
Poldermans D, Boersma E (2005) Beta-blocker therapy in noncardiac surgery. N Engl J Med 4:412
Polkey HJ, Vynalek WJ (1933) Spontaneous non-traumatic perirenal and renal hematomas: an experimental and clinical study. Arch Surg 26:196
Pollack HM, Wein AJ (1989) Imaging of renal trauma. Radiology 172:297
Pollen JJ, Funckes C (1982) Traumatic dislocation of the testes. J Trauma 22:247

Pomer S, Karcher G, Simon W (1983) Cutaneous ureterostomy as last resort treatment of intractable haemorrhagic cystitis following radiation. Br J Urol 55:392
Pontes JE, Pierce JM Jr (1978) Anterior urethral injuries: four years of experience at the Detroit General Hospital. J Urol 120:563
Poole GV et al (1991) Pelvic fracture from major blunt trauma. Outcome is determined by associated injuries. Ann Surg 213:532; discussion 538
Poole GV et al (1992) Complications of pelvic fractures from blunt trauma. Am Surg 58:225
Poole GV Jr (1985) Mechanical factors in abdominal wound closure: the prevention of fascial dehiscence. Surgery 97:631
Porodenko VA (1999) Specific features of kidney injuries altered by disease. Sud Med Ekspert 42:18
Porter JM, Singh Y (1998) Value of computed tomography in the evaluation of retroperitoneal organ injury in blunt abdominal trauma. Am J Emerg Med 16:225
Porter JR (2004) Management of intra- and postoperative complications. In: Cadeddu JA (ed) Laparoscopic urologic oncology. Humana Press, Totowa, p 329
Porter JR, Takayama TK, Defalco AJ (1997) Traumatic posterior urethral injury and early realigment using magnetic urethral catheters. J Urol 158:425
Potter SR, Kavoussi LR, Jackman SV (2001) Management of diaphragmatic injury during laparoscopic nephrectomy. J Urol 165:1203
Powell MA, Nicholas JM et al (1999) Blunt ureteropelvic junction disruption. J Trauma 47:186
Praveen BV, Sankaranarayanan A, Vaidyanathan S (1992) A comparative study of intravesical instillation of 15(s) 15 Me alpha and alum in the management of persistent hematuria of vesical origin. Int J Clin Pharmacol Ther Toxicol 30:7
Preminger GM, Assimos DG, Lingeman JE et al (2005) Chapter 1: AUA guideline on management of staghorn calculi: diagnosis and treatment recommendations. J Urol 173:1991
Presti JC Jr, Carroll PR, McAninch JW (1989) Ureteral and renal pelvic injuries from external trauma: diagnosis and management. J Trauma 29:370
Pretorius ES, Siegelman ES, Ramchandani P, Banner MP (2001) MR imaging of the penis. Radiographics 21:S283; discussion S2989
Price FV, Resnik E, Heller KA et al (1991) Placenta previa percreta involving the urinary bladder: a report of two cases and review of the literature. Obstet Gynecol 78:508
Prieto Chaparro L, Silmi Moyano A et al (1992) Renal injury on a pathological kidney. Incidence, management, and results of treatment. Arch Esp Urol 45:407
Prins MH, Hutten BA, Koopman MM, Buller HR (1999) Long-term treatment of venous thromboembolic disease. Thromb Haemost 82:892
Propst AM, Thorp JM Jr (1998) Traumatic vulvar hematomas: conservative versus surgical management. South Med J 91:144
Pruthi RS, Issa MM et al (1998) Renal masses presenting 25 and 50 years following blunt renal trauma. Urol Int 61:43
Pruthi RS, Chun, Richman M (2004) The use of a fibrin tissue sealant during laparoscopic partial nephrectomy. BJU Int 93:813
Pulsion Technology. PiCCO-System, Pulsion Technology, http://www.pulsion.com. Cited 6 Novemer 2006
Pumphrey RS (2000) Lessons for management of anaphylaxis from a study of fatal reactions. Clin Exp Allergy 30:1144
Puppo P, Ricciotti G, Bozzo W, Introini C (1999) Primary endoscopic treatment of ureteric calculi. A review of 378 cases. Eur Urol 36:48
Purdie KJ, Pennington J et al (1999) The promoter of a novel human papillomavirus (HPV77) associated with skin cancer displays UV responsiveness, which is mediated through a consensus p53 binding sequence. EMBO J 18:5359
Purohit OP, Radstone CR, Anthony C et al (1995) A randomised double-blind comparison of intravenous pamidronate and clodronate in the hypercalcaemia of malignancy. Br J Cancer 72:1289
Pusajo JF, Bumaschny EB, Doglio GR, Cherjovsky MR, Lipinszki AI, Hernandez MS, Egurrola MA (1993) Postoperative intra-abdominal sepsis requiring reoperation. Arch Surg 128:218
Puskar D, Balagovic I, Filipovic A et al (2001) Symptomatic physiologic hydronephrosis in pregnancy: incidence, complications, and treatment. Eur Urol 39:260
Pycha A, Lodde M, Lusuardi L, Palermo S, Signorello D, Galantini A, Mian C, Hohenfellner R (2003) Teaching transurethral resection of the bladder: still a challenge? Urology 62:46
Qiang W, Jianchen W, MacDonald R, Monga M, Wilt TJ (2005) Antibiotic prophylaxis for transurethral prostatic resection in men with preoperative urine containing less than 100,000 bacteria per ml: a systematic review. J Urol 173:1175
Qin R, Shao G et al (1996) The diagnosis and treatment of blunt renal trauma. Zhonghua Wai Ke Za Zhi 34:505
Qin R, Wang P et al (2002) Diagnosis and treatment of renal trauma in 298 patients. Chin J Traumatol 5:21
Quackels R (1964) Cure of patient suffering from priapism by cavernospongiosal anastomosis. Acta Urol Belg 32:5
Quartey JKM (1983) One-stage penile/preputial cutaneous island flap urethroplasty for urethral stricture : a preliminary report. J Urol 129:284
Quatan N, Kirby RS (2004) Improving outcomes in Fournier's gangrene. BJU Int 93:691
Quek ML, Stein JP, Skinner DG (2001) Surgical approaches to venous tumor thrombus. Sem Uro Onc 19:88
Quigley M, Fawcett DP (1999) Thrombophilia and priapism. BJU Int 83:155
Quillin SP, Darcy MD, Picus D (1994) Angiographic evaluation and therapy of ureteroarterial fistulas. Am J Roentgenol 162:873
Quinlan DM, Gearhart JP (1990) Blunt renal trauma in childhood. Features indicating severe injury. Br J Urol 66:526
Quinn JA, DeAngelis LM (2000) Neurologic emergencies in the cancer patient. Semin Oncol 27:311
Quinones-Baldrich WJ, Panetta TF et al (1999) Repair of type IV thoracoabdominal aneurysm with a combined endovascular and surgical approach. J Vasc Surg 30:555
Quint JH, Stanisic TH (1993) Above and below delayed endoscopic treatment of traumatic posterior urethral disruption. J Urol 149:484
Raad II, Sabbagh MF (1992) Optimal duration of therapy for catheter-related Staphylococcus aureus bacteremia: a study of 55 cases and review. Clin Infect Dis 14:75
Rabelo EA, Oliveira EA, Diniz JS, Silva JM, Filgueiras MT, Pezzuti IL et al (2004) Natural history of multicystic kidney conservatively managed: a prospective study. Pediatr Nephrol 19:1102
Rabii R, Joual A et al (2000) Stab wound to the left solitary kidney: report of a case. Ann Urol (Paris) 34:232
Rabinovici R, Ovadia P et al (1999) Abdominal injuries associated with lumbar spine fractures in blunt trauma. Injury 30:471
Radmayr C, Oswald J et al (2002) Blunt renal trauma in children:26 years clinical experience in an alpine region. Eur Urol 42:297
Radovic M, Ostric V et al (1996) Validity of prediction scores in acute renal failure due to polytrauma. Ren Fail 18:615
Rafique M, MH Arif (2002) Management of iatrogenic ureteric injuries associated with gynecological surgery. Int Urol Nephrol 34:31

Ragde H, McInnes GF (1969) Transpubic repair of the severed prostatomembranous urethra. J Urol 101:335
Raj GV, Peterson AC, Toh KL, Webster GD (2005) Outcomes following revisions and secondary implantation of the artificial urinary sphincter. J Urol 173:1242
Ramani AP, Desai MM, Steinberg AP, Ng CS, Abreu SC, Kaouk JH, Finelli A, Novick AC, Gill IS (2005) Complications of laparoscopic partial nephrectomy in 200 cases. J Urol 173:42
Ramchandani P, Cardella JF, Grassi CJ, Roberts AC, Sacks D, Schwartzberg MS, Lewis CA; SCVIR Standards of Practice Committee (2003) Quality improvement guidelines for percutaneous nephrostomy. J Vasc Interv Radiol 14:S277
Ramirez OM, Ruas E, Dellon AL (1990) „Components separation" method for closure of abdominal-wall defects: an anatomic and clinical study. Plast Reconstr Surg 86:519
Rampaul MS, Hosking SW (1998) Testicular torsion: most delay occurs outside hospital. Ann R Coll Surg Engl 80:169
Rane A, Cahill D, Saleemi A, Montgomery B, Palfrey E (2001) The issue of prophylactic antibiotics prior to flexible cystoscopy. Eur Urol 39:212
Rankin WR, Herman JR (2002) Rapidly progressive transitional cell carcinoma associated with dermatomyositis. J Urol 167:639
Rao PN, Dube DA, Weightman NC, Oppenheim BA, Morris J (1991) Prediction of septicemia following endourological manipulation for stones in the upper urinary tract. J Urol 146:955
Rapp DE, Cohn AB, Gottlieb LJ, Lyon MB, Bales GT (2005) Use of tissue expansion for scrotal sac reconstruction after scrotal skin loss. Urology 65:1216
Rappaport W, Haynes K (1990) The retained surgical sponge following intra-abdominal surgery. A continuing problem. Arch Surg 125:405
Rasanen J, Jouppila P (1995) Fetal cardiac function and ductus arteriosus during indomethacin and sulindac therapy for threatened preterm labor: a randomised study. Am J Obstet Gynecol 173:20
Raschke RA, Gollihare B, Peirce JC (1996) The effectiveness of implementing the weight-based heparin nomogram as a practice guideline. Arch Intern Med 156:1645
Rashad Net University (2006) The Jehovah Witness Patient. Published online by the Rashad Net University, Santa Monica, California, USA. http://www.rashaduniversity.com. Cited 6 November 2006
Rassweiler J, Stolzenburg J, Sulser T, Deger S, Zumbe J, Hofmockel G, John H, Janetschek G, Fehr JL, Hatzinger M, Probst M, Rothenberger KH, Poulakis V, Truss M, Popken G, Westphal J, Alles U, Fornara P (2006) Laparoscopic radical prostatectomy – the experience of the german laparoscopic working group. Eur Urol 49:113
Rathaus V, Pomeranz A et al (2004) Isolated severe renal injuries after minimal blunt trauma to the upper abdomen and flank: CT findings. Emerg Radiol 10:190
Ratner LE, Montgomery RA, Kavoussi LR (1999) Laparoscopic live donor nephrectomy: the four years John Hopkins University experience. Nephrol Dial Transplant 14:2090
Raves JJ, Slifkin M, Diamond DLA (1984) bacteriologic study comparing closed suction and simple conduit drainage. Am J Surg 148:618
Rawlins MC, Hefty TL, Brown SL, Biehl TR (2002) Learning laparoscopic donor nephrectomy safety: a report on 100 cases. Arch Surg 137:531
Raz R, Almog D, Elhanan G, Shental J (1994) The use of ceftriaxone in the prevention of urinary tract infection in patients undergoing transurethral resection of the prostate (TUR-P). Infection 22:347
Rebassa Llull MJ, Munoz Velez D et al (2000) Foreign body as renal pseudotumor in a patient with renal polycystic kidney. Arch Esp Urol 53:831
Reed MH (1976) Pelvic fractures in children. J Can Assoc Radiol 27:255
Regel G, Grotz M et al (1996) Pattern of organ failure following severe trauma. World J Surg 20:422
Rehm CG et al (1991) Blunt traumatic bladder rupture: the role of retrograde cystogram. Ann Emerg Med 20:845
Rehman J, Samadi D, Ricciardi R Jr, Kreutzer E (1998) Early endoscopic realignment as primary therapy for complete posterior urethral disruptions. J Endourol 12:283
Reich H (1992) Laparoscopic bowel injury. Surg Laparosc Endosc 2:74
Reichard SA et al (1980) Pelvic fractures in children-review of 120 patients with a new look at general management. J Pediatr Surg 15:727
Reilly KJ, Shapiro MB et al (1996) Angiographic embolization of a penetrating traumatic renal arteriovenous fistula. J Trauma 41:763
Reinhart K, Hüttemann E, Meier-Hellmann A (2004) Sepsis. In: Burchardi H, Larsen R, Schuster H-P, Suter PM (eds) Die Intensivmedizin. Springer Berlin Heidelberg New York, p 851
Reisman EM, Kennedy TJ, Roehrborn CG et al (1991) A prospective study of urologist-performed sonographic evaluation of the urinary tract in patients with prostatism. J Urol 145:1186
Reiter WJ, Schon-Pernerstorfer H, Dorfinger K et al (1999) Frequency of urolithiasis in individuals seropositive for human immunodeficiency virus treated with indinavir is higher than previously assumed. J Urol 161:1082
Rengel M, Gomes-Da-Silva G, Inchaustegui L, Lampreave JL, Robledo R, Echenagusia A, Vallejo JL, Valderrabano F (1998) Renal artery stenosis after kidney transplantation: diagnostic and therapeutic approach. Kidney Int Suppl 68:S99
Rengo M, Bianchi G et al (1997) Renal injury in childhood. G Chir 18:359
Resel Folkersma LE, Belon Lopez Tomasetti JA, Isorna Martinez de la Riva S et al (1999) Complications of endovesical treatment with BCG in a series of 200 patients. Arch Esp Urol 52:957
Rezkella SH (2003) Contrast nephropathy. Clin Med Res 1:301
Reznichek RC, Brosman SA, Rhodes DB (1973) Ureteral avulsion from blunt trauma. J Urol 109:812
Rhee P, Nunley MK, Demetriades D, Velmahos G, Doucet JJ (2005) Tetanus and trauma: a review and recommendations. J Trauma 58:1082
Rhen T, Cidlowski JA (2005) Anti-inflammatory action of glucocorticoids – new mechanisms for old drugs. N Engl J Med 353:1711
Ricard J, Richard L et al (1994) Lesions of the renal pedicle in blunt abdominal trauma in children. 7 cases. Prog Urol 4:76
Ricci G, Gentili A, Di Lorenzo F, Righetti F, Pigna A, Masi M, DeCastro R (1999) Latex allergy in subjects who had undergone multiple surgical procedures for bladder exstrophy: relationship with clinical intervention and atopic diseases. BJU Int 84:1058
Richardson JD, Trinkle JK (1976) Hemodynamics and respiratory alterations with increased intra-abdominal pressure. J Surg Res 20:401
Richter ER, Shriver CD (2001) Delayed nephrectomy in grade V renal injury with two interesting anatomic variations. Urology 58:607
Richter F, Schnorr D, Deger S, Trk I, Roigas J, Wille A, Loening SA (2003) Improvement of hemostasis in open and laparoscopically performed partial nephrectomy using a gelatin matrix-thrombin tissue sealant (FloSeal). Urology 61:73
Rickards D (2002) Non-traumatic abdominal emergencies: imaging and intervention in acute urinary conditions. Eur Radiol 12:2435

Rickman T, Garmany R, Doherty T, Benson D, Okusa MD (2001) Hypokalemia, metabolic alkalosis, and hypertension: Cushing's syndrome in a patient with metastatic prostate adenocarcinoma Am J Kidney Dis 37:838

Ridings PC, Bloomfield GL, Blocher CR, Sugerman HJ (1995) Cardiopulmonary effects of raised intra-abdominal pressure before and after intravascular volume expansion. J Trauma 39:1071

Rigaud J, Hetet JF, Bouchot I (2004) Management of radiation cystitis. Prog Urol 14:568

Rigg KM, Proud G, Taylor RM (1994) Urological complications following renal transplantation: a study of 1016 consecutive transplants from a single center. Transplant Int 7:120

Riggs BL Jr, Sprague RG (1961) Association of Cushing's syndrome and neoplastic disease: observations in 232 cases of Cushing's syndrome and review of the literature. Arch Intern Med 108:841

Rignault DP (1992) Recent progress in surgery for the victims of disaster, terrorism, and war – Introduction. World J Surg 16:885

Rijkmans BG, Bakker DJ, Dabhoiwala NF et al (1989) Successful treatment of radiation cystitis with hyperbaric oxygen. Eur Urol 16:354

Ring J, Messmer K (1977) Incidence and severity of anaphylactoid reactions to colloid volume substitutes. Lancet 1:466–469

Rini JN, Bhargava KK, Tronco GG, Singer C, Caprioli R, Marwin SE, Richardson HL, Nichols KJ, Pugliese PV, Palestro CJ (2006) PET with FDG-labeled leukocytes versus scintigraphy with 111In-oxine-labeled leukocytes for detection of infection. Radiology 238:978

Rios Gonzalez E, Ramon de Fata Chillon F et al (2002) Iatrogenic injury of the lumbar ureter and iliac vessels after lumbar discectomy: urologic treatment using kidney autotransplantation. Actas Urol Esp 26:504

Riou JP, Cohen JR, Johnson J (1992) Factors influencing wound dehiscence. Am J Surg 163:324

Rischmann P, Desgrandchamps F, Malavaud B et al (2000) BCG intravesical instillations: recommendations for side-effects management. Eur Urol 37 [Suppl 1]:33

Ritchey ML, Kelalis PP, Breslow N, Offord KP, Shochat SJ, D'Angio GJ (1988) Intracaval and atrial involvement with nephroblastoma: review of National Wilms Tumor Study-3. J Urol, 140:1113

Rittenberg M, Bagley D (1988) Ureteroscopic diagnosis and treatment of urinary calculi during pregnancy. Urology 32:427

Rivers E, Nguyen B, Havstad S et al (2001) Early goal-directed therapy in the treatment of severe sepsis and septic shock. N Engl J Med 345:1368

Rivers M, Nguyen B, Havstad S et al (2001) Early goal directed therapy in the treatment of severe sepsis and septic shock. N Engl J Med 19:1368

Rober PE, Smith JB, Pierce JM Jr (1990) Gunshot injuries of the ureter. J Trauma 30:83

Robert M, Drianno N et al (1996) Management of major blunt renal lacerations: surgical or nonoperative approach? Eur Urol 30:335

Roberts DB, Hester LL Jr (1972) Progressive synergistic bacterial gangrene arising from an abscess of the vulva and Bartholin's gland duct. Am J Obstet Gynecol 114:285

Roberts HR (1998) Clinical experience with activated factor VII focus on safety aspects. Blood Coagul Fibrinolysis 9 [Suppl 1]:S115

Robles JE, Rosell D (1996) Experimental applications of shock waves. Rev Med Univ Navarra 40:25

Roca B, Cunat E, Simon E (1998) HIV infection presenting with Fournier's gangrene. Neth J Med 53:168

Rodichok LD, Harper GR, Ruckdeschel JC (1981) Early diagnosis of spinal epidural metastases. Am J Med 70:1181

Rodoplu U, Arnold JL, Tokyay R et al (2005) Impact of the terrorist bombings of the Neve Shalom and Beth Israel synagogues on a hospital in Istanbul, Turkey. Acad Emerg Med 12:135

Rodriguez Alonso A, Suarez Pascual G e t al (2004) Iatrogenic rupture of the ureter following extracorporeal shock wave lithotripsy. Actas Urol Esp 28:530

Rodriguez-Patron RR, Sanz ME, Gomez GI et al (2003) Hypogastric artery embolization as a palliative treatment for bleeding secondary to intractable bladder or prostate disease. Arch Esp Urol 56:111

Roehrborn CG (2006) Alfuzosin 10 mg once daily prevents overall clinical progression of benign prostatic hyperplasia but not acute urinary retention: results of a 2-year placebo-controlled study. BJU Int 97:734

Roehrborn CG (2006) Definition of at-risk patients: baseline variables. BJU Int 97 [Suppl 2]:7

Roehrborn CG, McConnell JD, Saltzman B et al (2002) Storage (irritative) and voiding (obstructive) symptoms as predictors of benign prostatic hyperplasia progression and related outcomes. Eur Urol 42:1

Rogers CG, Knight V, MacUra KJ, Ziegfeld S, Paidas CN, Mathews RI (2004) High-grade renal injuries in children–is conservative management possible? Urology 64:574

Rogers CJ, Barber DB et al (1996) Spontaneous bladder perforation in paraplegia as a late complication of augmentation enterocystoplasty: case report. Arch Phys Med Rehabil 77:1198

Rogers FB (2001) Venous thromboembolism in trauma patients: a review. Surgery 130:1

Romero FR, Broglio M, Pires SR et al (2005) Indications for percutaneous nephrostomy in patients with obstructive uropathy due to malignant urogenital neoplasias. Int Braz J Urol 31:117

Rommens PM, Lacroix H et al (1996) Three vascular lesions in one patient. Injury 27:509

Ronkainen J, Nuutinen M, Koskimies O (2002) The adult kidney 24 years after childhood Henoch-Schönlein purpura: a retrospective cohort study. Lancet 360:666

Root RK, Lodato RF, Cade JF, Fotheringham N, Milwee S, Vincernt JL, Torres S, Rello J, Nelson S (2003) Multicenter, double-blind, placebo-controlled study of the use of filgrastim in patients hospitalized with pneumonia and sever sepsis. Crit Care Med 31:367

Rosales A, Arango O et al (1992) The use of ultrasonography as the initial diagnostic exploration in blunt renal trauma. Urol Int 48:134

Rosario DJ, Becker M, Anderson JB (2000) The changing pattern of mortality and morbidity from radical cystectomy. BJU Int 85:427

Rose BD (2006) Diagnosis and treatment of thromboembolic renal infarction. http://www.uptodateonline.com/utd/content/topic.do?topicKey=renldis/17093&type=A&selectedTitle=1~18 Cited 13 April 2006

Rose M, Fisher M (2001) Rocuronium: high risk for anaphylaxis? Br J Anaesth 86:678

Rosen M, Walsh RM, Goldblum JR (2004) Application of a new collagen-based sealant for the treatment of pancreatic injury. Surg Laparosc Endosc Percutan Tech 14:181

Rosen MA, McAninch JW (1994) Management of combined renal and pancreatic trauma. J Urol 152:22

Rosendaal FR (1999) Venous thrombosis: a multicausal disease. Lancet 353:1167

Rosenthal MA, Rosen D, Raghavan D et al (1992) Spinal cord compression in prostate cancer. A 10-year experience. Br J Urol 69:530

Rosol TJ, Capen CC (1992) Mechanisms of cancer-induced hypercalcemia. Lab Invest 67:690

Rotariu P, Yohannes P, Alexianu M et al (2001) Management of malignant extrinsic compression of the ureter by simultaneous placement of two ipsilateral ureteral stents. J Endourol 15:979

Rotondo MF, Schwab CW, McGonigal MD et al (1993) 'Damage control': an approach for improved survival in exsanguinating penetrating abdominal injury. Trauma 35:375

Rourke KF, Fischler AH, Jordan GH (2002) Treatment of recurrent idiopathic priapism with oral baclofen. J Urol 168:2552

Rowbotham JL, Eyre RC (1998) Urinary stoma. In: Libertino JA (ed) Recontructive urologic surgery, 3rd edn. Mosby, St. Louis, p 433

Rowe SA et al (2004) Pelvic ring fractures: implications of vehicle design, crash type, and occupant characteristics. Surgery 136:842

Rowen JL, Tate JM (1998) Management of neonatal candidiasis. Neonatal Candidiasis Study Group. Pediatr Infect Dis J 17:1007

Rowland JL, Kuhn M et al (2001) Accuracy of emergency department bedside ultrasonography. Emerg Med (Fremantle) 13:305

Rowland R (1995) Complications of continent cutaneous reservoirs and neobladders-series using contemporary techniques. AUA Update Ser 14:202

Roy C, Saussine A, Jahn C et al (1995) Fast imaging MR assessment of ureterohydronephrosis during pregnancy. Magn Reson Imaging 13:767

Roy C, Tuchmann C et al (2000) Helical CT of urinary tract: clinical applications. J Radiol 81 [9 Suppl]:1071

Roy C, Tuchmann C et al (2001) Post-traumatic rupture in ureteropelvic junction obstruction syndrome: two case reports. J Radiol 82:171

Ruberto U, D'Eufemia P, Martino F, Giardini O (1989) Amoxycillin and clavulanic acid in the treatment of urinary tract infections in children. J Int Med Res 17:168

Rubin MS, Schoetz DJ, Matthews JB (1994) Parastomal hernia. Is stoma relocation superior to fascial repair? Arch Surg 129:413

Rubin RH, Shapiro ED, Andriole VT, Davis RJ, Stamm WE (1992) Evaluation of new anti-infective drugs for the treatment of urinary tract infection. Infectious Diseases Society of America and the Food and Drug Administration. Clin Infect Dis 15 [Suppl 1]:S216

Rubulotta S, Garagozzo G et al (1997) Thrombosis of the renal artery of traumatic origin. Minerva Chir 52:309

Rucinski J, Margolis M, Panagopoulos G, Wise L (2001) Closure of the abdominal midline fascia: meta-analysis delineates the optimal technique. Am Surg 67:421

Rucker CM, Menias CO, Bhalla S (2004) Mimics of renal colic: alternative diagnoses at unenhanced helical CT. Radiographics 24:S11

Rudnick DM, Bennett PM, Dretler SP (1999) Retrograde renoscopic fragmentation of moderate-size (1.5–3.0-cm) renal cystine stones. J Endourol 13:483

Ruesch D, Happe W, Wulf H (1999) Is TIVA with remifentanil/propofol superior to sevoflurane/N2O regarding PONV in children undergoing strabismus surgery. Anaesthesist 48:80

Ruffion A, Manel A, Valignat C, Lopez JG, Perrin-Fayolle O, Perrin P (2000) Successful use of Samarium 153 for emergency treatment of disseminated intravascular coagulation due to metastatic hormone refractory prostate cancer. J Urol 164:782

Ruiz-Santana S, Ortiz E, Gonzalez B, Bolanos J, Ruiz-Santana AJ, Manzano JL (1991) Stress-induced gastroduodenal lesions and total parenteral nutrition in critically ill patients: frequency, complications, and the value of prophylactic treatment. A prospective, randomized study. Crit Care Med 19:887

Rusch MD, Gould LJ, Dzwierzynski WW et al (2002) Psychological impact of traumatic injuries: what the surgeon can do. Plast Reconstr Surg 109:18

Rushton HG, Woodard JR, Parrott TS, Jeffs RD, Gearhart JP (1988) Delayed bladder rupture after augmentation enterocystoplasty. J Urol 140:344

Russel JA (2006) Management of sepsis. N Engl J Med 355:1699

Russell RS, Gomelsky A et al (2001) Management of grade IV renal injury in children. J Urol 166:1049

Russo P (2000) Urologic emergencies in the cancer patient. Semin Oncol 27:284

Rutherford EJ, Skeete DA, Brasel KJ (2004) Management of the patient with an open abdomen: techniques in temporary and definitive closure. Curr Probl Surg 41 8:5

Rutsky EA, Dubovsky EV et al (1991) Long-term follow-up of a human subject with a remnant kidney. Am J Kidney Dis 18:509

Sacco WJ, Copes WS et al (1993) Effect of preinjury illness on trauma patient survival outcome. J Trauma 35:538; discussion 542

Sachse H (1974) Zur behandlung der Harnrohrenstriktur: Die transuretrale schlitzung unter Sicht mit scharfem Schinitt. Fortschr Med 92:12

Sacks SA, Rhodes DB, Malkasian DR, Rosenbloom AA (1975) Prostatic carcinoma producing syndrome of inappropriate secretion of antidiuretic hormone. Urology 6:489

Sadeghi-Nejad H, Kavoussi LR, Peters CA (1994) Bowel injury in open technique laparoscopic cannula placement. Urology 43:559

Sadeghi-Nejad H, Seftel AD (2002) The etiology, diagnosis, and treatment of priapism: review of the American Foundation for Urologic Disease Consensus Panel report. Curr Urol Rep 3:492

Saengsirisuwan V, Phadungkij S et al (1998) Renal and liver functions and muscle injuries during training and after competition in Thai boxers. Br J Sports Med 32:304

Safir MH, McAninch JW (1999) Diagnosis and management of trauma to the kidney. Curr Opin Urol 9:227

Sagalowsky AI, McConnell JD et al (1983) Renal trauma requiring surgery: an analysis of 185 cases. J Trauma 23:128

Sagalowsky AI, Peters PC (1998) Genitourinary trauma. In: Walsh PC, Retik AB, Vaughn ED, Wein AJ (eds) Campbell's urology, 7th edn. WB Saunders, Philadelphia, p 3116

Saggi BH, Bloomfield GK, Sugerman HJ, Blocher CR, Hull JP, Maramarou AP, Bullock MR (1999) Treatment of intracranial hypertension using nonsurgical abdominal decompression. J Trauma 46:646

Saggi BH, Sugerman HJ, Bloomfield GL (1999) Multisystem organ failure secondary to increased intraabdominal pressure. 27:61

Sahin H, Bircan MK, Akay AF, Gocmen M, Bilici A (1998) Endoscopic treatment of complete posterior urethral obliteration. Acta Urol Belg 66:21

Sahin H, Akay AF et al (2004) Retrospective analysis of 135 renal trauma cases. Int J Urol 11:332

Saidi A, Bocqueraz F et al (2003) Early revascularization by stent in renal pedicle trauma. Prog Urol 13:123

Saidi A, Bocqueraz F et al (2004) Blunt kidney trauma: a ten-year experience. Prog Urol 14:1125

Saidi A, Delaporte V, Lechevallier E (2005) Problèmes urologiques rencontrés au cours de la grossesse. Prog Urol 15:1

Saika T, Manabe D et al (1998) Clinical studies on renal trauma. Hinyokika Kiyo 44:697

Sairanen J, Isotalo T et al (2001) Treatment of a renal artery stab wound with selective embolization. Duodecim 117:959

Sakai Y (1999) A case of idiopathic retroperitoneal fibrosis

with renal subcapsular urinoma resolved by steroid therapy. Hinyokika Kiyo 45:249
Salam TA, Lumsden AB, Martin LG (1993) Local infusion of fibrinolytic agents for acute renal artery thromboembolism: report of ten cases.Ann Vasc Surg 7:21
Salant RL, Cohen MS, Warner RS (1990) Neodymium:YAG laser treatment of postoperative bladder neck contractures. Urology 35:385
Salom EM, Schey D, Penalver M, Gomez-Marin O, Lambrou N, Almeida Z, Mendez L (2003) The safety of incidental appendectomy at the time of abdominal hysterectomy. Am J Obstet Gynecol 189:1563; discussion 1567
Salvatierra O, Bucklew WB, Morrow JW (1967) Perinephric abscess: a report of 71 cases. J Urol 98:296
Salvatierra O Jr, Rigdon WO, Norris DM, Brady TW (1969)Vietnam experience with 252 urological war injuries. J Urol 101:615
Salzano A, De Rosa A et al (1999) Gunshot wounds of the abdomen studied by computed tomography. The authors' personal experience in 30 cases. Radiol Med (Torino) 98:168
Sanchez de la Nieta MD, Sanchez-Fructuoso AI, Alcazar R, Perez-Contin MJ, Prats D, Grimalt J, Blanco J (2004) Higher graft salvage rate in renal allograft rupture associated with acute tubular necrosis. Transplant Proc 36:3016
Sandell J, Ramanan R, Shah D (2002) Penile involvement in Henoch-Schönlein purpura. Indian J Pediatr 69:529
Sandfeldt L, Riddez L, Rajs J, Ewaldsson C, Piros D, Hahn RG (2001) High-dose intravenous infusion of irrigating fluids containing glycine and mannitol in the pig. J Surg Res 95:114
Sandhu C, Anson KM, Patel U (2003) Urinary tract stones: Part I: role of radiological imaging in diagnosis and treatment planning. Clin Radiol 58:415
Sandhu C, Anson KM, Patel U (2003) Urinary tract stones: Part II: current status of treatment. Clin Radiol 58:422
Sandhu DP, Mayor PE, Sambrook PA et al (1992) Outcome and prognostic factors in patients with advanced prostate cancer and obstructive uropathy. Br J Urol 70:412
Sandhu SS, Goldstraw M, Woodhouse CR (2004) The management of haemorrhagic cystitis with sodium pentosan polysulphate. BJU Int 94:845
Sandler CM et al (1981) Radiology of the bladder and urethra in blunt pelvic trauma. Radiol Clin North Am 19:195
Sandler CM et al (1986) Bladder injury in blunt pelvic trauma. Radiology 158:633
Sandler CM et al (1998) Lower urinary tract trauma. World J Urol 16:69
Sandler CM, Amis ES Jr et al (2000) Diagnostic approach to renal trauma. American College of Radiology. ACR Appropriateness Criteria. Radiology 215 [Suppl]:727
Sandler SG, Mallory D, Malamut D, Eckrich R (1995) IgA anaphylactic transfusion reactions. Transfus Med Rev 9:1
Santiago L, Bellman GC et al (1998) Small bowel and splenic injury during percutaneous renal surgery. J Urol 159:2071; discussion 2072
Santora T, Rukstalis DB (2001) Fournier's gangrene. www.emedicine.com/med/UROLOGY.htm. Cited 6 November 2006
Santos JFM et al (2002) Urinary tract infections in pregnant women. Int Urogynecol J 13:204
Santoshi N, Gaitonde K, Patil N, Goyal A, Srinivas V (2002) Incidental appendectomy during radical cystectomy–is it necessary? Urology 59:678
Santucci RA, Krieger JN (2000) Gentamicin for the praticing urologist: review of efficacy, singne daily dosing and „switch therapy". J Urol 163:1076
Santucci RA, McAninch JW (2000) Diagnosis and management of renal trauma: past, present, and future. J Am Coll Surg 191:443
Santucci RA, McAninch JM (2001) Grade IV renal injuries: evaluation, treatment, and outcome. World J Surg 25:1565
Santucci RA, McAninch JW et al (2001) Validation of the American Association for the Surgery of Trauma organ injury severity scale for the kidney. J Trauma 50:195
Santucci RA, Mario LA, McAninch JW (2002) Anastomotic urethroplasty for bulbar urethral stricture: analysis of 168 patients. J Urol 167:1715
Santucci RA, Deng D, Carney J (2004) Removal of metal penile foreign body with a widely available emergency-medical-services-provided air-driven grinder. Urology 63:1183
Santucci RA, Langenburg SE et al (2004) Traumatic hematuria in children can be evaluated as in adults. J Urol 171:822
Santucci RA, Wessells H et al (2004) Evaluation and management of renal injuries: consensus statement of the renal trauma subcommittee. BJU Int 93:937
Santucci RA, Fisher MB (2005) The literature increasingly supports expectant (conservative) management of renal trauma–a systematic review. J Trauma 59:493
Saposhkoff KJ (1922) Über den Zutritt zur Prostata und Samenblasen. Verhand. d. XV Kongr Russ Chir St Petersburg Sept. br.
Sarig G, Michaeli Y, Lanir N (2005) Mechanisms for acquired activated protein C resistance in cancer patients. J Thromb Hemost 3:589
Sarkisian AE, Khondkarian RA et al (1991) Sonographic screening of mass casualties for abdominal and renal injuries following the 1988 Armenian earthquake. J Trauma 31:247
Sartorelli KH, Frumiento C et al (2000) Nonoperative management of hepatic, splenic, and renal injuries in adults with multiple injuries. J Trauma 49:56; discussion 61
Sato M, Yoshii H (2004) Reevaluation of ultrasonography for solid-organ injury in blunt abdominal trauma. J Ultrasound Med 23:1583
Sato M, Grasser W, Endo N et al (1991) Bisphosphonate action. Alendronate localization in rat bone and effects on osteoclast ultrastructure. J Clin Invest 88:2095
Saunders F, Argall J (2002) Investigating microscopic haematuria in blunt abdominal trauma. Emerg Med J 19:322
Saunders MD, Kimmey MB (2005) Systematic review: acute colonic pseudo-obstruction. Aliment Pharmacol Ther 22:917
Sautter T, Haueisen H, Stierli P, Kwiatkowski M, Recker F (2001) A severe complication of retroperitoneoscopic nephrectomy. J Urol 165:515
Savage C, Reabe S et al (2003) Imaging of bilateral ureteropelvic junction laceration from blunt trauma. Emerg Radiol 10:99
Savoca G, Pietropaolo F, Scieri F, Bertolotto M, Mucelli FP, Belgrano E (2004) Sexual function after highly selective embolization of cavernous artery in patients with high flow priapism: long-term follow up. J Urol 172:644
Sawczuk I (1996) Renal cell carcinoma–local recurrence/splenic injury. J Urol 155:37
Saye WB, Miller W, Hertzmann P (1991) Electrosurgery thermal injury. Myth or misconception? Surg Laparosc Endosc 1:223
Sayers RD, Thompson MM et al (1997) Surgical management of 671 abdominal aortic aneurysms: a 13 year review from a single centre. Eur J Vasc Endovasc Surg 13:322
Scarpa RM, De Lisa A, Usai E (1996) Diagnosis and treatment of ureteral calculi during pregnancy with rigid ureteroscopes. J Urol 155:875
Schafer M, Lauper M, Krahenbuhl L (2001) Trocar and Veress needle injuries during laparoscopy. Surg Endosc 15:275
Schatz M (1984) Skin testing and incremental challenge in the evaluation of adverse reactions to local anesthetics. J Allergy Clin Immunol 74:606

Schein M, Ivatury R (1998) Intra-abdominal hypertension and the abdominal compartment syndrome. Br J Surg 85:1027

Scheinert D, Braunlich S, Nonnast-Daniel B, Schroeder M, Schmidt A, Biamino G, Daniel WG, Ludwig J (2001) Transradial approach for renal artery stenting. Catheter Cardiovasc Interv 54:442

Schell SR, Barbul A (1998) Coagulopathy. In: Cameron JL (ed) Current Surgical Therapy, 6th edn. Mosby, St. Louis, p 1146

Schild HH, Günther R, Thelen M (1994) Transrenal ureteral occlusion: results and problems. J Vasc Interv Radiol 5:321

Schimpff SC (1986) Empiric antibiotic therapy for granulocytopenic cancer patients. Am J Med 80:13

Schmidlin FR, Schmid P et al (1996) Force transmission and stress distribution in a computer-simulated model of the kidney: an analysis of the injury mechanisms in renal trauma. J Trauma 40:791

Schmidlin FR, Rohner S et al (1997) The conservative treatment of major kidney injuries. Ann Urol (Paris) 31:246

Schmidlin F, Farshad M et al (1998) Biomechanical analysis and clinical treatment of blunt renal trauma. Swiss Surg:237

Schmidlin FR, Iselin CE et al (1998) The higher injury risk of abnormal kidneys in blunt renal trauma. Scand J Urol Nephrol 32:388

Schmidt A, Rassweiler J, Gumpinger R, Mayer R, Eisenberger F (1990) Minimally invasive treatment of ureteric calculi using modern techniques. Br J Urol 65:242

Schmiedl UP, Carter S et al (1999) Sonographic detection of acute parenchymal injury in an experimental porcine model of renal hemorrhage: gray-scale imaging using a sonographic contrast agent. AJR Am J Roentgenol 173:1289

Schnarkowski P, Brecht-Krauss D et al (1992) Abdominal sonography in primary diagnosis of blunt abdominal trauma. Ultraschall Med 13:102

Schneider RE (1993) Genitourinary trauma. Emerg Med Clin North Am 11:137

Scholz HS, Petru E, Benedicic C, Haas J, Tamussino K (2002) Winter R Fibrin application for preventing lymphocysts after retroperitoneal lymphadenectomy in patients with gynecologic malignancies. Gynecol Oncol 84:43

Schouten O, Shaw L, Boersma E et al (2006) A meta-analysis of safety and effectiveness of perioperative beta-blocker use for the prevention of cardiac events in different types of non-cardiac surgery. Coron Artery Dis 2:173

Schreyer HH, Uggowitzer MM et al (2002) Helical CT of the urinary organs. Eur Radiol 12:575

Schroeder PL, Francisco LL (1990) Evaluating hematuria in children. Where to start and how to proceed. Postgrad Med 88:171

Schroeder-Printzen I, Vosshenrich R, Weidner R et al (1994) Malignant priapism in a patient with metastatic prostate adenocarcinoma. Urol Int 52:52

Schulam PG, Hedican SP, Docimo SG (1999) Radially dilating trocar system for open laparoscopic access. Urology 54:727

Schulman CI, Cohn SM, Blackbourne L, Soffer D, Hoskins N, Bowers N, Habib F, Crookes B, Benjamin B, Pizano LR (2005) How long should you wait for a chest radiograph after placing a chest tube on water seal? A prospective study. J Trauma 59:92

Schulman ML (1973) Reanastomosis of the amputated penis. J Urol 109:432

Schulman S (2003) Clinical practice. Care of patients receiving long-term anticoagulant therapy. N Engl J Med 349:675

Schultz ES, Diepgen TL, von den Driesch P et al (1995) Systemic corticosteroids are important in the treatment of Fournier's gangrene: a case report. Br J Dermatol 133:633

Schultz RE, Hanno PM, Wein AJ, Levin RM, Pollack HM, Van Arsdalen KN (1983) Percutaneous ultrasonic lithotripsy: choice of irrigant. J Urol 130:858

Schumpelick V, Riesener KP (1993) Peritoneovenous shunt–indications, limits, results. Chirurg 64:11

Schunk K, Schild H, Wandel E, Schinzel H, Weingartner K (1990) Local fibrinolysis in renal artery occlusion. Rofo 152:147

Schuster TG, Hollenbeck BK, Faerber GJ, Wolf JS Jr (2001) Complications of ureteroscopy: analysis of predictive factors. J Urol 166:538

Schwartz BF, Swanzy S, Thrasher JB (1996) A randomized prospective comparison of antibiotic tissue levels in the corpora cavernosa of patients undergoing penile prosthesis implantation using gentamicin plus cefazolin versus an oral fluoroquinolone for prophylaxis. J Urol 156:991

Schweitzer I (1990) Genital self-amputation and the Klingsor syndrome. Aust N Z J Psychiatry 24:566

Schweizer RT, Bartus SA, Kahn CS (1977) Fibrosis of a renal transplant ureter. J Urol 117:125

Scolapio JS (2004) A review of the trends in the use of enteral and parenteral nutrition support. J Clin Gastroenterol 38:403

Sebastia MC, Perez-Molina MO, Alvarez-Castells A et al (1997) CT evaluation of underlying cause in spontaneous subcapsular and perirenal hemorrhage. Eur Radiol 7:686

Sebastia MC, Rodriguez-Dobao M et al (1999) Renal trauma in occult ureteropelvic junction obstruction: CT findings. Eur Radiol 9:611

Secil M, Arslan D, Goktay AY et al (2001) The prediction of papaverine induced priapism by color Doppler sonography. J Urol 165:416

See WA, Monk TG, Weldon BC (1993) Complications of laparoscopy: strategies for prevention and treatment. In: Clayman RV, M E.M (eds) Laparoscopic Urology. Quality Medical, St. Louis

Segal BH, Walsh TJ, Gea-Banacloche JC, Holland SM (2005) Infections in the cancer patient. In: DeVita VT Jr, Hellman S, Rosenberg SA (eds) Cancer principles and practice of oncology. Lippincott Williams and Wilkins, Philadelphia

Segura JW, Preminger GM, Assimos DG, Dretler SP, Kahn RI, Lingeman JE, Macaluso JN Jr (1997) Ureteral Stones Clinical Guidelines Panel summary report on the management of ureteral calculi. The American Urological Association. J Urol 158:1915

Sehgal A, Mandhani A, Gupta N et al (2005) Can the need for palliative transurethral prostatic resection in patients with advanced carcinoma of the prostate be predicted? J Endourol 19:546

Sekiguchi Y, Miyai K et al (1998) Nonoperative management of major blunt renal lacerations with urinary extravasation: report of two cases. Hinyokika Kiyo 44:875

Selikowitz SM (1977) Penetrating high-velocity genitourinary injuries. Part II: Ureteral, lower tract, and genital wounds. Urology 9:493

Selzman AA, Spirnak JP (1996) Iatrogenic ureteral injuries: a 20-year experience in treating 165 injuries. J Urol 155:878

Senado-Lara I, Castro-Mendoza A et al (2004) Experience in management of trauma-related acute abdomen at the General Ignacio Zaragoza Regional Hospital in Mexico City. Cir Cir 72:93

Sengoku A, Yamashita M, Umezu K (1990) A case of Fournier's gangrene: was it triggered by prostatic massage (in Japanese)? Hinyokika Kiyo 36:1097

Serretta V, Morgia G, Fondacaro L, Curto G, Lo Bianco A, Pirritano D, Melloni D, Orestano F, Motta M, Pavone-Macaluso M (2002) Open prostatectomy for benign prostatic enlargement in southern Europe in the late 1990s: a contemporary series of 1800 interventions. Urology 60:623

Sessler CN, Gosnell MS, Grap MJ et al (2002) The Richmond Agitation-Sedation Scale – validity and reliability in adult

intensive care unit patients. Am J Respir Crit Care Med 166:1338
Sessler DI (1997) Mild perioperative hypothermia. N Engl J Med 336:1730
Sevitt S (1968) Fatal road accidents. Injuries, complications, and causes of death in 250 subjects. Br J Surg 55:481
Sexton DJ, Spelman D (2003) Current best practices and guidelines. Assessment and management of complications in infective endocarditis. Cardiol Clin 21:273, vii–viii
Sexton WJ, Wood CG, Kim R, Pisters LL (2003) Repeat retroperitoneal lymph node dissection for metastatic testis cancer. J Urol 169:1353
Shafizadeh SF, Daily PP, Baliga P, Rogers J, Baillie GM, Rajagopolan PR, Chavin KD (2002) Chylous ascites secondary to laparoscopic donor nephrectomy. Urology 60:345
Shah HN, Kausik VB, Hegde SS, Shah JN, Bansal MB (2005) Tubeless percutaneous nephrolithotomy: a prospective feasibility study and review of previous reports. BJU Int 96:879
Shahrokh H, Rasouli H, Zargar MA, Karimi K, Zargar K (2005) Spontaneous kidney allograft rupture. Transplant Proc 37: 3079
Shalev M, Buchumensky V et al (1997) Protective nephrostomy in the treatment of blunt trauma to a congenital hydronephrotic kidney: experience in three patients. Br J Urol 79:643
Shaloner E (2005) Blast injury in enclosed spaces. BMJ 331:119
Shanmuganathan K, Mirvis SE et al (2004) Penetrating torso trauma: triple-contrast helical CT in peritoneal violation and organ injury–a prospective study in 200 patients. Radiology 231:775
Shantha TR, Finnerty DP, Rodriquez AP (1989) Treatment of persistent penile erection and priapism using terbutaline. J Urol 141:1427
Shapiro MB, Nance ML et al (2001) Nonoperative management of solid abdominal organ injuries from blunt trauma: impact of neurologic impairment. Am Surg 67:793
Sharafuddin MJ, Hicks ME (1997) Current status of percutaneous mechanical thrombectomy. Part I. General principles. J Vasc Interv Radiol 8:911
Sharafuddin MJ, Hicks ME (1998a) Current status of percutaneous mechanical thrombectomy. Part II. Devices and mechanisms of action. J Vasc Interv Radiol 9:15
Sharafuddin MJ, Hicks ME (1998b) Current status of percutaneous mechanical thrombectomy. Part III. Present and future applications. J Vasc Interv Radiol 9:209
Sharp DS, Ross JH e t al (2002) Attitudes of pediatric urologists regarding sports participation by children with a solitary kidney. J Urol 168:1811; discussion 1815
Sharples EJ, Sobeh M et al (2002) Renal artery dissection after blunt abdominal trauma: a rare cause of acute cortical necrosis. Am J Kidney Dis 40:e11
Sheafor DH, Hertzberg BS, Freed KS et al (2000) Nonenhanced helical CT and US in the emergency evaluation of patients with renal colic: prospective comparison. Radiology 217:792
Shefi S, Mor Y, Dotan ZA, Ramon J (1999) Traumatic testicular dislocation: a case report and review of published reports. Urology 54:744
Shehadi (1982) WH Contrast media adverse reactions: occurrence, recurrence, and distribution patterns. Radiology 143:11
Shekarris B, Stoller ML (2002) The use of fibrin sealant in urology. J Urol 167:1218
Shekarriz B, Stoller ML (2002) The use of fibrin sealant in urology. J Urol 167:1218
Shekarriz B, Shekarriz H, Upadhyay J et al (1999) Outcome of palliative urinary diversion in the treatment of advanced malignancies. Cancer 85:998
Sheldon T (2005) Dutch doctors should tackle female genital mutilation. BMJ 330:922
Shemer J, Shapira SC (2001) Terror and medicine – the challenge. Isr Med Assoc J 3:799
Shepherd JD, Pringle LE, Barnett MJ et al (1991) Mesna versus hyperhydration for the prevention of cyclophosphamide-induced hemorrhagic cystitis in bone marrow transplantation. J Clin Oncol 9:2016
Sherer DM, Kendig JW, Sickel JZ, Salafia CM, Donahue ML (1994) In utero adrenal hemorrhage associated with fetal distress, subsequent transient neonatal hypertension, and a nonfunctioning ipsilateral kidney. Am J Perinatol 11:302
Shergill IS, Arya M, Hamid R, Khastgir J, Patel HR, Shah PJ (2004) The importance of autonomic dysreflexia to the urologist. BJU Int. 93:923
Shiba T, Higashi N, Nishimura Y (1998) Hyperglycaemia due to insulin resistance caused by interferon-gamma. Diabet Med 15:435
Shima H, Nosaka S et al (1997) Diagnostic imaging of renal pedicle injury. Nippon Igaku Hoshasen Gakkai Zasshi 57:5
Shimada T, Mizutani S, Muto T et al (2001) Cloning and characterization of FGF23 as a causative factor of tumor-induced osteomalacia. Proc Natl Acad Sci U S A 22:6500
Shimizu T, Yamazaki Y et al (1998) Giant retroperitoneal hematoma in a patient with von Recklinghausen's disease. Nippon Hinyokika Gakkai Zasshi 89:846
Shin M, Momohara C et al (2003) Traumatic rupture of giant hydronephrosis due to ureteral stone: a case report. Hinyokika Kiyo 49:679
Shingleton WB, Terrell F, Renfroe DL et al (1999) A randomized prospective study of laser ablation of the prostate versus transurethral resection of the prostate in men with benign prostatic hyperplasia. Urology 54:1017
Shinojima T, Nakajima Y et al (2004) Evaluation of 115 consecutive patients with blunt renal trauma by using the classification for renal injury of Japanese Association for the Surgery of Trauma. Nippon Hinyokika Gakkai Zasshi 95:783
Shipley WU, Prout GR Jr, Coachman NM et al (1988) Radiation therapy for localized prostate carcinoma: Experience at the Massachusetts General Hospital (1973–1981) J Natl Cancer Inst Monogr 7:67
Shiraishi J, Higaki Y, Oguni A, Inoue M, Tatsumi T, Azuma A, Matsubara H (2005) Transradial renal artery angioplasty and stenting in a patient with Leriche syndrome. Int Heart J 46:557
Shiramizu M, Katsuoka Y, Grodberg J, Koury ST, Fletcher JA, Davis KL, Sytkowski AJ (1994) Constitutive secretion of erythropoietin by human renal adenocarcinoma cells in vivo and in vitro. Exp Cell Res 215:249
Shnider SM, Webster GM (1965) Maternal and fetal hazards of surgery during pregnancy. Am J Obstet Gynecol 92:891
Shokeir AA, Mutabagani H (1998) Rigid ureteroscopy in pregnant women. Br J Urol 81:678
Shokeir AA, El-Diasty TA, Ghoneim MA (1993) Endouroligic management of ureteric complications after live-donor kidney transplantation. J Endourol 7:487
Shokeir AA, El-Diasty TA, Ghoneim MA (1993) Percutanous treatment of lymphocele in renal transplant recipients. J Endourol 7:481
Shokeir AA, Shamaa MA, Bakr MA, El-Diast TA, Ghoneim MA (1993) Salvage of difficult transplant urinary fistulae by ileal substitution of the ureter. Scand J Urol Nephrol 27:537
Shokeir AA, Mahran MR, Abdulmaamoud A (2000) Renal colic in pregnant women: role of renal resistive index. Urology 55:344
Shokeir AA, Shoma AM, Essam A et al (2002) Recoverability of renal function after relief of acute complete ureteral obstruction: clinical prospective study of the role of renal resistive index. Urology 59:506–510
Shokeir AA, Shoma AM, Mosbah A et al (2002) Noncontrast

computed tomography in obstructive anuria: a prospective study. Urology 59:861
Shokeir AA, El-Diasty T, Eassa W et al (2004) Diagnosis of ureteral obstruction in patients with compromised renal function: the role of noninvasive imaging modalities. J Urol 171:2303
Shokeir AA, El-Sherbiny MT, Gad HM, Dawaba M, Hafez AT, Taha MA et al (2005) Postnatal unilateral pelviureteral junction obstruction: impact of pyeloplasty and conservative management on renal function. Urology 65:980
Shoskes DA, Cecka JM (1997) Effect of delayed graft function on short and long-term kidney graft survival In: Clinical Transplant (JM Cecka and PL Terasaki, eds) P 297, UCLA Tissue Typing Laboratory. Los Angeles
Shoskes DA, Radzinski CA, Struthers NW, Honey RJ (1992) Aluminum toxicity and death following intravesical alum irrigation in a patient with renal impairment. J Urol 147:697
Shu T, Green JM, Orihuela E (2004) Renal and perirenal abscesses in patients with otherwise anatomically normal urinary tracts. J Urol 172:148
Shuford MD, McDougall EM, Chang SS, LaFleur BJ, Smith JA Jr, Cookson MS (2004) Complications of contemporary radical nephrectomy: comparison of open vs. laparoscopic approach. Urol Oncol 22:121
Shukla AR, Woodard C, Carr MC, Huff DS, Canning DA, Zderic SA et al (1999) Experience with testis sparing surgery for testicular teratoma. J Urol 171:161
Shupak A, Shoshani O, Goldenberg I et al (1995) Necrotizing fasciitis: an indication for hyperbaric oxygenation therapy? Surgery 118:873
Shurafa M, Shumaker E, Cronin S (1987) Prostaglandin F2-alpha bladder irrigation for control of intractable cyclophosphamide-induced hemorrhagic cystitis. J Urol 137:1230
Siablis D, Liatsikos EN, Kalogeropoulou CP, Zabakis P, Tsota I, Karnabatidis D, Fokaefs E, Barbalias GA (2002) Arterioureteral fistula – a rare complication of ureterolithotomy: treatment with embolization. J Endourol 16:97
Siablis D, Liatsikos EN, Goumenos D, Karnabatidis D, Voudoukis T, Barbalias G, Vlahogiannis J (2005) Percutaneous rheolytic thrombectomy for treatment of acute renal-artery thrombosis. J Endourol 19:68
Sibert L, Descargues G, Scotte M, Planet M, Thoumas D, Annoot M, Boillot B, Grise P (1994) Laparoscopic drainage of a lymphocele after radical prostatectomy. Ann Urol (Paris) 28:202
Siddins M, Rao MM et al (2001) Late laparoscopic nephrectomy following renal trauma. Aust N Z J Surg 71:618
Siebels M, Andrassy K et al (1998) Spontaneous splenic and renal rupture in polyarteritis nodosa. Aktuelle Radiol 8:236
Siegal T, Siegal T, Robin G et al (1982) Anterior decompression of the spine for metastatic epidural cord compression: a promising avenue of therapy. Ann Neurol 11:28–34
Siegal T, Tigva P, Siegal T et al (1985) Vertebral body resection for epidural compression by malignant tumors. J Bone Joint Surg 67:375
Siegel JF, Smith A, Moldwin R (1996) Minimally invasive treatment of renal abscess. J Urol 155:52
Siegel JH et al (1993) Safety belt restraints and compartment intrusions in frontal and lateral motor vehicle crashes: mechanisms of injuries, complications, and acute care costs. J Trauma 34:736; discussion 758
Siegel JH, Dalal SA, Burgess AR (1990) Pattern of organ injuries in pelvic fracture: Impact force implications for survival and death in motor vehicle injuries. Accid Anal Prev 22:457
Siegman-Igra Y, Anglim AM, Shapiro DE, Adal KA, Strain BA, Farr BM (1997) Diagnosis of vascular catheter-related bloodstream infection: a meta-analysis. J Clin Microbiol 35:928
Siegmeth A et al (2000) Associated injuries in severe pelvic trauma. Unfallchirurg 103:572
Siezenga MA, van Overhagen H, van Buren M (2005) Acute occlusion of the renal artery treated by means of rheolytic thrombectomy. Ned Tijdschr Geneeskd 149:2413
Silberzweig JE, Tey S et al (1998) Percutaneous renal biopsy complicated by renal capsular artery pseudoaneurysm. Am J Kidney Dis 31:533
Silfen R, Hudson DA, McCulley S (2000) Penile lengthening for traumatic penile amputation due to ritual circumcision: a case report. Ann Plast Surg 44:311
Silverstein A, Donatucci CF (2003) Bacterial biofilms and implantable prosthetic devices. Int J Impot Res 15 [Suppl 5]:S150
Silverstein MD, Heit JA, Mohr DN, Petterson TM, O'Fallon WM, Melton LJ 3rd (1998) Trends in the incidence of deep vein thrombosis and pulmonary embolism: a 25-year population-based study. Arch Intern Med 158:585
Silvert MA, Meares EM Jr (1976) Rationale of incidental appendectomy. Urology 7:129
Simckes AM, Chen SS, Osorio AV et al (1999) Ketorolac-induced irreversible renal failure in sickle cell disease: a case report. Pediatr Nephrol 13:63
Simerville JA, Maxted WC, Pahira JJ (2005) Urinalysis: a comprehensive review. Am Fam Physician 71:1153
Singer FR, Minoofar PN (1995) Bisphosphonates in the treatment of disorders of mineral metabolism. Adv Endocrinol Metab 6:259
Singer P, Cohen JD, Stein M (2005) Conventional terrorism and critical care. Crit Care Med 33:S61
Singh D, Gill IS (2005) Renal artery pseudoaneurysm following laparoscopic partial nephrectomy. J Urol 174:2256
Singh M, Blandy JP (1976) The pathology of urethral stricture. J Urol 115:673
Singh S, Choong S (2004) Rupture and perforation of urinary reservoirs made from bowel. World J Urol 22:222
Singh S, Devidayal Kumar L, Joshi K, Minz RW, Datta U (2002) Severe Henoch-Schönlein nephritis: resolution with azathioprine and steroids. Rheumatol Int 22:133
Singh TM, Hung R et al (2005) Endovascular repair of traumatic aortic pseudoaneurysm with associated celiacomesenteric trunk. J Endovasc Ther 12:138
Singh-Grewal D, Macdessi J, Craig J (2005) Circumcision for the prevention of urinary tract infection in boys: a systematic review of randomised trials and observational studies. Arch Dis Child 90:853
Sipsas NV, Bodey GP, Kontoyiannis DP (2005) Perspectives for the management of febrile neutropenic patients with cancer in the 21st century. Cancer 103:1103
Siqueira TM Jr, Kuo RL, Gardner TA, Paterson RF, Stevens LH, Lingeman JE, Koch MO, Shalhav AL (2002) Major complications in 213 laparoscopic nephrectomy cases: the Indianapolis experience. J Urol 168:1361
Siragusa S, Cosmi B, Piovella F, Hirsh J, Ginsberg JS (1996) Low-molecular-weight heparins and unfractionated heparin in the treatment of patients with acute venous thromboembolism: results of a meta-analysis. Am J Med 100:269
Sivit CJ, Taylor GA et al (1991) Blunt trauma in children: significance of peritoneal fluid. Radiology 178:185
Skari H, Bjornland K, Bjornstad-Ostensen A, Haugen G, Emblem R (1998) Consequences of prenatal ultrasound diagnosis: a preliminary report on neonates with congenital malformations. Acta Obstet Gynecol Scand 77:635
Skinner DG (1970) Complications of lymph node dissection. In: Smith RB, Skinner DG (eds) Complications of urologic surgery: prevention and management. WB Saunders, Philadelphia, p 422
Skinner DG, Calvin RB, Vermillion CD et al (1971) Diagnosis and management of renal cell carcinoma. Cancer 28:1165

Skolarikos A, Chrisofos M, Ferakis N, Papatsoris A, Dellis A, Deliveliotis C (2005) Does the management of bladder perforation during transurethral resection of superficial bladder tumors predispose to extravesical tumor recurrence? J Urol 173:1908
Skowvron O, Descotes JL et al (1995) Kidney injuries due to skiing. Prog Urol 5:361
Slater MS, Trunkey DD (1997) Terrorism in America. An evolving threat. Arch Surg. 132:1059
Slaton JW, Kropp KA (1996) Proximal ureteral stent migration: an avoidable complication? J Urol 155:58
Small MP (1978) Small-Carrion penile prosthesis: a report on 160 cases and review of the literature. J Urol 119:365
Smith CS, Ferrara LP (1992) Placenta previa percreta with bladder invasion presenting as incarcerated hernia. Urology 29:371
Smith D, Graham JB, Prystowski JB et al (1992) The effects of ultrasound-guided shock waves early in pregnancy in Sprague-Dawley rats. J Urol 147:1197
Smith DP, Klein FA (1997) Renal injury in a child with airbag deployment. J Trauma 42:341
Smith GL, Bunker CB, Dinneen MD (1998) Fournier's gangrene. Br J Urol 81:347
Smith J (1968) The measurement and significance of the urinary flow rate. Br J Urol 38:701
Smith JK, Kenney PJ (2003) Imaging of renal trauma. Radiol Clin North Am 41:1019
Smith M, Johnston B et al (2003) Trauma cases from Harborview Medical Center. Rupture of a ureteropelvic junction-obstructed kidney in a 15-year-old football player. AJR Am J Roentgenol 180:504
Smith RC, Levine J, Dalrymple NC et al (1999) Acute flank pain: a modern approach to diagnosis and management. Semin Ultrasound CT MR 20:108
Smith SD, Gardner MJ et al (1993) Renal artery occlusion in pediatric blunt abdominal trauma–decreasing the delay from injury to treatment. J Trauma 35:861
Snedeker JG, Barbezat M et al (2005) Strain energy density as a rupture criterion for the kidney: impact tests on porcine organs, finite element simulation, and a baseline comparison between human and porcine tissues. J Biomech 38:993
Snow JC, SH, Kripke BJ, Freed MM, Shah NK, Schlesinger RM (1978) Autonomic hyperreflexia during cystoscopy in patients with high spinal cord injuries. Paraplegia 15:327
Soderdahl DW, Henderson SR, Hansberry KL et al (1997) A comparison of intermittent pneumatic compression of the calf and whole leg in preventing deep venous thrombosis in urological surgery. J Urol 157:1774
Sofer M, Kaver I, Kluger Y et al (2001) Conservative management of an uncommon renal foreign body secondary to explosion injury. J Trauma 51:594
Sofocleous CT, C Hinrichs et al (2005) Angiographic findings and embolotherapy in renal arterial trauma. Cardiovasc Intervent Radiol 28:39
Sogani PC, Watson RC, Whitmore WF Jr (1981) Lymphocele after pelvic lymphadenectomy for urologic cancer. Urology 17:39
Sohn M, Kistler D, Kindler J et al (1989) Fournier's gangrene in hypersensitivity vasculitis. J Urol 142:823
Solberg A, Angelsen A, Bergan U, Haugen OA, Viset T, Klepp O (2003) Frequency of lymphoceles after open and laparoscopic pelvic lymph node dissection in patients with prostate cancer. Scand J Urol Nephrol 37:218
Soler Soler JL, Nogueras Ocana M et al (1994) Renal trauma in children: our experience and review of the literature. Arch Esp Urol 47:51
Soliman SM, Hafie E, Hassan TA et al (2003) Hair coil induced penile tourniquet injury. Saudi Med J 24:S55
Sollinger HW (1995) for the US Renal Transplant Mycophenolate Mofetil Study Group. Mycophenolate mofetil for the prevention of acute rejection in primary cadaveric renal allograft recipients. Transplantation 60:225
Solon AA, Gilbert CS, Meyer C (1994) Myopathy as a paraneoplastic manifestation of renal cell carcinoma Am J Med 97:491
Somekh E, Gorenstein A, Serour F (2004) Acute epididymitis in boys: evidence of a post-infectious etiology. J Urol 171:391
Sorensen S, Borgesen SE, Rohde K et al (1990) Metastatic epidural spinal cord compression. Results of treatment and survival. Cancer 65:1502
Sorensen S, Helweg-Larsen S, Mouridsen H et al (1994) Effect of high-dose dexamethasone in carcinomatous metastatic spinal cord compression treated with radiotherapy: a randomised trial. Eur J Cancer 30A:22
Sotto LSJ, Collins RJ (1958) Perigenital Hematomas. Obstet Gynecol 12:259
Soudack M et al (2004) Experience with focused abdominal sonography for trauma (FAST) in 313 pediatric patients. J Clin Ultrasound 32:53
Soulie M, Cuvillier X, Benaissa A et al (2001) The tension-free transvaginal tape procedure in the treatment of female urinary stress incontinence: a French prospective multicentre study. Eur Urol 39:709; discussion 715
Soulie M, Salomon L, Seguin P, Mervant C, Mouly P, Hoznek A, Antiphon P, Plante P, Abbou CC (2001) Multi-institutional study of complications in 1085 laparoscopic urologic procedures. Urology 58:899
Spencer JA (2000) Early report: comparison of breath-hold MR excretory urography, Doppler ultrasound and isotope renography in evaluation of symptomatic hydronephrosis in pregnancy. Clin Radiol 55:446
Spies JB, Bakal CW, Burke DR, Cardella JF, Drooz A, Edwards ME, Husted JW, Palestrant AM, Pentecost MJ, Roberts AC, Rogers WF, Spencer MC, Weyman PJ; Society of Interventional Radiology Standards of Practice Committee (2003) Angioplasty standard of practice. J Vasc Interv Radiol 14:S219
Spira RM, Reissman P, Goldberg S et al (2006) Evacuation of trauma patients solely to level 1 centers: Is the question patient or trauma center survival? Irs Med Assoc J 8:131
Spirnak JP, Resnick MI, Hampel N, Persky L (1984) Fournier's gangrene: report of 20 patients. J Urol 131:289
Spirnak JP, Hampel N, Resnick MI (1989) Ureteral injuries complicating vascular surgery: is repair indicated? J Urol 141:13
Spycher MA, Hauri D (1986) The ultrastructure of the erectile tissue in priapism. J Urol 135:142
Squadrone V, Coha M, Cerutti E, Schellino MM, Biolino P, Occella P, Belloni G, Vilianis G, Fiore G, Cavallo F et al (2005) Continuous positive airway pressure for treatment of postoperative hypoxemia: a randomized controlled trial. JAMA 293:589
Srinivasan V, Brown CH, Turner AG (1994) A comparison of two radiotherapy regimens for the treatment of symptoms from advanced bladder cancer. Clin Oncol (R Coll Radiol) 6:11
St Lezin MA, Stoller ML (1991) Surgical ureteral injuries. Urology 38:497
Stables DP (1982) Percutaneous nephrostomy: techniques, indications, and results. Urol Clin North Am 9:15
Stackl W, Marberger M (1986) Late sequelae of the management of ureteral calculi with the ureterorenoscope. J Urol 136:386
Stadler M, Bardieu F, Seidel L et al (2003) Difference in risk factors for postoperative nausea and vomiting. Anaesthesiology 98:46
Stalker HP, Kaufman RA et al (1990) The significance of hema-

turia in children after blunt abdominal trauma. AJR Am J Roentgenol 154:569
Stamboulian D, Carbone E (1997) Recognition, management and prophylaxis of endocarditis. Drugs 54:730
Stamm WE (2003) Urinary tract infections. Infect Dis Clin North Am 17:xiii-xiv
Stampfer DS (1997) Free intraperitoneal rupture of hydronephrotic kidney. J Urol 157:2242
Starkman JS, Santucci RA (2005) Comparison of bipolar transurethral resection of the prostate with standard transurethral prostatectomy: shorter stay, earlier catheter removal and fewer complications. BJU Int 95:69
Stauffer MH (1961) Nephrogenic hepatosplenomegaly (abstract). Gastroenterology 40:694
Stawicki SP, Hoff WS et al (2005) Human immunodeficiency virus infection in trauma patients: where do we stand? J Trauma 58:88
Stefanini M, English HA, Taylor AE (1990) Safe and effective, prolonged administration of epsilon aminocaproic acid in bleeding from the urinary tract. J Urol 143:559
Steffens J, Humke U, Ziegler M, Siemer S (2005) Partial nephrectomy with perfusion cooling for imperative indications: a 24-year experience. BJU Int 96:608
Steffens MG, Bode PJ et al (1996) Selective embolization of pseudo-aneurysms of the renal artery after blunt abdominal injury in a patient with a single kidney. Injury 27:219
Stein JP, Kaji DM et al (1994) Blunt renal trauma in the pediatric population: indications for radiographic evaluation. Urology 44:406
Stein JP, Skinner DG (2004) Surgical atlas radical cystectomy. B J Urol 94:197
Stein JP, Lieskovsky G, Cote R, Groshen S, Feng AC, Boyd S, Skinner E, Bochner B, Thangathurai D, Mikhail M et al (2001) Radical cystectomy in the treatment of invasive bladder cancer: long-term results in 1,054 patients. J Clin Oncol 19:666
Stein JP et al (2001) Contemporary surgical techniques for continent urinary diversion continence and potency preservation. Atlas Urol Clin of N Am 9:147
Stein JP, Dunn MD, Quek ML, Miranda G, Skinner DG (2004) The orthotopic T pouch ileal neobladder: experience with 209 patients. J Urol 172:584
Stein KL (2001) Scoring systems and outcome prediction. In: O'Donnell JM, Nacul FE (eds) Surgical intensive care medicine. Kluwer, Boston, p 853
Stein M (2006) Evacuation to a trauma center or non-trauma center? Is there any doubt? Isr Med Assoc J 8: 134
Stein M, Hirshberg A (1999) Medical consequences of terrorism. The conventional weapon threat. Surg Clin North Am 79:1537
Steinberg DL, Jeffrey RB et al (1984) The computerized tomography appearance of renal pedicle injury. J Urol 132:1163
Steinberg J, Eyre RC (1995) Management of recurrent priapism with epinephrine self-injection and gonadotropin-releasing hormone analogue. J Urol 153:152
Stella N, Rolli A, Catalano A, Udini M (2001) Simultaneous urokinase perfusion in renal artery and vein in a case of renal vein thrombosis. Minerva Cardioangiol 49:273
Stephenian E, Matas AJ, Gores P (1992) Sutherland DER, Najarian JS Retransplantation as a risk factor for lymphocele formation. Transplantation 53:676
Stephens BJ, Lathrop JC, Rice WT et al (1993) Fournier's gangrene: historic (1764) versus contemporary (1979) differences in etiology and clinical importance. Am Surg 59:149
Stephenson et al (2004) Morbidity and functional outcomes of salvage radical prostatectomy for locally recurrent prostate cancer after radiation therapy. J Urol 172:2239
Sternbergh WC 3rd, Ramee SR, DeVun DA, Money SR (2000) Endovascular treatment of multiple visceral artery paradoxical emboli with mechanical and pharmacological thrombolysis. J Endovasc Ther 7:155
Stevenson J, Battistella FD (1994) The 'one-shot' intravenous pyelogram: is it indicated in unstable trauma patients before celiotomy? J Trauma 36:828; discussion 833
Stewart A (1973) The carcinogenic effects of low-level radiation: a reappraisal of epidemiologists, methods and observations. Health Phys 24:223
Stewart AF (2005) Clinical practice. Hypercalcemia associated with cancer. N Engl J Med 352:373
Stewart DE, Lowery MR (1980) Replantation surgery following self-inflicted amputation. Can J Psychiatry 25:143
Stine RJ et al (1988) Diagnostic and therapeutic urologic procedures. Emerg Med Clin North Am 6:547
Stoller ML, Wolf JS (1996) Endoscopic ureteral injuries. In: McAninch JW (ed) Traumatic and reconstructive urology. WB Saunders, Philadelphia, p 199
Stoller ML, Wolf JS Jr, Hofmann R, Marc B (1992) Ureteroscopy without routine balloon dilation: an outcome assessment. J Urol 147:1238
Stone HH, Haney BB, Kolb LD, Geheber CE, Hooper CA (1979) Prophylactic and preventive antibiotic therapy: timing, duration and economics. Ann Surg 189:691
Stone MJ, Waterman MR, Harimoto D, Murray G, Willson N, Platt MR, Blomqvist G, Willerson JT (1977) Serum myoglobin level as diagnostic test in patients with acute myocardial infarction. Br Heart J 39:375
Stone NN, Stock RG (2002) Complications following permanent prostate brachytherapy. Eur Urol 41:427
Stothers L, Lee LM (1992) Renal colic in pregnancy. J Urol 148:1383
Strauch B, Sharzer LA, Petro J et al (1983) Replantation of amputated parts of the penis, nose, ear, and scalp. Clin Plast Surg 10:115
Strewler GJ, Wronski TJ, Halloran BP, Miller SC, Leung SC, Williams RD, Nissenson RA (1986) Pathogenesis of hypercalcemia in nude mice bearing a human renal carcinoma. Endocrinology 119:303
Strimling BS (1996) Partial amputation of glans penis during Mogen clamp circumcision. Pediatrics 97:906
String A, Berber E, Foroutani A, Macho JR, Pearl JM, Siperstein AE (2001) Use of the optical access trocar for safe and rapid entry in various laparoscopic procedures. Surg Endosc 15:570
Strohmaier WL, Lahme S et al (1999) Reduction of high-energy shock-wave-induced renal tubular injury by selenium. Urol Res 27:382
Studer U, Burkhard F, Schumacher M, Kessler T, Thoeny H, Fleischmann A et al (2006) Twenty years experience with an ileal orthotopic low pressure bladder substitute – Lessons to be learned. J Urol 176:161
Stumpe KD, Dazzi H, Schaffner A, von Schulthess GK (2000) Infection imaging using whole-body FDG-PET. Eur J Nucl Med 27:822
Subramaniam MH, Liscum KR, Hirshberg A (2002) The floating stoma: a new technique for controlling exposed fistulae in abdominal trauma. J Trauma 53:386
Subramonian K, Sundaram SK, MacDonald Hull SP (2000) Carcinoma of the prostate associated with dermatomyositis. BJU Int 86:401
Sufrin G, Mirand EA, Moore RH, Chu TM, Murphy GP (1977) Hormones in renal cancer. J Urol 117:433
Sugawara Y, Braun DK, Kison PV, Russo JE, Zasadny KR, Wahl RL (1998) Rapid detection of human infections with fluorine-18 fluorodeoxyglucose and positron emission tomography: preliminary results. Eur J Nucl Med 25:1238
Sullivan MJ, Stables DP (1972) Renal artery occlusion from trauma. JAMA 221:1282

Sullivan NM, Sutter VL, Mims MM, Marsh VH, Finegold SM (1973) Clinical aspects of bacteremia after manipulation of the genitourinary tract. J Infect Dis 127:49
Sullivan P (2002) Infant's death: another nail in circumcision's coffin, group says. CMAJ, 167:789
Sulser T, Reich O, Wyler S et al (2004) Photoselective KTP laser vaporization of the prostate: first experiences with 65 procedures. J Endourol 18:976
Sundaresan N, Galicich JH, Bains MS et al (1984) Vertebral body resection in the treatment of cancer involving the spine. Cancer 53:1393
Sundaresan N, Galicich JH, Lane JM (1985) Treatment of neoplastic epidural cord compression by vertebral body resection and stabilization. J Neurosurg 63:676
Sur RL, Kane CJ (2000) Sildenafil citrate-associated priapism. Urology 55:950
Surana R, Khan A et al (1995) Scarring following renal trauma in children. Br J Urol 75:663
Surlan M, Popovic P (2003) The role of interventional radiology in management of patients with end-stage renal disease. Eur J Radiol 46:96
Sutherland RS, Spees EK, Jones JW, Fink DW (1993) Renal artery stenosis after renal transplantation: The impact of the hypogastric artery anastomosis. J Urol 149:980
Sutphen SK (2005) Blast injuries: a review. http://www.medscape.com/viewarticle/516117. Cited 27 January 2006
Suzuki N, Mori I et al (1995) Analysis of 42 patients with renal trauma–radiographic assessment of surgical application. Hinyokika Kiyo 41:965
Suzuki S, Shinohara N, Harabayashi T et al (2002) Complications of bacillus Calmette-Guerin therapy in superficial urothelial cancer: clinical analysis and implications. Int J Clin Oncol 7:289
Suzuki T, Mehta RH, Ince H, Nagai R, Sakomura Y, Weber F, Sumiyoshi T, Bossone E, Trimarchi S, Cooper JV, Smith DE, Isselbacher EM, Eagle KA, Nienaber CA; International Registry of Aortic Dissection (2003) Clinical profiles and outcomes of acute type B aortic dissection in the current era: lessons from the International Registry of Aortic Dissection (IRAD). Circulation 108 [Suppl 1]:II312
Swain R, Ross D (1999) Lower extremity compartment syndrome. When to suspect acute or chronic pressure buildup. Postgrad Med 105:159
Swan MC, Banwell PE (2005) The open abdomen: aetiology, classification and current management strategies. J Wound Care 14:7
Swana HS, Cohn SM et al (1996) Renal artery pseudoaneurysm after blunt abdominal trauma: case report and literature review. J Trauma 40:459
Swischuk, LE (1999) I fell today and then there was blood in my urine. Pediatr Emerg Care 15:457
Sy WM, Seo IS et al (1999) A patient with three kidneys: a correlative imaging case report. Clin Nucl Med 24:264
Symbas PN (1989) Chest drainage tubes. Surg Clin North Am 69:41
Syrjala MT, Valtonen V, Liewendahl K, Myllyla G (1987) Diagnostic significance of indium-111 granulocyte scintigraphy in febrile patients. J Nucl Med 28:155
Szasz G, McLoughlin MG, Warren RJ (1990) Return of sexual functioning following penile replant surgery. Arch Sex Behav. 19343
Tachibana M, Miyakawa A, Tazaki H et al (1995) Autocrine growth of transitional cell carcinoma of the bladder induced by granulocyte-colony stimulating factor. Cancer Res 55:3438
Tachibana M, Miyakawa A, Uchida A et al (1997) Granulocyte colony-stimulating factor receptor expression on human transitional cell carcinoma of the bladder. Br J Cancer 75:1489
Tacyildiz I, Aldemir M (2004) The mistakes of surgeons: „gossypiboma". Acta Chir Belg 104:71
Tagaya N, Kasama K, Suzuki N, Taketsuka S, Horie K, Furihata M, Kubota K (2003) Laparoscopic resection of the pancreas and review of the literature. Surg Endosc 17:201
Tahan H, Randrianantenaina A, Michel F (1999) Treatment of complete rupture of the posterior urethra by endoscopic treatment. Prog Urol 9:489
Tahmaz L, Yalcin O et al (2000) Isolated ureteropelvic junction laceration following blunt body trauma. Ulus Travma Derg 6:266
Takamoto S, Sakura N, Namera A et al (2004) Monitoring of urinary acrolein concentration in patients receiving cyclophosphamide and ifosphamide. J Chromatogr B Analyt Technol Biomed Life Sci 806:59
Takeda M, Katayama Y et al (1994) Value of dimercaptosuccinic acid single photon emission computed tomography and magnetic resonance imaging in detecting renal injury in pediatric patients with vesicoureteral reflux. Comparison with dimercaptosuccinic acid planar scintigraphy and intravenous pyelography. Eur Urol 25:320
Takeyama K, Matsukawa M, Kunishima Y, Takahashi S, Hotta H, Nishiyama N, Tsukamoto T (2005) Incidence of and risk factors for surgical site infection in patients with radical cystectomy with urinary diversion. J Infect Chemother 11:177
Takhar S, Rosenthal MH (2001) Shock. In: O'Donnell JM, Nacul FE (eds) Surgical intensive care medicine. Kluwer, Boston, p 71
Talar-Williams C, Hijazi YM, Walther MM et al (1996) Cyclophosphamide-induced cystitis and bladder cancer in patients with Wegener granulomatosis. Ann Intern Med 124:477
Tallai B, Flasko T, Gyorgy T, Ponyi A, Andras C, Toth C, Danko K (2006) Prostate cancer underlying acute, definitive dermatomyositis: successful treatment with radical perineal prostatectomy. Clin Rheumatol 25:119
Tamai S, Nakamura Y, Motomiya Y (1977) Microsurgical replantation of a completely amputated penis and scrotum. Plast Reconstr Surg 60:287
Tambyah PA (2004) Catheter-associated urinary tract infections: diagnosis and prophylaxis. Int J Antimicrob Agents 24 [Suppl 1]:S44
Tambyah PA, Maki DG (2000) Catheter-associated urinary tract infection is rarely symptomatic: a prospective study of 1,497 catheterized patients. Arch Intern Med 160:678
Tamussino KF et al (2001) Tension-free vaginal tape operation: results of the Austrian registry. Obstet Gynecol 98:732
Tan AH, Al-Omar M, Denstedt JD, Razvi H (2005) Ureteroscopy for pediatric urolithiasis: an evolving first-line therapy. Urology 65:153
Tan LB, Chiang CP, Huang CH, Chou YH, Wang CJ (1991) Transvesical prostatectomy for benign prostatic hyperplasia–a 364 cases analysis. Gaoxiong Yi Xue Ke Xue Za Zhi 7:599
Tanaka M, Ozono S et al (1994) Clinical studies of renal trauma. Hinyokika Kiyo 40:975
Tang E, Berne TV (1994) Intravenous pyelography in penetrating trauma. Am Surg 60:384
Tanner J, Woodings D, Moncaster K (2006) Preoperative hair removal to reduce surgical site infection. Cochrane Database Syst Rev CD004122
Tarman GJ et al (2002) Lower genitourinary injury and pelvic fractures in pediatric patients. Urology 59:123; discussion 126
Taviloglu K, Gunay K et al (1998) Abdominal stab wounds: the role of selective management. Eur J Surg 164:17
Taylor JS, Erkek E (2004)Latex allergy:diagnosis and management. Dermatologic Therapy 17:289

Tazi H, Manunta A, Rodriguez A et al (2003) Spinal cord compression in metastatic prostate cancer. Eur Urol 44:527
Tazi K, el Fassi J et al (2000) Major renal trauma: report of 18 cases. Ann Urol (Paris) 34:249
Teber D, Egey A, Gozen AS et al (2005) Ureteral injuries Diagnostic and treatment algorithm.. Urologe A 44:870
Tegnell A, Aren C, Ohman L (2002) Wound infections after cardiac surgery–a wound scoring system may improve early detection. Scand Cardiovasc J 36:60
Teichman JM, Champion PC, Wollin TA, Denstedt JD (1998) Holmium: YAG lithotripsy of uric acid calculi. J Urol 160:2130
Teichman JM, Vassar GJ, Glickman RD et al (1998) Holmium: YAG lithotripsy: photothermal mechanism converts uric acid calculi to cyanide. J Urol 160:320
Teo REC et al (1996) Placenta percreta involving urinary bladder. BJU 78:140
Terk MD, Stock RG, Stone NN (1998) Identification of patients at increased risk for prolonged urinary retention following radioactive seed implantation of the prostate. J Urol 160: 1379
Ternamian AM (1997) Laparoscopy without trocars. Surg Endosc 11:815
Teruel JL, Escobar EM, Quereda C, Mayayo T, Ortuno J (1983) A simple and safe method for management of lymphocele after renal transplantation. J Urol 130:1058
Teschendorf P (2006) Standard Operating Procedure – Perioperative Beta-Blockers. Department of Anaesthesia, University Hospital of Heidelberg, Germany
Textor HJ, Wilhelm K, Strunk H, Layer G, Dolitzsch C, Schild HH (2000) Locoregional chemoperfusion with mitoxantrone for palliative therapy in bleeding bladder cancer compared with embolization. Rofo 172:462
Thall EH, Stone NN et al (1996) Conservative management of penetrating and blunt Type III renal injuries. Br J Urol 77:512
Theiss M, Hofmockel G, Frohmuller HG (1995) Fournier's gangrene in a patient with erectile dysfunction following use of a mechanical erection aid device. J Urol 153:1921
Thiel R, Adams JB, Schulam PG, Moore RG, Kavoussi LR (1996) Venous dissection injuries during laparoscopic urological surgery. J Urol 155:1874
Thiermann E (1952) Sakrale Prostatektomie bei Hypertrophie der Vorsteherdrüse. Z Urol 45:742
Thomas K, Chow K, Kirby RS (2004) Acute urinary retention: a review of the aetiology and management. Prostate Cancer Prostatic Dis 7:32
Thomas R, Steele R, Ahuja S (1996) Complications of urological laparoscopy: a standardized 1 institution experience. J Urol 156:469
Thomason RB, Julian JS et al (1989) Microscopic hematuria after blunt trauma. Is pyelography necessary? Am Surg 55:145
Thompson A, Balser JR (2004) Perioperative cardiac arrhythmias. Br J Anaesth 93:86
Thompson BH, Wheeless CR Jr (1973) Gastrointestinal complications of laparoscopy sterilization. Obstet Gynecol 41:669
Thompson IM, Flaherty SF, Morey AF (1998) Battlefield urologic injuries: the Gulf War experience. J Am Coll Surg 187:139
Thompson JS, Baxter BT, Allison JG, Johnson FE, Lee KK, Park WY (2003) Temporal patterns of postoperative complications. Arch Surg 138:596; discussion 602
Thompson-Fawcett M, Kolbe A (1996) Paediatric renal trauma: caution with conservative management of major injuries. Aust N Z J Surg 66:435
Thomsen HS, Morcos SK (2004) Contrast Media Safety Committee of European Society of Urogenital Radiology. Management of acute adverse reactions to contrast media. Eur Radiol 14:476
Thomsen TW, Brown DF et al (2004) Blunt renal trauma. J Emerg Med 26:331
Thong BY-H, Yeow-Chan (2004) Anaphylaxis during surgical and interventional procedures. Ann Allergy Asthma Immunol 92:619
Thorelius L (2004) Contrast-enhanced ultrasound in trauma. Eur Radiol 14 [Suppl 8]:P43
Thurlow JP, Gelpi J, Schwaitzberg SD, Rohrer RJ (1996) Laparoscopic peritoneal fenestration and internal drainage of lymphoceles after renal transplantation. Surg Laparosc Endosc 6:290
Tiguert R, Harb JF, Hurley PM, Gomes De Oliveira J, Castillo-Frontera RJ, Triest JA, Gheiler EL (2000) Management of shotgun injuries to the pelvis and lower genitourinary system. Urology 55:193
Tile M (1988) Pelvic ring fractures: should they be fixed? J Bone Joint Surg Br 70:1
Tile M (1996) Acute pelvic fractures: I causation and classification. J Am Acad Orthop Surg 4:143
Tile M (1999) The management of unstable injuries of the pelvic ring. J Bone Joint Surg Br 81:941
Tile M, Pennal GF (1980) Pelvic disruptions: Principles of management. Clin Orthop 151:56
Tillou A, Romero J et al (2001) Renal vascular injuries. Surg Clin North Am 81:1417
Tissot E, Woronoff-Lemsi MC, Cornette C, Plesiat P, Jacquet M, Capellier G (2001) Cost-effectiveness of urinary dipsticks to screen asymptomatic catheter-associated urinary infections in an intensive care unit. Intensive Care Med 27:1842
Titton RL, Gervais DA et al (2002) Renal trauma: radiologic evaluation and percutaneous treatment of nonvascular injuries. AJR Am J Roentgenol 178:1507
Titton RL, Gervais DA, Hahn PF, Harisinghani MG, Arellano RS, Mueller PR (2003) Urine leaks and urinomas: diagnosis and imaging-guided intervention. Radiographics 23:1133
Tligui M, Khadime MR, Tchala K et al (2003) Emergency extracorporeal shock wave lithotripsy (ESWL) for obstructing ureteral stones. Eur Urol 43:552
Tobin CE, Benjamin JA (1949) Anatomic and clinical re-evaluation of scrotum. Surg Gynec Obstet 88:545
Tolhurst SR, Rapp DE, O'Connor RC, Lyon MB, Orvieto MA, Steinberg GD (2005) Complications after cystectomy and urinary diversion in patients previously treated for localized prostate cancer. Urology 66:824
Tomita T, Galicich JH, Sundaresan N (1983) Radiation therapy for spinal epidural metastases with complete block. Acta Radiol Oncol 22:135
Tong YC, Chun JS et al (1992) Use of hematoma size on computerized tomography and calculated average bleeding rate as indications for immediate surgical intervention in blunt renal trauma. J Urol 147:984
Torgerson EL, Khalili R, Dobkin BH, Reiter RE (1999) Myasthenia gravis as a paraneoplastic syndrome associated with renal cell carcinoma. J Urol 162:154
Torode I, Zieg D (1985) Pelvic fractures in children. J Pediatr Orthop 5:76
Touiti D, Paparel P et al (2001) Retroperitoneal foreign body mimicking pararenal tumor. Ann Urol (Paris) 35:151
Touma NJ, Izawa JI, Chin JL (2005) Current status of loc l salvage therapies following radiation failure for prostate cancer. J Urol 173:373
Toutouzas KG, Karaiskakis M et al (2002) Nonoperative management of blunt renal trauma: a prospective study. Am Surg 68:1097
Townsend CM Jr (ed) (2004) Sabiston textbook of surgery, 17th edn. Saunders Elsevier, Philadelphia

Trachtenberg J (1984) Ketoconazole therapy in advanced prostatic cancer. J Urol 132:61

Trachtenberg J, Gittleman M, Steidle M et al (2002) A phase 3, multicenter, open label, randomized study of abarelix versus leuprolide plus daily antiandrogen in men with prostate cancer. J Urol 167:1670

Trainavicius K, Siaurusevicius B et al (2002) Renal trauma in children. Medicina (Kaunas) 38 [Suppl 1]:18

Traxer O, Lottmann H et al (1999) Extracorporeal lithotripsy in children. Study of its efficacy and evaluation of renal parenchymal damage by DMSA-Tc 99m scintigraphy: a series of 39 children. Arch Pediatr 6:251

Traxer O, Smith TG 3rd et al (2001) Renal parenchymal injury after standard and mini percutaneous nephrostolithotomy. J Urol 165:1693

Tricontinental Mycophenolate Mofetil Renal Transplantation Study Group (1996) A blinded, randomized clinical trial of mycophenolate mofetil for the prevention of acute rejection on cadaveric renal transplantation. Transplantation 61:1029

Trigg ME, O'Reilly J, Rumelhart S et al (1990) Prostaglandin E1 bladder instillations to control severe hemorrhagic cystitis. J Urol 143:92

Trinh-Duc P, Wintrebert P, Boulfroy D et al (1992) Comparison of the effects of epsilon-aminocaproic acid and aprotinin on intra- and postoperative bleeding in heart surgery. Ann Chir 46:677

Trivez Boned MA, Oliva Encina J et al (2001) Thrombosis of the renal artery secondary to closed abdominal trauma. Actas Urol Esp 25:295

Troisi R, Hesse UJ et al (1999) Functional, life-threatening disorders and splenectomy following liver transplantation. Clin Transplant 13:380

Troppmann C, Pierce JL, Gandhi MM, Gallay BJ, McVicar JP, Perez RV (2003) Higher surgical wound complication rates with sirolimus immunosuppression after kidney transplantation: A matched-pair pilot study. Transplantation 76:426

Trouillet JL, Chastre J, Vuagnat A, Joly-Guillou ML, Combaux D, Dombret MC, Gibert C (1998) Ventilator-associated pneumonia caused by potentially drug-resistant bacteria. Am J Respir Crit Care Med 157:531

Troxel SA, Low RK (2002) Renal intrapelvic pressure during percutaneous nephrolithotomy and its correlation with the development of postoperative fever. J Urol 168:1348.

Trunkey DD (2000) History and development of trauma care in the United States. Clin Orthop Relat Res (374):36

Tsang T, Demby AM (1992) Penile fracture with urethral injury. J Urol 147:466

Tsukamoto T, Kumamoto Y, Miyao N, Masumori N, Takahashi A, Yanase M (1992) Interleukin-6 in renal cell carcinoma. J Urol 148:1778

Tucak A, Lukacevic T, Kuvezdic H et al (1995) Urogenital wounds during the war in Croatia in 1991/1992. J Urol 153:121

Tucak A, Lukacevic T, Kuvezdic H, Petek Z, Novak R (1995) Urogenital wounds during the war in Croatia in 1991/1992. J Urol 153:121

Tuerk M, Weir WH Jr (1971) Successful replantation of a traumatically amputated glans penis. Plast Reconstr Surg 48:499

Tuncel A, Uzun B, Eruyar T et al (2005) Do prostatic infarction, prostatic inflammation and prostate morphology play a role in acute urinary retention? Eur Urol 48:277

Turi DC, Peerschke EI (1986) Sensitivity of three activated partial thromboplastin time reagents to coagulation factor deficiencies. Am J Clin Pathol 85:43

Turner S, Marosszeky B, Timms I et al (1993) Malignant spinal cord compression: a prospective evaluation. Int J Radiat Oncol Biol Phys 26:141

Turner-Warwick R (1973) Observations on the treatment of traumatic urethral injuries and the value of the fenestrated urethral catheter. Br J Surg 60:775

Turner-Warwick R (1977) Complex traumatic posterior urethral strictures. J Urol 118:564

Turner-Warwick R (1989) Prevention of complications resulting from pelvic fracture urethral injuries – and from their surgical management. Urol Clin North Am 16:335

Turnock RR, Sprigg A et al (1993) Computed tomography in the management of blunt abdominal trauma in children. Br J Surg 80:982

Turone F (2004) Controversy surrounds proposed Italian alternative to female genital mutilation. BMJ 328:247

Ubhi CS, Lam FT, Mavor AI, Giles GR (1989) Subcutaneous heparin therapy for cyclosporine-immunosupprised renal allograft recipients. Transplantation 48:886

Uchida T, Adachi K, Ao T, Fujino A, Omata T, Yoshizawa K, Kurokawa J, Kadowaki K, Shoji K, Yokoyama E et al (1993) Preoperative, operative and postoperative complications in 2266 cases of transurethral resection of the prostate. Nippon Hinyokika Gakkai Zasshi 84:897

Uchida T, Ohori M, Soh S, Sato T, Iwamura M, Ao T, Koshiba K (1999) Factors influencing morbidity in patients undergoing transurethral resection of the prostate. Urology 53:98

Udekwu PO, Gurkin B et al (1996) The use of computed tomography in blunt abdominal injuries. Am Surg 62:56

Uder M, Gohl D, Takahashi M, Derouet H, Defreyne L, Kramann B, Schneider G (2002) MRI of penile fracture: diagnosis and therapeutic follow-up. Eur Radiol 12:113

Uflacker R, Paolini RM, Lima S (1984) Management of traumatic hematuria by selective renal artery embolization. J Urol 132:662

Ugras M, Gunes A et al (2002) Severe renal bleeding caused by a ruptured renal sheath: case report of a rare complication of percutaneous nephrolithotomy. BMC Urol 2:10

Ulmsten U (2001) An introduction to tension-free vaginal tape (TVT)–a new surgical procedure for treatment of female urinary incontinence. Int Urogynecol J Pelvic Floor Dysfunct 12 [Suppl 2]:S3

Ulrich J, York JP, Koff SA (1995) The renal vascular response to acutely elevated intrapelvic pressure: resistive index measurements in experimental urinary obstruction. J Urol 154:1202

Ulvik NM, Bakke A, Hoisaeter PA (1995) Ureteroscopy in pregnancy. J Urol 154:1660

Ungania S (2003) Conservative... and non conservative... treatment of renal blunt injuries. Ann Ital Chir 74:445

UpToDate (2006) Contraindications to thrombolytic therapy in pulmonary embolism. http://www.uptodateonline.com/utd/content/image.do?imageKey=pulm_pix/contra15.gif. Cited 13 April 2006

Ure KJ, Amstutz HC, Nasser S, Schmalzried TP (1998) Direct-exchange arthroplasty for the treatment of infection after total hip replacement. An average ten-year follow-up. J Bone Joint Surg Am 80:961

Uribe CA, Castellanos RI et al (2002) Unusual cause of a mass in the superior pole of the kidney: report of a case. Arch Esp Urol 55:958

Uthappa MC, Cowan NC (2005) Retrograde or antegrade double-pigtail stent placement for malignant ureteric obstruction? Clin Radiol 60:608

Utikal P, Drac P, Bachleda P, Klein J, Kral V, Hrabalova M (2004) Peritoneovenous shunt – modification with the use of long saphenous vein. Biomed Pap Med Fac Univ Palacky Olomouc Czech Repub 148:89

Vaccaro JP, Brody JM (2000) CT cystography in the evaluation of major bladder trauma. Radiographics 20:1373

Vahasarja VJ, Hellstrom PA, Serlo W et al (1993) Treatment of penile incarceration by the string method: 2 case reports. J Urol 149:372

Vakili B, Chesson RR, Kyle BL, Shobeiri SA, Echols KT, Gist R, Zheng YT, Nolan TE (2005) The incidence of urinary tract injury during hysterectomy: a prospective analysis based on universal cystoscopy. Am J Obstet Gynecol 192:1599

Valeri CR, Feingold H, Cassidy G, Ragno G, Khuri S, Altschule MD (1987) Hypothermia-induced reversible platelet dysfunction. Ann Surg 205:175

Valkema R, Pauwels SA et al (2005) Long-term follow-up of renal function after peptide receptor radiation therapy with (90)Y-DOTA(0),Tyr(3)-octreotide and (177)Lu-DOTA(0), Tyr(3)-octreotate. J Nucl Med 46 [Suppl 1]:83S

Vallancien G, Capdeville R, Veillon B, Charton M, Brisset JM (1985) Colonic perforation during percutaneous nephrolithotomy. J Urol 134:1185

Vallancien G, Cathelineau X, Baumert H, Doublet JD, Guillonneau B (2002) Complications of transperitoneal laparoscopic surgery in urology: review of 1,311 procedures at a single center. J Urol 168:23

Van Amersfoort ES, Van Berkel TJC, Kuiper J (2003) Receptors, mediators, and mechanisms involved in bacterial sepsis and septic shock. Clin Microbiol Rev 16:379

Van Blerk M, Maes V, Huyghens L, Derde MP, Meert R, Gorus FK (1992) Analytical and clinical evaluation of creatine kinase MB mass assay by IMx: comparison with MB isoenzyme activity and serum myoglobin for early diagnosis of myocardial infarction. Clin Chem 38:2380

Van de Ven PJ, Kaatee R, Beutler JJ, Beek FJ, Woittiez AJ, Buskens E, Koomans HA, Mali WP (1999) Arterial stenting and balloon angioplasty in ostial atherosclerotic renovascular disease: a randomised trial. Lancet 353:282

Van den Berg JC, de Valois JC, Go PM et al (1999) Detection of groin hernia with physical examination, ultrasound, and MRI compared with laparoscopic findings. Invest Radiol 34:739

Van den Berghe G, Wouters P, Weekers F, Verwaest C, Bruyninckx F, Schetz M, Vlasselaers D, Ferdinande P, Lauwers P, Bouillon R (2001) Intensive insulin therapy in critically ill patients. N Engl J Med 345:1359

Van der Horst C, Martinez Portillo FJ, Seif C, Groth W, Jünemann KP (2004) Male genital injury: diagnosis and treatment. Br J Urol Int 93:927

Van der Linden YM, Dijkstra SP, Vonk EJ et al (2005) Prediction of survival in patients with metastases in the spinal column: results based on a randomized trial of radiotherapy. Cancer 103:320

Van der Voort M, Heijnsdijk EA, Gouma DJ (2004) Bowel injury as a complication of laparoscopy. Br J Surg 91:1253

Van Lieburg AF, de Jong MC, Hoitsma AJ, Buskens FG, Schroder CH, Monnens LA (1995) Renal transplant thrombosis in children. J Pediatr Surg 30:615

Van Marter LJ, Leviton A, Allred EN et al (1996) Persistent pulmonary hypertension of the newborn and smoking and aspirin and nonsteroidal anti-inflammatory drug consumption during pregnancy. Pediatrics 97:658

Van Poppel H, Dilen K, Baert L (2001) Incidental renal cell carcinoma and nephron sparing surgery. Curr Opin Urol 11:281

Varga A, Salah M et al (2001) Renal tumor-like pyonephrosis with foreign body. J Urol 165:891

Varkarakis I, Jarrett T, Ramakumar S (2005) Gallbladder, pancreas and splenic injuries. In: Ramakumar S, Jarrett T (eds) Complications of urologic laparoscopic surgery. Taylor & Francis, Boca Raton

Varkarakis IM, Allaf ME, Bhayani SB, Inagaki T, Su LM, Kavoussi LR, Jarrett TW (2004) Pancreatic injuries during laparoscopic urologic surgery. Urology 64:1089

Varkarakis I, Jarrett T, Ramakumar S (2005) Gallbladder, pancreas and splenic injuries. In: Ramakumar S, Jarrett T (eds) Complications of urologic laparoscopic surgery. Taylor & Francis, Boca Raton, p 67

Varol C, Studer UE (2004) Managing patients after an ileal orthotopic bladder substitution. BJU Int 93:266

Vasile M, Bellin MF et al (2000) Imaging evaluation of renal trauma. Abdom Imaging 25:424

Vastag B (2003) Living-donor transplants reexamined: Experts cite growing concerns about safety of donors. JAMA 290:181

Veenstra DL, Best JH et al (1999) Incidence and long-term cost of steroid-related side effects after renal transplantation. Am J Kidney Dis 33:829

Veerasarn V, Khorprasert C, Lorvidhaya V et al (2004) Reduced recurrence of late hemorrhagic radiation cystitis by WF10 therapy in cervical cancer patients: a multicenter, randomized, two-arm, open-label trial. Radiother Oncol 73:179

Veerasarn V, Boonnuch W, Kakanaporn C et al (2006) A phase II study to evaluate WF10 in patients with late hemorrhagic radiation cystitis and proctitis. Gynecol Oncol 100:179

Velaphi SC, Perlman JM (2001) Neonatal adrenal hemorrhage: clinical and abdominal sonographic findings. Clin Pediatr (Phila) 40:545

Velazquez OC, Bavaria JE et al (1999) Emergency repair of thoracoabdominal aortic aneurysms with immediate presentation. J Vasc Surg 30:996

Velmahos GC, Degiannis E (1997) The management of urinary tract injuries after gunshot wounds of the anterior and posterior abdomen. Injury 28:535

Velmahos GC, Demetriades D et al (1998) Selective management of renal gunshot wounds. Br J Surg 85:1121

Velmahos GC, Kamel E, Berne TV, Yassa N, Ramicone E, Song Z, Demetriades D (1999) Abdominal computed tomography for the diagnosis of intra-abdominal sepsis in critically injured patients: fishing in murky waters. Arch Surg 134:831; discussion 836

Velmahos GC, Chahwan S, Fallabella A et al (2000) Angiographic embolization for intraperitoneal and retroperitoneal injuries. World J Surg 24:539

Velmahos GC, Chahwan S, Hanks SE, Murray JA, Berne TV, Asensio J, Demetriades D (2000) Angiographic embolization of bilateral internal iliac arteries to control life-threatening hemorrhage after blunt trauma to the pelvis. Am Surg 66:858

Velmahos GC, Toutouzas KG et al (2003) Nonoperative treatment of blunt injury to solid abdominal organs: a prospective study. Arch Surg 138:844

Venkatasubramaniam AK, Mehta T, Chetter IC et al (2004) The value of abdominal examination in the diagnosis of abdominal aortic aneurysm. Eur J Vasc Endovasc Surg 27:56

Venn SN, Mundy AR (1998) Immediate management of major trauma to the urinary tract. Eur Urol 33:1

Venn SN, Greenwell TJ, Mundy AR (2000) The long-term outcome of artificial urinary sphincters. J Urol 164:702

Verhaeghe R, Stockx L, Lacroix H, Vermylen J, Baert AL (1997) Catheter-directed lysis of iliofemoral vein thrombosis with use of rt-PA. Eur Radiol 7:996

Veroux M, Veroux P, Puliatti C, Fiamingo P, Macarone M, Cappello D (2003) Renal allograft rupture caused by acute tubular necrosis. Chir Ital 55:753

Vest JM, Warden SS (1990) Ureteroscopic stone manipulation during pregnancy. Urology 35:250

Videtic GM, Ago CT, Winquist EW (1997) Hypercalcemia and carcinoma of the penis. Med Pediatr Oncol 29:576

Vieira MM, Brito GA, Belarmino-Filho JN et al (2003) Use of dexamethasone with mesna for the prevention of ifosfamide-induced hemorrhagic cystitis. Int J Urol 10:595

Vieweg J, Weber HM, Miller K, Hautmann R (1992) Female fertility following extracorporeal shock wave lithotripsy of distal ureteral calculi. J Urol 148:1007

Vignali C, Lonzi S, Bargellini I, Cioni R, Petruzzi P, Caramella D, Bartolozzi C (2004) Vascular injuries after percutaneous

renal procedures: treatment by transcatheter embolization. Eur Radiol 14:723
Villard J (1997) Atheromatous aneurysms of the thoracic aorta. Arch Mal Coeur Vaiss 90 [Suppl]:1741
Villas PA, Cohen G et al (1999) Wallstent placement in a renal artery after blunt abdominal trauma. J Trauma 46:1137
Virgili A, Bianchi A, Mollica G, Corazza M (2000) Serious hematoma of the vulva from a bicycle accident. A case report. J Reprod Med 45:662
Viterbo R, Greenberg RE, Al-Saleem T, Uzzo RG (2005) Prior abdominal surgery and radiation do not complicate the retroperitoneoscopic approach to the kidney or adrenal gland. J Urol 174:446
Voegeli TA, Effert PJ (2005) Pentaethylene-terephthalate (PET) bottles: a new device for autoerotic strangulation of the penis causing serious injury. Arch Sex Behav 34:469
Voelcker F (1919) Die Prostatektomie als gut übersichtliche Operation. Z Urol. Chir 4:253
Vogelzang NJ (1999) Re: Radiation induced renal cell cancer: a report of 4 cases and review of the literature. J Urol 162:1388
Voisard R, von Eicken J et al (1999) A human arterial organ culture model of postangioplasty restenosis: results up to 56 days after ballooning. Atherosclerosis 144:123
Volpe MA et al (1999) Is there a difference in outcome when treating traumatic intraperitoneal bladder rupture with or without a suprapubic tube? J Urol 161:1103
Von der Maase H, Hansen SW, Roberts JT et al (2000) Gemcitabine and cisplatin versus methotrexate, vinblastine, doxorubicin, and cisplatin in advanced or metastatic bladder cancer: results of a large, randomized, multinational, multicenter, phase III study. J Clin Oncol 18:3068
Von Kuenssberg Jehle D et al (2003) Sensitivity in detecting free intraperitoneal fluid with the pelvic views of the FAST exam. Am J Emerg Med 21:476
Vorwerk D, Günther RW, Keulers P, Jakse G (1993) Superselective kidney artery embolization as therapy of choice in bleeding of benign origin. Dtsch Med Wochenschr 118:325
Voyles CR, Madden B (1998) The floppy diaphragm sign with laparoscopic-associated pneumothorax. JSLS 2:71
Voyles CR, Tucker RD (1992) Education and engineering solutions for potential problems with laparoscopic monopolar electrosurgery. Am J Surg 164:57
Vrijland W, Tseng LN, Eijkman HJ, Hop WC, Jakimowicz JJ, Leguit P, Stassem LP, Swank DJ, Haverlag R, Bonjer HJ, Jeekel H (2002) Fewer intraperitoneal adhesions with the use of hyaluronic acid-carboxymethycellulose membrane: a randomized clinical trial. Ann Surg 235:193
Vuckovic I, Tucak A, Gotovac J et al (1995) Croatian experience in the treatment of 629 urogenital war injuries. J Trauma 39:733
Wachsberg R (1998) Unilateral absence of ureteral jets in the third trimester of pregnancy: pitfall in color Doppler US diagnosis of urinary obstruction. Radiology 209:279
Wadhwa SN, Chahal R, Hemal AK, Gupta NP, Dogra PN, Seth A (1998) Management of obliterative posttraumatic posterior urethral strictures after failed initial urethroplasty. J Urol 159:1898
Wagenlehner FM, Wagenlehner C, Schinzel S, Naber KG (2005) Prospective, randomized, multicentric, open, comparative study on the efficacy of a prophylactic single dose of 500 mg levofloxacin versus 1920 mg trimethoprim/sulfamethoxazole versus a control group in patients undergoing TUR of the prostate. Eur Urol 47:549
Wagner GW (1926) Studies on intra-abdominal pressure. Am J Med 171:697
Wah TM, Spencer JA (2001) The role of CT in the management of adult urinary tract trauma. Clin Radiol 56:268
Wahlgren CM, Wahlberg E (2005) Management of thoracoabdominal aneurysm type IV Eur J Vasc Endovasc Surg 29:116
Waldrop J, Ciraulo DL et al (2005) A comparison of continuous renal replacement therapy to intermittent dialysis in the management of renal insufficiency in the acutely III surgical patient. Am Surg 71:36
Walker L, Cassidy MT, Hutchison AG, Abel BJ, Lewi HJ (1984) Fournier's gangrene and urethral problems. Br J Urol 56:509
Walker TG, Grant PW, Goldstein I, Krane RJ, Greenfield AJ (1990) „High-flow" priapism: treatment with superselective transcatheter embolization. Radiology 174:1053
Walsh PC, Donker PJ (1982) Impotence following radical prostatectomy: Insight into etiology and prevention. J Urol 128:492
Walsh RM, Pracy JP, Huggon AM et al (1995) Bomb blast injuries to the ear: the London Bridge incident series. J Accid Emerg Med 12:194
Walther MM, Patel B, Choyke PL et al (1997) Hypercalcemia in patients with metastatic renal cell carcinoma: effect of nephrectomy and metabolic evaluation. J Urol 158:733
Walther MM, Johnson B, Culley D et al (1998) Serum interleukin-6 levels in metastatic renal cell carcinoma before treatment with interleukin-2 correlates with paraneoplastic syndromes but not patient survival J Urol 159:718
Walther PJ, Andriani RT, Maggio MI, Carson CC 3rd (1987) Fournier's gangrene: a complication of penile prosthetic implantation in a renal transplant patient. J Urol 137:299
Waltzman ML, Shannon M, Bowen AP, Bailey MC (1999) Monkeybar injuries: complications of play. Pediatrics 103:e58
Wang D, Zheng H, Deng F (2003) Spermatogenesis after scrotal reconstruction. Br J Plast Surg 56:484
Wang DJ, Forslund C, Persson U, Wiholm BE (1998) Drug-attributed anaphylaxis. Pharmacoepidemiol Drug Saf 7:269
Wang HT, Sax HC (2001) Incidental appendectomy in the era of managed care and laparoscopy. J Am Coll Surg 192:182
Wang KT, Hou CJ et al (1998) Late development of renal arteriovenous fistula following gunshot trauma–a case report. Angiology 49:415
Wanner A, Landa JF, Nieman RE Jr, Vevaina J, Delgado I (1973) Bedside bronchofiberscopy for atelectasis and lung abscess. JAMA 224:1281
Warkentin TE, Levine MN, Hirsh J, Horsewood P, Roberts RS, Gent M, Kelton JG (1995) Heparin-induced thrombocytopenia in patients treated with low-molecular-weight heparin or unfractionated heparin. N Engl J Med 332:1330
Warrell RP Jr (1997) Gallium nitrate for the treatment of bone metastases. Cancer 80 [8 Suppl]:1680
Warrell RP Jr, Bockman RS, Coonley CJ et al (1984) Gallium nitrate inhibits calcium resorption from bone and is effective treatment for cancer-related hypercalcemia. J Clin Invest 73:1487
Warrell RP Jr, Israel R, Frisone M et al (1988) Gallium nitrate for acute treatment of cancer-related hypercalcemia. A randomized, double-blind comparison to calcitonin. Ann Intern Med 108:669
Warrell RP Jr, Murphy WK, Schulman P et al (1991) A randomized double-blind study of gallium nitrate compared with etidronate for acute control of cancer-related hypercalcemia. J Clin Oncol 9:1467
Washecka R, Behling A (2002) Urologic complications of placenta percreta invading the urinary bladder: a case report and review of the literature. Hawaii Med J 61:66
Wasko R, Goldstein AG (1966) Traumatic rupture of the testicle. J Urol 95:721
Watanobe H, Yoshioka M, Takebe K (1988) Ectopic ACTH syndrome due to Grawitz tumor. Horm Metab Res 20:453
Watkins BP, Kothari SN, Landercasper J (2004) Stump appendicitis: case report and review. Surg Laparosc Endosc Percutan Tech 14:167
Watterson JD, Mahoney JE et al (1998) Iatrogenic ureteric inju-

ries: approaches to etiology and management. Can J Surg 41:379
Watterson JD, Girvan AR, Beiko DT et al (2002) Ureteroscopy and holmium:YAG laser lithotripsy: an emerging definitive management strategy for symptomatic ureteral calculi in pregnancy. Urology 60:383
Waugh AC (1986) Autocastration and biblical delusions in schizophrenia. Br J Psychiatry 149:656
Wazny LD, Daghigh B (2001) Desensitization protocols for vancomycin hypersensitivity. Ann Pharmacother 35:1458
Weatherall M, Harwood M (2002) The accuracy of clinical assessment of bladder volume. Arch Phys Med Rehabil 83:1300
Webb DR, Fitzpatrick JM (1985) Percutaneous nephrolithotripsy: a functional and morphological study. J Urol 134:587
Weber S et al (1987) Transurethral prostatectomy complicated by intraperitoneal extravasation of irrigating fluid. Can J Anaesth 34:193
Webster C, Bukkapatnam R, Seigne JD, Pow-Sang J, Hoffman M, Helal M et al (2003) Continent colonic urinary reservoir (Florida pouch): long-term surgical complications (greater than 11 years). J Urol 169:174
Webster GD (1987) The management of complex posterior urethral strictures. Prob Uro 1:226
Webster GD (1989) Perineal repair of membranous urethral stricture. Urol Clin North Am 16:303
Webster GD (1990) Impotence following delayed repair of prostatomembranous urethral disruption. Editorial comment. J Urol 144:678
Webster GD, Ramon J (1991) Repair of pelvic fracture posterior urethral defects using an elaborated perineal approach. J Urol 145:744
Webster GD, Mathes GL, Selli C (1983) Prostatomembranous urethral injuries. A review of the literature and a rational approach to their management. J Urol 130:898
Webster GD, Ramon J, Kreder K (1990) Salvage posterior urethroplasty after failed initial repair of pelvic fracture membranous urethral defects. J Urol 144:1370
Weems WL (1979) Management of genitourinary injuries in patients with pelvic fractures. Ann Surg 189:717
Wei FC, McKee NH, Huerta FJ et al (1983) Microsurgical replantation of a completely amputated penis. Ann Plast Surg 20:317
Weigand MA, Hofer S, Plachky J (2004) Heidelberg sepsis pathway – Recommendations for the therapy of sepsis. University Hospital Heidelberg, Germany
Weighlt JA, Krantz BE, Ali J et al (1997) Advanced Trauma Life Support Student Course Manual. American College of Surgeons Committee on Trauma, 6th edn. Chicago
Weinstein EC, Geraa JE, Greene LF (1961) Hypernephroma presenting as fever of obscure origin. Proc Mayo Clinic 36:12
Weis N, Jorgensen PE, Bruun E (1987) TUR syndrome after transurethral resection of the prostate using suprapubic drainage. Int Urol Nephrol 19:165
Weiss CA 3rd Statz CL, Dahms RA, Remucal MJ, Dunn DL, Beilman GJ (1999) Six years of surgical wound infection surveillance at a tertiary care center: review of the microbiologic and epidemiological aspects of 20,007 wounds. Arch Surg 134:1041
Weiss RM, George NJR, O'Reilly PH (2001) Comprehensive urology. Mosby, London
Weissglas M, Schamhart D, Lowik C, Papapoulos S, Vos P, Kurth KH (1995) Hypercalcemia and cosecretion of interleukin-6 and parathyroid hormone related peptide by a human renal cell carcinoma implanted into nude mice. J Urol 153:854
Welling RE, Kremchek TE et al (1989) Blunt arterial injuries associated with multiple trauma. Ann Vasc Surg 3:345
Welsby IJ, Monroe DM, Lawson JH, Hoffmann M (2005) Recombinant activated factor VII and the anaesthetist. Anaesthesia 60:1203
Werkman HA et al (1991) Urinary tract injuries in multiply-injured patients: a rational guideline for the initial assessment. Injury 22:471
Wessells H (2002) Evaluation and management of renal trauma in the 21st century. AUA Update Series, XXI, 30:234
Wessells H, McAninch JW (1996) Effect of colon injury on the management of simultaneous renal trauma. J Urol 155:1852
Wessells H, Deirmenjian J, McAninch JW (1997) Preservation of renal function after reconstruction for trauma: quantitative assessment with radionuclide scintigraphy. J Urol 157:1583
Wessells H, McAninch JW, Meyer A et al (1997) Criteria for nonoperative treatment of significant penetrating renal lacerations. J Urol 157:24
Wessells H, Suh D et al (2003) Renal injury and operative management in the United States: results of a population-based study. J Trauma 54:423
West OC, Anderson J et al (2002) Patterns of diagnostic error in trauma abdominal CT. Emerg Radiol 9:195
Wheeler AP, Bernard GR (1999) Treating patients with severe sepsis. N Engl J Med 340:207
Whelan C, Stewart J, Schwartz BF (2005) Mechanics of wound healing and importance of vaccum assisted closure in urology. J Urol May 173:1463
White KS, Grossman H (1991) Wilms' and associated renal tumors of childhood. Pediatr Radiol 21:81
Whitfield HN (1999) The management of ureteric stones. Part II: therapy. BJU Int 84:916
Whitmore WF Jr, Marner JA, Thompson IM Jr (1991) Expectant management of localized prostatic cancer. Cancer 67:1091
Wicky S, Wintermark M et al (2000) Imaging of blunt chest trauma. Eur Radiol 10:1524
Wightman JM, Gladish SL (2001) Explosions and blast injuries. Ann Emerg Med 37:664
Wilkinson AG, Haddock G et al (1999) Separation of renal fragments by a urinoma after renal trauma: percutaneous drainage accelerates healing. Pediatr Radiol 29:503
Wilkinson D, Doolette D (2004) Hyperbaric oxygen treatment and survival from necrotizing soft tissue infection. Arch Surg 139:1339
Wille AH, Roigas J, Deger S, Tullmann M, Turk I, Loening SA (2004) Laparoscopic radical nephrectomy: techniques, results and oncological outcome in 125 consecutive cases. Eur Urol 45:483; discussion 488
Williams DM, Lee DY, Hamilton BH, Marx MV, Narasimham DL, Kazanjian SN, Prince MR, Andrews JC, Cho KJ, Deeb GM (1997) The dissected aorta: percutaneous treatment of ischemic complications–principles and results. J Vasc Interv Radiol 8:605
Williams G (1993) Stents in the lower urinary tract. Am Urol Assoc Update Ser 12:26
Williams JM, Racadio JM, Johnson ND, Donnelly LF, Bissler JJ (2006) Embolization of renal angiomyolipomata in patients with tuberous sclerosis complex. Am J Kidney Dis 47:95
Willis LR, Evan AP et al (1999) Relationship between kidney size, renal injury, and renal impairment induced by shock wave lithotripsy. J Am Soc Nephrol 10:1753
Willmann JK, Roos JE et al (2002) Multidetector CT: detection of active hemorrhage in patients with blunt abdominal trauma. AJR Am J Roentgenol 179:437
Wilson JR, Urwin GH, Stower MJ (2005) The role of percutaneous nephrostomy in malignant ureteric obstruction. Ann R Coll Surg Engl 87:21
Wilson M, Seymour R, Henderson B (1998) Bacterial perturbation of cytokine networks. Infect Immun 66:2401

Wilson RF (1994) Pre-existing peripheral arterial disease in trauma. Crit Care Clin 10:567

Wilson SK, Delk JR 2nd (1995) Inflatable penile implant infection: predisposing factors and treatment suggestions. J Urol 153:659

Wilson TS, Lemack GE, Dmochowski RR (2002) UroLume stents: lessons learned. J Urol 167:2477

Wing DA, Hendershott CM, Dubuque L, Miller LK (1999) Outpatient treatment of acute pyelonephritis in pregnancy after 24 weeks. Obstet Gynecol 94:683

Wisplinghoff H, Seifert H, Wenzel RP et al (2003) Current trends in the epidemiology of nosocomial bloodstream infections in patients with hematological malignancies and solid neoplasms in hospitals in the United States. Clin Infect Dis 36:1103

Witt MA, Goldstein I, Saenz de Tejada I et al (1990) Traumatic laceration of intracavernosal arteries: the pathophysiology of non-ischemic, high flow, arterial priapism. J Urol 143:129

Wittmann DH, Iskander GA (2000) The compartment syndrome of the abdominal cavity: a state of the art review. J Inten Care Med 15:201

Wittmann DH, Schein M (1996) Let us shorten antibiotic prophylaxis and therapy in surgery. Am J Surg 172:S26–S32

Wittmann DH, Schein M, Condon RE (1996) Management of secondary peritonitis. Ann Surg 224:10

Wolchok JD, Herr HW, Kelly WK (1998) Localized squamous cell carcinoma of the bladder causing hypercalcemia and inhibition of PTH secretion. Urology 51:489

Wolf JS Jr, Stoller ML (1994) The physiology of laparoscopy: basic principles, complications and other considerations. J Urol 152:294

Wolfman NT, Bechtold RE et al (1992) Blunt upper abdominal trauma: evaluation by CT. AJR Am J Roentgenol 158:493

Wolk DJ et al (1985) Extraperitoneal bladder rupture without pelvic fracture. J Urol 134:1199

Wong J, Brown G (1996) Does once-daily dosing of aminoglycosides affect neuromuscular function ? J Clin Pharm Ther 21:407

Wong YC, Wang LJ et al (2000) Mortality after successful transcatheter arterial embolization in patients with unstable pelvic fractures: rate of blood transfusion as a predictive factor. J Trauma 49:71

Wood DP Jr, Bianco FJ Jr, Pontes JE, Heath MA, DaJusta D (2003) Incidence and significance of positive urine cultures in patients with an orthotopic neobladder. J Urol 169:2196

Woodside J, Schwarz H, Bergreen P (1976) Peripheral embolisation complicating bilateral renal infarction with Gelfoam. Am J Roentgenol 126:1033

World Health Organization (2000) Fact sheet No. 241, June 2000

Wu CL, Chou MC (1993) Surgical management of blunt renal trauma. Zhonghua Yi Xue Za Zhi (Taipei) 52:184

Wu CT, Chiang YJ, Liu KL, Chu SH (2004) Laparoscopic donor nephrectomy: new combination of hand-assisted and standard approaches. Transplant Proc 36:1909

Xeroulis G, Inaba K, Stewart TC, Lannigan R, Gray D, Malthaner R, Parry NG, Girotti M (2005) Human immunodeficiency virus, hepatitis B, and hepatitis C seroprevalence in a Canadian trauma population. J Trauma 59:105

Xu DM, Xu QM et al (2000) Evaluation of organ function monitoring and supporting during the treatment of multiple trauma. Hunan Yi Ke Da Xue Xue Bao 25:288

Yablon CM, Banner MP, Ramchandani P, Rovner ES (2004) Complications of prostate cancer treatment: spectrum of imaging findings. Radiographics 24 [Suppl 1]:S181

Yadin O (1994) Hematuria in children. Pediatr Ann 23:474

Yalcin S, Erman M, Tekuzman G, Ruacan S (2000) Syndrome of inappropriate antidiuretic hormone secretion (SIADH) associated with prostatic carcinoma. Am J Clin Oncol 23:384

Yamano Y, Tanaka H (1984) Replantation of a completely amputated penis by the microsurgical technique: A case report. Microsurgery 5:40

Yamazaki T, Suzuki H, Tobe T et al (2001) Prostate adenocarcinoma producing syndrome of inappropriate secretion of antidiuretic hormone. Int J Urol 8:513

Yang DM, Jung DH, Kim H, Kang JH, Kim SH, Kim JH, Hwang HY (2004) Retroperitoneal cystic masses: CT, clinical, and pathologic findings and literature review. Radiographics 24:1353

Yang SS, Tsai YC, Wu CC, Liu SP, Wang CC (2005) Highly potent and moderately potent topical steroids are effective in treating phimosis: a prospective randomized study. J Urol 173:1361

Yao DC, Jeffrey RB Jr et al (2002) Using contrast-enhanced helical CT to visualize arterial extravasation after blunt abdominal trauma: incidence and organ distribution. AJR Am J Roentgenol 178:17

Yasuda T, Yamanishi T, Isaka S, Okano T, Masai M, Shimazaki J (1991) Endoscopic re-establishment of membranous urethral disruption. J Urol 145:977

Yataco JC, Dweik RA (2005) Pleural effusions: evaluation and management. Cleve Clin J Med 72:854, 858, 862 passim

Yaycioglu O (2005) Delayed complications. In: Ramakumar S, Jarrett T (eds) Complications of urologic laparoscopic surgery. Taylor & Francis, Boca Raton, p 149

Yaycioglu O, Ramakumar S, Kavoussi LR, Jarrett TW (2002) Early repeated exploration after laparoscopic urologic surgery: comparison of clinical, radiologic, and surgical findings. Urology 59:190

Yeniyol CO, Yener H, Kececi Y, Ayder AR (2002) Microvascular replantation of a self-amputated penis. Int Urol Nephrol 33:117

Yeniyol CO, Suelozgen T, Arslan M et al (2004) Fournier's gangrene: experience with 25 patients and use of Fournier's gangrene severity index score. Urology 64:218

Yeong CT, Lim TL, Tan KH (1998) Ureteral injuries in an obstetric and gynaecology teaching hospital. Med J Malaysia 53:51

Yerkes EB, Robertson FM, Gitlin J, Kaefer M, Cain MP, Rink RC (2005) Management of perinatal torsion: today, tomorrow or never? J Urol 174:1579

Ying-Hao S, Chuan-Liang X, Xu G, Guo-Qiang L, Jian-Guo H (2000) Urethroscopic realignment of ruptured bulbar urethra. J Urol 164:1543

Yip KH, Peh WC, Tam PC (1998) Spontaneous rupture of renal tumours: the role of imaging in diagnosis and management. Br J Radiol 71:146

Yoon GH, Stein JP, Skinner DG (2005) Retroperitoneal lymph node dissection in the treatment of low-stage nonseminomatous mixed germ cell tumors of the testicle: An update. Urol Oncol 23:168

Yoshii H et al (1998) Usefulness and limitations of ultrasonography in the initial evaluation of blunt abdominal trauma. J Trauma 45:45; discussion 50

Yoshimura K, Utsunomiya N, Ichioka K et al (2005) Emergency drainage for urosepsis associated with upper urinary tract calculi. J Urol 173:458

Yoshinaga A, Hayashi T, Ishii N, Ohno R, Watanabe T, Yamada T (2005) Successful cure of dermatomyositis after treatment of nonseminomatous testicular cancer. Int J Urol 12:593

Yossepowitch O, Lifshitz DA, Dekel et al (2001) Predicting the success of retrograde stenting for managing ureteral obstruction. J Urol 166:1746

Yossepowitch O et al (2004) Urological injuries during cesarean section: intraoperative diagnosis and management. J Urol 172:196

Young HH, Stone HB (1913) An operation for urethro-rectal

fistula. report of three cases. Trans Am Assoc Genito Urin Surg 8:270
Young JW et al (1986) Lateral compression fractures of the pelvis: the importance of plain radiographs in the diagnosis and surgical management. Skeletal Radiol 15:103
Young JW, Resnik CS (1990) Fracture of the pelvis: current concepts of classification. AJR Am J Roentgenol 155:1169
Yu NC, Raman SS et al (2004) Fistulas of the genitourinary tract: a radiologic review. Radiographics 24:1331
Yurkanin P, Park E, Ramakumar S (2005) Major vascular injuries of urologic laparoscopic surgery. In: Ramakumar S, Jarrett T (eds) Complications of urologic laparoscopic surgery. Taylor & Francis, Boca Raton, p 33
Zacharias SR et al (1999) Damage control surgery. AACN Clin Issues 10:95; quiz 141
Zagoria RJ, Dyer RB, Assimos DG et al (1991) Spontaneous perinephric hemorrhage: imaging and management. J Urol 145:468
Zanetta G, Trio D, Lissoni A, Dalla Valle C, Rangoni G, Pittelli M, Marzola M, Pellegrino A (1993) Early and short-term complications after US-guided puncture of gynecologic lesions: evaluation after 1,000 consecutive cases. Radiology 189:161
Zaontz MR, Hatch DA, Firlit CF (1988) Urological complications in pediatric renal transplantation: Management and prevention. J Urol 140:1123
Zargooshi J (2000) Priapism as a complication of high dose testosterone therapy in a man with hypogonadism. J Urol 163:907
Zeisberg M, Shah AA et al (2005) Bone morphogenic protein-7 induces mesenchymal to epithelial transition in adult renal fibroblasts and facilitates regeneration of injured kidney. J Biol Chem 280:8094
Zekri J, Ahmed N, Coleman RE et al (2001) The skeletal metastatic complications of renal cell carcinoma. Int J Oncol 19:379
Zenn MR, Carson CC 3rd, Patel MP (2000) Replantation of the penis: a patient report. Ann Plast Surg 44:214
Zerres K, Rudnik-Schoneborn S, Steinkamm C, Becker J, Mucher G (1998) Autosomal recessive polycystic kidney disease. J Mol Med 76:303
Zhang JQ, Fielding JR, Zou KH (2002) Etiology of spontaneous perirenal hemorrhage: a meta-analysis. J Urol 167:1593
Zhang P, Zheng SB et al (2003) Selection of the imaging modalities for diagnosis of renal trauma: experience with 74 cases. Di Yi Jun Yi Da Xue Xue Bao 23:872
Zheng W, Denstedt J (2000) Intracorporeal lithotripsy. Urol Clin North Am 27:301
Zielger EJ, Fisher CJ, Sprung CL, Straube RC, Sadoff JC, Foulke GE, Wortel CH, Fink MP, Teng NN (1991) Treatment of Gram-negative bacteremia and septic shock with HA-1A human monoclonal antibody against endotoxin. A randomized, double-blind, placebo controlled trial. The HA-1A Sepsis Study Group. N Engl J Med 324:429
Zimmern PE, Cukier J (1985) Prostatic and membranous urethrorectal fistulas: a new technique of surgical closure. J Urol 134:355
Zink RA, Muller-Mattheis V et al (1990) Results of the West German multicenter study Urological traumatology. Urologe A 29:243
Zinman L, Libertino JA (1988) Control of bleeding in upper urinary tract and retroperitoneal surgery. Urol Clin North Am 15:139
Zinman LN (1997) The management of traumatic posterior urethral distraction defects. Editorial. J Urol 157:511
Zisman A, Lindner A (1993) Recurrent intermittent priapism following priapism (translation). Harefuah 125:85
Zojer N, Keck AV, Pecherstofer M (1999) Comparative tolerability of drug therapies for hypercalcaemia of malignancy. Drug Saf 21:389
Zorgniotti AW, Lefleur RS (1985) Auto-injection of the corpus cavernosum with a vasoactive drug combination for vasculogenic impotence. J Urol 133:39
Zorn G (1960) Beckenbruche mit Harnrohrenverletzungen, ihre Behandlung und Ergebnisse. Beitr Klin Chir 1960:147
Zozikov B, Naoumov N et al (2002) Associated trauma with urinary tract injuries. Ann Urol (Paris) 36:290
Zuckerman AM, Martin LG, Silverstein MI (1993) Emergent renal artery revascularization for acute anuria. J Vasc Interv Radiol 4:489
Zwergel T, Lindenmeyer T, Wullich B (1996) Management of acute hydronephrosis in pregnancy by ureteral stenting. Eur Urol 29:292
Zygun DA, Kortbeek JB et al (2005) Non-neurologic organ dysfunction in severe traumatic brain injury. Crit Care Med 33:654

Subject Index